Guyton & Hall
Textbook of Medical Physiology

Guyton & Hall
Textbook of Medical Physiology

SECOND SOUTH ASIA EDITION

John E. Hall, PhD

Arthur C. Guyton Professor and Chair
Department of Physiology and Biophysics
Associate Vice Chancellor for Research
University of Mississippi Medical Center
Jackson, MS, United States

Adaptation Editors

Mario Vaz, MD

Professor, Department of Physiology
St. John's Medical College
Bangalore, India

Anura Kurpad, MD, PhD

Professor, Department of Physiology
St. John's Medical College
Bangalore, India

Tony Raj, MD

Professor, Department of Physiology
St. John's Medical College
Bangalore, India

ELSEVIER

ELSEVIER

RELX India Pvt. Ltd.

Registered Office: 818, 8th floor, Indraprakash Building, 21, Barakhamba Road, New Delhi-110 001
Corporate Office: 14th Floor, Building No. 10B, DLF Cyber City, Phase II, Gurgaon-122 002, Haryana, India

Guyton and Hall Textbook of Medical Physiology, 13e by John E. Hall

ISBN: 978-1-4557-7005-2

This adaptation of **Guyton and Hall Textbook of Medical Physiology, 13e by John E. Hall** was undertaken by RELX India Private Limited and is published by arrangement with Elsevier Inc.

Guyton and Hall Textbook of Medical Physiology, Second South Asia Edition
Adaptation Editors: Mario Vaz, Anura Kurpad, Tony Raj

Copyright © 2016 RELX India Private Limited.
Adaptation ISBN: 978-81-312-4466-1
eISBN: 978-81-312-4665-8

First Printed in India 2016, Reprinted 2017 (twice)

Sr Project Manager—Education Solutions: Shabina Nasim
Manager—Content Strategist: Renu Rawat
Manager—Education Solutions (Digital): Smruti Snigdha
Content Strategist (Digital): Nabajyoti Kar
Project Manager: Ranjjiet Varhmen
Cover Designer: Raman Kumar

Typeset by Thomson Digital

Printed in India by Replika Press Pvt. Ltd.

To our Teachers and Families,
for their support through the years

PREFACE TO THE SECOND SOUTH ASIA EDITION

Guyton and Hall's Textbook of Medical Physiology continues to have at its core a conceptual and integrative framework that serves the needs not only of preclinical students but also of post-graduate students and practitioners. Advances in medicine and physiology continue to occur at an unabated pace; sometimes new information can be overwhelming when it remains just that—information, without a context or synthesis into existing models of body function. This is what sets *Guyton and Hall's Textbook of Medical Physiology* apart—the continued endeavor to provide a cohesive, readable narrative in the face of change. We have been overwhelmed by the response from students and faculty, to the adapted First South Asia Edition that we under-took about 3 years ago. A new 13th International Edition of *Guyton and Hall's Textbook of Medical Physiology* prompted a revision of the South Asia Edition. In this edition we have taken the opportunity to ensure that the adaptation of the original

textbook continues to faithfully mirror the changes in the new international edition, within the limitations of the original parameters of adaptation. Based on the feedback that we have received, we have added new diagrams, tables, and clarifications in the text. Another important enhancement to this edition are the videos, animations ▶ and assessments ⓜ available as on-line resources. We believe these will equip you better to develop understanding of key concepts and mechanisms of the body. We are truly grateful to all those of you—students and teachers—who sent in your comments. We encourage you to continue to do so—a textbook that is unresponsive to its readership would serve a very limited purpose.

Mario Vaz
Anura Kurpad
Tony Raj

PREFACE TO THE FIRST SOUTH ASIA EDITION

Guyton & Hall Textbook of Medical Physiology has served generations of students and teachers of human physiology extremely well. It is characterized by very lucid explanations of complex phenomena in the human body and is integrative in its approach allowing students to have a broad general understanding of human biology across organ systems. For the medical student and health practitioner who sees a patient not as a collection of symptoms or a deranged organ but rather as a whole being, this approach to human physiology is particularly helpful.

The early editions of the textbook were authored by Dr. Guyton alone. His tragic death was a loss not only to those who knew him but also to those who had grown in their understanding and appreciation of human physiology by reading his textbook and his research papers. Many students will attest to the fact that they find Guyton's textbook particularly easy to read. This, indeed, has been the intent, as Professor Hall who coedited the later editions with Guyton and then did this alone following his tragic death notes in his preface, "I have the same goal as for previous editions—to explain, in language easily understood by students, how the different cells, tissues, and organs of the human body work together to maintain life."

It was therefore with some reluctance that we approached this task of editing *Guyton & Hall Textbook of Medical Physiology*. The need to edit was driven by several factors. First, due to a curriculum change, the time allocated for human physiology in the Indian medical curriculum has been reduced—students are now under considerable pressure to complete a course and understand it in approximately 10 months while they also study anatomy and biochemistry and several other subjects and adjust to the new environs of a medical school. Second, an increasing number of students come from schools where they have studied in the vernacular and for them, reading a large textbook is particularly daunting. The examination system has also changed with shorter questions, more factually than conceptually oriented.

In the process of editing, we have shortened the textbook by approximately 20%. It has been our endeavor to do this without disrupting the explanatory narrative that characterizes the textbook so well. We have also rearranged the chapters and split chapters in some instances so that they might more closely reflect the sequence of lectures that teachers are likely to take. We have included boxes, tables, and flow diagrams at various points in the text to help students with their understanding and as aids to memory. Each chapter is preceded by broad learning objectives and a glossary of terms.

Throughout this process of editing, we have tried to remain true to the original intent of Guyton and Hall. Shortening the text has been difficult and has necessitated choices about what we felt was essential for undergraduate medical students to know in this constrained curriculum. Whether we have succeeded in this, time will tell, and we certainly would look for feedback from students and teachers alike.

Mario Vaz
Anura Kurpad
Tony Raj

PREFACE TO THE 13TH EDITION

The first edition of the *Textbook of Medical Physiology* was written by Arthur C. Guyton almost 60 years ago. Unlike most major medical textbooks, which often have 20 or more authors, the first 8 editions of the *Textbook of Medical Physiology* were written entirely by Dr. Guyton, with each new edition arriving on schedule for nearly 40 years. Dr. Guyton had a gift for communicating complex ideas in a clear and interesting manner that made studying physiology fun. He wrote the book to help students learn physiology, not to impress his professional colleagues.

I worked closely with Dr. Guyton for almost 30 years and had the privilege of writing parts of the 9th and 10th editions. After Dr. Guyton's tragic death in an automobile accident in 2003, I assumed responsibility for completing the subsequent editions.

For the 13th edition of the *Textbook of Medical Physiology*, I have the same goal as for previous editions—to explain, in language easily understood by students, how the different cells, tissues, and organs of the human body work together to maintain life.

This task has been challenging and fun because our rapidly increasing knowledge of physiology continues to unravel new mysteries of body functions. Advances in molecular and cellular physiology have made it possible to explain many physiology principles in the terminology of molecular and physical sciences rather than in merely a series of separate and unexplained biological phenomena.

The *Textbook of Medical Physiology*, however, is not a reference book that attempts to provide a compendium of the most recent advances in physiology. This is a book that continues the tradition of being written for students. It focuses on the basic principles of physiology needed to begin a career in the health care professions, such as medicine, dentistry, and nursing, as well as graduate studies in the biological and health sciences. It should also be useful to physicians and health care professionals who wish to review the basic principles needed for understanding the pathophysiology of human disease.

I have attempted to maintain the same unified organization of the text that has been useful to students in the past and to ensure that the book is comprehensive enough that students will continue to use it during their professional careers.

My hope is that this textbook conveys the majesty of the human body and its many functions and that it stimulates students to study physiology throughout their careers. Physiology is the link between the basic sciences and medicine. The great beauty of physiology is that it integrates the individual functions of all the body's different cells, tissues, and organs into a functional whole, the human body. Indeed, the human body is much more than the sum of its parts, and life relies on this total function, not just on the function of individual body parts in isolation from the others.

This brings us to an important question: How are the separate organs and systems coordinated to maintain proper function of the entire body? Fortunately, our bodies are endowed with a vast network of feedback controls that achieve the necessary balances without which we would be unable to live. Physiologists call this high level of internal bodily control *homeostasis*. In disease states, functional balances are often seriously disturbed and homeostasis is impaired. When even a single disturbance reaches a limit, the whole body can no longer live. One of the goals of this text, therefore, is to emphasize the effectiveness and beauty of the body's homeostasis mechanisms as well as to present their abnormal functions in disease.

Another objective is to be as accurate as possible. Suggestions and critiques from many students, physiologists, and clinicians throughout the world have checked factual accuracy as well as balance in the text. Even so, because of the likelihood of error in sorting through many thousands of bits of information, I wish to issue a further request to all readers to send along notations of error or inaccuracy. Physiologists understand the importance of feedback for proper function of the human body; so, too, is feedback important for progressive improvement of a textbook of physiology. To the many persons who have already helped, I express sincere thanks. Your feedback has helped to improve the text.

A brief explanation is needed about several features of the 13th edition. Although many of the chapters have been revised to include new principles of physiology and new figures to illustrate these principles, the text length has been closely monitored to limit the book size so that it can be used effectively in physiology courses for medical students and health care professionals. Many of the figures have also been redrawn and are in full color. New references have been chosen primarily for their presentation of physiological principles, for the quality of their own references, and for their easy accessibility. The selected bibliography at the end of the chapters lists papers mainly from recently published scientific journals that can be freely accessed from the PubMed site at http://www.ncbi.nlm.nih.gov/pubmed/. Use of these references, as well as cross-references from them, can give the student almost complete coverage of the entire field of physiology.

The effort to be as concise as possible has, unfortunately, necessitated a more simplified and dogmatic presentation of many physiological principles than I normally would have desired. However, the bibliography can be used to learn more about the controversies and unanswered questions that remain in understanding the complex functions of the human body in health and disease.

Another feature is that the print is set in two sizes. The material in large print constitutes the fundamental physiological information that students will require in virtually all of their medical activities and studies. The material in small print and highlighted with a pale blue background is of several different kinds: (1) anatomic, chemical, and other information that is needed for immediate discussion but that most students will learn in more detail in other courses; (2) physiological information of special importance to certain fields of clinical medicine; and (3) information that will be of value to those students who may wish to study particular physiological mechanisms more deeply.

I wish to express sincere thanks to many persons who have helped to prepare this book, including my colleagues in the Department of Physiology and Biophysics at the University of Mississippi Medical Center who provided valuable suggestions. The members of our faculty and a brief description of the research and educational activities of the department can be found at http://physiology.umc.edu/. I am also grateful to Stephanie Lucas for excellent secretarial services and to James Perkins for excellent illustrations. Michael Schenk and Walter (Kyle) Cunningham also contributed to many of the illustrations. I also thank Elyse O'Grady, Rebecca Gruliow, Carrie Stetz, and the entire Elsevier team for continued editorial and production excellence.

Finally, I owe an enormous debt to Arthur Guyton for the great privilege of contributing to the *Textbook of Medical Physiology* for the past 25 years, for an exciting career in physiology, for his friendship, and for the inspiration that he provided to all who knew him.

John E. Hall

CONTENTS

SECTION IV Cardiovascular Physiology
MARIO VAZ

SECTION V Respiratory Physiology
TONY RAJ

SECTION VI Gastrointestinal Physiology
TONY RAJ

SECTION VII Renal Physiology
ANURA KURPAD

SECTION VIII The Endocrine System
TONY RAJ

SECTION IX Reproductive Physiology
MARIO VAZ

SECTION X Central Nervous System

PART I
Sensory System   703
ANURA KURPAD

PART II
Special Senses   741
ANURA KURPAD

General Physiology

MARIO VAZ

1

Functional Organization of the Human Body and Control of the "Internal Environment"

LEARNING OBJECTIVES

- Compare intracellular and extracellular fluid.
- Define homeostasis.
- Describe the regulation systems in the body.
- Describe the process of negative and positive feedback using simple examples.

GLOSSARY OF TERMS

- **Homeostasis:** Maintenance of near-constant conditions in the internal environment

- **Negative feedback:** Feedback that reduces (hence negative) the output of a given system, for example, high circulating levels of a hormone reduce the further secretion of that hormone

- **Positive feedback:** Feedback that increases (hence positive) the output of a system, for example, injury resulting in bleeding results in the release of clotting factors that themselves increase the clotting process

Physiology is the science that seeks to explain the physical and chemical mechanisms that are responsible for the origin, development, and progression of life. Each type of life, from the simplest virus to the largest tree or the complicated human being, has its own functional characteristics. Therefore, the vast field of physiology can be divided into *viral physiology, bacterial physiology, cellular physiology, plant physiology, invertebrate physiology, vertebrate physiology, mammalian physiology, human physiology,* and many more subdivisions.

Human Physiology. The science of *human physiology* attempts to explain the specific characteristics and mechanisms of the human body that make it a living being. The fact that we remain alive is the result of complex control systems; hunger makes us seek food and fear makes us seek refuge. Sensations of cold make us look for warmth. Other forces cause us to seek fellowship and to reproduce. The fact that we are sensing, feeling, and knowledgeable beings is part of this automatic sequence of life; these special attributes allow us to exist under widely varying conditions, which otherwise would make life impossible.

Cells Are the Living Units of the Body

The basic living unit of the body is the cell. Each organ is an aggregate of many different cells held together by intercellular supporting structures.

Each type of cell is specially adapted to perform one or a few particular functions. For instance, the red blood cells, numbering about 25 trillion in each human being, transport oxygen from the lungs to the tissues. Although the red blood cells are the most abundant of any single type of cell in the body, about 75 trillion additional cells of other types perform functions different from those of the red blood cell. The entire body, then, contains about 100 trillion cells.

Although the many cells of the body often differ markedly from one another, all of them have certain basic characteristics that are alike. For instance, oxygen reacts with carbohydrate, fat, and protein to release the energy required for all cells to function. Further, the general chemical mechanisms for changing nutrients into energy are basically the same in all cells, and all cells deliver products of their chemical reactions into the surrounding fluids.

Almost all cells also have the ability to reproduce additional cells of their own kind. Fortunately, when cells of a particular type are destroyed, the remaining cells of this type usually generate new cells until the supply is replenished.

Extracellular Fluid—The "Internal Environment"

About 60% of the adult human body is fluid, mainly a water solution of ions and other substances. Although most of this fluid is inside the cells and is called *intracellular fluid*, about one-third is in the spaces outside the cells and is called *extracellular fluid*. This extracellular fluid is in constant motion throughout the body. It is transported rapidly in the circulating blood and then mixed between the blood and the tissue fluids by diffusion through the capillary walls.

In the extracellular fluid are the ions and nutrients needed by the cells to maintain life. Thus, all cells live in essentially the same environment—the extracellular fluid. For this reason, the extracellular fluid is also called the *internal environment* of the body, or the *milieu intérieur*, a term introduced more than 150 years ago by the great 19th-century French physiologist Claude Bernard.

Cells are capable of living, and performing their special functions as long as the proper concentrations of oxygen, glucose, different ions, amino acids, fatty substances, and other constituents are available in this internal environment.

Differences Between Extracellular and Intracellular Fluids. The extracellular fluid contains large amounts of *sodium, chloride*, and *bicarbonate ions* plus nutrients for the cells, such as *oxygen, glucose, fatty acids*, and *amino acids*. It also contains *carbon dioxide* that is being transported from the cells to the lungs to be excreted, plus other cellular waste products that are being transported to the kidneys for excretion.

The intracellular fluid differs significantly from the extracellular fluid; for example, it contains large amounts of *potassium, magnesium*, and *phosphate ions* instead of the sodium and chloride ions found in the extracellular fluid. These differences are highlighted in Figure 5-2. Special mechanisms for transporting ions through the cell membranes maintain the ion concentration differences between the extracellular and intracellular fluids. These transport processes are discussed in Chapter 4.

Homeostasis—Maintenance of a Nearly Constant Internal Environment

HOMEOSTASIS

In 1929, the American physiologist Walter Cannon coined the term *homeostasis* to describe the *maintenance of nearly constant conditions in the internal environment*. Essentially all organs and tissues of the body perform functions that help maintain these relatively constant conditions. For instance, the lungs provide oxygen to the extracellular fluid to replenish the oxygen used by the cells, the kidneys maintain constant ion concentrations, and the gastrointestinal system provides nutrients.

A large segment of this text is concerned with how each organ or tissue contributes to homeostasis. Normal body functions require the integrated actions of cells, tissues, organs, and the multiple nervous, hormonal, and local control systems that together contribute to homeostasis and good health.

Disease is often considered to be a state of disrupted homeostasis. However, even in the presence of disease, homeostatic mechanisms continue to operate and maintain vital functions through multiple compensations. The discipline of *pathophysiology* seeks to explain how the various physiological processes are altered in diseases or injury.

This chapter outlines the different functional systems of the body and their contributions to homeostasis; we then briefly discuss the basic theory of the body's control systems that allow the functional systems to operate in support of one another.

EXTRACELLULAR FLUID TRANSPORT AND MIXING SYSTEM—THE BLOOD CIRCULATORY SYSTEM

Extracellular fluid is transported through the body in two stages. The first stage is movement of blood through the body in the blood vessels, and the second is movement of fluid between the blood capillaries and the *intercellular spaces* between the tissue cells.

Figure 1-1 shows the overall circulation of blood. All the blood in the circulation traverses the entire circulatory circuit, an average of once each minute when the body is at rest and as many as six times each minute when a person is extremely active.

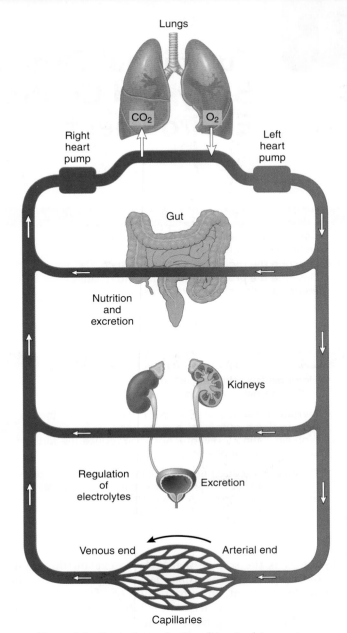

Figure 1-1   General organization of the circulatory system.

As blood passes through the blood capillaries, continual exchange of extracellular fluid also occurs between the plasma portion of the blood and the interstitial fluid that fills the intercellular spaces. This process is shown in Figure 1-2. The walls of the capillaries are permeable to most molecules in the plasma of the blood, with the exception of plasma proteins, which are too large to readily pass through the capillaries. Therefore, large amounts of fluid and its dissolved constituents *diffuse* back and forth between the blood and the tissue spaces, as shown by the arrows. This process of diffusion is caused by kinetic motion of the molecules in both the plasma and the interstitial fluid. That is, the fluid and dissolved molecules are continually moving and bouncing in all directions within the plasma and the fluid in the intercellular spaces, as well as through the capillary pores. Few cells are located more than 50 μm from a capillary, which ensures diffusion of almost any

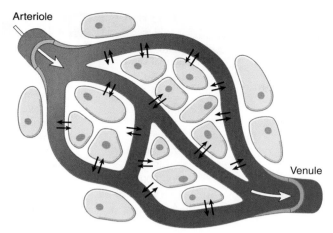

Arteriole

Venule

Figure 1-2 Diffusion of fluid and dissolved constituents through the capillary walls and through the interstitial spaces.

substance from the capillary to the cell within a few seconds. Thus, the extracellular fluid everywhere in the body—both that of the plasma and that of the interstitial fluid—is continually being mixed, thereby maintaining homogeneity of the extracellular fluid throughout the body.

REGULATION OF BODY FUNCTIONS

Nervous System. The nervous system is composed of three major parts: the *sensory input portion*, the *central nervous system* (or *integrative portion*), and the *motor output portion*. Sensory receptors detect the state of the body or the state of the surroundings. For instance, receptors in the skin alert us whenever an object touches the skin at any point. The eyes are sensory organs that give us a visual image of the surrounding area. The ears are also sensory organs. The central nervous system is composed of the brain and spinal cord. The brain can store information, generate thoughts, create ambition, and determine reactions that the body performs in response to the sensations. Appropriate signals are then transmitted through the motor output portion of the nervous system to carry out one's desires.

An important segment of the nervous system is called the *autonomic system.* It operates at a subconscious level and controls many functions of the internal organs, including the level of pumping activity by the heart, movements of the gastrointestinal tract, and secretion by many of the body's glands.

Hormone Systems. Located in the body are eight major endocrine glands and several organs and tissues that secrete chemical substances called hormones. Hormones are transported in the extracellular fluid to other parts of the body to help regulate cellular function. For instance, thyroid hormone increases the rate of most chemical reactions in all cells, thus helping to set the tempo of bodily activity. Insulin controls glucose metabolism; adrenocortical hormones control sodium and potassium ions, and protein metabolism; and parathyroid hormone controls bone calcium and phosphate. Thus, the hormones provide a system for regulation that complements the nervous system. The nervous system regulates many muscular and secretory activities of the body, whereas the hormonal system regulates many metabolic functions.

PROTECTION OF THE BODY

Immune System. The immune system consists of the white blood cells, tissue cells derived from white blood cells, the thymus, lymph nodes, and lymph vessels that protect the body from pathogens such as bacteria, viruses, parasites, and fungi. The immune system provides a mechanism for the body to (1) distinguish its own cells from foreign cells and substances, and (2) destroy the invader by *phagocytosis* or by producing *sensitized lymphocytes* or specialized proteins (eg, *antibodies*) that either destroy or neutralize the invader.

Integumentary System. The skin and its various appendages (including the hair, nails, glands, and other structures) cover, cushion, and protect the deeper tissues and organs of the body, and generally provide a boundary between the body's internal environment and the outside world. The integumentary system is also important for temperature regulation and excretion of wastes, and it provides a sensory interface between the body and the external environment. The skin generally comprises about 12–15% of body weight.

REPRODUCTION

Sometimes reproduction is not considered a homeostatic function. It does, however, help maintain homeostasis by generating new beings to take the place of those that are dying. This may sound like a permissive usage of the term *homeostasis*, but it illustrates that, in the final analysis, essentially all body structures are organized such that they help maintain the automaticity and continuity of life.

Control Systems of the Body

The human body has thousands of control systems. Some of the most intricate of these systems are the genetic control systems that operate in all cells to help control intracellular and extracellular functions. This subject is discussed in Chapter 3.

Many other control systems operate *within the organs* to control functions of the individual parts of the organs; others operate throughout the entire body *to control the interrelations between the organs*. For instance, the respiratory system, operating in association with the nervous system, regulates the concentration of carbon dioxide in the extracellular fluid. The liver and pancreas regulate the concentration of glucose in the extracellular fluid, and the kidneys regulate concentrations of hydrogen, sodium, potassium, phosphate, and other ions in the extracellular fluid.

Normal Ranges and Physical Characteristics of Important Extracellular Fluid Constituents

Table 1-1 lists some of the important constituents and physical characteristics of extracellular fluid, along with their normal values, normal ranges, and maximum limits without causing death. Note the narrowness of the normal range for each one. Values outside these ranges are often caused by illness, injury, or major environmental challenges.

Most important are the limits beyond which abnormalities can cause death. For example, an increase in the body temperature of only 11°F (7°C) above normal can lead to a vicious cycle of increasing cellular metabolism that destroys the cells. Note also the narrow range for acid–base balance in the body, with a normal pH value of 7.4 and lethal values only about 0.5 on either side of normal. Another important factor is the potassium ion

TABLE 1-1	Important Constituents and Physical Characteristics of Extracellular Fluid			
	Normal Value	Normal Range	Approximate Short-Term Nonlethal Limit	Unit
Oxygen (venous)	40	35–45	10–1000	mmHg
Carbon dioxide (venous)	45	35–45	5–80	mmHg
Sodium ion	142	138–146	115–175	mmol/L
Potassium ion	4.2	3.8–5.0	1.5–9.0	mmol/L
Calcium ion	1.2	1.0–1.4	0.5–2.0	mmol/L
Chloride ion	106	103–112	70–130	mmol/L
Bicarbonate ion	24	24–32	8–45	mmol/L
Glucose	90	75–95	20–1500	mg/dL
Body temperature	98.4 (37.0)	98–98.8 (37.0)	65–110 (18.3–43.3)	°F (°C)
Acid–base	7.4	7.3–7.5	6.9–8.0	pH

concentration because whenever it decreases to less than one-third of normal, a person is likely to be paralyzed as a result of the inability of nerves to carry signals. Alternatively, if potassium ion concentration increases to two or more times the normal, the heart muscle is likely to be severely depressed. Also, when calcium ion concentration falls below about one-half of normal, a person is likely to experience tetanic contraction of muscles throughout the body because of the spontaneous generation of excess nerve impulses in the peripheral nerves. When glucose concentration falls below one-half of normal, a person frequently exhibits extreme mental irritability and sometimes even has convulsions.

These examples should give one an appreciation for the extreme value and even the necessity of the vast numbers of control systems that keep the body operating in health; in the absence of any one of these controls, serious body malfunction or death can result.

CHARACTERISTICS OF CONTROL SYSTEMS

The aforementioned examples of homeostatic control mechanisms are only a few of the many thousands in the body, all of which have certain characteristics in common as explained in this section.

Negative Feedback Nature of Most Control Systems

Most control systems of the body act by *negative feedback*, which can best be explained by reviewing some of the homeostatic control systems mentioned previously. In the regulation of carbon dioxide concentration a high concentration of carbon dioxide in the extracellular fluid increases pulmonary ventilation. This, in turn, decreases the extracellular fluid carbon dioxide concentration because the lungs expire greater amounts of carbon dioxide from the body. In other words, the high concentration of carbon dioxide initiates events that decrease the concentration toward normal, which is *negative* to the initiating stimulus. Conversely, a carbon dioxide concentration that falls too low results in feedback to increase the concentration. This response is also negative to the initiating stimulus.

In the arterial pressure-regulating mechanisms a high pressure causes a series of reactions that promote a lowered pressure, or a low pressure causes a series of reactions that promote an elevated pressure. In both instances these effects are negative with respect to the initiating stimulus.

Therefore, in general, if some factor becomes excessive or deficient, a control system initiates *negative feedback*, which

consists of a series of changes that return the factor toward a certain mean value, thus maintaining homeostasis.

"Gain" of a Control System. The degree of effectiveness with which a control system maintains constant conditions is determined by the *gain* of the negative feedback. For instance, let us assume that a large volume of blood is transfused into a person whose baroreceptor pressure control system is not functioning, and the arterial pressure rises from the normal level of 100 mmHg up to 175 mmHg. Then, let us assume that the same volume of blood is injected into the same person when the baroreceptor system is functioning, and this time the pressure increases only 25 mmHg. Thus, the feedback control system has caused a "correction" of −50 mmHg—that is, from 175 to 125 mmHg. There remains an increase in pressure of +25 mmHg, called the "error," which means that the control system is not 100% effective in preventing change. The gain of the system is then calculated by using the following formula:

$$\text{Gain} = \frac{\text{correction}}{\text{error}}$$

Thus, in the baroreceptor system example, the correction is −50 mmHg and the error persisting is +25 mmHg. Therefore, the gain of the person's baroreceptor system for control of arterial pressure is −50 divided by +25, or −2. That is, a disturbance that increases or decreases the arterial pressure does so only one-third as much as would occur if this control system were not present.

The gains of some other physiological control systems are much greater than that of the baroreceptor system. For instance, the gain of the system controlling internal body temperature when a person is exposed to moderately cold weather is about −33. Therefore, one can see that the temperature control system is much more effective than the baroreceptor pressure control system.

Positive Feedback Can Sometimes Cause Vicious Cycles and Death

Why do most control systems of the body operate by negative feedback rather than positive feedback? If one considers the nature of positive feedback, it is obvious that positive feedback leads to instability rather than stability and, in some cases, can cause death.

Figure 1-3 shows an example in which death can ensue from positive feedback. This figure depicts the pumping effectiveness of the heart, showing that the heart of a healthy human being pumps about 5 L of blood per minute. If the person is suddenly

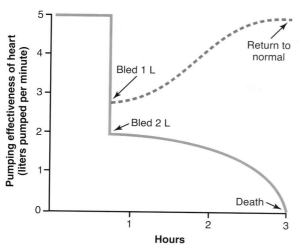

Figure 1-3 Recovery of heart pumping caused by *negative feedback* after 1 L of blood is removed from the circulation. Death is caused by *positive feedback* when 2 L of blood is removed.

bled 2 L, the amount of blood in the body is decreased to such a low level that not enough blood is available for the heart to pump effectively. As a result the arterial pressure falls and the flow of blood to the heart muscle through the coronary vessels diminishes. This scenario results in weakening of the heart, further diminished pumping, a further decrease in coronary blood flow, and still more weakness of the heart; the cycle repeats itself again and again until death occurs. Note that each cycle in the feedback results in further weakening of the heart. In other words, the initiating stimulus causes more of the same, which is *positive feedback*.

Positive feedback is better known as a "vicious cycle," but a mild degree of positive feedback can be overcome by the negative feedback control mechanisms of the body and the vicious cycle then fails to develop. For instance, if the person in the aforementioned example is bled only 1 L instead of 2 L, the normal negative feedback mechanisms for controlling cardiac output and arterial pressure can counterbalance the positive feedback and the person can recover, as shown by the dashed curve of Figure 1-3.

Positive Feedback Can Sometimes Be Useful. In some instances, the body uses positive feedback to its advantage. Blood clotting is an example of a valuable use of positive feedback. When a blood vessel is ruptured and a clot begins to form, multiple enzymes called *clotting factors* are activated within the clot. Some of these enzymes act on other inactivated enzymes of the immediately adjacent blood, thus causing more blood clotting. This process continues until the hole in the vessel is plugged and bleeding no longer occurs. On occasion, this mechanism can get out of hand and cause formation of unwanted clots. In fact, this is what initiates most acute heart attacks, which can be caused by a clot beginning on the inside surface of an atherosclerotic plaque in a coronary artery and then growing until the artery is blocked.

Childbirth is another instance in which positive feedback is valuable. When uterine contractions become strong enough for the baby's head to begin pushing through the cervix, stretching of the cervix sends signals through the uterine muscle back to the body of the uterus, causing even more powerful contractions. Thus, the uterine contractions stretch the cervix and the cervical stretch causes stronger contractions. When this process

becomes powerful enough, the baby is born. If it is not powerful enough, the contractions usually die out and a few days pass before they begin again.

Another important use of positive feedback is for the generation of nerve signals. That is, stimulation of the membrane of a nerve fiber causes slight leakage of sodium ions through sodium channels in the nerve membrane to the fiber's interior. The sodium ions entering the fiber then change the membrane potential, which in turn causes more opening of channels, more change of potential, still more opening of channels, and so forth. Thus, a slight leak becomes an explosion of sodium entering the interior of the nerve fiber, which creates the nerve action potential. This action potential in turn causes electrical current to flow along both the outside and the inside of the fiber and initiates additional action potentials. This process continues again and again until the nerve signal goes all the way to the end of the fiber.

In each case in which positive feedback is useful, the positive feedback is part of an overall negative feedback process. For example, in the case of blood clotting the positive feedback clotting process is a negative feedback process for maintenance of normal blood volume. Also, the positive feedback that causes nerve signals allows the nerves to participate in thousands of negative feedback nervous control systems.

More Complex Types of Control Systems— Adaptive Control

Later in this text, when we study the nervous system, we shall see that this system contains great numbers of interconnected control mechanisms. Some are simple feedback systems similar to those already discussed. Many are not. For instance, some movements of the body occur so rapidly that there is not enough time for nerve signals to travel from the peripheral parts of the body all the way to the brain and then back to the periphery again to control the movement. Therefore, the brain uses a principle called *feed-forward control* to cause required muscle contractions. That is, sensory nerve signals from the moving parts apprise the brain whether the movement is performed correctly. If not, the brain corrects the feed-forward signals that it sends to the muscles the *next* time the movement is required. Then, if still further correction is necessary, this process will be performed again for subsequent movements. This process is called *adaptive control*. Adaptive control, in a sense, is delayed negative feedback.

Thus, one can see how complex the feedback control systems of the body can be. A person's life depends on all of them. Therefore, a major share of this text is devoted to discussing these life-giving mechanisms.

Summary—Automaticity of the Body

The purpose of this chapter has been to point out, first, the overall organization of the body and, second, the means by which the different parts of the body operate in harmony. To summarize, the body is actually a *social order of about 100 trillion cells* organized into different functional structures, some of which are called *organs*. Each functional structure contributes its share to the maintenance of homeostatic conditions in the extracellular fluid, which is called the *internal environment*. As long as normal conditions are maintained in this internal environment, the cells of the body continue to live and function properly. Each cell benefits from homeostasis, and, in turn, each cell contributes its share toward the maintenance of homeostasis. This reciprocal interplay provides continuous automaticity of the body until one or more functional systems lose their ability to contribute their share of function. When this happens, all the cells of the body suffer. Extreme dysfunction leads to death; moderate dysfunction leads to sickness.

BIBLIOGRAPHY

Adolph EF: Physiological adaptations: hypertrophies and superfunctions, *Am. Sci.* 60:608, 1972.

Bernard C: *Lectures on the Phenomena of Life Common to Animals and Plants*, Springfield, IL, 1974, Charles C. Thomas.

Cannon WB: Organization for physiological homeostasis, *Physiol. Rev.* 9(3):399, 1929.

Chien S: Mechanotransduction and endothelial cell homeostasis: the wisdom of the cell, *Am. J. Physiol. Heart Circ. Physiol.* 292:H1209, 2007.

Csete ME, Doyle JC: Reverse engineering of biological complexity, *Science* 295:1664, 2002.

DiBona GF: Physiology in perspective: the wisdom of the body. Neural control of the kidney, *Am. J. Physiol. Regul. Integr. Comp. Physiol.* 289:R633, 2005.

Dickinson MH, Farley CT, Full RJ, et al: How animals move: an integrative view, *Science* 288:100, 2000.

Eckel-Mahan K, Sassone-Corsi P: Metabolism and the circadian clock converge, *Physiol. Rev.* 93:107, 2013.

Gao Q, Horvath TL: Neuronal control of energy homeostasis, *FEBS Lett.* 582:132, 2008.

Guyton AC: *Arterial Pressure and Hypertension*, Philadelphia, 1980, W.B. Saunders.

Herman MA, Kahn BB: Glucose transport and sensing in the maintenance of glucose homeostasis and metabolic harmony, *J. Clin. Invest.* 116:1767, 2006.

Krahe R, Gabbiani F: Burst firing in sensory systems, *Nat. Rev. Neurosci.* 5:13, 2004.

Orgel LE: The origin of life on the earth, *Sci. Am.* 271:76, 1994.

Sekirov I, Russell SL, Antunes LC, Finlay BB: Gut microbiota in health and disease, *Physiol. Rev.* 90:859, 2010.

Smith HW: *From Fish to Philosopher*, New York, 1961, Doubleday.

Srinivasan MV: Honeybees as a model for the study of visually guided flight, navigation, and biologically inspired robotics, *Physiol. Rev.* 91:413, 2011.

Tjian R: Molecular machines that control genes, *Sci. Am.* 272:54, 1995.

2 The Cell and Its Functions

LEARNING OBJECTIVES

- List the components of a cell and describe their functions.
- Describe the structure of the cell membrane and the function of its various components.

GLOSSARY OF TERMS

- **Cell membrane:** A lipid bilayer that envelopes the cell, within which proteins are embedded, the so-called "Fluid Mosaic Model"
- **Endoplasmic reticulum:** A network of tubular and flat vesicular structures in the cytoplasm [the granular endoplasmic reticulum (closely approximated to ribosomes) is involved in protein synthesis; the agranular (smooth) endoplasmic reticulum helps in lipid synthesis]
- **Golgi body:** Intracytoplasmic vesicles involved in intracellular secretions and modification of proteins
- **Nucleus:** The control center of the cell containing large quantities of DNA, which are the *genes* (these genes determine the characteristics of the cell's proteins, and also control and promote reproduction of the cell itself)
- **Oxidative phosphorylation:** The process by which ATP is synthesized in the mitochondria by the respiratory enzymes
- **Phagocytosis:** Ingestion of large particles
- **Pinocytosis:** Ingestion of minute particles that form vesicles of extracellular fluid and particulate constituents inside the cell cytoplasm

Each of the 100 trillion cells in a human being is a living structure that can survive for months or years, provided its surrounding fluids contain appropriate nutrients. Cells are the building blocks of the body, providing structure for the body's tissues and organs, ingesting nutrients and converting them to energy, and performing specialized functions. Cells also contain the body's hereditary code that controls the substances synthesized by the cells and permits them to make copies of themselves. To understand the function of organs and other structures of the body it is essential that we first understand the basic organization of the cell and the functions of its component parts.

Organization of the Cell

A typical cell, as seen by the light microscope, is shown in Figure 2-1. Its two major parts are the *nucleus* and the *cytoplasm*. The nucleus is separated from the cytoplasm by a *nuclear membrane* and the cytoplasm is separated from the surrounding fluids by a *cell membrane*, also called the *plasma membrane*.

The different substances that make up the cell are collectively called *protoplasm*. Protoplasm is composed mainly of five basic substances: water, electrolytes, proteins, lipids, and carbohydrates.

The principal fluid medium of the cell is water, which is present in most cells, except for fat cells, in a concentration of 70–85%. Important ions in the cell include *potassium, magnesium, phosphate, sulfate, bicarbonate*, and smaller quantities of *sodium, chloride*, and *calcium*. These are all discussed in more detail in Chapter 6, which considers the interrelations between the intracellular and extracellular fluids.

Proteins. After water, the most abundant substances in most cells are proteins that normally constitute 10–20% of the cell mass. These proteins can be divided into two types: *structural proteins* and *functional proteins*.

Structural proteins are present in the cell mainly in the form of long filaments that are polymers of many individual protein molecules. A prominent use of such intracellular filaments is to form *microtubules* that provide the "cytoskeletons" of such cellular organelles as cilia, nerve axons, the mitotic spindles of cells undergoing mitosis, and a tangled mass of thin filamentous tubules that hold the parts of the cytoplasm and nucleoplasm together in their respective compartments. Fibrillar proteins are found outside the cell especially in the collagen and elastin fibers of connective tissue and in blood vessel walls, tendons, ligaments, and so forth.

The *functional proteins* are an entirely different type of protein, and are usually composed of combinations of a few molecules in tubular–globular form. These proteins are mainly the *enzymes* of the cell and, in contrast to the fibrillar proteins, are often mobile in the cell fluid. Also, many of them are adherent to membranous structures inside the cell. The enzymes come into direct contact with other substances in the cellular fluid and catalyze specific intracellular chemical reactions. For instance, the chemical reactions that split glucose into its component parts and then combine these with oxygen to form carbon dioxide and water while simultaneously providing energy for cellular function are all catalyzed by a series of protein enzymes.

Lipids. Lipids are several types of substances that are grouped together because of their common property of being soluble in fat solvents. Especially important lipids are *phospholipids* and

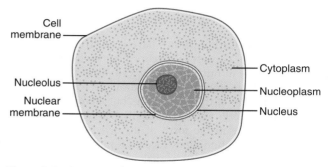

Figure 2-1 Structure of the cell as seen with the light microscope.

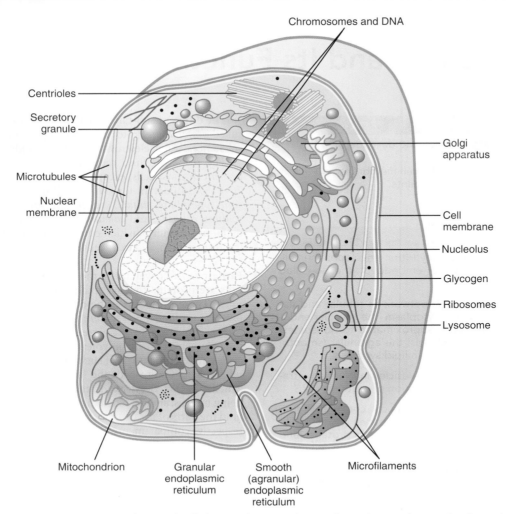

Figure 2-2   Reconstruction of a typical cell, showing the internal organelles in the cytoplasm and in the nucleus.

cholesterol, which together constitute only about 2% of the total cell mass. The significance of phospholipids and cholesterol is that they are mainly insoluble in water and, therefore, are used to form the cell membrane and intracellular membrane barriers that separate the different cell compartments.

In addition to phospholipids and cholesterol, some cells contain large quantities of *triglycerides*, also called *neutral fat*. In the *fat cells* triglycerides often account for as much as 95% of the cell mass. The fat stored in these cells represents the body's main storehouse of energy-giving nutrients that can later be used to provide energy wherever in the body it is needed.

Carbohydrates. Carbohydrates have little structural function in the cell except as parts of glycoprotein molecules, but they play a major role in nutrition of the cell. Most human cells do not maintain large stores of carbohydrates; the amount usually averages about 1% of their total mass but increases to as much as 3% in muscle cells and, occasionally, 6% in liver cells. However, carbohydrate in the form of dissolved glucose is always present in the surrounding extracellular fluid so that it is readily available to the cell. Also, a small amount of carbohydrate is stored in the cells in the form of *glycogen*, which is an insoluble polymer of glucose that can be depolymerized and used rapidly to supply the cells' energy needs.

Physical Structure of the Cell

The cell contains highly organized physical structures called *intracellular organelles*. The physical nature of each organelle is as important as the cell's chemical constituents for cell function. For instance, without one of the organelles, the *mitochondria*, more than 95% of the cell's energy release from nutrients would cease immediately. The most important organelles and other structures of the cell are shown in Figure 2-2.

MEMBRANOUS STRUCTURES OF THE CELL

Most organelles of the cell are covered by membranes composed primarily of lipids and proteins. These membranes include the *cell membrane, nuclear membrane, membrane of the endoplasmic reticulum*, and *membranes of the mitochondria, lysosomes*, and *Golgi apparatus.*

The lipids in the membranes provide a barrier that impedes movement of water and water-soluble substances from one cell compartment to another because water is not soluble in lipids. However, protein molecules in the membrane often penetrate all the way through the membrane, thus providing specialized pathways, often organized into actual *pores*, for passage of specific substances through the membrane. Also, many other

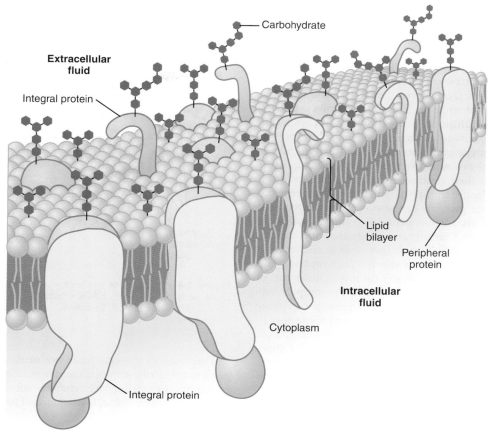

Figure 2-3 Structure of the cell membrane, showing that it is composed mainly of a lipid bilayer of phospholipid molecules, but with large numbers of protein molecules protruding through the layer. Also, carbohydrate moieties are attached to the protein molecules on the outside of the membrane and to additional protein molecules on the inside. *Modified from Lodish, H.F., Rothman, J.E., 1979. The assembly of cell membranes. Sci. Am. 240, 48. Copyright George V. Kevin.*

membrane proteins are *enzymes* that catalyze a multitude of different chemical reactions, discussed here and in subsequent chapters.

Cell Membrane

The cell membrane (also called the *plasma membrane*) envelops the cell, and is a thin, pliable, elastic structure only 7.5–10 nm thick. It is composed almost entirely of proteins and lipids. The approximate composition is proteins, 55%; phospholipids, 25%; cholesterol, 13%; other lipids, 4%; and carbohydrates, 3%.

The Cell Membrane Lipid Barrier Impedes Penetration by Water-Soluble Substances. Figure 2-3 shows the structure of the cell membrane. Its basic structure is a *lipid bilayer*, which is a thin, double-layered film of lipids—each layer only one molecule thick—that is continuous over the entire cell surface. Interspersed in this lipid film are large globular proteins.

The basic lipid bilayer is composed of three main types of lipids: *phospholipids*, *sphingolipids*, and *cholesterol*. Phospholipids are the most abundant of the cell membrane lipids. One end of each phospholipid molecule is soluble in water; that is, it is *hydrophilic*. The other end is soluble only in fats; that is, it is *hydrophobic*. The phosphate end of the phospholipid is hydrophilic and the fatty acid portion is hydrophobic.

Because the hydrophobic portions of the phospholipid molecules are repelled by water but are mutually attracted to one another, they have a natural tendency to attach to one another in the middle of the membrane, as shown in Figure 2-3. The hydrophilic phosphate portions then constitute the two surfaces of the complete cell membrane, in contact with *intracellular* water on the inside of the membrane and *extracellular* water on the outside surface.

The lipid layer in the middle of the membrane is impermeable to the usual water-soluble substances, such as ions, glucose, and urea. Conversely, fat-soluble substances, such as oxygen, carbon dioxide, and alcohol, can penetrate this portion of the membrane with ease.

Sphingolipids, derived from the amino alcohol *sphingosine*, also have hydrophobic and hydrophilic groups and are present in small amounts in the cell membranes, especially nerve cells. Complex sphingolipids in cell membranes are thought to serve several functions, including protection from harmful environmental factors, signal transmission, and as adhesion sites for extracellular proteins.

The cholesterol molecules in the membrane are also lipids because their steroid nuclei are highly fat soluble. These molecules, in a sense, are dissolved in the bilayer of the membrane. They mainly help determine the degree of permeability (or impermeability) of the bilayer to water-soluble constituents of body fluids. Cholesterol controls much of the fluidity of the membrane as well.

Integral and Peripheral Cell Membrane Proteins. Figure 2-3 also shows globular masses floating in the lipid bilayer. These membrane proteins are mainly *glycoproteins*. This model of the cell membrane is often referred to as the "Fluid Mosaic Model."

There are two types of cell membrane proteins: *integral proteins* that protrude all the way through the membrane and *peripheral proteins* that are attached only to one surface of the membrane and do not penetrate all the way through.

Many of the integral proteins provide structural *channels* (or *pores*) through which water molecules and water-soluble substances, especially ions, can diffuse between the extracellular and intracellular fluids. These protein channels also have selective properties that allow preferential diffusion of some substances over others.

Other integral proteins act as *carrier proteins* for transporting substances that otherwise could not penetrate the lipid bilayer. Sometimes these carrier proteins even transport substances in the direction opposite to their electrochemical gradients for diffusion, which is called "active transport." Still others act as *enzymes*.

Integral membrane proteins can also serve as *receptors* for water-soluble chemicals, such as peptide hormones, which do not easily penetrate the cell membrane. Interaction of cell membrane receptors with specific *ligands* that bind to the receptor causes conformational changes in the receptor protein. This process, in turn, enzymatically activates the intracellular part of the protein or induces interactions between the receptor and proteins in the cytoplasm that act as *second messengers*, relaying the signal from the extracellular part of the receptor to the interior of the cell. In this way integral proteins spanning the cell membrane provide a means of conveying information about the environment to the cell interior.

Peripheral protein molecules are often attached to the integral proteins. These peripheral proteins function almost entirely as enzymes or as controllers of transport of substances through the cell membrane "pores."

Membrane Carbohydrates—The Cell "Glycocalyx". Membrane carbohydrates occur almost invariably in combination with proteins or lipids in the form of glycoproteins or glycolipids. In fact, most of the integral proteins are glycoproteins and about one-tenth of the membrane lipid molecules are glycolipids. The "glyco" portions of these molecules almost invariably protrude to the outside of the cell, dangling outward from the cell surface. Many other carbohydrate compounds called proteoglycans—which are mainly carbohydrate substances bound to small protein cores—are loosely attached to the outer surface of the cell as well. Thus, the entire outside surface of the cell often has a loose carbohydrate coat called the glycocalyx.

The carbohydrate moieties attached to the outer surface of the cell have several important functions:

1. Many of them have a negative electrical charge, which gives most cells an overall negative surface charge that repels other negatively charged objects.
2. The glycocalyx of some cells attaches to the glycocalyx of other cells, thus attaching cells to one another.
3. Many of the carbohydrates act as *receptor substances* for binding hormones, such as insulin; when bound, this combination activates attached internal proteins that, in turn, activate a cascade of intracellular enzymes.
4. Some carbohydrate moieties enter into immune reactions, as discussed in Chapter 25.

CYTOPLASM AND ITS ORGANELLES

The cytoplasm is filled with both minute and large dispersed particles and organelles. The jelly-like fluid portion of the cytoplasm in which the particles are dispersed is called *cytosol*, and contains mainly dissolved proteins, electrolytes, and glucose.

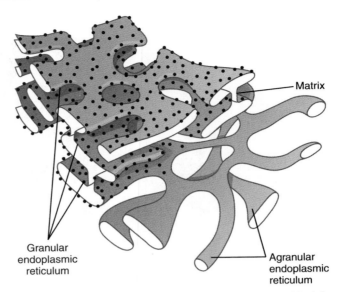

Figure 2-4   Structure of the endoplasmic reticulum. *Modified from DeRobertis, E.D.P., Saez, F.A., DeRobertis, E.M.F., 1975. Cell Biology, 6th ed. Philadelphia: W.B. Saunders.*

Dispersed in the cytoplasm are neutral fat globules, glycogen granules, ribosomes, secretory vesicles, and five especially important organelles: the *endoplasmic reticulum*, the *Golgi apparatus*, *mitochondria*, *lysosomes*, and *peroxisomes*.

Endoplasmic Reticulum

Figure 2-2 shows a network of tubular and flat vesicular structures in the cytoplasm, which is the *endoplasmic reticulum*. This organelle helps process molecules made by the cell and transports them to their specific destinations inside or outside the cell. The tubules and vesicles interconnect. Also, their walls are constructed of lipid bilayer membranes that contain large amounts of proteins, similar to the cell membrane. The total surface area of this structure in some cells—the liver cells, for instance—can be as much as 30–40 times the cell membrane area.

The detailed structure of a small portion of endoplasmic reticulum is shown in Figure 2-4. The space inside the tubules and vesicles is filled with *endoplasmic matrix*, a watery medium that is different from the fluid in the cytosol outside the endoplasmic reticulum. Electron micrographs show that the space inside the endoplasmic reticulum is connected with the space between the two membrane surfaces of the nuclear membrane.

Substances formed in some parts of the cell enter the space of the endoplasmic reticulum and are then directed to other parts of the cell. Also, the vast surface area of this reticulum and the multiple enzyme systems attached to its membranes provide machinery for a major share of the metabolic functions of the cell.

Ribosomes and the Granular Endoplasmic Reticulum. Attached to the outer surfaces of many parts of the endoplasmic reticulum are large numbers of minute granular particles called *ribosomes*. Where these particles are present, the reticulum is called the *granular endoplasmic reticulum*. The ribosomes are composed of a mixture of RNA and proteins, and they function to synthesize new protein molecules in the cell, as discussed later in this chapter and in Chapter 3.

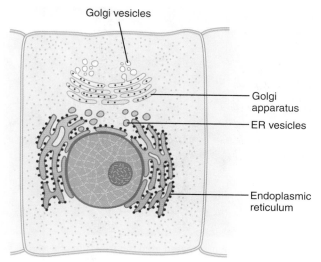

Figure 2-5 A typical Golgi apparatus and its relationship to the endoplasmic reticulum (ER) and the nucleus.

Agranular Endoplasmic Reticulum. Part of the endoplasmic reticulum has no attached ribosomes. This part is called the *agranular* or *smooth endoplasmic reticulum*. The agranular reticulum functions for the synthesis of lipid substances and for other processes of the cells promoted by intrareticular enzymes.

Golgi Apparatus

The Golgi apparatus, shown in Figure 2-5, is closely related to the endoplasmic reticulum. It has membranes similar to those of the agranular endoplasmic reticulum. The Golgi apparatus is usually composed of four or more stacked layers of thin, flat, enclosed vesicles lying near one side of the nucleus. This apparatus is prominent in secretory cells, where it is located on the side of the cell from which the secretory substances are extruded.

The Golgi apparatus functions in association with the endoplasmic reticulum. As shown in Figure 2-5, small "transport vesicles" (also called endoplasmic reticulum vesicles or *ER vesicles*) continually pinch off from the endoplasmic reticulum and shortly thereafter fuse with the Golgi apparatus. In this way, substances entrapped in the ER vesicles are transported from the endoplasmic reticulum to the Golgi apparatus. The transported substances are then processed in the Golgi apparatus to form lysosomes, secretory vesicles, and other cytoplasmic components that are discussed later in this chapter.

Lysosomes

Lysosomes, shown in Figure 2-2, are vesicular organelles that form by breaking off from the Golgi apparatus and then dispersing throughout the cytoplasm. The lysosomes provide an *intracellular digestive system* that allows the cell to digest (1) damaged cellular structures, (2) food particles that have been ingested by the cell, and (3) unwanted matter such as bacteria. The lysosome is quite different in various cell types, but it is usually 250–750 nm in diameter. It is surrounded by a typical lipid bilayer membrane and is filled with large numbers of small granules 5–8 nm in diameter, which are protein aggregates of as many as 40 different *hydrolase (digestive) enzymes*. A hydrolytic enzyme is capable of splitting an organic compound into two or more parts by combining hydrogen from a water molecule with one part of the compound and combining the hydroxyl portion of the water molecule with the other part of the compound. For instance, protein is hydrolyzed to form amino acids, glycogen is hydrolyzed to form glucose, and lipids are hydrolyzed to form fatty acids and glycerol.

Hydrolytic enzymes are highly concentrated in lysosomes. Ordinarily, the membrane surrounding the lysosome prevents the enclosed hydrolytic enzymes from coming in contact with other substances in the cell and, therefore, prevents their digestive actions. However, some conditions of the cell break the membranes of some of the lysosomes, allowing release of the digestive enzymes. These enzymes then split the organic substances with which they come in contact into small, highly diffusible substances such as amino acids and glucose. Some of the specific functions of lysosomes are discussed later in the chapter.

Peroxisomes

Peroxisomes are similar physically to lysosomes, but they are different in two important ways. First, they are believed to be formed by self-replication (or perhaps by budding off from the smooth endoplasmic reticulum) rather than from the Golgi apparatus. Second, they contain oxidases rather than hydrolases. Several of the oxidases are capable of combining oxygen with hydrogen ions derived from different intracellular chemicals to form hydrogen peroxide (H_2O_2). Hydrogen peroxide is a highly oxidizing substance and is used in association with *catalase*, another oxidase enzyme present in large quantities in peroxisomes, to oxidize many substances that might otherwise be poisonous to the cell. For instance, about half the alcohol a person drinks is detoxified into acetaldehyde by the peroxisomes of the liver cells in this manner. A major function of peroxisomes is to catabolize long-chain fatty acids.

Secretory Vesicles

One of the important functions of many cells is secretion of special chemical substances. Almost all such secretory substances are formed by the endoplasmic reticulum–Golgi apparatus system and are then released from the Golgi apparatus into the cytoplasm in the form of storage vesicles called *secretory vesicles* or *secretory granules*. Figure 2-6 shows typical secretory vesicles inside pancreatic acinar cells; these vesicles store protein proenzymes (enzymes that are not yet activated). The proenzymes are secreted later through the outer cell membrane into the pancreatic duct and thence into the duodenum, where they become activated and perform digestive functions on the food in the intestinal tract.

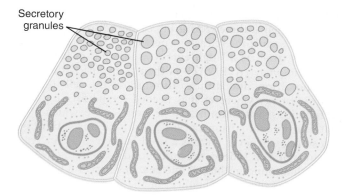

Figure 2-6 Secretory granules (secretory vesicles) in acinar cells of the pancreas.

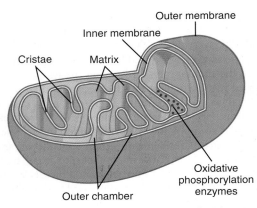

Figure 2-7   Structure of a mitochondrion. *Modified from DeRobertis, E.D.P., Saez, F.A., DeRobertis, E.M.F., 1975. Cell Biology, 6th ed. Philadelphia: W.B. Saunders.*

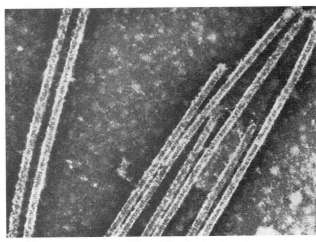

Figure 2-8   Microtubules teased from the flagellum of a sperm. *From Wolstenholme, G.E.W., O'Connor, M., and the publisher, J.A. Churchill, 1967. Figure 4, p. 314. Copyright the Novartis Foundation, formerly the Ciba Foundation.*

Mitochondria

The mitochondria, shown in Figures 2-2 and 2-7, are called the "powerhouses" of the cell. Without them cells would be unable to extract enough energy from the nutrients, and essentially all cellular functions would cease.

Mitochondria are present in all areas of each cell's cytoplasm, but the total number per cell varies from less than a hundred up to several thousand, depending on the amount of energy required by the cell. The cardiac muscle cells (cardiomyocytes), for example, use large amounts of energy and have far more mitochondria than do fat cells (adipocytes), which are much less active and use less energy. Further, the mitochondria are concentrated in those portions of the cell that are responsible for the major share of its energy metabolism. They are also variable in size and shape. Some mitochondria are only a few hundred nanometers in diameter and are globular in shape, whereas others are elongated and are as large as 1 μm in diameter and 7 μm long; still others are branching and filamentous.

The basic structure of the mitochondrion, shown in Figure 2-7, is composed mainly of two lipid bilayer–protein membranes: an *outer membrane* and an *inner membrane*. Many infoldings of the inner membrane form *shelves* or tubules called *cristae* onto which oxidative enzymes are attached. The cristae provide a large surface area for chemical reactions to occur. In addition, the inner cavity of the mitochondrion is filled with a *matrix* that contains large quantities of dissolved enzymes that are necessary for extracting energy from nutrients. These enzymes operate in association with the oxidative enzymes on the cristae to cause oxidation of the nutrients, thereby forming carbon dioxide and water, and at the same time releasing energy. The liberated energy is used to synthesize a "high-energy" substance called *adenosine triphosphate* (ATP). ATP is then transported out of the mitochondrion, and diffuses throughout the cell to release its own energy wherever it is needed for performing cellular functions. Mitochondria are self-replicative, which means that one mitochondrion can form a second one, a third one, and so on, whenever there is a need in the cell for increased amounts of ATP. Indeed, the mitochondria contain *DNA* similar to that found in the cell nucleus. In Chapter 3 we will see that DNA is the basic chemical of the nucleus that controls replication of the cell. The DNA of the mitochondrion plays a similar role, controlling replication of the mitochondrion.

Cells that are faced with increased energy demands—which occur, for example, in skeletal muscles subjected to chronic exercise training—may increase the density of mitochondria to supply the additional energy required.

Cell Cytoskeleton—Filament and Tubular Structures

The cell cytoskeleton is a network of fibrillar proteins organized into filaments or tubules. These originate as precursor protein molecules synthesized by ribosomes in the cytoplasm. The precursor molecules then polymerize to form *filaments*. As an example, large numbers of actin filaments frequently occur in the outer zone of the cytoplasm, called the *ectoplasm*, to form an elastic support for the cell membrane. Also, in muscle cells, actin and myosin filaments are organized into a special contractile machine that is the basis for muscle contraction, as is discussed in detail in Chapter 14.

A special type of stiff filament composed of polymerized *tubulin* molecules is used in all cells to construct strong tubular structures, the *microtubules*. Figure 2-8 shows typical microtubules from the flagellum of a sperm. Also, both the *centrioles* and the *mitotic spindle* of the mitosing cell are composed of stiff microtubules.

Thus, a primary function of microtubules is to act as a *cytoskeleton*, providing rigid physical structures for certain parts of cells. The cytoskeleton of the cell not only determines cell shape but also participates in cell division, allows cells to move, and provides a track-like system that directs the movement of organelles within the cells.

NUCLEUS

The nucleus, which is the control center of the cell, sends messages to the cell to grow and mature, to replicate, or to die. Briefly, the nucleus contains large quantities of DNA, which comprise the *genes*. The genes determine the characteristics of the cell's proteins, including the structural proteins as well as the intracellular enzymes that control cytoplasmic and nuclear activities.

The genes also control and promote reproduction of the cell. The genes first reproduce to create two identical sets of genes; then the cell splits by a special process called *mitosis* to form

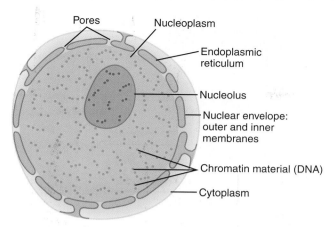

Pores
Nucleoplasm
Endoplasmic reticulum
Nucleolus
Nuclear envelope: outer and inner membranes
Chromatin material (DNA)
Cytoplasm

Figure 2-9 Structure of the nucleus.

two daughter cells, each of which receives one of the two sets of DNA genes. All these activities of the nucleus are considered in detail in Chapter 3.

Unfortunately, the appearance of the nucleus under the microscope does not provide many clues to the mechanisms by which the nucleus performs its control activities. Figure 2-9 shows the light microscopic appearance of the *interphase* nucleus (during the period between mitoses), revealing darkly staining *chromatin material* throughout the nucleoplasm. During mitosis the chromatin material organizes in the form of highly structured *chromosomes*, which can then be easily identified using the light microscope, as illustrated in Chapter 3.

NUCLEAR MEMBRANE

The *nuclear membrane*, also called the *nuclear envelope*, is actually two separate bilayer membranes, one inside the other. The outer membrane is continuous with the endoplasmic reticulum of the cell cytoplasm, and the space between the two nuclear membranes is also continuous with the space inside the endoplasmic reticulum, as shown in Figure 2-9.

The nuclear membrane is penetrated by several thousand *nuclear pores.* Large complexes of protein molecules are attached at the edges of the pores so that the central area of each pore is only about 9 nm in diameter. Even this size is large enough to allow molecules up to 44,000 molecular weight to pass through with reasonable ease.

NUCLEOLI AND FORMATION OF RIBOSOMES

The nuclei of most cells contain one or more highly staining structures called *nucleoli*. The nucleolus, unlike most other organelles discussed here, does not have a limiting membrane. Instead, it is simply an accumulation of large amounts of RNA and proteins of the types found in ribosomes. The nucleolus becomes considerably enlarged when the cell is actively synthesizing proteins.

Formation of the nucleoli (and of the ribosomes in the cytoplasm outside the nucleus) begins in the nucleus. First, specific DNA genes in the chromosomes cause RNA to be synthesized. Some of this synthesized RNA is stored in the nucleoli, but most of it is transported outward through the nuclear pores into cytoplasm. Here, it is used in conjunction with specific proteins to assemble "mature" ribosomes that play an essential role in forming cytoplasmic proteins, as discussed more fully in Chapter 3.

Functional Systems of the Cell

In the remainder of this chapter, we discuss several representative functional systems of the cell that make it a living organism.

INGESTION BY THE CELL—ENDOCYTOSIS

If a cell is to live and grow and reproduce, it must obtain nutrients and other substances from the surrounding fluids. Most substances pass through the cell membrane by *diffusion* and *active transport*.

Diffusion involves simple movement through the membrane caused by the random motion of the molecules of the substance; substances move either through cell membrane pores or, in the case of lipid-soluble substances, through the lipid matrix of the membrane.

Active transport involves the actual carrying of a substance through the membrane by a physical protein structure that penetrates all the way through the membrane. These active transport mechanisms are so important to cell function that they are presented in detail in Chapter 4.

Very large particles enter the cell by a specialized function of the cell membrane called *endocytosis*. The principal forms of endocytosis are *pinocytosis* and *phagocytosis*. Pinocytosis means ingestion of minute particles that form vesicles of extracellular fluid and particulate constituents inside the cell cytoplasm. Phagocytosis means ingestion of large particles, such as bacteria, whole cells, or portions of degenerating tissue.

Pinocytosis. Pinocytosis occurs continually in the cell membranes of most cells, but it is especially rapid in some cells. For instance, it occurs so rapidly in macrophages that about 3% of the total macrophage membrane is engulfed in the form of vesicles each minute. Even so, the pinocytotic vesicles are so small—usually only 100–200 nm in diameter—that most of them can be seen only with an electron microscope.

Pinocytosis is the only means by which most large macromolecules, such as most protein molecules, can enter cells. In fact, the rate at which pinocytotic vesicles form is usually enhanced when such macromolecules attach to the cell membrane.

Figure 2-10 demonstrates the successive steps of pinocytosis showing three molecules of protein attaching to the membrane. These molecules usually attach to specialized protein *receptors* on the surface of the membrane that are specific for the type of protein that is to be absorbed. The receptors generally are concentrated in small pits on the outer surface of the cell membrane, called *coated pits*. On the inside of the cell membrane beneath these pits is a latticework of fibrillar protein called *clathrin*, as well as other proteins, perhaps including contractile filaments of *actin* and *myosin*. Once the protein molecules have bound with the receptors, the surface properties of the local membrane change in such a way that the entire pit invaginates inward and the fibrillar proteins surrounding the invaginating pit cause its borders to close over the attached proteins as well as over a small amount of extracellular fluid. Immediately thereafter, the invaginated portion of the membrane breaks away from the surface of the cell, forming a *pinocytotic vesicle* inside the cytoplasm of the cell.

What causes the cell membrane to go through the necessary contortions to form pinocytotic vesicles is still unclear. This process requires energy from within the cell, which is supplied by ATP. This process also requires the presence of calcium ions in the extracellular fluid, which probably react with contractile

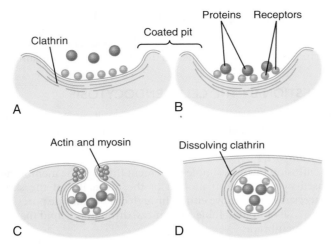

Figure 2-10   Mechanism of pinocytosis. (A) Three protein molecules and the receptors on a coated pit; (B) binding of protein molecules with the receptors; (C) invagination of the coated pit; (D) formation of the pinocytic vesicle.

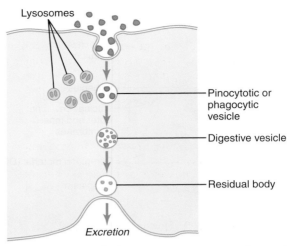

Figure 2-11   Digestion of substances in pinocytotic or phagocytic vesicles by enzymes derived from lysosomes.

protein filaments beneath the coated pits to provide the force for pinching the vesicles away from the cell membrane.

Phagocytosis. Phagocytosis occurs in much the same way as pinocytosis occurs, except that it involves large particles rather than molecules. Only certain cells have the capability of phagocytosis, most notably the tissue macrophages and some white blood cells.

Phagocytosis is initiated when a particle such as a bacterium, a dead cell, or tissue debris binds with receptors on the surface of the phagocyte. In the case of bacteria, each bacterium is usually already attached to a specific antibody, and it is the antibody that attaches to the phagocyte receptors, dragging the bacterium along with it. This intermediation of antibodies is called *opsonization*.

PINOCYTOTIC AND PHAGOCYTIC FOREIGN SUBSTANCES ARE DIGESTED INSIDE THE CELL BY LYSOSOMES

Almost immediately after a pinocytotic or phagocytic vesicle appears inside a cell, one or more *lysosomes* become attached to the vesicle and empty their *acid hydrolases* to the inside of the vesicle, as shown in Figure 2-11. Thus, a *digestive vesicle* is formed inside the cell cytoplasm in which the vesicular hydrolases begin hydrolyzing the proteins, carbohydrates, lipids, and other substances in the vesicle. The products of digestion are small molecules of amino acids, glucose, phosphates, and so forth that can diffuse through the membrane of the vesicle into the cytoplasm. What is left of the digestive vesicle, called the *residual body*, represents indigestible substances. In most instances, the residual body is finally excreted through the cell membrane by a process called *exocytosis*, which is essentially the opposite of endocytosis.

Thus, the pinocytotic and phagocytic vesicles containing lysosomes can be called the *digestive organs* of the cells.

Regression of Tissues and Autolysis of Damaged Cells. Tissues of the body often regress to a smaller size. For instance, this regression occurs in the uterus after pregnancy, in muscles during long periods of inactivity, and in mammary glands at the end of lactation. Lysosomes are responsible for much of this regression.

Another special role of the lysosomes is removal of damaged cells or damaged portions of cells from tissues. Damage to the

cell—caused by heat, cold, trauma, chemicals, or any other factor—induces lysosomes to rupture. The released hydrolases immediately begin to digest the surrounding organic substances. If the damage is slight, only a portion of the cell is removed and the cell is then repaired. If the damage is severe, the entire cell is digested, a process called *autolysis*. In this way the cell is completely removed and a new cell of the same type ordinarily is formed by mitotic reproduction of an adjacent cell to take the place of the old one.

The lysosomes also contain bactericidal agents that can kill phagocytized bacteria before they can cause cellular damage. These agents include (1) *lysozyme* that dissolves the bacterial cell membrane; (2) *lysoferrin* that binds iron and other substances before they can promote bacterial growth; and (3) acid at pH of about 5.0 that activates the hydrolases and inactivates bacterial metabolic systems.

Recycling of Cell Organelles—Autophagy. Lysosomes play a key role in the process of autophagy, which literally means "to eat oneself." Autophagy is a housekeeping process by which obsolete organelles and large protein aggregates are degraded and recycled. Worn-out cell organelles are transferred to lysosomes by double-membrane structures called *autophagosomes* that are formed in the cytosol. Invagination of the lysosomal membrane and the formation of vesicles provide another pathway for cytosolic structures to be transported into the lumen of the lysosomes. Once inside the lysosomes, the organelles are digested and the nutrients are reused by the cell. Autophagy contributes to the routine turnover of cytoplasmic components and is a key mechanism for tissue development, for cell survival when nutrients are scarce, and for maintaining homeostasis. In liver cells, for example, the average mitochondrion normally has a life span of only about 10 days before it is destroyed.

SYNTHESIS OF CELLULAR STRUCTURES BY ENDOPLASMIC RETICULUM AND GOLGI APPARATUS

Specific Functions of the Endoplasmic Reticulum

The extensiveness of the endoplasmic reticulum and the Golgi apparatus in secretory cells has already been emphasized. These structures are formed primarily of lipid bilayer membranes similar to the cell membrane, and their walls are loaded with protein enzymes that catalyze the synthesis of many substances required by the cell.

Most synthesis begins in the endoplasmic reticulum. The products formed there are then passed on to the Golgi apparatus, where they are further processed before being released into the cytoplasm. First, however, let us note the specific products that are synthesized in specific portions of the endoplasmic reticulum and the Golgi apparatus.

Proteins Are Formed by the Granular Endoplasmic Reticulum. The granular portion of the endoplasmic reticulum is characterized by large numbers of ribosomes attached to the outer surfaces of the endoplasmic reticulum membrane. As discussed in Chapter 3, protein molecules are synthesized within the structures of the ribosomes. The ribosomes extrude some of the synthesized protein molecules directly into the cytosol, but they also extrude many more through the wall of the endoplasmic reticulum to the interior of the endoplasmic vesicles and tubules, into the endoplasmic matrix.

Synthesis of Lipids by the Smooth Endoplasmic Reticulum. The endoplasmic reticulum also synthesizes lipids, especially phospholipids and cholesterol. These lipids are rapidly incorporated into the lipid bilayer of the endoplasmic reticulum itself, thus causing the endoplasmic reticulum to grow more extensive. This process occurs mainly in the smooth portion of the endoplasmic reticulum.

To keep the endoplasmic reticulum from growing beyond the needs of the cell small vesicles called *ER vesicles* or *transport vesicles* continually break away from the smooth reticulum; most of these vesicles then migrate rapidly to the Golgi apparatus.

Specific Functions of the Golgi Apparatus

Synthetic Functions of the Golgi Apparatus. Although the major function of the Golgi apparatus is to provide additional processing of substances already formed in the endoplasmic reticulum, it also has the capability of synthesizing certain carbohydrates that cannot be formed in the endoplasmic reticulum. This is especially true for the formation of large saccharide polymers bound with small amounts of protein; important examples include hyaluronic acid and chondroitin sulfate.

A few of the many functions of hyaluronic acid and chondroitin sulfate in the body are as follows: (1) they are the major components of proteoglycans secreted in mucus and other glandular secretions; (2) they are the major components of the *ground substance*, or nonfibrous components of the extracellular matrix, outside the cells in the interstitial spaces, acting as fillers between collagen fibers and cells; (3) they are principal components of the organic matrix in both cartilage and bone; and (4) they are important in many cell activities including migration and proliferation.

Processing of Endoplasmic Secretions by the Golgi Apparatus—Formation of Vesicles. Figure 2-12 summarizes the major functions of the endoplasmic reticulum and Golgi apparatus. As substances are formed in the endoplasmic reticulum, especially the proteins, they are transported through the tubules toward portions of the smooth endoplasmic reticulum that lie nearest the Golgi apparatus. At this point small transport vesicles composed of small envelopes of smooth endoplasmic reticulum continually break away and diffuse to the deepest layer of the Golgi apparatus. Inside these vesicles are the synthesized proteins and other products from the endoplasmic reticulum.

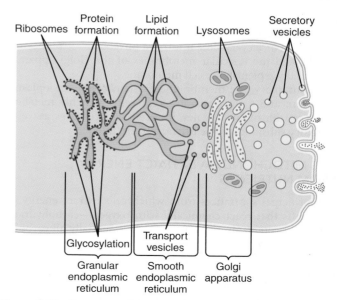

Figure 2-12 Formation of proteins, lipids, and cellular vesicles by the endoplasmic reticulum and Golgi apparatus.

The transport vesicles instantly fuse with the Golgi apparatus and empty their contained substances into the vesicular spaces of the Golgi apparatus. Here, additional carbohydrate moieties are added to the secretions. Also, an important function of the Golgi apparatus is to compact the endoplasmic reticular secretions into highly concentrated packets. As the secretions pass toward the outermost layers of the Golgi apparatus the compaction and processing proceed. Finally, both small and large vesicles continually break away from the Golgi apparatus, carrying with them the compacted secretory substances, and, in turn, the vesicles diffuse throughout the cell.

The following example provides an idea of the timing of these processes: When a glandular cell is bathed in radioactive amino acids, newly formed radioactive protein molecules can be detected in the granular endoplasmic reticulum within 3–5 minutes. Within 20 minutes, newly formed proteins are already present in the Golgi apparatus, and within 1–2 hours the proteins are secreted from the surface of the cell.

Types of Vesicles Formed by the Golgi Apparatus—Secretory Vesicles and Lysosomes. In a highly secretory cell the vesicles formed by the Golgi apparatus are mainly *secretory vesicles* containing protein substances that are to be secreted through the surface of the cell membrane. These secretory vesicles first diffuse to the cell membrane, and then fuse with it and empty their substances to the exterior by the mechanism called *exocytosis*. Exocytosis, in most cases, is stimulated by the entry of calcium ions into the cell; calcium ions interact with the vesicular membrane in some way that is not understood and cause its fusion with the cell membrane, followed by exocytosis—that is, opening of the membrane's outer surface and extrusion of its contents outside the cell. Some vesicles, however, are destined for intracellular use.

Use of Intracellular Vesicles to Replenish Cellular Membranes. Some of the intracellular vesicles formed by the Golgi apparatus fuse with the cell membrane or with the membranes of intracellular structures such as the mitochondria and even the endoplasmic reticulum. This fusion increases the expanse of these membranes and thereby replenishes the membranes as they are used up. For instance, the cell membrane loses much of its substance every time it forms a phagocytic or pinocytotic vesicle, and the vesicular membranes of the Golgi apparatus continually replenish the cell membrane.

In summary, the membranous system of the endoplasmic reticulum and Golgi apparatus represents a highly metabolic organ capable of forming new intracellular structures, as well as secretory substances to be extruded from the cell.

THE MITOCHONDRIA EXTRACT ENERGY FROM NUTRIENTS

The principal substances from which cells extract energy are foodstuffs that react chemically with oxygen—carbohydrates, fats, and proteins. In the human body, essentially all carbohydrates are converted into *glucose* by the digestive tract and liver before they reach the other cells of the body. Similarly, proteins are converted into *amino acids* and fats are converted into *fatty acids*. Figure 2-13 shows oxygen and the foodstuffs—glucose, fatty acids, and amino acids—all entering the cell. Inside the cell, the foodstuffs react chemically with oxygen under the influence of enzymes that control the reactions and channel the energy released in the proper direction. Briefly, almost all these oxidative reactions occur inside the mitochondria and the energy that is released is used to form the high-energy compound *ATP*. This process is called *oxidative phosphorylation*. Then, ATP, not the original foodstuffs, is used throughout the cell to energize almost all the subsequent intracellular metabolic reactions.

Functional Characteristics of ATP

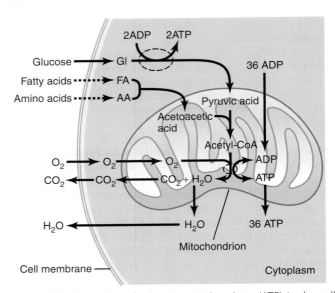

Figure 2-13 Formation of adenosine triphosphate (ATP) in the cell, showing that most of the ATP is formed in the mitochondria. *ADP,* adenosine diphosphate; *CoA,* coenzyme A.

ATP is a nucleotide composed of (1) the nitrogenous base *adenine,* (2) the pentose sugar *ribose,* and (3) three *phosphate radicals.* The last two phosphate radicals are connected with the remainder of the molecule by so-called *high-energy phosphate bonds,* which are represented in the formula shown by the symbol ~. *Under the physical and chemical conditions of the body,* each of these high-energy bonds contains about 12,000 cal of energy per mole of ATP, which is many times greater than the energy stored in the average chemical bond, thus giving rise to the term *high-energy bond.* Further, the high-energy phosphate bond is very labile so that it can be split instantly on demand whenever energy is required to promote other intracellular reactions.

When ATP releases its energy, a phosphoric acid radical is split away and *adenosine diphosphate* (ADP) is formed. This released energy is used to energize many of the cell's other functions, such as synthesis of substances and muscular contraction.

To reconstitute the cellular ATP as it is used up, energy derived from the cellular nutrients causes ADP and phosphoric acid to recombine to form new ATP, and the entire process is repeated over and over again. For these reasons, ATP has been called the *energy currency* of the cell because it can be spent and remade continually, having a turnover time of only a few minutes.

Chemical Processes in the Formation of ATP—Role of the Mitochondria. Upon entry into the cells, glucose is subjected to enzymes in the *cytoplasm* that convert it into *pyruvic acid* (a process called *glycolysis*). A small amount of ADP is changed into ATP by the energy released during this conversion, but this amount accounts for less than 5% of the overall energy metabolism of the cell.

About 95% of the cell's ATP formation occurs in the mitochondria. The pyruvic acid derived from carbohydrates, fatty acids from lipids, and amino acids from proteins are eventually converted into the compound *acetyl-coenzyme A (CoA)* in the matrix of the mitochondria. This substance, in turn, is further dissoluted (for the purpose of extracting its energy) by another series of enzymes in the mitochondrion matrix, undergoing dissolution in a sequence of chemical reactions called the *citric acid cycle* or *Krebs cycle.* In this citric acid cycle, acetyl-CoA is split into its component parts, *hydrogen atoms* and *carbon dioxide.* The carbon dioxide diffuses out of the mitochondria and eventually out of the cell; finally, it is excreted from the body through the lungs.

The hydrogen atoms, conversely, are highly reactive, and they combine with oxygen that has also diffused into the mitochondria. This combination releases a tremendous amount of energy, which is used by the mitochondria to convert large amounts of ADP to ATP. The processes of these reactions are complex, requiring the participation of many protein enzymes that are integral parts of mitochondrial *membranous shelves* that protrude into the mitochondrial matrix. The initial event is removal of an electron from the hydrogen atom, thus converting it to a hydrogen ion. The terminal event is combination of hydrogen ions with oxygen to form water plus release of tremendous amounts of energy to large globular proteins that protrude like knobs from the membranes of the mitochondrial shelves; this process is called *ATP synthetase*. Finally, the enzyme ATP synthetase uses the energy from the hydrogen ions to cause the conversion of ADP to ATP. The newly formed ATP is transported out of the mitochondria into all parts of the cell cytoplasm and nucleoplasm, where its energy is used to energize multiple cell functions.

This overall process for formation of ATP is called the *chemiosmotic mechanism* of ATP formation.

Uses of ATP for Cellular Function. Energy from ATP is used to promote three major categories of cellular functions: (1) *transport* of substances through multiple membranes in the cell, (2) *synthesis of chemical compounds* throughout the cell, and (3) *mechanical work*. These uses of ATP are illustrated by examples in Figure 2-14: (1) to supply energy for the transport of sodium through the cell membrane, (2) to promote protein synthesis by the ribosomes, and (3) to supply the energy needed during muscle contraction.

In addition to membrane transport of sodium, energy from ATP is required for membrane transport of potassium ions, calcium ions, magnesium ions, phosphate ions, chloride ions, urate ions, hydrogen ions, and many other ions and various organic substances. Membrane transport is so important to cell function that some cells—the renal tubular cells, for instance—use as much as 80% of the ATP that they form for this purpose alone.

In addition to synthesizing proteins, cells make phospholipids, cholesterol, purines, pyrimidines, and a host of other substances. Synthesis of almost any chemical compound requires energy. For instance, a single protein molecule might be composed of as many as several thousand amino acids attached to one another by peptide linkages. The formation of each of these linkages requires energy derived from the breakdown of four high-energy bonds; thus, many thousand ATP molecules must release their energy as each protein molecule is formed. Indeed, some cells use as much as 75% of all the ATP formed in the cell simply to synthesize new chemical compounds, especially protein molecules; this is particularly true during the growth phase of cells.

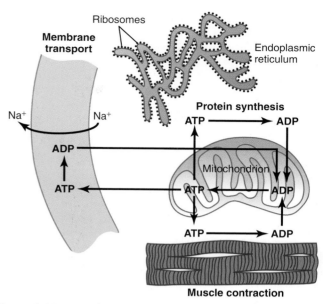

Figure 2-14 Use of adenosine triphosphate (ATP) (formed in the mitochondrion) to provide energy for three major cellular functions: membrane transport, protein synthesis, and muscle contraction. *ADP*, adenosine diphosphate.

The final major use of ATP is to supply energy for special cells to perform mechanical work. We see in Chapter 14 that each contraction of a muscle fiber requires expenditure of tremendous quantities of ATP energy. Other cells perform mechanical work in other ways, especially by *ciliary* and *ameboid motion*. The source of energy for all these types of mechanical work is ATP.

In summary, ATP is always available to release its energy rapidly and almost explosively wherever in the cell it is needed. To replace the ATP used by the cell, much slower chemical reactions break down carbohydrates, fats, and proteins and use the energy derived from these processes to form new ATP. More than 95% of this ATP is formed in the mitochondria, which accounts for the mitochondria being called the "powerhouses" of the cell.

BIBLIOGRAPHY

Alberts B, Johnson A, Lewis J, et al: *Molecular Biology of the Cell*, sixth ed., New York, 2007, Garland Science.
Bohdanowicz M, Grinstein S: Role of phospholipids in endocytosis, phagocytosis, and macropinocytosis, *Physiol. Rev.* 93:69, 2013.
Boya P, Reggiori F, Codogno P: Emerging regulation and functions of autophagy, *Nat. Cell Biol.* 15:713, 2013.
Brandizzi F, Barlowe C: Organization of the ER–Golgi interface for membrane traffic control, *Nat. Rev. Mol. Cell Biol.* 14:382, 2013.
Chen S, Novick P, Ferro-Novick S: ER structure and function, *Curr. Opin. Cell Biol.* 25:428, 2013.
Drummond IA: Cilia functions in development, *Curr. Opin. Cell Biol.* 24:24, 2012.
Edidin M: Lipids on the frontier: a century of cell-membrane bilayers, *Nat. Rev. Mol. Cell Biol.* 4:414, 2003.

Guerriero CJ, Brodsky JL: The delicate balance between secreted protein folding and endoplasmic reticulum-associated degradation in human physiology, *Physiol. Rev.* 92:537, 2012.
Hamasaki M, Shibutani ST, Yoshimori T: Up-to-date membrane biogenesis in the autophagosome formation, *Curr. Opin. Cell Biol.* 25:455, 2013.
Hla T, Dannenberg AJ: Sphingolipid signaling in metabolic disorders, *Cell Metab.* 16:420, 2012.
Insall R: The interaction between pseudopods and extracellular signalling during chemotaxis and directed migration, *Curr. Opin. Cell Biol.* 25:526, 2013.
Jin T: Gradient sensing during chemotaxis, *Curr. Opin. Cell Biol.* 25:532, 2013.
Kikkawa M: Big steps toward understanding dynein, *J. Cell Biol.* 202:15, 2013.

Lamb CA, Yoshimori T, Tooze SA: The autophagosome: origins unknown, biogenesis complex, *Nat. Rev. Mol. Cell Biol.* 14:759, 2013.
Marzetti E, Csiszar A, Dutta D, et al: Role of mitochondrial dysfunction and altered autophagy in cardiovascular aging and disease: from mechanisms to therapeutics, *Am. J. Physiol. Heart Circ. Physiol.* 305:H459, 2013.
Nakamura N, Wei JH, Seemann J: Modular organization of the mammalian Golgi apparatus, *Curr. Opin. Cell Biol.* 24:467, 2012.
Nixon RA: The role of autophagy in neurodegenerative disease, *Nat. Med.* 19:983, 2013.
Smith JJ, Aitchison JD: Peroxisomes take shape, *Nat. Rev. Mol. Cell Biol.* 14:803, 2013.
van der Zand A, Tabak HF: Peroxisomes: offshoots of the ER, *Curr. Opin. Cell Biol.* 25:449, 2013.

Genetic Control of Protein Synthesis, Cell Function, and Cell Reproduction

LEARNING OBJECTIVES

- List the steps that are involved in the genetic control of protein synthesis.
- Describe how gene expression is regulated.
- Describe how intracellular function is controlled by enzymes.
- Describe the basis of tests that are used to evaluate genetic function.
- List the steps that are involved in mitosis.
- Define apoptosis.

GLOSSARY OF TERMS

- **Apoptosis:** Programmed cell death
- **Gene:** A sequence of DNA that codes for a protein or a cellular trait
- **Transcription:** Assembly of the RNA chain from activated nucleotides using the DNA strand as a template
- **Translation:** The process by which the genetic information on the messenger RNA is used to make proteins in the ribosome

Almost everyone knows that the genes, which are located in the nuclei of all cells of the body, control heredity from parents to children, but many people do not realize that these same genes also control the day-to-day function of all the body's cells. The genes control cell function by determining which substances are synthesized within the cell—which structures, which enzymes, and which chemicals.

Figure 3-1 shows the general scheme of genetic control. Each gene, which is composed of *deoxyribonucleic acid* (DNA), controls the formation of another nucleic acid, *ribonucleic acid* (RNA); this RNA then spreads throughout the cell to control the formation of a specific protein. The entire process, from *transcription* of the genetic code in the nucleus to *translation* of the RNA code and the formation of proteins in the cell cytoplasm, is often referred to as *gene expression*.

Because there are approximately 30,000 different genes in each cell, it is theoretically possible to form a large number of different cellular proteins. In fact, RNA molecules transcribed from the same segment of DNA (ie, the same gene) can be processed in more than one way by the cell, giving rise to alternate versions of the protein. The total number of different proteins produced by the various cell types in humans is estimated to be at least 100,000.

Some of the cellular proteins are *structural proteins* that, in association with various lipids and carbohydrates, form the structures of the various intracellular organelles discussed in

Chapter 2. However, the majority of the proteins are *enzymes* that catalyze the different chemical reactions in the cells. For instance, enzymes promote all the oxidative reactions that supply energy to the cell, along with synthesis of all the cell chemicals, such as lipids, glycogen, and adenosine triphosphate (ATP).

Genes in the Cell Nucleus Control Protein Synthesis

In the cell nucleus, large numbers of genes are attached end-on-end in extremely long double-stranded helical molecules of DNA having molecular weights measured in the billions. A very short segment of such a molecule is shown in Figure 3-2. This molecule is composed of several simple chemical compounds bound together in a regular pattern, the details of which are explained in the next few paragraphs.

Basic Building Blocks of DNA. Figure 3-3 shows the basic chemical compounds involved in the formation of DNA. These compounds include (1) *phosphoric acid*, (2) a sugar called *deoxyribose*, and (3) four nitrogenous *bases* (two purines, *adenine* and *guanine*; and two pyrimidines, *thymine* and *cytosine*). The phosphoric acid and deoxyribose form the two helical strands that are the backbone of the DNA molecule and the nitrogenous bases lie between the two strands and connect them, as illustrated in Figure 3-6.

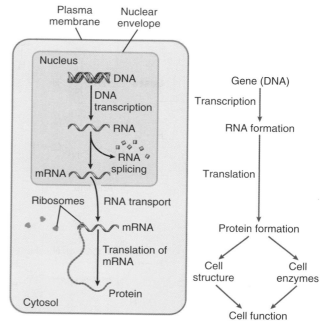

Figure 3-1 General scheme by which the genes control cell function. mRNA, messenger RNA.

Nucleotides. The first stage of DNA formation is to combine one molecule of phosphoric acid, one molecule of deoxyribose, and one of the four bases to form an acidic nucleotide. Four separate nucleotides are thus formed, one for each of the four bases: *deoxyadenylic, deoxythymidylic, deoxyguanylic,* and *deoxycytidylic acids.* Figure 3-4 shows the chemical structure of deoxyadenylic acid, and Figure 3-5 shows simple symbols for the four nucleotides that form DNA.

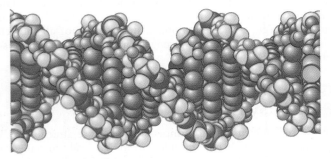

Figure 3-2 The helical, double-stranded structure of the gene. The outside strands are composed of phosphoric acid and the sugar deoxyribose. The internal molecules connecting the two strands of the helix are purine and pyrimidine bases; these determine the "code" of the gene.

Nucleotides Are Organized to Form Two Strands of DNA Loosely Bound to Each Other. Figure 3-6 shows the manner in which multiple numbers of nucleotides are bound together to form two strands of DNA. The two strands are, in turn, loosely bonded with each other by weak cross-linkages, as illustrated in Figure 3-6 by the central dashed lines. Note that the backbone of each DNA strand is composed of alternating phosphoric acid and deoxyribose molecules. In turn, purine and pyrimidine bases are attached to the sides of the deoxyribose molecules. Then, by means of loose *hydrogen bonds* (dashed lines) between the purine and pyrimidine bases, the two respective DNA strands are held together. Note the following caveats, however:

1. Each purine base *adenine* of one strand always bonds with a pyrimidine base *thymine* of the other strand.
2. Each purine base *guanine* always bonds with a pyrimidine base *cytosine.*

Thus, *in* Figure 3-6, the sequence of complementary pairs of bases is CG, CG, GC, TA, CG, TA, *GC, AT,* and AT. Because of the looseness of the hydrogen bonds, the two strands can pull apart with ease, and they do so many times during the course of their function in the cell.

To put the DNA of Figure 3-6 into its proper physical perspective, one could merely pick up the two ends and twist them into a helix. Ten pairs of nucleotides are present in each full turn of the helix in the DNA molecule, as shown in Figure 3-2.

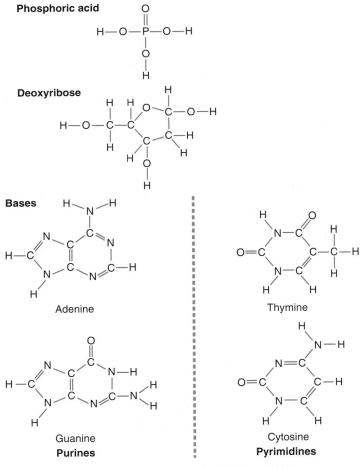

Figure 3-3 The basic building blocks of DNA.

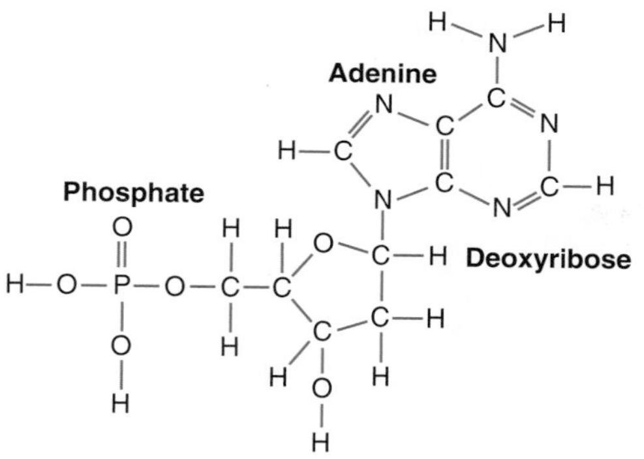

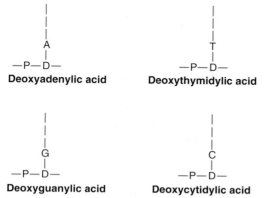

Figure 3-4   Deoxyadenylic acid, one of the nucleotides that make up DNA.

Deoxyadenylic acid

Deoxythymidylic acid

Deoxyguanylic acid

Deoxycytidylic acid

Figure 3-5   Symbols for the four nucleotides that combine to form DNA. Each nucleotide contains phosphoric acid (*P*), deoxyribose (*D*), and one of the four nucleotide bases: *A*, adenine; *T*, thymine; *G*, guanine; or *C*, cytosine.

GENETIC CODE

The importance of DNA lies in its ability to control the formation of proteins in the cell, which it achieves by means of a *genetic code*. That is, when the two strands of a DNA molecule are split apart, the purine and pyrimidine bases projecting to the side of each DNA strand are exposed, as shown by the top strand in Figure 3-7. It is these projecting bases that form the genetic code.

The genetic code consists of successive "triplets" of bases—that is, each three successive bases is a *code word*. The successive triplets eventually control the sequence of amino acids in a protein molecule that is to be synthesized in the cell. Note in Figure 3-6 that the top strand of DNA, reading from left to right, has the genetic code GGC, AGA, CTT,

with the triplets being separated from one another by the arrows. As we follow this genetic code through Figures 3-7 and 3-8, we see that these three respective triplets are responsible for successive placement of the three amino acids, *proline*, *serine*, and *glutamic acid*, in a newly formed molecule of protein.

The DNA Code in the Cell Nucleus Is Transferred to RNA Code in the Cell Cytoplasm—The Process of Transcription

Because the DNA is located in the nucleus of the cell, yet most of the functions of the cell are carried out in the cytoplasm, there must be some means for the DNA genes of the nucleus to control the chemical reactions of the cytoplasm. This control is achieved through the intermediary of another type of nucleic acid, RNA, the formation of which is controlled by the DNA of the nucleus. Thus, as shown in Figure 3-7, the code is transferred to the RNA in a process called *transcription*. The RNA, in turn, diffuses from the nucleus through nuclear pores into the cytoplasmic compartment, where it controls protein synthesis.

RNA IS SYNTHESIZED IN THE NUCLEUS FROM A DNA TEMPLATE

During synthesis of RNA, the two strands of the DNA molecule separate temporarily; one of these strands is used as a template for synthesis of an RNA molecule. The code triplets in the DNA cause formation of *complementary* code triplets (called *codons*) in the RNA. These codons, in turn, will control the sequence of amino acids in a protein to be synthesized in the cell cytoplasm.

Basic Building Blocks of RNA. The basic building blocks of RNA are almost the same as those of DNA, except for two differences. First, the sugar deoxyribose is not used in the formation of RNA. In its place is another sugar of slightly different composition, *ribose*, that contains an extra hydroxyl ion appended to the ribose ring structure. Second, thymine is replaced by another pyrimidine, *uracil*.

Formation of RNA Nucleotides. The basic building blocks of RNA form *RNA nucleotides*, exactly as previously described for DNA synthesis. Here again, four separate nucleotides are used in the formation of RNA. These nucleotides contain the bases *adenine*, *guanine*, *cytosine*, and *uracil*. Note that these bases are the same bases as in DNA, except that uracil in RNA replaces thymine in DNA.

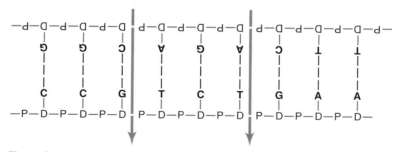

Figure 3-6   Arrangement of deoxyribose nucleotides in a double strand of DNA.

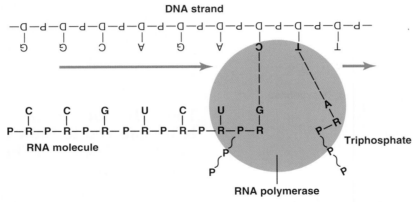

Figure 3-7   Combination of ribose nucleotides with a strand of DNA to form a molecule of RNA that carries the genetic code from the gene to the cytoplasm. The *RNA polymerase* enzyme moves along the DNA strand and builds the RNA molecule.

"Activation" of the RNA Nucleotides. The next step in the synthesis of RNA is "activation" of the RNA nucleotides by an enzyme, *RNA polymerase*. This activation occurs by adding two extra phosphate radicals to each nucleotide to form triphosphates (shown in Figure 3-7 by the two RNA nucleotides to the far right during RNA chain formation). These last two phosphates are combined with the nucleotide by *high-energy phosphate bonds* derived from ATP in the cell.

The result of this activation process is that large quantities of ATP energy are made available to each of the nucleotides. This energy is used to promote the chemical reactions that add each new RNA nucleotide at the end of the developing RNA chain.

ASSEMBLY OF THE RNA CHAIN FROM ACTIVATED NUCLEOTIDES USING THE DNA STRAND AS A TEMPLATE—THE PROCESS OF "TRANSCRIPTION"

As shown in Figure 3-7, assembly of the RNA molecule is accomplished under the influence of an enzyme *RNA polymerase*. This large protein enzyme has many functional properties necessary for formation of the RNA molecule, which are listed as follows:

1. In the DNA strand immediately ahead of the gene to be transcribed is a sequence of nucleotides called the *promoter*. The RNA polymerase has an appropriate complementary structure that recognizes this promoter and becomes attached to it, which is the essential step for initiating formation of the RNA molecule.
2. After the RNA polymerase attaches to the promoter, the polymerase causes unwinding of about two turns of the DNA helix and separation of the unwound portions of the two strands.
3. The polymerase then moves along the DNA strand, temporarily unwinding and separating the two DNA strands at each stage of its movement. As it moves along, at each stage it adds a new activated RNA nucleotide to the end of the newly forming RNA chain through the following steps:
   a. First, it causes a hydrogen bond to form between the end base of the DNA strand and the base of an RNA nucleotide in the nucleoplasm.
   b. Then, one at a time, the RNA polymerase breaks two of the three phosphate radicals away from each of these RNA nucleotides, liberating large amounts of energy

from the broken high-energy phosphate bonds; this energy is used to cause covalent linkage of the remaining phosphate on the nucleotide with the ribose on the end of the growing RNA chain.
   c. When the RNA polymerase reaches the end of the DNA gene, it encounters a new sequence of DNA nucleotides called the *chain-terminating sequence*; this causes the polymerase and the newly formed RNA chain to break away from the DNA strand. The polymerase can then be used again and again to form still more new RNA chains.
   d. As the new RNA strand is formed, its weak hydrogen bonds with the DNA template break away, because the DNA has a high affinity for rebonding with its own complementary DNA strand. Thus, the RNA chain is forced away from the DNA and is released into the nucleoplasm.

Thus, the code that is present in the DNA strand is eventually transmitted in *complementary* form to the RNA chain. The ribose nucleotide bases always combine with the deoxyribose bases in the following manner:

DNA Base		RNA Base
Guanine	....	Cytosine
Cytosine	....	Guanine
Adenine	....	Uracil
Thymine	....	Adenine

There Are Several Different Types of RNA. As research on RNA has continued to advance, many different types of RNA have been discovered. Some types of RNA are involved in protein synthesis, whereas other types serve gene regulatory functions or are involved in posttranscriptional modification of RNA. The functions of some types of RNA, especially those that do not appear to code for proteins, are still mysterious. The following six types of RNA play independent and different roles in protein synthesis:

1. *Precursor messenger RNA* (pre-mRNA) is a large immature single strand of RNA that is processed in the nucleus to form mature messenger RNA (mRNA). The pre-RNA includes two different types of segments called *introns*, which are removed by a process called splicing, and *exons*, which are retained in the final mRNA.

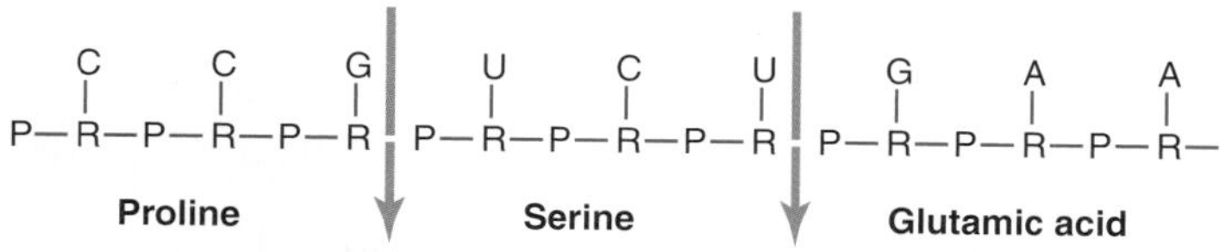

Figure 3-8 Portion of an RNA molecule, showing three RNA "codons"—CCG, UCU, and GAA—that control attachment of the three amino acids, *proline*, *serine*, and *glutamic acid*, respectively, to the growing RNA chain.

2. *Small nuclear RNA* (snRNA) directs the splicing of pre-mRNA to form mRNA.
3. *mRNA* carries the genetic code to the cytoplasm for controlling the type of protein formed.
4. *Transfer RNA* (tRNA) transports activated amino acids to the ribosomes to be used in assembling the protein molecule.
5. *Ribosomal RNA*, along with about 75 different proteins, forms *ribosomes*, the physical and chemical structures on which protein molecules are actually assembled.
6. *MicroRNAs* (miRNAs) are single-stranded RNA molecules of 21–23 nucleotides that can regulate gene transcription and translation.

MESSENGER RNA—THE CODONS

mRNA molecules are long, single RNA strands that are suspended in the cytoplasm. These molecules are composed of several hundred to several thousand RNA nucleotides in unpaired strands, and they contain *codons* that are exactly complementary to the code triplets of the DNA genes. Figure 3-8 shows a small segment of mRNA. Its codons are CCG, UCU, and GAA, which are the codons for the amino acids proline, serine, and glutamic acid. The transcription of these codons from the DNA molecule to the RNA molecule is shown in Figure 3-7.

RNA Codons for the Different Amino Acids. Table 3-1 lists the RNA codons for the 22 common amino acids found in protein molecules. Note that most of the amino acids are represented by more than one codon; also, one codon represents the signal "start manufacturing the protein molecule," and three codons represent "stop manufacturing the protein molecule." In Table 3-1 these two types of codons are designated CI for "chain-initiating" or "start" codon and CT for "chain-terminating" or "stop" codon.

TRANSFER RNA—THE ANTICODONS

Another type of RNA that plays an essential role in protein synthesis is called *tRNA* because it transfers amino acid molecules to protein molecules as the protein is being synthesized. Each type of tRNA combines specifically with 1 of the 20 amino acids that are to be incorporated into proteins. The tRNA then acts as a *carrier* to transport its specific type of amino acid to the ribosomes, where protein molecules are forming. In the ribosomes, each specific type of tRNA recognizes a particular codon on the mRNA (described later) and thereby delivers the appropriate amino acid to the appropriate place in the chain of the newly forming protein molecule.

tRNA, which contains only about 80 nucleotides, is a relatively small molecule in comparison with mRNA. It is a folded chain of nucleotides with a cloverleaf appearance similar to that shown in Figure 3-9. At one end of the molecule there is always an adenylic acid to which the transported amino acid attaches at a hydroxyl group of the ribose in the adenylic acid.

Because the function of tRNA is to cause attachment of a specific amino acid to a forming protein chain, it is essential that each type of tRNA also have specificity for a particular codon in the mRNA. The specific code in the tRNA that allows it to recognize a specific codon is again a triplet of nucleotide bases and is called an *anticodon*. This anticodon is located approximately in the middle of the tRNA molecule (at the bottom of the cloverleaf configuration shown in Figure 3-9). During formation of the protein molecule, the anticodon bases combine loosely by hydrogen bonding with the codon bases of the mRNA. In this way, the respective amino acids are lined up one after another along the mRNA chain, thus establishing the appropriate sequence of amino acids in the newly forming protein molecule.

RIBOSOMAL RNA

The third type of RNA in the cell is ribosomal RNA, which constitutes about 60% of the *ribosome*. The remainder of the ribosome is protein including about 75 types of proteins that are both structural proteins and enzymes needed in the manufacture of protein molecules.

The ribosome is the physical structure in the cytoplasm on which protein molecules are actually synthesized. However, it

TABLE 3-1	RNA Codons for Amino Acids and for Start and Stop				
Amino Acid	**RNA Codons**				
Alanine	GCU	GCC	GCA	GCG	
Arginine	CGU	CGC	CGA	CGG	AGA	AGG
Asparagine	AAU	AAC			
Aspartic acid	GAU	GAC			
Cysteine	UGU	UGC			
Glutamic acid	GAA	GAG			
Glutamine	CAA	CAG			
Glycine	GGU	GGC	GGA	GGG	
Histidine	CAU	CAC			
Isoleucine	AUU	AUC	AUA		
Leucine	CUU	CUC	CUA	CUG	UUA	UUG
Lysine	AAA	AAG			
Methionine	AUG				
Phenylalanine	UUU	UUC			
Proline	CCU	CCC	CCA	CCG	
Serine	UCU	UCC	UCA	UCG	AGC	AGU
Threonine	ACU	ACC	ACA	ACG	
Tryptophan	UGG				
Tyrosine	UAU	UAC			
Valine	GUU	GUC	GUA	GUG	
Start (CI)	AUG				
Stop (CT)	UAA	UAG	UGA		

CI, chain-initiating; CT, chain-terminating.

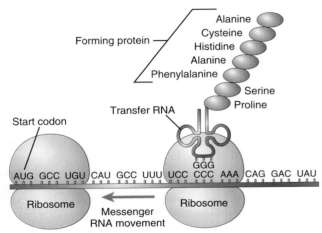

Figure 3-9 A messenger RNA strand is moving through two ribosomes. As each "codon" passes through an amino acid is added to the growing protein chain, which is shown in the right-hand ribosome. The transfer RNA molecule transports each specific amino acid to the newly forming protein.

always functions in association with the other two types of RNA: *tRNA* transports amino acids to the ribosome for incorporation into the developing protein molecule, whereas *mRNA* provides the information necessary for sequencing the amino acids in proper order for each specific type of protein to be manufactured.

Thus, the ribosome acts as a manufacturing plant in which the protein molecules are formed.

Formation of Ribosomes in the Nucleolus. The DNA genes for formation of ribosomal RNA are located in five pairs of chromosomes in the nucleus. Each of these chromosomes contains many duplicates of these particular genes because of the large amounts of ribosomal RNA required for cellular function.

As the ribosomal RNA forms, it collects in the *nucleolus*, a specialized structure lying adjacent to the chromosomes. When large amounts of ribosomal RNA are being synthesized, as occurs in cells that manufacture large amounts of protein, the nucleolus is a large structure, whereas in cells that synthesize little protein the nucleolus may not even be seen. Ribosomal RNA is specially processed in the nucleolus, where it binds with "ribosomal proteins" to form granular condensation products that are primordial subunits of ribosomes. These subunits are then released from the nucleolus and transported through the large pores of the nuclear envelope to almost all parts of the cytoplasm. After the subunits enter the cytoplasm, they are assembled to form mature, functional ribosomes. Therefore, proteins are formed in the cytoplasm of the cell, but not in the cell nucleus, because the nucleus does not contain mature ribosomes.

miRNA AND SMALL INTERFERING RNA

A fourth type of RNA in the cell is *miRNA*. miRNAs are short (21–23 nucleotides), single-stranded RNA fragments that regulate gene expression (Figure 3-10). The miRNAs are encoded from the transcribed DNA of genes, but they are not translated into proteins and are therefore often called *noncoding RNA*. The miRNAs are processed by the cell into molecules that are complementary to mRNA and act to decrease gene expression. Generation of miRNAs involves special processing of longer primary precursor RNAs called *pri-miRNAs*, which are the

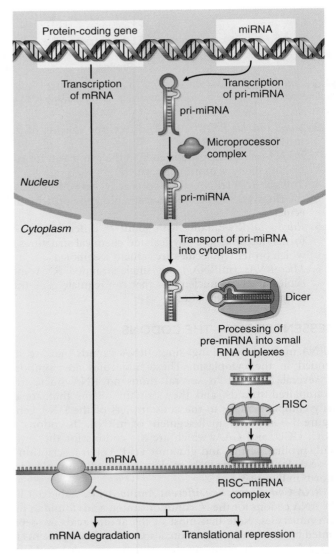

Figure 3-10 Regulation of gene expression by microRNA (miRNA). Primary miRNA (pri-miRNA), the primary transcripts of a gene processed in the cell nucleus by the microprocessor complex to pre-miRNAs. These pre-miRNAs are then further processed in the cytoplasm by *dicer*, an enzyme that helps assemble an RISC and generates miRNAs. The miRNAs regulate gene expression by binding to the complementary region of the RNA and repressing translation or promoting degradation of the mRNA before it can be translated by the ribosome. *RISC*, RNA-induced silencing complex.

primary transcripts of the gene. The pri-miRNAs are then processed in the cell nucleus by the *microprocessor complex* to pre-miRNAs, which are 70-nucleotide stem-loop structures. These pre-miRNAs are then further processed in the cytoplasm by a specific *dicer enzyme* that helps assemble an *RNA-induced silencing complex* (RISC) and generates miRNAs.

The miRNAs regulate gene expression by binding to the complementary region of the RNA and promoting repression of translation or degradation of the mRNA before it can be translated by the ribosome. miRNAs are believed to play an important role in the normal regulation of cell function, and alterations in miRNA function have been associated with diseases such as cancer and heart disease.

Another type of miRNA is *small interfering RNA* (siRNA), also called *silencing RNA* or *short interfering RNA*. The siRNAs are short, double-stranded RNA molecules, 20–25 nucleotides in length that interfere with the expression of specific genes. siRNAs generally refer to synthetic miRNAs and can be administered to silence expression of specific genes. They are designed to avoid the nuclear processing by the microprocessor complex, and after the siRNA enters the cytoplasm it activates the RISC silencing complex, blocking the translation of mRNA. Because siRNAs can be tailored for any specific sequence in the gene, they can be used to block translation of any mRNA and therefore expression by any gene for which the nucleotide sequence is known. Researchers have proposed that siRNAs may become useful therapeutic tools to silence genes that contribute to the pathophysiology of diseases.

FORMATION OF PROTEINS ON THE RIBOSOMES—THE PROCESS OF "TRANSLATION"

When a molecule of mRNA comes in contact with a ribosome, it travels through the ribosome, beginning at a predetermined end of the RNA molecule specified by an appropriate sequence of RNA bases called the "chain-initiating" codon. Then, as shown in Figure 3-9, while the mRNA travels through the ribosome a protein molecule is formed—a process called *translation*. Thus, the ribosome reads the codons of the mRNA in much the same way that a tape is "read" as it passes through the playback head of a tape recorder. Then, when a "stop" (or "chain-terminating") codon slips past the ribosome, the end of a protein molecule is signaled and the protein molecule is freed into the cytoplasm.

Polyribosomes. A single mRNA molecule can form protein molecules in several ribosomes at the same time because the initial end of the RNA strand can pass to a successive ribosome as it leaves the first, as shown at the bottom left in Figures 3-9 and 3-11. The protein molecules are in different stages of development in each ribosome. As a result, clusters of ribosomes frequently occur with 3–10 ribosomes being attached to a single mRNA at the same time. These clusters are called *polyribosomes*.

It is especially important to note that an mRNA can cause the formation of a protein molecule in any ribosome; that is, there is no specificity of ribosomes for given types of protein. The ribosome is simply the physical manufacturing plant in which the chemical reactions take place.

Many Ribosomes Attach to the Endoplasmic Reticulum. In Chapter 2, it was noted that many ribosomes become attached to the endoplasmic reticulum. This attachment occurs because the initial ends of many forming protein molecules have amino acid sequences that immediately attach to specific receptor sites on the endoplasmic reticulum, causing these molecules to penetrate the reticulum wall and enter the endoplasmic reticulum matrix. This process gives a granular appearance to the portions of the reticulum where proteins are being formed and are entering the matrix of the reticulum.

Figure 3-11 shows the functional relation of mRNA to the ribosomes and the manner in which the ribosomes attach to the membrane of the endoplasmic reticulum. Note the process of translation occurring in several ribosomes at the same time in response to the same strand of mRNA. Note also the newly forming polypeptide (protein) chains passing through the endoplasmic reticulum membrane into the endoplasmic matrix.

It should be noted that except in glandular cells in which large amounts of protein-containing secretory vesicles are formed most proteins synthesized by the ribosomes are released directly into the cytosol instead of into the endoplasmic reticulum. These proteins are enzymes and internal structural proteins of the cell.

Chemical Steps in Protein Synthesis. Some of the chemical events that occur in the synthesis of a protein molecule are shown in Figure 3-12. This figure shows representative reactions for three separate amino acids, AA1, AA2, and AA20. The stages of the reactions are as follows:

1. Each amino acid is *activated* by a chemical process in which ATP combines with the amino acid to form an *adenosine monophosphate complex with the amino acid*, giving up two high-energy phosphate bonds in the process.

2. The activated amino acid, having an excess of energy, then *combines with its specific tRNA to form an amino acid–tRNA complex* and, at the same time, releases the adenosine monophosphate.

3. The tRNA carrying the amino acid complex then comes in contact with the mRNA molecule in the ribosome, where the anticodon of the tRNA attaches temporarily to its specific codon of the mRNA, thus lining up the amino acid in appropriate sequence to form a protein molecule. Then, under the influence of the enzyme *peptidyl transferase* (one of the proteins in the ribosome) *peptide bonds* are

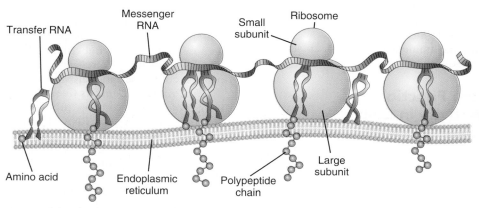

Figure 3-11 Physical structure of the ribosomes as well as their functional relation to messenger RNA, transfer RNA, and the endoplasmic reticulum during the formation of protein molecules.

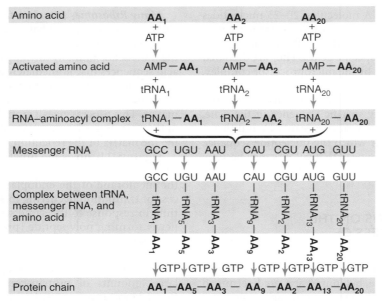

Figure 3-12 Chemical events in the formation of a protein molecule. AMP, adenosine monophosphate; ATP, adenosine triphosphate; tRNA, transfer RNA.

formed between the successive amino acids, thus adding progressively to the protein chain. These chemical events require energy from two additional high-energy phosphate bonds, making a total of four high-energy bonds used for each amino acid added to the protein chain. Thus the synthesis of proteins is one of the most energy-consuming processes of the cell.

Peptide Linkage. The successive amino acids in the protein chain combine with one another according to the following typical reaction:

$$R - \underset{\underset{NH_2}{|}}{C} - \underset{\underset{O}{\|}}{C} - OH + H - \underset{\underset{H}{|}}{N} - \underset{\underset{R}{|}}{C} - COOH \longrightarrow$$

$$R - \underset{\underset{NH_2}{|}}{C} - \underset{\underset{O}{\|}}{C} - \underset{\underset{H}{|}}{N} - \underset{\underset{R}{|}}{C} - COOH + H_2O$$

In this chemical reaction, a hydroxyl radical (OH^-) is removed from the COOH portion of the first amino acid and hydrogen (H^+) of the NH_2 portion of the other amino acid is removed. These combine to form water and the two reactive sites left on the two successive amino acids bond with each other resulting in a single molecule. This process is called *peptide linkage*. As each additional amino acid is added, an additional peptide linkage is formed.

Control of Gene Function and Biochemical Activity in Cells

From our discussion thus far, it is clear that the genes control both the physical and chemical functions of the cells. However, the degree of activation of respective genes must also be controlled; otherwise, some parts of the cell might overgrow or some chemical reactions might overact until they kill the cell. Each cell has powerful internal feedback control mechanisms that keep the various functional operations of the cell in step

with one another. For each gene (approximately 30,000 genes in all) at least one such feedback mechanism exists.

There are basically two methods by which the biochemical activities in the cell are controlled: (1) *genetic regulation*, in which the degree of activation of the genes and the formation of gene products are themselves controlled; and (2) *enzyme regulation*, in which the activity levels of already formed enzymes in the cell are controlled.

GENETIC REGULATION

Genetic regulation, or regulation of *gene expression*, covers the entire process from transcription of the genetic code in the nucleus to the formation of proteins in the cytoplasm. Regulation of gene expression provides all living organisms with the ability to respond to changes in their environment. In animals that have many different types of cells, tissues, and organs, differential regulation of gene expression also permits the many different cell types in the body to each perform their specialized functions. Although a cardiac myocyte contains the same genetic code as a renal tubular epithelia cell, many genes are expressed in cardiac cells that are not expressed in renal tubular cells. The ultimate measure of gene "expression" is whether (and how much of) the gene products (proteins) are produced because proteins carry out cell functions specified by the genes. Regulation of gene expression can occur at any point in the pathways of transcription, RNA processing, and translation.

The Promoter Controls Gene Expression. Synthesis of cellular proteins is a complex process that starts with the transcription of DNA into RNA. The transcription of DNA is controlled by regulatory elements found in the promoter of a gene (Figure 3-13). In eukaryotes, which includes all mammals, the basal promoter consists of a sequence of seven bases (TATAAAA) called the *TATA box*, the binding site for the *TATA-binding protein* and several other important *transcription factors* that are collectively referred to as the *transcription factor IID complex*. In addition to the transcription factor IID complex,

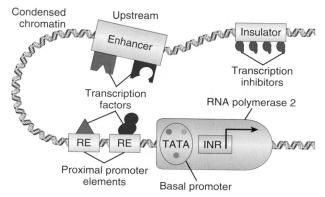

Figure 3-13 Gene transcription in eukaryotic cells. A complex arrangement of multiple clustered enhancer modules interspersed with insulator elements, which can be located either upstream or downstream of a basal promoter containing TATA box (*TATA*), proximal promoter elements (response elements, *RE*), and initiator sequences (*INR*).

1. A promoter is frequently controlled by transcription factors located elsewhere in the genome. That is, the regulatory gene causes the formation of a regulatory protein that in turn acts either as an activator or a repressor of transcription.

2. Occasionally, many different promoters are controlled at the same time by the same regulatory protein. In some instances, the same regulatory protein functions as an activator for one promoter and as a repressor for another promoter.

3. Some proteins are controlled not at the starting point of transcription on the DNA strand but farther along the strand. Sometimes the control is not even at the DNA strand itself but during the processing of the RNA molecules in the nucleus before they are released into the cytoplasm; control may also occur at the level of protein formation in the cytoplasm during RNA translation by the ribosomes.

4. In nucleated cells, the nuclear DNA is packaged in specific structural units, the *chromosomes*. Within each chromosome, the DNA is wound around small proteins called *histones*, which in turn are held tightly together in a compacted state by still other proteins. As long as the DNA is in this compacted state, it cannot function to form RNA. However, multiple control mechanisms are being discovered that can cause selected areas of chromosomes to become decompacted one part at a time so that partial RNA transcription can occur. Even then, specific *transcription factors* control the actual rate of transcription by the promoter in the chromosome. Thus, still higher orders of control are used to establish proper cell function. In addition, signals from outside the cell, such as some of the body's hormones, can activate specific chromosomal areas and specific transcription factors, thus controlling the chemical machinery for function of the cell.

Because there are more than 30,000 different genes in each human cell, the large number of ways in which genetic activity can be controlled is not surprising. The gene control systems are especially important for controlling intracellular concentrations of amino acids, amino acid derivatives, and intermediate substrates and products of carbohydrate, lipid, and protein metabolism.

Environmental factors can switch genes on and off—a phenomenon called *epigenetics*. In South Asia where intrauterine growth retardation is a major problem along with low birth weight, there has been interest in determining whether the intrauterine environment switches certain genes on and off and contributes to a greater propensity for noncommunicable diseases in later life.

Control of Intracellular Function by Enzyme Regulation

In addition to control of cell function by genetic regulation, cell activities are also controlled by intracellular inhibitors or activators that act directly on specific intracellular enzymes. Thus, enzyme regulation represents a second category of mechanisms by which cellular biochemical functions can be controlled.

Enzyme Inhibition. Some chemical substances formed in the cell have direct feedback effects to inhibit the specific enzyme systems that synthesize them. Almost always the synthesized product acts on the first enzyme in a sequence, rather than on the subsequent enzymes, usually binding directly with the

this region is where transcription factor IIB binds to both the DNA and RNA polymerase 2 to facilitate transcription of the DNA into RNA. This basal promoter is found in all protein-coding genes and the polymerase must bind with this basal promoter before it can begin traveling along the DNA strand to synthesize RNA. The *upstream promoter* is located further upstream from the transcription start site and contains several binding sites for positive or negative transcription factors that can affect transcription through interactions with proteins bound to the basal promoter. The structure and transcription factor binding sites in the upstream promoter vary from gene to gene to give rise to the different expression patterns of genes in different tissues.

Transcription of genes in eukaryotes is also influenced by *enhancers*, which are regions of DNA that can bind transcription factors. Enhancers can be located a great distance from the gene they act on or even on a different chromosome. They can also be located either upstream or downstream of the gene that they regulate. Although enhancers may be located far away from their target gene, they may be relatively close when DNA is coiled in the nucleus. It is estimated that there are 110,000 gene enhancer sequences in the human genome.

In the organization of the chromosome, it is important to separate active genes that are being transcribed from genes that are repressed. This separation can be challenging because multiple genes may be located close together on the chromosome. This separation is achieved by chromosomal *insulators*. These insulators are gene sequences that provide a barrier so that a specific gene is isolated against transcriptional influences from surrounding genes. Insulators can vary greatly in their DNA sequence and the proteins that bind to them. One way an insulator activity can be modulated is by *DNA methylation*, which is the case for the mammalian insulin-like growth factor 2 (IGF-2) gene. The mother's allele has an insulator between the enhancer and the promoter of the gene that allows for the binding of a transcriptional repressor. However, the paternal DNA sequence is methylated such that the transcriptional repressor cannot bind to the insulator and the IGF-2 gene is expressed from the paternal copy of the gene.

Other Mechanisms for Control of Transcription by the Promoter. Variations in the basic mechanism for control of the promoter have been rapidly discovered in the past two decades. Without giving details, let us list some of them:

enzyme and causing an allosteric conformational change that inactivates it. One can readily recognize the importance of inactivating the first enzyme because this prevents buildup of intermediary products that are not used.

Enzyme inhibition is another example of negative feedback control; it is responsible for controlling intracellular concentrations of multiple amino acids, purines, pyrimidines, vitamins, and other substances.

Enzyme Activation. Enzymes that are normally inactive often can be activated when needed. An example of this phenomenon occurs when most of the ATP has been depleted in a cell. In this case, a considerable amount of cyclic adenosine monophosphate (cAMP) begins to be formed as a breakdown product of ATP; the presence of this cAMP, in turn, immediately activates the glycogen-splitting enzyme phosphorylase, liberating glucose molecules that are rapidly metabolized with their energy used for replenishment of the ATP stores. Thus, cAMP acts as an enzyme activator for the enzyme phosphorylase and thereby helps control intracellular ATP concentration.

Another interesting instance of both enzyme inhibition and enzyme activation occurs in the formation of the purines and pyrimidines. These substances are needed by the cell in approximately equal quantities for formation of DNA and RNA. When purines are formed, they *inhibit* the enzymes that are required for formation of additional purines. However, they *activate* the enzymes for formation of pyrimidines. Conversely, the pyrimidines inhibit their own enzymes but activate the purine enzymes. In this way, there is continual cross-feed between the synthesizing systems for these two substances, resulting in almost exactly equal amounts of the two substances in the cells at all times.

Summary. There are two principal mechanisms by which cells control proper proportions and quantities of different cellular constituents: (1) genetic regulation and (2) enzyme regulation. The genes can be either activated or inhibited, and, likewise, the enzyme systems can be either activated or inhibited. These regulatory mechanisms most often function as feedback control systems that continually monitor the cell's biochemical composition and make corrections as needed. However, on occasion, substances from without the cell (especially some of the hormones discussed throughout this text) also control the intracellular biochemical reactions by activating or inhibiting one or more of the intracellular control systems.

Genetic Testing

Genetic tests can be done for a variety of reasons. Among these are the following:

- to determine the presence of genetic defects in an unborn baby;
- to find if people carrying a genetic disease can pass it on to their children;
- to confirm a diagnosis in individuals who show symptoms/features of a genetic disorder;
- to assess the risk of an individual for disease or to determine the likely response to treatment.

Genetic testing may involve tests of the following:

- *Chromosomes*: For example, in Down syndrome babies have three copies of chromosome 21 in each cell instead of the normal two, a condition called trisomy 21.
- *Genes*: The approach to altered genes linked to disease may take the form of simple tests that assess a mutation to gene sequencing.
- *Proteins*: Since genes code for proteins, evaluation of the gene product—that is, the protein—can be done.

The DNA–Genetic System Controls Cell Reproduction

Cell reproduction is another example of the ubiquitous role that the DNA–genetic system plays in all life processes. The genes and their regulatory mechanisms determine the growth characteristics of the cells and also when or whether these cells will divide to form new cells. In this way, the all-important genetic system controls each stage in the development of the human being, from the single-cell fertilized ovum to the whole functioning body. Thus, if there is any central theme to life, it is the DNA–genetic system.

Life Cycle of the Cell. The life cycle of a cell is the period from cell reproduction to the next cell reproduction. When mammalian cells *are not inhibited and are reproducing as rapidly as they can*, this life cycle may be as little as 10–30 hours. It is terminated by a series of distinct physical events called *mitosis* that cause division of the cell into two new daughter cells. The events of mitosis are shown in Figure 3-14 and are described later. The actual stage of mitosis, however, lasts for only about 30 minutes, and thus more than 95% of the life cycle of even rapidly reproducing cells is represented by the interval between mitosis called *interphase.*

Except in special conditions of rapid cellular reproduction inhibitory factors almost always slow or stop the uninhibited life cycle of the cell. Therefore, different cells of the body actually have life cycle periods that vary from as little as 10 hours for highly stimulated bone marrow cells to an entire lifetime of the human body for most nerve cells.

CELL REPRODUCTION BEGINS WITH REPLICATION OF DNA

As is true of almost all other important events in the cell, reproduction begins in the nucleus. The first step is *replication (duplication) of all DNA in the chromosomes*. It is only after this replication has occurred that mitosis take place.

The DNA begins to be duplicated approximately 5–10 hours before mitosis, and the duplication is completed in 4–8 hours. The net result is two exact *replicas* of all DNA. These replicas become the DNA in the two new daughter cells that will be formed at mitosis. After replication of the DNA there is another period of 1–2 hours before mitosis begins abruptly. Even during this period preliminary changes that will lead to the mitotic process are beginning to take place.

Chemical and Physical Events of DNA Replication. DNA is replicated in much the same way that RNA is transcribed from DNA, except for a few important differences:

1. Both strands of the DNA in each chromosome are replicated, not simply one of them.
2. Both entire strands of the DNA helix are replicated from end to end, rather than small portions of them, as occurs in the transcription of RNA.
3. The principal enzymes for replicating DNA are a complex of multiple enzymes called *DNA polymerase*, which is comparable to RNA polymerase. DNA polymerase attaches to and moves along the DNA template strand while

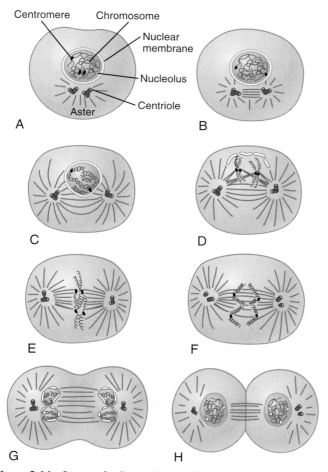

Centromere   Chromosome

Nuclear membrane

Nucleolus

Centriole

Aster

A   B   C   D   E   F   G   H

Figure 3-14   Stages of cell reproduction. (A–C) Prophase; (D) prometaphase; (E) metaphase; (F) anaphase; (G and H) telophase.

another enzyme, *DNA ligase*, causes bonding of successive DNA nucleotides to one another, using high-energy phosphate bonds to energize these attachments.

4. Formation of each new DNA strand occurs simultaneously in hundreds of segments along each of the two strands of the helix until the entire strand is replicated. Then the ends of the subunits are joined together by the DNA ligase enzyme.

5. Each newly formed strand of DNA remains attached by loose hydrogen bonding to the original DNA strand that was used as its template. Therefore, two DNA helixes are coiled together.

6. Because the DNA helixes in each chromosome are approximately 6 cm in length and have millions of helix turns, it would be impossible for the two newly formed DNA helixes to uncoil from each other were it not for some special mechanism. This uncoiling is achieved by enzymes that periodically cut each helix along its entire length, rotate each segment enough to cause separation, and then resplice the helix. Thus, the two new helixes become uncoiled.

DNA Repair, DNA "Proofreading," and "Mutation". During the hour or so between DNA replication and the beginning of mitosis there is a period of active repair and "proofreading" of the DNA strands. Wherever inappropriate DNA nucleotides have been matched up with the nucleotides of the original template strand, special enzymes cut out the defective areas and replace them with appropriate complementary nucleotides. This repair process, which is achieved by the same DNA polymerases and DNA ligases that are used in replication, is referred to as *DNA proofreading*.

Because of repair and proofreading, mistakes are rarely made in the transcription process. When a mistake is made, it is called a *mutation*. The mutation causes formation of some abnormal protein in the cell rather than a needed protein, often leading to abnormal cellular function and sometimes even cell death. Yet given that 30,000 or more genes exist in the human genome and that the period from one human generation to another is about 30 years, one would expect as many as 10 or many more mutations in the passage of the genome from parent to child. As a further protection, however, each human genome is represented by two separate sets of chromosomes with almost identical genes. Therefore, one functional gene of each pair is almost always available to the child despite mutations.

CHROMOSOMES AND THEIR REPLICATION

The DNA helixes of the nucleus are packaged in chromosomes. The human cell contains 46 chromosomes arranged in 23 pairs. Most of the genes in the two chromosomes of each pair are identical or almost identical to each other, so it is usually stated that the different genes also exist in pairs, although occasionally this is not the case.

In addition to DNA in the chromosome, there is a large amount of protein in the chromosome composed mainly of many small molecules of electropositively charged *histones*. The histones are organized into vast numbers of small, bobbin-like cores. Small segments of each DNA helix are coiled sequentially around one core after another.

The histone cores play an important role in the regulation of DNA activity because as long as the DNA is packaged tightly, it cannot function as a template for either the formation of RNA or the replication of new DNA. Further, some of the regulatory proteins have been shown to *decondense* the histone packaging of the DNA and allow small segments at a time to form RNA.

Several nonhistone proteins are also major components of chromosomes, functioning both as chromosomal structural proteins and, in connection with the genetic regulatory machinery, as activators, inhibitors, and enzymes.

Replication of the chromosomes in their entirety occurs during the next few minutes after replication of the DNA helixes has been completed; the new DNA helixes collect new protein molecules as needed. The two newly formed chromosomes remain attached to each other (until time for mitosis) at a point called the *centromere* located near their center. These duplicated but still attached chromosomes are called *chromatids*.

CELL MITOSIS

The actual process by which the cell splits into two new cells is called *mitosis*. Once each chromosome has been replicated to form the two chromatids, in many cells, mitosis follows automatically within 1 or 2 hours.

Mitotic Apparatus: Function of the Centrioles. One of the first events of mitosis takes place in the cytoplasm; it occurs during the latter part of interphase in or around the small structures called *centrioles*. As shown in Figure 3-14, two pairs of centrioles lie close to each other near one pole of the nucleus.

These centrioles, like the DNA and chromosomes, are also replicated during interphase, usually shortly before replication of the DNA. Each centriole is a small cylindrical body about 0.4 μm long and about 0.15 μm in diameter, consisting mainly of nine parallel tubular structures arranged in the form of a cylinder. The two centrioles of each pair lie at right angles to each other. Each pair of centrioles, along with attached *pericentriolar material*, is called a *centrosome*.

Shortly before mitosis is to take place, the two pairs of centrioles begin to move apart from each other. This movement is caused by polymerization of protein microtubules growing between the respective centriole pairs and actually pushing them apart. At the same time, other microtubules grow radially away from each of the centriole pairs, forming a spiny star called the *aster* in each end of the cell. Some of the spines of the aster penetrate the nuclear membrane and help separate the two sets of chromatids during mitosis. The complex of microtubules extending between the two new centriole pairs is called the *spindle*, and the entire set of microtubules plus the two pairs of centrioles is called the *mitotic apparatus*.

Prophase. The first stage of mitosis called *prophase* is shown in Figure 3-14A–C. While the spindle is forming the chromosomes of the nucleus (which in interphase consist of loosely coiled strands) become condensed into well-defined chromosomes.

Prometaphase. During the prometaphase stage (see Figure 3-14D), the growing microtubular spines of the aster fragment the nuclear envelope. At the same time, multiple microtubules from the aster attach to the chromatids at the centromeres, where the paired chromatids are still bound to each other; the tubules then pull one chromatid of each pair toward one cellular pole and its partner toward the opposite pole.

Metaphase. During the metaphase stage (see Figure 3-14E), the two asters of the mitotic apparatus are pushed farther apart. This pushing is believed to occur because the microtubular spines from the two asters, where they interdigitate with each other to form the mitotic spindle, actually push each other away. Minute contractile protein molecules called *molecular motors*, which are perhaps composed of the muscle protein *actin*, extend between the respective spines and, using a stepping action as in muscle, actively slide the spines in a reverse direction along each other. Simultaneously, the chromatids are pulled tightly by their attached microtubules to the very center of the cell, lining up to form the *equatorial plate* of the mitotic spindle.

Anaphase. During the anaphase phase (see Figure 3-14F), the two chromatids of each chromosome are pulled apart at the centromere. All 46 pairs of chromatids are separated forming 2 separate sets of 46 *daughter chromosomes.* One of these sets is pulled toward one mitotic aster and the other is pulled toward the other aster as the two respective poles of the dividing cell are pushed still farther apart.

Telophase. In the telophase stage (see Figure 3-14G and H) the two sets of daughter chromosomes are pushed completely apart. Then the mitotic apparatus dissolutes and a new nuclear membrane develops around each set of chromosomes. This membrane is formed from portions of the endoplasmic reticulum that are already present in the cytoplasm. Shortly thereafter, the cell pinches in two, midway between the two nuclei. This pinching is caused by formation of a contractile ring of *microfilaments* composed of *actin* and probably *myosin* (the two contractile proteins of muscle) at the juncture of the newly developing cells that pinches them off from each other.

CONTROL OF CELL GROWTH AND CELL REPRODUCTION

Some cells grow and reproduce all the time such as the blood-forming cells of the bone marrow, the germinal layers of the skin, and the epithelium of the gut. Many other cells, however, such as smooth muscle cells, may not reproduce for many years. A few cells, such as the neurons and most striated muscle cells, do not reproduce during the entire life of a person, except during the original period of fetal life.

In certain tissues, an insufficiency of some types of cells causes them to grow and reproduce rapidly until appropriate numbers of these cells are again available. For instance, in some young animals, seven-eighths of the liver can be removed surgically, and the cells of the remaining one-eighth will grow and divide until the liver mass returns to almost normal. The same phenomenon occurs for many glandular cells and most cells of the bone marrow, subcutaneous tissue, intestinal epithelium, and almost any other tissue except highly differentiated cells such as nerve and muscle cells.

The mechanisms that maintain proper numbers of the different types of cells in the body are still poorly understood. However, experiments have shown at least three ways in which growth can be controlled. First, growth often is controlled by *growth factors* that come from other parts of the body. Some of these growth factors circulate in the blood, but others originate in adjacent tissues. For instance, the epithelial cells of some glands, such as the pancreas, fail to grow without a growth factor from the underlying connective tissue of the gland. Second, most normal cells stop growing when they have run out of space for growth. This phenomenon occurs when cells are grown in tissue culture; the cells grow until they contact a solid object, and then growth stops. Third, cells grown in tissue culture often stop growing when minute amounts of their own secretions are allowed to collect in the culture medium. This mechanism, too, could provide a means for negative feedback control of growth.

Telomeres Prevent the Degradation of Chromosomes. A telomere is a region of repetitive nucleotide sequences located at each end of a chromatid (Figure 3-15). Telomeres serve as protective caps that prevent the chromosome from deterioration during cell division. During cell division, a short piece of "primer" RNA attaches to the DNA strand to start the replication. However, because the primer does not attach at the very end of the DNA strand, the copy is missing a small section of the DNA. With each cell division, the copied DNA loses additional nucleotides from the telomere region. The nucleotide sequences provided by the telomeres therefore prevent the degradation of genes near the ends of chromosomes. Without telomeres, the genomes would progressively lose information and be truncated after each cell division. Thus, the telomeres can be considered to be disposable chromosomal buffers that help maintain stability of the genes but are gradually consumed during repeated cell divisions.

Each time a cell divides, an average person loses 30–200 base pairs from the ends of that cell's telomeres. In human blood cells, the length of telomeres ranges from 8000 base pairs at birth to as low as 1500 in elderly people. Eventually, when the telomeres shorten to a critical length, the chromosomes become unstable and the cells die. This process of telomere shortening is believed to be an important reason for some of the physiological changes associated with aging. Telomere erosion can also occur as a result of diseases, especially those associated with oxidative stress and inflammation.

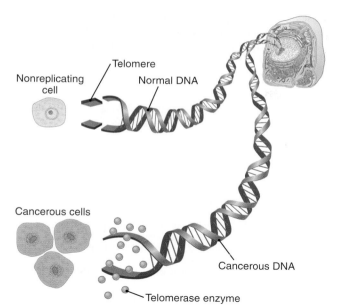

Figure 3-15 Control of cell replication by telomeres and telomerase. The cells' chromosomes are capped by telomeres, which, in the absence of telomerase activity, shorten with each cell division until the cell stops replicating. Therefore, most cells of the body cannot replicate indefinitely. In cancer cells, telomerase is activated and telomere length is maintained so that the cells continue to replicate themselves uncontrollably.

In some cells, such as stem cells of the bone marrow or skin that must be replenished throughout life, or the germ cells in the ovaries and testes, the enzyme *telomerase* adds bases to the ends of the telomeres so that many more generations of cells can be produced. However, telomerase activity is usually low in most cells of the body, and after many generations the descendent cells will inherit defective chromosomes, become *senescent*, and cease dividing. This process of telomere shortening is important in regulating cell proliferation and maintaining gene stability. In cancer cells telomerase activity is abnormally activated so that telomere length is maintained, making it possible for the cells to replicate over and over again uncontrollably (Figure 3-15). Some scientists have therefore proposed that telomere shortening protects us from cancer and other proliferative diseases.

Regulation of Cell Size. Cell size is determined almost entirely by the amount of functioning DNA in the nucleus. If replication of the DNA does not occur, the cell grows to a certain size and thereafter remains at that size. Conversely, use of the chemical *colchicine* makes it possible to prevent formation of the mitotic spindle and therefore to prevent mitosis, even though replication of the DNA continues. In this event, the nucleus contains far greater quantities of DNA than it normally does, and the cell grows proportionally larger. It is assumed that this cell growth results from increased production of RNA and cell proteins, which in turn cause the cell to grow larger.

Cell Differentiation

A special characteristic of cell growth and cell division is *cell differentiation*, which refers to changes in physical and functional properties of cells as they proliferate in the embryo to form the different bodily structures and organs.

It has become clear that differentiation results not from loss of genes but from selective repression of different gene promoters.

In fact, electron micrographs suggest that some segments of DNA helixes that are wound around histone cores become so condensed that they no longer uncoil to form RNA molecules. One explanation for this scenario is as follows: It has been supposed that the cellular genome begins at a certain stage of cell differentiation to produce a regulatory *protein* that forever after represses a select group of genes. Therefore, the repressed genes never function again. Regardless of the mechanism mature human cells produce a maximum of about 8000–10,000 proteins rather than the potential 30,000 or more that would have been produced if all genes were active.

Embryological experiments show that certain cells in an embryo control differentiation of adjacent cells. For instance, the *primordial chordamesoderm* is called the *primary organizer* of the embryo because it forms a focus around which the remainder of the embryo develops. It differentiates into a *mesodermal axis* that contains segmentally arranged *somites* and, as a result of *inductions* in the surrounding tissues, causes formation of essentially all the organs of the body.

Another instance of induction occurs when the developing eye vesicles come in contact with the ectoderm of the head and cause the ectoderm to thicken into a lens plate that folds inward to form the lens of the eye. Therefore, a large share of the embryo develops as a result of such inductions, one part of the body affecting another part, and this part affecting still other parts.

Thus, although our understanding of cell differentiation is still hazy, we are aware of many control mechanisms by which differentiation *could* occur.

Apoptosis—Programmed Cell Death

The 100 trillion cells of the body are members of a highly organized community in which the total number of cells is regulated not only by controlling the rate of cell division but also by controlling the rate of cell death. When cells are no longer needed or become a threat to the organism, they undergo a suicidal *programmed cell death* or *apoptosis*. This process involves a specific proteolytic cascade that causes the cell to shrink and condense, disassemble its cytoskeleton, and alter its cell surface so that a neighboring phagocytic cell such as a macrophage can attach to the cell membrane and digest the cell.

In contrast to programmed death, cells that die as a result of an acute injury usually swell and burst due to loss of cell membrane integrity, a process called cell *necrosis*. Necrotic cells may spill their contents, causing inflammation and injury to neighboring cells. Apoptosis, however, is an orderly cell death that results in disassembly and phagocytosis of the cell before any leakage of its contents occurs, and neighboring cells usually remain healthy.

Apoptosis is initiated by activation of a family of proteases called *caspases*, which are enzymes that are synthesized and stored in the cell as inactive *procaspases*. The mechanisms of activation of caspases are complex, but once activated the enzymes cleave and activate other procaspases, triggering a cascade that rapidly breaks down proteins within the cell. The cell thus dismantles itself, and its remains are rapidly digested by neighboring phagocytic cells.

A tremendous amount of apoptosis occurs in tissues that are being remodeled during development. Even in adult humans, billions of cells die each hour in tissues such as the intestine and bone marrow, and are replaced by new cells. Programmed cell death, however, is normally balanced by the formation of new cells in healthy adults. Otherwise, the body's tissues would shrink or grow excessively. Recent studies suggest that abnormalities of apoptosis may play a key role in neurodegenerative diseases such as Alzheimer disease, as well as in cancer and autoimmune disorders. Some drugs that have been used successfully for chemotherapy appear to induce apoptosis in cancer cells.

BIBLIOGRAPHY

Alberts B, Johnson A, Lewis J, et al: *Molecular Biology of the Cell*, fifth ed., New York, 2008, Garland Science.

Ameres SL, Zamore PD: Diversifying microRNA function, *Nat. Rev. Mol. Cell Biol.* 14:475, 2013.

Armanios M: Telomeres and age-related disease: how telomere biology informs clinical paradigms, *J. Clin. Invest.* 123:996, 2013.

Bickmore WA, van Steensel B: Genome architecture: domain organization of interphase chromosomes, *Cell* 152:1270, 2013.

Cairns BR: The logic of chromatin architecture and remodelling at promoters, *Nature* 461:193, 2009.

Castel SE, Martienssen RA: RNA interference in the nucleus: roles for small RNAs in transcription, epigenetics and beyond, *Nat. Rev. Genet.* 14:100, 2013.

Clift D, Schuh M: Restarting life: fertilization and the transition from meiosis to mitosis, *Nat. Rev. Mol. Cell Biol.* 14:549, 2013.

Dawson MA, Kouzarides T, Huntly BJ: Targeting epigenetic readers in cancer, *N. Engl. J. Med.* 367:647, 2012.

Frazer KA, Murray SS, Schork NJ, Topol EJ: Human genetic variation and its contribution to complex traits, *Nat. Rev. Genet.* 10:241, 2009.

Fuda NJ, Ardehali MB, Lis JT: Defining mechanisms that regulate RNA polymerase II transcription in vivo, *Nature* 461:186, 2009.

Hoeijmakers JH: DNA damage, aging, and cancer, *N. Engl. J. Med.* 361:1475, 2009.

Hotchkiss RS, Strasser A, McDunn JE, Swanson PE: Cell death, *N. Engl. J. Med.* 361:1570, 2009.

Kim N, Jinks-Robertson S: Transcription as a source of genome instability, *Nat. Rev. Genet.* 13:204, 2012.

Kong J, Lasko P: Translational control in cellular and developmental processes, *Nat. Rev. Genet.* 13:383, 2012.

Müller-McNicoll M, Neugebauer KM: How cells get the message: dynamic assembly and function of mRNA–protein complexes, *Nat. Rev. Genet.* 14:275, 2013.

Papamichos-Chronakis M, Peterson CL: Chromatin and the genome integrity network, *Nat. Rev. Genet.* 14:62, 2013.

Sayed D, Abdellatif M: MicroRNAs in development and disease, *Physiol. Rev.* 91:827, 2011.

Smith ZD, Meissner A: DNA mammalian development, *Nat. Rev. Genet.* 14:204, 2013.

Zhu H, Belcher M, van der Harst P: Healthy aging and disease: role for telomere biology? *Clin. Sci. (Lond.)* 120:427, 2011.

Transport of Substances Through Cell Membranes

LEARNING OBJECTIVES

- List the different types of transport across the cell membrane and give examples of each.
- Describe the features of each form of transport.
- Differentiate between diffusion and active transport.

GLOSSARY OF TERMS

- **Active transport:** When molecules are moved against a concentration gradient with the expenditure of energy
- **Diffusion:** Movement of molecules from an area of high concentration to an area of low concentration
- **Facilitated diffusion (*carrier-mediated diffusion*):** Substances being transported by diffusion through a membrane using a specific carrier protein
- **Osmolality:** A solution having *1 osm of solute dissolved in each kilogram of water* said to have an *osmolality of 1 osm/kg* (one osmole is 1 g molecular weight of osmotically active solute)
- **Osmolarity:** The osmolar concentration expressed as *osmoles per liter of solution* rather than osmoles per kilogram of water
- **Osmosis:** The net diffusion of water across a selectively permeable membrane from a region of high water concentration to one that has a lower water concentration

Figure 4-1 lists the approximate concentrations of important electrolytes and other substances in the *extracellular fluid* and *intracellular fluid*. The structure of the membrane covering the outside of every cell of the body is discussed in Chapter 2 and illustrated in Figures 2-3 and 4-2. This membrane not only consists almost entirely of a *lipid bilayer* but also contains large numbers of protein molecules in the lipid, many of which penetrate all the way through the membrane.

The lipid bilayer is not miscible with either the extracellular fluid or the intracellular fluid. Therefore, it constitutes a barrier against movement of water molecules and water-soluble substances between the extracellular and intracellular fluid compartments. However, as demonstrated in Figure 4-2 by the leftmost arrow, lipid-soluble substances can penetrate this lipid bilayer, diffusing directly through the lipid substance itself.

The protein molecules in the membrane have entirely different properties for transporting substances. Their molecular structures interrupt the continuity of the lipid bilayer, constituting an alternative pathway through the cell membrane. Many of these penetrating proteins can function as *transport proteins*. Different proteins function differently. Some proteins have watery spaces all the way through the molecule and allow free movement of water as well as selected ions or molecules; these proteins are called *channel proteins*. Other proteins, called *carrier proteins*, bind with molecules or ions that are to be transported; conformational changes in the protein molecules then move the substances through the interstices of the protein to the other side of the membrane. Channel proteins and the carrier proteins are usually selective for the types of molecules or ions that are allowed to cross the membrane.

"Diffusion" Versus "Active Transport". Transport through the cell membrane, either directly through the lipid bilayer or through the proteins, occurs via one of two basic processes: *diffusion* or *active transport*.

Although many variations of these basic mechanisms exist, diffusion means random molecular movement of substances molecule by molecule, either through intermolecular spaces in the membrane or in combination with a carrier protein. The energy that causes diffusion is the energy of the normal kinetic motion of matter.

In contrast, active transport means movement of ions or other substances across the membrane in combination with a carrier protein in such a way that the carrier protein causes the substance to move against an energy gradient, such as from a

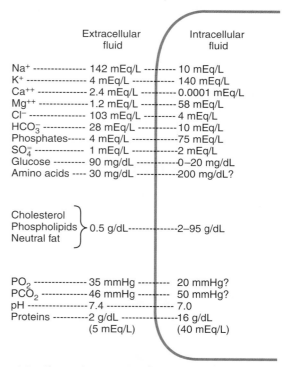

Figure 4-1 Chemical compositions of extracellular and intracellular fluids. The question mark indicates that precise values for intracellular fluid are unknown. The red line indicates the cell membrane.

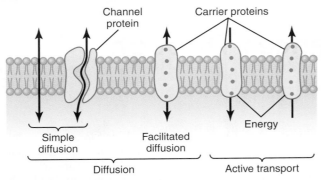

Figure 4-2 Transport pathways through the cell membrane, and the basic mechanisms of transport.

low-concentration state to a high-concentration state. This movement requires an additional source of energy besides kinetic energy. A more detailed explanation of the basic physics and physical chemistry of these two processes is provided in this chapter.

Diffusion

All molecules and ions in the body fluids, including water molecules and dissolved substances, are in constant motion, with each particle moving its separate way. The motion of these particles is what physicists call "heat"—the greater the motion, the higher is the temperature—and the motion never ceases except at absolute zero temperature. When a moving molecule, A, approaches a stationary molecule, B, the electrostatic and other nuclear forces of molecule A repel molecule B, transferring some of the energy of motion of molecule A to molecule B. Consequently, molecule B gains kinetic energy of motion, while molecule A slows down, losing some of its kinetic energy. As shown in Figure 4-3, a single molecule in a solution bounces among the other molecules first in one direction, then another, then another, and so forth, randomly bouncing thousands of times each second. This continual movement of molecules among one another in liquids or in gases is called *diffusion*.

Ions diffuse in the same manner as whole molecules, and even suspended colloid particles diffuse in a similar manner, except that the colloids diffuse far less rapidly than do molecular substances because of their large size.

DIFFUSION THROUGH THE CELL MEMBRANE

Diffusion through the cell membrane is divided into two subtypes called *simple diffusion* and *facilitated diffusion*. Simple

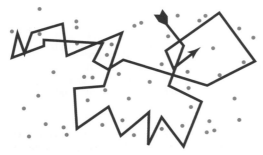

Figure 4-3 Diffusion of a fluid molecule during one-thousandth of a second.

diffusion means that kinetic movement of molecules or ions occurs through a membrane opening or through intermolecular spaces without any interaction with carrier proteins in the membrane. The rate of diffusion is determined by the amount of substance available, the velocity of kinetic motion, and the number and sizes of openings in the membrane through which the molecules or ions can move.

Facilitated diffusion requires interaction of a carrier protein. The carrier protein aids passage of the molecules or ions through the membrane by binding chemically with them and shuttling them through the membrane in this form.

Simple diffusion can occur through the cell membrane by two pathways: (1) through the interstices of the lipid bilayer if the diffusing substance is lipid soluble and (2) through watery channels that penetrate all the way through some of the large transport proteins, as shown to the left in Figure 4-2.

Diffusion of Lipid-Soluble Substances Through the Lipid Bilayer. An important factor that determines how rapidly a substance diffuses through the lipid bilayer is the *lipid solubility* of the substance. For instance, the lipid solubilities of oxygen, nitrogen, carbon dioxide, and alcohols are high, and all these substances can dissolve in the lipid bilayer and diffuse through the cell membrane in the same manner that diffusion of water solutes occurs in a watery solution. The rate of diffusion of each of these substances through the membrane is directly proportional to its lipid solubility. Especially large amounts of oxygen can be transported in this way; therefore, oxygen can be delivered to the interior of the cell almost as though the cell membrane did not exist.

Diffusion of Water and Other Lipid-Insoluble Molecules Through Protein Channels. Even though water is highly insoluble in the membrane lipids, it readily passes through channels in protein molecules that penetrate all the way through the membrane. Many of body's cell membranes contain "pores" called aquaporins that selectively permit passage of water through the cell membrane. The aquaporins are highly specialized, and there are at least 13 different types in various cells of mammals.

The rapidity with which water molecules can diffuse through most cell membranes is astounding. For example, the total amount of water that diffuses in each direction through the red blood cell membrane during each second is about 100 times as great as the volume of the red blood cell itself.

Other lipid-insoluble molecules can pass through the protein pore channels in the same way as water molecules if they are water soluble and small enough. However, as they become larger, their penetration falls off rapidly. For instance, the diameter of the urea molecule is only 20% greater than that of water, yet its penetration through the cell membrane pores is about 1000 times less than that of water. Even so, given the astonishing rate of water penetration, this amount of urea penetration still allows rapid transport of urea through the membrane within minutes.

DIFFUSION THROUGH PROTEIN PORES AND CHANNELS—SELECTIVE PERMEABILITY AND "GATING" OF CHANNELS

Computerized three-dimensional reconstructions of protein pores and channels have demonstrated tubular pathways all the way from the extracellular to the intracellular fluid. Therefore, substances can move by simple diffusion directly along these pores and channels from one side of the membrane to the other.

Pores are composed of integral cell membrane proteins that form open tubes through the membrane and are always open. However, the diameter of a pore and its electrical charges provide selectivity that permits only certain molecules to pass through. For example, protein pores called *aquaporins* or *water channels* permit rapid passage of water through cell membranes but exclude other molecules. At least 13 different types of aquaporins have been found in various cells of the human body. Aquaporins have a narrow pore that permits water molecules to diffuse through the membrane in single file. The pore is too narrow to permit passage of any hydrated ions. The density of some aquaporins (eg, aquaporin-2) in cell membranes is not static but is altered in different physiological conditions.

Selective Permeability of Protein Channels. Many of the protein channels are highly selective for transport of one or more specific ions or molecules. This selectivity results from the characteristics of the channel, such as its diameter, its shape, and the nature of the electrical charges and chemical bonds along its inside surfaces.

Potassium channels permit passage of potassium ions across the cell membrane about 1000 times more readily than they permit passage of sodium ions. This high degree of selectivity cannot be explained entirely by the molecular diameters of the ions because potassium ions are slightly larger than sodium ions. What is the mechanism for this remarkable ion selectivity? This question was partially answered when the structure of a *bacterial potassium channel* was determined by X-ray crystallography. Potassium channels were found to have a *tetrameric structure* consisting of four identical protein subunits surrounding a central pore (Figure 4-4). At the top of the channel pore are *pore loops* that form a narrow *selectivity filter*. Lining the selectivity filter are *carbonyl oxygens*. When hydrated potassium ions enter the selectivity filter, they interact with the carbonyl oxygens and shed most of their bound water molecules, permitting the dehydrated potassium ions to pass through the channel. The carbonyl oxygens are too far apart, however, to enable them to interact closely with the smaller sodium ions, which are therefore effectively excluded by the selectivity filter from passing through the pore.

Different selectivity filters for the various ion channels are believed to determine, in large part, the specificity of the various channels for cations or anions or for particular ions, such as sodium (Na^+), potassium (K^+), and calcium (Ca^{++}) that gain access to the channels.

One of the most important of the protein channels, the *sodium channel*, is only 0.3×0.5 nm in diameter, but more important, the inner surfaces of this channel are lined with amino acids that are *strongly negatively charged*, as shown by the negative signs inside the channel proteins in the top panel of Figure 4-5. These strong negative charges can pull small *dehydrated* sodium ions into these channels, actually pulling the sodium ions away from their hydrating water molecules. Once in the channel, the sodium ions diffuse in either direction according to the usual laws of diffusion. Thus, the sodium channel is specifically highly selective for passage of sodium ions.

Gating of Protein Channels

Gating of protein channels provides a means of controlling ion permeability of the channels. This mechanism is shown in both panels of Figure 4-5 for selective gating of sodium and potassium ions. It is believed that some of the gates are actual gate-like

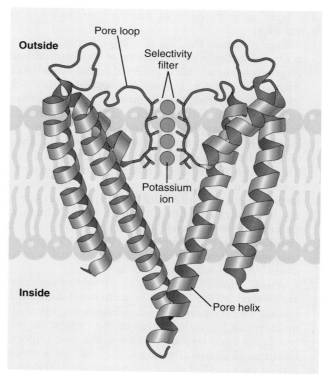

Figure 4-4 The structure of a potassium channel. The channel is composed of four subunits (only two of which are shown), each with two transmembrane helices. A narrow selectivity filter is formed from the pore loops and carbonyl oxygens line the walls of the selectivity filter, forming sites for transiently binding dehydrated potassium ions. The interaction of the potassium ions with carbonyl oxygens causes the potassium ions to shed their bound water molecules, permitting the dehydrated potassium ions to pass through the pore.

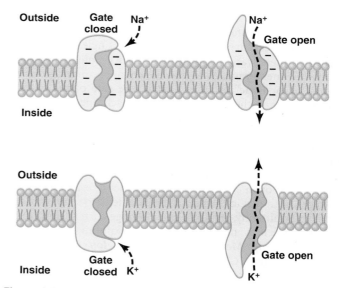

Figure 4-5 Transport of sodium and potassium ions through protein channels. Also shown are conformational changes in the protein molecules to open or close "gates" guarding the channels.

extensions of the transport protein molecule, which can close the opening of the channel or can be lifted away from the opening by a conformational change in the shape of the protein molecule itself.

The opening and closing of gates are controlled in two principal ways:

1. *Voltage gating*: In the case of voltage gating, the molecular conformation of the gate or of its chemical bonds responds to the electrical potential across the cell membrane. For instance, in the top panel of Figure 4-5, a strong negative charge on the inside of the cell membrane could cause the outside sodium gates to remain tightly closed; conversely, when the inside of the membrane loses its negative charge, these gates would open suddenly and allow sodium to pass inward through the sodium pores. This process is the basic mechanism for eliciting action potentials in nerves that are responsible for nerve signals. In the bottom panel of Figure 4-5, the potassium gates are on the intracellular ends of the potassium channels, and they open when the inside of the cell membrane becomes positively charged. The opening of these gates is partly responsible for terminating the action potential, a process discussed more fully in Chapter 9.

2. *Chemical (ligand) gating*: Some protein channel gates are opened by the binding of a chemical substance (a ligand) with the protein, which causes a conformational or chemical bonding change in the protein molecule that opens or closes the gate. One of the most important instances of chemical gating is the effect of acetylcholine on the so-called *acetylcholine channel*. Acetylcholine opens the gate of this channel, providing a negatively charged pore of about 0.65 nm in diameter that allows uncharged molecules or positive ions smaller than this diameter to pass through. This gate is exceedingly important for the transmission of nerve signals from one nerve cell to another (see Chapter 101) and from nerve cells to muscle cells to cause muscle contraction (see Chapter 12).

Open State Versus Closed State of Gated Channels. Figure 4-6A displays an interesting characteristic of most voltage-gated channels. This figure shows two recordings of electrical current flowing through a single sodium channel when there was an approximate 25-mV potential gradient across the membrane. Note that the channel conducts current "in an all-or-none" fashion. That is, the gate of the channel snaps open and then snaps close, with each open state lasting for only a fraction of a millisecond up to several milliseconds demonstrating the rapidity with which changes can occur during the opening and closing of the protein molecular gates. At one voltage potential, the channel may remain closed all the time or almost all the time, whereas at another voltage level, it may remain open either all or most of the time. At in-between voltages, as shown in the figure, the gates tend to snap open and close intermittently, resulting in an average current flow somewhere between the minimum and the maximum.

Patch-Clamp Method for Recording Ion Current Flow Through Single Channels. The patch-clamp method for recording ion current flow through single protein channels is illustrated in Figure 4-6A and B. A micropipette, with a tip diameter of only 1 or 2 μm, is abutted against the outside of a cell membrane. Suction is then applied inside the pipette to pull the membrane against the tip of the pipette, which creates a seal where the edges of the pipette touch the cell membrane. The result is a minute membrane "patch" at the tip of the pipette through which electrical current flow can be recorded.

Alternatively, as shown at the bottom right in Figure 4-6B, the small cell membrane patch at the end of the pipette can be

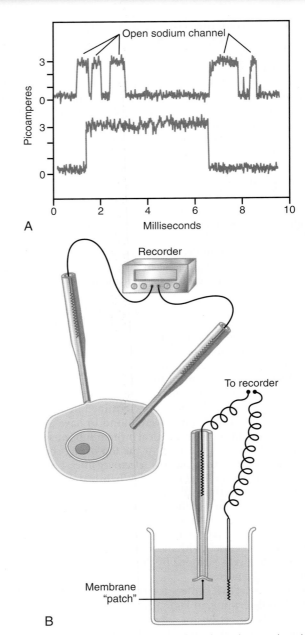

Figure 4-6 (A) A recording of current flow through a single voltage-gated sodium channel, demonstrating the "all-or-none" principle for opening and closing of the channel. (B) The "patch-clamp" method for recording current flow through a single protein channel. To the left, recording is performed from a "patch" of a living cell membrane. To the right, recording is from a membrane patch that has been torn away from the cell.

torn away from the cell. The pipette with its sealed patch is then inserted into a free solution, which allows the concentrations of ions both inside the micropipette and in the outside solution to be altered as desired. Also, the voltage between the two sides of the membrane can be set or "clamped" to a given voltage.

FACILITATED DIFFUSION REQUIRES MEMBRANE CARRIER PROTEINS

Facilitated diffusion is also called *carrier-mediated diffusion* because a substance transported in this manner diffuses through the membrane with the help of a specific carrier protein.

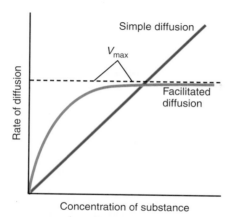

Figure 4-7 The effect of concentration of a substance on the rate of diffusion through a membrane by simple diffusion and facilitated diffusion. This graph shows that facilitated diffusion approaches a maximum rate called the V_{max}.

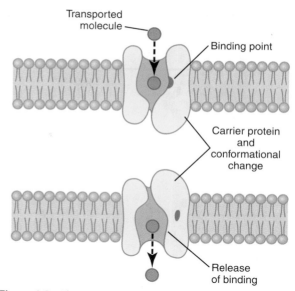

Figure 4-8 The postulated mechanism for facilitated diffusion.

Facilitated diffusion differs from simple diffusion in the following important way: Although the rate of simple diffusion through an open channel increases proportionately with the concentration of the diffusing substance, in facilitated diffusion the rate of diffusion approaches a maximum, called V_{max}, as the concentration of the diffusing substance increases. This difference between simple diffusion and facilitated diffusion is demonstrated in Figure 4-7. The figure shows that as the concentration of the diffusing substance increases the rate of simple diffusion continues to increase proportionately, but in the case of facilitated diffusion the rate of diffusion cannot rise greater than the V_{max} level.

What is it that limits the rate of facilitated diffusion? A probable answer is the mechanism illustrated in Figure 4-8. This figure shows a carrier protein with a pore large enough to transport a specific molecule partway through. It also shows a binding "receptor" on the inside of the protein carrier. The molecule to be transported enters the pore and becomes bound. Then, in a fraction of a second, a conformational or chemical change occurs in the carrier protein, so the pore now opens to the opposite side of the membrane. Because the binding force of the receptor is weak, the thermal motion of the attached molecule causes it to break away and be released on the opposite side of the membrane. The rate at which molecules can be transported by this mechanism can never be greater than the rate at which the carrier protein molecule can undergo change back and forth between its two states. Note specifically, though, that this mechanism allows the transported molecule to move—that is, to "diffuse"—in either direction through the membrane.

Among the many important substances that cross cell membranes by facilitated diffusion are *glucose* and most of the *amino acids*. In the case of glucose at least 14 members of a family of membrane proteins (called GLUT) that transport glucose transporter molecules have been discovered in various tissues. Some of these GLUT can also transport other monosaccharides that have structures similar to that of glucose, including galactose and fructose. One of these, glucose transporter 4 (GLUT4), is activated by insulin, which can increase the rate of facilitated diffusion of glucose as much as 10- to 20-fold in insulin-sensitive tissues. This is the principal mechanism by which insulin controls glucose use in the body, as discussed in Chapter 93.

A comparison of simple and facilitated diffusion is summarized in Table 4-1.

FACTORS THAT AFFECT NET RATE OF DIFFUSION

By now it is evident that many substances can diffuse through the cell membrane. What is usually important is the *net* rate of diffusion of a substance in the desired direction. This net rate is determined by several factors.

Net Diffusion Rate Is Proportional to the Concentration Difference Across a Membrane. Figure 4-9A shows a cell membrane with a high concentration of a substance on the outside and a low concentration on the inside. The rate at which the substance diffuses *inward* is proportional to the concentration of molecules on the *outside* because this concentration determines how many molecules strike the outside of the membrane each second. Conversely, the rate at which molecules diffuse *outward* is proportional to their concentration *inside* the membrane.

TABLE 4-1	Comparison of Simple and Facilitated Diffusion	
	Simple Diffusion	**Facilitated Diffusion**
Movement	Along concentration gradient	Along concentration gradient
Energy required	No	No
Carrier protein required	No	Yes
Saturation kinetics	No	Yes
Type of molecules transported	Small, lipid soluble	Large, lipid insoluble

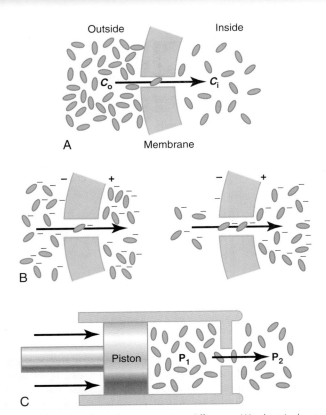

Figure 4-9 The effect of concentration difference (A), electrical potential difference affecting negative ions (B), and pressure difference (C) to cause diffusion of molecules and ions through a cell membrane.

$$\text{EMF (in millivolts)} = \pm 61 \log \frac{C_1}{C_2}$$

where EMF is the electromotive force (voltage) between side 1 and side 2 of the membrane, C_1 is the concentration on side 1, and C_2 is the concentration on side 2. This equation is extremely important in understanding the transmission of nerve impulses and is discussed in the context of the generation of the resting membrane potential in Chapter 7 and in the propagation of the nerve impulse in Chapter 10.

Effect of a Pressure Difference Across the Membrane. At times, considerable pressure difference develops between the two sides of a diffusible membrane. This pressure difference occurs, for instance, at the blood capillary membrane in all tissues of the body. The pressure is about 20 mmHg greater inside the capillary than outside.

Pressure actually means the sum of all the forces of the different molecules striking a unit surface area at a given instant. Therefore, having a higher pressure on one side of a membrane than on the other side means that the sum of all the forces of the molecules striking the channels on that side of the membrane is greater than on the other side. In most instances, this situation is caused by greater numbers of molecules striking the membrane per second on one side than on the other side. The result is that increased amounts of energy are available to cause net movement of molecules from the high-pressure side toward the low-pressure side. This effect is demonstrated in Figure 4-9C, which shows a piston developing high pressure on one side of a "pore," thereby causing more molecules to strike the pore on this side and, therefore, more molecules to "diffuse" to the other side.

OSMOSIS ACROSS SELECTIVELY PERMEABLE MEMBRANES—"NET DIFFUSION" OF WATER

By far the most abundant substance that diffuses through the cell membrane is water. Enough water ordinarily diffuses in each direction through the red blood cell membrane per second to equal about *100 times the volume of the cell itself*. Yet normally the amount that diffuses in the two directions is balanced so precisely that zero net movement of water occurs. Therefore, the volume of the cell remains constant. However, under certain conditions, a *concentration difference for water* can develop across a membrane. When this concentration gradient for water develops, net movement of water does occur across the cell membrane, causing the cell to either swell or shrink, depending on the direction of the water movement. This process of net movement of water caused by a concentration difference of water is called *osmosis*.

To illustrate osmosis, let us assume the conditions shown in Figure 4-10, with pure water on one side of the cell membrane and a solution of sodium chloride on the other side. Water molecules pass through the cell membrane with ease, whereas sodium and chloride ions pass through only with difficulty. Therefore, sodium chloride solution is actually a mixture of permeant water molecules and nonpermeant sodium and chloride ions, and the membrane is said to be *selectively permeable* to water but much less so to sodium and chloride ions. Yet the presence of the sodium and chloride has displaced some of the water molecules on the side of the membrane where these ions are present and, therefore, has reduced the concentration of water molecules to less than that of pure water. As a result, in the example of Figure 4-10, more water molecules strike the channels

Therefore, the rate of net diffusion into the cell is proportional to the concentration on the outside *minus* the concentration on the inside, or:

$$\text{Net diffusion} \propto C_o - C_i$$

where C_o is concentration outside and C_i is concentration inside.

Effect of Membrane Electrical Potential on Diffusion of Ions—The "Nernst Potential". If an electrical potential is applied across the membrane, as shown in Figure 4-9B, the electrical charges of the ions cause them to move through the membrane even though no concentration difference exists to cause movement. Thus, in the left panel of Figure 4-9B, the concentration of *negative* ions is the same on both sides of the membrane, but a positive charge has been applied to the right side of the membrane and a negative charge has been applied to the left, creating an electrical gradient across the membrane. The positive charge attracts the negative ions, whereas the negative charge repels them. Therefore, net diffusion occurs from left to right. After some time large quantities of negative ions have moved to the right, creating the condition shown in the right panel of Figure 4-9B, in which a concentration difference of the ions has developed in the direction opposite to the electrical potential difference. The concentration difference now tends to move the ions to the left, while the electrical difference tends to move them to the right. When the concentration difference rises high enough, the two effects balance each other. At normal body temperature (37°C), the electrical difference that will balance a given concentration difference of *univalent* ions—such as Na^+ ions—can be determined from the following formula, called the *Nernst equation*:

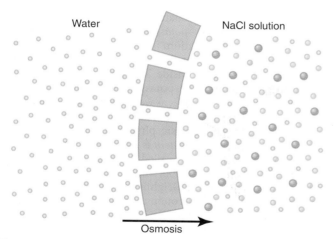

Figure 4-10 Osmosis at a cell membrane when a sodium chloride solution is placed on one side of the membrane and water is placed on the other side.

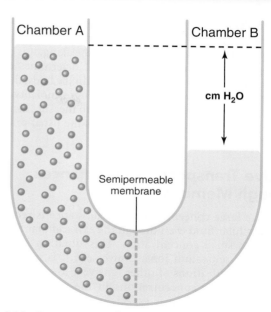

Figure 4-11 Demonstration of osmotic pressure caused by osmosis at a semipermeable membrane.

on the left side, where there is pure water, than on the right side, where the water concentration has been reduced. Thus, net movement of water occurs from left to right—that is, *osmosis* occurs from the pure water into the sodium chloride solution.

Osmotic Pressure

If in Figure 4-10 pressure was applied to the sodium chloride solution, osmosis of water into this solution would be slowed, stopped, or even reversed. The amount of pressure required to stop osmosis is called the *osmotic pressure* of the sodium chloride solution.

The principle of a pressure difference opposing osmosis is demonstrated in Figure 4-11, which shows a selectively permeable membrane separating two columns of fluid, one containing pure water and the other containing a solution of water and any solute that will not penetrate the membrane. Osmosis of water from chamber B into chamber A causes the levels of the fluid columns to become farther and farther apart, until eventually a pressure difference develops between the two sides of the membrane great enough to oppose the osmotic effect. The pressure difference across the membrane at this point is equal to the osmotic pressure of the solution that contains the nondiffusible solute.

Importance of Number of Osmotic Particles (Molar Concentration) in Determining Osmotic Pressure. The osmotic pressure exerted by particles in a solution, whether they are molecules or ions, is determined by the *number* of particles per unit volume of fluid, *not by the mass* of the particles. The reason for this is that each particle in a solution, regardless of its mass, exerts, on average, the same amount of pressure against the membrane. That is, large particles, which have greater mass (m) than do small particles, move at slower velocities (v). The small particles move at higher velocities in such a way that their average kinetic energies (k), determined by the equation:

$$k = \frac{mv^2}{2}$$

are the same for each small particle as for each large particle. Consequently, the factor that determines the osmotic pressure

of a solution is the concentration of the solution in terms of number of particles (which is the same as its *molar concentration* if it is a nondissociated molecule), not in terms of mass of the solute.

"Osmolality"—The Osmole. To express the concentration of a solution in terms of numbers of particles the unit called the *osmole* is used in place of grams.

One osmole is 1 g molecular weight of osmotically active solute. Thus, 180 g of glucose, which is 1 g molecular weight of glucose, is equal to 1 osm of glucose because glucose does not dissociate into ions. If a solute dissociates into two ions, 1 g molecular weight of the solute will become 2 osm because the number of osmotically active particles is now twice as great as is the case for the nondissociated solute. Therefore, when fully dissociated, 1 g molecular weight of sodium chloride, 58.5 g, is equal to 2 osm.

Thus, a solution that has *1 osm of solute dissolved in each kilogram of water* is said to have an *osmolality of 1 osm/kg*, and a solution that has 1/1000 osm dissolved per kilogram has an osmolality of 1 mOsm/kg. The normal osmolality of the extracellular and intracellular fluids is about *300 mOsm/kg of water*.

Relation of Osmolality to Osmotic Pressure. At normal body temperature, 37°C, a concentration of 1 osm/L will cause *19,300 mmHg* osmotic pressure in the solution. Likewise, *1 mOsm/L* concentration is equivalent to *19.3 mmHg* osmotic pressure. Multiplying this value by the 300-mOsm concentration of the body fluids gives a total calculated osmotic pressure of the body fluids of 5790 mmHg. The measured value for this, however, averages only about 5500 mmHg. The reason for this difference is that many of the ions in the body fluids, such as sodium and chloride ions, are highly attracted to one another; consequently, they cannot move entirely unrestrained in the fluids and create their full osmotic pressure potential. Therefore, on average, the actual osmotic pressure of the body fluids is about 0.93 times the calculated value.

The Term "Osmolarity". *Osmolarity* is the osmolar concentration expressed as *osmoles per liter of solution* rather than osmoles per kilogram of water. Although, strictly speaking, it is osmoles per kilogram of water (osmolality) that determines osmotic pressure for dilute solutions such as those in the body, the quantitative differences between osmolarity and osmolality are less than 1%. Because it is far more practical to measure osmolarity than osmolality, measuring osmolarity is the usual practice in almost all physiological studies.

"Active Transport" of Substances Through Membranes

At times, a large concentration of a substance is required in the intracellular fluid even though the extracellular fluid contains only a small concentration. This situation is true, for instance, for potassium ions. Conversely, it is important to keep the concentrations of other ions very low inside the cell even though their concentrations in the extracellular fluid are great. This situation is especially true for sodium ions. Neither of these two effects could occur by simple diffusion because simple diffusion eventually equilibrates concentrations on the two sides of the membrane. Instead, some energy source must cause excess movement of potassium ions to the inside of cells and excess movement of sodium ions to the outside of cells. When a cell membrane moves molecules or ions "uphill" against a concentration gradient (or "uphill" against an electrical or pressure gradient), the process is called *active transport*.

Different substances that are actively transported through at least some cell membranes include sodium, potassium, calcium, iron, hydrogen, chloride, iodide, and urate ions, several different sugars, and most of the amino acids.

Primary Active Transport and Secondary Active Transport. Active transport is divided into two types according to the source of the energy used to facilitate the transport: *primary active transport* and *secondary active transport*. In primary active transport, the energy is derived directly from breakdown of adenosine triphosphate (ATP) or some other high-energy phosphate compound. In secondary active transport, the energy is derived secondarily from energy that has been stored in the form of ionic concentration differences of secondary molecular or ionic substances between the two sides of a cell membrane, created originally by primary active transport. In both instances, transport depends on *carrier proteins* that penetrate through the cell membrane, as is true for facilitated diffusion. However, in active transport, the carrier protein functions differently from the carrier in facilitated diffusion because it is capable of imparting energy to the transported substance to move it against the electrochemical gradient. The following sections provide some examples of primary active transport and secondary active transport, with more detailed explanations of their principles of function.

PRIMARY ACTIVE TRANSPORT

Sodium–Potassium Pump Transports Sodium Ions Out of Cells and Potassium Ions into Cells

Among the substances that are transported by primary active transport are sodium, potassium, calcium, hydrogen, chloride, and a few other ions.

The active transport mechanism that has been studied in greatest detail is the *sodium–potassium* (Na^+–K^+) pump, a transport process that pumps sodium ions outward through the cell membrane of all cells and at the same time pumps potassium ions from the outside to the inside. This pump is responsible for maintaining the sodium and potassium concentration differences across the cell membrane, as well as for establishing a negative electrical voltage inside the cells as discussed in Chapter 7.

Figure 4-12 shows the basic physical components of the Na^+–K^+ pump. The *carrier protein* is a complex of two separate globular proteins: a larger one called the α subunit, with a molecular weight of about 100,000, and a smaller one called the β subunit, with a molecular weight of about 55,000. Although the function of the smaller protein is not known (except that it might anchor the protein complex in the lipid membrane), the larger protein has three specific features that are important for the functioning of the pump:

1. It has three *binding sites for sodium ions* on the portion of the protein that protrudes to the inside of the cell.
2. It has two *binding sites for potassium ions* on the outside.
3. The inside portion of this protein near the sodium binding sites has adenosine triphosphatse (ATPase) activity.

When two potassium ions bind on the outside of the carrier protein and three sodium ions bind on the inside, the ATPase function of the protein becomes activated. Activation of the ATPase function leads to cleavage of one molecule of ATP, splitting it to adenosine diphosphate (ADP) and liberating a high-energy phosphate bond of energy. This liberated energy is then believed to cause a chemical and conformational change in the protein carrier molecule, extruding the three sodium ions to the outside and the two potassium ions to the inside.

As with other enzymes, the Na^+–K^+ ATPase pump can run in reverse. If the electrochemical gradients for Na^+ and K^+ are experimentally increased to the degree that the energy stored in their gradients is greater than the chemical energy of ATP hydrolysis, these ions will move down their concentration gradients and the Na^+–K^+ pump will synthesize ATP from ADP and phosphate. The phosphorylated form of the Na^+–K^+ pump, therefore, can either donate its phosphate to ADP to produce ATP or use the energy to change its conformation and pump Na^+ out of the cell and K^+ into the cell. The relative concentrations of ATP, ADP, and phosphate, as well as the electrochemical gradients for Na^+ and K^+, determine the direction of the enzyme reaction. For some cells, such as electrically active nerve

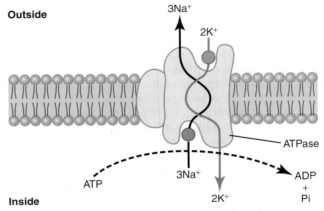

Figure 4-12 The postulated mechanism of the sodium–potassium pump. *ADP*, adenosine diphosphate; *ATP*, adenosine triphosphate; *Pi*, phosphate ion.

cells, 60–70% of the cells' energy requirement may be devoted to pumping Na^+ out of the cell and K^+ into the cell.

The Na^+–K^+ Pump Is Important for Controlling Cell Volume.

One of the most important functions of the Na^+–K^+ pump is to control the volume of each cell. Without function of this pump, most cells of the body would swell until they burst. The mechanism for controlling the volume is as follows: Inside the cell are large numbers of proteins and other organic molecules that cannot escape from the cell. Most of these proteins and other organic molecules are negatively charged and therefore attract large numbers of potassium, sodium, and other positive ions as well. All these molecules and ions then cause osmosis of water to the interior of the cell. Unless this process is checked, the cell will swell indefinitely until it bursts. The normal mechanism for preventing this outcome is the Na^+–K^+ pump. Note again that this device pumps three Na^+ ions to the outside of the cell for every two K^+ ions pumped to the interior. Also, the membrane is far less permeable to sodium ions than it is to potassium ions, and thus once the sodium ions are on the outside, they have a strong tendency to stay there. This process thus represents a net loss of ions out of the cell, which initiates osmosis of water out of the cell as well.

If a cell begins to swell for any reason, the Na^+–K^+ pump is automatically activated, moving still more ions to the exterior and carrying water with them. Therefore, the Na^+–K^+ pump performs a continual surveillance role in maintaining normal cell volume.

Electrogenic Nature of the Na^+–K^+ Pump.

The fact that the Na^+–K^+ pump moves three Na^+ ions to the exterior for every two K^+ ions that are moved to the interior means that a net of one positive charge is moved from the interior of the cell to the exterior for each cycle of the pump. This action creates positivity outside the cell but results in a deficit of positive ions inside the cell; that is, it causes negativity on the inside. Therefore, the Na^+–K^+ pump is said to be *electrogenic* because it creates an electrical potential across the cell membrane. As discussed in Chapter 7 this electrical potential is a basic requirement in nerve and muscle fibers for transmitting nerve and muscle signals.

SECONDARY ACTIVE TRANSPORT— COTRANSPORT AND COUNTERTRANSPORT

When sodium ions are transported out of cells by primary active transport, a large concentration gradient of sodium ions across the cell membrane usually develops with high concentration outside the cell and low concentration inside. This gradient represents a storehouse of energy because the excess sodium outside the cell membrane is always attempting to diffuse to the interior. Under appropriate conditions, this diffusion energy of sodium can pull other substances along with the sodium through the cell membrane. This phenomenon, called *cotransport*, is one form of *secondary active transport*.

For sodium to pull another substance along with it, a coupling mechanism is required, which is achieved by means of still another carrier protein in the cell membrane. The carrier in this instance serves as an attachment point for both the sodium ion and the substance to be cotransported. Once both of them are attached, the energy gradient of the sodium ion causes both the sodium ion and the other substance to be transported together to the interior of the cell.

In *countertransport*, sodium ions again attempt to diffuse to the interior of the cell because of their large concentration gradient. However, this time, the substance to be transported is on the inside of the cell and must be transported to the outside. Therefore, the sodium ion binds to the carrier protein where it projects to the exterior surface of the membrane, while the substance to be countertransported binds to the interior projection of the carrier protein. Once both have become bound, a conformational change occurs, and energy released by the action of the sodium ion moving to the interior causes the other substance to move to the exterior.

Cotransport of Glucose and Amino Acids Along with Sodium Ions

Glucose and many amino acids are transported into most cells against large concentration gradients; the mechanism of this action is entirely by cotransport, as shown in Figure 4-13. Note that the transport carrier protein has two binding sites on its exterior side, one for sodium and one for glucose. Also, the concentration of sodium ions is high on the outside and low inside, which provides energy for the transport. A special property of the transport protein is that a conformational change to allow sodium movement to the interior will not occur until a glucose molecule also attaches. When both of them become attached, the conformational change takes place, and the sodium and glucose are transported to the inside of the cell at the same time. Hence, this is a *sodium–glucose cotransport* mechanism. Sodium–glucose cotransporters are especially important mechanisms in transporting glucose across renal and intestinal epithelial cells, as discussed in Chapters 70 and 78.

Sodium cotransport of the amino acids occurs in the same manner as for glucose, except that it uses a different set of transport proteins. At least five *amino acid transport proteins* have been identified, each of which is responsible for transporting one subset of amino acids with specific molecular characteristics.

Sodium cotransport of glucose and amino acids occurs especially through the epithelial cells of the intestinal tract and the renal tubules of the kidneys to promote absorption of these substances into the blood. This is discussed in later chapters.

Other important cotransport mechanisms in at least some cells include cotransport of chloride, iodine, iron, and urate ions.

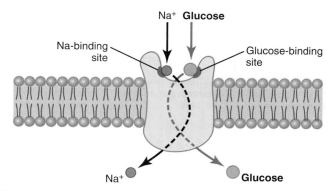

Figure 4-13 The postulated mechanism for sodium cotransport of glucose.

ACTIVE TRANSPORT THROUGH CELLULAR SHEETS

At many places in the body, substances must be transported all the way through a cellular sheet instead of simply through the cell membrane. Transport of this type occurs through the (1) intestinal epithelium, (2) epithelium of the renal tubules, (3) epithelium of all exocrine glands, (4) epithelium of the gallbladder, and (5) membrane of the choroid plexus of the brain, along with other membranes.

The basic mechanism for transport of a substance through a cellular sheet is (1) *active transport* through the cell membrane *on one side* of the transporting cells in the sheet, and then (2) either *simple diffusion* or *facilitated diffusion* through the membrane *on the opposite side* of the cell.

Figure 4-14 shows a mechanism for transport of sodium ions through the epithelial sheet of the intestines, gallbladder, and renal tubules. This figure shows that the epithelial cells are connected together tightly at the luminal pole by means of junctions. The brush border on the luminal surfaces of the cells is permeable to both sodium ions and water. Therefore, sodium and water diffuse readily from the lumen into the interior of the cell. Then, at the basal and lateral membranes of the cells, sodium ions are actively transported into the extracellular fluid of the surrounding connective tissue and blood vessels. This action creates a high sodium ion concentration gradient across these membranes, which in turn causes osmosis of water as well. Thus, active transport of sodium ions at the basolateral sides of the epithelial cells results in transport not only of sodium ions but also of water.

It is through these mechanisms that almost all nutrients, ions, and other substances are absorbed into the blood from the intestine. These mechanisms are also the way the same substances are reabsorbed from the glomerular filtrate by the renal tubules.

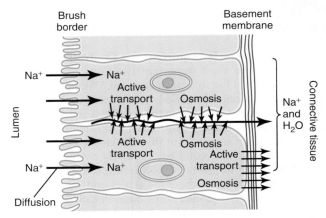

Figure 4-14 The basic mechanism of active transport across a layer of cells.

VESICULAR TRANSPORT

In addition to the examples of transport described above, there is also a need to transport large molecules (macromolecules). This is achieved by two processes: endocytosis and exocytosis.

1. Endocytosis is the process by which large molecules are transported from the extracellular space into the cell by the invagination of the cell membrane around the molecule. The molecule can then be released inside the cell. Pinocytosis and phagocytosis are examples of endocytosis.
2. Exocytosis is the process by which large molecules are released to the exterior of the cell following fusion of a vesicle with the cell membrane. Hormone and neurotransmitter release are examples of exocytosis.

Numerous examples of the different types of transport discussed in this chapter are provided throughout this text.

BIBLIOGRAPHY

Agre P, Kozono D: Aquaporin water channels: molecular mechanisms for human diseases, *FEBS Lett.* 555:72, 2003.

Blaustein MP, Zhang J, Chen L, et al: The pump, the exchanger, and endogenous ouabain: signaling mechanisms that link salt retention to hypertension, *Hypertension* 53:291, 2009.

Bröer S: Amino acid transport across mammalian intestinal and renal epithelia, *Physiol. Rev.* 88:249, 2008.

DeCoursey TE: Voltage-gated proton channels: molecular biology, physiology, and pathophysiology of the H(V) family, *Physiol. Rev.* 93:599, 2013.

DiPolo R, Beaugé L: Sodium/calcium exchanger: influence of metabolic regulation on ion carrier interactions, *Physiol. Rev.* 86:155, 2006.

Drummond HA, Jernigan NL, Grifoni SC: Sensing tension: epithelial sodium channel/acid-sensing ion channel proteins in cardiovascular homeostasis, *Hypertension* 51:1265, 2008.

Eastwood AL, Goodman MB: Insight into DEG/ENaC channel gating from genetics and structure, *Physiology (Bethesda)* 27:282, 2012.

Fischbarg J: Fluid transport across leaky epithelia: central role of the tight junction and supporting role of aquaporins, *Physiol. Rev.* 90:1271, 2010.

Gadsby DC: Ion channels versus ion pumps: the principal difference, in principle, *Nat. Rev. Mol. Cell Biol.* 10:344, 2009.

Jentsch TJ, Stein V, Weinreich F, Zdebik AA: Molecular structure and physiological function of chloride channels, *Physiol. Rev.* 82:503, 2002.

Mueckler M, Thorens B: The SLC2 (GLUT) family of membrane transporters, *Mol. Aspects Med.* 34:121, 2013.

Orlov SN, Platonova AA, Hamet P, Grygorczyk R: Cell volume and monovalent ion transporters: their role in cell death machinery triggering and progression, *Am. J. Physiol. Cell Physiol.* 305:C361, 2013.

Papadopoulos MC, Verkman AS: Aquaporin water channels in the nervous system, *Nat. Rev. Neurosci.* 14:265, 2013.

Sachs F: Stretch-activated ion channels: what are they? *Physiology* 25:50, 2010.

Schiöth HB, Roshanbin S, Hägglund MG, Fredriksson R: Evolutionary origin of amino acid transporter families SLC32, SLC36 and SLC38 and physiological, pathological and therapeutic aspects, *Mol. Aspects Med.* 34:571, 2013.

Schwab A, Fabian A, Hanley PJ, Stock C: Role of ion channels and transporters in cell migration, *Physiol. Rev.* 92:1865, 2012.

Sherwood TW, Frey EN, Askwith CC: Structure and activity of the acid-sensing ion channels, *Am. J. Physiol.* 303:C699, 2012.

Tian J, Xie ZJ: The Na–K-ATPase and calcium-signaling microdomains, *Physiology (Bethesda)* 23:205, 2008.

Wright EM, Loo DD, Hirayama BA: Biology of human sodium glucose transporters, *Physiol. Rev.* 91:733, 2011.

The Body Fluid Compartments

The maintenance of a relatively constant volume and a stable composition of the body fluids is essential for homeostasis. Some of the most common and important problems in clinical medicine arise because of abnormalities in the control systems that maintain this relative constancy of the body fluids. In this chapter and in Section VII, we discuss the overall regulation of body fluid volume, constituents of the extracellular fluid, acid–base balance, and control of fluid exchange between extracellular and intracellular compartments.

Fluid Intake and Output Are Balanced During Steady-State Conditions

The relative constancy of the body fluids is remarkable because there is continuous exchange of fluid and solutes with the external environment, as well as within the different body compartments. For example, fluid intake is highly variable and must be carefully matched by equal output of water from the body to prevent body fluid volumes from increasing or decreasing.

DAILY INTAKE OF WATER

Water is added to the body by two major sources: (1) it is ingested in the form of liquids or water in food, which together normally adds about 2100 mL/day to the body fluids, and (2) it is synthesized in the body by oxidation of carbohydrates, adding about 200 mL/day. These mechanisms provide a total water intake of about 2300 mL/day (Table 5-1). However, intake of water is highly variable among different people and even within the same person on different days, depending on climate, habits, and level of physical activity.

DAILY LOSS OF BODY WATER

Insensible Water Loss. Some water losses cannot be precisely regulated. For example, humans experience a continuous loss of water by evaporation from the respiratory tract and diffusion through the skin, which together account for about 700 mL/day of water loss under normal conditions. This loss is termed *insensible water loss* because we are not consciously aware of it, even though it occurs continually in all living humans.

Insensible water loss through the skin occurs independently of sweating and is present even in people who are born without sweat glands; the average water loss by diffusion through the skin is about 300–400 mL/day. This loss is minimized by the cholesterol-filled cornified layer of the skin, which provides a barrier against excessive loss by diffusion. When the cornified layer becomes denuded, as occurs with extensive burns, the rate of evaporation can increase as much as 10-fold, to 3–5 L/day. For this reason, persons with burns must be given large amounts of fluid, usually intravenously, to balance fluid loss.

Insensible water loss through the respiratory tract averages about 300–400 mL/day. As air enters the respiratory tract, it becomes saturated with moisture to a vapor pressure of about 47 mmHg before it is expelled. Because the vapor pressure of the inspired air is usually less than 47 mmHg, water is continuously lost through the lungs with respiration. In cold weather, the atmospheric vapor pressure decreases to nearly 0, causing an even greater loss of water from the lungs as the temperature decreases. This process explains the dry feeling in the respiratory passages in cold weather.

Fluid Loss in Sweat. The amount of water lost by sweating is highly variable depending on physical activity and environmental temperature. The volume of sweat normally is about 100 mL/day, but in very hot weather or during heavy exercise fluid loss occasionally increases to 1–2 L/hour. This fluid loss would rapidly deplete the body fluids if intake were not also increased by activating the thirst mechanism discussed in Chapter 80.

Water Loss in Feces. Only a small amount of water (100 mL/day) normally is lost in the feces. This loss can increase to several liters a day in people with severe diarrhea. For this reason, severe diarrhea can be life threatening if not corrected within a few days.

Water Loss by the Kidneys. The remaining water loss from the body occurs in the urine excreted by the kidneys. Multiple mechanisms control the rate of urine excretion. In fact, the most important means by which the body maintains a balance between water intake and output, as well as a balance between intake and output of most electrolytes in the body, is by controlling the rates at which the kidneys excrete these substances. For example, urine volume can be as low as 0.5 L/day in a dehydrated person or as high as 20 L/day in a person who has been drinking tremendous amounts of water.

This variability of intake is also true for most of the electrolytes of the body, such as sodium, chloride, and potassium. In some people, sodium intake may be as low as 20 mEq/day, whereas in

TABLE 5-1	Daily Intake and Output of Water (mL/Day)		
		Normal	Prolonged, Heavy Exercise
INTAKE			
Fluids ingested		2100	?
From metabolism		200	200
Total intake		2300	?
OUTPUT			
Insensible—skin		350	350
Insensible—lungs		350	650
Sweat		100	5000
Feces		100	100
Urine		1400	500
TOTAL OUTPUT		2300	6600

others, sodium intake may be as high as 300–500 mEq/day. The kidneys are faced with the task of adjusting the excretion rate of water and electrolytes to match precisely the intake of these substances, as well as compensating for excessive losses of fluids and electrolytes that occur in certain disease states. In Section VII, Chapters 79–82, we discuss the mechanisms that allow the kidneys to perform these remarkable tasks.

Body Fluid Compartments

The total body fluid is distributed mainly between two compartments: the *extracellular fluid* and the *intracellular fluid* (Figure 5-1). The extracellular fluid is divided into the *interstitial fluid* and the blood *plasma*.

There is another small compartment of fluid that is referred to as *transcellular fluid*. This compartment includes fluid in the synovial, peritoneal, pericardial, and intraocular spaces, as well as the cerebrospinal fluid; it is usually considered to be a specialized type of extracellular fluid, although in some cases its composition

may differ markedly from that of the plasma or interstitial fluid. All the transcellular fluids together constitute about 12 L.

In a 70-kg adult man, the total body water is about 60% of the body weight or about 42 L. This percentage depends on age, gender, and degree of obesity. As a person grows older, the percentage of total body weight that is fluid gradually decreases. This decrease is due in part to the fact that aging is usually associated with an increased percentage of the body weight being fat, which decreases the percentage of water in the body.

Because women normally have a greater percentage of body fat compared with men, their total body water averages about 50% of the body weight. In premature and newborn babies, the total body water ranges from 70 to 75% of body weight. Therefore, when discussing "average" body fluid compartments, we should realize that variations exist, depending on age, gender, and percentage of body fat.

INTRACELLULAR FLUID COMPARTMENT

About 28 of the 42 L of fluid in the body is inside the 100 trillion cells and is collectively called the *intracellular fluid*. Thus, the intracellular fluid constitutes about 40% of the total body weight in an "average" person.

The fluid of each cell contains its individual mixture of different constituents, but the concentrations of these substances are similar from one cell to another. In fact, the composition of cell fluids is remarkably similar even in different animals, ranging from the most primitive microorganisms to humans. For this reason, the intracellular fluid of all the different cells together is considered to be one large fluid compartment.

EXTRACELLULAR FLUID COMPARTMENT

All the fluids outside the cells are collectively called the *extracellular fluid*. Together these fluids account for about 20% of the body weight or about 14 L in a 70-kg man. The two largest compartments of the extracellular fluid are the *interstitial fluid*, which makes up more than three-fourths (11 L) of the extracellular fluid, and the *plasma* that makes up almost one-fourth of the extracellular fluid or about 3 L. The plasma is the noncellular part of the blood; it exchanges substances continuously with the interstitial fluid through the pores of the capillary membranes. These pores are highly permeable to almost all solutes in the extracellular fluid except the proteins. Therefore, the extracellular fluids are constantly mixing, so the plasma and interstitial fluids have about the same composition except for proteins that have a higher concentration in the plasma.

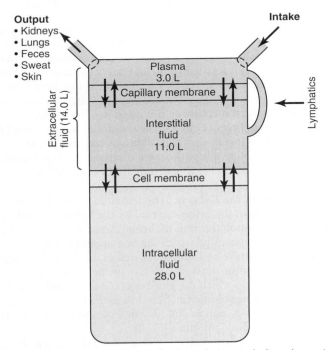

Figure 5-1 Summary of body fluid regulation, including the major body fluid compartments and the membranes that separate these compartments. The values shown are for an average 70-kg adult man.

Blood Volume

Blood contains both extracellular fluid (the fluid in plasma) and intracellular fluid (the fluid in the red blood cells). However, blood is considered to be a separate fluid compartment because it is contained in a chamber of its own, the circulatory system. The blood volume is especially important in the control of cardiovascular dynamics.

The average blood volume of adults is about 7% of body weight, or about 5 L. About 60% of the blood is plasma and 40% is red blood cells, but these percentages can vary considerably in different people, depending on gender, weight, and other factors.

Hematocrit (Packed Red Blood Cell Volume). The hematocrit is the fraction of the blood composed of red blood cells, as determined by centrifuging blood in a "hematocrit tube" until the cells become tightly packed in the bottom of the tube. Because the centrifuge does not completely pack the red blood cells together, about 3–4% of the plasma remains entrapped among the cells, and the true hematocrit is only about 96% of the measured hematocrit.

In men, the measured hematocrit is normally about 0.40, and in women, it is about 0.36. In people with severe *anemia*, the hematocrit may fall as low as 0.10, a value that is barely sufficient to sustain life. Conversely, in people with excessive production of red blood cells (*polycythemia*) the hematocrit can rise to 0.65.

Constituents of Extracellular and Intracellular Fluids

Comparisons of the composition of the extracellular fluid, including the plasma and interstitial fluid, and the intracellular fluid are shown in Figures 5-2 and 5-3 and in Table 6-1.

IONIC COMPOSITION OF PLASMA AND INTERSTITIAL FLUID IS SIMILAR

Because the plasma and interstitial fluid are separated only by highly permeable capillary membranes, their ionic composition is similar. The most important difference between these two compartments is the higher concentration of protein in the plasma; because the capillaries have a low permeability to the plasma proteins, only small amounts of proteins are leaked into the interstitial spaces in most tissues.

Because of the *Donnan effect*, the concentration of positively charged ions (cations) is slightly greater (~2%) in the plasma than in the interstitial fluid. The plasma proteins have a net negative charge and, therefore, tend to bind cations, such as sodium and potassium ions, thus holding extra amounts of these cations in the plasma along with the plasma proteins. Conversely, negatively charged ions (anions) tend to have a slightly higher concentration in the interstitial fluid compared with the plasma because the negative charges of the plasma proteins repel the negatively charged anions. For practical purposes, however, the concentration of ions in the interstitial fluid and in the plasma is considered to be about equal.

Referring again to Figure 5-2, one can see that the extracellular fluid, including the plasma and the interstitial fluid, contains large amounts of sodium and chloride ions, and reasonably large amounts of bicarbonate ions, but only small quantities of potassium, calcium, magnesium, phosphate, and organic acid ions.

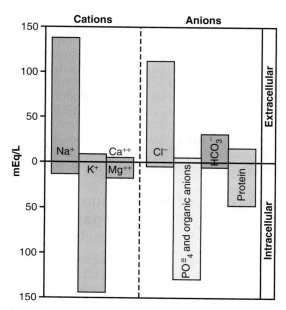

Figure 5-2 Major cations and anions of the intracellular and extracellular fluids. The concentrations of Ca^{++} and Mg^{++} represent the sum of these two ions. The concentrations shown represent the total of free ions and complexed ions.

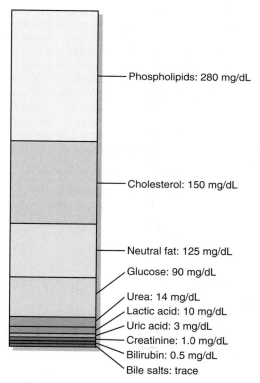

Phospholipids: 280 mg/dL
Cholesterol: 150 mg/dL
Neutral fat: 125 mg/dL
Glucose: 90 mg/dL
Urea: 14 mg/dL
Lactic acid: 10 mg/dL
Uric acid: 3 mg/dL
Creatinine: 1.0 mg/dL
Bilirubin: 0.5 mg/dL
Bile salts: trace

Figure 5-3 Nonelectrolytes of the plasma.

The composition of extracellular fluid is carefully regulated by various mechanisms, but especially by the kidneys, as discussed later. This regulation allows the cells to remain continually bathed in a fluid that contains the proper concentration of electrolytes and nutrients for optimal cell function.

INTRACELLULAR FLUID CONSTITUENTS

The intracellular fluid is separated from the extracellular fluid by a cell membrane that is highly permeable to water but is not permeable to most of the electrolytes in the body.

In contrast to the extracellular fluid, the intracellular fluid contains only small quantities of sodium and chloride ions and almost no calcium ions. Instead, it contains large amounts of potassium and phosphate ions plus moderate quantities of magnesium and sulfate ions, all of which have low concentrations in the extracellular fluid. Also, cells contain large amounts of protein, almost four times as much as in the plasma.

Measurement of Fluid Volumes in the Different Body Fluid Compartments— The Indicator–Dilution Principle

The volume of a fluid compartment in the body can be measured by placing an indicator substance in the compartment, allowing it to disperse evenly throughout the compartment's fluid, and then analyzing the extent to which the substance becomes diluted. Figure 5-4 shows this "indicator–dilution" method of measuring the volume of a fluid compartment. This method is based on the conservation of mass principle, which means that the total mass of a substance after dispersion in the fluid compartment will be the same as the total mass injected into the compartment.

In the example shown in Figure 5-4, a small amount of dye or other substance contained in the syringe is injected into a chamber and the substance is allowed to disperse throughout the chamber until it becomes mixed in equal concentrations in all areas. Then a sample of fluid containing the dispersed substance is removed and the concentration is analyzed chemically, photoelectrically, or by other means. If none of the substance leaks out of the compartment, the total mass of substance in the compartment (volume B × concentration B) will equal the total mass of the substance injected (volume A × concentration A). By simple rearrangement of the equation, one can calculate the unknown volume of chamber B as follows:

$$\text{Volume B} = \frac{\text{volume A} \times \text{concentration A}}{\text{concentration B}}$$

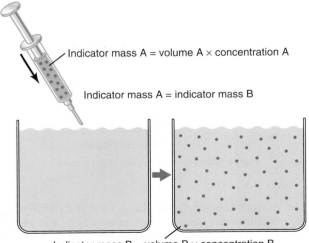

Indicator mass A = volume A × concentration A

Indicator mass A = indicator mass B

Indicator mass B = volume B × concentration B

Volume B = indicator mass B/concentration B

Figure 5-4   Indicator–dilution method for measuring fluid volumes.

Note that all one needs to know for this calculation is (1) the total amount of substance injected into the chamber (the numerator of the equation) and (2) the concentration of the fluid in the chamber after the substance has been dispersed (the denominator).

For example, if 1 mL of a solution containing 10 mg/mL of dye is dispersed into chamber B and the final concentration in the chamber is 0.01 mg for each milliliter of fluid, the unknown volume of the chamber can be calculated as follows:

$$\text{Volume B} = \frac{1 \text{ mL} \times 10 \text{ mg/mL}}{0.01 \text{ mg/mL}} = 1000 \text{ mL}$$

This method can be used to measure the volume of virtually any compartment in the body as long as:

1. The indicator disperses evenly throughout the compartment.
2. The indicator disperses only in the compartment that is being measured.
3. The indicator is not metabolized or excreted for a sufficient duration to allow its equilibration within the compartment of interest. If the indicator is metabolized or excreted, correction must be made for loss of the indicator from the body.
4. The indicator can be easily and accurately measured.
5. The indicator is nontoxic.

These are the features of an "ideal" indicator.

Determination of Volumes of Specific Body Fluid Compartments

Measurement of Total Body Water. Radioactive water (tritium, ^3H_2O) or heavy water (deuterium, ^2H_2O) can be used to measure total body water. These forms of water mix with the total body water within a few hours after being injected into the blood, and the dilution principle can be used to calculate total body water (Table 5-2). Another substance that has been used to measure total body water is *antipyrine*, which is very lipid soluble and can rapidly penetrate cell membranes and distribute itself uniformly throughout the intracellular and extracellular compartments.

Measurement of Extracellular Fluid Volume. The volume of extracellular fluid can be estimated using any of several substances that disperse in the plasma and interstitial fluid but do not readily permeate the cell membrane. They include radioactive sodium, radioactive chloride, radioactive iothalamate, thiosulfate ion, and inulin. When any one of these substances is injected into the blood, it usually disperses almost completely throughout the extracellular fluid within 30–60 minutes. Some of these substances, however, such as radioactive sodium, may diffuse into the cells in small amounts. Therefore, one frequently speaks of the *sodium space* or the *inulin space*, instead of calling the measurement the true extracellular fluid volume.

Calculation of Intracellular Volume. The intracellular volume cannot be measured directly. However, it can be calculated as follows:

Intracellular volume = total body water − extracellular volume

TABLE 5-2	Measurement of Body Fluid Volumes
Volume	Indicators
Total body water	^3H_2O, ^2H_2O, antipyrine
Extracellular fluid	^{22}Na, ^{125}I-iothalamate, thiosulfate, inulin
Intracellular fluid	Calculated as: (total body water) − (extracellular fluid volume)
Plasma volume	^{125}I-albumin, Evans blue dye (T-1824)
Blood volume	^{51}Cr-labeled red blood cells or calculated as: (blood volume) = (plasma volume)/(1 − hematocrit)
Interstitial fluid	Calculated as: (extracellular fluid volume) − (plasma volume)

Measurement of Plasma Volume. To measure plasma volume, a substance must be used that does not readily penetrate capillary membranes but remains in the vascular system after injection. One of the most commonly used substances for measuring plasma volume is serum albumin labeled with radioactive iodine (^{125}I-albumin). Also, dyes that avidly bind to the plasma proteins, such as *Evans blue dye* (also called *T-1824*), can be used to measure plasma volume.

Calculation of Interstitial Fluid Volume. Interstitial fluid volume cannot be measured directly, but it can be calculated as follows:

$$\text{Interstitial fluid volume} = \text{extracellular fluid volume} - \text{plasma volume}$$

Measurement of Blood Volume. If one measures plasma volume using the methods described earlier, blood volume can also be calculated if one knows the *hematocrit* (the fraction of the total blood volume composed of cells), using the following equation:

$$\text{Total blood volume} = \frac{\text{plasma volume}}{1 - \text{hematocrit}}$$

For example, if plasma volume is 3 L and hematocrit is 0.40, then total blood volume would be calculated as follows:

$$\frac{3\,L}{1 - 0.4} = 5\,L$$

Another way to measure blood volume is to inject into the circulation red blood cells that have been labeled with radioactive material. After these get mixed in the circulation, the radioactivity of a mixed blood sample can be measured and the total blood volume can be calculated using the indicator–dilution principle. A substance frequently used to label the red blood cells is radioactive chromium (^{51}Cr), which binds tightly with the red blood cells.

BIBLIOGRAPHY

Aukland K: Why don't our feet swell in the upright position? *News Physiol. Sci.* 9:214, 1994.

Bhave G, Neilson EG: Body fluid dynamics: back to the future, *J. Am. Soc. Nephrol.* 22:2166, 2011.

Guyton AC, Granger HJ, Taylor AE: Interstitial fluid pressure, *Physiol. Rev.* 51:527, 1971.

Halperin ML, Bohn D: Clinical approach to disorders of salt and water balance: emphasis on integrative physiology, *Crit. Care Clin.* 18:249, 2002.

Loh JA, Verbalis JG: Disorders of water and salt metabolism associated with pituitary disease, *Endocrinol. Metab. Clin. North Am.* 37:213, 2008.

Intracellular and Extracellular Fluid Compartments and Edema

A frequent problem in treating seriously ill patients is maintaining adequate fluids in one or both of the intracellular and extracellular compartments. As discussed in Chapter 39 and in this chapter, the relative amounts of extracellular fluid distributed between the plasma and interstitial spaces are determined mainly by the balance of hydrostatic and colloid osmotic forces across the capillary membranes.

The distribution of fluid between intracellular and extracellular compartments, in contrast, is determined mainly by the osmotic effect of the smaller solutes—especially sodium, chloride, and other electrolytes—acting across the cell membrane. The reason for this is that the cell membranes are highly permeable to water but relatively impermeable to even small ions such as sodium and chloride. Therefore, water moves across the cell membrane rapidly and the intracellular fluid remains isotonic with the extracellular fluid.

In the next section, we discuss the interrelations between intracellular and extracellular fluid volumes and the osmotic factors that can cause shifts of fluid between these two compartments.

Basic Principles of Osmosis and Osmotic Pressure

The basic principles of osmosis and osmotic pressure were presented in Chapter 4. Because cell membranes are relatively impermeable to most solutes but are highly permeable to water (ie, they are selectively permeable), whenever there is a higher concentration of solute on one side of the cell membrane, water diffuses across the membrane toward the region of higher solute concentration. Thus, if a solute such as sodium chloride is added to the extracellular fluid, water rapidly diffuses from the cells through the cell membranes into the extracellular fluid until the water concentration on both sides of the membrane becomes equal. Conversely, if a solute such as sodium chloride is removed from the extracellular fluid, water diffuses from the extracellular fluid through the cell membranes and into the cells. The rate of diffusion of water is called the *rate of osmosis*.

In Table 6-1, we note the approximate osmolarity of the various osmotically active substances in plasma, interstitial fluid, and intracellular fluid. About 80% of the total osmolarity of the interstitial fluid and plasma is due to sodium and chloride ions, whereas for intracellular fluid almost half the osmolarity is due to potassium ions and the remainder is divided among many other intracellular substances.

As shown in Table 6-1, the total osmolarity of each of the three compartments is about 300 mOsm/L, with that of the plasma being about 1 mOsm/L greater than that of the interstitial and intracellular fluids. The slight difference between plasma and interstitial fluid is caused by the osmotic effects of the plasma proteins, which maintain about 20 mmHg greater pressure in the capillaries than in the surrounding interstitial spaces, as discussed in Chapter 39.

Corrected Osmolar Activity of the Body Fluids. At the bottom of Table 6-1 are shown *corrected osmolar activities* of plasma, interstitial fluid, and intracellular fluid. The reason for these corrections is that cations and anions exert interionic attraction, which can cause a slight decrease in the osmotic "activity" of the dissolved substance.

Osmotic Equilibrium Is Maintained Between Intracellular and Extracellular Fluids

Large osmotic pressures can develop across the cell membrane with relatively small changes in the concentrations of solutes in the extracellular fluid. As discussed earlier, for each milliosmole concentration gradient of an *impermeant solute* (one that will not permeate the cell membrane), about 19.3 mmHg of osmotic pressure is exerted across the cell membrane. If the

TABLE 6-1	Osmolar Substances in Extracellular and Intracellular Fluids		
	Plasma (mOsm/L H₂O)	Interstitial (mOsm/L H₂O)	Intracellular (mOsm/L H₂O)
Na^+	142	139	14
K^+	4.2	4.0	140
Ca^{++}	1.3	1.2	0
Mg^{++}	0.8	0.7	20
Cl^-	106	108	4
HCO_3^-	24	28.3	10
$HPO_4^=, H_2PO_4^-$	2	2	11
$SO_4^=$	0.5	0.5	1
Phosphocreatine			45
Carnosine			14
Amino acids	2	2	8
Creatine	0.2	0.2	9
Lactate	1.2	1.2	1.5
Adenosine triphosphate			5
Hexose monophosphate			3.7
Glucose	5.6	5.6	
Protein	1.2	0.2	4
Urea	4	4	4
Others	4.8	3.9	10
Total (mOsm/L)	299.8	300.8	301.2
Corrected osmolar activity (mOsm/L)	282.0	281.0	281.0
Total osmotic pressure at 37°C (mmHg)	5441	5423	5423

cell membrane is exposed to pure water and the osmolarity of intracellular fluid is 282 mOsm/L, the potential osmotic pressure that can develop across the cell membrane is more than 5400 mmHg. This demonstrates the large force that can move water across the cell membrane when the intracellular and extracellular fluids are not in osmotic equilibrium. As a result of these forces, relatively small changes in the concentration of impermeant solutes in the extracellular fluid can cause large changes in cell volume.

Isosmotic, Hyperosmotic, and Hypoosmotic Fluids. The terms *isotonic*, *hypotonic*, and *hypertonic* refer to whether solutions will cause a change in cell volume. The tonicity of solutions depends on the concentration of impermeant solutes. Some solutes, however, can permeate the cell membrane. Solutions with an osmolarity the same as the cell are called *iso-osmotic*, regardless of whether the solute can penetrate the cell membrane.

The terms *hyperosmotic* and *hypoosmotic* refer to solutions that have a higher or lower osmolarity, respectively, compared with the normal extracellular fluid, without regard for whether the solute permeates the cell membrane. If a cell is placed in a *hypertonic* solution having a higher concentration of impermeant solutes, water will flow out of the cell into the extracellular fluid causing it to shrink. If a cell is placed into a *hypotonic* solution that has a lower concentration of impermeant solutes (<282 mOsm/L), water will diffuse into the cell, causing it to swell. Highly permeating substances, such as urea, can cause transient shifts in fluid volume between the intracellular and extracellular fluids, but given enough time, the concentrations of these substances eventually become equal in the two compartments and have little effect on intracellular volume under steady-state conditions.

Osmotic Equilibrium Between Intracellular and Extracellular Fluids Is Rapidly Attained. The transfer of fluid across the cell membrane occurs so rapidly that any differences in osmolarities between these two compartments are usually corrected within seconds or, at the most, minutes. This rapid movement of water across the cell membrane does not mean that complete equilibrium occurs between the intracellular and extracellular compartments throughout the whole body within the same short period. The reason for this is that fluid usually enters the body through the gut and must be transported by the blood to all tissues before complete osmotic equilibrium can occur. It usually takes about 30 minutes to achieve osmotic equilibrium everywhere in the body after drinking water.

Volume and Osmolality of Extracellular and Intracellular Fluids in Abnormal States

Some of the different factors that can cause extracellular and intracellular volumes to change markedly are excess ingestion or renal retention of water, dehydration, intravenous infusion of different types of solutions, loss of large amounts of fluid from the gastrointestinal tract, and loss of abnormal amounts of fluid by sweating or through the kidneys.

One can calculate both the changes in intracellular and extracellular fluid volumes and the types of therapy that should be instituted if the following basic principles are kept in mind:

1. *Water moves rapidly across cell membranes*; therefore, the osmolarities of intracellular and extracellular fluids remain almost exactly equal to each other except for a few minutes after a change in one of the compartments.

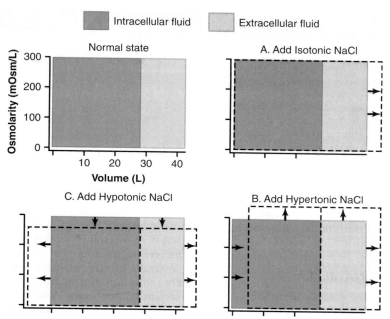

Figure 6-1   Effect of adding (A) isotonic, (B) hypertonic, and (C) hypotonic solutions to the extracellular fluid after osmotic equilibrium. The normal state is indicated by the solid lines, and the shifts from normal are shown by the shaded areas. The volumes of intracellular and extracellular fluid compartments are shown in the abscissa of each diagram, and the osmolarities of these compartments are shown on the ordinates.

2. *Cell membranes are almost completely impermeable to many solutes*, such as sodium and chloride; therefore, the number of osmoles in the extracellular or intracellular fluid generally remains constant unless solutes are added to or lost from the extracellular compartment.

With these basic principles in mind, we can analyze the effects of different abnormal fluid conditions on extracellular and intracellular fluid volumes and osmolarities.

EFFECT OF ADDING SALINE SOLUTION TO THE EXTRACELLULAR FLUID

If *isotonic* saline is added to the extracellular fluid compartment, the osmolarity of the extracellular fluid does not change; therefore, no osmosis occurs through the cell membranes. The only effect is an increase in extracellular fluid volume (Figure 6-1A).

If a *hypertonic* solution is added to the extracellular fluid, the extracellular osmolarity increases and causes osmosis of water out of the cells into the extracellular compartment (see Figure 6-1B). Again, almost all the added sodium chloride remains in the extracellular compartment and fluid diffuses from the cells into the extracellular space to achieve osmotic equilibrium. The net effect is an increase in extracellular volume (greater than the volume of fluid added), a decrease in intracellular volume, and a rise in osmolarity in both compartments.

If a *hypotonic* solution is added to the extracellular fluid, the osmolarity of the extracellular fluid decreases and some of the extracellular water diffuses into the cells until the intracellular and extracellular compartments have the same osmolarity (see Figure 6-1C). Both the intracellular and the extracellular volumes are increased by the addition of hypotonic fluid, although the intracellular volume increases to a greater extent.

Clinical Abnormalities of Fluid Volume Regulation: Hyponatremia and Hypernatremia

A measurement that is readily available to the clinician for evaluating a patient's fluid status is the plasma sodium concentration. Plasma osmolarity is not routinely measured, but because sodium and its associated anions (mainly chloride) account for more than 90% of the solute in the extracellular fluid, plasma sodium concentration is a reasonable indicator of plasma osmolarity under many conditions. When plasma sodium concentration is reduced more than a few milliequivalents below normal (about 142 mEq/L), a person is said to have *hyponatremia*. When plasma sodium concentration is elevated above normal, a person is said to have *hypernatremia*.

CAUSES OF HYPONATREMIA: EXCESS WATER OR LOSS OF SODIUM

Decreased plasma sodium concentration can result from loss of sodium chloride from the extracellular fluid or addition of excess water to the extracellular fluid (Table 6-2). A primary loss of sodium chloride usually results in *hyponatremia and dehydration* and is associated with decreased extracellular fluid volume. Conditions that can cause hyponatremia as a result of loss of sodium chloride include *diarrhea* and *vomiting*. Overuse of *diuretics* that inhibit the ability of the kidneys to conserve sodium and certain types of sodium-wasting kidney diseases can also cause modest degrees of hyponatremia. Finally, *Addison disease*, which results from decreased secretion of the hormone aldosterone, impairs the ability of the kidneys to reabsorb sodium and can cause a modest degree of hyponatremia.

Hyponatremia can also be associated with excess water retention, which dilutes the sodium in the extracellular fluid, a condition that is referred to as *hyponatremia—overhydration*.

TABLE 6-2	Abnormalities of Body Fluid Volume Regulation: Hyponatremia and Hypernatremia			
Abnormality	Cause	Plasma Na+ Concentration	Extracellular Fluid Volume	Intracellular Fluid Volume
Hyponatremia—dehydration	Adrenal insufficiency; overuse of diuretics	↓	↓	↑
Hyponatremia—overhydration	Excess ADH (SIADH); bronchogenic tumors	↓	↑	↑
Hypernatremia—dehydration	Diabetes insipidus; excessive sweating	↑	↓	↓
Hypernatremia—overhydration	Cushing disease; primary aldosteronism	↑	↑	↓

ADH, antidiuretic hormone; SIADH, syndrome of inappropriate ADH.

For example, *excessive secretion of antidiuretic hormone*, which causes the kidney tubules to reabsorb more water, can lead to hyponatremia and overhydration.

CONSEQUENCES OF HYPONATREMIA: CELL SWELLING

Rapid changes in cell volume as a result of hyponatremia can have profound effects on tissue and organ function, especially the brain. A rapid reduction in plasma sodium concentration, for example, can cause brain cell edema and neurological symptoms, including headache, nausea, lethargy, and disorientation. If plasma sodium concentration rapidly falls below 115–120 mmol/L, brain swelling may lead to seizures, coma, permanent brain damage, and death. Because the skull is rigid, the brain cannot increase its volume by more than about 10% without it being forced down the neck (*herniation*), which can lead to permanent brain injury and death.

When hyponatremia evolves more slowly over several days, the brain and other tissues respond by transporting sodium, chloride, potassium, and organic solutes, such as glutamate, from the cells into the extracellular compartment. This response attenuates osmotic flow of water into the cells and swelling of the tissues (Figure 6-2).

Transport of solutes from the cells during slowly developing hyponatremia, however, can make the brain vulnerable to injury if the hyponatremia is corrected too rapidly. When hypertonic solutions are added too rapidly to correct hyponatremia, this intervention can outpace the brain's ability to recapture the solutes lost from the cells and may lead to osmotic injury of the neurons that is associated with *demyelination*, a loss of the myelin sheath from nerves. This osmotic-mediated demyelination of neurons can be avoided by limiting the correction of chronic hyponatremia to less than 10–12 mmol/L in 24 hours and to less than 18 mmol/L in 48 hours. This slow rate of correction permits the brain to recover the lost osmoles that have occurred as a result of adaptation to chronic hyponatremia.

Hyponatremia is the most common electrolyte disorder encountered in clinical practice and may occur in up to 15–25% of hospitalized patients.

CAUSES OF HYPERNATREMIA: WATER LOSS OR EXCESS SODIUM

Increased plasma sodium concentration, which also causes increased osmolarity, can be due to either loss of water from the extracellular fluid, which concentrates the sodium ions, or excess sodium in the extracellular fluid. Primary loss of water from the extracellular fluid results in *hypernatremia and dehydration*.

This condition can occur from an inability to secrete antidiuretic hormone, which is needed for the kidneys to conserve water. As a result of lack of antidiuretic hormone, the kidneys excrete large amounts of dilute urine (a disorder referred to as *"central" diabetes insipidus*), causing dehydration and increased concentration of sodium chloride in the extracellular fluid. In certain types of renal diseases, the kidneys cannot respond to antidiuretic hormone, causing a type of *"nephrogenic" diabetes insipidus*. A more common cause of hypernatremia associated with decreased extracellular fluid volume is simple *dehydration* caused by water intake that is less than water loss, as can occur with sweating during prolonged, heavy exercise.

Hypernatremia can also occur when excessive sodium chloride is added to the extracellular fluid. This often results in *hypernatremia—overhydration* because excess extracellular sodium chloride is usually associated with at least some degree of water retention by the kidneys as well. For example, *excessive secretion of the sodium-retaining hormone aldosterone* can cause a mild degree of hypernatremia and overhydration. The reason that the hypernatremia is not more severe is that the sodium retention caused by increased aldosterone secretion also increases the secretion of antidiuretic hormone and causes the kidneys to also reabsorb greater amounts of water.

Thus, in analyzing abnormalities of plasma sodium concentration and deciding on proper therapy, one should first determine whether the abnormality is caused by a primary loss or gain of sodium or a primary loss or gain of water.

CONSEQUENCES OF HYPERNATREMIA: CELL SHRINKAGE

Hypernatremia is much less common than hyponatremia, and severe symptoms usually occur only with rapid and large increases in the plasma sodium concentration above 158–160 mmol/L. One reason for this phenomenon is that hypernatremia promotes intense thirst and stimulates secretion of antidiuretic hormone, which protect against a large increase in both plasma and extracellular fluid sodium, as discussed in Chapter 80. However, severe hypernatremia can occur in patients with hypothalamic lesions that impair their sense of thirst, in infants who may not have ready access to water, in elderly patients with altered mental status, or in persons with diabetes insipidus.

Correction of hypernatremia can be achieved by administering hypoosmotic sodium chloride or dextrose solutions. However, it is prudent to correct the hypernatremia slowly in patients who have had chronic increases in plasma sodium concentration because hypernatremia also activates defense mechanisms that protect the cell from changes in volume. These

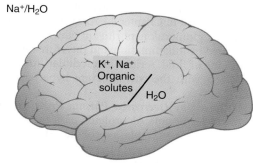

Na⁺/H₂O

K⁺, Na⁺
Organic
solutes

H₂O

Normonatremia

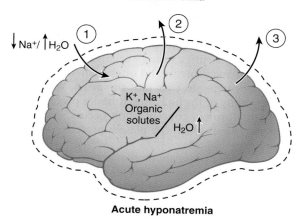

↓Na⁺/↑H₂O

K⁺, Na⁺
Organic
solutes

H₂O ↑

Acute hyponatremia

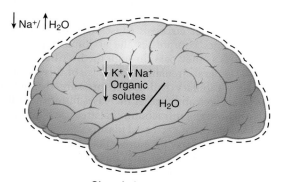

↓Na⁺/↑H₂O

↓K⁺, ↓Na⁺
Organic
↓solutes

H₂O

Chronic hyponatremia

Figure 6-2 Brain cell volume regulation during hyponatremia. During acute hyponatremia, caused by loss of Na⁺ or excess H₂O, there is diffusion of H₂O into the cells (1) and swelling of the brain tissue (indicated by the *dashed lines*). This process stimulates transport of Na⁺, K⁺, and organic solutes out of the cells (2), which then causes water diffusion out of the cells (3). With chronic hyponatremia, the brain swelling is attenuated by the transport of solutes from the cells.

defense mechanisms are opposite to those that occur for hyponatremia and consist of mechanisms that increase the intracellular concentration of sodium and other solutes.

Edema: Excess Fluid in the Tissues

Edema refers to the presence of excess fluid in the body tissues. In most instances, edema occurs mainly in the extracellular fluid compartment, but it can involve intracellular fluid as well.

INTRACELLULAR EDEMA

Three conditions are especially prone to cause intracellular swelling: (1) hyponatremia, as discussed earlier; (2) depression

of the metabolic systems of the tissues; and (3) lack of adequate nutrition to the cells. For example, when blood flow to a tissue is decreased, the delivery of oxygen and nutrients is reduced. If the blood flow becomes too low to maintain normal tissue metabolism, the cell membrane ionic pumps become depressed. When the pumps get depressed, sodium ions that normally leak into the interior of the cell can no longer be pumped out of the cells and the excess intracellular sodium ions cause osmosis of water into the cells. Sometimes this process can increase intracellular volume of a tissue area—even of an entire ischemic leg, for example—to two to three times normal. When such an increase in intracellular volume occurs, it is usually a prelude to death of the tissue.

Intracellular edema can also occur in inflamed tissues. Inflammation usually increases cell membrane permeability, allowing sodium and other ions to diffuse into the interior of the cell, with subsequent osmosis of water into the cells.

EXTRACELLULAR EDEMA

Extracellular fluid edema occurs when excess fluid accumulates in the extracellular spaces. There are two general causes of extracellular edema: (1) abnormal leakage of fluid from the plasma to the interstitial spaces across the capillaries and (2) failure of the lymphatics to return fluid from the interstitium back into the blood, often called *lymphedema*. The most common clinical cause of interstitial fluid accumulation is excessive capillary fluid filtration.

Factors that Can Increase Capillary Filtration

To understand the causes of excessive capillary filtration, it is useful to review the determinants of capillary filtration discussed in Chapter 39. Mathematically, capillary filtration rate can be expressed as follows:

$$\text{Filtration} = K_f \times (P_c - P_{if} - \pi_c + \pi_{if})$$

where K_f is the capillary filtration coefficient (the product of the permeability and surface area of the capillaries), P_c is the capillary hydrostatic pressure, P_{if} is the interstitial fluid hydrostatic pressure, π_c is the capillary plasma colloid osmotic pressure, and π_{if} is the interstitial fluid colloid osmotic pressure. From this equation, one can see *that any one of the following changes can increase the capillary filtration rate*:

- increased capillary filtration coefficient
- increased capillary hydrostatic pressure
- decreased plasma colloid osmotic pressure

SUMMARY OF CAUSES OF EXTRACELLULAR EDEMA

A large number of conditions can cause fluid accumulation in the interstitial spaces by abnormal leaking of fluid from the capillaries or by preventing the lymphatics from returning fluid from the interstitium back to the circulation. The following is a partial list of conditions that can cause extracellular edema by these two types of abnormalities:

I. increased capillary pressure
   A. excessive kidney retention of salt and water
      1. acute or chronic kidney failure
      2. mineralocorticoid excess
   B. high venous pressure and venous constriction
      1. heart failure
      2. venous obstruction

3. failure of venous pumps
    (a) paralysis of muscles
    (b) immobilization of parts of the body
    (c) failure of venous valves
C. decreased arteriolar resistance
    1. excessive body heat
    2. insufficiency of sympathetic nervous system
    3. vasodilator drugs
II. decreased plasma proteins
A. loss of proteins in urine (nephrotic syndrome)
B. loss of protein from denuded skin areas
    1. burns
    2. wounds
C. failure to produce proteins
    1. liver disease (eg, cirrhosis)
    2. serious protein or caloric malnutrition
III. increased capillary permeability
A. immune reactions that cause release of histamine and other immune products
B. toxins
C. bacterial infections
D. vitamin deficiency, especially vitamin C
E. prolonged ischemia
F. burns
IV. blockage of lymph return
A. cancer
B. infections (eg, filarial nematodes)
C. surgery
D. congenital absence or abnormality of lymphatic vessels

Edema Caused by Heart Failure. One of the serious and most common causes of edema is heart failure. In heart failure the heart fails to pump blood normally from the veins into the arteries, which raises venous pressure and capillary pressure, causing increased capillary filtration. In addition, the arterial pressure tends to fall, causing decreased excretion of salt and water by the kidneys, which causes still more edema. Also, blood flow to the kidneys is reduced in persons with heart failure and this reduced blood flow stimulates secretion of renin, causing increased formation of angiotensin II and increased secretion of aldosterone, both of which cause additional salt and water retention by the kidneys. Thus, in persons with untreated heart failure, all these factors acting together cause serious generalized extracellular edema.

In patients with left-sided heart failure, but without significant failure of the right side of the heart, blood is pumped into the lungs normally by the right side of the heart but cannot escape easily from the pulmonary veins to the left side of the heart because this part of the heart has been greatly weakened. Consequently, all the pulmonary vascular pressures, including pulmonary capillary pressure, rise far above normal, causing serious and life-threatening pulmonary edema. When left untreated, fluid accumulation in the lungs can rapidly progress, causing death within a few hours.

Edema Caused by Decreased Kidney Excretion of Salt and Water. Most sodium chloride added to the blood remains in the extracellular compartment, and only small amounts enter the cells. Therefore, in kidney diseases that compromise urinary excretion of salt and water large amounts of sodium chloride and water are added to the extracellular fluid. Most of this salt and water leaks from the blood into the interstitial spaces, but some remains in the blood. The main effects of this are (1) widespread increases in interstitial fluid volume (extracellular

edema) and (2) hypertension because of the increase in blood volume, as explained in Chapter 44. As an example, in children who have acute glomerulonephritis, in which the renal glomeruli are injured by inflammation and therefore fail to filter adequate amounts of fluid, serious extracellular fluid edema also develops; along with the edema severe hypertension usually develops.

Edema Caused by Decreased Plasma Proteins. Failure to produce normal amounts of proteins or leakage of proteins from the plasma causes the plasma colloid osmotic pressure to fall. This leads to increased capillary filtration throughout the body and extracellular edema.

One of the most important causes of decreased plasma protein concentration is loss of proteins in the urine in certain kidney diseases, a condition referred to as *nephrotic syndrome*. Multiple types of renal diseases can damage the membranes of the renal glomeruli, causing the membranes to become leaky to the plasma proteins and often allowing large quantities of these proteins to pass into the urine. When this loss exceeds the ability of the body to synthesize proteins, a reduction in plasma protein concentration occurs. Serious generalized edema occurs when the plasma protein concentration falls below 2.5 g/100 mL.

Cirrhosis of the liver is another condition that causes a reduction in plasma protein concentration. Cirrhosis means development of large amounts of fibrous tissue among the liver parenchymal cells. One result is failure of these cells to produce sufficient plasma proteins, leading to decreased plasma colloid osmotic pressure and the generalized edema that goes with this condition.

Another way liver cirrhosis causes edema is that the liver fibrosis sometimes compresses the abdominal portal venous drainage vessels as they pass through the liver before emptying back into the general circulation. Blockage of this portal venous outflow raises capillary hydrostatic pressure throughout the gastrointestinal area and further increases filtration of fluid out of the plasma into the intraabdominal areas. When this occurs, the combined effects of decreased plasma protein concentration and high portal capillary pressures cause transudation of large amounts of fluid and protein into the abdominal cavity, a condition referred to as *ascites*.

SAFETY FACTORS THAT NORMALLY PREVENT EDEMA

Even though many disturbances can cause edema, usually the abnormality must be severe before serious edema develops. The reason the abnormality must be severe is that three major safety factors prevent excessive fluid accumulation in the interstitial spaces: (1) low compliance of the interstitium when interstitial fluid pressure is in the negative pressure range, (2) the ability of lymph flow to increase 10- to 50-fold, and (3) wash down of interstitial fluid protein concentration, which reduces interstitial fluid colloid osmotic pressure as capillary filtration increases.

Safety Factor Caused by Low Compliance of the Interstitium in the Negative Pressure Range

Interstitial fluid hydrostatic pressure in most loose subcutaneous tissues of the body is slightly less than atmospheric pressure, averaging about −3 mmHg. This slight suction in the tissues helps hold the tissues together. Figure 6-3 shows the approximate relations between different levels of interstitial fluid

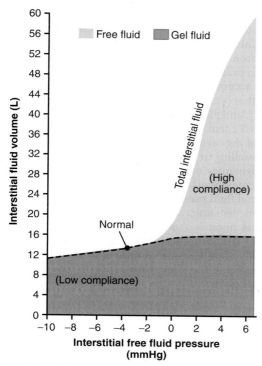

Figure 6-3 Relation between interstitial fluid hydrostatic pressure and interstitial fluid volumes, including total volume, free fluid volume, and gel fluid volume, for loose tissues such as skin. Note that significant amounts of free fluid occur only when the interstitial fluid pressure becomes positive. *Modified from Guyton, A.C., Granger, H.J., Taylor, A.E., 1971. Interstitial fluid pressure. Physiol. Rev. 51, 527.*

pressure and interstitial fluid volume, as extrapolated to the human being from animal studies. Note that in Figure 6-3 as long as the interstitial fluid pressure is in the negative range small changes in interstitial fluid volume are associated with relatively large changes in interstitial fluid hydrostatic pressure. Therefore, in the negative pressure range, the *compliance* of the tissues, defined as the change in volume per millimeter of mercury pressure change, is low.

How does the low compliance of the tissues in the negative pressure range act as a safety factor against edema? To answer this question, recall the determinants of capillary filtration discussed previously. When interstitial fluid hydrostatic pressure increases, this increased pressure tends to oppose further capillary filtration. Therefore, as long as the interstitial fluid hydrostatic pressure is in the negative pressure range, small increases in interstitial fluid volume cause relatively large increases in interstitial fluid hydrostatic pressure, opposing further filtration of fluid into the tissues.

Because the normal interstitial fluid hydrostatic pressure is −3 mmHg, the interstitial fluid hydrostatic pressure must increase by about 3 mmHg before large amounts of fluid will begin to accumulate in the tissues. Therefore, the safety factor against edema is a change of interstitial fluid pressure of about 3 mmHg.

Once interstitial fluid pressure rises above 0 mmHg, the compliance of the tissues increases markedly, allowing large amounts of fluid to accumulate in the tissues with relatively small additional increases in interstitial fluid hydrostatic pressure. Thus, in the positive tissue pressure range, this safety factor against edema is lost because of the large increase in compliance of the tissues.

Increased Lymph Flow as a Safety Factor Against Edema

A major function of the lymphatic system is to return to the circulation the fluid and proteins filtered from the capillaries into the interstitium. Without this continuous return of the filtered proteins and fluid to the blood the plasma volume would be rapidly depleted, and interstitial edema would occur.

The lymphatics act as a safety factor against edema because lymph flow can increase 10- to 50-fold when fluid begins to accumulate in the tissues. This increased lymph flow allows the lymphatics to carry away large amounts of fluid and proteins in response to increased capillary filtration, preventing the interstitial pressure from rising into the positive pressure range. The safety factor caused by increased lymph flow has been calculated to be about 7 mmHg.

"Wash Down" of the Interstitial Fluid Protein as a Safety Factor Against Edema

As increased amounts of fluid are filtered into the interstitium the interstitial fluid pressure increases, causing increased lymph flow. In most tissues the protein concentration of the interstitium decreases as lymph flow is increased, because larger amounts of protein are carried away than can be filtered out of the capillaries; the reason for this phenomenon is that the capillaries are relatively impermeable to proteins, compared with the lymph vessels. Therefore, the proteins are "washed out" of the interstitial fluid as lymph flow increases.

Because the interstitial fluid colloid osmotic pressure caused by the proteins tends to draw fluid out of the capillaries, decreasing the interstitial fluid proteins lowers the net filtration force across the capillaries and tends to prevent further accumulation of fluid. The safety factor from this effect has been calculated to be about 7 mmHg.

SUMMARY OF SAFETY FACTORS THAT PREVENT EDEMA

Putting together all the safety factors against edema, we find the following:
1. The safety factor caused by low tissue compliance in the negative pressure range is about 3 mmHg.
2. The safety factor caused by increased lymph flow is about 7 mmHg.
3. The safety factor caused by wash down of proteins from the interstitial spaces is about 7 mmHg.

Therefore, the total safety factor against edema is about 17 mmHg. This means that the capillary pressure in a peripheral tissue could theoretically rise by 17 mmHg, or approximately double the normal value, before marked edema would occur.

Fluids in the "Potential Spaces" of the Body

Some examples of "potential spaces" are the pleural cavity, pericardial cavity, peritoneal cavity, and synovial cavities, including both the joint cavities and the bursae. Virtually all these potential spaces have surfaces that almost touch each other, with only a thin layer of fluid in between, and the surfaces slide over each other. To facilitate the sliding, a viscous proteinaceous fluid lubricates the surfaces.

Fluid Is Exchanged Between the Capillaries and the Potential Spaces. The surface membrane of a potential space usually does not offer significant resistance to the passage of fluids, electrolytes, or even proteins, which all move back and forth between the space and the interstitial fluid in the surrounding tissue with relative ease. Therefore, each potential space is in reality a large tissue space. Consequently, fluid in the capillaries adjacent to the potential space diffuses not only into the interstitial fluid but also into the potential space.

Lymphatic Vessels Drain Protein from the Potential Spaces. Proteins collect in the potential spaces because of leakage out of the capillaries, similar to the collection of protein in the interstitial spaces throughout the body. The protein must be removed through lymphatics or other channels and returned to the circulation. Each potential space is either directly or indirectly connected with lymph vessels. In some cases, such as the pleural cavity and peritoneal cavity, large lymph vessels arise directly from the cavity itself.

Edema Fluid in the Potential Spaces Is Called "Effusion". When edema occurs in the subcutaneous tissues adjacent to the potential space, edema fluid usually collects in the potential space as well and this fluid is called *effusion*. Thus, lymph blockage or any of the multiple abnormalities that can cause excessive capillary filtration can cause effusion in the same way that interstitial edema is caused. The abdominal cavity is especially prone to collect effusion fluid, and in this instance, the effusion is called *ascites*. In serious cases, 20 L or more of ascitic fluid can accumulate.

The other potential spaces, such as the pleural cavity, pericardial cavity, and joint spaces, can become seriously swollen when generalized edema is present. Also, injury or local infection in any one of the cavities often blocks the lymph drainage, causing isolated swelling in the cavity.

The dynamics of fluid exchange in the pleural cavity are mainly representative of all the other potential spaces as well. The normal fluid pressure in most or all of the potential spaces in the nonedematous state is *negative* in the same way that this pressure is negative (subatmospheric) in loose subcutaneous tissue. For instance, the interstitial fluid hydrostatic pressure is normally about -7 to -8 mmHg in the pleural cavity, -3 to -5 mmHg in the joint spaces, and -5 to -6 mmHg in the pericardial cavity.

BIBLIOGRAPHY

Adrogué HJ, Madias NE: The challenge of hyponatremia, *J. Am. Soc. Nephrol.* 23:1140, 2012.

Aukland K: Why don't our feet swell in the upright position? *News Physiol. Sci.* 9:214, 1994.

Guyton AC, Granger HJ, Taylor AE: Interstitial fluid pressure, *Physiol. Rev.* 51:527, 1971.

Lindner G, Funk GC: Hypernatremia in critically ill patients, *J. Crit. Care* 28:216e11, 2013.

Loh JA, Verbalis JG: Disorders of water and salt metabolism associated with pituitary disease, *Endocrinol. Metab. Clin. North Am.* 37:213, 2008.

Parker JC: Hydraulic conductance of lung endothelial phenotypes and Starling safety factors against edema, *Am. J. Physiol. Lung Cell Mol. Physiol.* 292:L378, 2007.

Reynolds RM, Padfield PL, Seckl JR: Disorders of sodium balance, *Br. Med. J.* 332:702, 2006.

Sam R, Feizi I: Understanding hypernatremia, *Am. J. Nephrol.* 36:97, 2012.

Schrier RW, Sharma S, Shchekochikhin D: Hyponatraemia: more than just a marker of disease severity? *Nat. Rev. Nephrol.* 9:37, 2013.

Sterns RH, Hix JK, Silver SM: Management of hyponatremia in the ICU, *Chest* 144:672, 2013.

Trayes KP, Studdiford JS, Pickle S, Tully AS: Edema: diagnosis and management, *Am. Fam. Physician* 88:102, 2013.

Verbalis JG, Goldsmith SR, Greenberg A, et al: Diagnosis, evaluation, and treatment of hyponatremia: expert panel recommendations, *Am. J. Med.* 126(10 Suppl. 1):S1, 2013.

Resting Membrane Potential

LEARNING OBJECTIVES

- Describe the Nernst potential.
- List the elements of the Goldman equation for multiple ion movements.
- Explain the contribution of different ion movements to the development of the resting membrane potential.

GLOSSARY OF TERMS

- **Gibbs–Donnan equilibrium:** The inequitable distribution of diffusible ions across the cell membrane because of the presence of nondiffusible ions on one side

- **Nernst potential:** When a biological membrane is permeable to a single ion species, the potential developed at which point there is no net movement of the ion across the membrane is referred to as Nernst potential for that ion

- **Resting membrane potential:** The relatively stable membrane potential (inside of the cell membrane) of a cell in a quiescent (unstimulated) state

Electrical potentials exist across the membranes of virtually all cells of the body. Some cells such as nerve and muscle cells generate rapidly changing electrochemical impulses at their membranes, and these impulses are used to transmit signals along the nerve or muscle membranes. In other types of cells, such as glandular cells, macrophages, and ciliated cells, local changes in membrane potentials also activate many of the cells' functions.

Basic Physics of Membrane Potentials

MEMBRANE POTENTIALS CAUSED BY ION CONCENTRATION

Differences Across a Selectively Permeable Membrane. In Figure 7-1A, the potassium concentration is great *inside* a nerve fiber membrane but very low *outside* the membrane. Let us assume that the membrane in this instance is permeable to the potassium ions but not to any other ions. Because of the large potassium concentration gradient from inside toward outside, there is a strong tendency for extra numbers of potassium ions to diffuse outward through the membrane. As they do so, they carry positive electrical charges to the outside, thus creating electropositivity outside the membrane and electronegativity inside because of negative anions that remain behind and do not diffuse outward with the potassium. Within a millisecond

or so, the potential difference between the inside and outside, called the *diffusion potential*, becomes great enough to block further net potassium diffusion to the exterior, despite the high potassium ion concentration gradient. In the normal mammalian nerve fiber, *the potential difference is about 94 mV, with negativity inside the fiber membrane*.

Figure 7-1B shows the same phenomenon as in Figure 7-1A, but this time with a high concentration of sodium ions *outside* the membrane and a low concentration of sodium ions *inside*. These ions are also positively charged. This time, the membrane is highly permeable to the sodium ions but is impermeable to all other ions. Diffusion of the positively charged sodium ions to the inside creates a membrane potential of opposite polarity to that in Figure 7-1A, with negativity outside and positivity inside. Again, the membrane potential rises high enough within milliseconds to block further net diffusion of sodium ions to the inside; however, this time, in the mammalian nerve fiber, *the potential is about +61 mV inside the fiber*.

Thus, in both parts of Figure 7-1, we see that a concentration difference of ions across a selectively permeable membrane can, under appropriate conditions, create a membrane potential.

The Nernst Equation Describes the Relation of Diffusion Potential to the Ion Concentration Difference Across a Membrane. The diffusion potential level across a membrane that exactly opposes the net diffusion of a particular ion through the membrane is called the *Nernst potential* for that ion, a term that was introduced in Chapter 4. The magnitude of the Nernst potential is determined by the *ratio* of the concentrations of that specific ion on the two sides of the membrane. The greater this ratio, the greater is the tendency for the ion to diffuse in one direction, and therefore the greater is the Nernst potential required to prevent additional net diffusion. The following equation, called the *Nernst equation*, can be used to calculate the Nernst potential for any univalent ion at the normal body temperature of 98.6°F (37°C):

$$\text{EMF (millivolts)} = \pm \frac{61}{z} \times \log \frac{\text{concentration inside}}{\text{concentration outside}}$$

where EMF is electromotive force and z is the electrical charge of the ion (eg, +1 for K^+).

When using this formula, it is usually assumed that the potential in the extracellular fluid outside the membrane remains at zero potential, and the Nernst potential is the potential inside the membrane. Also, the sign of the potential is positive (+) if the ion diffusing from inside to outside is a negative ion, and it is negative (−) if the ion is positive. Thus, when the concentration of positive potassium ions on the inside is 10 times that on the outside, the log of 10 is 1, so the Nernst potential calculates to be −61 mV inside the membrane.

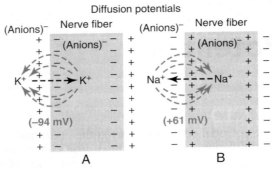

Diffusion potentials

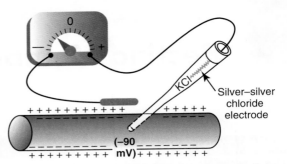

Figure 7-1 (A) Establishment of a "diffusion" potential across a nerve fiber membrane caused by diffusion of potassium ions from inside the cell to outside through a membrane that is selectively permeable only to potassium. (B) Establishment of a "diffusion potential" when the nerve fiber membrane is permeable only to sodium ions. Note that the internal membrane potential is negative when potassium ions diffuse and positive when sodium ions diffuse because of opposite concentration gradients of these two ions.

The Goldman Equation Is Used to Calculate the Diffusion Potential when the Membrane Is Permeable to Several Different Ions

When a membrane is permeable to several different ions, the diffusion potential that develops depends on three factors:

1. the polarity of the electrical charge of each ion,
2. the permeability of the membrane (P) to each ion, and
3. the concentrations (C) of the respective ions on the inside (i) and outside (o) of the membrane.

Thus, the following formula, called the *Goldman equation* or the *Goldman–Hodgkin–Katz equation*, gives the calculated membrane potential on the *inside* of the membrane when two univalent positive ions, sodium (Na^+) and potassium (K^+), and one univalent negative ion, chloride (Cl^-), are involved:

$$\text{EMF (millivolts)} = -61 \times \log \frac{C_{Na_i^+}P_{Na^+} + C_{K_i^+}P_{K^+} + C_{Cl_o^-}P_{Cl^-}}{C_{Na_o^+}P_{Na^+} + C_{K_o^+}P_{K^+} + C_{Cl_i^-}P_{Cl^-}}$$

Several key points become evident from the Goldman equation. First, sodium, potassium, and chloride ions are the most important ions involved in the development of membrane potentials in nerve and muscle fibers, as well as in the neuronal cells in the nervous system. The concentration gradient of each of these ions across the membrane helps determine the voltage of the membrane potential.

Second, the quantitative importance of each of the ions in determining the voltage is proportional to the membrane permeability for that particular ion. That is, if the membrane has zero permeability to potassium and chloride ions, the membrane potential becomes entirely dominated by the concentration gradient of sodium ions alone, and the resulting potential will be equal to the Nernst potential for sodium. The same holds for each of the other two ions if the membrane should become selectively permeable for either one of them alone.

Third, a positive ion concentration gradient from *inside* the membrane to the *outside* causes electronegativity inside the membrane. The reason for this phenomenon is that excess positive ions diffuse to the outside when their concentration is higher inside than outside. This diffusion carries positive charges to the outside but leaves the nondiffusible negative anions on the inside, thus creating electronegativity on the inside. The

opposite effect occurs when there is a gradient for a negative ion. That is, a chloride ion gradient from the *outside to the inside* causes negativity inside the cell because excess negatively charged chloride ions diffuse to the inside, while leaving the nondiffusible positive ions on the outside.

Measuring the Membrane Potential

The method for measuring the membrane potential is simple in theory but often difficult in practice because of the small size of most of the fibers. Figure 7-2 shows a small pipette filled with an electrolyte solution. The pipette is impaled through the cell membrane to the interior of the fiber. Another electrode, called the "indifferent electrode," is then placed in the extracellular fluid, and the potential difference between the inside and outside of the fiber is measured using an appropriate voltmeter. For recording rapid *changes* in the membrane potential during transmission of nerve impulses the microelectrode is connected to an oscilloscope, as explained later in the chapter.

The lower part of Figure 7-2 shows the electrical potential that is measured at each point in or near the nerve fiber membrane, beginning at the left side of the figure and passing to the right. As long as the electrode is outside the nerve membrane the recorded potential is zero, which is the potential of the extracellular fluid. Then, as the recording electrode passes through the voltage change area at the cell membrane (called the *electrical dipole layer*), the potential decreases abruptly to −90 mV. Moving across the center of the fiber, the potential remains at a steady −90-mV level but reverses back to zero the instant it passes through the membrane on the opposite side of the fiber.

To create a negative potential inside the membrane, only enough positive ions to develop the electrical dipole layer at the membrane itself must be transported outward. All the remaining ions inside the nerve fiber can be both positive and negative, as shown in the upper panel of Figure 7-3. Therefore, transfer of an incredibly small number of ions through the membrane can establish the normal "resting potential" of −90 mV inside the nerve fiber, which means that only about 1/3,000,000 to 1/100,000,000 of the total positive charges inside the fiber must be transferred. Also, an equally small number of positive ions moving from outside to inside the fiber can reverse the potential from −90 mV to as much as +35 mV within as little as 1/10,000 of a second. Rapid shifting of ions in this manner causes the nerve signals discussed in subsequent sections of this chapter.

Figure 7-2 Measurement of the membrane potential of the nerve fiber using a microelectrode.

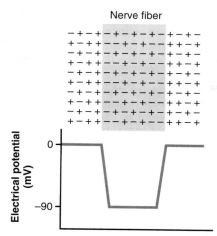

Figure 7-3 Distribution of positively and negatively charged ions in the extracellular fluid surrounding a nerve fiber and in the fluid inside the fiber. Note the alignment of negative charges along the inside surface of the membrane and positive charges along the outside surface. The lower panel displays the abrupt changes in membrane potential that occur at the membranes on the two sides of the fiber.

Resting Membrane Potential of Neurons

The resting membrane potential of large nerve fibers when they are not transmitting nerve signals is about −90 mV. That is, the potential *inside the fiber* is 90 mV more negative than the potential in the extracellular fluid on the outside of the fiber. In the next few paragraphs, the transport properties of the resting nerve membrane for sodium and potassium, and the factors that determine the level of this resting potential are explained.

Active Transport of Sodium and Potassium Ions Through the Membrane—The Sodium–Potassium (Na⁺-K⁺) Pump. All cell membranes of the body have a powerful Na⁺-K⁺ pump that continually transports sodium ions to the outside of the cell and potassium ions to the inside, as illustrated on the left side in Figure 7-4. Note that this is an *electrogenic pump* because more positive charges are pumped to the outside than to the inside (three Na⁺ ions to the outside for each two K⁺ ions to the inside), leaving a net deficit of positive ions on the inside and causing a negative potential inside the cell membrane.

The Na⁺-K⁺ pump also causes large concentration gradients for sodium and potassium across the resting nerve membrane. These gradients are as follows:

$$Na^+ \text{ (outside): } 142 \text{ mEq/L}$$
$$Na^+ \text{ (inside): } 14 \text{ mEq/L}$$
$$K^+ \text{ (outside): } 4 \text{ mEq/L}$$
$$K^+ \text{ (inside): } 140 \text{ mEq/L}$$

The ratios of these two respective ions from the inside to the outside are as follows:

$$\frac{Na^+_{inside}}{Na^+_{outside}} = 0.1$$

$$\frac{K^+_{inside}}{K^+_{outside}} = 35.0$$

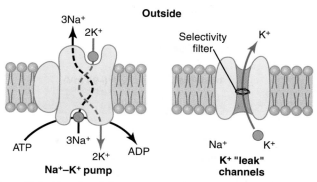

Figure 7-4 Functional characteristics of the Na⁺-K⁺ pump and of the K⁺ "leak" channels. The K⁺ "leak" channels also leak Na⁺ ions into the cell slightly, but are much more permeable to K⁺. *ADP*, adenosine diphosphate; *ATP*, adenosine triphosphate.

Leakage of Potassium Through the Nerve Cell Membrane. The right side of Figure 7-4 shows a channel protein, sometimes called a "*tandem pore domain*," *potassium channel*, or *potassium (K⁺) "leak" channel*, in the nerve membrane through which potassium can leak even in a resting cell. These K⁺ leak channels may also leak sodium ions slightly, but are far more permeable to potassium than to sodium, normally about 100 times as permeable. As discussed later, this differential in permeability is a key factor in determining the level of the normal resting membrane potential.

ORIGIN OF THE NORMAL RESTING MEMBRANE POTENTIAL

Figure 7-5 shows the important factors in the establishment of the normal resting membrane potential of −90 mV. They are as follows.

Contribution of the Potassium Diffusion Potential. In Figure 7-5A, we assume that the only movement of ions through the membrane is diffusion of potassium ions, as demonstrated by the open channels between the potassium symbols (K⁺) inside and outside the membrane. Because of the high ratio of potassium ions inside to outside, 35:1, the Nernst potential corresponding to this ratio is −94 mV because the logarithm of 35 is 1.54, and this multiplied by −61 mV is −94 mV. Therefore, if potassium ions were the only factor causing the resting potential, the resting potential *inside the fiber* would be equal to −94 mV, as shown in the figure.

Contribution of Sodium Diffusion Through the Nerve Membrane. Figure 7-5B shows the addition of slight permeability of the nerve membrane to sodium ions, caused by the minute diffusion of sodium ions through the K⁺-Na⁺ leak channels. The ratio of sodium ions from inside to outside the membrane is 0.1, which gives a calculated Nernst potential for the inside of the membrane of +61 mV. Also shown in Figure 7-5B is the Nernst potential for potassium diffusion of −94 mV. How do these interact with each other, and what will be the summated potential? This question can be answered by using the Goldman equation described previously. Intuitively, one can see that if the membrane is highly permeable to potassium but only slightly permeable to sodium, it is logical that the diffusion of potassium contributes far more to the membrane potential than does the diffusion of sodium. In the normal

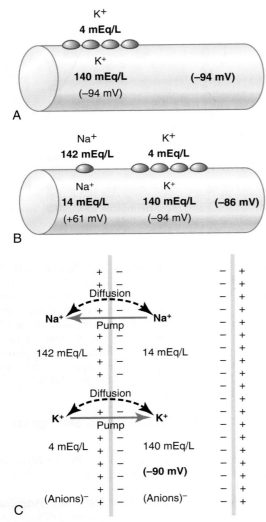

Figure 7-5 Establishment of resting membrane potentials in nerve fibers under three conditions: (A) when the membrane potential is caused entirely by potassium diffusion alone; (B) when the membrane potential is caused by diffusion of both sodium and potassium ions; and (C) when the membrane potential is caused by diffusion of both sodium and potassium ions plus pumping of both these ions by the Na^+–K^+ pump.

nerve fiber the permeability of the membrane to potassium is about 100 times as great as its permeability to sodium. Using this value in the Goldman equation gives a potential inside the membrane of −86 mV, which is near the potassium potential shown in the figure.

Contribution of the Na⁺–K⁺ Pump. In Figure 7-5C, the Na^+–K^+ pump is shown to provide an additional contribution to the resting potential. This figure shows that there is continuous pumping of three sodium ions to the outside for each two potassium ions pumped to the inside of the membrane. The pumping of more sodium ions to the outside than the pumping of potassium ions to the inside causes continual loss of positive charges from inside the membrane, creating an additional degree of negativity (about −4 mV additional) on the inside beyond that, which can be accounted for by diffusion alone. Therefore, as shown in Figure 7-5C, the net membrane potential when all these factors are operative at the same time is about −90 mV.

In summary, the diffusion potentials alone caused by potassium and sodium diffusion would give a membrane potential of about −86 mV, with almost all of this being determined by potassium diffusion. An additional −4 mV is then contributed to the membrane potential by the continuously acting electrogenic Na^+–K^+ pump, giving a net membrane potential of −90 mV.

Impermeant Anions (the Gibbs–Donnan Phenomenon)

Inside the cell are many negatively charged ions that cannot pass through the membrane channels. They include the anions of protein molecules and of many organic phosphate compounds and sulfate compounds. Because these ions cannot leave the interior of the cell, any deficit of positive ions inside the membrane leaves an excess of these impermeant anions. Therefore, these impermeant negative ions contribute to the negative charge inside the cell when there is a net deficit of positively charged potassium ions and other positive ions.

BIBLIOGRAPHY

Alberts B, Johnson A, Lewis J, et al: *Molecular Biology of the Cell*, fifth ed., New York, 2008, Garland Science.

Hodgkin AL, Huxley AF: Quantitative description of membrane current and its application to conduction and excitation in nerve, *J. Physiol. (Lond.)* 117:500, 1952.

Kandel ER, Schwartz JH, Jessell TM: *Principles of Neural Science*, fifth ed., New York, 2012, McGraw-Hill.

Vacher H, Mohapatra DP, Trimmer JS: Localization and targeting of voltage-dependent ion channels in mammalian central neurons, *Physiol. Rev.* 88:1407, 2008.

Nerve and Muscle Physiology

MARIO VAZ

Stimulus and Excitability of Nerve

Characteristics of a Stimulus

All living cells are excitable, that is, they are capable of responding to a change in the environment (stimulus). When they do so, the potential at the cell membrane changes and this electrical response precedes the biological response. The biological response varies from cell to cell based on its function. Some cells, such as nerve and muscle cells, are capable of generating rapidly changing electrochemical impulses at their membranes, and these impulses are used to transmit signals along the nerve or muscle membranes. In other types of cells, such as glandular cells, macrophages, and ciliated cells, local changes in membrane potentials also activate many of the cells' functions.

Stimuli can be extremely variable; they may be physical (as in pressure or temperature), chemical, or electrical. Much of the experimental work on nerve and muscle has involved the use of electrical stimuli since they are more easily and precisely controlled in terms of strength and duration.

Excitation—The Process of Eliciting the Action Potential

The structure of a typical nerve is shown in Figure 8-1. Basically, any factor that causes sodium ions to begin to diffuse inward through the membrane of the nerve in sufficient numbers can set off automatic regenerative opening of the sodium channels, and results in a change of the membrane potential (see Chapter 9). This automatic regenerative opening can result from *mechanical* disturbance of the membrane, *chemical* effects on the membrane, or passage of *electricity* through the membrane. All these approaches are used at different points in the body to elicit nerve or muscle action potentials: mechanical pressure to excite sensory nerve endings in the skin, chemical neurotransmitters to transmit signals from one neuron to the next in the brain, and electrical current to transmit signals between successive muscle cells in the heart and intestine. For the purpose of understanding the excitation process, let us begin by discussing the principles of electrical stimulation.

Excitation of a Nerve Fiber by a Negatively Charged Metal Electrode. The usual means for exciting a nerve or muscle in the experimental laboratory is to apply electricity to the nerve or muscle surface through two small electrodes, one of which is negatively charged and the other positively charged. When electricity is applied in this manner, the excitable membrane becomes stimulated at the negative electrode.

This effect occurs because the action potential is initiated by the opening of voltage-gated sodium channels. This is discussed in detail in Chapter 9. These voltage-gated sodium channels are opened by a decrease in the normal resting electrical voltage across the membrane, that is, negative current from the electrode decreases the voltage on the outside of the membrane to a negative value nearer to the voltage of the negative potential inside the fiber. This effect decreases the electrical voltage across the membrane and allows the sodium channels to open, resulting in an action potential. Conversely, at the positive electrode, the injection of positive charges on the outside of the nerve membrane heightens the voltage difference across the

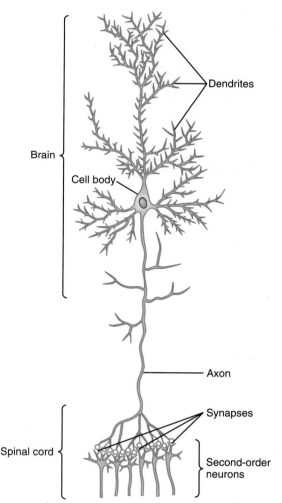

Figure 8-1 Structure of a large neuron in the brain, showing its important functional parts. *Modified from Guyton, A.C., 1987. Basic Neuroscience: Anatomy and Physiology. W.B. Saunders, Philadelphia.*

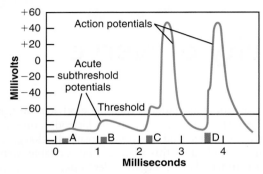

Figure 8-2   Effect of stimuli of increasing voltages to elicit an action potential. Note development of "acute subthreshold potentials" when the stimuli are below the threshold value required for eliciting an action potential.

membrane rather than lessening it. This effect causes a state of hyperpolarization, which actually decreases the excitability of the fiber rather than causing an action potential.

Threshold for Excitation, and "Acute Local Potentials". A weak negative electrical stimulus may not be able to excite a fiber. However, when the voltage of the stimulus is increased, there comes a point at which excitation does take place. Figure 8-2 shows the effects of successively applied stimuli of progressing strength. A weak stimulus at point A causes the membrane potential to change from −90 to −85 mV, but this is not sufficient for the automatic regenerative processes of the action potential to develop. At point B, the stimulus is greater, but the intensity is still not enough. The stimulus does, however, disturb the membrane potential locally for as long as 1 ms or more after both

of these weak stimuli. These local potential changes are called *acute local potentials*, and when they fail to elicit an action potential, they are called *acute subthreshold potentials*.

At point C in Figure 8-2, the stimulus is even stronger. Now the local potential has barely reached the level required to elicit an action potential called the *threshold level*, but this occurs only after a short "latent period." At point D, the stimulus is still stronger, the acute local potential is also stronger, and the action potential occurs after less of a latent period.

Thus, this figure shows that even a weak stimulus causes a local potential change at the membrane, but the intensity of the local potential must rise to a threshold level before the action potential is set off.

INHIBITION OF EXCITABILITY—"STABILIZERS" AND LOCAL ANESTHETICS

In contrast to the factors that increase nerve excitability, still others, called *membrane-stabilizing factors, can decrease excitability*. For instance, *a high extracellular fluid calcium ion concentration* decreases membrane permeability to sodium ions and simultaneously reduces excitability. Therefore, calcium ions are said to be a "stabilizer."

Local Anesthetics. Among the most important stabilizers are the many substances used clinically as local anesthetics, including *procaine* and *tetracaine*. Most of these substances act directly on the activation gates of the sodium channels, making it much more difficult for these gates to open, thereby reducing membrane excitability. When excitability has been reduced so low that the ratio of *action potential strength to excitability threshold* (called the "safety factor") is reduced below 1.0, nerve impulses fail to pass along the anesthetized nerves.

BIBLIOGRAPHY

Alberts B, Johnson A, Lewis J, et al: *Molecular Biology of the Cell*, fifth ed., New York, 2008, Garland Science.
Dai S, Hall DD, Hell JW: Supramolecular assemblies and localized regulation of voltage-gated ion channels, *Physiol. Rev.* 89:411, 2009.

Hodgkin AL, Huxley AF: Quantitative description of membrane current and its application to conduction and excitation in nerve, *J. Physiol. (Lond.)* 117:500, 1952.
Kandel ER, Schwartz JH, Jessell TM: *Principles of Neural Science*, fifth ed., New York, 2012, McGraw-Hill.

Vacher H, Mohapatra DP, Trimmer JS: Localization and targeting of voltage-dependent ion channels in mammalian central neurons, *Physiol. Rev.* 88:1407, 2008.

Action Potential of the Nerve

GLOSSARY OF TERMS

- **Absolute refractory period:** The period during the action potential where the nerve cannot respond to a second stimulus, no matter how strong it is

- **Action potential:** The electrical response of the membrane to a threshold or greater than threshold stimulus

- **Depolarization:** A change in the resting membrane potential toward zero as a result of the influx of positive ions into the cell

- **Hyperpolarization:** A membrane potential that is even more negative than the potential at rest (in an unexcited state)

- **Local response (potential):** The potential that is developed at the cell membrane in response to a subthreshold stimulus

- **Relative refractory period:** The period during the action potential where the nerve can respond to a second stimulus, provided it is greater than threshold strength

- **Repolarization:** The process by which the cell membrane potential is returned to its resting state after excitation

- **Threshold stimulus:** The minimum stimulus that results in the generation of an action potential

Nerve signals are transmitted by *action potentials*, which are rapid changes in the membrane potential that spread rapidly along the nerve fiber membrane. Each action potential begins with a sudden change from the normal resting negative membrane potential to a positive potential and ends with an almost equally rapid change back to the negative potential. The duration of the nerve action potential as indicated in Figure 9-1 is 0.3 ms. To conduct a nerve signal, the action potential moves along the nerve fiber until it comes to the fiber's end.

The upper panel of Figure 9-1 shows the changes that occur at the membrane during the action potential, with the transfer of positive charges to the interior of the fiber at its onset and the return of positive charges to the exterior at its end. The lower panel shows graphically the successive changes in membrane potential over a few ten-thousandths of a second, illustrating the explosive onset of the action potential and the almost equally rapid recovery.

The successive stages of the action potential are as follows.

Resting Stage. The resting stage is the resting membrane potential before the action potential begins. The membrane is said to be "polarized" during this stage because of the −90 mV negative membrane potential that is present.

Depolarization Stage. At this time, the membrane suddenly becomes permeable to sodium ions, allowing tremendous numbers of positively charged sodium ions to diffuse to the interior of the axon. The normal "polarized" state of −90 mV is immediately neutralized by the inflowing positively charged sodium ions, with the potential rising rapidly in the positive direction, a process called *depolarization*. In large nerve fibers, the great excess of positive sodium ions moving to the inside causes the membrane potential to actually "overshoot" beyond the zero level and to become somewhat positive. In some smaller fibers, as well as in many central nervous system neurons, the potential merely approaches the zero level and does not overshoot to the positive state.

Repolarization Stage. Within a few ten-thousandths of a second after the membrane becomes highly permeable to sodium ions, the sodium channels begin to close and the potassium

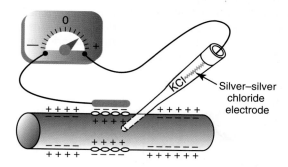

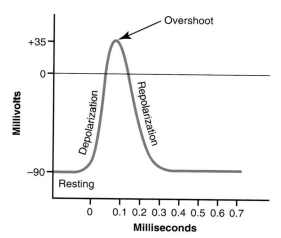

Figure 9-1 Typical action potential recorded by the method shown in the upper panel of the figure.

channels open to a greater degree than normal. Then, rapid diffusion of potassium ions to the exterior reestablishes the normal negative resting membrane potential, which is called *repolarization* of the membrane.

To explain more fully the factors that cause both depolarization and repolarization, we will describe the special characteristics of two other types of transport channels through the nerve membrane: the voltage-gated sodium and potassium channels.

Rectification. The return of the membrane to its original ionic state is achieved through the continued action of the sodium–potassium electrogenic pump.

Voltage-Gated Sodium and Potassium Channels

The necessary factor in causing both depolarization and repolarization of the nerve membrane during the action potential is the *voltage-gated sodium channel*. A *voltage-gated potassium channel* also plays an important role in increasing the rapidity of repolarization of the membrane. *These two voltage-gated channels are in addition to the Na⁺–K⁺ pump and the K⁺ leak channels.*

ACTIVATION AND INACTIVATION OF THE VOLTAGE-GATED SODIUM CHANNEL

The upper panel of Figure 9-2 shows the voltage-gated sodium channel in three separate states. This channel has two *gates*—one near the outside of the channel called the *activation gate* and another near the inside called the *inactivation gate*. The upper left of the figure depicts the state of these two gates in the normal resting membrane when the membrane potential is −90 mV. In this state, the activation gate is closed, which prevents any entry of sodium ions to the interior of the fiber through these sodium channels.

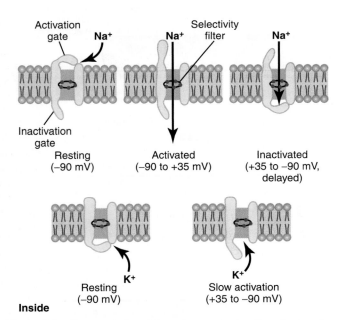

Figure 9-2   Characteristics of the voltage-gated sodium (*top*) and potassium (*bottom*) channels showing successive activation and inactivation of the sodium channels and delayed activation of the potassium channels when the membrane potential is changed from the normal resting negative value to a positive value.

Activation of the Sodium Channel

When the membrane potential becomes less negative than during the resting state, rising from −90 mV toward zero, it finally reaches a voltage—usually somewhere between −70 and −50 mV—that causes a sudden conformational change in the activation gate, flipping it all the way to the open position. During this *activated state* sodium ions can pour inward through the channel, increasing the sodium permeability of the membrane as much as from 500- to 5000-fold.

Inactivation of the Sodium Channel

The upper right panel of Figure 9-2 shows a third state of the sodium channel. The same increase in voltage that opens the activation gate also closes the inactivation gate. The inactivation gate, however, closes a few ten-thousandths of a second after the activation gate opens. That is, the conformational change that flips the inactivation gate to the closed state is a slower process than the conformational change that opens the activation gate. Therefore, after the sodium channel has remained open for a few ten-thousandths of a second, the inactivation gate closes, and sodium ions no longer can pour to the inside of the membrane. At this point, the membrane potential begins to return toward the resting membrane state, which is the repolarization process.

Another important characteristic of the sodium channel inactivation process is that the inactivation gate will not reopen until the membrane potential returns to or near the original resting membrane potential level. Therefore, it is usually not possible for the sodium channels to open again without first repolarizing the nerve fiber.

VOLTAGE-GATED POTASSIUM CHANNEL AND ITS ACTIVATION

The lower panel of Figure 9-2 shows the voltage-gated potassium channel in two states: during the resting state (left) and toward the end of the action potential (right). During the resting state, the gate of the potassium channel is closed and potassium ions are prevented from passing through this channel to the exterior. When the membrane potential rises from −90 mV toward zero, this voltage change causes a conformational opening of the gate and allows increased potassium diffusion outward through the channel. However, because of the slight delay in opening of the potassium channels, for the most part, they open just at the same time that the sodium channels are beginning to close because of inactivation. Thus, the decrease in sodium entry to the cell and the simultaneous increase in potassium exit from the cell combine to speed the repolarization process, leading to full recovery of the resting membrane potential within another few ten-thousandths of a second.

The "Voltage Clamp" Method for Measuring the Effect of Voltage on Opening and Closing of the Voltage-Gated Channels

The original research that led to quantitative understanding of the sodium and potassium channels was so ingenious that it led to Nobel Prizes for the scientists responsible, Hodgkin and Huxley. Figure 9-3 shows the *voltage clamp* method, which is used to measure the flow of ions through the different channels. Two electrodes are inserted into the nerve fiber. One of these electrodes is used to measure the voltage of the membrane potential, and the other is used to conduct electrical current into or out of the nerve fiber. The investigator decides which voltage

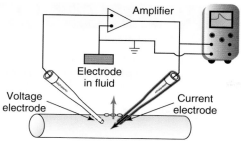

Figure 9-3 "Voltage clamp" method for studying flow of ions through specific channels.

to establish inside the nerve fiber. The electronic portion of the apparatus is then adjusted to the desired voltage, automatically injecting either positive or negative electricity through the current electrode at whatever rate is required to hold the voltage, as measured by the voltage electrode, at the level set by the operator. When the membrane potential is suddenly increased by this voltage clamp from −90 mV to zero, the voltage-gated sodium and potassium channels open and sodium and potassium ions begin to pour through the channels. To counterbalance the effect of these ion movements on the desired setting of the intracellular voltage, electrical current is injected automatically through the current electrode of the voltage clamp to maintain the intracellular voltage at the required steady zero level. To achieve this, the current injected must be equal to but of opposite polarity to the net current flow through the membrane channels. To measure how much current flow is occurring at each instance, the current electrode is connected to an oscilloscope that records the current flow, as demonstrated on the screen of the oscilloscope in Figure 9-3. Finally, the investigator adjusts the concentrations of the ions to other than normal levels both inside and outside the nerve fiber and repeats the study. This experiment can be performed easily when using large nerve fibers removed from some invertebrates, especially the giant squid axon, which in some cases is as large as 1 mm in diameter.

Another means for studying the flow of ions through an individual type of channel is to block one type of channel at a time. For instance, the sodium channels can be blocked by a toxin called *tetrodotoxin* when it is applied to the outside of the cell membrane where the sodium activation gates are located. Conversely, *tetraethylammonium ion* blocks the potassium channels when it is applied to the interior of the nerve fiber.

Summary of the Events that Cause the Action Potential

Figure 9-4 summarizes the sequential events that occur during and shortly after the action potential. The bottom of the figure shows the changes in membrane conductance for sodium and potassium ions. During the resting state, before the action potential begins, the conductance for potassium ions is 50–100 times as great as the conductance for sodium ions. This disparity is caused by much greater leakage of potassium ions than sodium ions through the leak channels. However, at the onset of the action potential, the sodium channels instantaneously become activated and allow up to a 5000-fold increase in sodium conductance. The inactivation process then closes the sodium channels within another fraction of a millisecond. The onset of the action potential also causes voltage gating of the potassium channels, causing them to begin opening more slowly a fraction

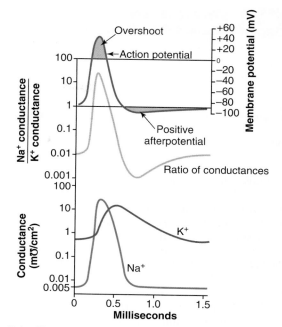

Figure 9-4 Changes in sodium and potassium conductance during the course of the action potential. Sodium conductance increases several thousand-fold during the early stages of the action potential, whereas potassium conductance increases only about 30-fold during the latter stages of the action potential and for a short period thereafter. (These curves were constructed from theory presented in papers by Hodgkin and Huxley but transposed from squid axon to apply to the membrane potentials of large mammalian nerve fibers.)

of a millisecond after the sodium channels open. At the end of the action potential, the return of the membrane potential to the negative state causes the potassium channels to close back to their original status, but again, only after an additional millisecond or more delay.

The middle portion of Figure 9-4 shows the ratio of sodium to potassium conductance at each instance during the action potential, and above this depiction is the action potential itself. During the early portion of the action potential, the ratio of sodium to potassium conductance increases more than 1000-fold. Therefore, far more sodium ions flow to the interior of the fiber than do potassium ions to the exterior. This is what causes the membrane potential to become positive at the onset of action potential. Then the sodium channels begin to close and the potassium channels begin to open, and thus the ratio of conductance shifts far in favor of high potassium conductance but low sodium conductance. This allows very rapid loss of potassium ions to the exterior but virtually zero flow of sodium ions to the interior. Consequently, the action potential quickly returns to its baseline level.

Roles of Other Ions During the Action Potential

Thus far, we have considered only the roles of sodium and potassium ions in the generation of the action potential. At least two other types of ions must be considered: negative anions and calcium ions.

Impermeant Negatively Charged Ions (Anions) Inside the Nerve Axon. Inside the axon are many negatively charged ions that cannot go through the membrane channels. They include the anions of protein molecules and of many organic phosphate

TABLE 9-1	Differences Between a Local Potential and an Action Potential	
	Local Potential	**Action Potential**
Nature of stimulus	Subthreshold	Threshold or suprathreshold
Type of potential change	Graded: depending on the strength of stimulus	Fixed amplitude (all-or-nothing principle)
	May be positive (depolarization, excitatory) or negative (hyperpolarization, inhibitory)	Always positive (depolarization)
Propagation	Conducted over short distances with a reduction in magnitude of potential	Conducted over the entire cell membrane
Summation	Can be summated	Cannot be summated

compounds, sulfate compounds, and so forth. Because these ions cannot leave the interior of the axon, any deficit of positive ions inside the membrane leaves an excess of these impermeant negative anions. Therefore, these impermeant negative ions are responsible for the negative charge inside the fiber when there is a net deficit of positively charged potassium ions and other positive ions.

Increased Permeability of the Sodium Channels when There Is a Deficit of Calcium Ions. The concentration of calcium ions in the extracellular fluid also has a profound effect on the voltage level at which the sodium channels become activated. When there is a deficit of calcium ions, the sodium channels become activated (opened) by a small increase of the membrane potential from its normal, very negative level. Therefore, the nerve fiber becomes highly excitable, sometimes discharging repetitively without provocation rather than remaining in the resting state. In fact, the calcium ion concentration needs to fall only 50% below normal before spontaneous discharge occurs in some peripheral nerves, often causing *muscle "tetany."* Muscle tetany is sometimes lethal because of tetanic contraction of the respiratory muscles.

The probable way in which calcium ions affect the sodium channels is as follows: These ions appear to bind to the exterior surfaces of the sodium channel protein molecule. The positive charges of these calcium ions in turn alter the electrical state of the sodium channel protein, thus altering the voltage level required to open the sodium gate.

INITIATION OF THE ACTION POTENTIAL

Up to this point, we have explained the changing sodium and potassium permeability of the membrane, as well as the development of the action potential itself, but we have not explained what initiates the action potential.

A Positive-Feedback Cycle Opens the Sodium Channels. First, as long as the membrane of the nerve fiber remains undisturbed, no action potential occurs in the normal nerve. However, if any event causes enough initial rise in the membrane potential from -90 mV toward the zero level, the rising voltage will cause many voltage-gated sodium channels to begin

opening. This occurrence allows rapid inflow of sodium ions, which causes a further rise in the membrane potential, thus opening still more voltage-gated sodium channels and allowing more streaming of sodium ions to the interior of the fiber. This process is a positive-feedback cycle that, once the feedback is strong enough, continues until all the voltage-gated sodium channels have become activated (opened). Then, within another fraction of a millisecond, the rising membrane potential causes closure of the sodium channels and opening of potassium channels and the action potential soon terminates.

Threshold for Initiation of the Action Potential. An action potential will not occur until the initial rise in membrane potential is great enough to create the positive feedback described in the preceding paragraph. This occurs when the number of Na^+ ions entering the fiber becomes greater than the number of K^+ ions leaving the fiber. A sudden rise in membrane potential of 15–30 mV is usually required. Therefore, a sudden increase in the membrane potential in a large nerve fiber from -90 mV up to about -65 mV usually causes the explosive development of an action potential. This level of -65 mV is said to be the *threshold* for stimulation.

Local Potentials

Not all stimuli result in an action potential. Small stimuli may result in local changes in the cell membrane potential that are below the threshold for the initiation of an action potential. These small changes in the cell membrane potential are called local responses and can be differentiated from action potentials as outlined in Table 9-1.

Refractory Period

The nerve cannot respond to a second stimulus during much of the action potential and even longer. This is referred to as the refractory period of the nerve. In fact, the refractory period is further divided into an absolute refractory period and a relative refractory period. The difference between these two is highlighted in Table 9-2.

TABLE 9-2	Difference Between Absolute Refractory Period and Relative Refractory Period	
	Absolute Refractory Period	**Relative Refractory Period**
Definition	The period during the action potential where the nerve cannot respond to a second stimulus, no matter how strong it is	The period during the action potential where the nerve can respond to a second stimulus, provided it is greater than threshold strength
Duration	Whole of depolarization and about one-third of repolarization	Remainder of repolarization and hyperpolarization phase
Mechanism	A large number of the Na^+ channels are inactivated and cannot open until the membrane returns to the resting state	In the initial part of the relative refractory period some Na^+ channels are still inactivated
		Throughout the relative refractory period, K^+ conductance is high, which opposes depolarization

BIBLIOGRAPHY

Alberts B, Johnson A, Lewis J, et al: Molecular Biology of the Cell, fifth ed., New York, 2008, Garland Science.

Biel M, Wahl-Schott C, Michalakis S, Zong X: Hyperpolarization-activated cation channels: from genes to function, *Physiol. Rev.* 89:847, 2009.

Blaesse P, Airaksinen MS, Rivera C, Kaila K: Cation-chloride cotransporters and neuronal function, *Neuron* 61:820, 2009.

Dai S, Hall DD, Hell JW: Supramolecular assemblies and localized regulation of voltage-gated ion channels, *Physiol. Rev.* 89:411, 2009.

Hodgkin AL, Huxley AF: Quantitative description of membrane current and its application to conduction and excitation in nerve, *J. Physiol. (Lond.)* 117:500, 1952.

Kandel ER, Schwartz JH, Jessell TM: *Principles of Neural Science*, fifth ed., New York, 2012, McGraw-Hill.

Vacher H, Mohapatra DP, Trimmer JS: Localization and targeting of voltage-dependent ion channels in mammalian central neurons, *Physiol. Rev.* 88:1407, 2008.

10 Propagation of the Nerve Impulse

LEARNING OBJECTIVES

- Describe the ionic basis for the propagation of a nerve impulse.
- State the all-or-nothing principle in relation to propagation of a nerve impulse.
- Describe how nerves are classified.
- Describe the ionic basis of saltatory conduction in myelinated fibers.

GLOSSARY OF TERMS

- **All-or-nothing principle:** Stating that once an action potential is elicited on a nerve fiber, it travels the entire length of the fiber
- **Antidromic conduction:** Conduction of a nerve impulse in a direction opposite to its normal direction, for example, toward a receptor for a sensory nerve
- **Nerve impulse:** Transmission of an action potential along a nerve
- **Orthodromic conduction:** Conduction of a nerve impulse in the normal direction, for example, from a receptor for a sensory nerve
- **Saltatory conduction:** The "jumping" of the nerve impulse from one node of Ranvier to another in a myelinated nerve fiber

In the preceding chapter, we discussed the action potential as it occurs at one spot on the membrane. However, an action potential elicited at any one point on an excitable membrane usually excites adjacent portions of the membrane, resulting in propagation of the action potential along the membrane. This mechanism is demonstrated in Figure 10-1. Figure 10-1A shows a normal resting nerve fiber, and Figure 10-1B shows a nerve fiber that has been excited in its midportion—that is, the midportion suddenly develops increased permeability to sodium. The arrows show a "local circuit" of current flow from the depolarized areas of the membrane to the adjacent resting membrane areas. That is, positive electrical charges are carried by the inward-diffusing sodium ions through the depolarized membrane and then for several millimeters in both directions along the core of the axon. These positive charges increase the voltage for a distance of 1–3 mm inside the large myelinated fiber to above the threshold voltage value for initiating an action potential. Therefore, the sodium channels in these new areas immediately open, as shown in Figure 10-1C and D, and the explosive action potential spreads. These newly depolarized areas produce still more local circuits of current flow farther along the membrane causing progressively more and more depolarization. Thus, the depolarization process travels along the entire length of the fiber. This transmission of the depolarization process along a nerve or muscle fiber is called a *nerve* or *muscle impulse.*

DIRECTION OF PROPAGATION

As demonstrated in Figure 10-1, an excitable membrane has no single direction of propagation but the action potential travels in all directions away from the stimulus—even along all branches of a nerve fiber—until the entire membrane has become depolarized. Thus when a nerve impulse is propagated in the normal direction, it is referred to as *orthodromic* conduction, while if the impulse is conducted in the opposite direction, it is referred to as *antidromic* conduction.

ALL-OR-NOTHING PRINCIPLE

Once an action potential has been elicited at any point on the membrane of a normal fiber, the depolarization process travels over the entire membrane if conditions are right but it does not travel at all if conditions are not right. This principle is called the *all-or-nothing principle*, and it applies to all normal excitable tissues. Occasionally, the action potential reaches a point on the membrane at which it does not generate sufficient voltage to stimulate the next area of the membrane. When this situation occurs, the spread of depolarization stops. Therefore, for continued propagation of an impulse to occur, the ratio of action potential to threshold for excitation must be at all times greater than 1. This "greater than 1" requirement is called the *safety factor* for propagation.

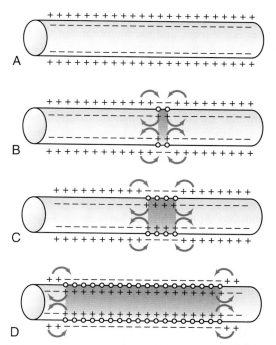

Figure 10-1 Propagation of action potentials in both directions along a conductive fiber. (A) Normal resting nerve fibre; (B) excitation of the nerve fibre in its mid portion; (C and D) spread of the action potential from its initial point of excitation.

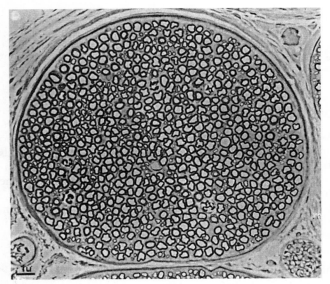

Figure 10-2 Cross-section of a small nerve trunk containing both myelinated and unmyelinated fibers.

Special Characteristics of Signal Transmission in Nerve Trunks

MYELINATED AND UNMYELINATED NERVE FIBERS

Figure 10-2 shows a cross-section of a typical small nerve revealing many large nerve fibers that constitute most of the cross-sectional area. However, a more careful look reveals many more small fibers lying between the large ones. The large fibers are *myelinated* and the small ones are *unmyelinated*. The average nerve trunk contains about twice as many unmyelinated fibers as myelinated fibers.

Figure 10-3 shows a typical myelinated fiber. The central core of the fiber is the *axon*, and the membrane of the axon is the membrane that actually conducts the action potential. The axon is filled in its center with *axoplasm*, which is a viscid intracellular fluid. Surrounding the axon is a *myelin sheath* that is often much thicker than the axon itself. About once every 1–3 mm along the length of the myelin sheath is a *node of Ranvier*.

The myelin sheath is deposited around the axon by Schwann cells in the following manner: The membrane of a Schwann cell first envelops the axon. The Schwann cell then rotates around the axon many times, laying down multiple layers of Schwann cell membrane containing the lipid substance *sphingomyelin*. This substance is an excellent electrical insulator that decreases ion flow through the membrane about 5000-fold. At the juncture between each two successive Schwann cells along the axon, a small uninsulated area only 2–3 μm in length remains where ions still can flow with ease through the axon membrane between the extracellular fluid and the intracellular fluid inside the axon. This area is called the *node of Ranvier*.

"SALTATORY" CONDUCTION IN MYELINATED FIBERS FROM NODE TO NODE

Even though almost no ions can flow through the thick myelin sheaths of myelinated nerves, they can flow with ease through the nodes of Ranvier. Therefore, action potentials occur *only at*

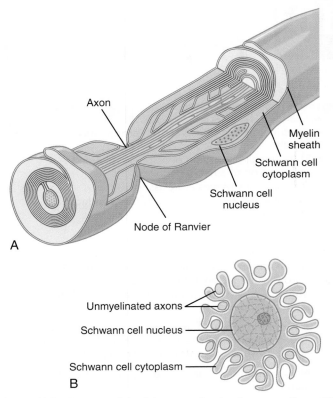

Figure 10-3 Function of the Schwann cell to insulate nerve fibers. (A) Wrapping of a Schwann cell membrane around a large axon to form the myelin sheath of the myelinated nerve fiber. (B) Partial wrapping of the membrane and cytoplasm of a Schwann cell around multiple unmyelinated nerve fibers (shown in cross-section). *(A) Modified from Leeson, T.S., Leeson, R., 1979. Histology. W.B. Saunders, Philadelphia.*

the nodes. Yet the action potentials are conducted from node to node, as shown in Figure 10-4; this is called *saltatory conduction.* That is, electrical current flows through the surrounding extracellular fluid outside the myelin sheath, as well as through the axoplasm inside the axon from node to node, exciting successive nodes one after another. Thus, the nerve impulse jumps along the fiber, which is the origin of the term "saltatory."

Saltatory conduction is of value for two reasons. First, by causing the depolarization process to jump long intervals along the axis of the nerve fiber, this mechanism increases the velocity of nerve transmission in myelinated fibers as much as 5- to 50-fold. Second, saltatory conduction conserves energy for the axon because only the nodes depolarize, allowing perhaps

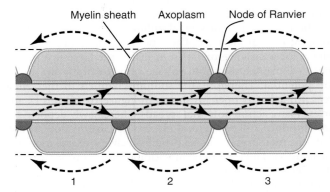

Figure 10-4 Saltatory conduction along a myelinated axon. Flow of electrical current from node to node is illustrated by the arrows 1–3.

| | Fiber Diameter | | Conduction Velocity | |
| TABLE 10-1 **Erlanger-Gasser Classification of Nerves Based on Their Diameter and Myelination, and the Conduction Velocity** | | | | |
Fiber Type	Fiber Diameter (μm)	Myelination	Conduction Velocity (m/second)	Type of Fiber/Receptor Supplied
Aα	16	Yes	100	Golgi tendon organ, muscle spindles, extrafusal muscle fibers
Aβ	8	Yes	50	Muscle spindles, skin mechanoreceptors
Aγ	5	Yes	25	Intrafusal muscle fibers
Aδ	4	Yes, but thin	15	Skin receptors
B	3	Yes	8	Preganglionic autonomic fibers
C	1	No	1	Postganglionic autonomic, skin receptors

A, B, and C fibers differ in their susceptibility to drugs and injury. For instance.

100 times less loss of ions than would otherwise be necessary, and therefore requiring little energy expenditure for reestablishing the sodium and potassium concentration differences across the membrane after a series of nerve impulses.

The excellent insulation afforded by the myelin membrane and the 50-fold decrease in membrane capacitance also allow repolarization to occur with little transfer of ions.

Erlanger and Gasser won the Nobel Prize in 1944 for their study of the characteristics of peripheral nerves and of conduction velocity. They classified nerves based on their diameter and myelination and the conduction velocity and a modification of this is depicted in Table 10-1. Thus the velocity of action potential conduction in nerve fibers varies from as little as 0.25 m/second in small unmyelinated fibers to as great as 100 m/second (more than the length of a football field in 1 second) in large myelinated fibers.

BIBLIOGRAPHY

Hodgkin AL, Huxley AF: Quantitative description of membrane current and its application to conduction and excitation in nerve, *J. Physiol. (Lond.)* 117:500, 1952.

Kandel ER, Schwartz JH, Jessell TM: *Principles of Neural Science*, fifth ed., New York, 2012, McGraw-Hill.

Poliak S, Peles E: The local differentiation of myelinated axons at nodes of Ranvier, *Nat. Rev. Neurosci.* 12:968, 2003.

11 Peripheral Nerve Damage

LEARNING OBJECTIVES

- Classify nerve injuries based on the degree of injury.
- Describe the process of Wallerian degeneration.
- Describe the use of strength–duration curves to assess nerve injury.
- Describe the process of nerve regeneration in peripheral nerves.

GLOSSARY OF TERMS

- **Chronaxie:** The duration that a stimulus twice the strength of rheobase needs to be applied in order to elicit a response

- **Denervation hypersensitivity (supersensitivity):** A heightened response of the target organ/tissue following denervation (nerve damage) due, in part, to an upregulation of receptors on the postsynaptic membrane

- **Rheobase:** The minimum strength of stimulus that can elicit a biological response in the strength–duration curve

- **Utilization time:** The duration for which a stimulus of rheobase strength needs to be applied in order to elicit a biological response

Peripheral nerves may be damaged due to a variety of reasons. The following list provides only a few of the many causes of peripheral nerve damage (peripheral neuropathy):

- nerve injury due to trauma
- systemic diseases such as diabetes
- nutritional deficiencies such as vitamin B_{12} deficiency
- infections such as leprosy or HIV–AIDS
- disruptions to the blood supply of nerves as occurs with vasculitis and arteriosclerosis
- side effects of drugs, for instance, some anticancer drugs

Nerve Injury

Peripheral nerves can be injured in different ways and this determines the severity of the nerve injury and the chances of recovery.

The least severe form of injury is called a *neurapraxia*. This is typically seen when the nerve is compressed or when the blood supply to the nerve is temporarily disrupted. The loss of function related to this type of injury is usually temporary and recovery can be rapid in the least severe forms, occurring within a few hours, although some forms of neurapraxia may need several months to recover.

In a more severe form of nerve injury, the axon itself is disrupted and this is called *axonotmesis*. It is in this form of nerve injury that Wallerian degeneration that is described later takes place.

The most severe form of nerve injury is *neurotmesis*. In this form of nerve injury, not only the axon but also the surrounding and encapsulating connective tissue is affected. This type of injury has the least chance of recovery.

Wallerian Degeneration

Over 150 years ago in 1850, Augustus Waller first described the changes that occurred when axons were physically separated (axotomy) from their cell bodies. This was further described in greater detail by the Nobel laureate, Cajal, and others.

The degenerative changes that occur in the distal segment (beyond the injury), which are highlighted in Figure 11-1, include the following:

- the formation of ovoids as Schwann cells begin to fragment the myelin sheaths and scavenge the myelin debris;
- a change in the Schwann cell properties, from myelinating to demyelinating;
- infiltration of leukocytes into the distal segments.

The degenerative changes in the nerve are mediated by calcium influx and the activation of axonal proteases.

In the proximal segment including the nerve cell body, the following changes are seen:

- The first node of Ranvier degenerates.
- *Chromatolysis* in the cell body, which includes the breakup of the rough endoplasmic reticulum and movement of the nucleus from the center of the cell body. The changes in the rough endoplasmic reticulum are part of the alterations in mRNA synthesis and gene expression that support neuronal recovery.

Nerve degeneration is associated with reduced/absent neurotransmitter release and an upregulation (increased number or affinity) of receptors on the postsynaptic membrane. Nerve regeneration or the exogenous administration of neurotransmitter agonists is associated with a heightened response because of the upregulation of the receptors, among other factors. This is called *denervation hypersensitivity*.

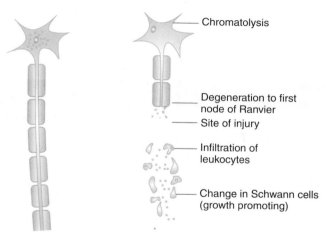

Figure 11-1 Wallerian degeneration.

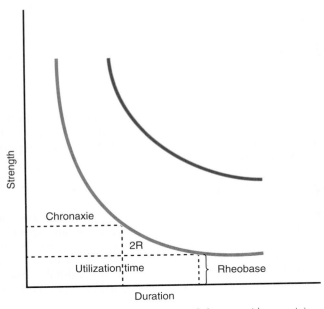

Figure 11-2   Strength–duration curve and changes with nerve injury.

Functional Assessment of Nerve Damage Using the Strength–Duration Curve

There are many ways that the functional status of nerves can be assessed. Motor nerves can be assessed clinically by evaluating the muscle strength of muscles they supply. Sensory nerves can be assessed by testing for sensation in the area of the specific nerve supply and there are a range of tests that assess autonomic nerve function. Nerve conduction studies can also be done that assess the speed of nerve conduction in motor and sensory nerves.

One of the tests that can be performed relies on varying the strength and duration of a stimulus applied to a nerve and evaluating the biological response. For instance, a small stimulating electrode can be placed over the point where a motor nerve enters a muscle. This point is called a "motor point" and there are readily available charts of motor points in the body that will guide the placement of such an electrode. Having placed this electrode, the strength (voltage) and duration (milliseconds) of the stimulus can be regulated until a biological response is achieved, in this case a muscle contraction. In this way a strength–duration curve can be elicited and this is depicted in Figure 11-2.

There are several parameters that can describe the red curve shown in Figure 11-2:
1. *Rheobase*: It is the minimum strength of stimulus that can elicit a biological response.
2. *Utilization time*: It is the duration for which a stimulus of rheobase strength needs to be applied in order to elicit a biological response.
3. *Chronaxie*: It is the duration that a stimulus twice the strength of rheobase needs to be applied in order to elicit a response.

In Figure 11-2, there is also a blue curve. This curve shows that rheobase is increased and utilization time and chronaxie are also prolonged compared to the red curve. This curve, which indicates reduced excitability in the nerve, represents a damaged nerve. The recovery of the nerve can be plotted using the strength–duration curve and recovery is associated with a gradual shift in the curve toward its normal state (the red line).

Nerve Regeneration

Although the process of "dedifferentiation" of the Schwann cells from a myelinating state to a demyelinating state and the infiltration of leukocytes into the distal segment might appear to aggravate the nerve injury, these processes are, in fact, critical to the recovery of nerves.

The recovery of nerves is mediated through several processes:
- The injury results in the activation and retrograde transport of injury-related signal molecules to the cell soma.
- These molecules help the nerve cell to express regeneration-associated genes (RAGs), the function of which are to support nerve growth and elongation as well as axonal guidance.
- Several neurotrophic factors including nerve growth factor (NGF) are upregulated in the dedifferentiated Schwann cells, which in fact are growth promoting.
- Macrophages and Schwann cells also release transforming growth factor-β (TGF-β).

Nerve regeneration is characterized by the development and prolongation of a growth cone from the proximal nerve stump and its extension along the surface of the Schwann cell column in the distal segment.

Injured nerves regenerate their axons in the peripheral nervous system but not in the central nervous system. Table 11-1 highlights some of the differences in the peripheral and central nervous systems that can be understood in the light of the processes involved in nerve degeneration and regeneration, which have been described earlier.

TABLE 11-1	Differences in Nerve Degeneration and Regeneration in the Peripheral and Central Nervous Systems	
	Peripheral Nervous System	**Central Nervous System**
Rate of removal of myelin debris	Relatively fast	Slow
Cytokine release	Relatively fast and in high concentrations	Slow and poor response
Regeneration-associated gene (RAG) expression	Relatively high	Low
Response of nonneuronal cells	Dedifferentiation of Schwann cells into "growth supporting" mode	No change in oligodendrocytes

BIBLIOGRAPHY

Abe N, Cavalli V: Nerve injury signaling, *Curr. Opin. Neurobiol.* 18(3):276-283, 2008.

Fenrich K, Gordon T: Axonal regeneration in the peripheral and central nervous systems—current issues and advances, *Can. J. Neurol. Sci.* 31:142-156, 2004.

Huebner EA, Strittmatter SM: Axon regeneration in the peripheral and central nervous systems, *Results Probl. Cell Differ.* 48:339-351, 2009.

Neuromuscular Transmission

LEARNING OBJECTIVES

- Draw and label a typical neuromuscular junction.
- Describe the sequence of events occurring at the neuromuscular junction.
- Classify drugs acting at the neuromuscular junction and describe their mechanisms of action.
- Describe the basis and features of myasthenia gravis.

GLOSSARY OF TERMS

- **End plate potential:** A local, positive potential on the postsynaptic membrane resulting from the entry of sodium via the acetylcholine receptor channels

- **Motor end plate (also called neuromuscular junction or myoneural junction):** The entire complex of the terminal axon and the muscle membrane that is in synaptic contact (some authors refer to this as the postsynaptic membrane alone)

Skeletal muscle fibers are innervated by large myelinated nerve fibers that originate from large motoneurons in the anterior horns of the spinal cord. Each nerve fiber, after entering the muscle belly, normally branches and stimulates three to several hundred skeletal muscle fibers. Each nerve ending makes a junction, called the *neuromuscular junction*, with the muscle fiber near its midpoint. The action potential initiated in the muscle fiber by the nerve impulse travels in both directions toward the muscle fiber ends. With the exception of about 2% of the muscle fibers, there is only one such junction per muscle fiber.

Physiological Anatomy of the Neuromuscular Junction— The Motor End Plate. Figure 12-1A and B shows the neuromuscular junction from a large myelinated nerve fiber to a skeletal muscle fiber. The nerve fiber forms a complex of *branching nerve terminals* that invaginate into the surface of the muscle fiber but lie outside the muscle fiber plasma membrane. The entire structure is called the *motor end plate*. It is covered by one or more Schwann cells that insulate it from the surrounding fluids.

Figure 12-1C shows the junction between a single axon terminal and the muscle fiber membrane. The invaginated membrane is called the *synaptic gutter* or *synaptic trough*, and the

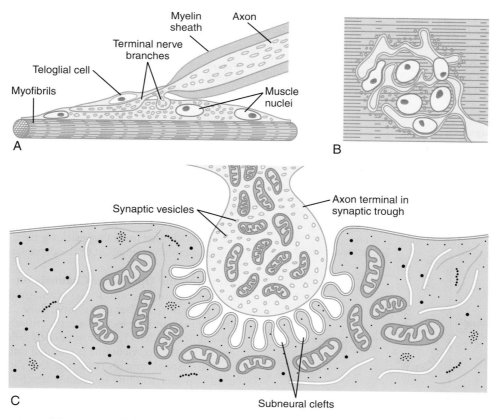

Figure 12-1 Different views of the motor end plate. (A) Longitudinal section through the end plate; (B) surface view of the end plate; (C) electron micrographic appearance of the contact point between a single axon terminal and the muscle fiber membrane. *Modified from Fawcett, D.W., as modified from Couteaux, R., in Bloom, W., Fawcett, D.W., 1986. A Textbook of Histology. W.B. Saunders, Philadelphia.*

space between the terminal and the fiber membrane is called the *synaptic space* or *synaptic cleft*. This space is 20–30 nm wide. At the bottom of the gutter are numerous smaller *folds* of the muscle membrane called *subneural clefts*, which greatly increase the surface area at which the synaptic transmitter can act.

In the axon terminal are many mitochondria that supply adenosine triphosphate (ATP), the energy source that is used for synthesis of an excitatory transmitter, *acetylcholine*. The acetylcholine in turn excites the muscle fiber membrane. Acetylcholine is synthesized in the cytoplasm of the terminal, but it is absorbed rapidly into many small *synaptic vesicles*, about 300,000 of which are normally in the terminals of a single end plate. In the synaptic space are large quantities of the enzyme *acetylcholinesterase*, which destroys acetylcholine a few milliseconds after it has been released from the synaptic vesicles.

Secretion of Acetylcholine by the Nerve Terminals

When a nerve impulse reaches the neuromuscular junction, about 125 vesicles of acetylcholine are released from the terminals into the synaptic space. Some of the details of this mechanism can be seen in Figure 12-2, which shows an expanded view of a synaptic space with the neural membrane above and the muscle membrane and its subneural clefts below.

On the inside surface of the neural membrane are linear *dense bars*, shown in cross-section in Figure 12-2. To each side of each dense bar are protein particles that penetrate the neural membrane; these are *voltage-gated calcium channels*. When an action potential spreads over the terminal, these channels open and allow calcium ions to diffuse from the synaptic space to the interior of the nerve terminal. The calcium ions are believed to activate Ca^{++}–*calmodulin-dependent protein kinase*, which, in turn, phosphorylates *synapsin* proteins that anchor on the acetylcholine vesicles to the cytoskeleton of the presynaptic terminal. This process frees the acetylcholine vesicles from the cytoskeleton and allows them to move to the *active zone* of the presynaptic neural

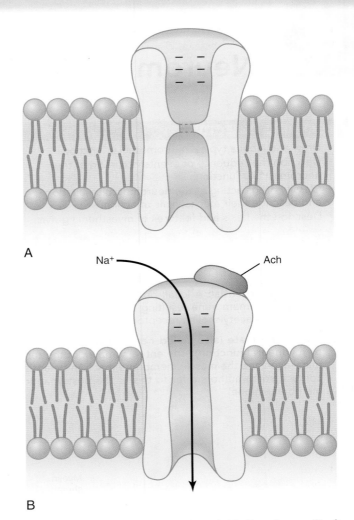

A

B

Figure 12-3   Acetylcholine-gated channel. (A) Closed state; (B) after acetylcholine (*Ach*) has become attached and a conformational change has opened the channel, allowing sodium ions to enter the muscle fiber and excite contraction. Note the negative charges at the channel mouth that prevent passage of negative ions such as chloride ions.

membrane adjacent to the dense bars. The vesicles then dock at the release sites, fuse with the neural membrane, and empty their acetylcholine into the synaptic space by the process of *exocytosis*.

Although some of the aforementioned details are speculative, it is known that the effective stimulus for causing acetylcholine release from the vesicles is entry of calcium ions and that acetylcholine from the vesicles is then emptied through the neural membrane adjacent to the dense bars.

Acetylcholine Opens Ion Channels on Postsynaptic Membranes. Figure 12-2 also shows many small *acetylcholine receptors* in the muscle fiber membrane; these are *acetylcholine-gated ion channels* and are located almost entirely near the mouths of the subneural clefts lying immediately below the dense bar areas, where the acetylcholine is emptied into the synaptic space.

The channel remains constricted, as shown in Figure 12-3A, until two acetylcholine molecules attach to the receptors. This attachment causes a conformational change that opens the channel, as shown in Figure 12-3B.

The acetylcholine-gated channel has a diameter of about 0.65 nm, which is large enough to allow the important positive ions—sodium (Na^+), potassium (K^+), and calcium (Ca^{++})—to

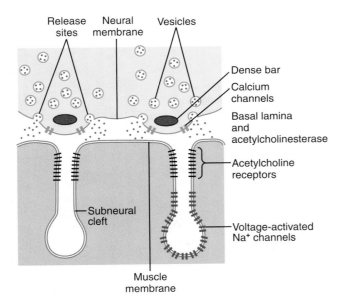

Figure 12-2   Release of acetylcholine from synaptic vesicles at the neural membrane of the neuromuscular junction. Note the proximity of the release sites in the neural membrane to the acetylcholine receptors in the muscle membrane at the mouths of the subneural clefts.

move easily through the opening. Patch-clamp studies have shown that one of these channels, when opened by acetylcholine, can transmit 15,000–30,000 sodium ions in 1 millisecond. Conversely, negative ions, such as chloride ions, do not pass through because of strong negative charges in the mouth of the channel that repel these negative ions.

In practice, far more sodium ions flow through the acetylcholine-gated channels than any other ions for two reasons. First, there are only two positive ions in large concentration: sodium ions in the extracellular fluid and potassium ions in the intracellular fluid. Second, the negative potential on the inside of the muscle membrane, −80 to −90 mV, pulls the positively charged sodium ions to the inside of the fiber, while simultaneously preventing efflux of the positively charged potassium ions when they attempt to pass outward.

As shown in Figure 12-3B, the principal effect of opening the acetylcholine-gated channels is to allow large numbers of sodium ions to pour to the inside of the fiber, carrying with them large numbers of positive charges. This action creates a local positive potential change inside the muscle fiber membrane, called the *end plate potential*. In turn, this end plate potential initiates an action potential that spreads along the muscle membrane and thus causes muscle contraction.

Destruction of the Released Acetylcholine by Acetylcholinesterase. The acetylcholine, once released into the synaptic space, continues to activate the acetylcholine receptors as long as the acetylcholine persists in the space. However, it is removed rapidly by two means: (1) Most of the acetylcholine is destroyed by the enzyme *acetylcholinesterase*; (2) a small amount of acetylcholine diffuses out of the synaptic space and is then no longer available to act on the muscle fiber membrane.

The short time that the acetylcholine remains in the synaptic space—a few milliseconds at most—normally is sufficient to excite the muscle fiber. Then the rapid removal of the acetylcholine prevents continued muscle reexcitation after the muscle fiber has recovered from its initial action potential.

End Plate Potential and Excitation of the Skeletal Muscle Fiber. The sudden insurgence of sodium ions into the muscle fiber when the acetylcholine-gated channels open causes the electrical potential inside the fiber at the *local area of the end plate* to increase in the positive direction as much as 50–75 mV, creating a *local potential* called the *end plate potential*. Recall from Chapter 9 that a sudden increase in nerve membrane potential of more than 20–30 mV is normally sufficient to initiate more and more sodium channel opening, thus initiating an action potential at the muscle fiber membrane.

Figure 12-4 shows the principle of an end plate potential initiating the action potential. This figure shows three separate end plate potentials. End plate potentials A and C are too weak to elicit an action potential, but they do produce weak local end plate voltage changes, as recorded in the figure. By contrast, end plate potential B is much stronger and causes enough sodium channels to open so that the self-regenerative effect of more and more sodium ions flowing to the interior of the fiber initiates an action potential.

Safety Factor for Transmission at the Neuromuscular Junction; Fatigue of the Junction. Ordinarily, each impulse that arrives at the neuromuscular junction causes about three times as much end plate potential as that required to stimulate the muscle fiber. Therefore, the normal neuromuscular junction

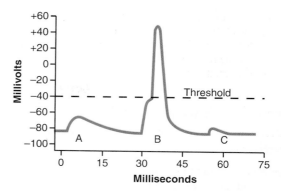

Figure 12-4 End plate potentials (in millivolts). (*A*) Weakened end plate potential recorded in a curarized muscle that is too weak to elicit an action potential; (*B*) normal end plate potential eliciting a muscle action potential; (*C*) weakened end plate potential caused by botulinum toxin that decreases end plate release of acetylcholine, again too weak to elicit a muscle action potential.

is said to have a high *safety factor*. However, stimulation of the nerve fiber at rates greater than 100 times per second for several minutes often diminishes the number of acetylcholine vesicles so much that impulses fail to pass into the muscle fiber. This situation is called *fatigue* of the neuromuscular junction, and it is the same effect that causes fatigue of synapses in the central nervous system when the synapses are overexcited. Under normal functioning conditions, measurable fatigue of the neuromuscular junction occurs rarely, and even then only at the most exhausting levels of muscle activity.

Molecular Biology of Acetylcholine Formation and Release

Formation and release of acetylcholine at the neuromuscular junction occur in the following stages:

1. Small vesicles, about 40 nm in size, are formed by the Golgi apparatus in the cell body of the motoneuron in the spinal cord. These vesicles are then transported by axoplasm all the way to the neuromuscular junction at the tips of the peripheral nerve fibers. About 300,000 of these small vesicles collect in the nerve terminals of a single skeletal muscle end plate.

2. Acetylcholine is synthesized in the cytosol of the nerve fiber terminal but is immediately transported through the membranes of the vesicles to their interior, where it is stored in highly concentrated form, about 10,000 molecules of acetylcholine in each vesicle.

3. When an action potential arrives at the nerve terminal, it opens many calcium channels in the membrane of the nerve terminal because this terminal has an abundance of voltage-gated calcium channels. As a result, the calcium ion concentration inside the terminal membrane increases about 100-fold, which in turn increases the rate of fusion of the acetylcholine vesicles with the terminal membrane about 10,000-fold. This fusion makes many of the vesicles rupture, allowing *exocytosis* of acetylcholine into the synaptic space. About 125 vesicles usually rupture with each action potential. Then, after a few milliseconds, the acetylcholine is split by acetylcholinesterase into acetate ion and choline and the choline is reabsorbed actively into the neural terminal to be reused to form new acetylcholine. This sequence of events occurs within a period of 5–10 milliseconds.

4. The number of vesicles available in the nerve ending is sufficient to allow transmission of only a few thousand nerve-to-muscle impulses. Therefore, for continued function of the neuromuscular junction, new vesicles need to be re-formed rapidly.

Drugs that Enhance or Block Transmission at the Neuromuscular Junction

Drugs that Prevent the Release of Acetylcholine. Botulinum toxin, a product of the bacterium *Clostridium botulinum*, prevents the acetylcholine vesicles from fusing with the presynaptic membrane, thus preventing the release of the neurotransmitter into the synaptic cleft.

Drugs that Stimulate the Muscle Fiber by Acetylcholine-Like Action and Block the Transmission. Many compounds, including *methacholine, carbachol,* and *nicotine,* have the same effect on the muscle fiber as does acetylcholine and act by causing localized areas of depolarization of the muscle fiber membrane at the motor end plate where the acetylcholine receptors are located. They cause initial muscle twitching and then paralysis due to persistent depolarization. The difference between these drugs and acetylcholine is that the drugs are not destroyed by cholinesterase or are destroyed so slowly that their action often persists for many minutes to several hours.

Drugs that Stimulate the Neuromuscular Junction by Inactivating Acetylcholinesterase. Three particularly well-known drugs, *neostigmine, physostigmine,* and *diisopropyl fluorophosphate,* inactivate acetylcholinesterase in the synapses so that it no longer hydrolyzes acetylcholine. Therefore, with each successive nerve impulse, additional acetylcholine accumulates and stimulates the muscle fiber repetitively. This activity causes *muscle spasm.* Unfortunately, it can also cause death as a result of laryngeal spasm, which smothers the person.

Neostigmine and physostigmine combine with acetylcholinesterase to inactivate the acetylcholinesterase for up to several hours, after which these drugs are displaced from the acetylcholinesterase so that the esterase once again becomes active. Conversely, diisopropyl fluorophosphate, which is a powerful "nerve" gas poison, inactivates acetylcholinesterase for weeks, which makes this poison particularly lethal.

Drugs that Block Transmission at the Neuromuscular Junction. A group of drugs known as *curariform drugs* can prevent passage of impulses from the nerve ending into the muscle. For instance, D-tubocurarine blocks the action of acetylcholine on the muscle fiber acetylcholine receptors, thus preventing sufficient increase in permeability of the muscle membrane channels to initiate an action potential.

Myasthenia Gravis

Myasthenia gravis is an autoimmune disease, which occurs in about 1 in every 20,000 persons, causing muscle weakness because of the inability of the neuromuscular junctions to transmit enough signals from the nerve fibers to the muscle fibers. Pathologically, antibodies that attack the acetylcholine receptors have been demonstrated in the blood of most patients with myasthenia gravis. The pathological changes that occur in the neuromuscular junction in myasthenia gravis are summarized in Figure 12-5. These changes demonstrate why neuromuscular transmission is compromised in these patients.

The end plate potentials that occur in the muscle fibers are mostly too weak to initiate opening of the voltage-gated sodium channels and thus muscle fiber depolarization does not occur. If the disease is intense enough, the patient may die of respiratory failure as a result of severe weakness of the respiratory muscles. The disease can usually be suppressed for several hours by administering *neostigmine* or some other anticholinesterase drug that allows larger than normal amounts of acetylcholine to accumulate in the synaptic space. Within minutes, some of these people can begin to function almost normally, until a new dose of neostigmine is required a few hours later.

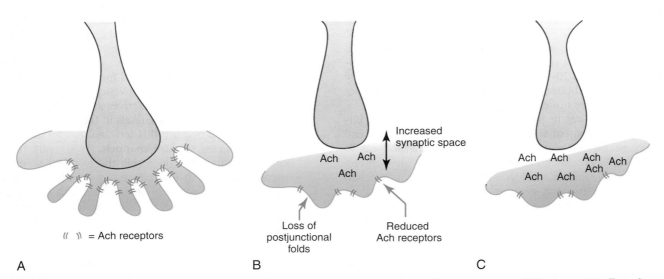

Figure 12-5   Pathological changes in myasthenia gravis. (A) Normal neuromuscular junction; (B) changes in myasthenia gravis; (C) effect of neostigmine in myasthenia gravis: Inhibition of cholinesterase increases the concentration of Ach and increases the chances of Ach–receptor interactions. *Ach,* acetylcholine.

Muscle Action Potential—Comparison with Nerve Action Potential

Almost everything discussed in Chapter 9 regarding initiation and conduction of action potentials in nerve fibers applies equally to skeletal muscle fibers, except for quantitative differences. A comparison of the nerve and muscle action potential is given in Table 12-1.

Figure 12-6 summarizes the structure of the neuromuscular junction, the events that occur at this site, and the various drugs that act on the neuromuscular junction.

TABLE 12-1 | Comparison of the Nerve and Muscle Action Potential

	Nerve Action Potential	Muscle Action Potential
Resting membrane potential (mV)	−90	−80 to −90
Duration of action potential (milliseconds)	0.2–0.3	1–5
Velocity of conduction (m/second)	70–120	3–5

Velocity of conduction refers to large myelinated nerves.

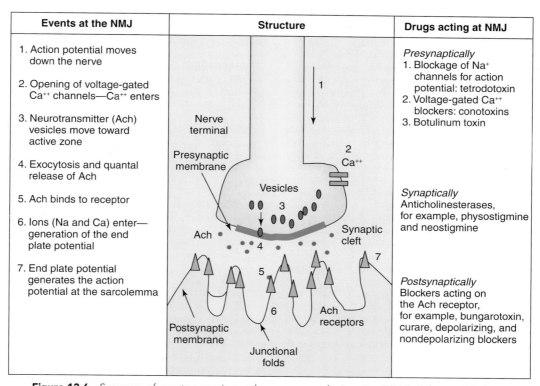

Events at the NMJ	Structure	Drugs acting at NMJ
1. Action potential moves down the nerve		*Presynaptically*
2. Opening of voltage-gated Ca++ channels—Ca++ enters		1. Blockage of Na+ channels for action potential: tetrodotoxin
3. Neurotransmitter (Ach) vesicles move toward active zone	Nerve terminal / Presynaptic membrane / Vesicles	2. Voltage-gated Ca++ blockers: conotoxins 3. Botulinum toxin
4. Exocytosis and quantal release of Ach	Ach / Synaptic cleft	
5. Ach binds to receptor		*Synaptically*
6. Ions (Na and Ca) enter—generation of the end plate potential	Ach receptors	Anticholinesterases, for example, physostigmine and neostigmine
7. End plate potential generates the action potential at the sarcolemma	Postsynaptic membrane / Junctional folds	*Postsynaptically* Blockers acting on the Ach receptor, for example, bungarotoxin, curare, depolarizing, and nondepolarizing blockers

Figure 12-6 Summary of events occurring at the neuromuscular junction (NMJ). *Ach*, acetylcholine.

BIBLIOGRAPHY

Cossins J, Belaya K, Zoltowska K, et al: The search for new antigenic targets in myasthenia gravis, *Ann. N. Y. Acad. Sci.* 1275:123, 2012.

Fagerlund MJ, Eriksson LI: Current concepts in neuromuscular transmission, *Br. J. Anaesth.* 103:108, 2009.

Farrugia ME, Vincent A: Autoimmune mediated neuromuscular junction defects, *Curr. Opin. Neurol.* 23:489, 2010.

Hirsch NP: Neuromuscular junction in health and disease, *Br. J. Anaesth.* 99:132, 2007.

Konieczny P, Swiderski K, Chamberlain JS: Gene and cell-mediated therapies for muscular dystrophy, *Muscle Nerve* 47:649, 2013.

Leite JF, Rodrigues-Pinguet N, Lester HA: Insights into channel function via channel dysfunction, *J. Clin. Invest.* 111:436, 2003.

Meriggioli MN, Sanders DB: Muscle autoantibodies in myasthenia gravis: beyond diagnosis? *Expert Rev. Clin. Immunol.* 8:427, 2012.

Rahimov F, Kunkel LM: The cell biology of disease: cellular and molecular mechanisms underlying muscular dystrophy, *J. Cell Biol.* 201:499, 2013.

Rekling JC, Funk GD, Bayliss DA, et al: Synaptic control of motoneuronal excitability, *Physiol. Rev.* 80:767, 2000.

Rosenberg PB: Calcium entry in skeletal muscle, *J. Physiol.* 587:3149, 2009.

Ruff RL: Endplate contributions to the safety factor for neuromuscular transmission, *Muscle Nerve* 44:854, 2011.

Sine SM: End-plate acetylcholine receptor: structure, mechanism, pharmacology, and disease, *Physiol. Rev.* 92:1189, 2012.

Van der Kloot W, Molgo J: Quantal acetylcholine release at the vertebrate neuromuscular junction, *Physiol. Rev.* 74:899, 1994.

Vincent A: Unraveling the pathogenesis of myasthenia gravis, *Nat. Rev. Immunol.* 10:797, 2002.

Excitation–Contraction Coupling

The skeletal muscle fiber is so large that action potentials spreading along its surface membrane cause almost no current flow deep within the fiber. Maximum muscle contraction, however, requires the current to penetrate deeply into the muscle fiber to the vicinity of the separate myofibrils. This penetration is achieved by transmission of action potentials along *transverse tubules* (T tubules) that penetrate all the way through the muscle fiber from one side of the fiber to the other, as illustrated in Figure 13-1. The T tubule action potentials cause release of calcium ions inside the muscle fiber in the immediate vicinity of the myofibrils, and these calcium ions then cause contraction. This overall process is called *excitation–contraction* coupling.

Transverse Tubule–Sarcoplasmic Reticulum System

Figure 13-1 shows myofibrils surrounded by the T tubule–sarcoplasmic reticulum system. The T tubules are small and run transverse to the myofibrils. They begin at the cell membrane and penetrate all the way from one side of the muscle fiber to the opposite side. *Where the T tubules originate from the cell membrane, they are open to the exterior of the muscle fiber.* Therefore, they communicate with the extracellular fluid surrounding the muscle fiber and contain extracellular fluid in their lumens. In other words, the T tubules are actually internal extensions of the cell membrane. Therefore, when an action potential spreads over a muscle fiber membrane, a potential change also spreads along the T tubules to the deep interior of the muscle fiber. The electrical currents surrounding these T tubules then elicit muscle contraction.

Figure 13-1 also shows a *sarcoplasmic reticulum*, in yellow. This sarcoplasmic reticulum is composed of two major parts: (1) large chambers called *terminal cisternae* that abut the T tubules and (2) long longitudinal tubules that surround all surfaces of the actual contracting myofibrils.

Release of Calcium Ions by the Sarcoplasmic Reticulum

One of the special features of the sarcoplasmic reticulum is that within its vesicular tubules is an excess of calcium ions in high concentration, and many of these ions are released from each vesicle when an action potential occurs in the adjacent T tubule.

Figures 13-2 and 13-3 show that the action potential of the T tubule causes current flow into the sarcoplasmic reticular cisternae where they abut the T tubule. As the action potential reaches the T tubule, the voltage change is sensed by *dihydropyridine receptors* that are linked to *calcium release channels*, also called *ryanodine receptor channels*, in the adjacent sarcoplasmic reticular cisternae (see Figure 13-2). Activation of dihydropyridine receptors triggers the opening of the calcium release channels in the cisternae, as well as in their attached longitudinal tubules. These channels remain open for a few milliseconds releasing calcium ions into the sarcoplasm surrounding the myofibrils and causing contraction, as discussed in Chapter 14.

A Calcium Pump Removes Calcium Ions from the Myofibrillar Fluid After Contraction Occurs. Once the calcium ions have been released from the sarcoplasmic tubules and have diffused among the myofibrils, muscle contraction continues as long as the calcium concentration remains high. However, a continually active calcium pump located in the walls of the sarcoplasmic reticulum pumps calcium ions away from the myofibrils back into the sarcoplasmic tubules (see Figure 13-2). This pump can concentrate the calcium ions about 10,000-fold inside the tubules. In addition, inside the reticulum is a protein called *calsequestrin* that can bind up to 40 times more calcium.

Excitatory "Pulse" Calcium Ions. The normal resting state concentration ($<10^{-7}$ mol/L) of calcium ions in the cytosol that bathes the myofibrils is too little to elicit contraction. Therefore, the troponin–tropomyosin complex keeps the actin filaments inhibited and maintains a relaxed state of the muscle.

Conversely, full excitation of the T tubule and sarcoplasmic reticulum system causes enough release of calcium ions to increase the concentration in the myofibrillar fluid to as high as 2×10^{-4} mol/L, a 500-fold increase, which is about 10 times the level required to cause maximum muscle contraction. Immediately thereafter, the calcium pump depletes the calcium ions again. The total duration of this calcium "pulse" in the usual *skeletal muscle* fiber lasts about one-twentieth of a second, although it may last several times as long in some fibers and

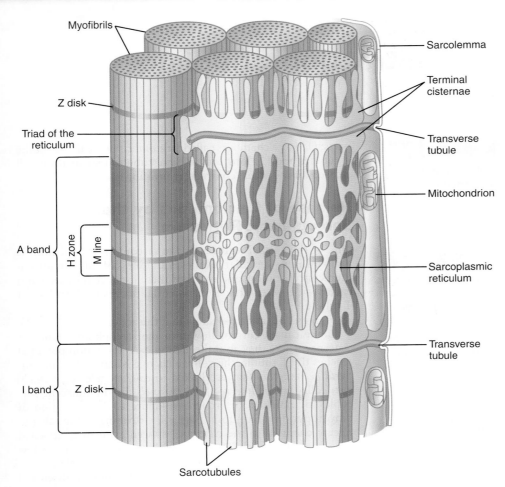

Myofibrils

Z disk

Triad of the reticulum

A band

H zone

M line

I band

Z disk

Sarcolemma

Terminal cisternae

Transverse tubule

Mitochondrion

Sarcoplasmic reticulum

Transverse tubule

Sarcotubules

Figure 13-1 Transverse (T) tubule–sarcoplasmic reticulum system. Note that the T tubules communicate with the outside of the cell membrane, and deep in the muscle fiber, each T tubule lies adjacent to the ends of longitudinal sarcoplasmic reticulum tubules that surround all sides of the actual myofibrils that contract. This illustration was drawn from frog muscle, which has one T tubule per sarcomere, located at the Z disk. A similar arrangement is found in mammalian heart muscle, but mammalian skeletal muscle has two T tubules per sarcomere, located at the A–I band junctions.

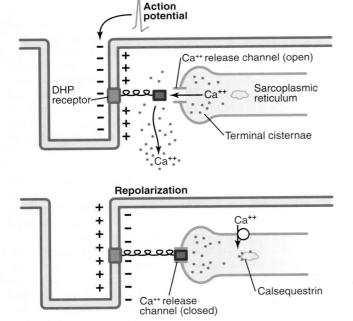

Action potential

Ca^{++} release channel (open)

DHP receptor

Ca^{++}

Sarcoplasmic reticulum

Terminal cisternae

Ca^{++}

Repolarization

Ca^{++}

Calsequestrin

Ca^{++} release channel (closed)

Figure 13-2 Excitation–contraction coupling in skeletal muscle. The *top panel* shows an action potential in the transverse tubule that causes a conformational change in the voltage-sensing dihydropyridine (*DHP*) receptors, opening the Ca^{++} release channels in the terminal cisternae of the sarcoplasmic reticulum and permitting Ca^{++} to rapidly diffuse into the sarcoplasm and initiate muscle contraction. During repolarization (*bottom panel*) the conformational change in the DHP receptor closes the Ca^{++} release channels and Ca^{++} is transported from the sarcoplasm into the sarcoplasmic reticulum by an adenosine triphosphate-dependent calcium pump.

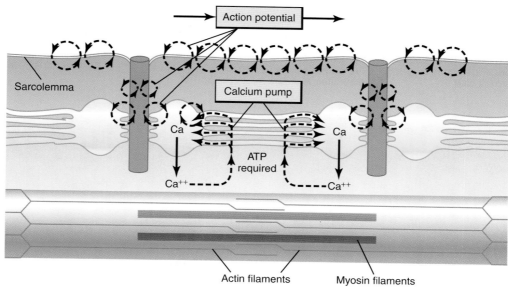

Figure 13-3   Excitation–contraction coupling in the muscle showing (1) an action potential that causes release of calcium ions from the sarcoplasmic reticulum and then (2) reuptake of the calcium ions by a calcium pump. ATP, adenosine triphosphate.

several times less in others. (In heart muscle, the calcium pulse lasts about one-third of a second because of the long duration of the cardiac action potential.)

During this calcium pulse, muscle contraction occurs. If the contraction is to continue without interruption for long intervals, a series of calcium pulses must be initiated by a continuous series of repetitive action potentials, as discussed in Chapter 16.

A summary of the entire process of excitation–contraction coupling is provided in Figure 13-4.

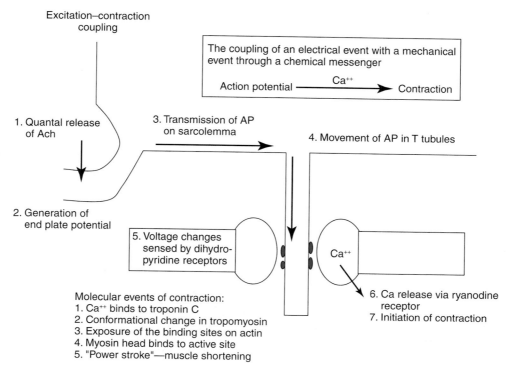

Figure 13-4   Summary of the entire process of excitation–contraction coupling. Ach, acetylcholine; AP, action potential.

BIBLIOGRAPHY

Cheng H, Lederer WJ: Calcium sparks, *Physiol. Rev.* 88:1491, 2008.

Dirksen RT: Checking your SOCCs and feet: the molecular mechanisms of Ca^{2+} entry in skeletal muscle, *J. Physiol.* 587:3139, 2009.

Rosenberg PB: Calcium entry in skeletal muscle, *J. Physiol.* 587:3149, 2009.

Toyoshima C, Nomura H, Sugita Y: Structural basis of ion pumping by Ca^{2+}-ATPase of sarcoplasmic reticulum, *FEBS Lett.* 555:106, 2003.

Treves S, Vukcevic M, Maj M, et al: Minor sarcoplasmic reticulum membrane components that modulate excitation–contraction coupling in striated muscles, J. Physiol. 587:3071, 2009.

14

Molecular Basis of Skeletal Muscle Contraction

LEARNING OBJECTIVES

- Describe the structure of skeletal muscle fibers.
- Describe the functional unit of the skeletal muscle—the sarcomere.
- Describe the steps involved in actin–myosin interactions and the generation of the power stroke.

GLOSSARY OF TERMS

- **Anisotropic:** Nonuniformity of physical properties in different directions (in phase microscopy it is doubly refractive, thus dark, since it contains both actin and myosin filaments)
- **Contractile proteins:** Proteins that contract or cause contraction in response to a suitable stimulus (in muscle these are actin and myosin)
- **Isotropic:** Uniformity of physical properties in all directions (in phase microscopy it is singly refractive, thus light, since it contains only actin filaments)
- **Myofibril:** A bundle of myofilaments each consisting of thin (actin) and thick (myosin) filaments arranged longitudinally along the muscle
- **Sarcolemma:** The thin membrane covering the muscle fiber (it consists of a true cell membrane covered by a coat of polysaccharide that contains thin collagen fibrils)
- **Sarcomere:** Repeating units along the length of a muscle fiber demarcated by two consecutive Z bands

About 40% of the body is skeletal muscle, and perhaps another 10% is smooth and cardiac muscle. Some of the same basic principles of contraction apply to all of these types of muscle. In this chapter, we focus on skeletal muscle.

Physiological Anatomy of Skeletal Muscle

SKELETAL MUSCLE FIBER

Figure 14-1 shows the organization of skeletal muscle, demonstrating that all skeletal muscles are composed of numerous fibers ranging from 10 to 80 μm in diameter. Each of these fibers is made up of successively smaller subunits, also shown in Figure 14-1 and described in subsequent paragraphs.

In most skeletal muscles, each fiber extends the entire length of the muscle. Except for about 2% of the fibers, each fiber is usually innervated by only one nerve ending, located near the middle of the fiber.

The Sarcolemma Is a Thin Membrane Enclosing a Skeletal Muscle Fiber. The sarcolemma consists of a true cell membrane, called the *plasma membrane*, and an outer coat made up of a thin layer of polysaccharide material that contains numerous thin collagen fibrils. At each end of the muscle fiber, this surface layer of the sarcolemma fuses with a tendon fiber. The tendon fibers in turn collect into bundles to form the muscle tendons that then connect the muscles to the bones.

Myofibrils Are Composed of Actin and Myosin Filaments. Each muscle fiber contains several hundred to several thousand *myofibrils*, which are illustrated in the cross-sectional view of Figure 14-1C. Each myofibril (Figure 14-1D and E) is composed of about 1500 adjacent *myosin filaments* and 3000 *actin filaments*, which are large polymerized protein molecules that are responsible for the actual muscle contraction. These filaments can be seen in longitudinal view in the electron micrograph of Figure 14-2 and are represented diagrammatically in Figure 14-1E–L. The thick filaments in the diagrams are *myosin* and the thin filaments are *actin*.

Note in Figure 14-1E that the myosin and actin filaments partially interdigitate and thus cause the myofibrils to have alternate light and dark bands, as illustrated in Figure 14-2. The light bands contain only actin filaments and are called *I bands* because they are *isotropic* to polarized light. The dark bands contain myosin filaments as well as the ends of the actin filaments where they overlap the myosin, and are called *A bands* because they are *anisotropic* to polarized light. Note also the small projections from the sides of the myosin filaments in Figure 14-1E and L. These projections are *cross-bridges*. It is the interaction between these cross-bridges and the actin filaments that causes contraction.

The Sarcomere. Figure 14-1E also shows that the ends of the actin filaments are attached to a so-called *Z disk*. From this disk, these filaments extend in both directions to interdigitate with the myosin filaments. The Z disk, which is composed of filamentous proteins different from the actin and myosin filaments, passes crosswise across the myofibril and also crosswise from myofibril to myofibril, attaching the myofibrils to one another all the way across the muscle fiber. Therefore, the entire muscle fiber has light and dark bands, as do the individual myofibrils. These bands give skeletal and cardiac muscle their striated appearance.

The portion of the myofibril (or of the whole muscle fiber) that lies between two successive Z disks is called a *sarcomere*. When the muscle fiber is contracted, as shown at the bottom of Figure 14-5, the length of the sarcomere is about 2 μm. At this length, the actin filaments completely overlap the myosin filaments, and the tips of the actin filaments are just beginning to overlap one another. As discussed later, at this length the muscle is capable of generating its greatest force of contraction.

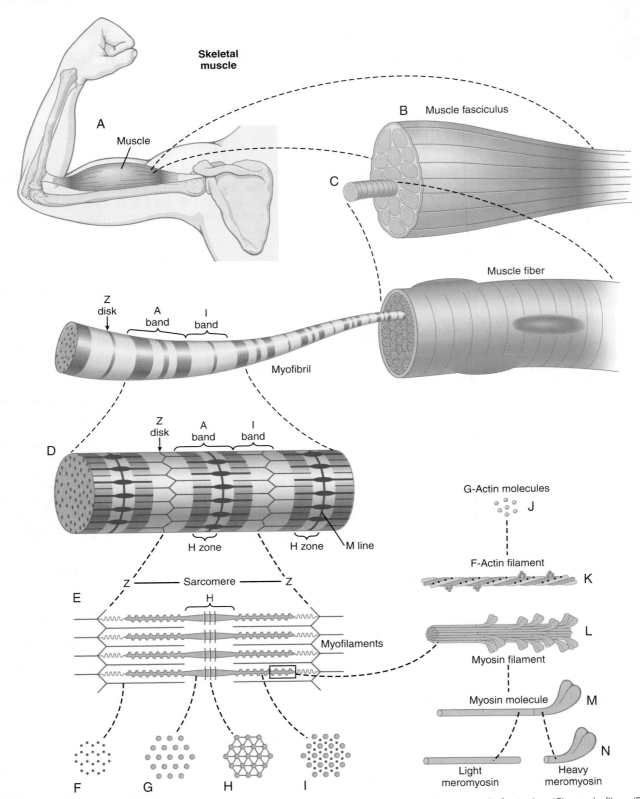

Figure 14-1 Organization of skeletal muscle from the gross to the molecular level. (A) Muscle; (B) muscle fasciculus; (C) muscle fiber; (D and E) arrangement of the sarcomere; (F–I) cross-sections at the levels indicated; (J–N) structure of the actin and myosin filaments.

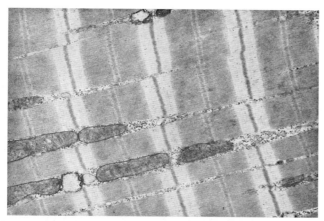

Figure 14-2 An electron micrograph of muscle myofibrils showing the detailed organization of actin and myosin filaments. Note the mitochondria lying between the myofibrils. *From Fawcett, D.W., 1981. The Cell. W.B. Saunders, Philadelphia.*

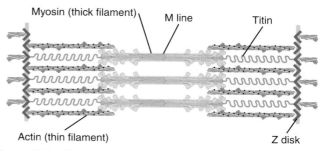

Figure 14-3 Organization of proteins in a sarcomere. Each titin molecule extends from the *Z disc* to the *M line*. Part of the titin molecule is closely associated with the myosin thick filament, whereas the rest of the molecule is springy and changes length as the sarcomere contracts and relaxes.

Titin Filamentous Molecules Keep the Myosin and Actin Filaments in Place. The side-by-side relationship between the myosin and actin filaments is maintained by a large number of filamentous molecules of a protein called *titin* (Figure 14-3). Each titin molecule has a molecular weight of about 3 million, which makes it one of the largest protein molecules in the body. Also, because it is filamentous, it is *very springy*. These springy titin molecules act as a framework that holds the myosin and actin filaments in place so that the contractile machinery of the sarcomere will work.

Sarcoplasm Is the Intracellular Fluid Between Myofibrils. The many myofibrils of each muscle fiber are suspended side-by-side in the muscle fiber. The spaces between the myofibrils are filled with intracellular fluid called *sarcoplasm*, containing large quantities of potassium, magnesium, and phosphate, plus multiple protein enzymes. Also present are tremendous numbers of *mitochondria* that lie parallel to the myofibrils. These mitochondria supply the contracting myofibrils with large amounts of energy in the form of adenosine triphosphate (ATP) formed by the mitochondria.

Sarcoplasmic Reticulum Is a Specialized Endoplasmic Reticulum of Skeletal Muscle. Also in the sarcoplasm surrounding the myofibrils of each muscle fiber is an extensive reticulum (Figure 14-4), called the *sarcoplasmic reticulum*. This reticulum has a special organization that is extremely important in regulating calcium storage, release, and reuptake and therefore muscle contraction, as discussed in Chapter 13. The rapidly contracting types of muscle fibers have especially extensive sarcoplasmic reticula.

General Mechanism of Muscle Contraction

The initiation and execution of muscle contraction occur in the following sequential steps:

1. An action potential travels along a motor nerve to its endings on muscle fibers.
2. At each ending, the nerve secretes a small amount of the neurotransmitter substance *acetylcholine*.
3. The acetylcholine acts on a local area of the muscle fiber membrane to open "acetylcholine-gated" cation channels through protein molecules floating in the membrane.
4. Opening of the acetylcholine-gated channels allows large quantities of sodium ions to diffuse to the interior of the

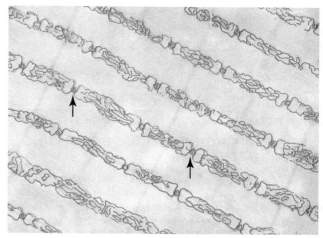

Figure 14-4 Sarcoplasmic reticulum in the extracellular spaces between the myofibrils showing a longitudinal system paralleling the myofibrils. Also shown in cross-section are T tubules (*arrows*) that lead to the exterior of the fiber membrane and are important for conducting the electrical signal into the center of the muscle fiber. *From Fawcett, D.W., 1981. The Cell. W.B. Saunders, Philadelphia.*

muscle fiber membrane. This action causes a local depolarization that leads to opening of voltage-gated sodium channels, which initiates an action potential at the membrane.
5. The action potential travels along the muscle fiber membrane in the same way that action potentials travel along nerve fiber membranes.
6. The action potential depolarizes the muscle membrane, and much of the action potential electricity flows through the center of the muscle fiber. Here it causes the sarcoplasmic reticulum to release large quantities of calcium ions that have been stored within this reticulum.
7. The calcium ions initiate attractive forces between the actin and myosin filaments, causing them to slide alongside each other, which is the contractile process.
8. After a fraction of a second, the calcium ions are pumped back into the sarcoplasmic reticulum by a Ca^{++} membrane pump and remain stored in the reticulum until a new muscle action potential comes along; this removal of calcium ions from the myofibrils causes the muscle contraction to cease.

We now describe the molecular machinery of the muscle contractile process.

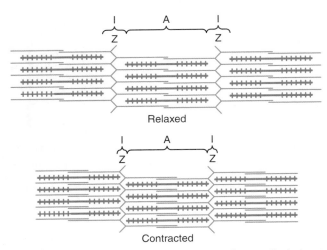

Figure 14-5 Relaxed and contracted states of a myofibril showing (*top*) sliding of the actin filaments (*pink*) into the spaces between the myosin filaments (*red*) and (*bottom*) pulling of the Z membranes toward each other.

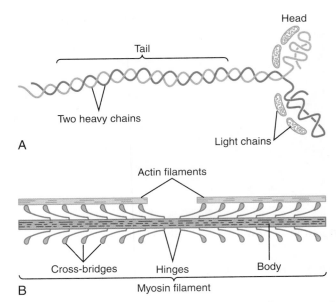

Figure 14-6 (A) Myosin molecule; (B) combination of many myosin molecules to form a myosin filament. Also shown are thousands of myosin *cross-bridges* and interaction between the *heads* of the cross-bridges with adjacent actin filaments.

Molecular Mechanism of Muscle Contraction

MUSCLE CONTRACTION OCCURS BY A SLIDING FILAMENT MECHANISM

Figure 14-5 demonstrates the basic mechanism of muscle contraction. It shows the relaxed state of a sarcomere (*top*) and the contracted state (*bottom*). In the relaxed state, the ends of the actin filaments extending from two successive Z disks barely overlap one another. Conversely, in the contracted state, these actin filaments have been pulled inward among the myosin filaments, so their ends overlap one another to their maximum extent. Also, the Z disks have been pulled by the actin filaments up to the ends of the myosin filaments. Thus, muscle contraction occurs by a *sliding filament mechanism.*

But what causes the actin filaments to slide inward among the myosin filaments? This action is caused by forces generated by interaction of the cross-bridges from the myosin filaments with the actin filaments. Under resting conditions, these forces are inactive but when an action potential travels along the muscle fiber, this causes the sarcoplasmic reticulum to release large quantities of calcium ions that rapidly surround the myofibrils. The calcium ions in turn activate the forces between the myosin and actin filaments, and contraction begins. However, energy is needed for the contractile process to proceed. This energy comes from high-energy bonds in the ATP molecule, which is degraded to adenosine diphosphate (ADP) to liberate the energy. In the next few sections, we describe these molecular processes of contraction.

MOLECULAR CHARACTERISTICS OF THE CONTRACTILE FILAMENTS

Myosin Filaments Are Composed of Multiple Myosin Molecules. Each of the myosin molecules, shown in Figure 14-6A, has a molecular weight of about 480,000. Figure 14-6B shows the organization of many molecules to form a myosin filament as well as interaction of this filament on one side with the ends of two actin filaments.

The *myosin molecule* (see Figure 14-6A) is composed of six polypeptide chains—two *heavy chains*, each with a molecular weight of about 200,000, and four *light chains* with molecular weights of about 20,000 each. The two heavy chains wrap spirally around each other to form a double helix, which is called the *tail* of the myosin molecule. One end of each of these chains is folded bilaterally into a globular polypeptide structure called a myosin *head.* Thus, there are two free heads at one end of the double-helix myosin molecule. The four light chains are also part of the myosin head, two to each head. These light chains help control the function of the head during muscle contraction.

The *myosin filament* is made up of 200 or more individual myosin molecules. The central portion of one of these filaments is shown in Figure 14-6B, displaying the tails of the myosin molecules bundled together to form the *body* of the filament, while many heads of the molecules hang outward to the sides of the body. Also, part of the body of each myosin molecule hangs to the side along with the head, thus providing an *arm* that extends the head outward from the body, as shown in the figure. The protruding arms and heads together are called *cross-bridges.* Each cross-bridge is flexible at two points called *hinges*—one where the arm leaves the body of the myosin filament and the other where the head attaches to the arm. The hinged arms allow the heads to be either extended far outward from the body of the myosin filament or brought close to the body. The hinged heads in turn participate in the actual contraction process, as discussed in the following sections.

The total length of each myosin filament is uniform, almost exactly 1.6 μm. Note, however, that there are no cross-bridge heads in the center of the myosin filament for a distance of about 0.2 μm because the hinged arms extend away from the center.

Now, to complete the picture, the myosin filament is twisted so that each successive pair of cross-bridges is axially displaced from the previous pair by 120 degrees. This twisting

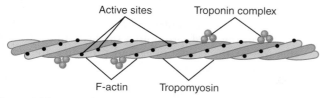

Figure 14-7 Actin filament composed of two helical strands of *F-actin* molecules and two strands of *tropomyosin* molecules that fit in the grooves between the actin strands. Attached to one end of each tropomyosin molecule is a *troponin* complex that initiates contraction.

ensures that the cross-bridges extend in all directions around the filament.

Adenosine Triphosphatase Activity of the Myosin Head. Another feature of the myosin head that is essential for muscle contraction is that it functions as an *ATPase enzyme.* As explained later, this property allows the head to cleave ATP and use the energy derived from the ATP's high-energy phosphate bond to energize the contraction process.

Actin Filaments Are Composed of Actin, Tropomyosin, and Troponin. The backbone of the actin filament is a double-stranded *F-actin protein molecule,* represented by the two lighter-colored strands in Figure 14-7. The two strands are wound in a helix in the same manner as the myosin molecule.

Each strand of the double F-actin helix is composed of polymerized *G-actin molecules,* each having a molecular weight of about 42,000. Attached to each one of the G-actin molecules is one molecule of ADP. These ADP molecules are believed to be the active sites on the actin filaments with which the cross-bridges of the myosin filaments interact to cause muscle contraction. The active sites on the two F-actin strands of the double helix are staggered, giving one active site on the overall actin filament about every 2.7 nm.

Each actin filament is about 1 μm long. The bases of the actin filaments are inserted strongly into the Z disks; the ends of the filaments protrude in both directions to lie in the spaces between the myosin molecules, as shown in Figure 14-5.

Tropomyosin Molecules. The actin filament also contains another protein, *tropomyosin.* Each molecule of tropomyosin has a molecular weight of 70,000 and a length of 40 nm. These molecules are wrapped spirally around the sides of the F-actin helix. In the resting state, the tropomyosin molecules lie on top of the active sites of the actin strands so that attraction cannot occur between the actin and myosin filaments to cause contraction.

Troponin and its Role in Muscle Contraction. Attached intermittently along the sides of the tropomyosin molecules are additional protein molecules called *troponin.* These are actually complexes of three loosely bound protein subunits, each of which plays a specific role in controlling muscle contraction. One of the subunits (troponin I) has a strong affinity for actin, another (troponin T) for tropomyosin, and a third (troponin C) for calcium ions. This complex is believed to attach the tropomyosin to the actin. The strong affinity of the troponin for calcium ions is believed to initiate the contraction process, as explained in the next section.

Interaction of One Myosin Filament, Two Actin Filaments, and Calcium Ions to Cause Contraction

Inhibition of the Actin Filament by the Troponin–Tropomyosin Complex. A pure actin filament without the presence of the troponin–tropomyosin complex (but in the presence of magnesium ions and ATP) binds instantly and strongly with the heads

of the myosin molecules. Then, if the troponin–tropomyosin complex is added to the actin filament, the binding between myosin and actin does not take place. Therefore, it is believed that the active sites on the normal actin filament of the relaxed muscle are inhibited or physically covered by the troponin–tropomyosin complex. Consequently, the sites cannot attach to the heads of the myosin filaments to cause contraction. Before contraction can take place, the inhibitory effect of the troponin–tropomyosin complex must itself be inhibited.

Activation of the Actin Filament by Calcium Ions. In the presence of large amounts of calcium ions, the inhibitory effect of the troponin–tropomyosin on the actin filaments is itself inhibited. The mechanism of this inhibition is not known, but one suggestion is as follows: When calcium ions combine with troponin C, each molecule of which can bind strongly with up to four calcium ions, the troponin complex supposedly undergoes a conformational change that in some way tugs on the tropomyosin molecule and moves it deeper into the groove between the two actin strands. This action "uncovers" the active sites of the actin, thus allowing these active sites to attract the myosin cross-bridge heads and cause contraction to proceed. Although this mechanism is hypothetical, it does emphasize that the normal relation between the troponin–tropomyosin complex and actin is altered by calcium ions, producing a new condition that leads to contraction.

Interaction of the "Activated" Actin Filament and the Myosin Cross-Bridges—The "Walk-Along" Theory of Contraction. As soon as the actin filament is activated by the calcium ions, the heads of the cross-bridges from the myosin filaments become attracted to the active sites of the actin filament, and this, in some way, causes contraction to occur. Although the precise manner in which this interaction between the cross-bridges and the actin causes contraction is still partly theoretical, one hypothesis for which considerable evidence exists is the "walk-along" (or "ratchet") theory of contraction.

Figure 14-8 demonstrates this postulated walk-along mechanism for contraction. The figure shows the heads of two cross-bridges attaching to and disengaging from active sites of an actin filament. When a head attaches to an active site, this attachment simultaneously causes profound changes in the intramolecular forces between the head and arm of its cross-bridge. The new alignment of forces causes the head to tilt toward the arm and to drag the actin filament along with it. This tilt of the head is called the *power stroke.* Immediately after tilting, the head then automatically breaks away from the active site. Next, the head returns to its extended direction. In this position, it combines with a new active site farther down along the actin filament; the head then tilts again to cause a new power stroke, and the actin filament moves another step. Thus, the heads of the cross-bridges bend back and forth and step by step walk along the actin filament, pulling the ends of two successive actin filaments toward the center of the myosin filament.

Each one of the cross-bridges is believed to operate independently of all others, each attaching and pulling in a continuous repeated cycle. Therefore, the greater the number of cross-bridges in contact with the actin filament at any given time, the greater is the force of contraction.

ATP as the Energy Source for Contraction—Chemical Events in the Motion of the Myosin Heads. When a muscle contracts, work is performed and energy is required. Large amounts of ATP are cleaved to form ADP during the contraction process and the greater the amount of work performed by the muscle, the greater is the amount of ATP that is cleaved; this phenomenon

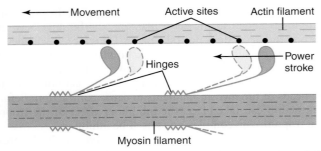

Figure 14-8 The "walk-along" mechanism for contraction of the muscle.

is called the *Fenn effect*. The following sequence of events is believed to be the means by which this effect occurs:

1. Before contraction begins, the heads of the cross-bridges bind with ATP. The ATPase activity of the myosin head immediately cleaves the ATP but leaves the cleavage products, ADP plus phosphate ion, bound to the head. In this state, the conformation of the head is such that it extends perpendicularly toward the actin filament but is not yet attached to the actin.

2. When the troponin–tropomyosin complex binds with calcium ions, active sites on the actin filament are uncovered and the myosin heads then bind with these sites, as shown in Figure 14-8.

3. The bond between the head of the cross-bridge and the active site of the actin filament causes a conformational change in the head, prompting the head to tilt toward the arm of the cross-bridge and providing the *power stroke* for pulling the actin filament. The energy that activates the power stroke is the energy already stored, like a "cocked" spring, by the conformational change that occurred in the head when the ATP molecule was cleaved earlier.

4. Once the head of the cross-bridge tilts, release of the ADP and phosphate ion that were previously attached to the head is allowed. At the site of release of the ADP, a new molecule of ATP binds. This binding of new ATP causes detachment of the head from the actin.

5. After the head has detached from the actin, the new molecule of ATP is cleaved to begin the next cycle, leading to a new power stroke. That is, the energy again "cocks" the head back to its perpendicular condition, ready to begin the new power stroke cycle.

6. When the cocked head (with its stored energy derived from the cleaved ATP) binds with a new active site on the actin filament, it becomes uncocked and once again provides a new power stroke.

Thus, the process proceeds again and again until the actin filaments pull the Z membrane up against the ends of the myosin filaments or until the load on the muscle becomes too great for further pulling to occur.

BIBLIOGRAPHY

Berchtold MW, Brinkmeier H, Muntener M: Calcium ion in skeletal muscle: its crucial role for muscle function, plasticity, and disease, *Physiol. Rev.* 80:1215, 2000.

Clausen T: Na$^+$–K$^+$ pump regulation and skeletal muscle contractility, *Physiol. Rev.* 83:1269, 2003.

Fitts RH: The cross-bridge cycle and skeletal muscle fatigue, *J. Appl. Physiol.* 104:551, 2008.

Gordon AM, Homsher E, Regnier M: Regulation of contraction in striated muscle, *Physiol. Rev.* 80:853, 2000.

Gunning P, O'Neill G, Hardeman E: Tropomyosin-based regulation of the actin cytoskeleton in time and space, *Physiol. Rev.* 88:1, 2008.

Heckman CJ, Enoka RM: Motor unit, *Compr. Physiol.* 2:2629, 2012.

Huxley AF, Gordon AM: Striation patterns in active and passive shortening of muscle, *Nature (London)* 193:280, 1962.

MacIntosh BR: Role of calcium sensitivity modulation in skeletal muscle performance, *News Physiol. Sci.* 18:222, 2003.

Treves S, Vukcevic M, Maj M, et al: Minor sarcoplasmic reticulum membrane components that modulate excitation–contraction coupling in striated muscles, *J. Physiol.* 587:3071, 2009.

15

Chemical Changes During Skeletal Muscle Contraction

Energetics of Muscle Contraction

WORK OUTPUT DURING MUSCLE CONTRACTION

When a muscle contracts against a load, it performs *work*. To perform work means that *energy* is transferred from the muscle to the external load to lift an object to a greater height or to overcome resistance to movement.

In mathematical terms, work is defined by the following equation:

$$W = L \times D$$

where W is the work output, L is the load, and D is the distance of movement against the load. The energy required to perform the work is derived from the chemical reactions in the muscle cells during contraction, as described in the following sections.

THREE SOURCES OF ENERGY FOR MUSCLE CONTRACTION

Most of energy required for muscle contraction is used to actuate the walk-along mechanism by which the cross-bridges pull the actin filaments, but small amounts are required for (1) pumping calcium ions from the sarcoplasm into the sarcoplasmic reticulum after the contraction is over and (2) pumping sodium and potassium ions through the muscle fiber membrane to maintain an appropriate ionic environment for propagation of muscle fiber action potentials.

The concentration of adenosine triphosphate (ATP) in the muscle fiber, about 4 mmol/L, is sufficient to maintain full contraction for only 1–2 seconds at most. The ATP is split to form adenosine diphosphate (ADP), which transfers energy from the ATP molecule to the contracting machinery of the muscle fiber. Then, as described in Chapter 2, the ADP is rephosphorylated to form new ATP within another fraction of a second, which allows the muscle to continue its contraction. There are three sources of the energy for this rephosphorylation.

The first source of energy that is used to reconstitute the ATP is the substance phosphocreatine, which carries a high-energy phosphate bond similar to the bonds of ATP. The high-energy phosphate bond of phosphocreatine has a slightly higher amount of free energy than that of each ATP bond. Therefore, phosphocreatine is instantly cleaved, and its released energy causes bonding of a new phosphate ion to ADP to reconstitute the ATP. However, the total amount of phosphocreatine in the muscle fiber is small—only about five times as great as the ATP. Therefore, the combined energy of both the stored ATP and the phosphocreatine in the muscle is capable of causing maximal muscle contraction for only 5–8 seconds.

The second important source of energy, which is used to reconstitute both ATP and phosphocreatine, is "glycolysis" of glycogen previously stored in the muscle cells. Rapid enzymatic breakdown of the glycogen to pyruvic acid and lactic acid liberates energy that is used to convert ADP to ATP; the ATP can then be used directly to energize additional muscle contraction and also to re-form the stores of phosphocreatine.

The importance of this glycolysis mechanism is twofold. First, the glycolytic reactions can occur even in the absence of oxygen, so muscle contraction can be sustained for many seconds and sometimes up to more than a minute, even when oxygen delivery from the blood is not available. Second, the rate of formation of ATP by the glycolytic process is about 2.5 times as rapid as ATP formation in response to cellular foodstuffs reacting with oxygen. However, so many end products of glycolysis accumulate in the muscle cells that glycolysis also loses its capability to sustain maximum muscle contraction after about 1 minute.

The third and final source of energy is oxidative metabolism, which means combining oxygen with the end products of glycolysis and with various other cellular foodstuffs to liberate ATP. More than 95% of all energy used by the muscles for sustained, long-term contraction is derived from oxidative phosphorylation. The foodstuffs that are consumed are carbohydrates, fats, and protein. For extremely long-term maximal muscle activity—over a period of many hours—by far the greatest proportion of energy comes from fats, but for periods of 2–4 hours, as much as one-half of the energy can come from stored carbohydrates.

TABLE 15-1	Nature of the Heat Production Depending on the Type of Contraction of Muscle		
Type of Heat	Phase of Muscle Contraction	Isometric Contraction	Isotonic Contraction
Resting	Prior to muscle contraction, that is, in the unstimulated muscle	+	+
Activation	Muscle is activated but has not started contracting	+	+
Shortening	Only seen during the actual process of shortening in isotonic contractions		+
Relaxation	Relaxation phase	+	+
Recovery	Associated with metabolic changes required to return muscle to its initial, resting state	+	+

Heat production in isotonic contraction is higher than in isometric contraction because of the absence of shortening heat in isometric contraction.

The importance of the different mechanisms of energy release during performance of different sports is discussed in Chapter 17.

EFFICIENCY OF MUSCLE CONTRACTION

The efficiency of an engine or a motor is calculated as the percentage of energy input that is converted into work instead of heat. The percentage of the input energy to muscle (the chemical energy in nutrients) that can be converted into work, even under the best conditions, is less than 25%, with the remainder becoming heat. The reason for this low efficiency is that about one-half of the energy in foodstuffs is lost during the formation of ATP, and even then, only 40–45% of the energy in the ATP itself can later be converted into work.

Maximum efficiency can be realized only when the muscle contracts at a moderate velocity. If the muscle contracts slowly or without any movement, small amounts of *maintenance heat* are released during contraction, even though little or no work is performed, thereby decreasing the conversion efficiency to as little as zero. Conversely, if contraction is too rapid, large proportions of the energy are used to overcome viscous friction within the muscle itself, and this, too, reduces the efficiency of contraction. Ordinarily, maximum efficiency is developed when the velocity of contraction is about 30% of maximum.

Fenn found that muscle uses extra energy in proportion to the work done; this was therefore called the *Fenn effect*.

HEAT PRODUCTION DURING MUSCLE CONTRACTION

As described earlier, in the process of contracting muscles produce heat. This was extensively studied by the Nobel laureate (1922), A.V. Hill. The nature of the heat production varies depending on whether the contraction of the muscle is isotonic or isometric. This is summarized in Table 15-1.

MUSCLE FATIGUE

The inability of skeletal muscle to sustain a given amplitude of contraction is called fatigue. This is best seen when there is prolonged and strong contraction of a muscle. There are many causes of fatigue:

1. A *reduction in the central command* (neural drive) to working muscles, possibly through a serotonergic mechanism, can cause fatigue.
2. Experiments have also shown that *transmission of the nerve signal through the neuromuscular junction* can diminish at least a small amount after intense prolonged muscle activity, thus further diminishing muscle contraction.
3. Studies in athletes have shown that muscle fatigue increases in almost direct proportion to the rate of *depletion of muscle glycogen*. Therefore, fatigue results mainly from inability of the contractile and metabolic processes of the muscle fibers to continue supplying the same work output.
4. *Interruption of blood flow through a contracting muscle* leads to almost complete muscle fatigue within 1 or 2 minutes because of the loss of nutrient supply, especially loss of oxygen.

RIGOR MORTIS

Several hours after death, all the muscles of the body go into a state of *contracture* called "rigor mortis"; that is, the muscles contract and become rigid even without action potentials. This rigidity results from loss of all the ATP, which is required to cause separation of the cross-bridges from the actin filaments during the relaxation process. The muscles remain in rigor until the muscle proteins deteriorate about 15–25 hours later, which presumably results from autolysis caused by enzymes released from lysosomes. All these events occur more rapidly at higher temperatures.

HEAT RIGOR

Muscle also undergoes shortening when it is exposed to heat, for instance, at around 50°C or greater during which there is coagulation of muscle proteins. This is readily demonstrated in isolated muscle preparations and is called *heat rigor*.

BIBLIOGRAPHY

Allen DG, Lamb GD, Westerblad H: Skeletal muscle fatigue: cellular mechanisms, *Physiol. Rev.* 88:287, 2008.

Cairns SP, Lindinger MI: Do multiple ionic interactions contribute to skeletal muscle fatigue? *J. Physiol.* 586:4039, 2008.

Fitts RH: The cross-bridge cycle and skeletal muscle fatigue, *J. Appl. Physiol.* 104:551, 2008.

Kent-Braun JA, Fitts RH, Christie A: Skeletal muscle fatigue, *Compr. Physiol.* 2:997, 2012.

MacIntosh BR, Holash RJ, Renaud JM: Skeletal muscle fatigue—regulation of excitation–contraction coupling to avoid metabolic catastrophe, *J. Cell Sci.* 125:2105, 2012.

Powers SK, Jackson MJ: Exercise-induced oxidative stress: cellular mechanisms and impact on muscle force production, *Physiol. Rev.* 88:1243, 2008.

Ranatunga KW, Coupland ME: Crossbridge mechanism(s) examined by temperature perturbation studies on muscle, *Adv. Exp. Med. Biol.* 682:247, 2010.

Sieck GC, Regnier M: Plasticity and energetic demands of contraction in skeletal and cardiac muscle, *J. Appl. Physiol.* 90:1158, 2001.

16

Characteristics of Skeletal Muscle Contraction

LEARNING OBJECTIVES

- Describe the relation between force of contraction and initial fiber length.
- Describe the relation between load and velocity of contraction.
- Differentiate between isometric and isotonic contractions.
- Differentiate between the characteristics of slow and fast skeletal muscle fibers.
- Describe the relation between frequency of stimulation and muscle contraction.

GLOSSARY OF TERMS

- **All-or-none law (for a motor unit):** States that a threshold or greater than threshold stimulus produces a contraction of similar amplitude

- **Isometric contraction:** A static contraction in which the length of the muscle does not change

- **Isotonic contraction:** A contraction in which tension remains unchanged and the muscle's length changes

- **Motor unit:** A single alpha motoneuron together with all the muscle fibers that it innervates

- **Starling law:** States that within physiological limits, the force of contraction is directly proportional to the initial length of the muscle fiber (although commonly referred to as Frank–Starling law of the heart, this is applicable to skeletal muscle as well)

- **Tetanus:** Sustained contraction of muscle at high frequencies of stimulation

In the previous chapter, we outlined the molecular basis of skeletal muscle contraction. In this chapter we will focus on the characteristics of skeletal muscle contraction.

The Amount of Actin and Myosin Filament Overlap Determines Tension Developed by the Contracting Muscle

Figure 16-1 shows the effect of sarcomere length and the amount of myosin–actin filament overlap on the active tension developed by a contracting muscle fiber. To the right are different degrees of overlap of the myosin and actin filaments at different sarcomere lengths. At point D on the diagram, the actin filament has pulled all the way out to the end of the myosin filament, with no actin–myosin overlap. At this point, the tension developed by the activated muscle is zero. Then, as the sarcomere

shortens and the actin filament begins to overlap the myosin filament, the tension increases progressively until the sarcomere length decreases to about 2.2 μm. At this point, the actin filament has already overlapped all the cross-bridges of the myosin filament but has not yet reached the center of the myosin filament. With further shortening, the sarcomere maintains full tension until point B is reached, at a sarcomere length of about 2 μm. At this point, the ends of the two actin filaments begin to overlap each other in addition to overlapping the myosin filaments. As the sarcomere length decreases from 2 μm down to about 1.65 μm, at point A, the strength of contraction decreases rapidly. At this point, the two Z disks of the sarcomere abut the ends of the myosin filaments. Then, as contraction proceeds to still shorter sarcomere lengths, the ends of the myosin filaments are crumpled and, as shown in the figure, the strength of contraction approaches zero, but the sarcomere has now contracted to its shortest length.

Effect of Muscle Length on Force of Contraction in the Whole Intact Muscle. The top curve of Figure 16-2 is similar to that in Figure 16-1, but the curve in Figure 16-2 depicts tension of the intact whole muscle rather than of a single muscle fiber. The whole muscle has a large amount of connective tissue in it; in addition, the sarcomeres in different parts of the muscle do not always contract the same amount. Therefore, the curve has somewhat different dimensions from those shown for the individual muscle fiber, but it exhibits the same general form for the slope *in the normal range of contraction*, as noted

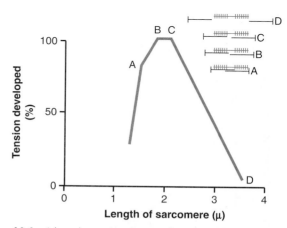

Figure 16-1 A length–tension diagram for a single fully contracted sarcomere, showing the maximum strength of contraction when the sarcomere is 2.0–2.2 μm in length. At the upper right are the relative positions of the actin and myosin filaments at different sarcomere lengths from *point A* to *point D. Modified from Gordon, A.M., Huxley, A.F., Julian, F.J., 1964. The length–tension diagram of single vertebrate striated muscle fibers. J. Physiol. 171, 28P.*

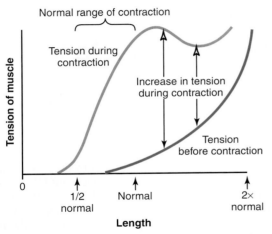

Figure 16-2 Relation of muscle length to tension in the muscle both before and during muscle contraction.

TABLE **16-1**	Characteristics of Isotonic and Isometric Contractions	
	Isotonic Contraction	Isometric Contraction
Shortening	Yes	No
Increase in tension	No	Yes
Amount of heat generated	Greater	Less
Work done	Yes	No
Example	Lifting a bucket off the floor	Pushing against a wall

in Figure 16-2. Thus, within physiological limits, the force of contraction is directly proportional to the initial length of the muscle fiber; this is referred to as Starling law.

Note in Figure 16-2 that when the muscle is at its normal *resting* length, which is at a sarcomere length of about 2 μm, it contracts upon activation with the approximate maximum force of contraction. However, the *increase* in tension that occurs during contraction, called *active tension*, decreases as the muscle is stretched beyond its normal length—that is, to a sarcomere length greater than about 2.2 μm. This phenomenon is demonstrated by the decreased length of the arrow in the figure at greater than normal muscle length.

Relation of Velocity of Contraction to Load

A skeletal muscle contracts rapidly when it contracts against no load—to a state of full contraction in about 0.1 second for the average muscle. When loads are applied, the velocity of contraction becomes progressively less as the load increases, as shown in Figure 16-3. That is, when the load has been increased to equal the maximum force that the muscle can exert, the velocity of contraction becomes zero and no contraction results despite activation of the muscle fiber.

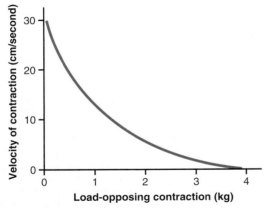

Figure 16-3 Relation of load to velocity of contraction in a skeletal muscle with a cross-section of 1 cm² and a length of 8 cm.

This decreasing velocity of contraction with load is because a load on a contracting muscle is a reverse force that opposes the contractile force caused by muscle contraction. Therefore, the net force that is available to cause velocity of shortening is reduced.

ISOMETRIC VERSUS ISOTONIC CONTRACTION

Muscle contraction is said to be *isometric* when the muscle does not shorten during contraction and *isotonic* when it does shorten but the tension on the muscle remains constant throughout the contraction. The characteristics of isotonic and isometric contractions are summarized in Table 16-1.

FAST VERSUS SLOW MUSCLE FIBERS

Every muscle of the body is composed of a mixture of so-called *fast* and *slow* muscle fibers, with still other fibers gradated between these two extremes. Muscles that react rapidly, including the anterior tibialis, are composed mainly of "fast" fibers with only small numbers of the slow variety. Conversely, muscles such as soleus that respond slowly but with prolonged contraction are composed mainly of "slow" fibers. The differences between these two types of fibers are described in the following sections.

Slow Fibers (Type 1, Red Muscle)

The following are the characteristics of slow fibers:
1. Slow fibers are smaller than fast fibers.
2. Slow fibers are also innervated by smaller nerve fibers.
3. Compared with fast fibers, slow fibers have a more extensive blood vessel system and more capillaries to supply extra amounts of oxygen.
4. Slow fibers have greatly increased numbers of mitochondria to support high levels of oxidative metabolism.
5. Slow fibers contain large amounts of myoglobin, an iron-containing protein similar to hemoglobin in red blood cells. Myoglobin combines with oxygen and stores it until needed; this greatly speeds oxygen transport to the mitochondria. The myoglobin gives the slow muscle a reddish appearance and hence the name *red muscle*.

Fast Fibers (Type II, White Muscle)

The following are the characteristics of fast fibers:
1. Fast fibers are large for greater strength of contraction.
2. Fast fibers have an extensive sarcoplasmic reticulum for the rapid release of calcium ions to initiate contraction.
3. Large amounts of glycolytic enzymes are present for the rapid release of energy by the glycolytic process.
4. Fast fibers have a less extensive blood supply than do slow fibers because oxidative metabolism is of secondary importance.

5. Fast fibers have fewer mitochondria than do slow fibers, because oxidative metabolism is secondary. A deficit of red myoglobin in fast muscle gives it the name *white muscle*.

Mechanics of Skeletal Muscle Contraction

MOTOR UNIT—ALL THE MUSCLE FIBERS INNERVATED BY A SINGLE NERVE FIBER

Each motoneuron that leaves the spinal cord innervates multiple muscle fibers, with the number of fibers innervated depending on the type of muscle. All the muscle fibers innervated by a single nerve fiber are called a *motor unit* (Figure 16-4). In general, small muscles that react rapidly and whose control must be exact have more nerve fibers for fewer muscle fibers (eg, as few as two or three muscle fibers per motor unit in some of the laryngeal muscles). Conversely, large muscles that do not require fine control, such as the soleus muscle, may have several hundred muscle fibers in a motor unit. An average figure for all the muscles of the body is questionable, but a good guess would be about 80–100 muscle fibers in a motor unit.

The muscle fibers in each motor unit are not all bunched together in the muscle but overlap other motor units in microbundles of 3–15 fibers. This interdigitation allows the separate motor units to contract in support of one another rather than entirely as individual segments.

MUSCLE CONTRACTIONS OF DIFFERENT FORCE—FORCE SUMMATION

Summation means the adding together of individual twitch contractions to increase the intensity of overall muscle contraction. Summation occurs in two ways: (1) by increasing the number of motor units contracting simultaneously, which is called *multiple fiber summation*, and (2) by increasing the frequency of contraction, which is called *frequency summation* and can lead to *tetanization*.

Multiple Fiber Summation

When the central nervous system sends a weak signal to contract a muscle, the smaller motor units of the muscle may be stimulated in preference to the larger motor units. Then, as the strength of the signal increases, larger and larger motor units begin to be excited as well, with the largest motor units often having as much as 50 times the contractile force of the smallest units. This phenomenon where larger motor units are recruited with increasing signal strength is called the *size principle*. It is important because it allows the gradations of muscle force during weak contraction to occur in small steps, whereas the steps become progressively greater when large amounts of force are required. This size principle occurs because the smaller motor units are driven by small motor nerve fibers, and the small motoneurons in the spinal cord are more excitable than the larger ones, so they are naturally excited first.

Another important feature of multiple fiber summation is that the different motor units are driven asynchronously by the spinal cord; as a result, contraction alternates among motor units one after the other, thus providing smooth contraction even at low frequencies of nerve signals.

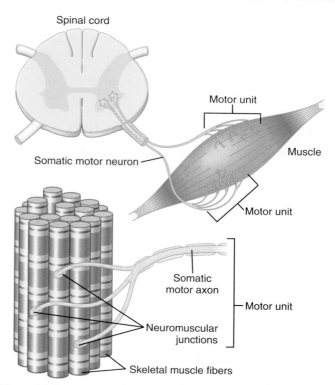

Figure 16-4   A motor unit consists of a motor neuron and the group of skeletal muscle fibers it innervates. A single motor axon may branch to innervate several muscle fibers that function together as a group. Although each muscle fiber is innervated by a single motor neuron, an entire muscle may receive input from hundreds of different motor neurons.

Frequency Summation and Tetanization

Figure 16-5 shows the principles of frequency summation and tetanization. Individual twitch contractions occurring one after another at low frequency of stimulation are displayed to the left. Then, as the frequency increases, there comes a point when each new contraction occurs before the preceding one is over. As a result, the second contraction is added partially to the first, and thus the total strength of contraction rises progressively with increasing frequency. When the frequency reaches a critical level, the successive contractions eventually become so rapid that they fuse together and the whole muscle contraction appears to be completely smooth and continuous, as shown in Figure 16-5. This process is called *tetanization*. At a slightly higher frequency, the strength of contraction reaches its maximum, and thus any

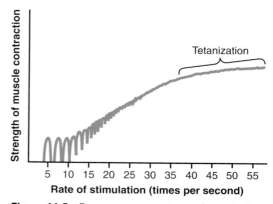

Figure 16-5   Frequency summation and tetanization.

additional increase in frequency beyond that point has no further effect in increasing contractile force. Tetany occurs because enough calcium ions are maintained in the muscle sarcoplasm, even between action potentials, so that full contractile state is sustained without allowing any relaxation between the action potentials.

MAXIMUM STRENGTH OF CONTRACTION

The maximum strength of tetanic contraction of a muscle operating at a normal muscle length averages between 3 and 4 kg/cm^2 of muscle, or 50 psi. Because a quadriceps muscle can have up to 16 (in.)^2 of muscle belly, as much as 800 lb of tension may be applied to the patellar tendon. Thus, one can readily understand how it is possible for muscles to pull their tendons out of their insertions in bone.

CHANGES IN MUSCLE STRENGTH AT THE ONSET OF CONTRACTION—THE STAIRCASE EFFECT (TREPPE)

When a muscle begins to contract after a long period of rest, its initial strength of contraction may be as little as one-half its strength, 10–50 muscle twitches later. That is, the strength of contraction increases to a plateau, a phenomenon called the *staircase effect*, or *treppe*.

Although all the possible causes of the staircase effect are not known, it is believed to be caused primarily by increasing calcium ions in the cytosol because of the release of more and more ions from the sarcoplasmic reticulum with each successive muscle action potential and failure of the sarcoplasm to recapture the ions immediately.

SKELETAL MUSCLE TONE

Even when muscles are at rest, a certain amount of tautness usually remains, which is called *muscle tone*. Because normal skeletal muscle fibers do not contract without an action potential to stimulate the fibers, skeletal muscle tone results entirely from a low rate of nerve impulses coming from the spinal cord. These nerve impulses, in turn, are controlled partly by signals transmitted from the brain to the appropriate spinal cord anterior motoneurons and partly by signals that originate in *muscle spindles* located in the muscle itself. Both of these signals are discussed in relation to muscle spindle and spinal cord function in Chapter 113.

BIBLIOGRAPHY

Berchtold MW, Brinkmeier H, Muntener M: Calcium ion in skeletal muscle: its crucial role for muscle function, plasticity, and disease, *Physiol. Rev.* 80:1215, 2000.

Cheng H, Lederer WJ: Calcium sparks, *Physiol. Rev.* 88:1491, 2008.

Clausen T: Na$^+$–K$^+$ pump regulation and skeletal muscle contractility, *Physiol. Rev.* 83:1269, 2003.

Huxley AF, Gordon AM: Striation patterns in active and passive shortening of muscle, *Nature (London)* 193:280, 1962.

Kjær M: Role of extracellular matrix in adaptation of tendon and skeletal muscle to mechanical loading, *Physiol. Rev.* 84:649, 2004.

Lieber RL, Ward SR: Skeletal muscle design to meet functional demands, *Philos. Trans. R. Soc. Lond. B Biol. Sci.* 366:1466, 2011.

MacIntosh BR: Role of calcium sensitivity modulation in skeletal muscle performance, *News Physiol. Sci.* 18:222, 2003.

Schiaffino S, Reggiani C: Fiber types in mammalian skeletal muscles, *Physiol. Rev.* 91:1447, 2011.

van Breemen C, Fameli N, Evans AM: Pan-junctional sarcoplasmic reticulum in vascular smooth muscle: nanospace Ca^{2+} transport for site- and function-specific Ca^{2+} signalling, *J. Physiol.* 591:2043, 2013.

17

Applied Skeletal Muscle Physiology

Very strenuous exercise is one of the most stressful conditions that the normal circulatory system faces. This is true because there is such a large amount of skeletal muscle in the body (approximately 40% of body weight), all of it requiring large amounts of blood flow.

Blood Flow Regulation in Skeletal Muscle at Rest and During Exercise

RATE OF BLOOD FLOW THROUGH THE MUSCLES

During rest, blood flow through skeletal muscle averages 3–4 mL/minute per 100 g of muscle. During extreme exercise in the well-conditioned athlete, this can increase 25- to 50-fold, rising to 100–200 mL/minute per 100 g of muscle. Peak blood flows as high as 400 mL/minute per 100 g of muscle have been reported in thigh muscles of endurance-trained athletes.

Blood Flow During Muscle Contractions. Figure 17-1 shows a record of blood flow changes in a calf muscle of a human leg during strong rhythmical muscular exercise. Note that the flow increases and decreases with each muscle contraction. At the end of the contractions, the blood flow remains very high for a few seconds but then returns toward normal during the next few minutes.

The cause of the lower flow during the muscle contraction phase of exercise is compression of the blood vessels by the contracted muscle. During strong tetanic contraction, which causes sustained compression of the blood vessels, the blood flow can be almost stopped, but this also causes rapid weakening of the contraction.

Increased Blood Flow in Muscle Capillaries During Exercise. During rest, some muscle capillaries have little or no flowing blood but during strenuous exercise, all the capillaries open. This opening of dormant capillaries diminishes the distance that oxygen and other nutrients must diffuse from the capillaries to the contracting muscle fibers and sometimes contributes a twofold to threefold increased capillary surface area through which oxygen and nutrients can diffuse from the blood to the tissues.

CONTROL OF BLOOD FLOW IN SKELETAL MUSCLES

Decreased Oxygen in Muscle Greatly Enhances Flow. The tremendous increase in muscle blood flow that occurs during skeletal muscle activity is caused mainly by chemicals acting directly on the muscle arterioles to cause dilation. One of the most important chemical effects is reduction of oxygen in the muscle tissues. When muscles are active, they use oxygen rapidly, thereby decreasing the oxygen concentration in the tissue fluids. This in turn causes local arteriolar vasodilation because the arteriolar walls cannot maintain contraction in the absence of oxygen and because oxygen deficiency causes release of vasodilator substances. Adenosine may be an important vasodilator substance, but experiments have shown that even large amounts of adenosine infused directly into a muscle artery cannot increase blood flow to the same extent as during intense exercise

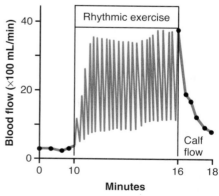

Figure 17-1 Effects of muscle exercise on blood flow in the calf of a leg during strong rhythmical contraction. The blood flow was much less during contractions than between contractions. *Adapted from Barcroft, H., Dornhorst, A.C., 1949. The blood flow through the human calf during rhythmic exercise. J. Physiol. 109, 402.*

and cannot sustain vasodilation in skeletal muscle for more than about 2 hours.

Fortunately, even after the muscle blood vessels have become insensitive to the vasodilator effects of adenosine, still other vasodilator factors continue to maintain increased capillary blood flow as long as the exercise continues. These factors include (1) potassium ions, (2) adenosine triphosphate (ATP), (3) lactic acid, and (4) carbon dioxide. We still do not know quantitatively how great a role each of these factors plays in increasing muscle blood flow during muscle activity.

Nervous Control of Muscle Blood Flow. In addition to local tissue vasodilator mechanisms, skeletal muscles are provided with sympathetic vasoconstrictor nerves and (in some species of animals) sympathetic vasodilator nerves as well.

Sympathetic Vasoconstrictor Nerves. The sympathetic vasoconstrictor nerve fibers secrete norepinephrine at their nerve endings. When maximally activated, this mechanism can decrease blood flow through resting muscles to as little as one-half to one-third of normal. This vasoconstriction is of physiological importance in attenuating decreases of arterial pressure in circulatory shock and during other periods of stress when it may even be necessary to increase arterial pressure.

In addition to the norepinephrine secreted at the sympathetic vasoconstrictor nerve endings, the medullae of the two adrenal glands also secrete large amounts of norepinephrine plus even more epinephrine into the circulating blood during strenuous exercise. The circulating norepinephrine acts on the muscle vessels to cause a vasoconstrictor effect similar to that caused by direct sympathetic nerve stimulation. The epinephrine, however, often has a slight vasodilator effect because epinephrine excites more of the beta-adrenergic receptors of the vessels, which are vasodilator receptors, in contrast to the alpha vasoconstrictor receptors excited especially by norepinephrine.

Muscles in Exercise

STRENGTH, POWER, AND ENDURANCE OF MUSCLES

The final common determinant of success in athletic events is what the muscles can do—that is, what strength they can give when it is needed, what power they can achieve in the performance of work, and how long they can continue their activity.

The strength of a muscle is determined mainly by its size, with a *maximal contractile force between 3 and 4 kg/cm²* of muscle cross-sectional area. Thus, a man who is well supplied with testosterone or who has enlarged his muscles through an exercise training program will have correspondingly increased muscle strength.

Mechanical work performed by a muscle is the amount of force applied by the muscle multiplied by the distance over which the force is applied. The *power* of muscle contraction is different from muscle strength because power is a measure of the total amount of work that the muscle performs in a unit period of time. Power is therefore determined not only by the strength of muscle contraction but also by its *distance of contraction* and the *number of times that it contracts each minute.* Muscle power is generally measured in *kilogram meters per minute.* That is, a muscle that can lift 1-kg weight to a height of 1 m or that can move some object laterally against a force of 1 kg for a distance of 1 m in 1 minute is said to have a power of 1 kg m/minute. The maximal power achievable by all the muscles in the body of a highly trained athlete with all the muscles working together is approximately the following:

	Kilogram Meters Per Minute
First 8–10 seconds	7000
Next 1 minute	4000
Next 30 minutes	1700

Thus, it is clear that a person has the capability of extreme power surges for short periods, such as during a 100-m dash that is completed entirely within 10 seconds, whereas for long-term endurance events, the power output of the muscles is only one-fourth as great as during the initial power surge.

This does not mean that one's athletic performance is four times as great during the initial power surge as it is for the next 30 minutes, because the *efficiency* for translation of muscle power output into athletic performance is often much less during rapid activity than during less rapid but sustained activity. Thus, the velocity of the 100-m dash is only 1.75 times as great as the velocity of a 30-minute race, despite the four-fold difference in short-term versus long-term muscle power capability.

Another measure of muscle performance is *endurance.* Endurance, to a great extent, depends on the nutritive support for the muscle—more than anything else it depends on the amount of glycogen that has been stored in the muscle before the period of exercise. A person who consumes a high-carbohydrate diet stores far more glycogen in muscles than does a person who consumes either a mixed diet or a high-fat diet. Therefore, endurance is enhanced by a high-carbohydrate diet. When athletes run at speeds typical for the marathon race, their endurance (as measured by the time that they can sustain the race until complete exhaustion) is approximately the following:

	Minutes
High-carbohydrate diet	240
Mixed diet	120
High-fat diet	85

The corresponding amounts of glycogen stored in the muscle before the race started explain these differences. The amounts stored are approximately the following:

	Gram Per Kilogram Muscle
High-carbohydrate diet	40
Mixed diet	20
High-fat diet	6

MUSCLE METABOLIC SYSTEMS IN EXERCISE

The basic metabolic systems in muscle are the (1) *phosphocreatine–creatine system,* (2) *glycogen–lactic acid system,* and (3) *aerobic system.*

Adenosine Triphosphate. The source of energy actually used to cause muscle contraction is ATP.

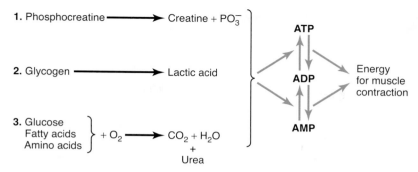

Figure 17-2 Important metabolic systems that supply energy for muscle contraction.

The amount of ATP present in the muscles, even in a well-trained athlete, is sufficient to sustain maximal muscle power for only about 3 seconds, which might be enough for one-half of a 50-m dash. Therefore, except for a few seconds at a time, it is essential that new ATP be formed continuously, even during the performance of short athletic events. Figure 17-2 shows the overall metabolic system, demonstrating the breakdown of ATP first to adenosine diphosphate (ADP) and then to adenosine monophosphate (AMP), with the release of energy to the muscles for contraction. The left-hand side of the figure shows the three metabolic systems that provide a continuous supply of ATP in the muscle fibers.

Phosphocreatine–Creatine System

Phosphocreatine (also called *creatine phosphate*) is another chemical compound that has a high-energy phosphate bond. A special characteristic of energy transfer from phosphocreatine to ATP is that it occurs within a small fraction of a second. Therefore, all the energy stored in muscle phosphocreatine is almost instantaneously available for muscle contraction, just as is the energy stored in ATP.

The combined amounts of cell ATP and cell phosphocreatine are called the *phosphagen energy system*. These substances together can provide maximal muscle power for 8–10 seconds, almost enough for the 100-m run. *Thus, the energy from the phosphagen system is used for maximal short bursts of muscle power.*

Glycogen–Lactic Acid System

The stored glycogen in muscle can be split into glucose and the glucose can then be used for energy. The initial stage of this process, called *glycolysis*, occurs without use of oxygen and, therefore, is said to be *anaerobic metabolism*. During glycolysis, each glucose molecule is split into two *pyruvic acid molecules*, and energy is released to form four ATP molecules for each original glucose molecule. Ordinarily, the pyruvic acid then enters the mitochondria of muscle cells and reacts with oxygen to form still many more ATP molecules. However, when there is insufficient oxygen for this second stage (the oxidative stage) of glucose metabolism to occur, most of the pyruvic acid then is converted into *lactic acid*, which diffuses out of the muscle cells into the interstitial fluid and blood. Therefore, much of the muscle glycogen is transformed to lactic acid, but in doing so, considerable amounts of ATP are formed entirely without consumption of oxygen.

Another characteristic of the glycogen–lactic acid system is that it can form ATP molecules about 2.5 times as rapidly as can the oxidative mechanism of mitochondria. Therefore, when large amounts of ATP are required for short to moderate periods of muscle contraction, this anaerobic glycolysis mechanism can be used as a rapid source of energy. However, it is only about one-half as rapid as the phosphagen system. Under optimal conditions, the glycogen–lactic acid system can provide 1.3–1.6 minutes of maximal muscle activity in addition to the 8–10 seconds provided by the phosphagen system, although at somewhat reduced muscle power.

Aerobic System

The aerobic system is the oxidation of foodstuffs in the mitochondria to provide energy. That is, as shown to the left in Figure 17-2, glucose, fatty acids, and amino acids from the foodstuffs—after some intermediate processing—combine with oxygen to release tremendous amounts of energy that are used to convert AMP and ADP into ATP.

In comparing this aerobic mechanism of energy supply with the glycogen–lactic acid system and the phosphagen system, the relative *maximal rates of power generation* in terms of moles of ATP generation per minute are the following:

	Moles of ATP Per Minute
Phosphagen system	4
Glycogen–lactic acid system	2.5
Aerobic system	1

When comparing the same systems for endurance, the relative values are the following:

	Time
Phosphagen system	8–10 seconds
Glycogen–lactic acid system	1.3–1.6 minutes
Aerobic system	Unlimited time (as long as nutrients last)

Thus, one can readily see that the phosphagen system is used by the muscle for power surges of a few seconds, and the aerobic system is required for prolonged athletic activity. In between is the glycogen–lactic acid system, which is especially important for providing extra power during such intermediate races as the 200- to 800-m runs.

What Types of Sports Use Which Energy Systems?

By considering the vigor of a sports activity and its duration, one can estimate closely which of the energy systems is used for each activity. Various approximations are presented in Table 17-1.

TABLE 17-1	Energy Systems Used in Various Sports

Phosphagen system, almost entirely

  100-m dash
  Jumping
  Weight lifting
  Diving
  Football dashes
  Baseball triple

Phosphagen and glycogen–lactic acid systems

  200-m dash
  Basketball
  Ice hockey dashes

Glycogen–lactic acid system, mainly

  400-m dash
  100-m swim
  Tennis
  Soccer

Glycogen–lactic acid and aerobic systems

  800-m dash
  200-m swim
  1500-m skating
  Boxing
  2000-m rowing
  1500-m run
  1-mile run
  400-m swim

Aerobic system

  10,000-m skating
  Cross-country skiing
  Marathon run (26.2 miles, 42.2 km)
  Jogging

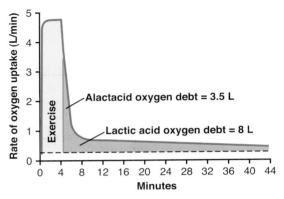

Figure 17-3   Rate of oxygen uptake by the lungs during maximal exercise for 4 minutes and then for about 40 minutes after the exercise is over. This figure demonstrates the principle of *oxygen debt.*

Recovery of the Muscle Metabolic Systems After Exercise

In the same way that the energy from phosphocreatine can be used to reconstitute ATP, energy from the glycogen–lactic acid system can be used to reconstitute both phosphocreatine and ATP. Energy from the oxidative metabolism of the aerobic system can then be used to reconstitute all the other systems—the ATP, phosphocreatine, and glycogen–lactic acid system.

Reconstitution of the lactic acid system means mainly the removal of the excess lactic acid that has accumulated in the body fluids. Removal of the excess lactic acid is especially important because *lactic acid causes extreme fatigue.* When adequate amounts of energy are available from oxidative metabolism, removal of lactic acid is achieved in two ways: (1) a small portion of it is converted back into pyruvic acid and then metabolized oxidatively by the body tissues, and (2) the remaining lactic acid is reconverted into glucose mainly in the liver, and the glucose in turn is used to replenish the glycogen stores of the muscles.

Recovery of the Aerobic System After Exercise

Even during the early stages of heavy exercise, a portion of one's aerobic energy capability is depleted. This depletion results from two effects: (1) the so-called *oxygen debt* and (2) *depletion of the glycogen stores* of the muscles.

Oxygen Debt

The body normally contains about 2 L of stored oxygen that can be used for aerobic metabolism even without breathing any new oxygen. This stored oxygen consists of the following: (1) 0.5 L in the air of the lungs, (2) 0.25 L dissolved in the body fluids, (3) 1 L combined with the hemoglobin of the blood, and (4) 0.3 L

stored in the muscle fibers, combined mainly with myoglobin, an oxygen-binding chemical similar to hemoglobin.

In heavy exercise, almost all this stored oxygen is used within a minute or so for aerobic metabolism. Then, after the exercise is over, this stored oxygen must be replenished by breathing extra amounts of oxygen over and above the normal requirements. In addition, about 9 L more oxygen must be consumed to reconstitute both the phosphagen system and the lactic acid system. All this extra oxygen that must be "repaid," about 11.5 L, is called the *oxygen debt.*

Figure 17-3 shows this principle of oxygen debt. During the first 4 minutes as depicted in the figure, the person exercises heavily, and the rate of oxygen uptake increases more than 15-fold. Then, even after the exercise is over, the oxygen uptake still remains above normal, at first very high while the body is reconstituting the phosphagen system and repaying the stored oxygen portion of the oxygen debt, and then for another 40 minutes at a lower level while the lactic acid is removed. The early portion of the oxygen debt is called the *alactacid oxygen debt* and amounts to about 3.5 L. The latter portion is called the *lactic acid oxygen debt* and amounts to about 8 L.

Recovery of Muscle Glycogen

Recovery from exhaustive muscle glycogen depletion is not a simple matter. This process often requires days, rather than the seconds, minutes, or hours required for recovery of the phosphagen and lactic acid metabolic systems. Figure 17-4 shows this recovery process under three conditions: first, in people who consume a high-carbohydrate diet; second, in people who consume a high-fat, high-protein diet; and third, in people who do not consume food. Note that for persons who consume a high-carbohydrate diet, full recovery occurs in about 2 days. Conversely, people who consume a high-fat, high-protein diet or who do not consume food at all show very little recovery even after as long as 5 days. The messages of this comparison are (1) it is important for athletes to consume a high-carbohydrate diet before a grueling athletic event and (2) athletes should not participate in exhaustive exercise during the 48 hours preceding the event.

NUTRIENTS USED DURING MUSCLE ACTIVITY

In addition to the use of a large amount of carbohydrates by the muscles during exercise, especially during the early stages of exercise, muscles use large amounts of fat for energy in the

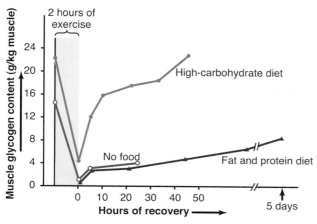

Figure 17-4 The effect of diet on the rate of muscle glycogen replenishment after prolonged exercise. *Modified from Fox, E.L., 1979. Sports Physiology. Saunders College Publishing, Philadelphia.*

form of *fatty acids* and *acetoacetic acid* as well as (to a much less extent) proteins in the form of *amino acids*. In fact, even under the best conditions, in endurance athletic events that last longer than 4–5 hours, the glycogen stores of the muscle become almost totally depleted and are of little further use for energizing muscle contraction. Instead, the muscle now depends on energy from other sources, mainly from fats.

Figure 17-5 shows the approximate relative usage of carbohydrates and fat for energy during prolonged exhaustive exercise under three dietary conditions: a high-carbohydrate diet, a mixed diet, and a high-fat diet. Note that most of the energy is derived from carbohydrates during the first few seconds or minutes of the exercise, but at the time of exhaustion, as much as 60–85% of the energy is being derived from fats, rather than carbohydrates.

Not all the energy from carbohydrates comes from the stored *muscle* glycogen. In fact, almost as much glycogen is stored in the *liver* as in the muscles, and this glycogen can be released into the blood in the form of glucose and then taken up by the

muscles as an energy source. In addition, glucose solutions given to an athlete to drink during the course of an athletic event can provide as much as 30–40% of the energy required during prolonged events such as marathon races.

Therefore, if muscle glycogen and blood glucose are available, they are the energy nutrients of choice for intense muscle activity. Even so, for a long-term endurance event, one can expect fat to supply more than 50% of the required energy after about the first 3–4 hours.

MUSCLE HYPERTROPHY

The average size of a person's muscles is determined to a great extent by heredity plus the level of testosterone secretion, which, in men, causes considerably larger muscles than in women. With training, however, the muscles can become hypertrophied perhaps an additional 30–60%. Most of this hypertrophy results from increased diameter of the muscle fibers rather than increased numbers of fibers. However, a very few greatly enlarged muscle fibers are believed to split down the middle along their entire length to form entirely new fibers, thus increasing the number of fibers slightly.

The changes that occur inside the hypertrophied muscle fibers include (1) increased numbers of myofibrils, proportionate to the degree of hypertrophy; (2) up to 120% increase in mitochondrial enzymes; (3) as much as 60–80% increase in the components of the phosphagen metabolic system, including both ATP and phosphocreatine; (4) as much as 50% increase in stored glycogen; and (5) as much as 75–100% increase in stored triglyceride (fat). Because of all these changes, the capabilities of both the anaerobic and the aerobic metabolic systems are increased, especially increasing the maximum oxidation rate and efficiency of the oxidative metabolic system as much as 45%.

HEREDITARY DIFFERENCES AMONG ATHLETES FOR FAST-TWITCH VERSUS SLOW-TWITCH MUSCLE FIBERS

Some people have considerably more fast-twitch than slow-twitch fibers, and others have more slow-twitch fibers; this factor could determine to some extent the athletic capabilities of different individuals. Athletic training has not been shown to change the relative proportions of fast-twitch and slow-twitch fibers, however much an athlete might want to develop one type of athletic prowess over another. Instead, the relative proportions of fast-twitch and slow-twitch fibers seem to be determined almost entirely by genetic inheritance, which in turn helps determine which area of athletics is most suited to each person: some people appear to be born to be marathoners, whereas others are born to be sprinters and jumpers. For example, the following values are recorded percentages of fast-twitch versus slow-twitch fiber in the quadriceps muscles of different types of athletes:

	Fast-Twitch	Slow-Twitch
Marathoners	18	82
Swimmers	26	74
Average male	55	45
Weight lifters	55	45
Sprinters	63	37
Jumpers	63	37

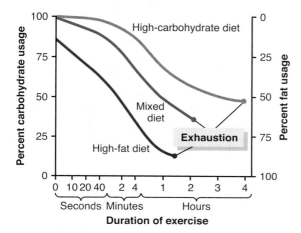

Figure 17-5 The effect of duration of exercise, as well as type of diet, on relative percentages of carbohydrate or fat used for energy by muscles. *Data from Fox, E.L., 1979. Sports Physiology. Saunders College Publishing, Philadelphia.*

Gender Differences in Athletic Performance

Most of the quantitative data that are given in this chapter are for the young male athlete, not because it is desirable to know only these values but because it is only in male athletes that relatively complete measurements have been made. However, for measurements that have been made in the female athlete, similar basic physiological principles apply, except for quantitative differences caused by differences in body size, body composition, and the presence or absence of the male sex hormone testosterone.

In general, most quantitative values for women—such as muscle strength, pulmonary ventilation, and cardiac output, all of which are related mainly to the muscle mass—vary between two-thirds and three-quarters of the values recorded in men, although there are many exceptions to this generalization. When measured in terms of strength per square centimeter of cross-sectional area, the female muscle can achieve almost exactly the same maximal force of contraction as that of the male muscle—between 3 and 4 kg/cm^2. Therefore, most of the difference in total muscle performance lies in the extra percentage of the male body that is muscle, which is caused by endocrine differences that we will discuss later.

The performance capabilities of the female versus male athlete are illustrated by the relative running speeds for a marathon race. In a comparison, the top female performer had a running speed that was 11% less than that of the top male performer. For other events, however, women have at times held records faster than men—for instance, for the two-way swim across the English Channel, for which the availability of extra fat seems to be an advantage for heat insulation, buoyancy, and extra long-term energy.

Testosterone secreted by the male testes has a powerful *anabolic effect* in causing greatly increased deposition of protein everywhere in the body, but especially in the muscles. In fact, even a male who participates in very little sports activity but who nevertheless has a normal level of testosterone will have muscles that grow about 40% larger than those of a comparable female without the testosterone.

The female sex hormone *estrogen* probably also accounts for some of the difference between female and male performance, although not nearly so much as testosterone. Estrogen increases the deposition of fat in the female, especially in the breasts, hips, and subcutaneous tissue. At least partly for this reason, the average nonathletic female has about 27% body fat composition, in contrast to the nonathletic male, who has about 15%. This increased body fat composition is a detriment to the highest levels of athletic performance in those events in which performance depends on speed or on the ratio of total body muscle strength to body weight.

Drugs and Athletes

Without belaboring this issue, let us list some of the effects of drugs in athletics.

First, some people believe that *caffeine* increases athletic performance. In one experiment performed by a marathon runner, running time for the marathon was improved by 7% through the judicious use of caffeine in amounts similar to those found in one to three cups of coffee. Yet experiments by other investigators have failed to confirm any advantage, thus leaving this issue in doubt.

Second, use of *male sex hormones (androgens)* or other anabolic steroids to increase muscle strength undoubtedly can increase athletic performance under some conditions, especially in women and even in men. However, anabolic steroids also greatly increase the risk of cardiovascular disease because they often cause hypertension, decreased high-density blood lipoproteins, and increased low-density lipoproteins, all of which promote heart attacks and strokes.

In men, any type of male sex hormone preparation also leads to decreased testicular function, including both decreased formation of sperm and decreased secretion of the person's own natural testosterone, with residual effects sometimes lasting at least for many months and perhaps indefinitely. In a woman, even more significant effects can occur such as facial hair, a bass voice, ruddy skin, and cessation of menses because she is not normally adapted to the male sex hormone.

Other drugs, such as *amphetamines* and *cocaine*, have been reputed to increase athletic performance. It is equally true that overuse of these drugs can lead to deterioration of performance. Furthermore, experiments have failed to prove the value of these drugs except as a psychic stimulant. Some athletes have been known to die during athletic events because of interaction between such drugs and the norepinephrine and epinephrine released by the sympathetic nervous system during exercise. One of the possible causes of death under these conditions is overexcitability of the heart, leading to ventricular fibrillation, which is lethal within seconds.

BIBLIOGRAPHY

Blair SN, LaMonte MJ, Nichaman MZ: The evolution of physical activity recommendations. How much is enough, *Am. J. Clin. Nutr.* 79:913S, 2004.

Casey DP, Joyner MJ: Compensatory vasodilatation during hypoxic exercise: mechanisms responsible for matching oxygen supply to demand, *J. Physiol.* 590:6321, 2012.

Joyner MJ, Green DJ: Exercise protects the cardiovascular system: effects beyond traditional risk factors, *J. Physiol.* 587:5551, 2009.

Quindry JC: Mechanisms of exercise-induced cardioprotection, *Physiology (Bethesda)* 29:27, 2014.

Rosner MH: Exercise-associated hyponatremia, *Semin. Nephrol.* 29:271, 2009.

Saltin B: Exercise hyperaemia: magnitude and aspects on regulation in humans, *J. Physiol.* 583:819, 2007.

Sandri M: Signaling in muscle atrophy and hypertrophy, *Physiology (Bethesda)* 23:160, 2008.

Schiaffino S, Dyar KA, Ciciliot S, et al: Mechanisms regulating skeletal muscle growth and atrophy, *FEBS J.* 280:4294, 2013.

Seals DR, Edward F: Adolph Distinguished Lecture: the remarkable anti-aging effects of aerobic exercise on systemic arteries, *J. Appl. Physiol.* 117:425, 2014.

Thompson D, Karpe F, Lafontan M, Frayn K: Physical activity and exercise in the regulation of human adipose tissue physiology, *Physiol. Rev.* 92:157, 2012.

Blood and Its Constituents

ANURA KURPAD

18

Introduction to Blood and Plasma Proteins

LEARNING OBJECTIVES

- Describe the formed elements of blood.
- Explain the difference between serum and plasma.
- Broadly describe the functions of blood.
- List the major plasma proteins in blood.
- Describe the functions of plasma proteins.
- Define plasmapheresis and its potential uses.

GLOSSARY OF TERMS

- **Colloid osmotic pressure:** Osmotic pressure exerted by plasma proteins
- **Pinocytosis:** A form of endocytosis in which small particles are brought into the cell suspended within small vesicles that are pinched off from the cell membrane
- **Plasma proteins:** Proteins that are present in the plasma and have a wide variety of functions

Blood makes up about 7–8% of the body weight, which amounts to about 5 L in the adult human. Blood is essential to life, and has several functions. First, it functvions to transport oxygen and nutrients to the tissues from the pulmonary and digestive systems while taking away waste products such as carbon dioxide from the tissues to the pulmonary system. In doing so, it performs an important role in maintaining the pH of the body fluids. Other waste products that are removed from tissues by the blood include lactic acid from muscles (during anaerobic respiration), as well as urea and ammonia. It is also important for maintaining body thermal equilibrium as well as in immunity. It is also a medium for the transport of hormones from their site of production to their site of action. The blood has an intrinsic ability to commence clotting and to reduce or stop blood loss from the body. The blood can be considered to be a specialized tissue composed of many different kinds of cellular and matrix components, such as the red blood cells, white blood cells, platelets, and plasma.

Red blood cells, or erythrocytes, are relatively large microscopic cells without nuclei and make up about half of the total blood volume. The red color of blood is primarily due to oxygenated red cells. White blood cells or leukocytes exist in variable numbers and types but make up a very small part of blood's volume, and are involved in the immune response. They occur outside the blood as well, in the spleen, liver, and lymph nodes. Platelets or thrombocytes are small anuclear bodies that stop bleeding and aid in the process of blood coagulation. The plasma is the cell-free fluid matrix of the blood, which is obtained after centrifugation of anticoagulant-treated blood. On the other hand, serum is the portion of blood after coagulation is complete, that is, it is the plasma without the proteins thvvat are used in coagulation. Plasma is light yellow in color, and

comprises about 55% of blood volume. Plasma contains the plasma proteins, blood clotting factors, sugars, lipids, vitamins, minerals, hormones, enzymes, and antibodies.

Functional Roles of the Plasma Proteins

The major types of protein present in the plasma are *albumin*, *globulin*, and *fibrinogen*. Table 18-1 lists some of the plasma proteins and their important functions.

A major function of *albumin* is to provide *colloid osmotic pressure* in the plasma, which prevents plasma loss from the capillaries, as discussed in Chapter 39.

The *globulins* perform a number of *enzymatic functions* in the plasma, but equally important, they are principally responsible for the body's both natural and acquired *immunity* against invading organisms, discussed in Chapter 25.

Fibrinogen polymerizes into long fibrin threads during blood coagulation, thereby *forming blood clots* that help repair leaks in the circulatory system, discussed in Chapter 27.

FORMATION OF THE PLASMA PROTEINS

Essentially all the albumin and fibrinogen of the plasma proteins, as well as 50–80% of the globulins, are formed in the liver. The remaining globulins are formed almost entirely in the lymphoid tissues. They are mainly the gamma globulins that constitute the antibodies used in the immune system.

The rate of plasma protein formation by the liver can be extremely high, as much as 30 g/day. Certain disease conditions cause rapid loss of plasma proteins; severe burns that denude large surface areas of the skin can cause the loss of several liters of plasma through the denuded areas each day. The rapid

TABLE 18-1	Some of the Plasma Proteins and their Important Functions
Albumin	Maintenance of osmotic pressure Carrier protein Buffering capacity for acid–base balance
Immunoglobulins	Humoral immunity
Transferrin	Iron transport
Ceruloplasmin	Copper transport
C-reactive protein	Acute phase reactant Inflammation
Fibrinogen	Blood coagulation Precursor of fibrin
Coagulation factors	Blood coagulation
Haptoglobin	Hemoglobin transport (outside the RBC)
Hemopexin	Heme binding and transport
Transthyretin	Formerly known as prealbumin Binding and transport of thyroid hormone and retinol

production of plasma proteins by the liver is valuable in preventing death in such states. Occasionally, a person with severe renal disease loses as much as 20 g of plasma protein in the urine each day for months, and it is continually replaced mainly by liver production of the required proteins.

In *cirrhosis of the liver*, large amounts of fibrous tissue develop among the liver parenchymal cells, causing a reduction in their ability to synthesize plasma proteins. As discussed in Chapter 5, this leads to decreased plasma colloid osmotic pressure, which causes generalized edema.

PROTEINS IN THE PLASMA CAUSE COLLOID OSMOTIC PRESSURE

In the basic discussion of osmotic pressure in Chapter 4, it was pointed out that only those molecules or ions that fail to pass through the pores of a semipermeable membrane exert osmotic pressure. Because the proteins are the only dissolved constituents in the plasma and interstitial fluids that do not readily pass through the capillary pores, it is the proteins of the plasma and interstitial fluids that are responsible for the osmotic pressures on the two sides of the capillary membrane. To distinguish this osmotic pressure from that which occurs at the cell membrane, it is called either *colloid osmotic pressure* or *oncotic pressure*. The term "colloid" osmotic pressure is derived from the fact that a protein solution resembles a colloidal solution despite the fact that it is actually a true molecular solution.

Normal Values for Plasma Colloid Osmotic Pressure

The colloid osmotic pressure of normal human plasma averages about 28 mmHg; 19 mmHg of this is caused by molecular effects of the dissolved protein and 9 mmHg by the *Donnan effect*—that is, extra osmotic pressure caused by sodium, potassium, and the other cations held in the plasma by the proteins.

Effect of the Different Plasma Proteins on Colloid Osmotic Pressure

The plasma proteins are a mixture that contains albumin, with an average molecular weight of 69,000; globulins, 140,000; and fibrinogen, 400,000. Thus, 1 g of globulin contains only half as many molecules as 1 g of albumin, and 1 g of fibrinogen contains only one-sixth as many molecules as 1 g of albumin. It should be recalled from the discussion of osmotic pressure in Chapter 4 that osmotic pressure is determined by the *number of molecules* dissolved in a fluid rather than by the mass of these molecules. Therefore, when corrected for number of molecules rather than mass, the following table gives both the relative mass concentrations (gram per deciliter) of the different types of proteins in normal plasma and their respective contributions to the total plasma colloid osmotic pressure (Πp):

	Grams Per Deciliter	Πp (mmHg)
Albumin	4.5	21.8
Globulins	2.5	6.0
Fibrinogen	0.3	0.2
Total	7.3	28.0

Thus, about 80% of the total colloid osmotic pressure of the plasma results from the albumin fraction, 20% from the globulins, and almost none from the fibrinogen. Therefore, from the point of view of capillary and tissue fluid dynamics, it is mainly albumin that is important.

PLASMA PROTEINS AS CARRIER PROTEINS

Some plasma proteins act as carriers for water-insoluble (lipophilic) substances. For example, albumin acts as a carrier of steroid hormones, fatty acids, and thyroid hormones. Other specific carrier proteins in the blood are also important in transporting lipophilic hormones to target cells. These carrier proteins include the sex hormone–binding globulin (SHBG), which binds estradiol and testosterone, corticosteroid-binding globulin (CBG), and thyroxine-binding globulin (TBG).

PLASMA PROTEINS AS A SOURCE OF AMINO ACIDS FOR THE TISSUES

When the tissues become depleted of proteins, the plasma proteins can act as a source of rapid replacement. Indeed, whole plasma proteins can be imbibed in toto by tissue macrophages through the process of pinocytosis; once in these cells, they are split into amino acids that are transported back into the blood and used throughout the body to build cellular proteins wherever needed. In this way, the plasma proteins function as a labile protein storage medium and represent a readily available source of amino acids whenever a particular tissue requires them.

REVERSIBLE EQUILIBRIUM BETWEEN THE PLASMA PROTEINS AND THE TISSUE PROTEINS

There is a constant state of equilibrium, as shown in Figure 18-1, among the plasma proteins, the amino acids of the plasma, and the tissue proteins. It has been estimated from radioactive tracer studies that normally about 400 g of body protein is synthesized and degraded each day as part of the continual state of flux of amino acids. This demonstrates the general principle of reversible exchange of amino acids among the different proteins of the body. Even during starvation or severe debilitating diseases, the ratio of total tissue proteins to total plasma proteins in the body remains relatively constant at about 33:1.

Because of this reversible equilibrium between plasma proteins and the other proteins of the body, one of the most effective therapies for severe, acute whole-body protein deficiency is

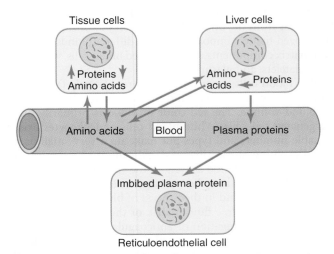

Figure 18-1 Reversible equilibrium among the tissue proteins, plasma proteins, and plasma amino acids.

intravenous transfusion of plasma protein. Within a few days, or sometimes within hours, the amino acids of the administered protein are distributed throughout the cells of the body to form new proteins as needed.

A reduction in plasma concentration of proteins because of either failure to produce normal amounts of proteins or leakage of proteins from the plasma causes the plasma colloid osmotic pressure to fall. This leads to increased capillary filtration throughout the body and extracellular edema.

Plasmapheresis

Plasmapheresis is a process in which plasma can be removed from the blood without removing the red blood cells. Blood is drawn from the patient and the plasma separated from it. The red blood cells are returned to the body of the patient such that there is no loss of these cells, yet some plasma was removed. The plasmapheresis process can be used on patients who have excess plasma proteins in their blood, making it viscous, or on those who have certain antibodies present in their blood.

BIBLIOGRAPHY

Anderson NL, Anderson NG: High resolution two-dimensional electrophoresis of human plasma proteins, *Proc. Natl. Acad. Sci. U. S. A.* 74:5421, 1977.

Anderson NL, Anderson NG: The human plasma proteome: history, character, and diagnostic prospects, *Mol. Cell. Proteomics* 1:845, 2002.

Prudent M, Tissot JD, Lion N: Proteomics of blood and derived products: what's next? *Expert Rev. Proteomics* 8:717, 2011.

19

Red Blood Cells (Erythrocytes)

GLOSSARY OF TERMS
- **Glucose-6-phosphate dehydrogenase (G6PD):** An enzyme in the pentose phosphate pathway [G6PD converts glucose-6-phosphate into 6-phosphoglucono-δ-lactone; this pathway maintains the level of the co-enzyme nicotinamide adenine dinucleotide phosphate (NADPH), which in turn maintains the supply of reduced glutathione, which prevents oxidative damage]
- **Hematocrit:** The proportion of whole blood that is red blood cells, typically about 42%
- **Kupffer cells:** Specialized macrophages located in the liver, lining the walls of the sinusoids (these cells form part of the reticuloendothelial system)

BOX 19-1   PHYSIOLOGICAL AND PATHOLOGICAL VARIATIONS IN RED BLOOD CELL COUNT
- Increased in response to hypoxia (physiological)
- Increased in polycythemia (pathological)
- Decreased in nutritional anemia
- Decreased in hemolytic anemia

A major function of red blood cells, also known as *erythrocytes*, is to transport *hemoglobin*, which in turn carries oxygen from the lungs to the tissues. In some lower animals, hemoglobin circulates as free protein in the plasma, not enclosed in red blood cells. When it is free in the plasma of the human being, about 3% of it leaks through the capillary membrane into the tissue spaces or through the glomerular membrane of the kidney into the glomerular filtrate each time the blood passes through the capillaries. Therefore, hemoglobin must remain inside red blood cells to effectively perform its functions in humans.

The red blood cells have other functions besides transport of hemoglobin. For instance, they contain a large quantity of *carbonic anhydrase*, an enzyme that catalyzes the reversible reaction between carbon dioxide (CO_2) and water to form carbonic acid (H_2CO_3), increasing the rate of this reaction several thousandfold. The rapidity of this reaction makes it possible for the water of the blood to transport enormous quantities of CO_2 in the form of bicarbonate ion (HCO_3^-) from the tissues to the lungs, where it is reconverted to CO_2 and expelled into the atmosphere as a body waste product. The hemoglobin in the cells is an excellent *acid–base buffer* (as is true of most proteins), so the red blood cells are responsible for most of the acid–base buffering power of whole blood.

Shape and Size of Red Blood Cells

Normal red blood cells, shown in Figure 20-3, are biconcave discs having a mean diameter of about 7.8 μm and a thickness of 2.5 μm at the thickest point and 1 μm or less in the center. The average volume of the red blood cell is 90–95 μm³.

The shapes of red blood cells can change remarkably as the cells squeeze through capillaries. Actually, the red blood cell is a "bag" that can be deformed into almost any shape. Furthermore, because the normal cell has a great excess of cell membrane for the quantity of material inside, deformation does not stretch the membrane greatly and, consequently, does not rupture the cell, as would be the case with many other cells.

Concentration of Red Blood Cells in the Blood

In healthy men, the average number of red blood cells per cubic millimeter is 5,200,000 (±300,000); in women, it is 4,700,000 (±300,000). Persons living at high altitudes have greater numbers of red blood cells, as discussed later (Box 19-1).

Quantity of Hemoglobin in the Cells

Red blood cells have the ability to concentrate hemoglobin in the cell fluid up to about 34 g in each 100 mL of cells. The concentration does not rise above this value because this is the metabolic limit of the cell's hemoglobin-forming mechanism. Furthermore, in normal people, the percentage of hemoglobin is almost always near the maximum in each cell. However, when hemoglobin formation is deficient, the percentage of hemoglobin in the cells may fall considerably below this value and the volume of the red cell may also decrease because of diminished hemoglobin to fill the cell.

When the hematocrit (the percentage of blood that is in cells—normally, 40–45%) and the quantity of hemoglobin in each respective cell are normal, the whole blood of men contains an average of 15 g of hemoglobin per 100 mL of cells; for women, it contains an average of 14 g per 100 mL.

As discussed in connection with blood transport of oxygen in Chapter 59, each gram of pure hemoglobin is capable of combining with 1.34 mL of oxygen. Therefore, in a normal man a maximum of about 20 mL of oxygen can be carried in combination with hemoglobin in each 100 mL of blood, and in a normal woman 19 mL of oxygen can be carried.

HEMATOCRIT

The proportion of the blood that is red blood cells is called the *hematocrit*. Thus, if a person has a hematocrit of 40, this means that 40% of the blood volume is made up of cells and the remainder is plasma. The hematocrit of adult men averages about 42, while that of women averages about 38. These values vary tremendously, depending on whether the person has anemia, on the degree of bodily activity, and on the altitude at which the person resides.

The hematocrit is the fraction of the blood composed of red blood cells, as determined by centrifuging blood in a "hematocrit tube" until the cells become tightly packed in the bottom of the tube. It is impossible to completely pack the red cells together; therefore, about 3–4% of the plasma remains entrapped among the cells, and the true hematocrit is only about 96% of the measured hematocrit.

In men, the measured hematocrit is normally about 0.40, and in women, it is about 0.36. In severe *anemia*, the hematocrit may fall as low as 0.10, a value that is barely sufficient to sustain life. Conversely, there are some conditions in which there is excessive production of red blood cells, resulting in *polycythemia*. In these conditions, the hematocrit can rise to 0.65.

Life Span of Red Blood Cells Is About 120 Days

When red blood cells are delivered from the bone marrow into the circulatory system, they normally circulate an average of 120 days before being destroyed. Even though mature red cells do not have a nucleus, mitochondria, or endoplasmic reticulum, they do have cytoplasmic enzymes that are capable of metabolizing glucose and forming small amounts of adenosine triphosphate (ATP). These enzymes also (1) maintain pliability of the cell membrane, (2) maintain membrane transport of ions, (3) keep the iron of the cells' hemoglobin in the ferrous form rather than ferric form, and (4) prevent oxidation of the proteins in the red cells. Even so, the metabolic systems of old red cells become progressively less active and the cells become more and more fragile, presumably because their life processes wear out.

Once the red cell membrane becomes fragile, the cell ruptures during passage through some tight spot of the circulation. Many of the red cells self-destruct in the spleen, where they squeeze through the red pulp of the spleen. There, the spaces between the structural trabeculae of the red pulp, through which most of the cells must pass, are only 3 μm wide, in comparison with the 8-μm diameter of the red cell. When the spleen is removed, the number of old abnormal red cells circulating in the blood increases considerably.

FRAGILITY OF RED BLOOD CELLS

The fragility of red blood cells is related to their shape, deformability, surface area/volume ratio, and intrinsic membrane properties. Since the biconcave shape and deformability of these cells allow them to squeeze through capillaries and the splenic pulp, a change in shape (to spherical, eg) would lead to their trapping and eventual destruction. Congenital hemolytic anemia, which occurs, for example, in hereditary spherocytosis, is suggested by a positive family history, and the triad of anemia, splenomegaly, and jaundice. Enzymatic deficiencies can also lead to hemolysis. Glucose-6-phosphate dehydrogenase (G6PD) deficiency leads to hemolysis of red blood cells when they are exposed to oxidative stress, since G6PD maintains levels of the important intracellular antioxidant glutathione.

DESTRUCTION OF HEMOGLOBIN

When red blood cells burst and release their hemoglobin, the hemoglobin is phagocytized almost immediately by macrophages in many parts of the body, but especially by the Kupffer cells of the liver and macrophages of the spleen and bone marrow. During the next few hours to days, the macrophages release iron from the hemoglobin and pass it back into the blood, to be carried by transferrin either to the bone marrow for the production of new red blood cells or to the liver and other tissues for storage in the form of ferritin. The porphyrin portion of the hemoglobin molecule is converted by the macrophages, through a series of stages, into the bile pigment *bilirubin*, which is released into the blood and later removed from the body by secretion through the liver into the bile; this is discussed in relation to liver function in Chapter 69.

Erythrocyte Sedimentation Rate

If a column of anticoagulated fresh blood is left to stand by itself without disturbance, the erythrocytes begin to settle at the bottom, leaving the clear plasma above. The rate of sedimentation of the erythrocytes is called the erythrocyte sedimentation rate (ESR). The ESR tends to be higher in women, with increasing age, and during pregnancy. When there is an increase in fibrinogen, immunoglobulins, or acute-phase reactants, the erythrocytes tend to cluster together to form stacks known as *rouleaux* and settle more quickly. Therefore, the ESR is higher in some disease conditions, such as infections, malignancies, and chronic disease states. However, it should be noted that this is a nondiscriminatory test for these conditions, and may perform poorly as a screening test in those individuals who have no symptoms. It is best used to follow the course of the disease as a prognostic test.

The ESR can be measured by the Wintrobe or Westergren method, but the values for ESR vary in both these methods because of differences in the tube length and shape. The ESR rate is given as millimeters per hour, and is up to 15 mm/hour in men and up to 20 mm/hour in women, measured by the Westergren method.

BIBLIOGRAPHY

Alayash AI: Oxygen therapeutics: can we tame haemoglobin? *Nat. Rev. Drug Discov.* 3:152, 2004.

Alleyne M, Horne MK, Miller JL: Individualized treatment for iron-deficiency anemia in adults, *Am. J. Med.* 121:943, 2008.

Claster S, Vichinsky EP: Managing sickle cell disease, *BMJ* 327:1151, 2003.

Coates D: Physiology and pathophysiology of iron in hemoglobin associated diseases, *Free Radic. Biol. Med.* 72C:23, 2014.

Elliott S, Pham E, Macdougall IC: Erythropoietins: a common mechanism of action, *Exp. Hematol.* 36:1573, 2008.

Fandrey J: Oxygen-dependent and tissue-specific regulation of erythropoietin gene expression, *Am. J. Physiol. Regul. Integr. Comp. Physiol.* 286: R977, 2004.

Hentze MW, Muckenthaler MU, Andrews NC: Balancing acts: molecular control of mammalian iron metabolism, *Cell* 117:285, 2004.

Kato GJ, Gladwin MT: Evolution of novel small-molecule therapeutics targeting sickle cell vasculopathy, *JAMA* 300:2638, 2008.

Lappin T: The cellular biology of erythropoietin receptors, *Oncologist* 8(Suppl. 1):15, 2003.

Maxwell P: HIF-1: an oxygen response system with special relevance to the kidney, *J. Am. Soc. Nephrol.* 14:2712, 2003.

Metcalf D: Hematopoietic cytokines, *Blood* 111:485, 2008.

Nangaku M, Eckardt KU: Hypoxia and the HIF system in kidney disease, *J. Mol. Med.* 85:1325, 2007.

Percy MJ, Rumi E: Genetic origins and clinical phenotype of familial and acquired erythrocytosis and thrombocytosis, *Am. J. Hematol.* 84:46, 2009.

Pietrangelo A: Hereditary hemochromatosis—a new look at an old disease, *N. Engl. J. Med.* 350:2383, 2004.

Platt OS: Hydroxyurea for the treatment of sickle cell anemia, *N. Engl. J. Med.* 27(358):1362, 2008.

20

Erythropoiesis

LEARNING OBJECTIVES

- Describe the stages of development of RBCs.
- Describe the factors regulating erythropoiesis.
- Describe the sources of erythropoietin and its role in erythropoiesis.

GLOSSARY OF TERMS

- **Sprue:** Tropical sprue, commonly found in the tropical areas, being a condition in which there is malabsorption of many nutrients from the small intestine due to abnormally flattened villi and inflammation of the small intestinal mucosa

- **Yolk sac:** Membranous sac attached to an embryo, providing early nourishment to the embryo

Areas of the Body that Produce Red Blood Cells

In the early weeks of embryonic life, primitive, nucleated red blood cells are produced in the *yolk sac*. During the middle trimester of gestation, the *liver* is the main organ for production of red blood cells, but reasonable numbers are also produced in the *spleen* and *lymph nodes*. Then, during the last month or so of gestation and after birth, red blood cells are produced exclusively in the *bone marrow*.

As demonstrated in Figure 20-1, the bone marrow of essentially all bones produces red blood cells until a person is 5 years old. The marrow of the long bones, except for the proximal portions of the humeri and tibiae, becomes quite fatty and produces no more red blood cells after about age 20 years. Beyond this age, most red cells continue to be produced in the marrow of the membranous bones, such as the vertebrae, sternum, ribs, and ilia. Even in these bones, the marrow becomes less productive as age increases.

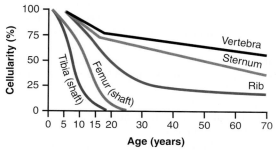

Figure 20-1 Relative rates of red blood cell production in the bone marrow of different bones at different ages.

Genesis of Blood Cells

PLURIPOTENTIAL HEMATOPOIETIC STEM CELLS, GROWTH INDUCERS, AND DIFFERENTIATION INDUCERS

The blood cells begin their lives in the bone marrow from a single type of cell called the *pluripotential hematopoietic stem cell*, from which all the cells of the circulating blood are eventually derived. Figure 20-2 shows the successive divisions of the pluripotential cells to form the different circulating blood cells. As these cells reproduce, a small portion of them remains exactly like the original pluripotential cells and is retained in the bone marrow to maintain a supply of these, although their numbers diminish with age. Most of the reproduced cells, however, differentiate to form the other cell types shown to the right in Figure 20-2. The intermediate-stage cells are very much like the pluripotential stem cells, even though they have already become committed to a particular line of cells and are called *committed stem cells*.

The different committed stem cells, when grown in culture, will produce colonies of specific types of blood cells. A committed stem cell that produces erythrocytes is called a *colony-forming unit-erythrocyte*, and the abbreviation CFU-E is used to designate this type of stem cell. Likewise, colony-forming units that form granulocytes and monocytes have the designation CFU-GM and so forth.

Growth and reproduction of the different stem cells are controlled by multiple proteins called *growth inducers*. At least four major growth inducers have been described, each having different characteristics. One of these, *interleukin-3*, promotes growth and reproduction of virtually all the different types of committed stem cells, whereas the others induce growth of only specific types of cells.

The growth inducers promote growth but not differentiation of the cells, which is the function of another set of proteins called *differentiation inducers*. Each of these differentiation inducers causes one type of committed stem cell to differentiate one or more steps toward a final adult blood cell.

Formation of the growth inducers and differentiation inducers is controlled by factors outside the bone marrow. For instance, in the case of erythrocytes (red blood cells), exposure of the blood to low oxygen for a long time causes growth induction, differentiation, and production of greatly increased numbers of erythrocytes, as discussed later in the chapter. In the case of some of the white blood cells, infectious diseases cause growth, differentiation, and eventual formation of specific types of white blood cells that are needed to combat each infection.

Stages of Differentiation of Red Blood Cells

The first cell that can be identified as belonging to the red blood cell series is the *proerythroblast*, shown at the starting point in Figure 20-3. Under appropriate stimulation, large numbers of these cells are formed from the CFU-E stem cells.

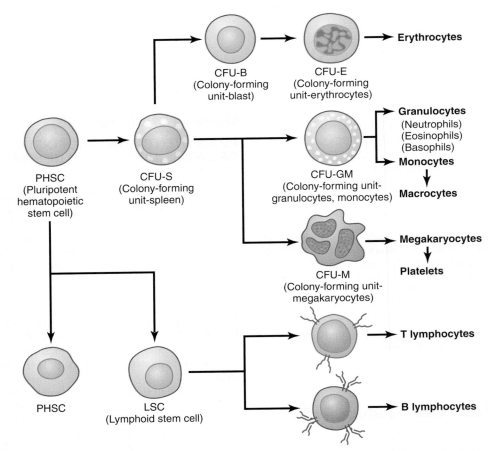

Figure 20-2   Formation of the multiple different blood cells from the original *pluripotent hematopoietic stem cell (PHSC)* in the bone marrow.

Once the proerythroblast has been formed, it divides multiple times, eventually forming many mature red blood cells. The first-generation cells are called *basophil erythroblasts* because they stain with basic dyes; the cell at this time has accumulated very little hemoglobin. In the succeeding generations, as shown in Figure 20-3, the cells become filled with hemoglobin to a concentration of about 34%, the nucleus condenses to a small size, and its final remnant is absorbed or extruded from the cell. At the same time, the endoplasmic reticulum is also reabsorbed. The cell at this stage is called a *reticulocyte* because it still contains a small amount of basophilic material, consisting of remnants of the Golgi apparatus, mitochondria, and a few other cytoplasmic organelles. During this reticulocyte stage, the cells pass from the bone marrow into the blood capillaries by *diapedesis* (squeezing through the pores of the capillary membrane).

The remaining basophilic material in the reticulocyte normally disappears within 1–2 days, and the cell is then a *mature erythrocyte*. Because of the short life of the reticulocytes, their concentration among all the red cells of the blood is normally slightly less than 1%.

Erythropoietin Regulates Red Blood Cell Production

The total mass of red blood cells in the circulatory system is regulated within narrow limits, so (1) an adequate red cells are always available to provide sufficient transport of oxygen from the lungs to the tissues, yet (2) the cells do not become so numerous that they impede blood flow. This control mechanism is diagrammed in Figure 20-4 and is as follows.

TISSUE OXYGENATION IS THE MOST ESSENTIAL REGULATOR OF RED BLOOD CELL PRODUCTION

Conditions that decrease the quantity of oxygen transported to the tissues ordinarily increase the rate of red blood cell production. Thus, when a person becomes extremely *anemic*, as a result of hemorrhage or any other condition, the bone marrow begins to produce large quantities of red blood cells. Also, destruction of major portions of the bone marrow, especially by X-ray therapy, causes hyperplasia of the remaining bone marrow, in an attempt to supply the demand for red blood cells in the body.

At very *high altitudes*, where the quantity of oxygen in the air is greatly decreased, insufficient oxygen is transported to the tissues and red cell production is greatly increased. In this case, it is not only the concentration of red blood cells in the blood that controls red cell production but also the amount of oxygen transported to the tissues in relation to tissue demand for oxygen.

Various diseases of the circulation that decrease tissue blood flow, and particularly those that cause failure of oxygen absorption by the blood as it passes through the lungs, can also increase the rate of red cell production. This result is especially apparent in prolonged *cardiac failure* and in many *lung diseases* because the tissue hypoxia resulting from these conditions increases red

Genesis of RBCs

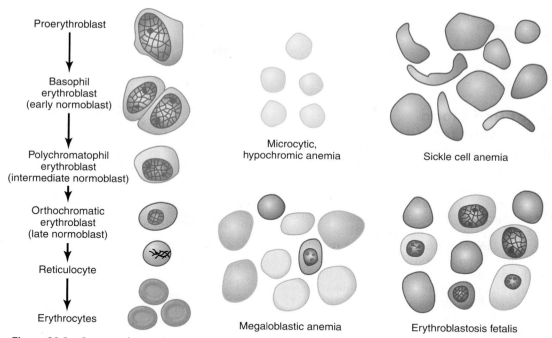

Figure 20-3 Genesis of normal red blood cells (RBCs) and characteristics of RBCs in different types of anemias.

cell production, with a resultant increase in hematocrit and usually total blood volume as well.

ERYTHROPOIETIN STIMULATES RED BLOOD CELL PRODUCTION, AND ITS FORMATION INCREASES IN RESPONSE TO HYPOXIA

The principal stimulus for red blood cell production in low oxygen states is a circulating hormone called *erythropoietin*, a glycoprotein with a molecular weight of about 34,000. In the absence of erythropoietin, hypoxia has little or no effect to stimulate red

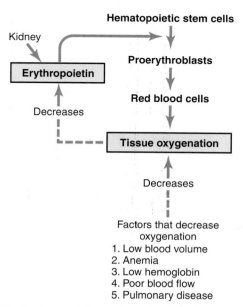

Figure 20-4 Function of the erythropoietin mechanism to increase production of red blood cells when tissue oxygenation decreases.

blood cell production. But when the erythropoietin system is functional, hypoxia causes a marked increase in erythropoietin production, and the erythropoietin in turn enhances red blood cell production until the hypoxia is relieved.

ERYTHROPOIETIN IS FORMED MAINLY IN THE KIDNEYS

Normally, about 90% of all erythropoietin is formed in the kidneys, and the remainder is formed mainly in the liver. It is not known exactly where in the kidneys the erythropoietin is formed. Some studies suggest that erythropoietin is secreted mainly by fibroblast-like interstitial cells surrounding the tubules in the cortex and outer medulla, where much of the kidney's oxygen consumption occurs. It is likely that other cells, including the renal epithelial cells, also secrete the erythropoietin in response to hypoxia.

Renal tissue hypoxia leads to increased tissue levels of *hypoxia-inducible factor-1* (HIF-1), which serves as a transcription factor for a large number of hypoxia-inducible genes, including the erythropoietin gene. HIF-1 binds to a *hypoxia response element* residing in the erythropoietin gene, inducing transcription of messenger RNA and, ultimately, increased erythropoietin synthesis.

At times, hypoxia in other parts of the body, but not in the kidneys, stimulates kidney erythropoietin secretion, which suggests that there might be some non-renal sensor that sends an additional signal to the kidneys to produce this hormone. In particular, both norepinephrine and epinephrine and several of the prostaglandins stimulate erythropoietin production.

When both kidneys are removed from a person or when the kidneys are destroyed by renal disease, the person invariably becomes very anemic because the 10% of the normal erythropoietin formed in other tissues (mainly in the liver) is sufficient to cause only one-third to one-half of the red blood cell formation needed by the body.

BOX 20-1   FACTORS AFFECTING ERYTHROPOIESIS AND MATURATION OF RBCs

- Hypoxia and erythropoietin
- Dietary protein and energy
- Vitamin B_{12}
- Folic acid
- Pyridoxine
- Riboflavin

- Niacin
- Ascorbic acid (vitamin C)
- Vitamin A
- Vitamin E
- Iron
- Copper

Maturation of Red Blood Cells—Requirement for Vitamin B_{12} (Cyanocobalamin) and Folic Acid

Because of the continuing need to replenish red blood cells, the erythropoietic cells of the bone marrow are among the most rapidly growing and reproducing cells in the entire body. Therefore, as would be expected, their maturation and rate of production are affected greatly by a person's nutritional status.

Especially important for final maturation of the red blood cells are two vitamins, *vitamin B_{12}* and *folic acid*. Both of these are essential for the synthesis of DNA because each, in a different way, is required for the formation of thymidine triphosphate, one of the essential building blocks of DNA. Therefore, lack of either vitamin B_{12} or folic acid causes abnormal and diminished DNA and, consequently, failure of nuclear maturation and cell division. Furthermore, the erythroblastic cells of the bone marrow, in addition to failing to proliferate rapidly, produce mainly larger than normal red cells called *macrocytes* and the cell itself has a flimsy membrane and is often irregular, large, and oval instead of the usual biconcave disc. These poorly formed cells, after entering the circulating blood, are capable of carrying oxygen normally, but their fragility causes them to have a short life, one-half to one-third normal. Therefore, it is said that deficiency of either vitamin B_{12} or folic acid causes *maturation failure* in the process of erythropoiesis (Box 20-1).

MATURATION FAILURE CAUSED BY POOR ABSORPTION OF VITAMIN B_{12} FROM THE GASTROINTESTINAL TRACT—PERNICIOUS ANEMIA

A common cause of red blood cell maturation failure is failure to absorb vitamin B_{12} from the gastrointestinal tract. This often occurs in the disease *pernicious anemia*, in which the basic abnormality is an *atrophic gastric mucosa* that fails to produce normal gastric secretions. The parietal cells of the gastric glands secrete a glycoprotein called *intrinsic factor*, which combines with vitamin B_{12} in food and makes it available for absorption by the gut. It does this in the following way: (1) Intrinsic factor binds tightly with the vitamin B_{12}. In this bound state, vitamin B_{12} is protected from digestion by the gastrointestinal secretions. (2) Still in the bound state, intrinsic factor binds to specific receptor sites on the brush border membranes of the mucosal cells in the ileum. (3) Then, vitamin B_{12} is transported into the blood during the next few hours by the process of pinocytosis, carrying intrinsic factor and the vitamin together through the membrane. Lack of intrinsic factor, therefore, decreases availability of vitamin B_{12} because of faulty absorption of the vitamin.

Once vitamin B_{12} has been absorbed from the gastrointestinal tract, it is first stored in large quantities in the liver and then released slowly as needed by the bone marrow. The minimum amount of vitamin B_{12} required each day to maintain normal red cell maturation is only 1–3 mcg, and the normal storage in the liver and other body tissues is about 1000 times this amount. Therefore, 3–4 years of defective vitamin B_{12} absorption are usually required to cause maturation failure anemia.

FAILURE OF MATURATION CAUSED BY DEFICIENCY OF FOLIC ACID (PTEROYLGLUTAMIC ACID)

Folic acid is a normal constituent of green vegetables, some fruits, and meats (especially liver). However, it is easily destroyed during cooking. Also, people with gastrointestinal absorption abnormalities, such as the frequently occurring small intestinal disease called *sprue*, often have serious difficulty absorbing both folic acid and vitamin B_{12}. Therefore, in many instances of maturation failure the cause is deficiency of intestinal absorption of both folic acid and vitamin B_{12}.

A summary of factors regulating erythropoiesis and maturation of RBCs is given as follows:

Hormones: Erythropoietin, androgens, thyroid hormone, corticosteroid hormones

Vitamins: Vitamin B_{12} (and intrinsic factor), folic acid, pyridoxine, vitamin C (helps iron absorption)

Minerals: iron, copper

BIBLIOGRAPHY

Elliott S, Pham E, Macdougall IC: Erythropoietins: a common mechanism of action, *Exp. Hematol.* 36:1573, 2008.

Fandrey J: Oxygen-dependent and tissue-specific regulation of erythropoietin gene expression, *Am. J. Physiol. Regul. Integr. Comp. Physiol.* 286:R977, 2004.

Lappin T: The cellular biology of erythropoietin receptors, *Oncologist* 8(Suppl. 1):15, 2003.

Maxwell P: HIF-1: an oxygen response system with special relevance to the kidney, *J. Am. Soc. Nephrol.* 14:2712, 2003.

Metcalf D: Hematopoietic cytokines, *Blood* 111:485, 2008.

Nangaku M, Eckardt KU: Hypoxia and the HIF system in kidney disease, *J. Mol. Med.* 85:1325, 2007.

21

Hemoglobin

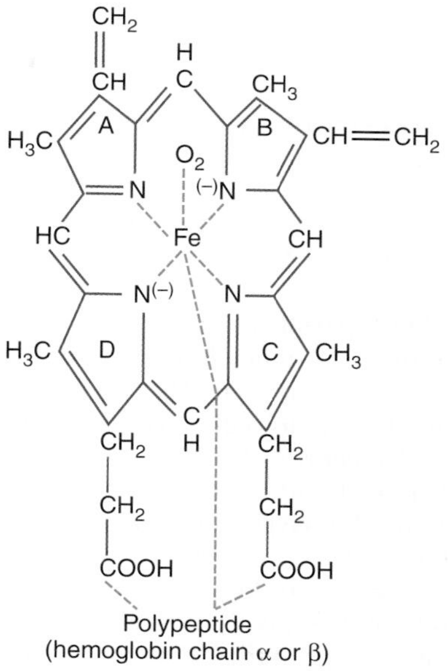

Figure 21-2 Basic structure of the hemoglobin molecule, showing one of the four heme chains that bind together to form the hemoglobin molecule.

Formation of Hemoglobin

Synthesis of hemoglobin begins in the proerythroblasts and continues even into the reticulocyte stage of the red blood cells. Therefore, when reticulocytes leave the bone marrow and pass into the bloodstream, they continue to form minute quantities of hemoglobin for another day or so until they become mature erythrocytes.

Figure 21-1 shows the basic chemical steps in the formation of hemoglobin. First, succinyl-CoA, formed in the Krebs metabolic cycle, binds with glycine to form a pyrrole molecule. In turn, four pyrroles combine to form protoporphyrin IX, which then combines with iron to form the *heme* molecule. Finally, each heme molecule combines with a long polypeptide chain, a *globin* synthesized by ribosomes, forming a subunit of hemoglobin called a *hemoglobin chain* (Figure 21-2). Each chain has a molecular weight of about 16,000; four of these in turn bind together loosely to form the whole hemoglobin molecule.

There are several slight variations in the different subunit hemoglobin chains, depending on the amino acid composition of the polypeptide portion. The different types of chains are designated *alpha chains*, *beta chains*, *gamma chains*, and *delta chains*. The most common form of hemoglobin in the adult human being, *hemoglobin A*, is a combination of *two alpha chains* and *two beta chains*. Hemoglobin A has a molecular weight of 64,458 (Table 21-1).

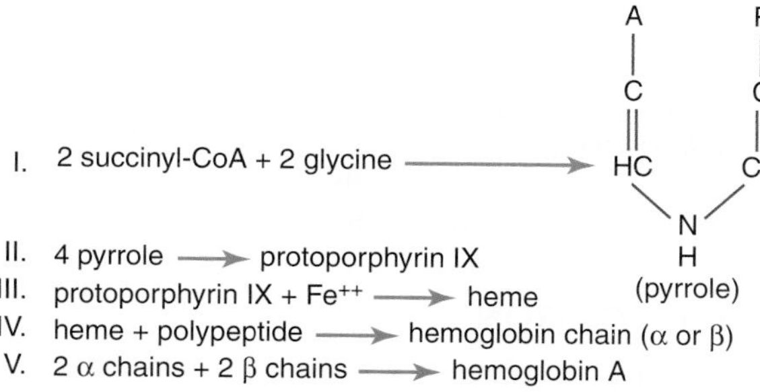

Because each hemoglobin chain has a heme prosthetic group containing an atom of iron, and because there are four hemoglobin chains in each hemoglobin molecule, one finds four iron atoms in each hemoglobin molecule; each of these can bind loosely with one molecule of oxygen, making a total of four molecules of oxygen (or eight oxygen atoms) that can be transported by each hemoglobin molecule.

The types of hemoglobin chains in the hemoglobin molecule determine the binding affinity of the hemoglobin for oxygen. Abnormalities of the chains can alter the physical characteristics of the hemoglobin molecule as well. For instance, in *sickle cell anemia*, the amino acid *valine* is substituted for *glutamic acid* at one point in each of the two beta chains (Table 21-1). When this type of hemoglobin is exposed to low oxygen, it forms elongated crystals inside the red blood cells that are sometimes 15 μm in length. These make it almost impossible for the cells to pass through many small capillaries, and the spiked ends of the crystals are likely to rupture the cell membranes, leading to sickle cell anemia.

COMBINATION OF HEMOGLOBIN WITH OXYGEN

The most important feature of the hemoglobin molecule is its ability to combine loosely and reversibly with oxygen. This ability is discussed in detail in Chapter 59 in relation to respiration because the primary function of hemoglobin in the body is to combine with oxygen in the lungs and then to release this

I.   2 succinyl-CoA + 2 glycine ⟶

II. 4 pyrrole ⟶ protoporphyrin IX

III. protoporphyrin IX + Fe++ ⟶ heme

IV. heme + polypeptide ⟶ hemoglobin chain (α or β)

V.   2 α chains + 2 β chains ⟶ hemoglobin A

Figure 21-1 Summary of formation of hemoglobin. *CoA*, coenzyme A.

TABLE 21-1	Inherited Disorders of Hemoglobin	
Condition	**Abnormality**	**Functional Abnormality**
Normal globin chains		
α-Thalassemia	Reduced or no production of α-globin chains	Dysfunctional Hb (HbB, Hb Barts)
β-Thalassemia	Reduced or no production of β-globin chains	Dysfunctional erythropoiesis
		Unstable RBC membrane

Condition	**Mutation (Position on β-Globin Chain)**	**Functional Abnormality**
Abnormal globin chains		
Hb S (sickle cell anemia)	Val → Glu (6)	Aggregation, shortened survival
Hb C	Lys → Glu (6)	Shortened RBC survival
Hb E	Glu → Lys (26)	Microcytosis
Hb M	Tyr → His (63)	Methemoglobin formation

oxygen readily in the peripheral tissue capillaries, where the gaseous tension of oxygen is much lower than in the lungs.

Oxygen *does not* combine with the two positive bonds of the iron in the hemoglobin molecule. Instead, it binds loosely with one of the so-called coordination bonds of the iron atom. This is an extremely loose bond, so the combination is easily reversible. Furthermore, the oxygen does not become ionic oxygen but is carried as molecular oxygen (composed of two oxygen atoms) to the tissues, where, because of the loose, readily reversible combination, it is released into the tissue fluids still in the form of molecular oxygen rather than ionic oxygen.

Iron Metabolism

Because iron is important for the formation not only of hemoglobin but also of other essential elements in the body (eg, *myoglobin, cytochromes, cytochrome oxidase, peroxidase, catalase*), it is important to understand the means by which iron is utilized in the body. The total quantity of iron in the body averages 4–5 g, about 65% of which is in the form of hemoglobin. About 4% is in the form of myoglobin, 1% is in the form of the various heme compounds that promote intracellular oxidation, 0.1% is combined with the protein transferrin in the blood plasma, and 15–30% is stored for later use, mainly in the reticuloendothelial system and liver parenchymal cells, principally in the form of ferritin.

TRANSPORT AND STORAGE OF IRON

Transport, storage, and metabolism of iron in the body are diagrammed in Figure 21-3 and can be explained as follows: When iron is absorbed from the small intestine, it immediately combines in the blood plasma with a beta globulin, *apotransferrin*, to form *transferrin*, which is then transported in the plasma. The iron is loosely bound in the transferrin and, consequently, can be released to any tissue cell at any point in the body. Excess iron in the blood is deposited *especially* in the liver hepatocytes and less in the reticuloendothelial cells of the bone marrow.

In the cell cytoplasm, iron combines mainly with a protein, *apoferritin*, to form *ferritin*. Apoferritin has a molecular weight of about 460,000, and varying quantities of iron can combine in clusters of iron radicals with this large molecule; therefore, ferritin may contain only a small amount of iron or a large amount. This iron stored as ferritin is called *storage iron*.

Smaller quantities of the iron in the storage pool are in an extremely insoluble form called *hemosiderin*. This is especially

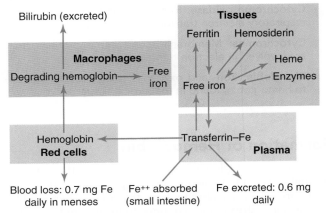

Figure 21-3   Iron transport and metabolism.

true when the total quantity of iron in the body is more than the apoferritin storage pool can accommodate. Hemosiderin collects in cells in the form of large clusters that can be observed microscopically as large particles. In contrast, ferritin particles are so small and dispersed that they usually can be seen in the cell cytoplasm only with the electron microscope.

When the quantity of iron in the plasma falls low, some of the iron in the ferritin storage pool is removed easily and transported in the form of transferrin in the plasma to the areas of the body where it is needed. A unique characteristic of the transferrin molecule is that it binds strongly with receptors in the cell membranes of erythroblasts in the bone marrow. Then, along with its bound iron, it is ingested into the erythroblasts by endocytosis. There the transferrin delivers the iron directly to the mitochondria, where heme is synthesized. In people who do not have adequate quantities of transferrin in their blood, failure to transport iron to the erythroblasts in this manner can cause severe *hypochromic anemia* (ie, red cells that contain much less hemoglobin than normal).

When red blood cells have lived their life span of about 120 days and are destroyed, the hemoglobin released from the cells is ingested by monocyte–macrophage cells. There, iron is liberated and is stored mainly in the ferritin pool to be used as needed for the formation of new hemoglobin.

DAILY LOSS OF IRON

A man excretes about 0.6 mg of iron each day mainly into the feces. Additional quantities of iron are lost when bleeding occurs. For a woman, additional menstrual loss of blood brings long-term iron loss to an average of about 1.3 mg/day.

ABSORPTION OF IRON FROM THE INTESTINAL TRACT

Iron is absorbed from all parts of the small intestine, mostly by the following mechanism. The liver secretes moderate amounts of *apotransferrin* into the bile, which flows through the bile duct into the duodenum. Here, the apotransferrin binds with free iron and also with certain iron compounds, such as hemoglobin and myoglobin from meat, two of the most important sources of iron in the diet. This combination is called *transferrin*. It, in turn, is attracted to and binds with receptors in the membranes of the intestinal epithelial cells. Then, by pinocytosis, the transferrin molecule, carrying its iron store, is absorbed into the epithelial cells and later released into the blood capillaries beneath these cells in the form of *plasma transferrin*.

Iron absorption from the intestines is extremely slow, at a maximum rate of only a few milligrams per day. This means that even when tremendous quantities of iron are present in the food, only small proportions can be absorbed.

Regulation of Total Body Iron by Controlling Rate of Absorption

When the body has become saturated with iron so that essentially all apoferritin in the iron storage areas is already combined with iron, the rate of additional iron absorption from the intestinal tract becomes greatly decreased. Conversely, when the iron stores have become depleted, the rate of absorption can accelerate probably five or more times normal. Thus, total body iron is regulated mainly by altering its rate of absorption. This regulation is performed by the iron-regulatory hormone hepcidin and its receptor ferroportin, which is the iron channel on the enterocyte. Hepcidin causes ferroportin internalization and degradation, thereby decreasing iron transfer into blood plasma from the duodenum. The formation of hepcidin is regulated by feedback of iron concentrations in plasma and the liver as well as by the erythropoietic demand for iron.

BIBLIOGRAPHY

Alayash AI: Oxygen therapeutics: can we tame haemoglobin? *Nat. Rev. Drug Discov.* 3:152, 2004.

Alleyne M, Horne MK, Miller JL: Individualized treatment for iron-deficiency anemia in adults, *Am. J. Med.* 121:943, 2008.

Claster S, Vichinsky EP: Managing sickle cell disease, *BMJ* 327:1151, 2003.

de Montalembert M: Management of sickle cell disease, *BMJ* 337:a1397, 2008.

Ganz T: Hepcidin and iron regulation, 10 years later, *Blood* 117:4425, 2011.

Hentze MW, Muckenthaler MU, Andrews NC: Balancing acts: molecular control of mammalian iron metabolism, *Cell* 117:285, 2004.

Kato GJ, Gladwin MT: Evolution of novel small-molecule therapeutics targeting sickle cell vasculopathy, *JAMA* 300:2638, 2008.

Pietrangelo A: Hereditary hemochromatosis—a new look at an old disease, *N. Engl. J. Med.* 350:2383, 2004.

Platt OS: Hydroxyurea for the treatment of sickle cell anemia, *N. Engl. J. Med.* 27:358, 2008.

22 Anemia and Polycythemia

Anemia

Anemia means deficiency of hemoglobin in the blood, which can be caused by either too few red blood cells or too little hemoglobin in the cells. Some types of anemia and their physiological causes classified on the basis of the red cell morphology are the following (Table 22-1).

Blood Loss Anemia. After rapid hemorrhage the body replaces the fluid portion of the plasma in 1–3 days, but this leaves a low concentration of red blood cells. If a second hemorrhage does not occur, the red blood cell concentration usually returns to normal within 3–6 weeks.

In chronic blood loss a person frequently cannot absorb enough iron from the intestines to form hemoglobin as rapidly as it is lost. Red cells that are much smaller than normal and have too little hemoglobin inside them are then produced, giving rise to *microcytic, hypochromic anemia*, which is shown in Figure 20-3.

Aplastic Anemia. *Bone marrow aplasia* means lack of functioning bone marrow. For instance, a person exposed to high-dose radiation or chemotherapy for cancer treatment can damage stem cells of the bone marrow, followed in a few weeks by anemia. Likewise, high doses of certain toxic chemicals, such as insecticides or benzene in gasoline, may cause the same effect. In autoimmune disorders, such as lupus erythematosus, the immune system begins attacking healthy cells such as bone marrow stem cells, which may lead to aplastic anemia. In about half of aplastic anemia cases the cause is unknown, a condition called *idiopathic aplastic anemia*.

People with severe aplastic anemia usually die unless treated with blood transfusions, which can temporarily increase the numbers of red blood cells, or by bone marrow transplantation.

Megaloblastic Anemia. Based on the earlier discussions of vitamin B$_{12}$, folic acid, and intrinsic factor from the stomach mucosa, one can readily understand that loss of any one of these can lead to slow reproduction of erythroblasts in the bone marrow. As a result, the red cells grow too large, with odd shapes, and are called *megaloblasts*. Thus, atrophy of the stomach mucosa, as occurs in *pernicious anemia*, or loss of the entire stomach after surgical total gastrectomy can lead to megaloblastic anemia. Also, patients who have intestinal sprue, in which folic acid, vitamin B$_{12}$, and other vitamin B compounds are poorly absorbed, often develop megaloblastic anemia. Because in these

TABLE 22-1	Morphological Classification of Anemias	
Macrocytic (MCV > 100)	**Normocytic (MCV 80–100)**	**Microcytic (MCV < 80)**
Vitamin B$_{12}$ deficiency (megaloblastic) • Dietary deficiency • Pernicious anemia • Gastric resection • Ileal disease • Tropical sprue • Fish tapeworm	Posthemorrhagic	Iron deficiency • Dietary deficiency • Inhibitory diet (high phytate) • Hookworm • Chronic bleeding • Infection
Folate deficiency (megaloblastic) • Dietary deficiency • Drug induced • Pregnancy • Tropical sprue	Endocrine disorders • Hypothyroidism • Addison disease • Hypopituitarism	Thalassemia
Hypothyroidism Alcoholism	Anemia of chronic disorders	Hemoglobinopathies (S, C, E) Anemia of chronic disorders, infection

MCV, mean corpuscular volume.

states the erythroblasts cannot proliferate rapidly enough to form normal numbers of red blood cells, those red cells that are formed are mostly oversized, have bizarre shapes, and have fragile membranes. These cells rupture easily, leaving the person in dire need of an adequate number of red cells.

Hemolytic Anemia. Different abnormalities of the red blood cells, many of which are hereditarily acquired, make the cells fragile, so they rupture easily as they go through the capillaries, especially through the spleen. Even though the number of red blood cells formed may be normal, or even much greater than normal in some hemolytic diseases, the life span of the fragile red cell is so short that the cells are destroyed faster than they can be formed and serious anemia results.

In *hereditary spherocytosis*, the red cells are very small and *spherical* rather than being biconcave discs. These cells cannot withstand compression forces because they do not have the normal loose, bag-like cell membrane structure of the biconcave discs. On passing through the splenic pulp and some other tight vascular beds, they are easily ruptured by even slight compression.

In *sickle cell anemia*, which is present in 0.3–1.0% of West African and American blacks, the cells have an abnormal type of hemoglobin called *hemoglobin S*, containing faulty beta chains in the hemoglobin molecule, as explained earlier in the chapter. When this hemoglobin is exposed to low concentrations of oxygen, it precipitates into long crystals inside the red blood cell. These crystals elongate the cell and give it the appearance of a sickle rather than a biconcave disc. The precipitated hemoglobin also damages the cell membrane, so the cells become highly fragile, leading to serious anemia. Such patients frequently experience a vicious circle of events called a sickle cell disease "crisis," in which low oxygen tension in the tissues causes sickling, which leads to ruptured red cells, which causes a further decrease in oxygen tension and still more sickling and red cell destruction. Once the process starts, it progresses rapidly, eventuating in a serious decrease in red blood cells within a few hours and, in some cases, death.

In *erythroblastosis fetalis*, Rh-positive red blood cells in the fetus are attacked by antibodies from an Rh-negative mother. These antibodies make the Rh-positive cells fragile, leading to rapid rupture and causing the child to be born with serious anemia. This is discussed in Chapter 28 in relation to the Rh factor of blood. The extremely rapid formation of new red cells to make up for the destroyed cells in erythroblastosis fetalis causes a large number of early *blast* forms of red cells to be released from the bone marrow into the blood.

EFFECTS OF ANEMIA ON FUNCTION OF THE CIRCULATORY SYSTEM

The viscosity of the blood depends largely on the blood concentration of red blood cells. In severe anemia, the blood viscosity may fall to as low as 1.5 times that of water rather than the normal value of about 3. This decreases the resistance to blood flow in the peripheral blood vessels, so far greater than normal quantities of blood flow through the tissues and return to the heart, thereby greatly increasing cardiac output. Moreover, hypoxia resulting from diminished transport of oxygen by the blood causes the peripheral tissue blood vessels to dilate, allowing a further increase in the return of blood to the heart and increasing the cardiac output to a still higher level—sometimes three to four times normal. Thus, one of the major effects of

anemia is greatly *increased cardiac output*, as well as *increased pumping workload on the heart*.

The increased cardiac output in anemia partially offsets the reduced oxygen-carrying effect of the anemia because even though each unit quantity of blood carries only small quantities of oxygen, the rate of blood flow may be increased enough that almost normal quantities of oxygen are actually delivered to the tissues. However, when a person with anemia begins to exercise, the heart is not capable of pumping much greater quantities of blood than it is already pumping. Consequently, during exercise, which greatly increases tissue demand for oxygen, extreme tissue hypoxia results and *acute cardiac failure* may ensue.

Polycythemia

Secondary Polycythemia. Whenever the tissues become hypoxic because of too little oxygen in the breathed air, such as at high altitudes, or because of failure of oxygen delivery to the tissues, such as in cardiac failure, the blood-forming organs automatically produce large quantities of extra red blood cells. This condition is called *secondary polycythemia*, and the red cell count commonly rises to 6–7 million/mm^3, about 30% above normal.

A common type of secondary polycythemia, called *physiological polycythemia*, occurs in natives who live at altitudes of 14,000–17,000 ft., where the atmospheric oxygen is very low. The blood count is generally 6–7 million/mm^3; this allows these people to perform reasonably high levels of continuous work even in a rarefied atmosphere.

Polycythemia Vera (Erythremia). In addition to those people who have physiological polycythemia, others have a pathological condition known as *polycythemia vera*, in which the red blood cell count may be 7–8 million/mm^3 and the hematocrit may be 60–70% instead of the normal 40–45%. Polycythemia vera is caused by a genetic aberration in the hemocytoblastic cells that produce the blood cells. The blast cells no longer stop producing red cells when too many cells are already present. This causes excess production of red blood cells in the same manner that a breast tumor causes excess production of a specific type of breast cell. It usually causes excess production of white blood cells and platelets as well.

In polycythemia vera, not only does the hematocrit increase, but the total blood volume also increases, on some occasions to almost twice normal. As a result, the entire vascular system becomes intensely engorged. Also, many blood capillaries become plugged by the viscous blood; the viscosity of the blood in polycythemia vera sometimes increases from the normal of 3 times the viscosity of water to 10 times that of water.

EFFECT OF POLYCYTHEMIA ON FUNCTION OF THE CIRCULATORY SYSTEM

Because of the greatly increased viscosity of the blood in polycythemia, blood flow through the peripheral blood vessels is often very sluggish. In accordance with the factors that regulate return of blood to the heart, as discussed in Chapter 36, increasing blood viscosity *decreases* the rate of venous return to the heart. Conversely, the blood volume is greatly increased in polycythemia, which tends to *increase* venous return. Actually, the cardiac output in polycythemia is not far from normal because these two factors more or less neutralize each other.

The arterial pressure is also normal in most people with polycythemia, although in about one-third of them the arterial pressure is elevated. This means that the blood pressure–regulating mechanisms can usually offset the tendency for increased blood viscosity to increase peripheral resistance and, thereby, increase arterial pressure. Beyond certain limits, however, these regulations fail and hypertension develops.

The color of the skin depends to a great extent on the quantity of blood in the skin subpapillary venous plexus. In polycythemia vera, the quantity of blood in this plexus is greatly increased. Further, because the blood passes sluggishly through the skin capillaries before entering the venous plexus, a larger than normal quantity of hemoglobin is deoxygenated. The blue color of all this deoxygenated hemoglobin masks the red color of the oxygenated hemoglobin. Therefore, a person with polycythemia vera ordinarily has a ruddy complexion with a bluish (cyanotic) tint to the skin.

BIBLIOGRAPHY

Banka S, Ryan K, Thomson W, et al: Pernicious anemia—genetic insights, *Autoimmun. Rev.* 10:455, 2011.

Lee FS, Percy MJ: The HIF pathway and erythrocytosis, *Annu. Rev. Pathol.* 6:165, 2011.

Milman N: Anemia—still a major health problem in many parts of the world! *Ann. Hematol.* 90:369, 2011.

Percy MJ, Rumi E: Genetic origins and clinical phenotype of familial and acquired erythrocytosis and thrombocytosis, *Am. J. Hematol.* 84:46, 2009.

23 Jaundice

LEARNING OBJECTIVES

- Define jaundice.
- Classify the different types of jaundice.
- Describe the biochemical tests done to investigate jaundice and how they can be interpreted.

GLOSSARY OF TERMS

- **Bilirubin:** Yellow breakdown product of heme from hemoglobin (it is responsible for the yellow color of urine and the yellow discoloration in jaundice)
- **Hemolytic jaundice:** An excess of unconjugated bilirubin in the blood due to excessive hemolysis
- **Obstructive jaundice:** An increase in conjugated bilirubin in the blood due to obstruction of biliary flow
- **Urobilinogen:** A colorless product of the reduction of bilirubin by bacteria in the intestine (it can be reabsorbed from the intestine into the circulation, for later excretion by the kidney, constituting an enterohepatic urobilinogen cycle)
- **van den Bergh reaction:** Test to measure the concentration of conjugated bilirubin in the blood

Jaundice refers to a yellowish tint to the body tissues, including a yellowness of the skin and deep tissues. The usual cause of jaundice is large quantities of bilirubin in the extracellular fluids, either unconjugated or conjugated bilirubin. The normal plasma concentration of bilirubin, which is almost entirely the unconjugated form, averages 0.5 mg/dL of plasma. In certain abnormal conditions, this can rise to as high as 40 mg/dL, and much of it can become the conjugated type. The skin usually begins to appear jaundiced when the concentration rises to about three times normal—that is, above 1.5 mg/dL.

The common causes of jaundice are (1) increased destruction of red blood cells, with rapid release of bilirubin into the blood, and (2) obstruction of the bile ducts or damage to the liver cells so that even the usual amounts of bilirubin cannot be excreted into the gastrointestinal tract. These two types of jaundice are called, respectively, *hemolytic jaundice* and *obstructive jaundice*. They differ from each other in the following ways.

Hemolytic Jaundice Is Caused by Hemolysis of Red Blood Cells

In hemolytic jaundice, the excretory function of the liver is not impaired, but red blood cells are hemolyzed so rapidly that the hepatic cells simply cannot excrete the bilirubin as quickly as it is formed. Therefore, the plasma concentration of free bilirubin rises to above-normal levels. Likewise, the rate of formation of *urobilinogen* in the intestine is greatly increased, and much of this is absorbed into the blood and later excreted in the urine.

Obstructive Jaundice Is Caused by Obstruction of Bile Ducts or Liver Disease

In obstructive jaundice, caused either by obstruction of the bile ducts (which most often occurs when a gallstone or cancer blocks the common bile duct) or by damage to the hepatic cells (which occurs in *hepatitis*), the rate of bilirubin formation is normal but the bilirubin formed cannot pass from the blood into the intestines. The unconjugated bilirubin still enters the liver cells and becomes conjugated in the usual way. This conjugated bilirubin is then returned to the blood, probably by rupture of the congested bile canaliculi and direct emptying of the bile into the lymph leaving the liver. Thus, *most of the bilirubin in the plasma becomes the conjugated type* rather than the unconjugated type.

Diagnostic Differences Between Hemolytic and Obstructive Jaundice

Chemical laboratory tests can be used to differentiate between unconjugated and conjugated bilirubin in the plasma. In hemolytic jaundice, almost all the bilirubin is in the "unconjugated" form; in obstructive jaundice, it is mainly in the "conjugated" form. A test called the *van den Bergh reaction* can be used to differentiate between the two (Table 23-1).

When there is total obstruction of bile flow, no bilirubin can reach the intestines to be converted into urobilinogen by bacteria. Therefore, no urobilinogen is reabsorbed into the blood, and none can be excreted by the kidneys into the urine. Consequently, in *total* obstructive jaundice, tests for urobilinogen in the urine are completely negative. Also, the stools become clay colored owing to a lack of stercobilin and other bile pigments.

Another major difference between unconjugated and conjugated bilirubin is that the kidneys can excrete small quantities of the highly soluble conjugated bilirubin but not the albumin-bound unconjugated bilirubin. Therefore, in severe obstructive jaundice significant quantities of conjugated bilirubin appear in the urine. This can be demonstrated simply by shaking the

TABLE 23-1	Tests for Jaundice

Serum unconjugated bilirubin (indirect van den Bergh test)
Serum conjugated bilirubin (direct van den Bergh test)
Urine urobilinogen
Liver function tests
Serum
- Alanine transaminase
- Aspartate transaminase
- Alkaline phosphatase
- Gamma-glutamyl transpeptidase
Coagulation tests
Prothrombin time

urine and observing the foam, which turns an intense yellow. Thus, by understanding the physiology of bilirubin excretion by the liver and by the use of a few simple tests, it is often possible to differentiate among multiple types of hemolytic diseases and liver diseases, as well as to determine the severity of the disease.

The spleen is the usual site for extravascular (normal) hemolysis. Bilirubin formed here is transported as "unconjugated bilirubin" in the plasma, to the liver. In the liver, it is conjugated to form a soluble bilirubin that is excreted into the bile (Figure 23-1).

Note that if there is excessive intravascular hemolysis, such as in hemolytic anemia, free Hb is present in the plasma and a part of it binds to haptoglobin for transport to the liver. The rest circulates as free hemoglobin, and can be filtered by the kidney out of the blood as a dimer, into the urine, where it can precipitate in the renal tubules. Otherwise, methemoglobin is formed, which breaks down to free heme, which is, in turn, bound by another plasma protein called hemopexin, or by albumin to yield methemalbumin. In both these instances, it is transported to the liver (marked with asterisk in the diagram) where a similar chain of events occurs leading to the formation of bilirubin.

The points marked 1, 2, and 3 indicate where problems that lead to excess bilirubin in the blood can occur. At point 1, due to increased hemolysis, excess unconjugated bilirubin can appear in the plasma (prehepatic jaundice). At point 2, due to hepatic dysfunction or blockage of intrahepatic biliary canaliculi (hepatic jaundice), conjugated bilirubin appears in the plasma, due to regurgitation. A similar scenario exists for point 3, where there is blockage of the bile duct, leading to posthepatic jaundice (Figure 23-1).

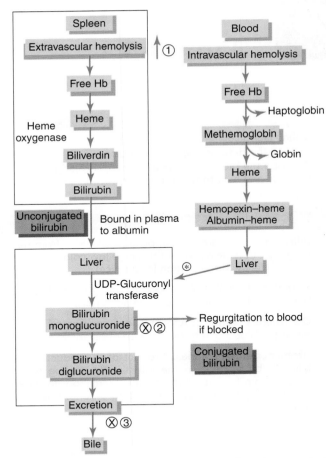

Figure 23-1   Fate of hemoglobin after extravascular or intravascular hemolysis, and points at which jaundice can occur. UDP, Uridine 5′-diphosphoglucuronyl transferase.

BIBLIOGRAPHY

Fevery J: Bilirubin in clinical practice: a review, *Liver Int.* 28:592-605, 2008.
Kosters A, Karpen SJ: The role of inflammation in cholestasis: clinical and basic aspects, *Semin. Liver Dis.* 30:186-194, 2010.

Maines MD: Biliverdin reductase: PKC interaction at the cross-talk of MAPK and PI3K signaling pathways, *Antioxid. Redox Signal.* 9:2187-2195, 2007.
Roche SP, Kobos R: Jaundice in the adult patient, *Am. Fam. Physician* 69:299-304, 2004.

Watson RL: Hyperbilirubinemia, *Crit. Care Nurs. Clin. North Am.* 21:97-120, 2009.
Winger J, Michelfelder A: Diagnostic approach to the patient with jaundice, *Prim. Care* 38:469-482, 2011.

24 White Blood Cells

Our bodies are exposed continually to bacteria, viruses, fungi, and parasites, all of which occur normally and to varying degrees in the skin, the mouth, the respiratory passageways, the intestinal tract, the lining membranes of the eyes, and even the urinary tract. Many of these infectious agents are capable of causing serious abnormal physiological function or even death if they invade the deeper tissues. We are also exposed intermittently to other highly infectious bacteria and viruses besides those that are normally present, and these agents can cause acute lethal diseases such as pneumonia, streptococcal infection, and typhoid fever.

Our bodies have a special system for combating the different infectious and toxic agents. This system is composed of blood leukocytes (white blood cells) and tissue cells derived from leukocytes. These cells work together in two ways to prevent disease: (1) by actually destroying invading bacteria or viruses by *phagocytosis* and (2) by forming *antibodies* and *sensitized lymphocytes*, which may destroy or inactivate the invader. This chapter is concerned with the first of these methods, and Chapter 25 is concerned with the second.

Leukocytes (White Blood Cells)

The leukocytes, also called *white blood cells*, are the *mobile units* of the body's protective system. They are formed partially in the bone marrow (*granulocytes* and *monocytes* and a few *lymphocytes*) and partially in the lymph tissue (*lymphocytes* and *plasma cells*). After formation, they are transported in the blood to different parts of the body where they are needed.

The real value of the white blood cells is that most of them are specifically transported to areas of serious infection and inflammation, thereby providing a rapid and potent defense against infectious agents. As we see later, the granulocytes and monocytes have a special ability to "seek out and destroy" a foreign invader.

GENERAL CHARACTERISTICS OF LEUKOCYTES

Types of White Blood Cells. Six types of white blood cells are normally present in the blood: *polymorphonuclear neutrophils, polymorphonuclear eosinophils, polymorphonuclear basophils, monocytes, lymphocytes,* and, occasionally, *plasma cells.* In addition, there are large numbers of *platelets,* which are fragments of another type of cell similar to the white blood cells found in the bone marrow, the *megakaryocyte.* The first three types of cells, the polymorphonuclear cells, have a granular appearance, as shown in cell numbers 7, 10, and 12 in Figure 24-1, and for this reason are called *granulocytes,* or, in clinical terminology, "polys," because of the multiple nuclei.

The granulocytes and monocytes protect the body against invading organisms by ingesting them (ie, by *phagocytosis*) or by releasing antimicrobial or inflammatory substances that have multiple effects that aid in destroying the offending organism (see Tables 24-1 and 24-2). The lymphocytes and plasma cells function mainly in connection with the immune system as is discussed in Chapter 25. Finally, the function of platelets is specifically to activate the blood clotting mechanism, which is discussed in Chapter 27. A list of the causes of physiological and pathological variations of white blood cells is given in Table 24-2.

Concentrations of the Different White Blood Cells in the Blood. The adult human being has about 7000 white blood cells per *microliter* of blood (in comparison with 5 million red blood cells). Of the total white blood cells, the normal percentages of the different types are approximately the following:

Polymorphonuclear neutrophils	62.0%
Polymorphonuclear eosinophils	2.3%
Polymorphonuclear basophils	0.4%
Monocytes	5.3%
Lymphocytes	30.0%

The number of platelets, which are only cell fragments, in each microliter of blood is normally about 300,000.

GENESIS OF WHITE BLOOD CELLS

Early differentiation of the pluripotential hematopoietic stem cell into the different types of committed stem cells is shown in Figure 20-2. Aside from the cells committed to form red blood cells, two major lineages of *white blood cells* are formed, the myelocytic and the lymphocytic lineages. The left side of Figure 24-1 shows the *myelocytic lineage*, beginning with the *myeloblast*; the right side shows the *lymphocytic lineage*, beginning with the *lymphoblast*.

The granulocytes and monocytes are formed only in the bone marrow. Lymphocytes and plasma cells are produced mainly in the various lymphogenous tissues—especially the lymph glands, spleen, thymus, tonsils, and various pockets of

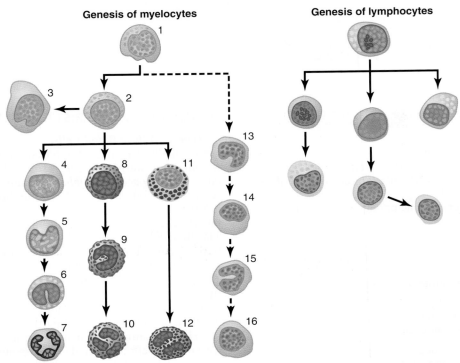

Figure 24-1   Genesis of white blood cells. The different cells of the myelocyte series are as follows: (*1*) myeloblast; (*2*) promyelocyte; (*3*) megakaryocyte; (*4*) neutrophil myelocyte; (*5*) young neutrophil metamyelocyte; (*6*) "band" neutrophil metamyelocyte; (*7*) polymorphonuclear neutrophil; (*8*) eosinophil myelocyte; (*9*) eosinophil metamyelocyte; (*10*) polymorphonuclear eosinophil; (*11*) basophil myelocyte; (*12*) polymorphonuclear basophil; (*13–16*) stages of monocyte formation.

TABLE 24-1	WBCs and their Functions	
Cell Type	**Percentage of Total**	**Functions**
MYELOID		
Neutrophils	50–70	Endothelial adhesion, chemotaxis, phagocytosis, antibacterial compounds in granules
Eosinophils	1–4	Interaction with T lymphocytes in allergy, helminth larvicidal
Basophils	<0.5	Inflammation, initiation of tissue repair after injury
LYMPHOID		
T lymphocytes	20–40	Cellular immunity (helper, memory and cytotoxic T cells)
B lymphocytes		Humoral immunity (plasma cells secreting immunoglobulins)
MONOCYTIC		
Monocytes	2–8	Immunoregulatory—antigen-presenting cells, phagocytic, chemotaxis

TABLE 24-2	Physiological and Pathological Variations in WBCs

Physiological
- Exercise
- Digestive
- Pregnancy
- Stress—linked to catecholamines

Pathological
- Bacterial, viral, and fungal infections
- Allergy
- Helminthic infestations

lymphoid tissue elsewhere in the body, such as in the bone marrow and in so-called Peyer's patches underneath the epithelium in the gut wall.

The white blood cells formed in the bone marrow are stored within the marrow until they are needed in the circulatory system. Then, when the need arises, various factors cause them to be released (these factors are discussed later). Normally, about three times as many white blood cells are stored in the marrow as circulate in the entire blood. This represents about a 6-day supply of these cells.

The lymphocytes are mostly stored in the various lymphoid tissues, except for a small number that are temporarily being transported in the blood.

As shown in Figure 24-1, megakaryocytes (cell 3) are also formed in the bone marrow. These megakaryocytes fragment in the bone marrow; the small fragments, known as *platelets* (or *thrombocytes*), then pass into the blood. They are very important in the initiation of blood clotting.

LIFE SPAN OF WHITE BLOOD CELLS

The life of the granulocytes after being released from the bone marrow is normally 4–8 hours circulating in the blood and another 4–5 days in tissues where they are needed. In times of serious tissue infection, this total life span is often shortened to only a few hours because the granulocytes proceed even more rapidly to the infected area, perform their functions, and, in the process, are themselves destroyed.

The monocytes also have a short transit time, 10–20 hours in the blood, before wandering through the capillary membranes into the tissues. Once in the tissues, they swell to much larger sizes to become *tissue macrophages*, and, in this form, they can live for months unless destroyed while performing phagocytic functions. These tissue macrophages are the basis of the *tissue macrophage system*, (discussed in greater detail later), which provides continuing defense against infection.

Lymphocytes enter the circulatory system continually, along with drainage of lymph from the lymph nodes and other lymphoid tissue. After a few hours, they pass out of the blood back into the tissues by diapedesis. Then they reenter the lymph and return to the blood again and again; thus, there is continual circulation of lymphocytes through the body. The lymphocytes have life spans of weeks or months, depending on the body's need for these cells.

The platelets in the blood are replaced about once every 10 days; in other words, about 30,000 platelets are formed each day for each microliter of blood.

Neutrophils and Macrophages Defend Against Infections

It is mainly the neutrophils and tissue macrophages that attack and destroy invading bacteria, viruses, and other injurious agents. The neutrophils are mature cells that can attack and destroy bacteria even in the circulating blood. Conversely, the tissue macrophages begin life as blood monocytes, which are immature cells while still in the blood and have little ability to fight infectious agents at that time. However, once they enter the tissues, they begin to swell—sometimes increasing their diameters as much as fivefold—to as great as 60–80 μm, a size that can barely be seen with the naked eye. These cells are now called *macrophages*, and they are extremely capable of combating disease agents in the tissues.

White Blood Cells Enter the Tissue Spaces by Diapedesis. Neutrophils and monocytes can squeeze through the pores of the blood capillaries by *diapedesis*. That is, even though a pore is much smaller than a cell, a small portion of the cell slides through the pore at a time; the portion sliding through is momentarily constricted to the size of the pore, as shown in Figure 24-2.

White Blood Cells Move Through Tissue Spaces by Ameboid Motion. Both neutrophils and macrophages can move through the tissues by ameboid motion, described in Chapter 2. Some cells move at velocities as great as 40 μm/minute, a distance as great as their own length each minute.

White Blood Cells Are Attracted to Inflamed Tissue Areas by Chemotaxis. Many different chemical substances in the tissues cause both neutrophils and macrophages to move toward the source of the chemical. This phenomenon, shown in Figure 24-2, is known as *chemotaxis*. When a tissue becomes inflamed, at least a dozen different products that can cause chemotaxis toward the inflamed area are formed. They include (1) some of the bacterial or viral toxins, (2) degenerative products of the inflamed tissues, (3) several reaction products of the "complement complex"

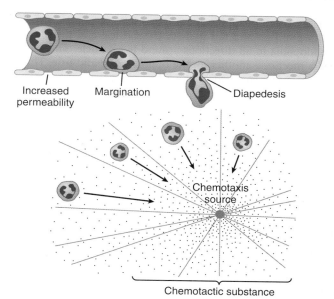

Figure 24-2   Movement of neutrophils by *diapedesis* through capillary pores and by *chemotaxis* toward an area of tissue damage.

(discussed in Chapter 25) activated in inflamed tissues, and (4) several reaction products caused by plasma clotting in the inflamed area, as well as other substances.

As shown in Figure 24-2, chemotaxis depends on the concentration gradient of the chemotactic substance. The concentration is greatest near the source, which directs the unidirectional movement of the white cells. Chemotaxis is effective up to 100 μm away from an inflamed tissue. Therefore, because almost no tissue area is more than 50 μm away from a capillary, the chemotactic signal can easily move hordes of white cells from the capillaries into the inflamed area.

PHAGOCYTOSIS

The most important function of the neutrophils and macrophages is *phagocytosis*, which means cellular ingestion of the offending agent. Phagocytes must be selective of the material that is phagocytized; otherwise, normal cells and structures of the body might be ingested. Whether phagocytosis will occur depends especially on three selective procedures.

First, most natural structures in the tissues have smooth surfaces, which resist phagocytosis. However if the surface is rough, the likelihood of phagocytosis is increased.

Second, most natural substances of the body have protective protein coats that repel the phagocytes. Conversely, most dead tissues and foreign particles have no protective coats, which make them subject to phagocytosis.

Third, the immune system of the body (described in Chapter 25) develops *antibodies* against infectious agents such as bacteria. The antibodies then adhere to the bacterial membranes and thereby make the bacteria especially susceptible to phagocytosis. To do this, the antibody molecule also combines with the C3 product of the *complement cascade*, which is an additional part of the immune system discussed in the next chapter. The C3 molecules, in turn, attach to receptors on the phagocyte membrane, thus initiating phagocytosis. This process by which a pathogen is selected for phagocytosis and destruction is called *opsonization*.

Phagocytosis by Neutrophils. The neutrophils entering the tissues are already mature cells that can immediately begin phagocytosis. On approaching a particle to be phagocytized, the neutrophil first attaches itself to the particle and then projects pseudopodia in all directions around the particle. The pseudopodia meet one another on the opposite side and fuse. This action creates an enclosed chamber that contains the phagocytized particle. Then the chamber invaginates to the inside of the cytoplasmic cavity and breaks away from the outer cell membrane to form a free-floating *phagocytic vesicle* (also called a *phagosome*) inside the cytoplasm. A single neutrophil can usually phagocytize 3–20 bacteria before the neutrophil becomes inactivated and dies.

Phagocytosis by Macrophages. Macrophages are the end-stage product of monocytes that enter the tissues from the blood. When activated by the immune system, as described in Chapter 25, they are much more powerful phagocytes than neutrophils, often capable of phagocytizing as many as 100 bacteria. They also have the ability to engulf much larger particles, even whole red blood cells or, occasionally, malarial parasites, whereas neutrophils are not capable of phagocytizing particles much larger than bacteria. Also, after digesting particles, macrophages can extrude the residual products and often survive and function for many more months.

Once Phagocytized, Most Particles Are Digested by Intracellular Enzymes. Once a foreign particle has been phagocytized, lysosomes and other cytoplasmic granules in the neutrophil or macrophage immediately come in contact with the phagocytic vesicle, and their membranes fuse, thereby dumping many digestive enzymes and bactericidal agents into the vesicle. Thus, the phagocytic vesicle now becomes a *digestive vesicle*, and digestion of the phagocytized particle begins immediately.

Both neutrophils and macrophages contain an abundance of lysosomes filled with *proteolytic enzymes* especially geared for digesting bacteria and other foreign protein matter. The lysosomes of macrophages (but not of neutrophils) also contain large amounts of *lipases*, which digest the thick lipid membranes possessed by some bacteria such as the tuberculosis bacillus.

Neutrophils and Macrophages Can Kill Bacteria. In addition to the digestion of ingested bacteria in phagosomes, neutrophils and macrophages contain *bactericidal agents* that kill most bacteria even when the lysosomal enzymes fail to digest them. This characteristic is especially important because some bacteria have protective coats or other factors that prevent their destruction by digestive enzymes. Much of the killing effect results from several powerful *oxidizing agents* formed by enzymes in the membrane of the phagosome or by a special organelle called the *peroxisome*. These oxidizing agents include large quantities of *superoxide* (O_2^-), *hydrogen peroxide* (H_2O_2), and *hydroxyl ions* (OH^-), all of which are lethal to most bacteria, even in small quantities. Also, one of the lysosomal enzymes, myeloperoxidase, catalyzes the reaction between H_2O_2 and chloride ions to form hypochlorite, which is exceedingly bactericidal.

Some bacteria, notably the tuberculosis bacillus, have coats that are resistant to lysosomal digestion and also secrete substances that partially resist the killing effects of the neutrophils and macrophages. These bacteria are responsible for many of the chronic diseases, an example of which is tuberculosis.

Monocyte–Macrophage Cell System (Reticuloendothelial System)

In the preceding paragraphs, we described the macrophages mainly as mobile cells that are capable of wandering through the tissues. However, after entering the tissues and becoming macrophages, another large portion of monocytes becomes attached to the tissues and remains attached for months or even years until they are called on to perform specific local protective functions. They have the same capabilities as the mobile macrophages to phagocytize large quantities of bacteria, viruses, necrotic tissue, or other foreign particles in the tissue. In addition, when appropriately stimulated, they can break away from their attachments and once again become mobile macrophages that respond to chemotaxis and all the other stimuli related to the inflammatory process. Thus, the body has a widespread "monocyte–macrophage system" in virtually all tissue areas.

The total combination of monocytes, mobile macrophages, fixed tissue macrophages, and a few specialized endothelial cells in the bone marrow, spleen, and lymph nodes is called the *reticuloendothelial system*. However, all or almost all these cells originate from monocytic stem cells; therefore, the reticuloendothelial system is almost synonymous with the monocyte–macrophage system. Because the term *reticuloendothelial system* is much better known in medical literature than the term *monocyte–macrophage system*, it should be remembered as a generalized phagocytic system located in all tissues, especially in the tissue areas where large quantities of particles, toxins, and other unwanted substances must be destroyed.

Tissue Macrophages in the Skin and Subcutaneous Tissues (Histiocytes). Although the skin is mainly impregnable to infectious agents, this is no longer true when the skin is broken. When infection begins in a subcutaneous tissue and local inflammation ensues, local tissue macrophages can divide in situ and form still more macrophages. Then they perform the usual functions of attacking and destroying the infectious agents, as described earlier.

Macrophages in the Lymph Nodes. Essentially no particulate matter that enters the tissues, such as bacteria, can be absorbed directly through the capillary membranes into the blood. Instead, if the particles are not destroyed locally in the tissues, they enter the lymph and flow to the lymph nodes located intermittently along the course of the lymph flow. The foreign particles are then trapped in these nodes in a meshwork of sinuses lined by *tissue macrophages*.

Figure 24-3 illustrates the general organization of the lymph node, showing lymph entering through the lymph node capsule by way of *afferent lymphatics*, then flowing through the *nodal medullary sinuses*, and finally passing out the *hilus* into *efferent lymphatics* that eventually empty into the venous blood.

Large numbers of macrophages line the lymph sinuses, and if any particles enter the sinuses by way of the lymph, the macrophages phagocytize them and prevent general dissemination throughout the body.

Alveolar Macrophages in the Lungs. Another route by which invading organisms frequently enter the body is through the lungs. Large numbers of tissue macrophages are present as integral components of the alveolar walls. They can phagocytize particles that become entrapped in the alveoli. If the particles are digestible, the macrophages can also digest them and release the digestive products into the lymph. If the particle is not digestible, the macrophages often form a "giant cell" capsule around the particle until such time—if ever—that it can be slowly dissolved. Such capsules are frequently formed around tuberculosis bacilli, silica dust particles, and even carbon particles.

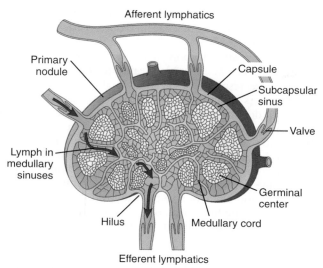

Figure 24-3 Functional diagram of a lymph node.

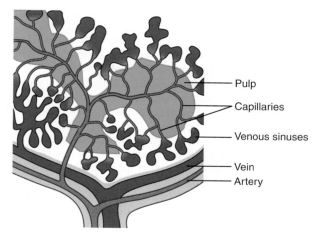

Figure 24-5 Functional structures of the spleen.

MACROPHAGES OF THE SPLEEN AND BONE MARROW

If an invading organism succeeds in entering the general circulation, there are other lines of defense by the tissue macrophage system, especially by macrophages of the spleen and bone marrow. In both these tissues, macrophages become entrapped by the reticular meshwork of the two organs, and when foreign particles come in contact with these macrophages, they are phagocytized.

The spleen is similar to the lymph nodes, except that blood, instead of lymph, flows through the tissue spaces of the spleen. Figure 24-5 shows a small peripheral segment of spleen tissue. Note that a small artery penetrates from the splenic capsule into the *splenic pulp* and terminates in small capillaries. The capillaries are highly porous, allowing whole blood to pass out of the capillaries into *cords of red pulp*. The blood then gradually *squeezes* through the trabecular meshwork of these cords and eventually returns to the circulation through the endothelial walls of the *venous sinuses*. The trabeculae of the red pulp and the venous sinuses are lined with vast numbers of macrophages. This peculiar passage of blood through the cords of the red pulp provides an exceptional means of phagocytizing unwanted debris in the blood, including especially old and abnormal red blood cells.

Macrophages (Kupffer Cells) in the Liver Sinusoids. Another route by which bacteria invade the body is through the gastrointestinal tract. Large numbers of bacteria from ingested food constantly pass through the gastrointestinal mucosa into the portal blood. Before this blood enters the general circulation, it passes through the liver sinusoids, which are lined with tissue macrophages called *Kupffer cells*, shown in Figure 24-4. These cells form such an effective particulate filtration system that almost none of the bacteria from the gastrointestinal tract pass from the portal blood into the general systemic circulation. Indeed, motion pictures of phagocytosis by Kupffer cells have demonstrated phagocytosis of a single bacterium in less than one-hundredth of a second.

Eosinophils

The eosinophils normally constitute about 2% of all the blood leukocytes. Eosinophils are weak phagocytes, and they exhibit chemotaxis, but in comparison with the neutrophils, it is doubtful that the eosinophils are significant in protecting against the usual types of infection.

Eosinophils, however, are often produced in large numbers in people with parasitic infections, and they migrate into tissues diseased by parasites. Although most parasites are too large to be phagocytized by eosinophils or any other phagocytic cells, eosinophils attach themselves to the parasites by way of special surface molecules and release substances that kill many of the parasites. For instance, one of the most widespread infections is *schistosomiasis*, a parasitic infection found in as many as one-third of the population of some developing countries in Asia, Africa, and South America; the parasite can invade any part of

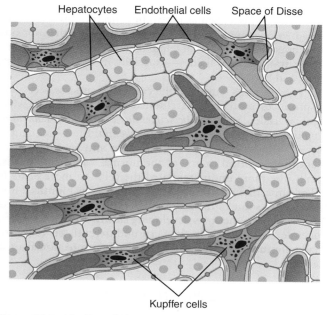

Figure 24-4 Kupffer cells lining the liver sinusoids, showing phagocytosis of India ink particles into the cytoplasm of the Kupffer cells.

the body. Eosinophils attach themselves to the juvenile forms of the parasite and kill many of them. They do so in several ways: (1) by releasing hydrolytic enzymes from their granules, which are modified lysosomes; (2) probably by also releasing highly reactive forms of oxygen that are especially lethal to parasites; and (3) by releasing from the granules a highly larvicidal polypeptide called *major basic protein*.

In a few areas of the world, another parasitic disease that causes eosinophilia is *trichinosis*. This disease results from invasion of the body's muscles by the *Trichinella* parasite ("pork worm") after a person eats undercooked infested pork.

Eosinophils also have a special propensity to collect in tissues in which allergic reactions occur, such as in the peribronchial tissues of the lungs in people with asthma and in the skin after allergic skin reactions. This action is caused at least partly by the fact that many mast cells and basophils participate in allergic reactions, as discussed in the next paragraph. The mast cells and basophils release an *eosinophil chemotactic factor* that causes eosinophils to migrate toward the inflamed allergic tissue. The eosinophils are believed to detoxify some of the inflammation-inducing substances released by the mast cells and basophils, and probably also to phagocytize and destroy allergen–antibody complexes, thus preventing excess spread of the local inflammatory process.

Basophils

The basophils in the circulating blood are similar to the large tissue *mast cells* located immediately outside many of the capillaries in the body. Both mast cells and basophils liberate *heparin* into the blood. Heparin is a substance that can prevent blood coagulation.

The mast cells and basophils also release *histamine*, as well as smaller quantities of *bradykinin* and *serotonin*. Indeed, it is mainly the mast cells in inflamed tissues that release these substances during inflammation.

The mast cells and basophils play an important role in some types of allergic reactions because the type of antibody that causes allergic reactions, the immunoglobulin E (IgE) type, has a special propensity to become attached to mast cells and basophils. Then, when the specific antigen for the specific IgE antibody subsequently reacts with the antibody, the resulting attachment of antigen to antibody causes the mast cell or basophil to rupture and release large quantities of *histamine, bradykinin, serotonin, heparin, slow-reacting substance of anaphylaxis* (a mixture of three *leukotrienes*), and a number of *lysosomal enzymes*. These substances cause local vascular and tissue reactions that cause many, if not most, of the allergic manifestations. These reactions are discussed in greater detail in Chapter 25.

Leukopenia

A clinical condition known as *leukopenia*, in which the bone marrow produces very few white blood cells, occasionally occurs. This condition leaves the body unprotected against many bacteria and other agents that might invade the tissues.

Normally, the human body lives in symbiosis with many bacteria because all the mucous membranes of the body are constantly exposed to large numbers of bacteria. The mouth almost always contains various spirochetal, pneumococcal, and streptococcal bacteria, and these same bacteria are present to a lesser extent in the entire respiratory tract. The distal gastrointestinal tract is especially loaded with colon bacilli. Furthermore, one can always find bacteria on the surfaces of the eyes, urethra, and vagina. Any decrease in the number of white blood cells immediately allows invasion of adjacent tissues by bacteria that are already present.

Within 2 days after the bone marrow stops producing white blood cells, ulcers may appear in the mouth and colon, or some form of severe respiratory infection might develop. Bacteria from the ulcers rapidly invade surrounding tissues and the blood might develop. Without treatment, death often ensues in less than a week after acute total leukopenia begins.

Irradiation of the body by X-rays or gamma rays, or exposure to drugs and chemicals that contain benzene or anthracene nuclei, is likely to cause aplasia of the bone marrow. Indeed, some common drugs, such as chloramphenicol (an antibiotic), thiouracil (used to treat thyrotoxicosis), and even various barbiturate hypnotics, on rare occasions cause leukopenia, thus setting off the entire infectious sequence of this malady.

After moderate irradiation injury to the bone marrow, some stem cells, myeloblasts, and hemocytoblasts may remain undestroyed in the marrow and are capable of regenerating the bone marrow, provided sufficient time is available. A patient properly treated with transfusions, plus antibiotics and other drugs to ward off infection, usually develops enough new bone marrow within weeks to months for blood cell concentrations to return to normal.

Leukemias

Uncontrolled production of white blood cells can be caused by cancerous mutation of a myelogenous or lymphogenous cell. This process causes *leukemia*, which is usually characterized by greatly increased numbers of abnormal white blood cells in the circulating blood.

TWO GENERAL TYPES OF LEUKEMIA

Lymphocytic and Myelogenous. The lymphocytic leukemias are caused by cancerous production of lymphoid cells, usually beginning in a lymph node or other lymphocytic tissue and spreading to other areas of the body. The second type of leukemia, myelogenous leukemia, begins by cancerous production of young myelogenous cells in the bone marrow and then spreads throughout the body so that white blood cells are produced in many extramedullary tissues—especially in the lymph nodes, spleen, and liver.

In myelogenous leukemia, the cancerous process occasionally produces partially differentiated cells, resulting in what might be called *neutrophilic leukemia, eosinophilic leukemia, basophilic leukemia,* or *monocytic leukemia.* More frequently, however, the leukemia cells are bizarre and undifferentiated and not identical to any of the normal white blood cells. Usually, the more undifferentiated the cell, the more *acute* is the leukemia, often leading to death within a few months if untreated. With some of the more differentiated cells, the process can be *chronic*, sometimes developing slowly over 10–20 years. Leukemic cells, especially the very undifferentiated cells, are usually nonfunctional for providing normal protection against infection.

EFFECTS OF LEUKEMIA ON THE BODY

The first effect of leukemia is metastatic growth of leukemic cells in abnormal areas of the body. Leukemic cells from the bone marrow may reproduce so greatly that they invade the surrounding bone, causing pain and, eventually, a tendency for bones to fracture easily.

Almost all leukemias eventually spread to the spleen, lymph nodes, liver, and other vascular regions, regardless of whether the origin of the leukemia is in the bone marrow or the lymph nodes. Common effects in leukemia are the development of infection, severe anemia, and a bleeding tendency caused by thrombocytopenia (lack of platelets). These effects result mainly from displacement of the normal bone marrow and lymphoid cells by the nonfunctional leukemic cells.

Finally, an important effect of leukemia on the body is excessive use of metabolic substrates by the growing cancerous cells. The leukemic tissues reproduce new cells so rapidly that tremendous demands are made on the body reserves for foodstuffs, specific amino acids, and vitamins. Consequently, the energy of the patient is greatly depleted, and excessive utilization of amino acids by the leukemic cells causes especially rapid deterioration of the normal protein tissues of the body. Thus, while the leukemic tissues grow, other tissues become debilitated. After metabolic starvation has continued long enough, this alone is sufficient to cause death.

BIBLIOGRAPHY

Alexander JS, Granger DN: Lymphocyte trafficking mediated by vascular adhesion protein-1: implications for immune targeting and cardiovascular disease, *Circ. Res.* 86:1190, 2000.

Blander JM, Medzhitov R: Regulation of phagosome maturation by signals from toll-like receptors, *Science* 304:1014, 2004.

Bromley SK, Mempel TR, Luster AD: Orchestrating the orchestrators: chemokines in control of T cell traffic, *Nat. Immunol.* 9:970, 2008.

Ferrajoli A, O'Brien SM: Treatment of chronic lymphocytic leukemia, *Semin. Oncol.* 31(Suppl. 4):60, 2004.

Huynh KK, Kay JG, Stow JL, et al: Fusion, fission, and secretion during phagocytosis, *Physiology (Bethesda)* 22:366, 2007.

Johnson LA, Jackson DG: Cell traffic and the lymphatic endothelium, *Ann. N. Y. Acad. Sci.* 1131:119, 2008.

Kinchen JM, Ravichandran KS: Phagosome maturation: going through the acid test, *Nat. Rev. Mol. Cell Biol.* 9:781, 2008.

Kunkel EJ, Butcher EC: Plasma-cell homing, *Nat. Rev. Immunol.* 3:822, 2003.

Kvietys PR, Sandig M: Neutrophil diapedesis: paracellular or transcellular? *News Physiol. Sci.* 16:15, 2001.

Medzhitov R: Origin and physiological roles of inflammation, *Nature* 24(454):428, 2008.

Ossovskaya VS, Bunnett NW: Protease-activated receptors: contribution to physiology and disease, *Physiol. Rev.* 84:579, 2004.

Pui CH, Relling MV, Downing JR: Acute lymphoblastic leukemia, *N. Engl. J. Med.* 350:1535, 2004.

Ricardo SD, van Goor H, Eddy AA: Macrophage diversity in renal injury and repair, *J. Clin. Invest.* 118:3522, 2008.

Sigmundsdottir H, Butcher EC: Environmental cues, dendritic cells and the programming of tissue-selective lymphocyte trafficking, *Nat. Immunol.* 9:981, 2008.

Smith KA, Griffin JD: Following the cytokine signaling pathway to leukemogenesis: a chronology, *J. Clin. Invest.* 118:3564, 2008.

Viola A, Luster AD: Chemokines and their receptors: drug targets in immunity and inflammation, *Annu. Rev. Pharmacol. Toxicol.* 48:171, 2008.

Werner S, Grose R: Regulation of wound healing by growth factors and cytokines, *Physiol. Rev.* 83:835, 2003.

Zullig S, Hengartner MO: Cell biology: tickling macrophages, a serious business, *Science* 304:1123, 2004.

Immunity and Allergy

The human body has the ability to resist almost all types of organisms or toxins that tend to damage the tissues and organs. This capability is called *immunity*. Much of immunity is *acquired immunity* that does not develop until after the body is first attacked by a bacterium, virus, or toxin, often weeks or months are required for the immunity to develop. An additional element of immunity that results from general processes, rather than from processes directed at specific disease organisms, is called *innate immunity*. It includes the following aspects:

1. phagocytosis of bacteria and other invaders by white blood cells and cells of the tissue macrophage system, as described in Chapter 24;
2. destruction of swallowed organisms by the acid secretions of the stomach and the digestive enzymes;
3. resistance of the skin to invasion by organisms;
4. presence, in the blood, of certain chemicals and cells that attach to foreign organisms or toxins and destroy them. Some of these are (a) *lysozyme*, a mucolytic polysaccharide that attacks bacteria and causes them to dissolute; (b) *basic polypeptides*, which react with and inactivate certain types of gram-positive bacteria; (c) *the complement complex* that is described later, a system of about 20 proteins that can be activated in various ways to destroy bacteria; and (d) *natural killer lymphocytes* that can recognize and destroy foreign cells, tumor cells, and even some infected cells.

This innate immunity makes the human body resistant to such diseases as some paralytic viral infections of animals, hog cholera, cattle plague, and distemper—a viral disease that kills a large percentage of dogs that become afflicted with it. Conversely, many animals are resistant or even immune to many human diseases, such as poliomyelitis, mumps, human cholera, measles, and syphilis, which are very damaging or even lethal to human beings.

Acquired (Adaptive) Immunity

In addition to its generalized innate immunity, the human body has the ability to develop extremely powerful specific immunity against individual invading agents such as lethal bacteria, viruses, toxins, and even foreign tissues from other animals. This ability is called *acquired* or *adaptive immunity*. Acquired immunity is caused by a special immune system that forms antibodies and/or activated lymphocytes that attack and destroy the specific invading organism or toxin. It is with this acquired immunity mechanism and some of its associated reactions, especially the allergies, that this chapter is concerned.

Acquired immunity can often bestow an extreme degree of protection. For instance, certain toxins, such as the paralytic botulinum toxin or the tetanizing toxin of tetanus, can be protected against in doses as high as 100,000 times the amount that would be lethal without immunity. It is for this reason that the treatment process known as *immunization* is so important in protecting human beings against disease and against toxins, as explained later in this chapter.

BASIC TYPES OF ACQUIRED IMMUNITY— HUMORAL AND CELL-MEDIATED

Two basic but closely allied types of acquired immunity occur in the body (Table 25-1). In one of these the body develops circulating antibodies, which are globulin molecules in the blood plasma that are capable of attacking the invading agent. This type of immunity is called *humoral immunity* or *B-cell immunity* (because B lymphocytes produce the antibodies). The second type of acquired immunity is achieved through the formation of large numbers of activated *T lymphocytes* that are specifically crafted in the lymph nodes to destroy the foreign agent. This type of immunity is called *cell-mediated immunity* or T-cell immunity (because the activated lymphocytes are T lymphocytes). We shall see shortly that both the antibodies and the activated lymphocytes are formed in the lymphoid tissues of the body. Let us discuss the initiation of the immune process by *antigens*.

BOTH TYPES OF ACQUIRED IMMUNITY ARE INITIATED BY ANTIGENS

Because acquired immunity does not develop until after invasion by a foreign organism or toxin, it is clear that the body must have some mechanism for recognizing this invasion. Each toxin or each type of organism almost always contains one or more specific chemical compounds in its makeup that are different from all other compounds. In general, these are proteins or large polysaccharides, and it is they that initiate the acquired immunity. These substances are called *antigens* (*antibody generations*).

TABLE 25-1	Comparison of Cellular and Humoral Immunity				
Cellular					**Humoral**
Uses T lymphocytes					Uses B lymphocytes
Primary encounter with foreign cell—cancer cell, virus infected cell, parasites, etc.					Primary encounter with antigen—bacteria, bacterial toxin, some viruses
↓					↓
Cytotoxic T cell	T-helper cell (CD4 cells), also called Th1 and Th2 cells	Memory T cell	Suppressor T cell		Plasma cells
↓	↓				↓
Directly attacks foreign cell (perforins)	• Secrete interleukins • Recruit macrophages and B cells	Quick secondary exposure response	• Suppresses immune response • Regulatory role		Antibodies—IgM, IgG, IgA, IgD, IgE Memory B cells—helps in a quick secondary exposure response

IgA, immunoglobulin A; *IgD,* immunoglobulin D; *IgE,* immunoglobulin E; *IgG,* immunoglobulin G; *IgM,* immunoglobulin M.

For a substance to be antigenic, it usually must have a high molecular weight, 8000 or greater. Furthermore, the process of antigenicity usually depends on regularly recurring molecular groups, called *epitopes*, on the surface of the large molecule. This factor also explains why proteins and large polysaccharides are almost always antigenic because both of these substances have this stereochemical characteristic.

LYMPHOCYTES ARE RESPONSIBLE FOR ACQUIRED IMMUNITY

Acquired immunity is the product of the body's lymphocytes. In people who have a genetic lack of lymphocytes or whose lymphocytes have been destroyed by radiation or chemicals, no acquired immunity can develop. Within days after birth, such a person dies of fulminating bacterial infection unless he or she is treated by heroic measures. Therefore, it is clear that the lymphocytes are essential to the survival of the human being.

The lymphocytes are located most extensively in the lymph nodes, but they are also found in special lymphoid tissues such as the spleen, submucosal areas of the gastrointestinal tract, thymus, and bone marrow. The lymphoid tissue is distributed advantageously in the body to intercept invading organisms or toxins before they can spread too widely.

In most instances, the invading agent first enters the tissue fluids and then is carried by lymph vessels to the lymph node or other lymphoid tissue. For instance, the lymphoid tissue of the gastrointestinal walls is exposed immediately to antigens invading from the gut. The lymphoid tissue of the throat and pharynx (the tonsils and adenoids) is well located to intercept antigens that enter by way of the upper respiratory tract. The lymphoid tissue in the lymph nodes is exposed to antigens that invade the peripheral tissues of the body, and finally, the lymphoid tissue of the spleen, thymus, and bone marrow plays the specific role of intercepting antigenic agents that have succeeded in reaching the circulating blood.

T and B Lymphocytes Promote "Cell-Mediated" Immunity or "Humoral" Immunity. Although most lymphocytes in normal lymphoid tissue look alike when studied under a microscope, these cells are distinctly divided into two major populations. One of the populations, the T lymphocytes, is responsible for forming the activated lymphocytes that provide "cell-mediated" immunity, and the other population, the B lymphocytes, is responsible for forming antibodies that provide "humoral" immunity.

Both types of lymphocytes are derived originally in the embryo from *pluripotent hematopoietic stem cells* that form *common lymphoid progenitor cells* as one of their most important offspring as they differentiate. Almost all of the lymphocytes that are formed eventually end up in the lymphoid tissue, but before doing so they are further differentiated or "preprocessed" in the following ways.

The lymphoid progenitor cells that are destined to eventually form activated T lymphocytes first migrate to and are preprocessed in the thymus gland, and thus they are called "T" lymphocytes to designate the role of the thymus. They are responsible for cell-mediated immunity.

The other population of lymphocytes—the B lymphocytes that are destined to form antibodies—are preprocessed in the liver during midfetal life and in the bone marrow in late fetal life and after birth. This population of cells was first discovered in birds that have a special preprocessing organ called the *bursa of Fabricius*. For this reason, these lymphocytes are called "B" lymphocytes to designate the role of the bursa, and they are responsible for humoral immunity. Figure 25-1 shows the two lymphocyte systems for the formation, respectively, of (1) the activated T lymphocytes and (2) the antibodies.

PREPROCESSING OF THE T AND B LYMPHOCYTES

Although all lymphocytes in the body originate from *lymphocyte-committed stem cells* of the embryo, these stem cells are incapable of forming directly either activated T lymphocytes or antibodies. Before they can do so, they must be further differentiated in appropriate processing areas as follows.

The Thymus Gland Preprocesses the T Lymphocytes. The T lymphocytes, after origination in the bone marrow, first migrate to the thymus gland. Here they divide rapidly and at the same time develop extreme diversity for reacting against different specific antigens. That is, one thymic lymphocyte develops specific reactivity against one antigen, and the next lymphocyte develops specificity against another antigen. This process continues until there are thousands of different types of thymic lymphocytes with specific reactivities against many thousands of different antigens. These different types of preprocessed T lymphocytes now leave the thymus and spread by way of the blood throughout the body to lodge in lymphoid tissue everywhere.

The thymus also makes certain that any T lymphocytes leaving the thymus will not react against proteins or other antigens that are present in the body's own tissues; otherwise, the T

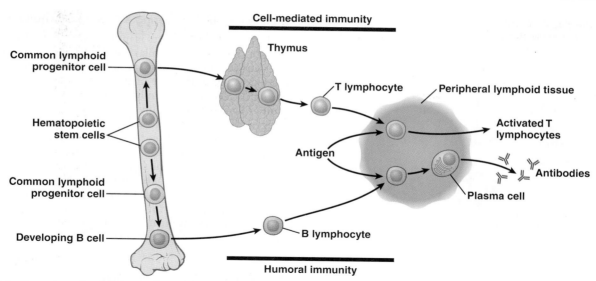

Figure 25-1 Formation of antibodies and sensitized lymphocytes by a lymph node in response to antigens. This figure also shows the origin of thymic (*T*) and bursal (*B*) lymphocytes that, respectively, are responsible for the cell-mediated and humoral immune processes.

lymphocytes would be lethal to the person's own body in only a few days. The thymus selects which T lymphocytes will be released by first mixing them with virtually all the specific "self-antigens" from the body's own tissues. If a T lymphocyte reacts, it is destroyed and phagocytized instead of being released. This happens to up to 90% of the cells. Thus, the only cells that are finally released are those that are nonreactive against the body's own antigens—they react only against antigens from an outside source, such as from a bacterium, a toxin, or even a transplanted tissue from another person.

Most of the preprocessing of T lymphocytes in the thymus occurs shortly before birth of a baby and for a few months after birth. Beyond this period, removal of the thymus gland diminishes (but does not eliminate) the T-lymphocytic immune system. However, removal of the thymus several months before birth can prevent development of all cell-mediated immunity. Because this cellular type of immunity is mainly responsible for rejection of transplanted organs, such as hearts and kidneys, one can transplant organs with much less likelihood of rejection if the thymus is removed from an animal a reasonable time before its birth.

Liver and Bone Marrow Preprocess the B Lymphocytes. Much less is known about the details for preprocessing B lymphocytes than for preprocessing T lymphocytes. In humans, B lymphocytes are known to be preprocessed in the liver during midfetal life and in the bone marrow during late fetal life and after birth.

B lymphocytes are different from T lymphocytes in two ways: First, instead of the whole cell developing reactivity against the antigen, as occurs for the T lymphocytes, the B lymphocytes actively secrete *antibodies* that are the reactive agents. These agents are large proteins that are capable of combining with and destroying the antigenic substance, which is explained elsewhere in this chapter and in Chapter 24. Second, the B lymphocytes have even greater diversity than the T lymphocytes, thus forming many millions of types of B-lymphocyte antibodies with different specific reactivities. After preprocessing, the B lymphocytes, like the T lymphocytes, migrate to lymphoid tissue throughout the body, where they lodge near but are slightly removed from the T lymphocyte areas.

T LYMPHOCYTES AND B-LYMPHOCYTE ANTIBODIES REACT HIGHLY SPECIFICALLY AGAINST SPECIFIC ANTIGENS—ROLE OF LYMPHOCYTE CLONES

When specific antigens come in contact with T and B lymphocytes in the lymphoid tissue, certain of the T lymphocytes become activated to form activated T cells and certain of the B lymphocytes become activated to form antibodies. The activated T cells and antibodies in turn react highly specifically against the particular types of antigens that initiated their development. The mechanism of this specificity is the following.

Millions of Specific Types of Lymphocytes Are Stored in the Lymphoid Tissue. Millions of different types of preformed B lymphocytes and preformed T lymphocytes that are capable of forming highly specific types of antibodies or T cells have been stored in the lymph tissue, as explained earlier. Each of these preformed lymphocytes is capable of forming only one type of antibody or one type of T cell with a single type of specificity, and only the specific type of antigen can activate it. Once the specific lymphocyte is activated by its antigen, it reproduces wildly, forming tremendous numbers of duplicate lymphocytes (Figure 25-2). If it is a B lymphocyte, its progeny will eventually secrete the specific type of antibody that then circulates throughout the body. If it is a T lymphocyte, its progeny are specific sensitized T cells that are released into the lymph and then carried to the blood and circulated through all the tissue fluids and back into the lymph, sometimes circulating around and around in this circuit for months or years.

All the different lymphocytes that are capable of forming one specific antibody or T cell are called a *clone of lymphocytes*. That is, the lymphocytes in each clone are alike and are derived originally from one or a few early lymphocytes of its specific type.

ORIGIN OF THE MANY CLONES OF LYMPHOCYTES

Only several hundred to a few thousand genes code for the millions of different types of antibodies and T lymphocytes. At

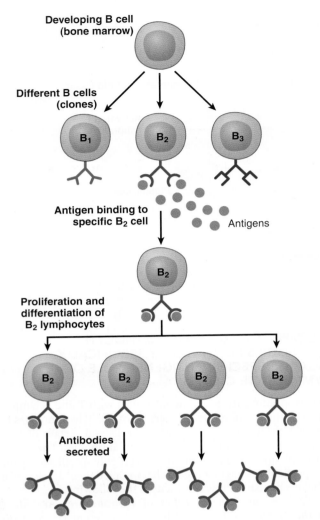

Developing B cell (bone marrow)

Different B cells (clones)

B₁ B₂ B₃

Antigen binding to specific B₂ cell

Antigens

B₂

Proliferation and differentiation of B₂ lymphocytes

B₂ B₂ B₂ B₂

Antibodies secreted

Figure 25-2 An antigen activates only the lymphocytes that have cell surface receptors that are complementary and recognize a specific antigen. Millions of different clones of lymphocytes exist (shown as B1, B2, and B3). When the lymphocyte clone (B2 in this example) is activated by its antigen, it reproduces to form large numbers of duplicate lymphocytes, which then secrete antibodies.

Mechanism for Activating a Clone of Lymphocytes

Each clone of lymphocytes is responsive to only a single type of antigen (or to several similar antigens that have almost exactly the same stereochemical characteristics). The reason for this is the following: In the case of the B lymphocytes, each of these has on its cell surface membrane about 100,000 antibody molecules that will react highly specifically with only one type of antigen. Therefore, when the appropriate antigen comes along, it immediately attaches to the antibody in the cell membrane; this leads to the activation process, which is described in more detail subsequently. In the case of the T lymphocytes, molecules similar to antibodies, called *surface receptor proteins* (or *T-cell markers*), are on the surface of the T-cell membrane, and these are also highly specific for one specified activating antigen. An antigen therefore stimulates only those cells that have complementary receptors for the antigen and are already committed to respond to it.

Role of Macrophages in the Activation Process. Aside from the lymphocytes in lymphoid tissue, literally millions of macrophages are also present in the same tissue. These macrophages line the sinusoids of the lymph nodes, spleen, and other lymphoid tissue, and they lie in apposition to many of the lymph node lymphocytes. Most invading organisms are first phagocytized and partially digested by the macrophages, and the antigenic products are liberated into the macrophage cytosol. The macrophages then pass these antigens by cell-to-cell contact directly to the lymphocytes, thus leading to activation of the specified lymphocytic clones. The macrophages, in addition, secrete a special activating substance, *interleukin-1*, that promotes still further growth and reproduction of the specific lymphocytes.

Role of the T Cells in Activation of the B Lymphocytes. Most antigens activate both T lymphocytes and B lymphocytes at the same time. Some of the T cells that are formed, called *T-helper cells*, secrete specific substances (collectively called *lymphokines*) that activate the specific B lymphocytes. Indeed, without the aid of these T-helper cells the quantity of antibodies formed by the B lymphocytes is usually slight. We discuss this cooperative relationship between T-helper cells and B cells after describing the mechanisms of the T-cell system of immunity.

SPECIFIC ATTRIBUTES OF THE B-LYMPHOCYTE SYSTEM—HUMORAL IMMUNITY AND THE ANTIBODIES

Formation of Antibodies by Plasma Cells. Before exposure to a specific antigen, the clones of B lymphocytes remain dormant in the lymphoid tissue. Upon entry of a foreign antigen, macrophages in lymphoid tissue phagocytize the antigen and then present it to adjacent B lymphocytes. In addition, the antigen is presented to T cells at the same time, and activated T-helper cells are formed. These helper cells also contribute to extreme activation of the B lymphocytes, as discussed later.

The B lymphocytes specific for the antigen immediately enlarge and take on the appearance of *lymphoblasts*. Some of the lymphoblasts further differentiate to form plasmablasts, which are precursors of plasma cells. In the *plasmablasts*, the cytoplasm expands and the rough endoplasmic reticulum vastly proliferates. The plasmablasts then begin to divide at a rate of about once every 10 hours for about 9 divisions, giving in 4 days a total

first, it was a mystery how it was possible for so few genes to code for the millions of different specificities of antibodies or T cells that can be produced by the lymphoid tissue. This mystery has now been solved.

The whole gene for forming each type of T cell or B cell is never present in the original stem cells from which the functional immune cells are formed. Instead, there are only "gene segments"—actually, hundreds of such segments—but not whole genes. During preprocessing of the respective T- and B-cell lymphocytes, these gene segments become mixed with one another in random combinations, in this way finally forming whole genes.

Because there are several hundred types of gene segments, as well as millions of different combinations in which the segments can be arranged in single cells, one can understand the millions of different cell gene types that can occur. For each functional T or B lymphocyte that is finally formed, the gene structure codes for only a single antigen specificity. These mature cells then become the highly specific T and B cells that spread to and populate the lymphoid tissue.

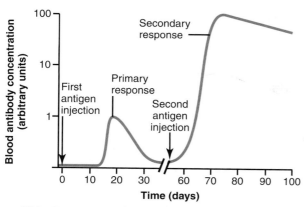

Figure 25-3 Time course of the antibody response in the circulating blood to a primary injection of antigen and to a secondary injection several weeks later.

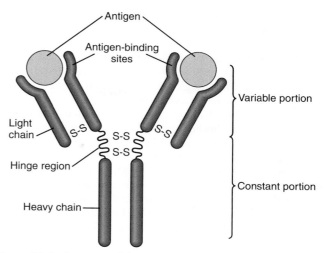

Figure 25-4 Structure of the typical IgG antibody, showing it to be composed of two heavy polypeptide chains and two light polypeptide chains. The antigen binds at two different sites on the variable portions of the chains. IgG, immunoglobulin G.

population of about 500 cells for each original plasmablast. The mature plasma cell then produces gamma globulin antibodies at an extremely rapid rate—about 2000 molecules/second for each plasma cell. In turn, the antibodies are secreted into the lymph and carried to the circulating blood. This process continues for several days or weeks until finally exhaustion and death of the plasma cells occur.

Formation of "Memory" Cells—Enhances the Antibody Response to Subsequent Antigen Exposure. A few of the lymphoblasts formed by activation of a clone of B lymphocytes do not go on to form plasma cells but instead form moderate numbers of new B lymphocytes similar to those of the original clone. In other words, the B-cell population of the specifically activated clone becomes greatly enhanced, and the new B lymphocytes are added to the original lymphocytes of the same clone. They also circulate throughout the body to populate all the lymphoid tissue; immunologically, however, they remain dormant until activated once again by a new quantity of the same antigen. These lymphocytes are called *memory cells.* Subsequent exposure to the same antigen will cause a much more rapid and much more potent antibody response this second time around because there are many more memory cells than there were original B lymphocytes of the specific clone.

Figure 25-3 shows the differences between the primary response for forming antibodies that occurs on first exposure to a specific antigen and the secondary response that occurs after second exposure to the same antigen. Note the 1-week delay in the appearance of the primary response, its weak potency, and its short life. The secondary response, by contrast, begins rapidly after exposure to the antigen (often within hours), is far more potent, and forms antibodies for many months rather than for only a few weeks. The increased potency and duration of the secondary response explains why immunization is usually accomplished by injecting antigen in multiple doses with periods of several weeks or several months between injections.

Nature of the Antibodies

Antibodies are gamma globulins called *immunoglobulins* (Ig), that have molecular weights between 160,000 and 970,000 and constitute about 20% of all the plasma proteins.

All the Igs are composed of combinations of *light* and *heavy polypeptide chains.* Most are a combination of two light and two heavy chains, as shown in Figure 25-4. However, some of the Igs

have combinations of as many as 10 heavy and 10 light chains, which give rise to high-molecular-weight Igs. Yet, in all Igs, each heavy chain is paralleled by a light chain at one of its ends, thus forming a heavy–light pair, and there are always at least 2 and as many as 10 such pairs in each Ig molecule.

Figure 25-4 shows a designated end of each light and heavy chain, called the *variable portion*; the remainder of each chain is called the *constant portion.* The variable portion is different for each specific antibody, and it is this portion that attaches specifically to a particular type of antigen. The constant portion of the antibody determines other properties of the antibody, establishing such factors as antibody diffusivity in the tissues, adherence of the antibody to specific structures within the tissues, attachment to the complement complex, ease with which the antibodies pass through membranes, and other biological properties of the antibody. A combination of noncovalent and covalent bonds (disulfide) holds the light and heavy chains together.

Specificity of Antibodies. Each antibody is specific for a particular antigen; this characteristic is caused by its unique structural organization of amino acids in the variable portions of both the light and heavy chains. The amino acid organization has a different steric shape for each antigen specificity, so when an antigen comes in contact with it, multiple prosthetic groups of the antigen fit as a mirror image with those of the antibody, thus allowing rapid and tight bonding between the antibody and the antigen. When the antibody is highly specific, there are so many bonding sites that the antibody–antigen coupling is exceedingly strong, held together by (1) hydrophobic bonding, (2) hydrogen bonding, (3) ionic attractions, and (4) van der Waals forces. It also obeys the thermodynamic mass action law:

$$K_a = \frac{\text{concentration of bound antibody} - \text{antigen}}{(\text{concentration of antibody}) \times (\text{concentration of antigen})}$$

K_a is called the *affinity constant* and is a measure of how tightly the antibody binds with the antigen.

Note, especially, in Figure 25-4 that there are two variable sites on the illustrated antibody for attachment of antigens, making this type of antibody bivalent. A small proportion of the antibodies, which consist of combinations of up to 10 light and 10 heavy chains, have as many as 10 binding sites.

Five General Classes of Antibodies. There are five general classes of antibodies, respectively, named *IgM, IgG, IgA, IgD,* and *IgE. Ig* stands for immunoglobulin and the other five respective letters designate the respective classes.

For the purpose of our present limited discussion, two of these classes of antibodies are of particular importance: IgG, which is a bivalent antibody and constitutes about 75% of the antibodies of the normal person, and IgE, which constitutes only a small percentage of the antibodies but is especially involved in allergy. The IgM class is also interesting because a large share of the antibodies formed during the primary response is of this type. These antibodies have 10 binding sites that make them exceedingly effective in protecting the body against invaders, even though there are not many IgM antibodies.

Mechanisms of Action of Antibodies

Antibodies act mainly in two ways to protect the body against invading agents: (1) by direct attack on the invader and (2) by activation of the "complement system" that then has multiple means of its own for destroying the invader.

Direct Action of Antibodies on Invading Agents. Figure 25-5 shows antibodies (designated by the red Y-shaped bars) reacting with antigens (designated by the shaded objects). Because of the bivalent nature of the antibodies and the multiple antigen sites on most invading agents, the antibodies can inactivate the invading agent in one of several ways, as follows:

1. *agglutination,* in which multiple large particles with antigens on their surfaces, such as bacteria or red cells, are bound together into a clump;
2. *precipitation,* in which the molecular complex of soluble antigen (eg, tetanus toxin) and antibody becomes so large that it is rendered insoluble and precipitates;
3. *neutralization,* in which the antibodies cover the toxic sites of the antigenic agent;

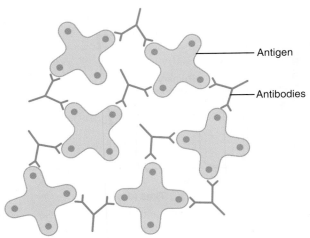

Figure 25-5 Binding of antigen molecules to one another by bivalent antibodies.

4. *lysis,* in which some potent antibodies are occasionally capable of directly attacking membranes of cellular agents and thereby cause rupture of the agent.

These direct actions of antibodies often are not strong enough to play a major role in protecting the body against the invader. Most of the protection comes through the amplifying effects of the complement system described next.

Complement System for Antibody Action

"Complement" is a collective term that describes a system of about 20 proteins, many of which are enzyme precursors. The principal actors in this system are 11 proteins designated C1–C9, B, and D, shown in Figure 25-6. All these are present normally among the plasma proteins in the blood, as well as among the proteins that leak out of the capillaries into the tissue spaces. The enzyme precursors are normally inactive, but they can be activated mainly by the so-called *classical pathway.*

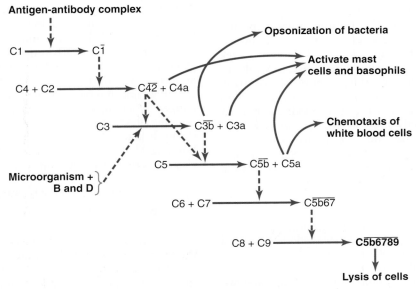

Figure 25-6 Cascade of reactions during activation of the classic pathway of complement.

Classical Pathway. The classic pathway is initiated by an antigen–antibody reaction. That is, when an antibody binds with an antigen, a specific reactive site on the "constant" portion of the antibody becomes uncovered or "activated," and this in turn binds directly with the C1 molecule of the complement system, setting into motion a "cascade" of sequential reactions, shown in Figure 25-6, beginning with activation of the proenzyme C1. The C1 enzymes that are formed then activate successively increasing quantities of enzymes in the later stages of the system so that from a small beginning, an extremely large "amplified" reaction occurs. Multiple end products are formed, as shown to the right in the figure, and several of these cause important effects that help to prevent damage to the body's tissues caused by the invading organism or toxin. Among the more important effects are the following:

1. *Opsonization and phagocytosis*: One of the products of the complement cascade, C3b, strongly activates phagocytosis by both neutrophils and macrophages, causing these cells to engulf the bacteria to which the antigen–antibody complexes are attached. This process is called *opsonization*. It often enhances the number of bacteria that can be destroyed by many hundredfold.

2. *Lysis*: One of the most important of all the products of the complement cascade is the lytic complex, which is a combination of multiple complement factors and designated C5b6789. This has a direct effect of rupturing the cell membranes of bacteria or other invading organisms.

3. *Agglutination*: The complement products also change the surfaces of the invading organisms, causing them to adhere to one another, thus promoting agglutination.

4. *Neutralization of viruses*: The complement enzymes and other complement products can attack the structures of some viruses and thereby render them nonvirulent.

5. *Chemotaxis*: Fragment C5a initiates chemotaxis of neutrophils and macrophages, thus causing large numbers of these phagocytes to migrate into the tissue area adjacent to the antigenic agent.

6. *Activation of mast cells and basophils*: Fragments C3a, C4a, and C5a activate mast cells and basophils, causing them to release histamine, heparin, and several other substances into the local fluids. These substances in turn cause increased local blood flow, increased leakage of fluid and plasma protein into the tissue, and other local tissue reactions that help inactivate or immobilize the antigenic agent. The same factors play a major role in inflammation (which was discussed in Chapter 24) and in allergy, as we discuss later.

7. *Inflammatory effects*: In addition to inflammatory effects caused by activation of the mast cells and basophils, several other complement products contribute to local inflammation. These products cause (a) the already increased blood flow to increase still further, (b) the capillary leakage of proteins to be increased, and (c) the interstitial fluid proteins to coagulate in the tissue spaces, thus preventing movement of the invading organism through the tissues.

SPECIAL ATTRIBUTES OF THE T-LYMPHOCYTE SYSTEM—ACTIVATED T CELLS AND CELL-MEDIATED IMMUNITY

Release of Activated T Cells from Lymphoid Tissue and Formation of Memory Cells. Upon exposure to the proper antigen, as presented by adjacent macrophages, the T lymphocytes of a specific lymphocyte clone proliferate and release large numbers of activated, specifically reacting T cells in ways that parallel antibody release by activated B cells. The principal difference is that instead of releasing antibodies, whole activated T cells are formed and released into the lymph. These T cells then pass into the circulation and are distributed throughout the body, passing through the capillary walls into the tissue spaces, back into the lymph and blood once again, and circulating again and again throughout the body, sometimes lasting for months or even years.

Also, *T lymphocyte memory cells* are formed in the same way that B memory cells are formed in the antibody system. That is, when a clone of T lymphocytes is activated by an antigen, many of the newly formed lymphocytes are preserved in the lymphoid tissue to become additional T lymphocytes of that specific clone; in fact, these memory cells even spread throughout the lymphoid tissue of the entire body. Therefore, on subsequent exposure to the same antigen anywhere in the body, release of activated T cells occurs far more rapidly and much more powerfully than during first exposure.

Antigen-Presenting Cells, MHC Proteins, and Antigen Receptors on the T Lymphocytes. T-cell responses are extremely antigen specific, like the antibody responses of B cells, and are at least as important as antibodies in defending against infection. In fact, acquired immune responses usually require assistance from T cells to begin the process, and T cells play a major role in helping to eliminate invading pathogens.

Although B lymphocytes recognize intact antigens, T lymphocytes respond to antigens only when they are bound to specific molecules called *major histocompatibility complex (MHC) proteins* on the surface of *antigen-presenting cells* in the lymphoid tissues (Figure 25-7). The three major types of antigen-presenting cells are *macrophages*, *B lymphocytes*, and *dendritic cells*. The dendritic cells, the most potent of the antigen-presenting cells, are located throughout the body, and their only known function is to present antigens to T cells. Interaction of cell adhesion proteins is critical in permitting the T cells to bind to antigen-presenting cells long enough to become activated.

The MHC proteins are encoded by a large group of genes called the *MHC*. The MHC proteins bind peptide fragments of

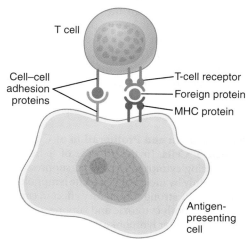

Figure 25-7 Activation of T cells requires interaction of T-cell receptors with an antigen (foreign protein) that is transported to the surface of the antigen-presenting cell by a MHC protein. Cell-to-cell adhesion proteins enable the T cell to bind to the antigen-presenting cell long enough to become activated. *MHC*, major histocompatibility complex.

antigen proteins that are degraded inside antigen-presenting cells and then transport them to the cell surface. There are two types of MHC proteins: (1) *MHC I proteins*, which present antigens to *cytotoxic T cells*, and (2) *MHC II proteins*, which present antigens to *T-helper cells*. The specific functions of cytotoxic and T-helper cells are discussed later.

The antigens on the surface of antigen-presenting cells bind with receptor molecules on the surfaces of T cells in the same way that they bind with plasma protein antibodies. These receptor molecules are composed of a variable unit similar to the variable portion of the humoral antibody, but its stem section is firmly bound to the cell membrane of the T lymphocyte. There are as many as 100,000 receptor sites on a single T cell.

SEVERAL TYPES OF T CELLS AND THEIR DIFFERENT FUNCTIONS

It has become clear that there are multiple types of T cells. They are classified into three major groups: (1) *T-helper cells*, (2) *cytotoxic T cells*, and (3) *suppressor T cells*. The functions of each of these T cells are distinct.

T-Helper Cells are the Most Numerous of the T Cells

The T-helper cells are by far the most numerous of the T cells, usually constituting more than three-quarters of all of them. As their name implies, they help in the functions of the immune system, and they do so in many ways. In fact, they serve as the major regulator of virtually all immune functions, as shown in Figure 25-8. They do this by forming a series of protein mediators, called *lymphokines*, that act on other cells of the immune system, as well as on bone marrow cells. Among the most important lymphokines secreted by the T-helper cells are the following:

- interleukin-2
- interleukin-3
- interleukin-4
- interleukin-5
- interleukin-6
- granulocyte–monocyte colony-stimulating factor
- interferon-γ

Specific Regulatory Functions of the Lymphokines. In the absence of the lymphokines from the T-helper cells, the remainder of the immune system is almost paralyzed. In fact, it is the T-helper cells that are inactivated or destroyed by the *human immunodeficiency virus* (*HIV*), which leaves the body almost totally unprotected against infectious disease, therefore leading to the now well-known debilitating and lethal effects of *acquired immunodeficiency syndrome* (*AIDS*). Some of the specific regulatory functions are described in the following sections.

Stimulation of Growth and Proliferation of Cytotoxic T Cells and Suppressor T Cells. In the absence of T-helper cells, the clones for producing cytotoxic T cells and suppressor T cells are activated only slightly by most antigens. The lymphokine interleukin-2 has an especially strong stimulatory effect in causing growth and proliferation of both cytotoxic and suppressor T cells. In addition, several of the other lymphokines have less potent effects.

Stimulation of B-Cell Growth and Differentiation to Form Plasma Cells and Antibodies. The direct actions of antigens to cause B-cell growth, proliferation, formation of plasma cells, and secretion of antibodies are also slight without the "help" of

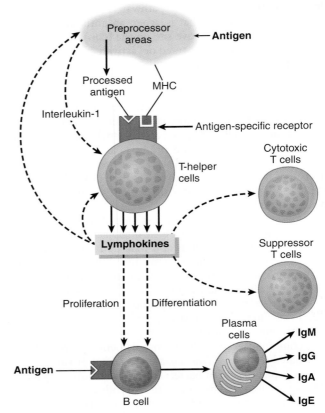

Figure 25-8 Regulation of the immune system, emphasizing a pivotal role of the T-helper cells. *IgA*, immunoglobulin A; *IgE*, immunoglobulin E; *IgG*, immunoglobulin G; *IgM*, immunoglobulin M; *MHC*, major histocompatibility complex.

the T-helper cells. Almost all the interleukins participate in the B-cell response, but especially interleukins 4, 5, and 6. In fact, these three interleukins have such potent effects on the B cells that they have been called B-cell–stimulating factors or B-cell growth factors.

Activation of the Macrophage System. The lymphokines also affect the macrophages. First, they slow or stop the migration of the macrophages after they have been chemotactically attracted into the inflamed tissue area, thus causing great accumulation of macrophages. Second, they activate the macrophages to cause far more efficient phagocytosis, allowing them to attack and destroy increasing numbers of invading bacteria or other tissue-destroying agents.

Feedback Stimulatory Effect on the T-Helper Cells. Some of the lymphokines, especially interleukin-2, have a direct positive feedback effect in stimulating activation of the T-helper cells themselves. This acts as an amplifier by further enhancing the helper cell response, as well as the entire immune response to an invading antigen.

Cytotoxic T Cells Are "Killer" Cells

The cytotoxic T cell is a direct-attack cell that is capable of killing microorganisms and, at times, even some of the body's own cells. For this reason, these cells are called *killer cells*. The receptor proteins on the surfaces of the cytotoxic cells cause them to bind tightly to the organisms or cells that contain the appropriate

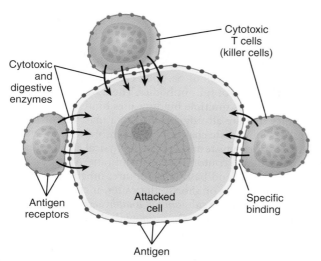

Figure 25-9 Direct destruction of an invading cell by sensitized lymphocytes (cytotoxic T cells).

binding-specific antigen. Then, they kill the attacked cell in the manner shown in Figure 25-9. After binding, the cytotoxic T cell secretes hole-forming proteins, called *perforins*, that literally punch round holes in the membrane of the attacked cell. Then fluid flows rapidly into the cell from the interstitial space. In addition, the cytotoxic T cell releases cytotoxic substances directly into the attacked cell. Almost immediately, the attacked cell becomes greatly swollen, and it usually dissolves shortly thereafter.

Of special importance is that these cytotoxic killer cells can pull away from the victim cells after they have punched holes and delivered cytotoxic substances, and then move on to kill more cells. Indeed, some of these cells persist for months in the tissues.

Some of the cytotoxic T cells are especially lethal to tissue cells that have been invaded by viruses because many virus particles become entrapped in the membranes of the tissue cells and attract T cells in response to the viral antigenicity. The cytotoxic cells also play an important role in destroying cancer cells, heart transplant cells, or other types of cells that are foreign to the person's own body.

Suppressor T Cells

Much less is known about the suppressor T cells than about the others, but they are capable of suppressing the functions of both cytotoxic and T-helper cells. These suppressor functions are believed to prevent the cytotoxic cells from causing excessive immune reactions that might be damaging to the body's own tissues. For this reason, the suppressor cells are classified, along with the T-helper cells, as *regulatory T cells*. It is probable that the suppressor T-cell system plays an important role in limiting the ability of the immune system to attack a person's own body tissues, called *immune tolerance*, as we discuss in the next section.

TOLERANCE OF THE ACQUIRED IMMUNITY SYSTEM TO ONE'S OWN TISSUES—ROLE OF PREPROCESSING IN THE THYMUS AND BONE MARROW

The process of acquired immunity would destroy the individual's own body if a person became immune to his or her own tissues. The immune mechanism normally "recognizes" a person's own tissues as being distinctive from bacteria or viruses, and the person's immunity system forms few antibodies or activated T cells against his or her own antigens.

Most Tolerance Results from Clone Selection During Preprocessing. Most tolerance is believed to develop during preprocessing of T lymphocytes in the thymus and of B lymphocytes in the bone marrow. The reason for this belief is that injecting a strong antigen into a fetus while the lymphocytes are being preprocessed in these two areas prevents development of clones of lymphocytes in the lymphoid tissue that are specific for the injected antigen. Experiments have shown that specific immature lymphocytes in the thymus, when exposed to a strong antigen, become lymphoblastic, proliferate considerably, and then combine with the stimulating antigen—an effect that is believed to cause the cells to be destroyed by the thymic epithelial cells before they can migrate to and colonize the total body lymphoid tissue.

It is believed that during the preprocessing of lymphocytes in the thymus and bone marrow, all or most of the clones of lymphocytes that are specific to damage the body's own tissues are self-destroyed because of their continual exposure to the body's antigens.

Failure of the Tolerance Mechanism Causes Autoimmune Diseases. Sometimes people lose immune tolerance of their own tissues. This phenomenon occurs to a greater extent the older a person becomes. It usually occurs after destruction of some of the body's own tissues, which releases considerable quantities of "self-antigens" that circulate in the body and presumably cause acquired immunity in the form of either activated T cells or antibodies.

Several specific diseases that result from autoimmunity include (1) *rheumatic fever*, in which the body becomes immunized against tissues in the joints and heart, especially the heart valves, after exposure to a specific type of streptococcal toxin that has an epitope in its molecular structure similar to the structure of some of the body's own self-antigens; (2) one type of *glomerulonephritis*, in which the person becomes immunized against the basement membranes of glomeruli; (3) *myasthenia gravis*, in which immunity develops against the acetylcholine receptor proteins of the neuromuscular junction, causing paralysis; and (4) *systemic lupus erythematosus (SLE)*, in which the person becomes immunized against many different body tissues at the same time, a disease that causes extensive damage and even death when SLE is severe.

IMMUNIZATION BY INJECTION OF ANTIGENS

Immunization has been used for many years to produce acquired immunity against specific diseases. A person can be immunized by injecting dead organisms that are no longer capable of causing disease but that still have some of their chemical antigens. This type of immunization is used to protect against typhoid fever, whooping cough, diphtheria, and many other types of bacterial diseases.

Immunity can be achieved against toxins that have been treated with chemicals so that their toxic nature has been destroyed even though their antigens for causing immunity are still intact. This procedure is used in immunizing against tetanus, botulism, and other similar toxic diseases.

And, finally, a person can be immunized by being infected with live organisms that have been "attenuated." That is, these organisms either have been grown in special culture media or have been passed through a series of animals until they have mutated enough that they will not cause disease but do still carry specific antigens required for immunization. This procedure is used to protect against smallpox, yellow fever, poliomyelitis, measles, and many other viral diseases.

PASSIVE IMMUNITY

Thus far, all the acquired immunity we have discussed has been *active immunity*. That is, the person's own body develops either antibodies or activated T cells in response to invasion of the body by a foreign antigen. However, temporary immunity can be achieved in a person without injecting any antigen. This temporary immunity is achieved by infusing antibodies, activated T cells, or both obtained from the blood of someone else or from some other animal that has been actively immunized against the antigen.

Antibodies last in the body of the recipient for 2–3 weeks, and during that time the person is protected against the invading disease. Activated T cells last for a few weeks if transfused from another person, but only for a few hours to a few days if transfused from an animal. Such transfusion of antibodies or T lymphocytes to confer immunity is called *passive immunity*.

Allergy and Hypersensitivity

An important undesirable side effect of immunity is the development, under some conditions, of allergy or other types of immune hypersensitivity. There are several types of allergy and other hypersensitivities, some of which occur only in people who have a specific allergic tendency.

ALLERGY CAUSED BY ACTIVATED T CELLS: DELAYED-REACTION ALLERGY

Delayed-reaction allergy is caused by activated T cells and not by antibodies. In the case of poison ivy, the toxin of poison ivy in itself does not cause much harm to the tissues. However, upon repeated exposure, it does cause the formation of activated helper and cytotoxic T cells. Then, after subsequent exposure to the poison ivy toxin, within a day or so, the activated T cells diffuse from the circulating blood in large numbers into the skin to respond to the poison ivy toxin. At the same time, these T cells elicit a cell-mediated type of immune reaction. Remembering that this type of immunity can cause release of many toxic substances from the activated T cells, as well as extensive invasion of the tissues by macrophages along with their subsequent effects, one can well understand that the eventual result of some delayed-reaction allergies can be serious tissue damage. The damage normally occurs in the tissue area where the instigating antigen is present, such as in the skin in the case of poison ivy, or in the lungs to cause lung edema or asthmatic attacks in the case of some airborne antigens.

"ATOPIC" ALLERGIES ASSOCIATED WITH EXCESS IgE ANTIBODIES

Some people have an "allergic" tendency. Their allergies are called *atopic allergies* because they are caused by a nonordinary response of the immune system. The allergic tendency is genetically passed from parent to child and is characterized by the presence of large quantities of IgE antibodies in the blood. These antibodies are called *reagins* or *sensitizing antibodies* to distinguish them from the more common IgG antibodies. When an *allergen* (defined as an antigen that reacts specifically with a specific type of IgE reagin antibody) enters the body, an allergen–reagin reaction takes place and a subsequent allergic reaction occurs.

A special characteristic of the IgE antibodies (the reagins) is a strong propensity to attach to mast cells and basophils. Indeed, a single mast cell or basophil can bind as many as half a million molecules of IgE antibodies. Then, when an antigen (an allergen) that has multiple binding sites binds with several IgE antibodies that are already attached to a mast cell or basophil, this causes immediate change in the membrane of the mast cell or basophil, perhaps resulting from a physical effect of the antibody molecules to contort the cell membrane. At any rate, many of the mast cells and basophils rupture; others release special agents immediately or shortly thereafter, including *histamine, protease, slow-reacting substance of anaphylaxis* (which is a mixture of toxic leukotrienes), *eosinophil chemotactic substance, neutrophil chemotactic substance, heparin,* and *platelet-activating factors*. These substances cause such effects as dilation of the local blood vessels, attraction of eosinophils and neutrophils to the reactive site, increased permeability of the capillaries with loss of fluid into the tissues, and contraction of local smooth muscle cells. Therefore, several different tissue responses can occur, depending on the type of tissue in which the allergen–reagin reaction occurs. Among the different types of allergic reactions caused in this manner are the following.

Anaphylaxis. When a specific allergen is injected directly into the circulation, the allergen can react with basophils of the blood and mast cells in the tissues located immediately outside the small blood vessels if the basophils and mast cells have been sensitized by attachment of IgE reagins. Therefore, a widespread allergic reaction occurs throughout the vascular system and closely associated tissues. This reaction is called *anaphylaxis*. Histamine is released into the circulation and causes body-wide vasodilation, as well as increased permeability of the capillaries with resultant marked loss of plasma from the circulation. Occasionally, a person who experiences this reaction dies of circulatory shock within a few minutes unless treated with epinephrine to oppose the effects of the histamine.

Also released from the activated basophils and mast cells is a mixture of leukotrienes called *slow-reacting substance of anaphylaxis*. These leukotrienes can cause spasm of the smooth muscle of the bronchioles, eliciting an asthma-like attack, sometimes causing death by suffocation.

Urticaria. Urticaria results from antigen entering specific skin areas and causing localized anaphylactoid reactions. Histamine released locally causes (1) vasodilation that induces an immediate red flare and (2) increased local permeability of the capillaries that leads to local circumscribed areas of swelling of the skin within another few minutes. The swellings are commonly called *hives*. Administration of antihistamine drugs to a person before exposure will prevent the hives.

Hay Fever. In hay fever, the allergen–reagin reaction occurs in the nose. Histamine released in response to the reaction causes local intranasal vascular dilation, with resultant increased capillary pressure and increased capillary permeability. Both these effects cause rapid fluid leakage into the nasal cavities and into associated deeper tissues of the nose, and the nasal linings become swollen and secretory. Here again, use of antihistamine drugs can prevent this swelling reaction. However, other products of the allergen–reagin reaction can still cause irritation of the nose, eliciting the typical sneezing syndrome.

Asthma. Asthma often occurs in the "allergic" type of person. In such a person, the allergen–reagin reaction occurs in the bronchioles of the lungs. Here, an important product released from the mast cells is believed to be the *slow-reacting substance of anaphylaxis* (a mixture of three leukotrienes), which causes spasm of the bronchiolar smooth muscle. Consequently, the person has difficulty breathing until the reactive products of the allergic reaction have been removed. Administration of antihistamine medication has less effect on the course of asthma because histamine does not appear to be the major factor eliciting the asthmatic reaction.

BIBLIOGRAPHY

Alberts B, Johnson A, Lewis J, et al: *Molecular Biology of the Cell*, fifth ed., New York, 2008, Garland Science.

Anderson GP: Endotyping asthma: new insights into key pathogenic mechanisms in a complex, heterogeneous disease, *Lancet* 372:1107, 2008.

Barton GM: A calculated response: control of inflammation by the innate immune system, *J. Clin. Invest.* 118:413, 2008.

Cossart P, Sansonetti PJ: Bacterial invasion: the paradigms of enteroinvasive pathogens, *Science* 304:242, 2004.

Dorshkind K, Montecino-Rodriguez E, Signer RA: The ageing immune system: is it ever too old to become young again? *Nat. Rev. Immunol.* 9:57, 2009.

Eisenbarth GS, Gottlieb PA: Autoimmune polyendocrine syndromes, *N. Engl. J. Med.* 350:2068, 2004.

Fanta CH: Asthma, *N. Engl. J. Med.* 360:1002, 2009.

Grossman Z, Min B, Meier-Schellersheim M, et al: Concomitant regulation of T-cell activation and homeostasis, *Nat. Rev. Immunol.* 4:387, 2004.

Kupper TS, Fuhlbrigge RC: Immune surveillance in the skin: mechanisms and clinical consequences, *Nat. Rev. Immunol.* 4:211, 2004.

Linton PJ, Dorshkind K: Age-related changes in lymphocyte development and function, *Nat. Immunol.* 5:133, 2004.

Mackay IR: Autoimmunity since the 1957 clonal selection theory: a little acorn to a large oak, *Immunol. Cell Biol.* 86:67, 2008.

Medzhitov R: Recognition of microorganisms and activation of the immune response, *Nature* 449:819, 2007.

Mizushima N, Levine B, Cuervo AM, et al: Autophagy fights disease through cellular self-digestion, *Nature* 45:1069, 2008.

Nabel GJ: Designing tomorrow's vaccines, *N. Engl. J. Med.* 368:551, 2013.

Rahman A, Isenberg DA: Systemic lupus erythematosus, *N. Engl. J. Med.* 358:929, 2008.

Vivier E, Anfossi N: Inhibitory NK-cell receptors on T cells: witness of the past, actors of the future, *Nat. Rev. Immunol.* 4:190, 2004.

Wahren-Herlenius M, Dorner T: Immunopathogenic mechanisms of systemic autoimmune disease, *Lancet* 382:819, 2012.

Welner RS, Pelayo R, Kincade PW: Evolving views on the genealogy of B cells, *Nat. Rev. Immunol.* 8:95, 2008.

26

Platelets

LEARNING OBJECTIVES

- Describe the development and morphology of platelets.
- List and describe platelet functions.
- Describe early events in hemostasis and the formation of the platelet plug.
- Describe thrombocytopenia.
- Define bleeding time.
- Describe thromboembolic conditions and principles of their treatment.

GLOSSARY OF TERMS

- **Autacoid:** Referring to local effects from chemicals that are not blood borne (usually these effects are on smooth muscle)
- **Myogenic:** Deriving from muscle (smooth) action
- **Pseudopods:** Meaning false feet—temporary projections of a cell
- **Punctate:** Pinpoint
- **Splenectomy:** Surgical removal of the spleen

Hemostasis Events

The term *hemostasis* means prevention of blood loss. Whenever a vessel is severed or ruptured, hemostasis is achieved by several mechanisms: (1) vascular constriction, (2) formation of a platelet plug, (3) formation of a blood clot as a result of blood coagulation, and (4) eventual growth of fibrous tissue into the blood clot to close the hole in the vessel permanently.

Vascular Constriction

Immediately after a blood vessel has been cut or ruptured, the trauma to the vessel wall causes smooth muscle in the wall contract; this instantaneously reduces the flow of blood from the ruptured vessel. The contraction results from (1) local myogenic spasm, (2) local autacoid factors from the traumatized tissues and blood platelets, and (3) nervous reflexes. The nervous reflexes are initiated by pain nerve impulses or other sensory impulses that originate from the traumatized vessel or nearby tissues. However, even more vasoconstriction probably results from local *myogenic contraction* of the blood vessels initiated by direct damage to the vascular wall. And, for the smaller vessels, the platelets are responsible for much of the vasoconstriction by releasing a vasoconstrictor substance, *thromboxane A_2*.

The more severely a vessel is traumatized, the greater is the degree of vascular spasm. The spasm can last for many minutes or even hours, during which time the processes of platelet plugging and blood coagulation can take place.

FORMATION OF THE PLATELET PLUG

If the cut in the blood vessel is very small—indeed, many very small vascular holes develop throughout the body each day—the cut is often sealed by a *platelet plug*, rather than by a blood clot. To understand this process, it is important that we first discuss the nature of platelets themselves.

BLOOD COAGULATION IN THE RUPTURED VESSEL

The third mechanism for hemostasis is formation of the blood clot. The clot begins to develop in 15–20 seconds if the trauma to the vascular wall has been severe, and in 1–2 minutes if the trauma has been minor. Activator substances from the traumatized vascular wall, from platelets, and from blood proteins adhering to the traumatized vascular wall initiate the clotting process. The physical events of this process are shown in Figure 26-1, and Table 26-1 lists the most important of the clotting factors.

Within 3–6 minutes after rupture of a vessel, the entire opening or broken end of the vessel is filled with clot if the vessel opening is not too large. After 20 minutes to an hour, the clot retracts which closes the vessel still further. Platelets also play an important role in this clot retraction, as is discussed later.

FIBROUS ORGANIZATION OR DISSOLUTION OF THE BLOOD CLOT

Once a blood clot has formed, it can follow one of two courses: (1) it can become invaded by *fibroblasts*, which subsequently form connective tissue all through the clot, or (2) it can dissolve. The usual course for a clot that forms in a small hole of a vessel wall is invasion by fibroblasts, beginning within a few hours

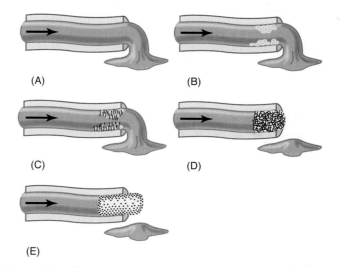

Figure 26-1 Clotting process in a traumatized blood vessel. (A) Severed vessel; (B) platelets agglutinate; (C) fibrin appears; (D) fibrin clot forms; (E) clot retraction occurs. *Modified from Seegers, W.H., 1948. Hemostatic Agents. Charles C. Thomas, Springfield, IL. Courtesy Charles C. Thomas, Publisher Ltd., Springfield, IL.*

TABLE 26-1	Clotting Factors in Blood and Their Synonyms
Clotting Factor	**Synonyms**
Fibrinogen	Factor I
Prothrombin	Factor II
Tissue factor	Factor III; tissue thromboplastin
Calcium	Factor IV
Factor V	Proaccelerin; labile factor; Ac-globulin (Ac-G)
Factor VII	Serum prothrombin conversion accelerator (SPCA); proconvertin; stable factor
Factor VIII	Antihemophilic factor (AHF); antihemophilic globulin (AHG); antihemophilic factor A
Factor IX	Plasma thromboplastin component (PTC); Christmas factor; antihemophilic factor B
Factor X	Stuart factor; Stuart–Prower factor
Factor XI	Plasma thromboplastin antecedent (PTA); antihemophilic factor C
Factor XII	Hageman factor
Factor XIII	Fibrin-stabilizing factor
Prekallikrein	Fletcher factor
High-molecular-weight kininogen	Fitzgerald factor; high-molecular-weight kininogen (HMWK)
Platelets	

after the clot is formed (which is promoted at least partially by *growth factor* secreted by platelets). This process continues to complete organization of the clot into fibrous tissue within about 1–2 weeks.

Conversely, when excess blood has leaked into the tissues and tissue clots have occurred where they are not needed, special substances within the clot itself usually become activated. These substances function as enzymes to dissolve the clot, as discussed later in the chapter.

PHYSICAL AND CHEMICAL CHARACTERISTICS OF PLATELETS

Platelets (also called *thrombocytes*) are minute discs 1–4 μm in diameter. They are formed in the bone marrow from *megakaryocytes*, which are extremely large hematopoietic cells in the marrow; the megakaryocytes fragment into the minute platelets either in the bone marrow or soon after entering the blood, especially as they squeeze through capillaries. The normal concentration of platelets in the blood is between 150,000 and 300,000/μL.

Platelets have many functional characteristics of whole cells, even though they do not have nuclei and cannot reproduce. In their cytoplasm are (1) *actin* and *myosin molecules*, which are contractile proteins similar to those found in muscle cells, and still another contractile protein, *thrombosthenin*, that can cause the platelets to contract; (2) residuals of both the *endoplasmic reticulum* and the *Golgi apparatus* that synthesize various enzymes and especially store large quantities of calcium ions; (3) mitochondria and enzyme systems that are capable of forming *adenosine triphosphate* (ATP) and *adenosine diphosphate* (ADP); (4) enzyme systems that synthesize *prostaglandins*, which are local hormones that cause many vascular and other local tissue reactions; (5) an important protein called *fibrin-stabilizing factor*, which we discuss later in relation to blood coagulation; and (6) a *growth factor* that causes vascular endothelial cells, vascular smooth muscle cells, and fibroblasts to multiply and grow, thus causing cellular growth that eventually helps repair damaged vascular walls.

On the platelet cell membrane surface is a coat of *glycoproteins* that repulses adherence to normal endothelium and yet causes adherence to *injured* areas of the vessel wall, especially to injured endothelial cells and even more so to any exposed collagen from deep within the vessel wall. In addition, the platelet membrane contains large amounts of *phospholipids* that activate multiple stages in the blood-clotting process, as we discuss later.

Thus, the platelet is an active structure. It has a half-life in the blood of 8–12 days, so over several weeks its functional processes run out; it is then eliminated from the circulation, mainly by the tissue macrophage system. More than one-half of the platelets are removed by macrophages in the spleen, where the blood passes through a latticework of tight trabeculae.

Mechanism of the Platelet Plug

Platelet repair of vascular openings is based on several important functions of the platelet. When platelets come in contact with a damaged vascular surface, especially with collagen fibers in the vascular wall, the platelets rapidly change their own characteristics drastically. They begin to swell; they assume irregular forms with numerous irradiating pseudopods protruding from their surfaces; their contractile proteins contract forcefully and cause the release of granules that contain multiple active factors; they become sticky so that they adhere to collagen in the tissues and to a protein called *von Willebrand factor* that leaks into the traumatized tissue from the plasma; they secrete large quantities of ADP; and their enzymes form *thromboxane A_2*. The ADP and thromboxane in turn act on nearby platelets to activate them as well, and the stickiness of these additional platelets causes them to adhere to the original activated platelets.

Therefore, at the site of a puncture in a blood vessel wall, the damaged vascular wall activates successively increasing numbers of platelets that attract more and more additional platelets, thus forming a *platelet plug*. This plug is loose at first, but it is usually successful in blocking blood loss if the vascular opening is small. Then, during the subsequent process of blood coagulation, *fibrin threads* form. These threads attach tightly to the platelets, thus constructing an unyielding plug (Box 26-1).

Importance of the Platelet Mechanism for Closing Vascular Holes. The platelet-plugging mechanism is extremely important for closing minute ruptures in very small blood vessels that occur many thousands of times daily. Indeed, multiple small holes through the endothelial cells themselves are often closed by platelets actually fusing with the endothelial cells to form additional endothelial cell membrane. Literally thousands of

---

BOX 26-1 FUNCTIONS OF PLATELETS

Mainly involved in thrombosis and formation of platelet plug
Also involved in promoting coagulation
Can be deduced from contents of platelet granules:
1. α-Granules contain the following:
   a. platelet factor 4—procoagulant
   b. fibronectin—helps in binding to trauma site
   c. thrombospondin—stabilization of platelet plug
   d. platelet-derived growth factor—promotes fibrosis and wound healing
2. Dense bodies—contain adenine nucleotides and serotonin
3. Lysosomes—contain enzymes like acid hydrolases
4. Microperoxisomes—contain catalase

small hemorrhagic areas develop each day under the skin and throughout the internal tissues of a person who has few blood platelets. This phenomenon does not occur in persons with normal numbers of platelets.

Thrombocytopenia

Thrombocytopenia means the presence of very low numbers of platelets in the circulating blood. People with thrombocytopenia have a tendency to bleed, as do hemophiliacs, except that the bleeding is usually from many small venules or capillaries, rather than from larger vessels, as in hemophilia. As a result, small punctate hemorrhages occur throughout all the body tissues. The skin of such a person displays many small, purplish blotches, giving the disease the name *thrombocytopenic purpura*. As stated earlier, platelets are especially important for repair of minute breaks in capillaries and other small vessels.

Ordinarily, bleeding will not occur until the number of platelets in the blood falls below 50,000/μL, rather than the normal 150,000–300,000. Levels as low as 10,000/μL are frequently lethal.

Even without making specific platelet counts in the blood, sometimes one can suspect the existence of thrombocytopenia if the person's blood clot fails to retract. As pointed out earlier, clot retraction is normally dependent on release of multiple coagulation factors from the large numbers of platelets entrapped in the fibrin mesh of the clot.

Most people with thrombocytopenia have the disease known as *idiopathic thrombocytopenia*, which means thrombocytopenia of unknown cause. In most of these people, it has been discovered that, for unknown reasons, specific antibodies have formed and react against the platelets to destroy them. Relief from bleeding for 1–4 days can often be effected in a patient with thrombocytopenia by giving *fresh whole blood transfusions* that contain large numbers of platelets. Also, *splenectomy* is often helpful, sometimes effecting almost complete cure because the spleen normally removes large numbers of platelets from the blood.

Thromboembolic Conditions

Thrombi and Emboli. An abnormal clot that develops in a blood vessel is called a *thrombus*. Once a clot has developed, continued flow of blood past the clot is likely to break it away from its attachment and cause the clot to flow with the blood; such freely flowing clots are known as *emboli*. Also, emboli that originate in large arteries or in the left side of the heart can flow peripherally and plug arteries or arterioles in the brain, kidneys, or elsewhere. Emboli that originate in the venous system or in the right side of the heart generally flow into the lungs to cause pulmonary arterial embolism.

Cause of Thromboembolic Conditions. The causes of thromboembolic conditions in the human being are usually twofold: (1) any *roughened endothelial surface of a vessel*—as may be caused by arteriosclerosis, infection, or trauma—is likely to initiate the clotting process, and (2) blood often clots *when it flows very slowly* through blood vessels, where small quantities of thrombin and other procoagulants are always being formed.

Use of t-PA in Treating Intravascular Clots. Genetically engineered tissue plasminogen activator (t-PA) is available. When delivered through a catheter to an area with a thrombus, it is effective in activating plasminogen to plasmin, which in turn can dissolve some intravascular clots. For instance, if used within the first hour or so after thrombotic occlusion of a coronary artery or after a stroke, the heart and the brain are often spared serious damage.

FEMORAL VENOUS THROMBOSIS AND MASSIVE PULMONARY EMBOLISM

Because clotting almost always occurs when blood flow is blocked for many hours in any vessel of the body, the immobility of patients confined to bed plus the practice of propping the knees with pillows often causes intravascular clotting because of blood stasis in one or more of the leg veins for hours at a time. Then the clot grows mainly in the direction of the slowly moving venous blood, sometimes growing the entire length of the leg veins and occasionally even up into the common iliac vein and inferior vena cava. Then, about 1 out of every 10 times, a large part of the clot disengages from its attachments to the vessel wall and flows freely with the venous blood through the right side of the heart and into the pulmonary arteries to cause massive blockage of the pulmonary arteries called *massive pulmonary embolism*. If the clot is large enough to occlude both pulmonary arteries at the same time, immediate death ensues. If only one pulmonary artery is blocked, death may not occur, or the embolism may lead to death a few hours to several days later because of further growth of the clot within the pulmonary vessels. However, again, t-PA therapy can be a lifesaver.

Bleeding Time

When a sharp-pointed knife is used to pierce the tip of the finger or lobe of the ear, bleeding ordinarily lasts for 1–6 minutes. The time depends largely on the depth of the wound and the degree of hyperemia in the finger or earlobe at the time of the test. Lack of any one of several of the clotting factors can prolong the bleeding time, but it is especially prolonged by lack of platelets.

BIBLIOGRAPHY

Andrews RK, Berndt MC: Platelet adhesion: a game of catch and release, *J. Clin. Invest.* 118:3009, 2008.

Blombery P, Scully M: Management of thrombotic thrombocytopenic purpura: current perspectives, *J. Blood Med.* 5:15, 2014.

Brass LF, Zhu L, Stalker TJ: Minding the gaps to promote thrombus growth and stability, *J. Clin. Invest.* 115:3385, 2005.

Furie B, Furie BC: Mechanisms of thrombus formation, *N. Engl. J. Med.* 359:938, 2008.

Jennings LK: Role of platelets in atherothrombosis, *Am. J. Cardiol.* 103(3 Suppl.):4A, 2009.

Koreth R, Weinert C, Weisdorf DJ, et al: Measurement of bleeding severity: a critical review, *Transfusion* 44:605, 2004.

Nachman RL, Rafii S: Platelets, petechiae, and preservation of the vascular wall, *N. Engl. J. Med.* 359:1261, 2008.

Pabinger I, Ay C: Biomarkers and venous thromboembolism, *Arterioscler. Thromb. Vasc. Biol.* 29:332, 2009.

Smyth SS, Woulfe DS, Weitz JI, 2008 Platelet Colloquium Participants: et al: G-protein-coupled receptors as signaling targets for antiplatelet therapy, *Arterioscler. Thromb. Vasc. Biol.* 29:449, 2009.

Tapson VF: Acute pulmonary embolism, *N. Engl. J. Med.* 358:1037, 2008.

Wells PS, Forgie MA, Rodger MA: Treatment of venous thromboembolism, *JAMA* 311:717, 2014.

27

Blood Coagulation

BASIC THEORY

More than 50 important substances that cause or affect blood coagulation have been found in the blood and in the tissues—some that promote coagulation are called *procoagulants*, and others that inhibit coagulation are called *anticoagulants*. Whether blood will coagulate depends on the balance between these two groups of substances. In the bloodstream, the anticoagulants normally predominate, so the blood does not coagulate while it is circulating in the blood vessels. However when a vessel is ruptured, procoagulants from the area of tissue damage become "activated" and override the anticoagulants, and then a clot does develop.

GENERAL MECHANISM

Clotting takes place in three essential steps: (1) In response to rupture of the vessel or damage to the blood itself, a complex cascade of chemical reactions occurs in the blood involving more than a dozen blood coagulation factors. The net result is formation of a complex of activated substances collectively called *prothrombin activator*. (2) The prothrombin activator catalyzes conversion of *prothrombin* into *thrombin*. (3) The thrombin acts as an enzyme to convert *fibrinogen* into *fibrin fibers* that enmesh platelets, blood cells, and plasma to form the clot.

We will first discuss the mechanism by which the blood clot itself is formed, beginning with conversion of prothrombin to thrombin, and then come back to the initiating stages in the clotting process by which prothrombin activator is formed.

Conversion of Prothrombin to Thrombin

First, prothrombin activator is formed as a result of rupture of a blood vessel or as a result of damage to special substances in the blood. Second, the prothrombin activator, in the presence of sufficient amounts of ionic calcium (Ca^{++}), causes conversion of prothrombin to thrombin (Figure 27-1). Third, the thrombin causes polymerization of fibrinogen molecules into fibrin fibers within another 10–15 seconds. Thus, the rate-limiting factor in causing blood coagulation is usually the formation of prothrombin activator and not the subsequent reactions beyond that point, because these terminal steps normally occur rapidly to form the clot.

Platelets also play an important role in the conversion of prothrombin to thrombin because much of the prothrombin first attaches to prothrombin receptors on the platelets already bound to the damaged tissue.

Prothrombin and Thrombin. Prothrombin is a plasma protein, an α2-globulin, having a molecular weight of 68,700. It is present in normal plasma in a concentration of about 15 mg/dL. It is an unstable protein that can split easily into smaller compounds, one of which is *thrombin*, which has a molecular weight of 33,700, almost exactly one-half that of prothrombin.

Prothrombin is formed continually by the liver, and it is continually being used throughout the body for blood clotting. If the liver fails to produce prothrombin, in a day or so prothrombin concentration in the plasma falls too low to provide normal blood coagulation.

Vitamin K is required by the liver for normal activation of prothrombin, as well as a few other clotting factors. Therefore,

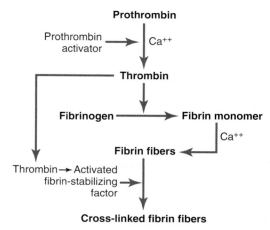

Figure 27-1 Schema for conversion of prothrombin to thrombin and polymerization of fibrinogen to form fibrin fibers.

either lack of vitamin K or the presence of liver disease that prevents normal prothrombin formation can decrease the prothrombin to such a low level that a bleeding tendency results.

Conversion of Fibrinogen to Fibrin— Formation of the Clot

Fibrinogen Formed in the Liver Is Essential for Clot Formation. Fibrinogen is a high-molecular-weight (HMW) protein (MW = 340,000) that occurs in the plasma in quantities of 100–700 mg/dL. Fibrinogen is formed in the liver, and liver disease can decrease the concentration of circulating fibrinogen, as it does the concentration of prothrombin, pointed out earlier.

Because of its large molecular size, little fibrinogen normally leaks from the blood vessels into the interstitial fluids, and because fibrinogen is one of the essential factors in the coagulation process, interstitial fluids ordinarily do not coagulate. Yet, when the permeability of the capillaries becomes pathologically increased, fibrinogen does leak into the tissue fluids in sufficient quantities to allow clotting of these fluids in much the same way that plasma and whole blood can clot.

Action of Thrombin on Fibrinogen to Form Fibrin. Thrombin is a protein *enzyme* with weak proteolytic capabilities. It acts on fibrinogen to remove four low-molecular-weight peptides from each molecule of fibrinogen, forming one molecule of *fibrin monomer* that has the automatic capability to polymerize with other fibrin monomer molecules to form fibrin fibers. Therefore, many fibrin monomer molecules polymerize within seconds into *long fibrin fibers* that constitute the *reticulum* of the blood clot.

In the early stages of polymerization, the fibrin monomer molecules are held together by weak noncovalent hydrogen bonding, and the newly forming fibers are not cross-linked with one another; therefore, the resultant clot is weak and can be broken apart with ease. However, another process occurs during the next few minutes that greatly strengthens the fibrin reticulum. This process involves a substance called *fibrin-stabilizing factor* that is present in small amounts in normal plasma globulins but is also released from platelets entrapped in the clot. Before fibrin-stabilizing factor can have an effect on the fibrin fibers, it must be activated. The same thrombin that causes fibrin formation also activates the fibrin-stabilizing factor. This activated substance then operates as an enzyme to cause *covalent bonds* between more and more of the fibrin monomer molecules, as well as multiple cross-linkages between adjacent fibrin fibers, thus adding tremendously to the three-dimensional strength of the fibrin meshwork.

Blood Clot. The clot is composed of a meshwork of fibrin fibers running in all directions and entrapping blood cells, platelets, and plasma. The fibrin fibers also adhere to damaged surfaces of blood vessels; therefore, the blood clot becomes adherent to any vascular opening and thereby prevents further blood loss.

Clot Retraction— and Expression of Serum. Within a few minutes after a clot is formed, it begins to contract and usually expresses most of the fluid from the clot within 20–60 minutes. The fluid expressed is called *serum* because all its fibrinogen and most of the other clotting factors have been removed; in this way, serum differs from plasma. Serum cannot clot because it lacks these factors.

Platelets are necessary for clot retraction to occur. Therefore, failure of clot retraction is an indication that the number of platelets in the circulating blood might be low. Electron micrographs of platelets in blood clots show that they become attached to the fibrin fibers in such a way that they actually bond different fibers together. Furthermore, platelets entrapped in the clot continue to release procoagulant substances, one of the most important of which is *fibrin-stabilizing factor*, which causes more and more cross-linking bonds between adjacent fibrin fibers. In addition, the platelets contribute directly to clot contraction by activating platelet thrombosthenin, actin, and myosin molecules, which are all contractile proteins in the platelets and cause strong contraction of the platelet spicules attached to the fibrin. This action also helps compress the fibrin meshwork into a smaller mass. The contraction is activated and accelerated by thrombin, as well as by calcium ions released from calcium stores in the mitochondria, endoplasmic reticulum, and Golgi apparatus of the platelets.

As the clot retracts, the edges of the broken blood vessel are pulled together, thus contributing still further to hemostasis.

Positive Feedback of Clot Formation

Once a blood clot has started to develop, it normally extends within minutes into the surrounding blood that is, the clot initiates a positive feedback to promote more clotting. One of the most important causes of this clot promotion is that the proteolytic action of thrombin allows it to act on many of the other blood-clotting factors in addition to fibrinogen. For instance, thrombin has a direct proteolytic effect on prothrombin, tending to convert this into still more thrombin, and it acts on some of the blood-clotting factors responsible for formation of prothrombin activator. (These effects, discussed in subsequent paragraphs, include acceleration of the actions of Factors VIII, IX, X, XI, and XII, and aggregation of platelets.) Once a critical amount of thrombin is formed, a positive feedback develops that causes still more blood clotting and more and more thrombin to be formed; thus, the blood clot continues to grow until blood leakage ceases.

Initiation of Coagulation: Formation of Prothrombin Activator

Now that we have discussed the clotting process, we turn to the more complex mechanisms that initiate clotting in the first place. These mechanisms are set into play by (1) trauma to the vascular wall and adjacent tissues, (2) trauma to the blood, or (3) contact of the blood with damaged endothelial cells or with collagen and other tissue elements outside the blood vessel. In each instance, this leads to the formation of *prothrombin activator*, which then causes prothrombin conversion to thrombin and all the subsequent clotting steps.

Prothrombin activator is generally considered to be formed in two ways, although, in reality, the two ways interact constantly with each other: (1) by the *extrinsic pathway* that begins with trauma to the vascular wall and surrounding tissues and (2) by the *intrinsic pathway* that begins in the blood.

In both the extrinsic and the intrinsic pathways, a series of different plasma proteins called *blood-clotting factors* plays a major role. Most of these proteins are *inactive* forms of proteolytic enzymes. When converted to the active forms, their enzymatic actions cause the successive, cascading reactions of the clotting process.

Most of the clotting factors, which are listed in Table 26-1, are designated by Roman numerals. To indicate the activated form of the factor, a small letter "a" is added after the Roman numeral, such as Factor VIIIa to indicate the activated state of Factor VIII.

EXTRINSIC PATHWAY FOR INITIATING CLOTTING

The extrinsic pathway for initiating the formation of prothrombin activator begins with a traumatized vascular wall or traumatized extravascular tissues that come in contact with the blood. This condition leads to the following steps, as shown in Figure 27-2:

1. *Release of tissue factor*: Traumatized tissue releases a complex of several factors called *tissue factor* or *tissue thromboplastin*. This factor is composed especially of *phospholipids* from the membranes of the tissue plus a *lipoprotein complex* that functions mainly as a *proteolytic enzyme*.

2. *Activation of Factor X—role of Factor VII and tissue factor*: The lipoprotein complex of tissue factor further complexes with blood coagulation Factor VII and, in the presence of calcium ions, acts enzymatically on Factor X to form *activated Factor X (Xa)*.

3. *Effect of Xa to form prothrombin activator—role of Factor V*: The activated Factor X combines immediately with tissue phospholipids that are part of tissue factors or with additional phospholipids released from platelets, as well as with Factor V to form the complex called *prothrombin activator*. Within a few seconds, in the presence of Ca^{++}, prothrombin is split to form thrombin, and the clotting process proceeds as already explained. At first, the Factor V in the prothrombin activator complex is inactive, but once clotting begins and thrombin begins to form, the proteolytic action of thrombin activates Factor V. This then becomes an additional strong accelerator of prothrombin activation. Thus, in the final prothrombin activator complex, activated Factor X is the actual protease that causes splitting of prothrombin to form

thrombin; activated Factor V greatly accelerates this protease activity, and platelet phospholipids act as a vehicle that further accelerates the process. Note especially the *positive feedback* effect of thrombin, acting through Factor V, to accelerate the entire process once it begins.

INTRINSIC PATHWAY FOR INITIATING CLOTTING

The second mechanism for initiating formation of prothrombin activator, and therefore for initiating clotting, *begins with trauma to the blood or exposure of the blood to collagen* from a traumatized blood vessel wall. Then the process continues through the series of cascading reactions shown in Figure 27-3:

1. *Blood trauma causes (a) activation of Factor XII and (b) release of platelet phospholipids.* Trauma to the blood or exposure of the blood to vascular wall collagen alters two important clotting factors in the blood: Factor XII and the platelets. When Factor XII is disturbed, such as by coming into contact with collagen or with a wettable surface such as glass, it takes on a new molecular configuration that converts it into a proteolytic enzyme called "activated Factor XII." Simultaneously, the blood trauma also damages the platelets because of adherence to either collagen or a wettable surface (or by damage in other ways), and this releases platelet phospholipids that contain the lipoprotein called *platelet factor 3*, which also plays a role in subsequent clotting reactions.

2. *Activation of Factor XI*: The activated Factor XII acts enzymatically on Factor XI to activate this factor as well, which is the second step in the intrinsic pathway. This reaction also requires *high-molecular-weight kininogen* and is accelerated by prekallikrein.

3. *Activation of Factor IX by activated Factor XI*: The activated Factor XI then acts enzymatically on Factor IX to activate this factor as well.

4. *Activation of Factor X—role of Factor VIII*: The activated Factor IX, acting in concert with activated Factor VIII and with the platelet phospholipids and Factor III from the traumatized platelets, activates Factor X. It is clear that when either Factor VIII or platelets are in short supply, this step is deficient. Factor VIII is the factor that is missing in a person who has classic *hemophilia*, for which reason it is called *antihemophilic factor*. Platelets are the clotting factor that is lacking in the bleeding disease called *thrombocytopenia*.

5. *Action of activated Factor X to form prothrombin activator—role of Factor V*: This step in the intrinsic pathway is the same as the last step in the extrinsic pathway. That is, activated Factor X combines with Factor V and platelet or tissue phospholipids to form the complex called *prothrombin activator*. The prothrombin activator in turn initiates within seconds the cleavage of prothrombin to form thrombin, thereby setting into motion the final clotting process, as described earlier.

ROLE OF CALCIUM IONS IN THE INTRINSIC AND EXTRINSIC PATHWAYS

Except for the first two steps in the intrinsic pathway, calcium ions are required for promotion or acceleration of all the blood-clotting reactions. Therefore, in the absence of calcium ions blood clotting by either pathway does not occur.

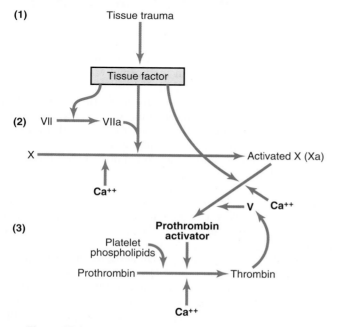

Figure 27-2 Extrinsic pathway for initiating blood clotting.

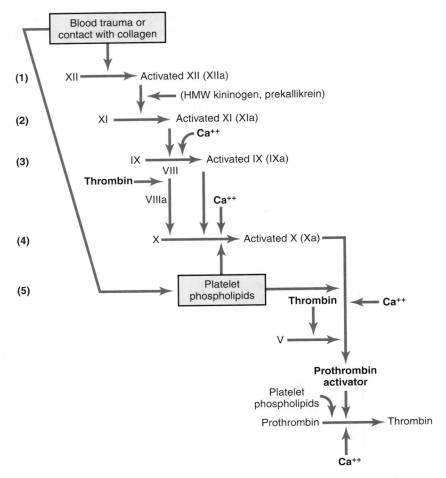

Figure 27-3 Intrinsic pathway for initiating blood clotting. *HMW*, high-molecular-weight.

In the living body, the calcium ion concentration seldom falls low enough to significantly affect the kinetics of blood clotting. However, when blood is removed from a person, it can be prevented from clotting by reducing the calcium ion concentration below the threshold level for clotting, either by deionizing the calcium by causing it to react with substances such as *citrate ion* or by precipitating the calcium with substances such as *oxalate ion*.

INTERACTION BETWEEN THE EXTRINSIC AND INTRINSIC PATHWAYS—SUMMARY OF BLOOD-CLOTTING INITIATION

It is clear from the schemas of the intrinsic and extrinsic systems that after blood vessels rupture, clotting occurs by both pathways simultaneously. Tissue factor initiates the extrinsic pathway, whereas contact of Factor XII and platelets with collagen in the vascular wall initiates the intrinsic pathway.

An especially important difference between the extrinsic and intrinsic pathways is that *the extrinsic pathway* can be explosive; once initiated, its speed of completion to the final clot is limited only by the amount of tissue factor released from the traumatized tissues and by the quantities of Factors X, VII, and V in the blood. With severe tissue trauma, clotting can occur in as little as 15 seconds. The intrinsic pathway is much slower to proceed, usually requiring 1–6 minutes to cause clotting.

Intravascular Anticoagulants Prevent Blood Clotting in the Normal Vascular System

Endothelial Surface Factors. Probably the most important factors for preventing clotting in the normal vascular system are (1) the *smoothness* of the endothelial cell surface, which prevents contact activation of the intrinsic clotting system; (2) a layer of *glycocalyx* on the endothelium (glycocalyx is a mucopolysaccharide adsorbed to the surfaces of the endothelial cells), which repels clotting factors and platelets, thereby preventing activation of clotting; and (3) a protein bound with the endothelial membrane, *thrombomodulin*, which binds thrombin. Not only does the binding of thrombin with thrombomodulin slow the clotting process by removing thrombin, but also the thrombomodulin–thrombin complex activates a plasma protein, *protein C*, that acts as an anticoagulant by *inactivating* activated Factors V and VIII.

When the endothelial wall is damaged, its smoothness and its glycocalyx–thrombomodulin layer are lost, which activates both Factor XII and the platelets, thus setting off the intrinsic pathway of clotting. If Factor XII and platelets come in contact with the subendothelial collagen, the activation is even more powerful.

Antithrombin Action of Fibrin and Antithrombin III. Among the most important *anticoagulants* in the blood are those that remove thrombin from the blood. The most powerful of these are (1) the *fibrin fibers* that are formed during the process of clotting and (2) an α-globulin called *antithrombin III* or *antithrombin–heparin cofactor*.

While a clot is forming, about 85–90% of the thrombin formed from the prothrombin becomes adsorbed to the fibrin fibers as they develop. This adsorption helps prevent the spread of thrombin into the remaining blood and, therefore, prevents excessive spread of the clot.

The thrombin that does not adsorb to the fibrin fibers soon combines with antithrombin III, which further blocks the effect of the thrombin on the fibrinogen and then also inactivates the thrombin itself during the next 12–20 minutes.

Heparin. Heparin is another powerful anticoagulant, but because its concentration in the blood is normally low, it has significant anticoagulant effects only under special physiological conditions. However, heparin is used widely as a pharmacological agent in medical practice in much higher concentrations to prevent intravascular clotting.

The heparin molecule is a highly negatively charged conjugated polysaccharide. By itself, it has little or no anticoagulant properties, but when it combines with antithrombin III the effectiveness of antithrombin III for removing thrombin increases by 100-fold to 1000-fold, and thus it acts as an anticoagulant. Therefore, in the presence of excess heparin, removal of free thrombin from the circulating blood by antithrombin III is almost instantaneous.

The complex of heparin and antithrombin III removes several other activated coagulation factors in addition to thrombin, further enhancing the effectiveness of anticoagulation. The others include activated Factors XII, XI, X, and IX.

Heparin is produced by many different cells of the body, but the largest quantities are formed by the basophilic *mast cells* located in the pericapillary connective tissue throughout the body. These cells continually secrete small quantities of heparin that diffuse into the circulatory system. The *basophil cells* of the blood, which are functionally almost identical to the mast cells, release small quantities of heparin into the plasma.

Mast cells are abundant in tissue surrounding the capillaries of the lungs and, to a lesser extent, capillaries of the liver. It is easy to understand why large quantities of heparin might be needed in these areas because the capillaries of the lungs and liver receive many embolic clots formed in slowly flowing venous blood; sufficient formation of heparin prevents further growth of the clots.

Plasmin Causes Lysis of Blood Clots

The plasma proteins contain a euglobulin called *plasminogen* (or *profibrinolysin*) that, when activated, becomes a substance called *plasmin* (or *fibrinolysin*). Plasmin is a proteolytic enzyme that resembles trypsin, the most important proteolytic digestive enzyme of pancreatic secretion. Plasmin digests fibrin fibers and some other protein coagulants such as fibrinogen, Factor V, Factor VIII, prothrombin, and Factor XII. Therefore, whenever plasmin is formed, it can cause lysis of a clot by destroying many of the clotting factors, thereby sometimes even causing hypocoagulability of the blood.

Activation of Plasminogen to Form Plasmin, then Lysis of Clots. When a clot is formed, a large amount of plasminogen is trapped in the clot along with other plasma proteins. This will not become plasmin or cause lysis of the clot until it is activated. The injured tissues and vascular endothelium very slowly release a powerful activator called *tissue plasminogen activator* (t-PA); a few days later, after the clot has stopped the bleeding, t-PA eventually converts plasminogen to plasmin, which in turn removes the remaining unnecessary blood clot. In fact, many small blood vessels in which blood flow has been blocked by clots are reopened by this mechanism. Thus, an especially important function of the plasmin system is to remove minute clots from millions of tiny peripheral vessels that eventually would become occluded were there no way to clear them.

Conditions that Cause Excessive Bleeding in Humans

Excessive bleeding can result from a deficiency of any one of the many blood-clotting factors. Three particular types of bleeding tendencies that have been studied to the greatest extent are discussed here: bleeding caused by (1) vitamin K deficiency, (2) hemophilia, and (3) thrombocytopenia (platelet deficiency).

DECREASED PROTHROMBIN, FACTOR VII, FACTOR IX, AND FACTOR X CAUSED BY VITAMIN K DEFICIENCY

With few exceptions, almost all the blood-clotting factors are formed by the liver. Therefore, diseases of the liver such as *hepatitis*, *cirrhosis*, and *acute yellow atrophy* (i.e., degeneration of the liver caused by toxins, infections, or other agents) can sometimes depress the clotting system so greatly that the patient experiences the development of a severe tendency to bleed.

Another cause of depressed formation of clotting factors by the liver is vitamin K deficiency. Vitamin K is an essential factor to a liver carboxylase that adds a carboxyl group to glutamic acid residues on five of the important clotting factors: *prothrombin*, *Factor VII*, *Factor IX*, *Factor X*, and *protein C*. Upon adding the carboxyl group to glutamic acid residues on the immature clotting factors, vitamin K is oxidized and becomes inactive. Another enzyme, *vitamin K epoxide reductase complex 1 (VKOR c1)*, reduces vitamin K back to its active form.

In the absence of active vitamin K, subsequent insufficiency of these coagulation factors in the blood can lead to serious bleeding tendencies.

Vitamin K is continually synthesized in the intestinal tract by bacteria, so vitamin K deficiency seldom occurs in healthy persons as a result of the absence of vitamin K from the diet (except in neonates before they establish their intestinal bacterial flora). However, in persons with gastrointestinal disease, vitamin K deficiency often occurs as a result of poor absorption of fats from the gastrointestinal tract because vitamin K is fat soluble and is ordinarily absorbed into the blood along with the fats.

One of the most prevalent causes of vitamin K deficiency is failure of the liver to secrete bile into the gastrointestinal tract (which occurs either as a result of obstruction of the bile ducts or as a result of liver disease). Lack of bile prevents adequate fat digestion and absorption and, therefore, depresses vitamin K absorption as well. Thus, liver disease often causes decreased production of prothrombin and some other clotting factors both because of poor vitamin K absorption and because of the diseased liver cells. As a result, vitamin K is injected into surgical patients with liver disease or with obstructed bile ducts before the surgical procedure is performed. Ordinarily, if vitamin K is given to a deficient patient 4–8 hours before the operation and the liver parenchymal cells are at least one-half normal in function, sufficient clotting factors will be produced to prevent excessive bleeding during the operation.

HEMOPHILIA

Hemophilia is a bleeding disease that occurs almost exclusively in males. In 85% of cases, it is caused by an *abnormality or deficiency of Factor VIII*; this type of hemophilia is called *hemophilia A* or *classic hemophilia*. About 1 of every 10,000 males in the United States has classic hemophilia. In the other 15% of patients with hemophilia, the bleeding tendency is caused by deficiency of Factor IX. Both of these factors are transmitted genetically by way of the female chromosome. Therefore, a woman will almost never have hemophilia because at least one of her two X chromosomes will have the appropriate genes. If one of her X chromosomes is deficient, she will be a *hemophilia carrier*, transmitting the disease to half of her male offspring and transmitting the carrier state to half of her female offspring.

The bleeding trait in hemophilia can have various degrees of severity, depending on the genetic deficiency. Bleeding usually does not occur except after trauma, but in some patients the degree of trauma required to cause severe and prolonged bleeding may be so mild that it is hardly noticeable. For instance, bleeding can often last for days after extraction of a tooth.

Factor VIII has two active components, a large component with a molecular weight in the millions and a smaller component with a molecular weight of about 230,000. The smaller component is most important in the intrinsic pathway for clotting, and it is deficiency of this part of Factor VIII that causes classic hemophilia. Another bleeding disease with somewhat different characteristics, called *von Willebrand disease*, results from loss of the large component.

When a person with classic hemophilia experiences severe prolonged bleeding, almost the only therapy that is truly effective is injection of purified Factor VIII. The cost of Factor VIII is high because it is gathered from human blood and only in extremely small quantities. However, increasing production and use of recombinant Factor VIII is making this treatment available to more patients with classic hemophilia.

DISSEMINATED INTRAVASCULAR COAGULATION

Occasionally the clotting mechanism becomes activated in widespread areas of the circulation, giving rise to the condition called *disseminated intravascular coagulation*. This condition often results from the presence of large amounts of traumatized or dying tissue in the body that releases great quantities of tissue factor into the blood. Frequently, the clots are small but numerous, and they plug a large share of the small peripheral blood vessels. This process occurs especially in patients with widespread septicemia, in which either circulating bacteria or bacterial toxins—especially *endotoxins*—activate the clotting mechanisms. Plugging of small peripheral vessels greatly diminishes delivery of oxygen and other nutrients to the tissues—a situation that leads to or exacerbates circulatory shock. It is partly for this reason that *septicemic shock* is lethal in 85% or more of patients.

A peculiar effect of disseminated intravascular coagulation is that the patient on occasion begins to bleed. The reason for this bleeding is that so many of the clotting factors are removed by the widespread clotting that too few procoagulants remain to allow normal hemostasis of the remaining blood.

Anticoagulants for Clinical Use

In some thromboembolic conditions, it is desirable to delay the coagulation process. Various anticoagulants have been developed for this purpose (Table 27-1). The ones most useful clinically are *heparin* and the *coumarins*.

HEPARIN AS AN INTRAVENOUS ANTICOAGULANT

Commercial heparin is extracted from several different animal tissues and prepared in almost pure form. Injection of relatively small quantities, about 0.5–1 mg/kg of body weight, causes the blood-clotting time to increase from a normal of about 6 to 30 or more minutes. Furthermore, this change in clotting time occurs instantaneously, thereby immediately preventing or slowing further development of a thromboembolic condition.

TABLE 27-1	Anticoagulant and Antiplatelet Agents		
	Mechanism of Action		**Usage**
ANTICOAGULANT AGENTS			
Heparin (including low-molecular-weight heparin)	Inactivates thrombin and Factor Xa		Intravenous Immediate action
Warfarin (coumarin analogs)	Inhibits vitamin K Synthesis of prothrombin, Factors VII, IX, and X inhibited		Oral Takes 4–5 days for complete response
ANTIPLATELET AGENTS			
Aspirin	Inhibits platelet cyclooxygenase, synthesis of thromboxane A2, platelet aggregation		Oral—used in low doses
Dipyridamole	Inhibits platelet phosphodiesterase		Oral
Ticlopidine	Inhibits platelet aggregation, prevents GP IIb–IIIa expression		Oral

GP, glycoprotein.

The action of heparin lasts about 1.5–4 hours. The injected heparin is destroyed by an enzyme in the blood known as *heparinase*.

COUMARINS AS ANTICOAGULANTS

When a coumarin, such as *warfarin*, is given to a patient, the amounts of active prothrombin and Factors VII, IX, and X, all formed by the liver, begin to fall. Warfarin causes this effect by inhibiting the enzyme, *VKOR c1*. As discussed previously, this enzyme converts the inactive, oxidized form of vitamin K to its active, reduced form. By inhibiting *VKOR c1*, warfarin decreases the available active form of vitamin K in the tissues. When this decrease occurs, the coagulation factors are no longer carboxylated and are biologically inactive. Over several days the body stores of the active coagulation factors degrade and are replaced by inactive factors. Although the coagulation factors continue to be produced, they have greatly decreased coagulant activity.

After administration of an effective dose of warfarin, the coagulant activity of the blood decreases to about 50% of normal by the end of 12 hours and to about 20% of normal by the end of 24 hours. In other words, the coagulation process is not blocked immediately but must await the degradation of the active prothrombin and the other affected coagulation factors already present in the plasma. Normal coagulation usually returns 1–3 days after discontinuing coumarin therapy.

PREVENTION OF BLOOD COAGULATION OUTSIDE THE BODY

Although blood removed from the body and held in a glass test tube normally clots in about 6 minutes, blood collected in *siliconized containers* often does not clot for 1 hour or more. The reason for this delay is that preparing the surfaces of the containers with silicone prevents contact activation of platelets and Factor XII, the two principal factors that initiate the intrinsic clotting mechanism. Conversely, untreated glass containers allow contact activation of the platelets and Factor XII, with rapid development of clots.

Heparin can be used for preventing coagulation of blood outside the body, as well as in the body. Heparin is especially used in surgical procedures in which the blood must be passed through a heart–lung machine or artificial kidney machine and then back into the person.

Various substances that *decrease the concentration of calcium ions* in the blood can also be used for preventing blood coagulation *outside* the body. For instance, a soluble *oxalate* compound mixed in a very small quantity with a sample of blood causes precipitation of calcium oxalate from the plasma and thereby decreases the ionic calcium level so much that blood coagulation is blocked.

Any substance that deionizes the blood calcium will prevent coagulation. The negatively charged *citrate ion* is especially valuable for this purpose, mixed with blood usually in the form of *sodium*, *ammonium*, or *potassium citrate*. The citrate ion combines with calcium in the blood to cause an unionized calcium compound, and the lack of *ionic* calcium prevents coagulation. Citrate anticoagulants have an important advantage over the oxalate anticoagulants because oxalate is toxic to the body, whereas moderate quantities of citrate can be injected intravenously. After injection, the citrate ion is removed from the blood within a few minutes by the liver and is polymerized into glucose or metabolized directly for energy. Consequently, 500 mL of blood that has been rendered incoagulable by citrate can ordinarily be transfused into a recipient within a few minutes without dire consequences. However, if the liver is damaged or if large quantities of citrated blood or plasma are given too rapidly (within fractions of a minute), the citrate ion may not be removed quickly enough, and the citrate can, under these conditions, greatly depress the level of calcium ion in the blood, which can result in tetany and convulsive death.

Blood Coagulation Tests
CLOTTING TIME

Many methods have been devised for determining blood-clotting times. The one most widely used is to collect blood in a chemically clean glass test tube and then to tip the tube back and forth about every 30 seconds until the blood has clotted. By this method, the normal clotting time is 6–10 minutes. Procedures using multiple test tubes have also been devised for determining clotting time more accurately.

Unfortunately, the clotting time varies widely, depending on the method used for measuring it, so it is no longer used in many clinics. Instead, measurements of the clotting factors themselves are made using sophisticated chemical procedures.

PROTHROMBIN TIME AND INTERNATIONAL NORMALIZED RATIO

Prothrombin time gives an indication of the concentration of prothrombin in the blood. Figure 27-4 shows the relation of prothrombin concentration to prothrombin time. The method for determining prothrombin time is the following.

Blood removed from the patient is immediately oxalated so that none of the prothrombin can change into thrombin. Then a large excess of calcium ion and tissue factor is quickly mixed with the oxalated blood. The excess calcium nullifies the effect of the oxalate and the tissue factor activates the prothrombin-to-thrombin reaction by means of the extrinsic clotting pathway. The time required for coagulation to take place is known

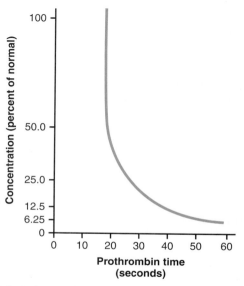

Figure 27-4 Relation of prothrombin concentration in the blood to "prothrombin time."

TABLE 27-2	Comparison of Bleeding and Clotting Disorders	
Test	Bleeding Disorder	Clotting Disorder
Family history	Rare	Usually present
Bleeding from superficial cuts	Profuse	Not unusually increased
Petechiae	Usual	Rare
Deep hematomas	Rare	Usual
Bleeding into joints (hemarthrosis)	Rare	Usual
Bleeding time	Prolonged	Normal
Clotting time	Normal	Prolonged

as the *prothrombin time*. The *shortness of the time* is determined mainly by prothrombin concentration. The normal prothrombin time is about 12 seconds. In each laboratory, a curve relating prothrombin concentration to prothrombin time, such as that shown in Figure 27-4, is drawn for the method used so that the prothrombin in the blood can be quantified.

The results obtained for prothrombin time may vary considerably even in the same individual if there are differences in activity of the tissue factor and the analytical system used to perform the test. Tissue factor is isolated from human tissues, such as placental tissue, and different batches may have different activity. The *international normalized ratio (INR)* was devised as a way to standardize measurements of prothrombin time. For each batch of tissue factor, the manufacturer assigns an international sensitivity index (ISI), which indicates the activity of the tissue factor with a standardized sample. The ISI usually varies between 1.0 and 2.0. The INR is the ratio of the person's prothrombin time (PT) to a normal control sample raised to the power of the ISI:

$$INR = \left(\frac{PT_{test}}{PT_{normal}} \right)^{ISI}$$

where PT is the prothrombin time. The normal range for INR in a healthy person is 0.9–1.3. A high INR level (eg, 4 or 5) indicates a high risk of bleeding, whereas a low INR (eg, 0.5) suggests that there is a chance of having a clot. Patients undergoing warfarin therapy usually have an INR of 2.0–3.0.

Another useful test is the partial thromboplastin time (PTT) or activated partial thromboplastin time (aPTT or APTT). This tests the efficacy of the intrinsic and the common coagulation pathways. Since the intrinsic pathway is activated by contact with collagen, this test is started by mixing calcium and a contact factor such as silica or kaolin with oxalated blood and observing the time taken for a clot to form. This test is often used to monitor treatment effects with anticoagulants. Other tests

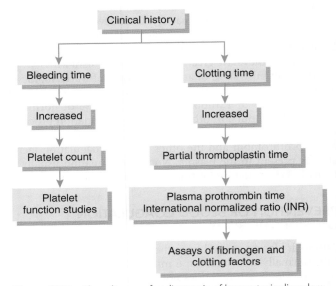

Figure 27-5 Flow diagram for diagnosis of hemostasis disorders.

similar to that for prothrombin time and INR have been devised to determine the quantities of other blood-clotting factors. In each of these tests, excesses of calcium ions and all the other factors *besides the one being tested* are added to oxalated blood all at once. Then the time required for coagulation is determined in the same manner as for prothrombin time. If the factor being tested is deficient, the coagulation time is prolonged. The time itself can then be used to quantitate the concentration of the factor. In general, the approach to a patient with disorders of hemostasis is a logical one, first to clinically define whether a bleeding or clotting disorder is present (Table 27-2), and then to define, through laboratory tests such as the INR and PTT (Figure 27-5), as well as more complex assays, the nature of the clotting disorder.

BIBLIOGRAPHY

Berntorp E, Shapiro AD: Modern hemophilia care, *Lancet* 379:1447, 2012.

Brass LF, Zhu L, Stalker TJ: Minding the gaps to promote thrombus growth and stability, *J. Clin. Invest.* 115:3385, 2005.

Crawley JT, Lane DA: The haemostatic role of tissue factor pathway inhibitor, *Arterioscler. Thromb. Vasc. Biol.* 28:233, 2008.

Furie B, Furie BC: Mechanisms of thrombus formation, *N. Engl. J. Med.* 359:938, 2008.

Gailani D, Renné T: Intrinsic pathway of coagulation and arterial thrombosis, *Arterioscler. Thromb. Vasc. Biol.* 27:2507, 2007.

Hunt BJ: Bleeding and coagulopathies in critical care, *N. Engl. J. Med.* 370:847, 2014.

Koreth R, Weinert C, Weisdorf DJ, et al: Measurement of bleeding severity: a critical review, *Transfusion* 44:605, 2004.

Pabinger I, Ay C: Biomarkers and venous thromboembolism, *Arterioscler. Thromb. Vasc. Biol.* 29:332, 2009.

Rijken DC, Lijnen HR: New insights into the molecular mechanisms of the fibrinolytic system, *J. Thromb. Haemost.* 7:4, 2009.

Schmaier AH: The elusive physiologic role of Factor XII, *J. Clin. Invest.* 118:3006, 2008.

28

Blood Groups

LEARNING OBJECTIVES

- Classify blood groups.
- Define Landsteiner's laws.
- Describe Rh incompatibility.
- Describe hemolytic diseases due to Rh incompatibility including erythroblastosis fetalis, and its treatment and prevention.
- List the indications for blood transfusion.
- Describe the different transfusion reactions.
- Describe the method of collection of blood, storage of blood, and the changes that occur in blood during storage.

GLOSSARY OF TERMS

- **Agglutinin:** The antibody corresponding to the agglutinogen; found in the plasma
- **Agglutinogen:** Antigen; referred to here as the antigen on RBCs that causes blood agglutination

Multiplicity of Antigens in the Blood Cells

At least 30 commonly occurring antigens and hundreds of other rare antigens, each of which can at times cause antigen–antibody reactions, have been found on the surfaces of the cell membranes of human blood cells. Most of the antigens are weak and therefore are of importance principally for studying the inheritance of genes to establish parentage.

Two particular types of antigens are much more likely than the others to cause blood transfusion reactions. They are the *O–A–B* system of antigens and the *Rh* system.

O–A–B Blood Types

A AND B ANTIGENS—AGGLUTINOGENS

Two antigens—type A and type B—occur on the surfaces of the red blood cells in a large proportion of human beings. It is these antigens (also called *agglutinogens* because they often cause blood cell agglutination) that cause most blood transfusion reactions. Because of the way these agglutinogens are inherited, people may have neither of them on their cells, they may have one, or they may have both simultaneously.

Major O–A–B Blood Types. In transfusing blood from one person to another, the blood of donors and that of recipients are normally classified into four major O–A–B blood types, as shown in Table 28-1, depending on the presence or absence of the two agglutinogens, the A and B agglutinogens. When neither A nor B agglutinogen is present, the blood is *type O*. When only type A agglutinogen is present, the blood is *type A*. When only type B agglutinogen is present, the blood is *type B*. When both A and B agglutinogens are present, the blood is *type AB*. The reciprocal relationship between agglutinogens on the red blood cells and agglutinins in the serum is at the core of Landsteiner's laws. The first law states that if an agglutinogen is present on the red cells, the corresponding agglutinin must be absent from the plasma. The second law states that if an agglutinogen is absent on the red cells, the corresponding agglutinin must be present in the plasma.

Genetic Determination of the Agglutinogens. The ABO blood group genetic locus has three *alleles*, which means three different forms of the same gene. These three alleles, I^A, I^B, and I^O, determine the three blood types. We typically call these alleles "A," "B," and "O," but geneticists often represent alleles of a gene by variations of the same symbol. In this case, the common symbol is the letter "I," which stands for "immunoglobulin."

The type O allele is either functionless or almost functionless, so it causes no significant type O agglutinogen on the cells. Conversely, the type A and type B alleles do cause strong agglutinogens on the cells. Thus, the O allele is recessive to both the A and B alleles, which show *co-dominance*.

Because each person has only two sets of chromosomes, only one of these alleles is present on each of the two chromosomes in any individual. However, the presence of three different alleles means that there are six possible combinations of alleles, as shown in Table 28-1, are OO, OA, OB, AA, BB, and AB. These combinations of alleles are known as the *genotypes*, and each person is one of the six genotypes.

One can also observe from Table 28-1 that a person with genotype OO produces no agglutinogens, and therefore the blood type is O. A person with genotype OA or AA produces type A agglutinogens and therefore has blood type A. Genotypes OB and BB give type B blood, and genotype AB gives type AB blood.

Relative Frequencies of the Different Blood Types. The prevalence of the different blood types among one group of persons studied was approximately the following:

O	47%
A	41%
B	9%
AB	3%

It is obvious from these percentages that the O and A genes occur frequently, whereas the B gene occurs infrequently.

TABLE 28-1	Blood Types with their Genotypes and their Constituent Agglutinogens and Agglutinins

Genotypes	Blood Types	Agglutinogens	Agglutinins
OO	O	—	Anti-A and Anti-B
OA or AA	A	A	Anti-B
OB or BB	B	B	Anti-A
AB	AB	A and B	—

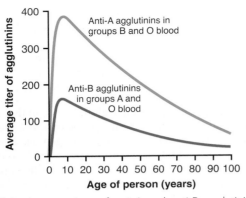

Figure 28-1 Average titers of anti-A and anti-B agglutinins in the plasmas of people with different blood types.

AGGLUTININS

When type A agglutinogen *is not present* in a person's red blood cells, antibodies known as *anti-A agglutinins* develop in the plasma. Also, when type B agglutinogen *is not present* in the red blood cells, antibodies known as *anti-B agglutinins* develop in the plasma.

Thus, referring once again to Table 28-1, note that type O blood, although containing no agglutinogens, does contain both *anti-A* and *anti-B agglutinins*. Type A blood contains type A agglutinogens and *anti-B agglutinins*, and type B blood contains type B agglutinogens and anti-A agglutinins. Finally, type AB blood contains both A and B agglutinogens but no agglutinins.

Titer of the Agglutinins at Different Ages. Immediately after birth, the quantity of agglutinins in the plasma is almost zero. Two to 8 months after birth, an infant begins to produce agglutinins—anti-A agglutinins when type A agglutinogens are not present in the cells, and anti-B agglutinins when type B agglutinogens are not present in the cells. Figure 28-1 shows the changing titers of the anti-A and anti-B agglutinins at different ages. A maximum titer is usually reached at 8–10 years of age, and this titer gradually declines throughout the remaining years of life.

Origin of Agglutinins in the Plasma. The agglutinins are gamma globulins, as are almost all antibodies, and they are produced by the same bone marrow and lymph gland cells that produce antibodies to any other antigens. Most of them are immunoglobulin M (IgM) and immunoglobulin G (IgG) molecules.

But why are these agglutinins produced in people who do not have the respective agglutinogens in their red blood cells? The answer to this question is that small amounts of type A and B antigens enter the body in food, in bacteria, and in other ways, and these substances initiate the development of the anti-A and anti-B agglutinins.

For instance, infusion of group A antigen into a recipient having a non-A blood type causes a typical immune response with formation of greater quantities of anti-A agglutinins than ever. Also, the neonate has few, if any, agglutinins, showing that agglutinin formation occurs almost entirely after birth.

AGGLUTINATION PROCESS IN TRANSFUSION REACTIONS

When bloods are mismatched so that anti-A or anti-B plasma agglutinins are mixed with red blood cells that contain A or B agglutinogens, respectively, the red cells agglutinate as a result of the agglutinins attaching themselves to the red blood cells. Because the agglutinins have 2 binding sites (IgG type) or 10 binding sites (IgM type), a single agglutinin can attach to two

or more red blood cells at the same time, thereby causing the cells to be bound together by the agglutinin. This binding causes the cells to clump, which is the process of "agglutination." Then these clumps plug small blood vessels throughout the circulatory system. During ensuing hours to days, either physical distortion of the cells or attack by phagocytic white blood cells destroys the membranes of the agglutinated cells, releasing hemoglobin into the plasma, which is called "*hemolysis*" of the red blood cells.

Acute Hemolysis Occurs in Some Transfusion Reactions. Sometimes, when recipient and donor bloods are mismatched, immediate hemolysis of red cells occurs in the circulating blood. In this case, the antibodies cause lysis of the red blood cells by activating the complement system, which releases proteolytic enzymes (the *lytic complex*) that rupture the cell membranes, as described in Chapter 25. *Immediate* intravascular hemolysis is far less common than agglutination followed by *delayed* hemolysis because not only does there have to be a high titer of antibodies for lysis to occur, but also a different type of antibody seems to be required, mainly the IgM antibodies; these antibodies are called *hemolysins*.

BLOOD TYPING

Before giving a transfusion to a person, it is necessary to determine the blood type of the recipient's blood and the blood type of the donor blood so that the bloods can be appropriately matched. This process is called *blood typing* and *blood matching*, and these procedures are performed in the following way: The red blood cells are first separated from the plasma and diluted with saline solution. One portion is then mixed with anti-A agglutinin and another portion with anti-B agglutinin. After several minutes, the mixtures are observed under a microscope. If the red blood cells have become clumped—that is, "agglutinated"— one knows that an antibody–antigen reaction has resulted.

Table 28-2 lists the presence (+) or absence (−) of agglutination of the four types of red blood cells. Type O red blood cells have no agglutinogens and therefore do not react with either the anti-A or the anti-B agglutinins. Type A blood has A agglutinogens and therefore agglutinates with anti-A agglutinins. Type B blood has B agglutinogens and agglutinates with anti-B agglutinins. Type AB blood has both A and B agglutinogens and agglutinates with both types of agglutinins.

RH Blood Types

Along with the O–A–B blood type system, the Rh blood type system is also important when transfusing blood. The major difference between the O–A–B system and the Rh system is the following: In the O–A–B system, the plasma agglutinins responsible for causing transfusion reactions develop spontaneously, whereas in the Rh system spontaneous agglutinins almost never

TABLE 28-2	Blood Typing, Showing Agglutination of Cells of the Different Blood Types with Anti-A or Anti-B Agglutinins in the Sera	
	Sera	
Red Blood Cell Types	**Anti-A**	**Anti-B**
O	−	−
A	+	−
B	−	+
AB	+	+

occur. Instead, the person must first be massively exposed to an Rh antigen, such as by transfusion of blood containing the Rh antigen, before enough agglutinins to cause a significant transfusion reaction will develop.

Rh Antigens—"Rh-Positive" and "Rh-Negative" People.

There are six common types of Rh antigens, each of which is called an *Rh factor*. These types are designated C, D, E, c, d, and e. A person who has a C antigen does not have the c antigen, but the person missing the C antigen always has the c antigen. The same is true for the D–d and E–e antigens. Also, because of the manner of inheritance of these factors, each person has one of each of the three pairs of antigens.

The type D antigen is widely prevalent in the population and considerably more antigenic than the other Rh antigens. Anyone who has this type of antigen is said to be *Rh-positive*, whereas a person who does not have type D antigen is said to be *Rh-negative*. However, it must be noted that even in Rh-negative people some of the other Rh antigens can still cause transfusion reactions, although the reactions are usually much milder.

About 85% of all white people are Rh-positive and 15% are Rh-negative. In American blacks, the percentage of Rh-positives is about 95%, whereas in African blacks, it is virtually 100%.

Rh IMMUNE RESPONSE

Formation of Anti-Rh Agglutinins. When red blood cells containing Rh factor are injected into a person whose blood does not contain the Rh factor—that is, into an Rh-negative person—anti-Rh agglutinins develop slowly, reaching maximum concentration of agglutinins about 2–4 months later. This immune response occurs to a much greater extent in some people than in others. With multiple exposures to the Rh factor, an Rh-negative person eventually becomes strongly "sensitized" to Rh factor.

Characteristics of Rh Transfusion Reactions. If an Rh-negative person has never before been exposed to Rh-positive blood, transfusion of Rh-positive blood into that person will likely cause no immediate reaction. However, anti-Rh antibodies can develop in sufficient quantities during the next 2–4 weeks to cause agglutination of the transfused cells that are still circulating in the blood. These cells are then hemolyzed by the tissue macrophage system. Thus, a *delayed* transfusion reaction occurs, although it is usually mild. Upon subsequent transfusion of Rh-positive blood into the same person, who is now already immunized against the Rh factor, the transfusion reaction is greatly enhanced and can be immediate and as severe as a transfusion reaction caused by mismatched type A or B blood.

Erythroblastosis Fetalis ("Hemolytic Disease of the Newborn"). Rh incompatibility is a condition that develops when an Rh-negative pregnant woman has a baby in her womb with Rh-positive blood. This leads to a condition called erythroblastosis fetalis, which is a disease of the fetus and newborn child characterized by agglutination and phagocytosis of the fetus's red blood cells. In most instances of erythroblastosis fetalis, the mother is Rh-negative and the father Rh-positive. The baby has inherited the Rh-positive antigen from the father, and the mother develops anti-Rh agglutinins from exposure to the fetus's Rh antigen. In turn, the mother's agglutinins diffuse through the placenta into the fetus and cause red blood cell agglutination (Figure 28-2). It is important to note that this condition does not affect the first child, since sensitization to the Rh antigen occurs during parturition of the first child. However, if the Rh-negative mother was earlier sensitized to the Rh antigen (by, eg,

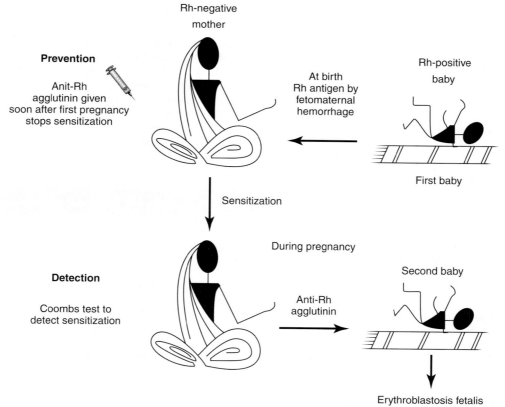

Figure 28-2 Mechanism of development of erythroblastosis fetalis and the utility of the Coombs test.

an earlier blood transfusion with Rh-positive blood), then even the first child can be affected.

Incidence of the Disease. An Rh-negative mother having her first Rh-positive child usually does not develop sufficient anti-Rh agglutinins to cause any harm. However, about 3% of second Rh-positive babies exhibit some signs of erythroblastosis fetalis; about 10% of third babies exhibit the disease; and the incidence rises progressively with subsequent pregnancies.

Effect of the Mother's Antibodies on the Fetus. After anti-Rh antibodies have formed in the mother, they diffuse slowly through the placental membrane into the fetus's blood. There they cause agglutination of the fetus's blood. The agglutinated red blood cells subsequently hemolyze, releasing hemoglobin into the blood. The fetus's macrophages then convert the hemoglobin into bilirubin, which causes the baby's skin to become yellow (jaundiced). The antibodies can also attack and damage other cells of the body.

Clinical Picture of Erythroblastosis. The jaundiced, erythroblastotic newborn baby is usually anemic at birth, and the anti-Rh agglutinins from the mother usually circulate in the infant's blood for another 1–2 months after birth, destroying more and more red blood cells.

The hematopoietic tissues of the infant attempt to replace the hemolyzed red blood cells. The liver and spleen become greatly enlarged and produce red blood cells in the same manner that they normally do during the middle of gestation. Because of the rapid production of red cells, many early forms of red blood cells, including many *nucleated blastic forms*, are passed from the baby's bone marrow into the circulatory system, and it is because of the presence of these nucleated blastic red blood cells that the disease is called *erythroblastosis fetalis*.

Although the severe anemia of erythroblastosis fetalis is usually the cause of death, many children who barely survive the anemia exhibit permanent mental impairment or damage to motor areas of the brain because of precipitation of bilirubin in the neuronal cells, causing destruction of many, a condition called *kernicterus*.

Treatment of Neonates with Erythroblastosis Fetalis. One treatment for erythroblastosis fetalis is to replace the neonate's blood with Rh-negative blood. About 400 mL of Rh-negative blood is infused over a period of 1.5 or more hours while the neonate's own Rh-positive blood is being removed. This procedure may be repeated several times during the first few weeks of life, mainly to keep the bilirubin level low and thereby prevent kernicterus. By the time these transfused Rh-negative cells are replaced with the infant's own Rh-positive cells, a process that requires 6 or more weeks, the anti-Rh agglutinins that had come from the mother will have been destroyed.

Prevention of Erythroblastosis Fetalis. The D antigen of the Rh blood group system is the primary culprit in causing immunization of an Rh-negative mother to an Rh-positive fetus. In the 1970s, a dramatic reduction in the incidence of erythroblastosis fetalis was achieved with the development of *Rh immunoglobulin globin, an anti-D antibody* that is administered to the expectant mother starting at 28–30 weeks of gestation. The anti-D antibody is also administered to Rh-negative women who deliver Rh-positive babies to prevent sensitization of the mothers to the D antigen. This greatly reduces the risk of developing large amounts of D antibodies during the second pregnancy.

The mechanism by which Rh immunoglobulin globin prevents sensitization of the D antigen is not completely understood, but one effect of the anti-D antibody is to inhibit antigen-induced B lymphocyte antibody production in the expectant mother. The administered anti-D antibody also attaches to D-antigen sites on Rh-positive fetal red blood cells that may cross the placenta and enter the circulation of the expectant mother, thereby interfering with the immune response to the D antigen.

TRANSFUSION REACTIONS RESULTING FROM MISMATCHED BLOOD TYPES

If donor blood of one blood type is transfused into a recipient who has another blood type, a transfusion reaction is likely to occur in which the red blood cells *of the donor blood* are agglutinated. It is rare that the transfused blood causes agglutination *of the recipient's cells*, for the following reason: The plasma portion of the donor blood immediately becomes diluted by all the plasma of the recipient, thereby decreasing the titer of the infused agglutinins to a level usually too low to cause agglutination. Conversely, the small amount of infused blood does not significantly dilute the agglutinins in the recipient's plasma. Therefore, the recipient's agglutinins can still agglutinate the mismatched donor cells.

All transfusion reactions eventually cause either immediate hemolysis resulting from hemolysins or later hemolysis resulting from phagocytosis of agglutinated cells. Transfusion reactions can be hemolytic or nonhemolytic (Table 28-3). In hemolytic transfusion reactions, the hemoglobin released from the red cells is then converted by the phagocytes into bilirubin and later excreted in the bile by the liver, as discussed in Chapter 69. The concentration of bilirubin in the body fluids often rises high enough to cause *jaundice*—that is, the person's internal tissues and skin become *colored with yellow bile pigment*. However if liver function is normal, the bile pigment will be excreted into the intestines by way of the liver bile, so jaundice usually does not appear in an adult person unless more than 400 mL of blood are hemolyzed in less than a day.

Acute Kidney Failure After Transfusion Reactions. One of the most lethal effects of transfusion reactions is *kidney failure*, which can begin within a few minutes to a few hours and continue until the person dies of acute renal failure.

The kidney shutdown seems to result from three causes: First, the antigen–antibody reaction of the transfusion reaction releases toxic substances from the hemolyzing blood that cause powerful renal vasoconstriction. Second, loss of circulating

TABLE 28-3	**Types of Transfusion Reactions**	
Type	**Cause**	**Clinical Features**
HEMOLYTIC		
Immediate	ABO incompatibility	Ranges from fever, chills to shock, renal failure
Delayed	Rh incompatibility, secondary or delayed response to RBC antigen	Recurrent anemia, may be fever
NONHEMOLYTIC		
Febrile reaction	Contamination of stored blood with endotoxin or due to cytokines that are released on storage	Fever and chills

BOX 28-1 EFFECTS OF STORAGE OF BLOOD ON RBCs

STRUCTURAL CHANGES

- RBCs tending to lose their shape and becoming spherical
- Loss of membrane flexibility—not deformable and likely to be removed quickly from circulation
- Loss of membrane stability

BIOCHEMICAL CHANGES

- Decreased glycolysis
- Reduced glutathione
- Depletion of ATP and adenine

red cells in the recipient, along with production of toxic substances from the hemolyzed cells and from the immune reaction, often causes circulatory shock. The arterial blood pressure falls very low, and renal blood flow and urine output decrease. Third, if the total amount of free hemoglobin released into the circulating blood is greater than the quantity that can bind with "*haptoglobin*" (a plasma protein that binds small amounts of hemoglobin), much of the excess leaks through the glomerular membranes into the kidney tubules. If this amount is still slight, it can be reabsorbed through the tubular epithelium into the blood and will cause no harm; if it is great, then only a small percentage is reabsorbed. Yet water continues to be reabsorbed, causing the tubular hemoglobin concentration to rise so high that the hemoglobin precipitates and blocks many of the kidney tubules. Thus, renal vasoconstriction, circulatory shock, and renal tubular blockage together cause acute renal shutdown. If the shutdown is complete and fails to resolve, the patient dies within a week to 12 days, as explained in Chapter 84, unless he or she is treated with an artificial kidney.

COLLECTION OF BLOOD FOR TRANSFUSION, ITS STORAGE, AND CHANGES THAT OCCUR DURING STORAGE

Blood is often collected from donors for transfusion into those that need it. Typically, about 450 mL of blood is collected from a vein (usually the antecubital vein) from a healthy donor who has been screened for diseases such as HIV, malaria, hepatitis, and syphilis, which could be transmitted during transfusion. When the blood that is collected is used for transfusion back into the donor (eg, after surgery), it is called an autologous donation. The blood is collected from the donor's vein into a flexible plastic bag, which already has a solution of chemicals in it. These chemicals are sodium citrate, which binds to calcium in the blood and prevents clotting, phosphate buffers to buffer the pH of the collected blood as well as to provide a source of phosphate, dextrose to provide an energy source, and adenine to provide the substrate for adenosine triphosphate (ATP) synthesis. By using these chemicals, the storage of blood can be prolonged to up to 35 days at 4°C.

However, blood that is stored in this fashion for several days does not escape changes. Several changes do occur: red blood cells can become spherical due to metabolic changes, with an associated change in cell rigidity, leading to a fairly large destruction of the transfused RBCs in the body of the recipient. Within the red blood cell, there is a reduction in ATP as well as 2,3-diphosphoglycerate levels. Granulocytes lose their phagocytic and bactericidal properties within 4–6 hours, while platelets could become nonfunctional within 36–48 hours. Other changes with regard to the level of clotting factors also occur. Finally, the potassium levels in the stored blood can also increase due to loss of potassium from the RBC into the plasma (Box 28-1).

BIBLIOGRAPHY

An X, Mohandas N: Disorders of red cell membrane, *Br. J. Haematol.* 141:367, 2008.

Avent ND, Reid ME: The Rh blood group system: a review, *Blood* 95:375, 2000.

Bowman J: Thirty-five years of Rh prophylaxis, *Transfusion* 43:1661, 2003.

Burton NM, Anstee DJ: Structure, function and significance of Rh proteins in red cells, *Curr. Opin. Hematol.* 15:625, 2008.

Horn KD: The classification, recognition and significance of polyagglutination in transfusion medicine, *Blood Rev.* 13:36, 1999.

Hunt SA, Haddad F: The changing face of heart transplantation, *J. Am. Coll. Cardiol.* 52:587, 2008.

Olsson ML, Clausen H: Modifying the red cell surface: towards an ABO-universal blood supply, *Br. J. Haematol.* 140:3, 2008.

Shimizu K, Mitchell RN: The role of chemokines in transplant graft arterial disease, *Arterioscler. Thromb. Vasc. Biol.* 28:1937, 2008.

Stroncek DF, Rebulla P: Platelet transfusions, *Lancet* 370:427, 2007.

Sumpter TL, Wilkes DS: Role of autoimmunity in organ allograft rejection: a focus on immunity to type V collagen in the pathogenesis of lung transplant rejection, *Am. J. Physiol. Lung Cell. Mol. Physiol.* 286:L1129, 2004.

Watchko JF, Tiribelli C: Bilirubin-induced neurologic damage—mechanisms and management approaches, *N. Engl. J. Med.* 369:2021, 2013.

Westhoff CM: The structure and function of the Rh antigen complex, *Semin. Hematol.* 44:42, 2007.

Yazer MH, Hosseini-Maaf B, Olsson ML: Blood grouping discrepancies between ABO genotype and phenotype caused by O alleles, *Curr. Opin. Hematol.* 15:618, 2008.

Cardiovascular Physiology

MARIO VAZ

29

Organization of the Cardiovascular System

The function of the circulation is to serve the needs of the body tissues—to transport nutrients to the body tissues, to transport waste products away, to transport hormones from one part of the body to another, and, in general, to maintain an appropriate environment in all the tissue fluids of the body for survival and optimal function of the cells.

The rate of blood flow through many tissues is controlled mainly in response to their need for nutrients. In some organs, such as the kidneys, the circulation serves additional functions. Blood flow to the kidney, for example, is far in excess of its metabolic requirements and is related to its excretory function, which requires that a large volume of blood be filtered each minute.

The heart and blood vessels, in turn, are controlled to provide the necessary cardiac output and arterial pressure to cause the needed tissue blood flow. What are the mechanisms for controlling blood volume and blood flow, and how does this process relate to the other functions of the circulation? These are some of the topics and questions that we discuss in this section on the circulation.

Physical Characteristics of the Circulation

The circulation, shown in Figure 29-1, is divided into the *systemic circulation* and the *pulmonary circulation*. Because the systemic circulation supplies blood flow to all the tissues of the body except the lungs, it is also called the *greater circulation* or

peripheral circulation. It is also clear from the figure that the heart is in fact two pumps in series. The right heart pumps blood into the pulmonary circulation while the left heart pumps blood into the systemic circulation.

Functional Parts of the Circulation. Before discussing the details of circulatory function, it is important to understand the role of each part of the circulation.

The function of the *arteries* is to transport blood *under high pressure* to the tissues. For this reason, the arteries have strong vascular walls and blood flows at a high velocity in the arteries.

The *arterioles* are the last small branches of the arterial system; they act as *control conduits* through which blood is released into the capillaries. Arterioles have strong muscular walls that can close the arterioles completely or can, by relaxing, dilate the vessels severalfold, thus having the capability of vastly altering blood flow in each tissue in response to its needs. These blood vessels are sometimes called *resistance vessels*.

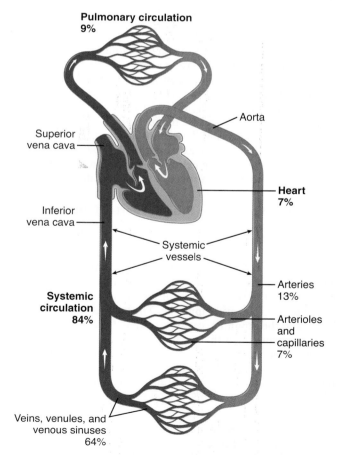

Figure 29-1 Distribution of blood (in percentage of total blood) in the different parts of the circulatory system.

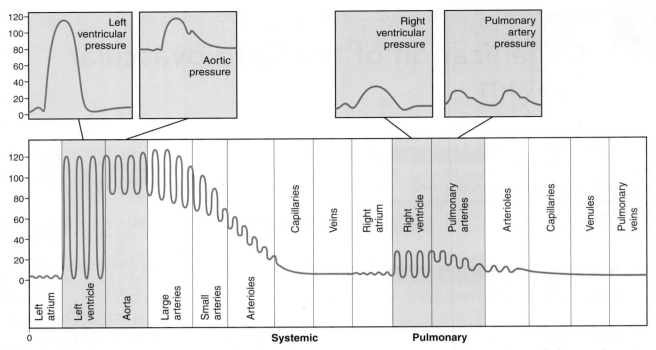

Figure 29-2 Normal blood pressures in the different portions of the circulatory system when a person is lying in the horizontal position.

The function of the *capillaries* is to exchange fluid, nutrients, electrolytes, hormones, and other substances between the blood and the interstitial fluid; they are therefore sometimes called *exchange vessels*. To serve this role, the capillary walls are thin and have numerous minute *capillary pores* permeable to water and other small molecular substances.

The *venules* collect blood from the capillaries and gradually coalesce into progressively larger veins.

The *veins* function as conduits for transport of blood from the venules back to the heart; equally important, they serve as a major reservoir of extra blood and are sometimes referred to as *capacitance vessels*. Because the pressure in the venous system is very low, the venous walls are thin. Even so, they are muscular enough to contract or expand and thereby serve as a controllable reservoir for the extra blood, either a small or a large amount, depending on the needs of the circulation.

Volumes of Blood in the Different Parts of the Circulation. Figure 29-1 gives an overview of the circulation and lists the percentage of the total blood volume in major segments of the circulation. For instance, about 84% of the entire blood volume of the body is in the systemic circulation and 16% is in the heart and lungs. Of the 84% in the systemic circulation, approximately 64% is in the veins, 13% is in the arteries, and 7% is in the systemic arterioles and capillaries. The heart contains 7% of the blood and the pulmonary vessels contain 9%.

Most surprising is the low blood volume in the capillaries. It is here, however, that the most important function of the circulation occurs, diffusion of substances back and forth between the blood and the tissues. This function is discussed in detail in Chapter 39.

Cross-Sectional Areas and Velocities of Blood Flow. If all the *systemic vessels* of each type were put side by side, their approximate total cross-sectional areas for the average human being would be as follows:

Vessel	Cross-Sectional Area (cm^2)
Aorta	2.5
Small arteries	20
Arterioles	40
Capillaries	2500
Venules	250
Small veins	80
Venae cavae	8

Note particularly that the cross-sectional areas of the veins are much larger than those of the arteries, averaging about four times those of the corresponding arteries. This difference explains the large blood storage capacity of the venous system in comparison with the arterial system.

Because the same volume of blood flow (F) must pass through each segment of the circulation each minute, the velocity of blood flow (v) is inversely proportional to vascular cross-sectional area (A):

$$v = \frac{F}{A}$$

Thus, under resting conditions, the velocity averages about 33 cm/second in the aorta but is only 1/1000 as rapid in the capillaries, about 0.3 mm/second. However, because the capillaries have a typical length of only 0.3–1 mm, the blood remains in the capillaries for only 1–3 seconds, which is surprising because all diffusion of nutrient food substances and electrolytes that occurs through the capillary walls must be performed in this short time.

Pressures in the Various Portions of the Circulation. Because the heart pumps blood continually into the aorta, the mean pressure in the aorta is high, averaging about 100 mmHg. Also, because heart pumping is pulsatile, the arterial pressure alternates between a *systolic pressure level* of 120 mmHg and a *diastolic pressure level* of 80 mmHg, as shown on the left side of Figure 29-2.

TABLE 29-1	Comparison Between Pulmonary and Systemic Circulations	
	Systemic Circulation	Pulmonary Circulation
Blood flow (L/minute)	5	5
Percentage of blood volume	84	9
Arterial blood pressure (mmHg)	120/80	25/8
Oxygen content of the arteries (PO_2; mmHg)	100	40

As the blood flows through the *systemic circulation*, its mean pressure falls progressively to about 0 mmHg by the time it reaches the termination of the superior and inferior venae cavae where they empty into the right atrium of the heart.

The pressure in the systemic capillaries varies from as high as 35 mmHg near the arteriolar ends to as low as 10 mmHg near the venous ends, but their average "functional" pressure in most vascular beds is about 17 mmHg, a pressure low enough that little of the plasma leaks through the minute *pores* of the capillary walls, even though nutrients can *diffuse* easily through these same pores to the outlying tissue cells.

Note at the far right side of Figure 29-2 the respective pressures in the different parts of the *pulmonary circulation*. In the pulmonary arteries, the pressure is pulsatile, just as in the aorta, but the pressure is far less: *pulmonary artery systolic pressure* averages about 25 mmHg and *diastolic pressure* averages about 8 mmHg, with a mean pulmonary arterial pressure of only 16 mmHg. The mean pulmonary capillary pressure averages only 7 mmHg. Yet the total blood flow through the lungs each minute is the same as through the systemic circulation. The low pressures of the pulmonary system are in accord with the needs of the lungs because all that is required is to expose the blood in the pulmonary capillaries to oxygen and other gases in the pulmonary alveoli.

Table 29-1 compares the pulmonary and systemic circulations.

Basic Principles of Circulatory Function

Although the details of circulatory function are complex, three basic principles underlie all functions of the system:

1. *Blood flow to most tissues is controlled according to the tissue need.* When tissues are active, they need a greatly increased supply of nutrients and therefore much more blood flow than when at rest—occasionally as much as 20–30 times the resting level. Yet the heart normally cannot increase its cardiac output more than four to seven times greater than resting levels. Therefore, it is not possible simply to increase blood flow everywhere in the body when a particular tissue demands increased flow. Instead, the microvessels of each tissue continuously monitor tissue needs, such as the availability of oxygen and other nutrients and the accumulation of carbon dioxide and other tissue waste products, and these microvessels in turn act directly on the local blood vessels, dilating or constricting them, to control local blood flow precisely to that level required for the tissue activity. Also, nervous control of the circulation from the central nervous system and hormones provide additional help in controlling tissue blood flow.

2. *Cardiac output is the sum of all the local tissue flows.* When blood flows through a tissue, it immediately returns by way of the veins to the heart. The heart responds automatically to this increased inflow of blood by pumping it immediately back into the arteries. Thus, the heart acts as an automaton, responding to the demands of the tissues. The heart, however, often needs help in the form of special nerve signals to make it pump the required amounts of blood flow.

3. *Arterial pressure regulation is generally independent of either local blood flow control or cardiac output control.* The circulatory system is provided with an extensive system for controlling the arterial blood pressure. For instance, if at any time the pressure falls significantly below the normal level of about 100 mmHg, within seconds a barrage of nervous reflexes elicits a series of circulatory changes to raise the pressure back toward normal. The nervous signals especially (a) increase the force of heart pumping, (b) cause contraction of the large venous reservoirs to provide more blood to the heart, and (c) cause constriction of the arterioles in many tissues so that more blood accumulates in the large arteries to increase the arterial pressure. Then, over more prolonged periods, hours and days, the kidneys play an additional major role in pressure control both by secreting pressure-controlling hormones and by regulating the blood volume.

BIBLIOGRAPHY

Badeer HS: Hemodynamics for medical students, *Am. J. Physiol. (Adv. Physiol. Educ.)* 25:44, 2001.

Guyton AC, Jones CE, Coleman TG: *Circulatory physiology: cardiac output and its regulation*, Philadelphia, 1963, W. B. Saunders.

Hall JE: Integration and regulation of cardiovascular function, *Am. J. Physiol. (Adv. Physiol. Educ.)* 22:S174, 1999.

30 Properties of Cardiac Muscle

LEARNING OBJECTIVES

- List the special anatomical and functional characteristics of cardiac muscle.
- Compare the structural and functional differences between cardiac, skeletal, and smooth muscles.
- List the properties of cardiac muscle that ensure its nonfatigability.

GLOSSARY OF TERMS

- **Bathmotropy:** Relating to excitability (a positively bathmotropic agent increases excitability, while a negatively bathmotropic agent reduces excitability)

- **Inotropy:** Relating to the force of contraction (a positively inotropic agent increases the force of contraction, while a negatively inotropic agent reduces the force of contraction)

- **Starling law of the heart:** Stating that the force of contraction of the heart is directly proportional to the end-diastolic volume (and pressure) within physiological limits

- **Syncytium:** A collection of cardiac muscle cells joined by intercalated discs that allows the entire collection to contract as a single unit (there are two syncytia: atrial and ventricular, separated from each other by a fibrous band)

The heart is composed of three major types of cardiac muscle: *atrial muscle*, *ventricular muscle*, and specialized *excitatory* and *conductive muscle* fibers. The atrial and ventricular types of muscle contract in much the same way as skeletal muscle, except that the duration of contraction is much longer. The specialized excitatory and conductive fibers of the heart, however, contract only feebly because they contain few contractile fibrils; instead, they exhibit either automatic rhythmical electrical discharge in the form of action potentials or conduction of the action potentials through the heart, providing an excitatory system that controls the rhythmical beating of the heart.

Anatomical Characteristics of Cardiac Muscle

Figure 30-1 shows the histology of cardiac muscle. This figure shows that:

- Cardiac muscle fibers are arranged in a latticework with the fibers dividing, recombining, and then spreading again.
- Cardiac muscle is *striated* in the same manner as in skeletal muscle. Further, cardiac muscle has typical myofibrils that contain *actin* and *myosin filaments* almost identical to those found in skeletal muscle; these filaments lie side by side and slide during contraction in the same manner as occurs in skeletal muscle (see Chapter 14). In other ways, however, cardiac muscle is quite different from skeletal muscle, as we shall see.

Physiological Characteristics of Cardiac Muscle

1. *Cardiac muscle is excitable.* Like all other living cells, cardiac muscle cells are excitable, that is, they have the ability to respond to a stimulus. The response to a stimulus is a change in the membrane potential and if the stimulus provided is of sufficient intensity, a biological response, that is, contraction, is obtained. Factors that affect the excitability of the heart are referred to as *bathmotropic factors*. Those factors that increase excitability are called positively bathmotropic while those that reduce excitability are called negatively bathmotropic.

2. *Autorhythmicity.* Cardiac muscle is self-excitatory, although this property can be modulated by nerves, hormones, and drugs. The ability of the heart to generate its own rhythm is discussed in greater detail in Chapters 31 and 32.

3. *Cardiac muscle is contractile.* This is self-explanatory. However, cardiac muscle contraction differs in important ways from skeletal muscle contraction and these are discussed later in the chapter. *Inotropy* refers to the force of muscle contraction. Factors that increase the force of contraction are called positively inotropic while those that reduce the force of contraction are called negatively inotropic.

4. *Cardiac muscle conducts electrical impulses.* The presence of intercalated discs (see later text) is especially important in allowing cardiac muscle to conduct electrical impulses. However, the speed with which impulses are conducted in cardiac muscle is relatively slow. The heart has in place a specialized conducting system, which is discussed in Chapter 32.

5. *Cardiac muscle is a syncytium.* The dark areas crossing the cardiac muscle fibers in Figure 30-1 are called *intercalated discs*. At each intercalated disc the cell membranes fuse with one another in such a way to form permeable

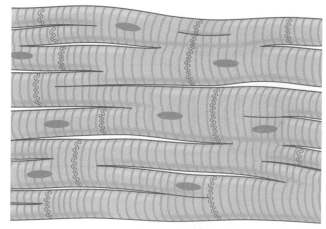

Figure 30-1 Syncytial, interconnecting nature of cardiac muscle fibers.

"communicating" junctions (gap junctions) that allow rapid diffusion of ions. Therefore, from a functional point of view, ions move with ease in the intracellular fluid so that action potentials travel easily from one cardiac muscle cell to the next, past the intercalated discs. Thus, cardiac muscle is a *syncytium* of many heart muscle cells in which the cardiac cells are so interconnected that when one cell becomes excited, the action potential spreads to all of them. The heart actually is composed of two syncytiums: the *atrial syncytium*, which constitutes the walls of the two atria, and the *ventricular syncytium*, which constitutes the walls of the two ventricles. The atria are separated from the ventricles by fibrous tissue that surrounds the atrioventricular (A-V) valvular openings between the atria and ventricles. Normally, potentials are not conducted from the atrial syncytium into the ventricular syncytium directly through this fibrous tissue. Instead, they are conducted only by way of a specialized conductive system called the *A-V bundle* (see Chapter 32).

This division of the muscle of the heart into two functional syncytiums allows the atria to contract a short time ahead of ventricular contraction; this allows the blood in the atria to empty into the ventricles before the ventricles begin contracting.

6. *The all-or-none law in the heart applies to the entire syncytium.* Earlier (Chapter 16) while discussing skeletal muscle contraction we talked about the all-or-none law. For skeletal muscle a stimulus that is of threshold or greater than threshold intensity applied to a motor nerve fiber will result in the contraction of all the muscle fibers supplied by the nerve, that is, the entire motor unit. In the case of the heart, because cardiac muscle behaves like a syncytium, a threshold or greater than threshold stimulus applied to any part of the syncytium will result in the contraction of the entire syncytium.

7. *The action potential in cardiac muscle is prolonged and has a long refractory period.* The *action potential* recorded in a ventricular muscle fiber is shown in Figure 30-2. After the initial *spike*, the membrane remains depolarized for about 0.2 second, exhibiting a *plateau*, followed at the end of the

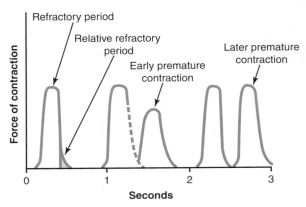

Figure 30-3 Force of ventricular heart muscle contraction, showing also duration of the refractory period and relative refractory period, plus the effect of premature contraction. Note that premature contractions do not cause wave summation, as occurs in skeletal muscle.

plateau by abrupt repolarization. The presence of this plateau in the action potential causes ventricular contraction to last as much as 15 times as long in cardiac muscle as in skeletal muscle. The details of the ionic basis of the cardiac muscle action potential are discussed in Chapter 31.

One of the characteristics of cardiac muscle, like all excitable tissue, is that it is refractory to restimulation during the action potential. Therefore, the refractory period of the heart is the interval of time, as shown to the left in Figure 30-3, during which a normal cardiac impulse cannot reexcite an already excited area of cardiac muscle. The normal refractory period of the ventricle is 0.25–0.30 second, which is about the duration of the prolonged plateau action potential. There is an additional *relative refractory period* of about 0.05 second during which the muscle is more difficult to excite than normal but nevertheless can be excited by a very strong excitatory signal, as demonstrated by the early "premature" contraction in the second example of Figure 30-3. The refractory period of atrial muscle is much shorter than that for the ventricles (about 0.15 second for the atria compared with 0.25–0.30 second for the ventricles). The long refractory period is one of the factors why cardiac muscle does not fatigue.

8. *Cardiac muscle requires calcium in the extracellular fluid to contract.* As is true for skeletal muscle, when an action potential passes over the cardiac muscle membrane, the action potential spreads to the interior of the cardiac muscle fiber along the membranes of the transverse (T) tubules. The T tubule action potentials in turn act on the membranes of the *longitudinal sarcoplasmic tubules* to cause release of calcium ions into the muscle sarcoplasm from the sarcoplasmic reticulum. In another few thousandths of a second, these calcium ions diffuse into the myofibrils and catalyze the chemical reactions that promote sliding of the actin and myosin filaments along one another, which produces the muscle contraction.

Thus far, this mechanism of excitation–contraction coupling is the same as that for skeletal muscle, but there is a second effect that is quite different. In addition to the calcium ions that are released into the sarcoplasm from the cisternae of the sarcoplasmic reticulum, calcium ions also diffuse into the sarcoplasm from the T tubules themselves at the time of the action potential, which opens voltage-dependent calcium channels in the membrane of

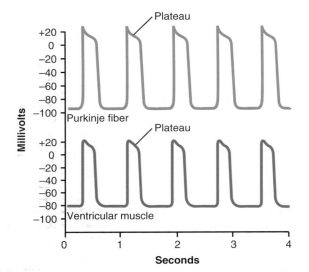

Figure 30-2 Rhythmical action potentials (in millivolts) from a Purkinje fiber and from a ventricular muscle fiber, recorded by means of microelectrodes.

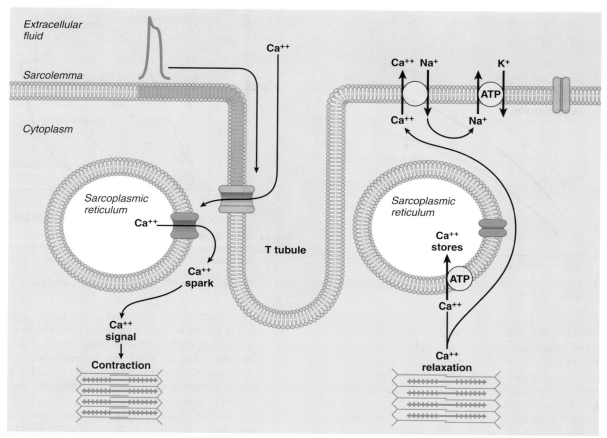

Figure 30-4 Mechanisms of excitation–contraction coupling and relaxation in cardiac muscle. *ATP*, adenosine triphosphate.

the T tubule (Figure 30-4). Calcium entering the cell then activates *calcium release channels*, also called *ryanodine receptor channels*, in the sarcoplasmic reticulum membrane, triggering the release of calcium into the sarcoplasm. Calcium ions in the sarcoplasm then interact with troponin to initiate cross-bridge formation and contraction by the same basic mechanism as described for skeletal muscle in Chapter 14.

Without the calcium from the T tubules, the strength of cardiac muscle contraction would be reduced considerably because the sarcoplasmic reticulum of cardiac muscle is less well developed than that of skeletal muscle and does not store enough calcium to provide full contraction. The T tubules of cardiac muscle, however, have a diameter 5 times greater than that of the skeletal muscle tubules, which means 25 times greater volume. Also, inside the T tubules is a large quantity of mucopolysaccharides that are electronegatively charged and bind an abundant store of calcium ions, keeping them available for diffusion to the interior of the cardiac muscle fiber when a T-tubule action potential appears.

The strength of contraction of cardiac muscle depends to a great extent on the concentration of calcium ions in the extracellular fluids. In fact, a heart placed in a calcium-free solution will quickly stop beating. The reason for this response is that the openings of the T tubules pass directly through the cardiac muscle cell membrane into the extracellular spaces surrounding the cells, allowing the same extracellular fluid that is in the cardiac muscle interstitium to percolate through the T tubules. Consequently,

the quantity of calcium ions in the T-tubule system (ie, the availability of calcium ions to cause cardiac muscle contraction) depends to a great extent on the extracellular fluid calcium ion concentration.

9. *Cardiac muscle contraction is dependent on the initial length of the muscle fiber (Frank–Starling law of the heart and concepts of preload and afterload).* The degree of tension on the muscle when it begins to contract is called the *preload*, while the load against which the muscle exerts its contractile force is called the *afterload*. For cardiac contraction, the *preload* is usually considered to be the end-diastolic pressure when the ventricle has become filled. The greater the end-diastolic volume (ventricular filling) and the greater the corresponding end-diastolic pressure, the greater is the stretch of the cardiac muscle. This increased initial length of the muscle results in a greater force of contraction within physiological limits and is referred to as Frank–Starling law of the heart.

The relationship of length to contractility is modified by the presence of inotropic factors as shown in Figure 30-5. For instance, intense sympathetic stimulation can increase the heart rate in young adult humans from the normal rate of 70 beats/minute up to 180–200 and, rarely, even 250 beats/minute. Sympathetic stimulation also increases the force of heart contraction to as much as double the normal value, thereby increasing the volume of blood pumped and increasing the ejection pressure. Thus, sympathetic stimulation often can increase the maximum cardiac output as much as twofold to threefold, in addition to the increased output caused

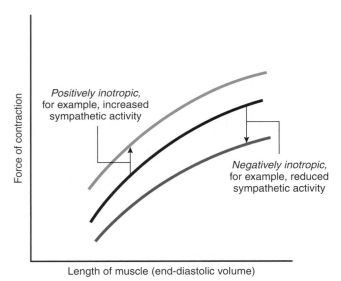

Figure 30-5 Modifications of the length and force of contraction relationship by inotropic factors.

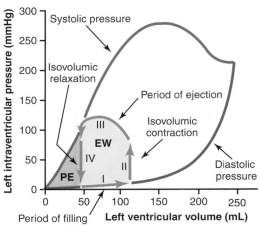

Figure 30-6 Relationship between left ventricular volume and intraventricular pressure during diastole and systole. Also shown by the heavy red lines is the "volume–pressure diagram," demonstrating changes in intraventricular volume and pressure during the normal cardiac cycle. *EW*, net external work; PE, potential energy.

by the Frank–Starling mechanism already discussed. Conversely, *inhibition* of the sympathetic nerves to the heart can decrease cardiac pumping to a moderate extent in the following way: Under normal conditions, the sympathetic nerve fibers to the heart discharge continuously at a slow rate that maintains pumping at about 30% above that with no sympathetic stimulation. Therefore, when the activity of the sympathetic nervous system is depressed below normal, this decreases both heart rate and strength of ventricular muscle contraction, thereby decreasing the level of cardiac pumping as much as 30%

below normal. The *afterload* of the ventricle is the pressure in the aorta leading from the ventricle. In Figure 30-6, this corresponds to the systolic pressure described by the phase III curve of the volume–pressure diagram. (Sometimes the afterload is loosely considered to be the resistance in the circulation rather than the pressure.)

The importance of the concepts of preload and afterload is that in many abnormal functional states of the heart or circulation, the pressure during filling of the ventricle (the preload), the arterial pressure against which the ventricle must contract (the afterload), or both are altered from normal to a severe degree.

TABLE 30-1	Comparison of Skeletal, Smooth, and Cardiac Muscles		
	Skeletal	**Smooth**	**Cardiac**
STRUCTURAL			
Striated	Yes	No	Yes
Distribution of myofilaments	Orderly—along myofibrils	Scattered	Orderly—along myofibrils
T tubules	Yes	No	Yes
Intercellular connections	No	Some gap junctions	Many intercalated discs
Types	Slow and fast	Unitary and multiunit	—
FUNCTIONAL FEATURES			
Source of Ca ions for activation	Sarcoplasmic reticulum	Sarcoplasmic reticulum and extracellular fluid	Sarcoplasmic reticulum and extracellular fluid
Spontaneous electrical activity and contraction	No	Yes	Yes
Duration of action potential	Few milliseconds (5 ms)	Hundreds of milliseconds with plateau (300 ms)	Variable: from 10-ms spike potentials to prolonged potentials with a plateau phase
Response to rapid multiple stimuli	Tetanization	Cannot be tetanized	Cannot be tetanized
Susceptibility to fatigue	High	Resistant to fatigue	Resistant to fatigue
REGULATORY			
Response to nerve stimulation	Excitation–contraction	Excitation or inhibition	Excitation or inhibition
Response to hormones	Small	Large	Large

10. *Cardiac muscle does not fatigue.* It is truly amazing that the heart continues to beat in a healthy individual with such regularity the entire life span of an individual without getting tired. Even the most well-trained skeletal muscle in the most elite of athletes cannot achieve this. There are several reasons why cardiac muscle does not get fatigued:

a. Cardiac muscle has a long refractory period. Thus cardiac muscle cannot be tetanized. While tetany allows for the generation of greater force, fatigue also sets in much faster.

b. Cardiac muscle has a rich blood supply. In context, cardiac muscle has a capillary density that is about four times greater than skeletal muscle.

c. Cardiac muscle undergoes aerobic metabolism. Thus, the accumulation of lactic acid, an important factor in the development of fatigue in anaerobically exercising muscles, plays no role in cardiac muscle.

d. Cardiac muscle is rich in mitochondria; mitochondria account for almost one-third of the cardiac muscle by weight and are best appreciated by an examination of the histology of cardiac muscle.

Table 30-1 compares the structural and functional differences between skeletal, smooth, and cardiac muscles.

BIBLIOGRAPHY

Bers DM: Calcium cycling and signaling in cardiac myocytes, Annu. Rev. Physiol. 70:23, 2008.

Chantler PD, Lakatta EG, Najjar SS: Arterial–ventricular coupling: mechanistic insights into cardiovascular performance at rest and during exercise, *J. Appl. Physiol.* 105:1342, 2008.

Ibrahim M, Gorelik J, Yacoub MH, Terracciano CM: The structure and function of cardiac t-tubules in health and disease, *Proc. Biol. Sci.* 278:2714, 2011.

Kho C, Lee A, Hajjar RJ: Altered sarcoplasmic reticulum calcium cycling—targets for heart failure therapy, *Nat. Rev. Cardiol.* 9:717, 2012.

Korzick DH: Regulation of cardiac excitation–contraction coupling: a cellular update, *Adv. Physiol. Educ.* 27:192, 2003.

Luo M, Anderson ME: Mechanisms of altered Ca^{2+} handling in heart failure, *Circ. Res.* 113:690, 2013.

Mangoni ME, Nargeot J: Genesis and regulation of the heart automaticity, *Physiol. Rev.* 88:919, 2008.

Sarnoff SJ: Myocardial contractility as described by ventricular function curves, *Physiol. Rev.* 35:107, 1955.

Starling EH: *The Linacre Lecture on the Law of the Heart*, London, 1918, Longmans Green.

ter Keurs HE: The interaction of Ca^{2+} with sarcomeric proteins: role in function and dysfunction of the heart, *Am. J. Physiol. Heart Circ. Physiol.* 302:H38, 2012.

31

Cardiac Action Potentials

LEARNING OBJECTIVES

- Describe the ionic basis of the low action potential of the SA node.
- Describe the cardiac muscle action potential in terms of:
  - phases of the action potential;
  - ion fluxes contributing to each phase of the action potential.
- Describe the actions of the sympathetic and parasympathetic nervous systems on the cardiac action potential.

GLOSSARY OF TERMS

- **Fast action potentials:** Refer to potentials seen in contractile and conducting cells that are characterized by rapid depolarization due to the opening of fast sodium channels

- **Pacemaker potentials:** Also called diastolic depolarization/prepotential (it is the slow increase in membrane potential to threshold level that occurs between the end of one potential and the start of another in the SA node)

- **Slow action potentials:** Are characterized by a slow upstroke because of influx of calcium, and are of lower amplitude and slower conduction than the fast action potentials; typically seen in the SA and A-V nodes

There are essentially two different types of potentials that are seen in the heart. Slow potentials are seen in the pacemaker areas, that is, the sinoatrial (SA) node and atrioventricular (A-V) node. Fast action potentials are seen in contractile and conducting cells. These two potentials differ in many ways, but one is the speed with which depolarization occurs, hence the names.

Membrane Potentials for the SA Node and Muscle Fibers

The sinus node (also called *SA node*) is a small, flattened, ellipsoid strip of specialized cardiac muscle about 3 mm wide, 15 mm long, and 1 mm thick. It is located in the superior posterolateral wall of the right atrium immediately below and slightly lateral to the opening of the superior vena cava.

While the sinus node has no true resting membrane potential, the lowest potential it achieves is about −55 to −60 mV in comparison with −85 to −90 mV resting membrane potential for the ventricular muscle fiber. Figure 31-1 shows action potentials recorded from inside a sinus nodal fiber for three heartbeats and, by comparison, a single ventricular muscle fiber

action potential. The cause of the lesser negativity in the sinus nodal fiber is that the cell membranes of the sinus fibers are naturally leaky to sodium and calcium ions, and positive charges of the entering sodium and calcium ions neutralize some of the intracellular negativity.

Ionic Basis of the Slow Action Potential of the SA Node. Because of the high sodium ion concentration in the extracellular fluid outside the nodal fiber, as well as a moderate number of already open sodium channels, positive sodium ions from outside the fibers normally tend to leak to the inside. Therefore, between heartbeats, influx of positively charged sodium ions causes a slow rise in the "resting" membrane potential in the positive direction. Thus, as shown in Figure 31-1, the "resting" potential gradually rises and becomes less negative between each two heartbeats. When the potential reaches a threshold voltage of about −40 mV, the L-type calcium channels become "activated," thus causing the action potential. Therefore, basically, the inherent leakiness of the sinus nodal fibers to sodium and calcium ions causes their self-excitation.

Why does this leakiness to sodium and calcium ions not cause the sinus nodal fibers to remain depolarized all the time? Two events occur during the course of the action potential to prevent such a constant state of depolarization. First, the L-type calcium channels become inactivated (ie, they close) within about 100–150 milliseconds after opening, and, second, at about the same time, greatly increased numbers of potassium channels open. Therefore, influx of positive calcium ions through the L-type calcium channels ceases, while at the same time large quantities of positive potassium ions diffuse out of the fiber. Both of these effects reduce the intracellular potential back to its negative resting level and therefore terminate the action potential. Furthermore, the potassium channels remain open for another few tenths of a second, temporarily continuing movement of positive charges out of the cell, with resultant excess negativity inside the fiber; this process is called *hyperpolarization*.

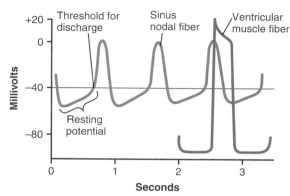

Figure 31-1 Rhythmical discharge of a sinus nodal fiber. Also, the sinus nodal action potential is compared with that of a ventricular muscle fiber.

The hyperpolarization state initially carries the "resting" membrane potential down to about −55 to −60 mV at the termination of the action potential.

Why is this new state of hyperpolarization not maintained forever? The reason is that during the next few tenths of a second after the action potential is over, progressively more and more potassium channels close. The hyperpolarization also causes the inward leak of sodium ions that once again overbalance the outward flux of potassium ions, and this causes the "resting" potential to drift upward once more, finally reaching the threshold level for discharge at a potential of about −40 mV. Since the inward leak of sodium ions is brought about by hyperpolarization rather than depolarization (which is the more usual process for the opening of channels), these channels are sometimes called "funny" channels. The entire process then begins again: self-excitation to cause the action potential, recovery from the action potential, hyperpolarization after the action potential is over, drift of the "resting" potential to threshold, and finally reexcitation to elicit another cycle. This process continues throughout a person's life.

IONIC BASIS OF THE FAST ACTION POTENTIAL IN CARDIAC MUSCLE

The *action potential* recorded in a ventricular muscle fiber rises from a very negative value, about −85 mV, rapidly to a slightly positive value, about +20 mV, during each beat (Figure 31-2). After the initial *spike*, the membrane remains depolarized exhibiting a *plateau* and is followed at the end of the plateau by abrupt repolarization. The presence of this plateau in the action potential causes ventricular contraction to last as much as 15 times as long in cardiac muscle as in skeletal muscle.

What Causes the Long Action Potential and the Plateau? In *cardiac muscle, the action potential* is caused by opening of two types of channels: (1) the same *fast voltage-gated sodium channels* as those in skeletal muscle and (2) another entirely different

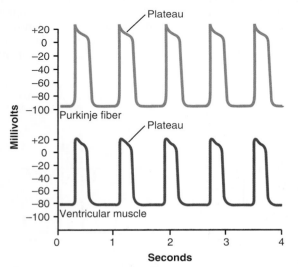

Figure 31-2   Rhythmical action potentials (in millivolts) from a Purkinje fiber and from a ventricular muscle fiber, recorded by means of microelectrodes.

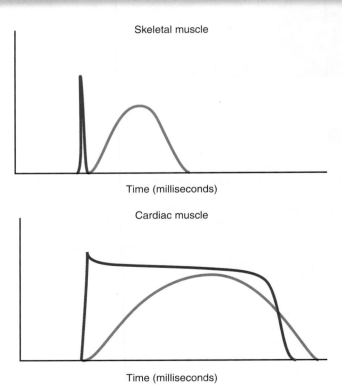

Figure 31-3   The temporal association between electrical (blue) and contractile (red) responses in skeletal and cardiac muscles.

population of *L-type calcium channels*. This second population of channels differs from the fast sodium channels in that they are slower to open and, even more important, remain open for several tenths of a second. During this time, a large quantity of both calcium and sodium ions flow through these channels to the interior of the cardiac muscle fiber, and this activity maintains a prolonged period of depolarization, *causing the plateau* in the action potential. Further, the calcium ions that enter during this plateau phase activate the muscle contractile process, whereas the calcium ions that cause skeletal muscle contraction are derived from the intracellular sarcoplasmic reticulum. A comparison of the temporal association of the action potentials and contractile responses in skeletal and cardiac muscles is provided in Figure 31-3.

Immediately after the onset of the action potential, the permeability of the cardiac muscle membrane for potassium ions *decreases* about fivefold, an effect that does not occur in skeletal muscle. This decreased potassium permeability may result from the excess calcium influx through the calcium channels just noted. Regardless of the cause, the decreased potassium permeability greatly decreases the outflux of positively charged potassium ions during the action potential plateau and thereby prevents early return of the action potential voltage to its resting level. When the L-type calcium channels do close at the end of 0.2–0.3 second and the influx of calcium and sodium ions ceases, the membrane permeability for potassium ions also increases rapidly; this rapid loss of potassium from the fiber immediately returns the membrane potential to its resting level, thus ending the action potential.

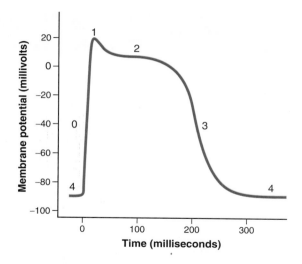

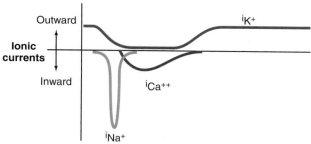

Figure 31-4 Phases of action potential of cardiac ventricular muscle cell and associated ionic currents for sodium ($^iNa^+$), calcium ($^iCa^{++}$), and potassium ($^iK^+$).

Summary of Phases of Cardiac Muscle Action Potential. Figure 31-4 summarizes the phases of the action potential in cardiac muscle and the ion flows that occur during each phase:

Phase 0 (depolarization), fast sodium channels open. When the cardiac cell is stimulated and depolarizes, the membrane potential becomes more positive. Voltage-gated sodium channels (fast sodium channels) open and permit sodium to rapidly flow into the cell and depolarize it. The membrane potential reaches about +20 mV before the sodium channels close.

Phase 1 (initial repolarization), fast sodium channels close. The sodium channels close, the cell begins to repolarize, and potassium ions leave the cell through open potassium channels.

Phase 2 (plateau), calcium channels open and fast potassium channels close. A brief initial repolarization occurs and the action potential then plateaus as a result of (1) increased calcium ion permeability and (2) decreased potassium ion permeability. The voltage-gated calcium ion channels open slowly during phases 1 and 0, and calcium enters the cell. Potassium channels then close, and the combination of decreased potassium ion efflux and increased calcium ion influx causes the action potential to plateau.

Phase 3 (rapid repolarization), calcium channels close and slow potassium channels open. The closure of calcium ion channels and increased potassium ion permeability, permitting potassium ions to rapidly exit the cell, ends the plateau and returns the cell membrane potential to its resting level.

Phase 4 (resting membrane potential) averages about −90 mV.

Control of Cardiac Action Potentials by the Sympathetic and Parasympathetic Nerves

SYMPATHETIC EFFECT

Stimulation of the sympathetic nerves releases the hormone *norepinephrine* at the sympathetic nerve endings. Norepinephrine in turn stimulates *beta-1 adrenergic receptors*, which mediate the effects on heart rate. The precise mechanism by which beta-1 adrenergic stimulation acts on cardiac muscle fibers is somewhat unclear, but the belief is that it increases the permeability of the fiber membrane to sodium and calcium ions. In the sinus node, an increase of sodium–calcium permeability causes a more positive resting potential and also causes an increased rate of upward drift of the diastolic membrane potential toward the threshold level for self-excitation, thus accelerating self-excitation and, therefore, increasing the heart rate.

In the A-V node and A-V bundles, increased sodium–calcium permeability makes it easier for the action potential to excite each succeeding portion of the conducting fiber bundles, thereby decreasing the conduction time from the atria to the ventricles.

The increase in permeability to calcium ions is at least partially responsible for the increase in contractile strength of the cardiac muscle under the influence of sympathetic stimulation, because calcium ions play a powerful role in exciting the contractile process of the myofibrils.

VAGAL (PARASYMPATHETIC) EFFECTS

The acetylcholine released at the vagal nerve endings greatly increases the permeability of the fiber membranes to potassium ions, which allows rapid leakage of potassium out of the conductive fibers. This process causes increased negativity inside the fibers, an effect called *hyperpolarization*, which makes this excitable tissue much less excitable.

In the sinus node, the state of hyperpolarization decreases the "resting" membrane potential of the sinus nodal fibers from −65 to −75 mV rather than the normal level of −55 to −60 mV. Therefore, the initial rise of the sinus nodal membrane potential caused by inward sodium and calcium leakage requires much longer to reach the threshold potential for excitation. This requirement greatly slows the rate of rhythmicity of these nodal fibers. If the vagal stimulation is strong enough, it is possible to stop entirely the rhythmical self-excitation of this node.

In the A-V node, a state of hyperpolarization caused by vagal stimulation makes it difficult for the small atrial fibers entering the node to generate enough electricity to excite the nodal fibers. Therefore, the safety factor for transmission of the cardiac impulse through the transitional fibers into the A-V nodal fibers decreases. A moderate decrease simply delays conduction of the impulse, but a large decrease blocks conduction entirely.

Effect of Drugs on the Cardiac Action Potential

It is beyond the scope of this chapter to discuss the comprehensive role of drugs acting on the cardiac action potential. Table 31-1, however, provides a framework for the actions of some drugs that the student will be able to relate to based on the ionic currents that have been discussed in this chapter.

TABLE 31-1	Effect of Some Drugs on the Cardiac Action Potential	
Channel/Receptor	**Nature of Action**	**Effect**
Sodium channel	Blocker	Reduce the maximum rise of the action potential and decrease in conduction through the conducting system and atrial and ventricular muscles
Beta receptor	Blocker	Reduces sodium–calcium entry in the SA and A-V nodes; reduces heart rate and slows conduction
Potassium channel	Blocker	Prolongation of the action potential duration
Calcium channel	Blocker	Depression of the plateau phase of the action potential; negative inotropism

A-V, atrioventricular; SA, sinoatrial.

BIBLIOGRAPHY

Clancy CE, Kass RS: Defective cardiac ion channels: from mutations to clinical syndromes, *J. Clin. Invest.* 110:1075, 2002.

Dobrzynski H, Boyett MR, Anderson RH: New insights into pacemaker activity: promoting understanding of sick sinus syndrome, *Circulation* 115:1921, 2007.

Hancox JC, Patel KCR, Jones JV: Antiarrhythmics—from cell to clinic: past, present, and future, *Heart* 84:14, 2000.

Hondeghem LM: Classification of antiarrhythmic agents and the two laws of pharmacology, *Cardiovasc. Res.* 45:57, 2000.

Mangoni ME, Nargeot J: Genesis and regulation of the heart automaticity, *Physiol. Rev.* 88:919, 2008.

Origin and Conduction of the Cardiac Impulse

- List in sequence the pathway of the electrical excitation of the heart.
- Describe the functional significance of A-V nodal delay.
- List the effects of sympathetic and parasympathetic nervous activity on the conduction of the cardiac impulse.
- Describe the consequences of aberrant excitation in the heart in relation to: (1) ectopic pacemaker and (2) Wolff–Parkinson–White syndrome.

GLOSSARY OF TERMS

- **A-V block:** Failure of the cardiac impulse to pass normally from the atria into the ventricles through the A-V nodal and bundle system
- **Chronotropy:** Related to the heart rate (factors that slow down the heart rate are called negatively chronotropic, while those factors that increase the heart rate are called positively chronotropic)
- **Dromotropy:** Related to the conduction of the cardiac impulse (factors that slow down the conduction of the cardiac impulse are called negatively dromotropic, while those factors that increase the conduction of the cardiac impulse are called positively dromotropic)
- **Stokes–Adams syndrome:** Sudden transient episodes of fainting caused by a reduction in cardiac output due to cardiac asystole or heart block resulting in a lack of blood flow to the brain
- **Ventricular escape:** Intense vagal stimulation resulting in A-V block being compensated for by a self-generated electrical discharge initiated by the ventricles of the heart
- **Wolff–Parkinson–White syndrome:** Abnormal atrioventricular transmission of the cardiac impulse through an aberrant pathway that does not have the impulse slowing property of the A-V node

The human heart has a special system for rhythmical self-excitation and repetitive contraction approximately 100,000 times each day, or 3 billion times in the average human lifetime. This impressive feat is performed by a system that (1) generates rhythmical electrical impulses to initiate rhythmical contraction of the heart muscle and (2) conducts these impulses rapidly through the heart.

While cardiac muscle can transmit electrical activity through the low-impedance intercalated disks, the heart is endowed with a special conducting system that:

1. generates rhythmical electrical impulses to cause rhythmical contraction of the heart muscle;
2. conducts these impulses rapidly through the heart;
3. enables the atria to contract about one-sixth of a second ahead of ventricular contraction, which allows filling of the ventricles before they pump the blood through the lungs and peripheral circulation;
4. allows all portions of the ventricles to contract almost simultaneously, which is essential for most effective pressure generation in the ventricular chambers.

Specialized Excitatory and Conductive System of the Heart

Figure 32-1 shows the specialized excitatory and conductive system of the heart that controls cardiac contractions.

SINUS (SINOATRIAL) NODE

The sinus node [also called *sinoatrial (S-A) node*] is a small, flattened, ellipsoid strip of specialized cardiac muscle about 3 mm wide, 15 mm long, and 1 mm thick. It is located in the superior posterolateral wall of the right atrium immediately below and slightly lateral to the opening of the superior vena cava. The sinus nodal fibers connect directly with the atrial muscle fibers so that any action potential that begins in the sinus node spreads immediately into the atrial muscle wall.

Automatic Electrical Rhythmicity of the Sinus Fibers

Some cardiac fibers have the capability of *self-excitation*, a process that can cause automatic rhythmical discharge and

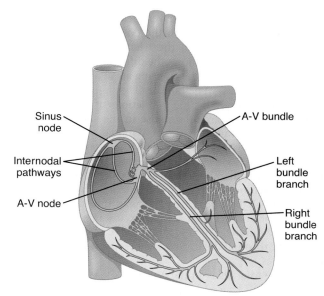

Figure 32-1 Sinus node and the Purkinje system of the heart showing also the atrioventricular node, atrial internodal pathways, and ventricular bundle branches. *A-V,* atrioventricular.

contraction. This capability is especially true for the fibers of the heart's specialized conducting system including the fibers of the sinus node. This self-generated electrical activity in the sinus node is a specific property of specialized cells called pacemaker (P) cells. The sinus node ordinarily controls the rate at which the entire heart beats. The spontaneous electrical potentials at the S-A node have been described earlier in Chapter 31.

INTERNODAL AND INTERATRIAL PATHWAYS TRANSMIT CARDIAC IMPULSES THROUGH THE ATRIA

The ends of the sinus nodal fibers connect directly with surrounding atrial muscle fibers. Therefore, action potentials originating in the sinus node travel outward into these atrial muscle fibers. In this way, the action potential spreads through the entire atrial muscle mass and, eventually, to the atrioventricular (A-V) node. The velocity of conduction in most atrial muscle is about 0.3 m/second but conduction is more rapid, about 1 m/second, in several small bands of atrial fibers. One of these bands, called the *anterior interatrial band*, passes through the anterior walls of the atria to the left atrium. In addition, three other small bands curve through the anterior, lateral, and posterior atrial walls and terminate in the A-V node, shown in Figures 32-1 and 32-2; these are called, respectively, the *anterior, middle, and posterior internodal pathways*. The cause of more rapid velocity of conduction in these bands is the presence of specialized conduction fibers. These fibers are similar to even more rapidly conducting "Purkinje fibers" of the ventricles, which are discussed as follows.

THE ATRIOVENTRICULAR NODE DELAYS IMPULSE CONDUCTION FROM THE ATRIA TO THE VENTRICLES

The atrial conductive system is organized so that the cardiac impulse does not travel from the atria into the ventricles too rapidly; this delay allows time for the atria to empty their blood into the ventricles before ventricular contraction begins. It is primarily the A-V node and its adjacent conductive fibers that delay this transmission into the ventricles.

The A-V node is located in the posterior wall of the right atrium immediately behind the tricuspid valve as shown in Figure 32-1. Figure 32-2 shows the different parts of this node, and its connections with the entering atrial internodal pathway fibers and the exiting A-V bundle. This figure also shows the approximate intervals of time in fractions of a second between initial onset of the cardiac impulse in the sinus node and its subsequent appearance in the A-V nodal system. Note that the impulse, after traveling through the internodal pathways, reaches the A-V node about 0.03 second after its origin in the sinus node. Then there is a delay of another 0.09 second in the A-V node itself before the impulse enters the penetrating portion of the A-V bundle, where it passes into the ventricles. A final delay of another 0.04 second occurs mainly in this penetrating A-V bundle, which is composed of multiple small fascicles passing through the fibrous tissue separating the atria from the ventricles.

Thus, the total delay in the A-V nodal and A-V bundle system is about 0.13 second. This delay, in addition to the initial conduction delay of 0.03 second from the sinus node to the A-V node, makes a total delay of 0.16 second before the excitatory signal finally reaches the contracting muscle of the ventricles.

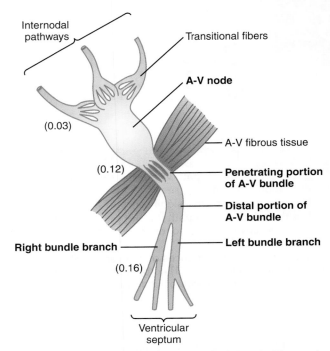

Figure 32-2 Organization of the atrioventricular node. The numbers represent the interval of time from the origin of the impulse in the sinus node. The values have been extrapolated to human beings. *A-V,* atrioventricular.

Cause of the Slow Conduction. The slow conduction in the transitional, nodal, and penetrating A-V bundle fibers is caused *mainly by diminished numbers of gap junctions between successive cells in the conducting pathways,* so there is great resistance to conduction of excitatory ions from one conducting fiber to the next. Therefore, it is easy to see why each succeeding cell is slow to be excited.

Wolff–Parkinson–White Syndrome. In some individuals, there is an abnormal pathway (called the bundle of Kent) between the atria and the ventricles. This pathway does not have the delaying properties of the A-V node—transmission into the ventricles is therefore faster. While most individuals are asymptomatic, abnormally fast rhythms generated in the atria will be conducted into the ventricles. The additional pathway can be destroyed by radio-frequency catheter ablation.

RAPID TRANSMISSION IN THE VENTRICULAR PURKINJE SYSTEM

Special Purkinje fibers lead from the A-V node through the A-V bundle into the ventricles. Except for the initial portion of these fibers, where they penetrate the A-V fibrous barrier, they have functional characteristics that are quite the opposite of those of the A-V nodal fibers. They are very large fibers, even larger than the normal ventricular muscle fibers, and they transmit action potentials at a velocity of 1.5–4.0 m/second, a velocity about six times that in the usual ventricular muscle and 150 times that in some of the A-V nodal fibers. This velocity allows almost instantaneous transmission of the cardiac impulse throughout the entire remainder of the ventricular muscle.

The rapid transmission of action potentials by Purkinje fibers is believed to be caused by a very high level of permeability of the gap junctions at the intercalated discs between the successive cells that make up the Purkinje fibers.

One-Way Conduction Through the A-V Bundle. A special characteristic of the A-V bundle is the inability, except in abnormal states, of action potentials to travel backward from the ventricles to the atria. This characteristic prevents reentry of cardiac impulses by this route from the ventricles to the atria, allowing only forward conduction from the atria to the ventricles.

Furthermore, it should be recalled that everywhere, except at the A-V bundle, the atrial muscle is separated from the ventricular muscle by a continuous fibrous barrier, a portion of which is shown in Figure 32-2. This barrier normally acts as an insulator to prevent passage of the cardiac impulse between atrial and ventricular muscles through any other route besides forward conduction through the A-V bundle.

Distribution of the Purkinje Fibers in the Ventricles—The Left and Right Bundle Branches. After penetrating the fibrous tissue between the atrial and ventricular muscles, the distal portion of the A-V bundle passes downward in the ventricular septum for 5–15 mm toward the apex of the heart, as shown in Figures 32-1 and 32-2. Then the bundle divides into left and right bundle branches that lie beneath the endocardium on the two respective sides of the ventricular septum. Each branch spreads downward toward the apex of the ventricle, progressively dividing into smaller branches. These branches in turn course sidewise around each ventricular chamber and back toward the base of the heart. The ends of the Purkinje fibers penetrate about one-third of the way into the muscle mass and finally become continuous with the cardiac muscle fibers.

The total elapsed time averages only 0.03 second from the time the cardiac impulse enters the bundle branches in the ventricular septum until it reaches the terminations of the Purkinje fibers. Therefore, once the cardiac impulse enters the ventricular Purkinje conductive system, it spreads almost immediately to the entire ventricular muscle mass.

TRANSMISSION OF THE CARDIAC IMPULSE IN THE VENTRICULAR MUSCLE

Once the impulse reaches the ends of the Purkinje fibers, it is transmitted through the ventricular muscle mass by the ventricular muscle fibers themselves. The velocity of transmission is now only 0.3–0.5 m/second, one-sixth of that in the Purkinje fibers.

The cardiac muscle wraps around the heart in a double spiral with fibrous septa between the spiraling layers; therefore, the cardiac impulse does not necessarily travel directly outward toward the surface of the heart but instead angulates toward the surface along the directions of the spirals. Because of this angulation, transmission from the endocardial surface to the epicardial surface of the ventricle requires as much as another 0.03 second, approximately equal to the time required for transmission through the entire ventricular portion of the Purkinje system. Thus, the total time for transmission of the cardiac impulse from the initial bundle branches to the last of the ventricular muscle fibers in the normal heart is about 0.06 second.

SUMMARY OF THE SPREAD OF THE CARDIAC IMPULSE THROUGH THE HEART

Figure 32-3 summarizes the transmission of the cardiac impulse through the human heart. The numbers on the figure

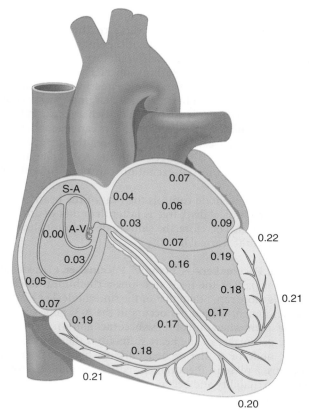

Figure 32-3 Transmission of the cardiac impulse through the heart showing the time of appearance (in fractions of a second after initial appearance at the sinoatrial node) in different parts of the heart. *A-V*, atrioventricular; *S-A*, sinoatrial.

represent the intervals of time, in fractions of a second, that lapse between the origin of the cardiac impulse in the sinus node and its appearance at each respective point in the heart. Note that the impulse spreads at moderate velocity through the atria but is delayed more than 0.1 second in the A-V nodal region before appearing in the ventricular septal A-V bundle. Once it has entered this bundle, it spreads very rapidly through the Purkinje fibers to the entire endocardial surfaces of the ventricles. Then the impulse once again spreads slightly less rapidly through the ventricular muscle to the epicardial surfaces.

Control of Excitation and Conduction in the Heart

THE SINUS NODE IS THE NORMAL PACEMAKER OF THE HEART

We have noted that the cardiac impulse normally arises in the sinus node. In some abnormal conditions, this is not the case. Other parts of the heart can also exhibit intrinsic rhythmical excitation in the same way that the sinus nodal fibers do; this capability is particularly true of the A-V nodal and Purkinje fibers.

The A-V nodal fibers, when not stimulated from some outside source, discharge at an intrinsic rhythmical rate of 40–60 times/minute and the Purkinje fibers discharge at a rate somewhere between 15 and 40 times/minute. These rates are in contrast to the normal rate of the sinus node of 70–80 times/minute.

Why then does the sinus node rather than the A-V node or the Purkinje fibers control the heart's rhythmicity? The answer is because the discharge rate of the sinus node is considerably faster than the natural self-excitatory discharge rate of either the A-V node or the Purkinje fibers. Each time the sinus node discharges, its impulse is conducted into both the A-V node and the Purkinje fibers, also discharging their excitable membranes. However, the sinus node discharges again before either the A-V node or the Purkinje fibers can reach their own thresholds for self-excitation. Therefore, the new impulse from the sinus node discharges both the A-V node and the Purkinje fibers before self-excitation can occur in either of these sites.

Thus, the sinus node controls the beat of the heart because its rate of rhythmical discharge is faster than that of any other part of the heart. Therefore, the sinus node is almost always the pacemaker of the normal heart.

Abnormal Pacemakers—"Ectopic" Pacemaker. Occasionally, some other part of the heart develops a rhythmical discharge rate that is more rapid than that of the sinus node. For instance, this development sometimes occurs in the A-V node or in the Purkinje fibers when one of these becomes abnormal. In either case, the pacemaker of the heart shifts from the sinus node to the A-V node or to the excited Purkinje fibers. Under rarer conditions, a place in the atrial or ventricular muscle develops excessive excitability and becomes the pacemaker.

A pacemaker elsewhere than the sinus node is called an *"ectopic" pacemaker*. An ectopic pacemaker causes an abnormal sequence of contraction of the different parts of the heart and can cause significant debility of heart pumping.

Another cause of shift of the pacemaker is blockage of transmission of the cardiac impulse from the sinus node to the other parts of the heart. The new pacemaker then occurs most frequently at the A-V node or in the penetrating portion of the A-V bundle on the way to the ventricles.

When A-V block occurs—that is, when the cardiac impulse fails to pass from the atria into the ventricles through the A-V nodal and bundle system—the atria continue to beat at the normal rate of rhythm of the sinus node, while a new pacemaker usually develops in the Purkinje system of the ventricles and drives the ventricular muscle at a new rate somewhere between 15 and 40 beats/minute. After sudden A-V bundle block, the Purkinje system does not begin to emit its intrinsic rhythmical impulses until 5–20 seconds later because, before the blockage, the Purkinje fibers had been "overdriven" by the rapid sinus impulses and, consequently, are in a suppressed state. During these 5–20 seconds, the ventricles fail to pump blood and the person faints after the first 4–5 seconds because of lack of blood flow to the brain. This delayed pickup of the heartbeat is called *Stokes–Adams syndrome*. If the delay period is too long, it can lead to death.

THE PURKINJE SYSTEM CAUSES SYNCHRONOUS CONTRACTION OF THE VENTRICULAR MUSCLE

The rapid conduction of the Purkinje system normally permits the cardiac impulse to arrive at almost all portions of the ventricles within a narrow span of time, exciting the first ventricular muscle fiber only 0.03–0.06 second ahead of excitation of the last ventricular muscle fiber. This timing causes all portions of the ventricular muscle in both ventricles to begin contracting at almost the same time and then to continue contracting for about another 0.3 second.

Effective pumping by the two ventricular chambers requires this synchronous type of contraction. If the cardiac impulse should travel through the ventricles slowly, much of the ventricular mass would contract before contraction of the remainder, in which case the overall pumping effect would be greatly depressed. Indeed, in some types of cardiac debilities, slow transmission does occur and the pumping effectiveness of the ventricles is decreased as much as 20–30%.

SYMPATHETIC AND PARASYMPATHETIC NERVES CONTROL HEART RHYTHMICITY AND IMPULSE CONDUCTION

The heart is supplied with both sympathetic and parasympathetic nerves. The parasympathetic nerves (the vagi) are distributed mainly to the S-A and A-V nodes, to a lesser extent to the muscle of the two atria, and very little directly to the ventricular muscle. The sympathetic nerves, conversely, are distributed to all parts of the heart, with strong representation to the ventricular muscle, as well as to all the other areas.

Parasympathetic (Vagal) Stimulation Slows the Cardiac Rhythm and Conduction. Stimulation of the parasympathetic nerves to the heart (the vagi) causes *acetylcholine* to be released at the vagal endings. This has two major effects on the heart. First, it decreases the rate of rhythm of the sinus node, and second, it decreases the excitability of the A-V junctional fibers between the atrial musculature and the A-V node, thereby slowing transmission of the cardiac impulse into the ventricles, that is, it is *negatively dromotropic*.

Weak to moderate vagal stimulation slows the rate of heart pumping, often to as little as one-half normal. Furthermore, strong stimulation of the vagi can stop completely the rhythmical excitation by the sinus node or block completely transmission of the cardiac impulse from the atria into the ventricles through the A-V node. In either case, rhythmical excitatory signals are no longer transmitted into the ventricles. The ventricles may stop beating for 5–20 seconds, but then some small area in the Purkinje fibers, usually in the ventricular septal portion of the A-V bundle, develops a rhythm of its own and causes ventricular contraction at a rate of 15–40 beats/minute. This phenomenon is called *ventricular escape*.

Sympathetic Stimulation Increases Cardiac Rhythm and Conduction. Sympathetic stimulation causes essentially the opposite effects on the heart to those caused by vagal stimulation as follows: First, it increases the rate of sinus nodal discharge (*positively chronotropic*). Second, it increases the rate of conduction (*positively dromotropic*), as well as the level of excitability (*positively bathmotropic*) in all portions of the heart. Third, it increases greatly the force of contraction (*positively inotropic*) of all the cardiac musculature, both atrial and ventricular, as discussed in Chapter 30.

In short, sympathetic stimulation increases the overall activity of the heart.

BIBLIOGRAPHY

Anderson RH, Boyett MR, Dobrzynski H, Moorman AF: The anatomy of the conduction system: implications for the clinical cardiologist, *J. Cardiovasc. Transl. Res.* 6:187, 2013.

Barbuti A, DiFrancesco D: Control of cardiac rate by "funny" channels in health and disease, *Ann. N. Y. Acad. Sci.* 1123:213, 2008.

Dobrzynski H, Boyett MR, Anderson RH: New insights into pacemaker activity: promoting understanding of sick sinus syndrome, *Circulation* 115:2007, 1921.

Fedorov VV, Glukhov AV, Chang R: Conduction barriers and pathways of the sinoatrial pacemaker complex: their role in normal rhythm and atrial arrhythmias, *Am. J. Physiol. Heart Circ. Physiol.* 302:H1773, 2012.

Kléber AG, Rudy Y: Basic mechanisms of cardiac impulse propagation and associated arrhythmias, *Physiol. Rev.* 84:431, 2004.

Leclercq C, Hare JM: Ventricular resynchronization: current state of the art, *Circulation* 109:296, 2004.

Mangoni ME, Nargeot J: Genesis and regulation of the heart automaticity, *Physiol. Rev.* 88:919, 2008.

Monfredi O, Maltsev VA, Lakatta EG: Modern concepts concerning the origin of the heartbeat, *Physiology (Bethesda)* 28:74, 2013.

Munshi NV: Gene regulatory networks in cardiac conduction system development, *Circ. Res.* 110:1525, 2012.

Roubille F, Tardif JC: New therapeutic targets in cardiology: heart failure and arrhythmia: HCN channels, *Circulation* 127:1986, 2013.

Smaill BH, Zhao J, Trew ML: Three-dimensional impulse propagation in myocardium: arrhythmogenic mechanisms at the tissue level, *Circ. Res.* 112:834, 2013.

Wickramasinghe SR, Patel VV: Local innervation and atrial fibrillation, *Circulation* 128:1566, 2013.

The Normal Electrocardiogram

When the cardiac impulse passes through the heart, electrical current also spreads from the heart into the adjacent tissues surrounding the heart. A small portion of the current spreads all the way to the surface of the body. If electrodes are placed on the skin on opposite sides of the heart, electrical potentials generated by the current can be recorded; the recording is known as an electrocardiogram (ECG). A normal ECG for two beats of the heart is shown in Figure 33-1.

Characteristics of the Normal Electrocardiogram

The normal ECG (see Figure 33-1) is composed of a P wave, a QRS complex, and a T wave. The QRS complex is often, but not always, three separate waves: the Q wave, the R wave, and the S wave.

The P wave is caused by electrical potentials generated when the atria depolarize before atrial contraction begins. The QRS complex is caused by potentials generated when the ventricles depolarize before contraction, that is, as the depolarization wave spreads through the ventricles. Therefore, both the P wave and the components of the QRS complex are *depolarization waves.* The atria repolarize about 0.15–0.20 second after termination of the P wave. This is also approximately when the QRS complex is being recorded in the ECG. Therefore, the atrial repolarization wave, known as the *atrial T wave*, is usually obscured by the much larger QRS complex. For this reason, an atrial T wave seldom is observed in the ECG.

The T wave is caused by potentials generated as the ventricles recover from the state of depolarization. This process normally occurs in ventricular muscle 0.25–0.35 second after depolarization. The T wave is known as a *repolarization wave.* Ordinarily, ventricular muscle begins to repolarize in some fibers about 0.20 second after the beginning of the depolarization wave (the QRS complex), but in many other fibers, it takes as long as 0.35 second. Thus, the process of ventricular repolarization extends over a long period, about 0.15 second. For this reason, the T wave in the normal ECG is a prolonged wave, but the voltage of the T wave is considerably less than the voltage of the QRS complex, partly because of its prolonged length.

Thus, the ECG is composed of both depolarization and repolarization waves. The principles of depolarization and repolarization are discussed in Chapter 9.

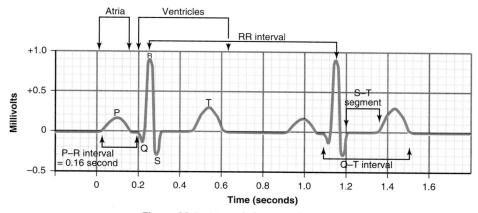

Figure 33-1 Normal electrocardiogram.

RELATION OF THE MONOPHASIC ACTION POTENTIAL OF VENTRICULAR MUSCLE TO THE QRS AND T WAVES IN THE STANDARD ELECTROCARDIOGRAM

The monophasic action potential of ventricular muscle, discussed in Chapter 31, normally lasts between 0.25 and 0.35 second. The top part of Figure 33-2 shows a monophasic action potential recorded from a microelectrode inserted to the inside of a single ventricular muscle fiber. The upsweep of this action potential is caused by depolarization and the return of the potential to the baseline is caused by repolarization.

The lower half of Figure 33-2 shows a simultaneous recording of the ECG from this same ventricle. Note that the QRS waves appear at the beginning of the monophasic action potential and the T wave appears at the end. Note especially that *no potential is recorded in the ECG when the ventricular muscle is either completely polarized or completely depolarized.* Only when the muscle is partly polarized and partly depolarized does current flow from one part of the ventricles to another part and therefore current also flows to the surface of the body to produce the ECG.

VOLTAGE AND TIME CALIBRATION OF THE ELECTROCARDIOGRAM

All recordings of ECG are made with appropriate calibration lines on the recording paper. Either these calibration lines are already ruled on the paper, as is the case when a pen recorder is used, or they are recorded on the paper at the same time that the ECG is recorded, which is the case with the photographic types of electrocardiographs.

As shown in Figure 33-1, the horizontal calibration lines are arranged so that 10 of the small line divisions upward or downward in the standard ECG represent 1 mV, with positivity in the upward direction and negativity in the downward direction.

The vertical lines on the ECG are time calibration lines. A typical ECG is run at a paper speed of 25 mm/second, although faster speeds are sometimes used. Therefore, each 25 mm in the horizontal direction is 1 second, and each 5-mm segment, indicated by the dark vertical lines, represents 0.20 second. The 0.20-second intervals are then broken into five smaller intervals by thin lines, each of which represents 0.04 second.

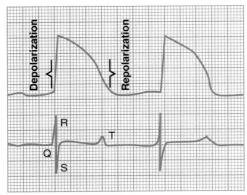

Figure 33-2   *(Top)* Monophasic action potential from a ventricular muscle fiber during normal cardiac function showing rapid depolarization and then repolarization occurring slowly during the plateau stage but rapidly toward the end. *(Bottom)* Electrocardiogram recorded simultaneously.

Normal Voltages in the Electrocardiogram. The recorded voltages of the waves in the normal ECG depend on the manner in which the electrodes are applied to the surface of the body and how close the electrodes are to the heart. When one electrode is placed directly over the ventricles and a second electrode is placed elsewhere on the body remote from the heart, the voltage of the QRS complex may be as great as 3–4 mV. Even this voltage is small in comparison with the monophasic action potential of 110 mV recorded directly at the heart muscle membrane. When ECGs are recorded from electrodes on the two arms or on one arm and one leg, the voltage of the QRS complex usually is 1.0–1.5 mV from the top of the R wave to the bottom of the S wave; the voltage of the P wave is between 0.1 and 0.3 mV; and the voltage of the T wave is between 0.2 and 0.3 mV.

P–Q or P–R Interval. The time between the beginning of the P wave and the beginning of the QRS complex is the interval between the beginning of electrical excitation of the atria and the beginning of excitation of the ventricles. This period is called the *P–Q interval*. The normal P–Q interval is about 0.16 second. (Often this interval is called the *P–R interval* because the Q wave is likely to be absent.)

Q–T Interval. Contraction of the ventricle lasts almost from the beginning of the Q wave (or R wave, if the Q wave is absent) to the end of the T wave. This interval is called the *Q–T interval* and ordinarily is about 0.35 second.

Rate of Heartbeat as Determined from the Electrocardiogram. The rate of the heartbeat can be determined easily from an ECG because the heart rate is the reciprocal of the time interval between two successive heartbeats. If the interval between two beats as determined from the time calibration lines is 1 second, the heart rate is 60 beats/minute. The normal interval between two successive QRS complexes in an adult person is about 0.83 second, which is a heart rate of 60/0.83 times/minute or 72 beats/minute.

Flow of Current Around the Heart During the Cardiac Cycle

RECORDING ELECTRICAL POTENTIALS FROM A PARTIALLY DEPOLARIZED MASS OF SYNCYTIAL CARDIAC MUSCLE

Figure 33-3 shows a syncytial mass of cardiac muscle that has been stimulated at its central-most point. Before stimulation,

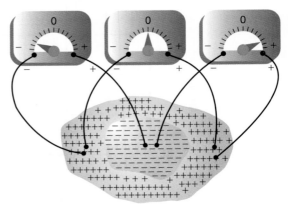

Figure 33-3   Instantaneous potentials develop on the surface of a cardiac muscle mass that has been depolarized in its center.

all the exteriors of the muscle cells had been positive and the interiors had been negative. As soon as an area of cardiac syncytium becomes depolarized, negative charges leak to the outsides of the depolarized muscle fibers, making this part of the surface electronegative, as represented by the minus signs in Figure 33-3. The remaining surface of the heart, which is still polarized, is represented by the plus signs. Therefore, a meter connected with its negative terminal on the area of depolarization and its positive terminal on one of the still-polarized areas, as shown to the right in the figure, records positively.

FLOW OF ELECTRICAL CURRENTS IN THE CHEST AROUND THE HEART

Figure 33-4 shows the ventricular muscle lying within the chest. Even the lungs, although mostly filled with air, conduct electricity to a surprising extent and fluids in other tissues surrounding the heart conduct electricity even more easily. Therefore, the heart is actually suspended in a conductive medium. When one portion of the ventricles depolarizes and therefore becomes electronegative with respect to the remainder, electrical current flows from the depolarized area to the polarized area in large circuitous routes, as noted in the figure.

It should be recalled from the discussion of the Purkinje system in Chapter 32 that the cardiac impulse first arrives in the ventricles in the septum and shortly thereafter spreads to the inside surfaces of the remainder of the ventricles, as shown by the red areas and the negative signs in Figure 33-4. This process provides electronegativity on the insides of the ventricles and electropositivity on the outer walls of the ventricles, with electrical current flowing through the fluids surrounding the ventricles along elliptical paths, as demonstrated by the curving arrows in the figure. If one algebraically averages all the lines of current flow (the elliptical lines), one finds that *the average current flow occurs with negativity toward the base of the heart and with positivity toward the apex.*

During most of the remainder of the depolarization process, current also continues to flow in this same direction, while depolarization spreads from the endocardial surface outward through the ventricular muscle mass. Then, immediately before depolarization has completed its course through the ventricles, the average direction of current flow reverses for about 0.01 second, flowing from the ventricular apex toward the base, because the last part of the heart to become depolarized is the outer walls of the ventricles near the base of the heart.

Thus, in normal heart ventricles, current flows from negative to positive primarily in the direction from the base of the heart toward the apex during almost the entire cycle of depolarization, except at the very end. If a meter is connected to electrodes on the surface of the body as shown in Figure 33-4, the electrode nearer the base will be negative, whereas the electrode nearer the apex will be positive, and the recording meter will show positive recording in the ECG.

Electrocardiographic Leads

THREE BIPOLAR LIMB LEADS

Figure 33-5 shows electrical connections between the patient's limbs and the electrocardiograph for recording ECGs from the so-called *standard bipolar limb leads.* The term "bipolar" means that the ECG is recorded from two electrodes located on different sides of the heart—in this case, on the limbs. Thus, a "lead" is not a single wire connecting from the body but a combination of two wires and their electrodes to make a complete circuit between the body and the electrocardiograph. The electrocardiograph in each instance is represented by an electrical meter in the diagram, although the actual electrocardiograph is a computer-based system with an electronic display.

Lead I. In recording limb lead I, the negative terminal of the electrocardiograph is connected to the right arm and the positive terminal is connected to the left arm. Therefore, when the point where the right arm connects to the chest is electronegative with respect to the point where the left arm connects, the electrocardiograph records positively, that is, above the zero voltage line in the ECG. When the opposite is true, the electrocardiograph records below the line.

Lead II. To record limb lead II, the negative terminal of the electrocardiograph is connected to the right arm and the positive terminal is connected to the left leg. Therefore, when the right arm is negative with respect to the left leg, the electrocardiograph records positively.

Lead III. To record limb lead III, the negative terminal of the electrocardiograph is connected to the left arm and the positive terminal is connected to the left leg. This configuration means that the electrocardiograph records positively when the left arm is negative with respect to the left leg.

Einthoven Triangle. In Figure 33-5, the triangle, called *Einthoven triangle,* is drawn around the area of the heart. This illustrates that the two arms and the left leg form apices of a triangle surrounding the heart. The two apices at the upper part of the triangle represent the points at which the two arms connect

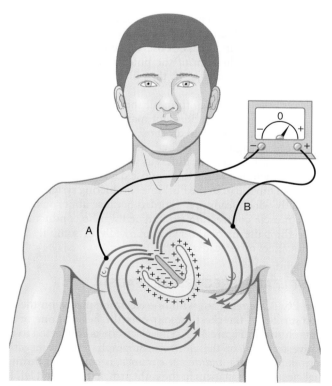

Figure 33-4 Flow of current in the chest around partially depolarized ventricles. *A* and *B*, electrodes.

electrically with the fluids around the heart, and the lower apex is the point at which the left leg connects with the fluids.

Einthoven Law. Einthoven law states that if the ECGs are recorded simultaneously with the three limb leads, the sum of the potentials recorded in leads I and III will equal the potential in lead II:

Lead I potential + lead III potential = lead II potential

In other words, if the electrical potentials of any two of the three bipolar limb electrocardiographic leads are known at any given instant, the third one can be determined by simply summing the first two. Note, however, that the positive and negative signs of the different leads must be observed when making this summation.

For instance, let us assume that momentarily, as noted in Figure 33-5, the right arm is −0.2 mV (negative) with respect to the average potential in the body, the left arm is +0.3 mV (positive), and the left leg is +1.0 mV (positive). Observing the meters in the figure, one can see that lead I records a positive potential of +0.5 mV because this is the difference between the −0.2 mV on the right arm and the +0.3 mV on the left arm. Similarly, lead III records a positive potential of +0.7 mV, and lead II records a positive potential of +1.2 mV because these are

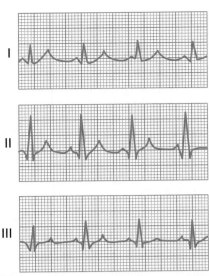

Figure 33-6 Normal electrocardiograms recorded from the three standard electrocardiographic leads.

the instantaneous potential differences between the respective pairs of limbs.

Now, note that the sum of the voltages in leads I and III equals the voltage in lead II; that is, 0.5 plus 0.7 equals 1.2. Mathematically, this principle, called Einthoven law, holds true at any given instant while the three "standard" bipolar ECGs are being recorded.

Normal Electrocardiograms Recorded from the Three Standard Bipolar Limb Leads. Figure 33-6 shows recordings of the ECGs in leads I, II, and III. It is obvious that the ECGs in these three leads are similar to one another because they all record positive P waves and positive T waves, and the major portion of the QRS complex is also positive in each ECG.

On analysis of the three ECGs, it can be shown, with careful measurements and proper observance of polarities, that at any given instant the sum of the potentials in leads I and III equals the potential in lead II, thus illustrating the validity of Einthoven law.

Because the recordings from all the bipolar limb leads are similar to one another, it does not matter greatly which lead is recorded when one wants to diagnose different cardiac arrhythmias, because diagnosis of arrhythmias depends mainly on the time relations between the different waves of the cardiac cycle. However, when one wants to diagnose damage in the ventricular or atrial muscle or in the Purkinje conducting system, it matters greatly which leads are recorded because abnormalities of cardiac muscle contraction or cardiac impulse conduction do change the patterns of the ECGs markedly in some leads yet may not affect other leads.

CHEST LEADS (PRECORDIAL LEADS)

Often ECGs are recorded with one electrode placed on the anterior surface of the chest directly over the heart at one of the points shown in Figure 33-7. This electrode is connected to the positive terminal of the electrocardiograph, and the negative electrode, called the *indifferent electrode*, is connected through equal electrical resistances to the right arm, left arm, and left leg all at the same time, as also shown in the figure. Usually six standard chest leads are recorded, one at a time, from the anterior

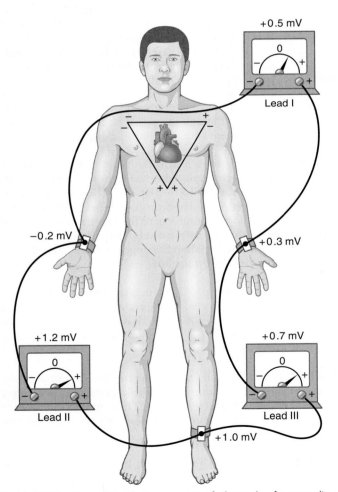

Figure 33-5 Conventional arrangement of electrodes for recording the standard electrocardiographic leads. Einthoven triangle is superimposed on the chest.

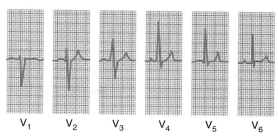

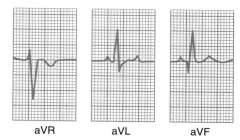

Figure 33-8 Normal electrocardiograms recorded from the six standard chest leads.

Figure 33-9 Normal electrocardiograms recorded from the three augmented unipolar limb leads.

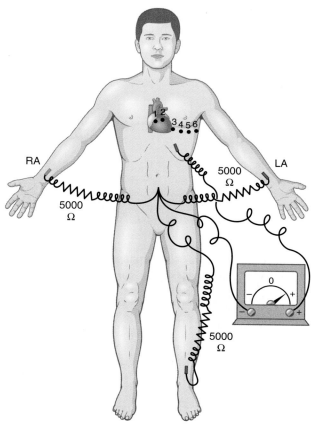

Figure 33-7 Connections of the body with the electrocardiograph for recording chest leads. *LA*, left arm; *RA*, right arm.

chest wall, with the chest electrode being placed sequentially at the six points shown in the diagram. The different recordings are known as leads V_1, V_2, V_3, V_4, V_5, and V_6.

Figure 33-8 illustrates the ECGs of the healthy heart as recorded from these six standard chest leads. Because the heart surfaces are close to the chest wall, each chest lead records mainly the electrical potential of the cardiac musculature immediately beneath the electrode. Therefore, relatively minute abnormalities in the ventricles, particularly in the anterior ventricular wall, can cause marked changes in the ECGs recorded from individual chest leads.

In leads V_1 and V_2, the QRS recordings of the normal heart are mainly negative because, as shown in Figure 33-7, the chest

electrode in these leads is nearer to the base of the heart than to the apex, and the base of the heart is the direction of electronegativity during most of the ventricular depolarization process. Conversely, the QRS complexes in leads V4, V5, and V6 are mainly positive because the chest electrode in these leads is nearer the heart apex, which is the direction of electropositivity during most of depolarization.

AUGMENTED UNIPOLAR LIMB LEADS

Another system of leads in wide use is the *augmented unipolar limb lead*. In this type of recording, two of the limbs are connected through electrical resistances to the negative terminal of the electrocardiograph, and the third limb is connected to the positive terminal. When the positive terminal is on the right arm, the lead is known as the aVR lead; when on the left arm, it is known as the aVL lead; and when on the left leg, it is known as the aVF lead.

Normal recordings of the augmented unipolar limb leads are shown in Figure 33-9. They are all similar to the standard limb lead recordings, except that the recording from the aVR lead is inverted.

BIBLIOGRAPHY

See bibliography for Chapter 34.

AUGMENTED UNIPOLAR LIMB LEADS

Clinical Applications of the Electrocardiogram

LEARNING OBJECTIVES

- Describe the changes in the ECG that occur with disturbances in the conducting system of the heart including common arrhythmias.
- Describe the principles of vectorial analysis of the ECG, and the way these can be applied to left and right ventricular hypertrophy.
- Describe the changes in the ECG that occur with myocardial ischemia and infarction.

GLOSSARY OF TERMS

- **Angina pectoris:** Chest pain due to the inadequate supply of oxygen to the cardiac muscle
- **Heart block:** A delay or complete block in the transmission of the cardiac impulse along the conducting pathway
- **Myocardial infarction:** Obstruction of the circulation to a part of the heart resulting in cell death (necrosis)
- **Palpitations:** A usually uncomfortable sensation in which a person is aware of an irregular, hard, or rapid heartbeat

A detailed discussion of the scope of the clinical applications of the electrocardiogram (ECG) is beyond the aims of this chapter and the interested student is referred to the many clinical textbooks of ECG for this.

Some of the most distressing types of heart malfunction occur because of abnormal rhythm of the heart. For instance, sometimes the beat of the atria is not coordinated with the beat of the ventricles, so the atria no longer function as primer pumps for the ventricles.

The purpose of this chapter is to discuss the physiology of common cardiac arrhythmias and their effects on heart pumping, as well as their diagnosis by electrocardiography. The causes of the cardiac arrhythmias are usually one or a combination of the following abnormalities in the rhythmicity–conduction system of the heart:

- abnormal rhythmicity of the pacemaker;
- shift of the pacemaker from the sinus node to another place in the heart;
- blocks at different points in the spread of the impulse through the heart;
- abnormal pathways of impulse transmission through the heart;
- spontaneous generation of spurious impulses in almost any part of the heart.

Abnormal Sinus Rhythms

TACHYCARDIA

The term "tachycardia" means *fast heart rate*, which is usually defined as faster than 100 beats/minute in an adult. An ECG recorded from a patient with tachycardia is shown in Figure 34-1. This ECG is normal except that the heart rate, as determined from the time intervals between QRS complexes, is about 150 beats/minute instead of the normal 72 beats/minute.

Some causes of tachycardia include increased body temperature, stimulation of the heart by the sympathetic nerves, or toxic conditions of the heart.

The heart rate increases about 10 beats/minute for each degree Fahrenheit (with an increase of 18 beats/minute per degree Celsius), up to a body temperature of about 105°F (40.5°C); beyond this, the heart rate may decrease because of progressive debility of the heart muscle as a result of the fever. Fever causes tachycardia because increased temperature increases the rate of metabolism of the sinus node, which in turn directly increases its excitability and rate of rhythm.

Many factors can cause the sympathetic nervous system to excite the heart, as we discuss at multiple points in this text. For instance, when a patient sustains severe blood loss, sympathetic reflex stimulation of the heart may increase the heart rate to 150–180 beats/minute.

Simple weakening of the myocardium usually increases the heart rate because the weakened heart does not pump blood into the arterial tree to a normal extent and this phenomenon causes reductions in blood pressure and elicits sympathetic reflexes to increase the heart rate.

BRADYCARDIA

The term "bradycardia" means a *slow heart rate*, usually defined as fewer than 60 beats/minute. Bradycardia is shown by the ECG in Figure 34-2.

Bradycardia in Athletes. The well-trained athlete's heart is often larger and considerably stronger than that of a normal person, which allows the athlete's heart to pump a large stroke volume output per beat even during periods of rest. When the athlete is at rest, excessive quantities of blood pumped into the arterial tree with each beat initiate feedback circulatory reflexes or other effects to cause bradycardia.

Vagal Stimulation Causes Bradycardia. Any circulatory reflex that stimulates the vagus nerves causes release of acetylcholine at the vagal endings in the heart, thus giving a parasympathetic effect. Perhaps the most striking example of this phenomenon occurs in patients with *carotid sinus syndrome.* In these patients, the pressure receptors (baroreceptors) in the carotid sinus region of the carotid artery walls are excessively sensitive. Therefore, even mild external pressure on the neck elicits a strong baroreceptor reflex causing intense vagal–acetylcholine

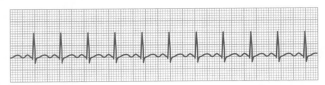

Figure 34-1   Sinus tachycardia (lead I).

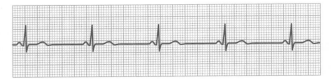

Figure 34-2   Sinus bradycardia (lead III).

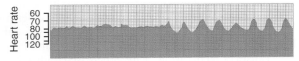

Figure 34-3   Sinus arrhythmia as recorded by a cardiotachometer. To the left is the record when the subject was breathing normally; to the right, when breathing deeply.

effects on the heart, including extreme bradycardia. Indeed, sometimes this reflex is so powerful that it actually stops the heart for 5–10 seconds.

SINUS ARRHYTHMIA

Figure 34-3 shows a *cardiotachometer* recording of the heart rate, at first during normal respiration and then (in the second half of the record) during deep respiration. A cardiotachometer is an instrument that records *by the height of successive spikes* the duration of the interval between the successive QRS complexes in the ECG. Note from this record that the heart rate increased and decreased not more than 5% during quiet respiration (shown on the left half of the record). Then, *during deep respiration*, the heart rate increased and decreased with each respiratory cycle by as much as 30%.

Sinus arrhythmia can result from any one of many circulatory conditions that alter the strengths of the sympathetic and parasympathetic nerve signals to the heart sinus node. The "respiratory" type of sinus arrhythmia, as shown in Figure 34-3, results mainly from "spillover" of signals from the medullary respiratory center into the adjacent vasomotor center during inspiratory and expiratory cycles of respiration. The spillover signals cause an alternate increase and decrease in the number of impulses transmitted through the sympathetic and vagus nerves to the heart.

Abnormal Rhythms that Result from Block of Heart Signals within the Intracardiac Conduction Pathways

SINOATRIAL BLOCK

In rare instances, the impulse from the sinus node is blocked before it enters the atrial muscle. This phenomenon is demonstrated in Figure 34-4, which shows sudden cessation of P waves with resultant standstill of the atria. However, the ventricles pick

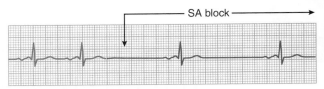

Figure 34-4   Sinoatrial nodal block with A-V nodal rhythm during the block period (lead III). *SA,* sinoatrial.

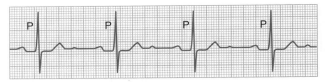

Figure 34-5   Prolonged P–R interval caused by first-degree A-V heart block (lead II).

up a new rhythm, with the impulse usually originating spontaneously in the atrioventricular (A-V) node, so the rate of the ventricular QRS–T complex is slowed but not otherwise altered.

ATRIOVENTRICULAR BLOCK

The only means by which impulses ordinarily can pass from the atria into the ventricles is through the *A-V bundle*, also known as the *bundle of His*. Conditions that can either decrease the rate of impulse conduction in this bundle or block the impulse entirely are as follows:

1. *Ischemia of the A-V node or A-V bundle fibers* often delays or blocks conduction from the atria to the ventricles. Coronary insufficiency can cause ischemia of the A-V node and bundle in the same way that it can cause ischemia of the myocardium.
2. *Compression of the A-V bundle* by scar tissue or by calcified portions of the heart can depress or block conduction from the atria to the ventricles.
3. *Inflammation of the A-V node or A-V bundle* can depress conduction from the atria to the ventricles. Inflammation results frequently from different types of myocarditis, caused, for example, by diphtheria or rheumatic fever.
4. *Extreme stimulation of the heart by the vagus nerves* in rare instances blocks impulse conduction through the A-V node. Such vagal excitation occasionally results from strong stimulation of the baroreceptors in people with *carotid sinus syndrome,* discussed earlier in relation to bradycardia.

INCOMPLETE ATRIOVENTRICULAR HEART BLOCK

Prolonged P–R (or P–Q) Interval—First-Degree Block. The usual lapse of time between the *beginning* of the P wave and the *beginning* of the QRS complex is about 0.16 second when the heart is beating at a normal rate. This so-called *P–R interval* usually decreases in length with faster heartbeat and increases with slower heartbeat. In general, when the P–R interval increases to greater than 0.20 second, the P–R interval is said to be prolonged and the patient is said to have *first-degree incomplete heart block.*

Figure 34-5 shows an ECG with prolonged P–R interval; the interval in this instance is about 0.30 second instead of the normal 0.20 or less. Thus, first-degree block is defined as a *delay* of conduction from the atria to the ventricles but not actual blockage of conduction. The P–R interval seldom increases above 0.35–0.45 second because, by that time, conduction through the A-V bundle is depressed so much that conduction stops entirely. One means for determining the severity of some heart diseases, such as *acute rheumatic heart disease*, is to measure the P–R interval.

Second-Degree Block. When conduction through the A-V bundle is slowed enough to increase the P–R interval to 0.25–0.45 second, the action potential is sometimes strong enough to pass through the bundle into the ventricles and sometimes not strong enough to do so. In this instance, there will be an atrial P wave but no QRS–T wave, and it is said that there are "dropped beats" of the ventricles. This condition is called *second-degree heart block*.

There are two types of second-degree A-V block: type I (also known as *Wenckebach periodicity*) and type II. Type I block is characterized by progressive prolongation of the P-R interval until a ventricular beat is dropped and is then followed by resetting of the P-R and repeating of the abnormal cycle. A type I block is almost always caused by abnormality of the A-V node. In most cases, this type of block is benign and no specific treatment is needed.

In type II block there is usually a fixed number of nonconducted P waves for every QRS complex. For example, a 2:1 block implies that there are two P waves for every QRS complex. At other times, rhythms of 3:2 or 3:1 may develop. Type II block is generally caused by an abnormality of the bundle of His–Purkinje system and may require implantation of a pacemaker to prevent progression to complete heart block and cardiac arrest.

Figure 34-6 shows P–R intervals of 0.30 second as well as one dropped ventricular beat as a result of failure of conduction from the atria to the ventricles.

Complete A-V Block (Third-Degree Block). When the condition causing poor conduction in the A-V node or A-V bundle becomes severe, complete block of the impulse from the atria into the ventricles occurs. In this case, the ventricles spontaneously establish their own signal, usually originating in the A-V node or A-V bundle distal to the block. Therefore, the P waves become dissociated from the QRS–T complexes, as shown in Figure 34-7. Note that the *rate of rhythm of the atria* in this ECG is about 100 beats/minute, whereas the *rate of ventricular beat* is less than 40 beats/minute. Furthermore, there is no relation between the rhythm of the P waves and that of the QRS–T complexes because the ventricles have "escaped" from control by the atria, and are beating at their own natural rate, controlled

most often by rhythmical signals distal to the A-V node or A-V bundle where the block occurred.

Stokes–Adams Syndrome—Ventricular Escape. In some patients with A-V block, the total block comes and goes; that is, impulses are conducted from the atria into the ventricles for a period of time and then suddenly impulses are not conducted. The duration of block may be a few seconds, a few minutes, a few hours, or even weeks or longer before conduction returns. This condition occurs in hearts with borderline ischemia of the conductive system.

Each time A-V conduction ceases, the ventricles often do not start their own beating until after a delay of 5–30 seconds. This delay results from the phenomenon called *overdrive suppression*. Overdrive suppression means that ventricular excitability is at first suppressed because the ventricles have been driven by the atria at a rate greater than their natural rate of rhythm. However, after a few seconds, some part of the Purkinje system beyond the block, usually in the distal part of the A-V node beyond the blocked point in the node, or in the A-V bundle, begins discharging rhythmically at a rate of 15–40 times/minute and acting as the pacemaker of the ventricles. This phenomenon is called *ventricular escape*.

Because the brain cannot remain active for more than 4–7 seconds without blood supply, most people faint a few seconds after complete block occurs because the heart does not pump any blood for 5–30 seconds, until the ventricles "escape." After escape, however, the slowly beating ventricles (typically beating less than 40 beats/minute) usually pump enough blood to allow rapid recovery from the faint and then to sustain the person. These periodic fainting spells are known as the *Stokes–Adams syndrome*.

Occasionally, the interval of ventricular standstill at the onset of complete block is so long that it becomes detrimental to the patient's health or even causes death. Consequently, most of these patients are provided with an *artificial pacemaker*, a small battery-operated electrical stimulator planted beneath the skin, with electrodes usually connected to the right ventricle. The pacemaker provides continued rhythmical impulses to the ventricles.

Premature Contractions

A premature contraction is a contraction of the heart before the time that normal contraction would have been expected. This condition is also called *extrasystole, premature beat*, or *ectopic beat*.

Causes of Premature Contractions. Most premature contractions result from *ectopic foci* in the heart, which emit abnormal impulses at odd times during the cardiac rhythm. Possible causes of ectopic foci are (1) local areas of ischemia; (2) small calcified plaques at different points in the heart, which press against the adjacent cardiac muscle so that some of the fibers are irritated; and (3) toxic irritation of the A-V node, Purkinje system, or myocardium caused by infection, drugs, nicotine, or caffeine. Mechanical initiation of premature contractions is also frequent during cardiac catheterization; large numbers of premature contractions often occur when the catheter enters the right ventricle and presses against the endocardium.

PREMATURE ATRIAL CONTRACTIONS

Figure 34-8 shows a single premature atrial contraction. The P wave of this beat occurred too soon in the heart cycle; the P–R interval is shortened indicating that the ectopic origin of the beat

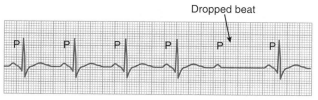

Dropped beat

Figure 34-6 Second-degree A-V block showing occasional failure of the ventricles to receive the excitatory signals (lead V₃).

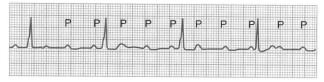

Figure 34-7 Complete A-V block (lead II).

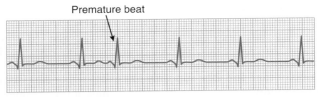

Figure 34-8 Atrial premature beat (lead I).

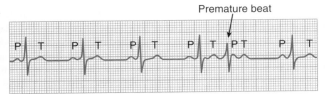

Figure 34-9 A-V nodal premature contraction (lead III).

is in the atria near the A-V node. Also, the interval between the premature contraction and the next succeeding contraction is slightly prolonged, which is called a *compensatory pause*. One of the reasons for this compensatory pause is that the premature contraction originated in the atrium some distance from the sinus node, and the impulse had to travel through a considerable amount of atrial muscle before it discharges the sinus node. Consequently, the sinus node discharges late in the premature cycle, which made the succeeding sinus node discharge also late in appearing.

A-V NODAL OR A-V BUNDLE PREMATURE CONTRACTIONS

Figure 34-9 shows a premature contraction that originated in the A-V node or in the A-V bundle. The P wave is missing from the electrocardiographic record of the premature contraction. Instead, the P wave is superimposed onto the QRS–T complex because the cardiac impulse traveled backward into the atria at the same time that it traveled forward into the ventricles; this P wave slightly distorts the QRS–T complex, but the P wave itself cannot be discerned as such. In general, A-V nodal premature contractions have the same significance and cause atrial premature contractions.

PREMATURE VENTRICULAR CONTRACTIONS

The ECG in Figure 34-10 shows a series of premature ventricular contractions (PVCs) alternating with normal contractions. PVCs cause specific effects in the ECG, as follows:

1. The QRS complex is usually considerably prolonged. The reason for this prolongation is that the impulse is conducted mainly through slowly conducting muscle of the ventricles rather than through the Purkinje system.
2. The QRS complex has a high voltage. When the normal impulse passes through the heart, it passes through both ventricles nearly simultaneously; consequently, in the normal heart, the depolarization waves of the two sides of the heart—mainly of opposite polarity to each other—partially neutralize each other in the ECG. When a PVC occurs, the impulse almost always travels in only one direction, so there is no such neutralization effect and one entire side or end of the ventricles is depolarized ahead of the other, which causes large electrical potentials, as shown for the PVCs in Figure 34-10.

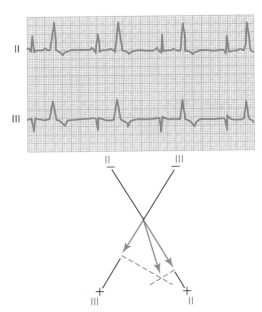

Figure 34-10 Premature ventricular contractions (PVCs) demonstrated by the large abnormal QRS–T complexes (leads II and III). Axis of the premature contractions is plotted in accordance with the principles of vectorial analysis; this shows the origin of the PVC to be near the base of the ventricles.

3. After almost all PVCs, the T wave has an electrical potential polarity exactly opposite to that of the QRS complex because the *slow conduction of the impulse* through the cardiac muscle causes the muscle fibers that depolarize first also to repolarize first.

Some PVCs are relatively benign in their effects on overall pumping by the heart; they can result from such factors as cigarettes, excessive intake of coffee, lack of sleep, various mild toxic states, and even emotional irritability. Conversely, many other PVCs result from stray impulses or reentrant signals that originate around the borders of infarcted or ischemic areas of the heart. The presence of such PVCs is not to be taken lightly. People with significant numbers of PVCs have a much higher than normal risk of developing spontaneous lethal ventricular fibrillation, presumably initiated by one of the PVCs. This development is especially true when the PVCs occur during the vulnerable period for causing fibrillation, just at the end of the T wave when the ventricles are coming out of refractoriness.

Paroxysmal Tachycardia

Some abnormalities in different portions of the heart, including the atria, the Purkinje system, or the ventricles, can occasionally cause rapid rhythmical discharge of impulses that spread in all directions throughout the heart. This phenomenon is believed to be caused most frequently by reentrant circus movement feedback pathways that set up local repeated self-reexcitation. Because of the rapid rhythm in the irritable focus, this focus becomes the pacemaker of the heart.

The term "paroxysmal" means that the heart rate becomes rapid in paroxysms, with the paroxysm beginning suddenly and lasting for a few seconds, a few minutes, a few hours, or much longer. The paroxysm usually ends as suddenly as it began, with the pacemaker of the heart instantly shifting back to the sinus node.

Paroxysmal tachycardia often can be stopped by eliciting a vagal reflex. A type of vagal reflex sometimes elicited for this purpose is to press on the neck in the regions of the carotid sinuses, which may cause enough of a vagal reflex to stop the paroxysm. Various drugs may also be used. Antiarrhythmic drugs may also be used to slow conduction or prolong the refractory period in cardiac tissues.

ATRIAL PAROXYSMAL TACHYCARDIA

Figure 34-11 demonstrates a sudden increase in the heart rate from about 95 to about 150 beats/minute in the middle of the record. On close study of the ECG, an inverted P wave is seen during the rapid heartbeat before each QRS–T complex and this P wave is partially superimposed onto the normal T wave of the preceding beat. This finding indicates that the origin of this paroxysmal tachycardia is in the atrium, but because the P wave is abnormal in shape, the origin is not near the sinus node.

VENTRICULAR PAROXYSMAL TACHYCARDIA

Figure 34-12 shows a typical short paroxysm of ventricular tachycardia. The ECG of ventricular paroxysmal tachycardia has the appearance of a series of ventricular premature beats occurring one after another without any normal beats interspersed.

Ventricular paroxysmal tachycardia is usually a serious condition for two reasons. First, this type of tachycardia usually does not occur unless considerable ischemic damage is present in the ventricles. Second, ventricular tachycardia frequently initiates the lethal condition of ventricular fibrillation because of rapid repeated stimulation of the ventricular muscle, as we discuss in the next section.

Sometimes intoxication from the heart treatment drug *digitalis* causes irritable foci that lead to ventricular tachycardia. Antiarrhythmic drugs such as *amiodarone* or *lidocaine* can be used to treat ventricular tachycardia. Lidocaine depresses the normal increase in sodium permeability of the cardiac muscle membrane during generation of the action potential, thereby often blocking the rhythmical discharge of the focal point that is causing the paroxysmal attack. Amiodarone has multiple actions such as prolonging the action potential and refractory period in cardiac muscle and slowing A-V conduction. In some cases, *cardioversion* with an electric shock to the heart is needed for restoration of normal heart rhythm.

Ventricular Fibrillation

The most serious of all cardiac arrhythmias is ventricular fibrillation, which, if not stopped within 1–3 minutes, is almost invariably fatal. Ventricular fibrillation results from cardiac impulses that have gone berserk within the ventricular muscle mass, stimulating first one portion of the ventricular muscle, then another portion, then another, and eventually feeding back onto itself to reexcite the same ventricular muscle over and over—never stopping. When this phenomenon occurs, many small portions of the ventricular muscle will be contracting at the same time, while equally as many other portions will be relaxing. Thus, there is never a coordinated contraction of all the ventricular muscle at once, which is required for a pumping cycle of the heart. Despite massive movement of stimulatory signals throughout the ventricles, the ventricular chambers neither enlarge nor contract but remain in an indeterminate stage of partial contraction, pumping either no blood or negligible amounts. Therefore, after fibrillation begins, unconsciousness occurs within 4–5 seconds because of lack of blood flow to the brain and irretrievable death of tissues begins to occur throughout the body within a few minutes.

Multiple factors can spark the beginning of ventricular fibrillation—a person may have a normal heartbeat one moment, but 1 second later, the ventricles are in fibrillation. Especially likely to initiate fibrillation are (1) sudden electrical shock of the heart or (2) ischemia of the heart muscle, of its specialized conducting system, or both.

PHENOMENON OF REENTRY—"CIRCUS MOVEMENTS" AS THE BASIS FOR VENTRICULAR FIBRILLATION

When the *normal* cardiac impulse in the normal heart has traveled through the extent of the ventricles, it has no place to go because all the ventricular muscle is refractory and cannot conduct the impulse farther. Therefore, that impulse dies, and the heart awaits a new action potential to begin in the atrial sinus node.

Under some circumstances, however, this normal sequence of events does not occur. Therefore, let us explain more fully the background conditions that can initiate reentry and lead to "circus movements," which in turn cause ventricular fibrillation.

Figure 34-13 shows several small cardiac muscle strips cut in the form of circles. If such a strip is stimulated at the 12-o'clock position so that the impulse travels in only one direction, the

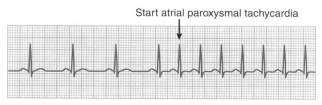

Start atrial paroxysmal tachycardia

Figure 34-11 Atrial paroxysmal tachycardia—onset in middle of record (lead I).

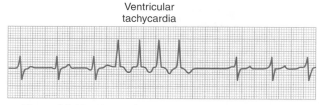

Ventricular tachycardia

Figure 34-12 Ventricular paroxysmal tachycardia (lead III).

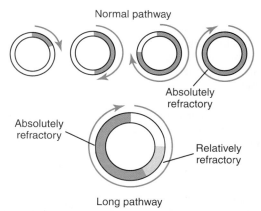

Normal pathway

Absolutely refractory

Absolutely refractory

Relatively refractory

Long pathway

Figure 34-13 Circus movement showing annihilation of the impulse in the short pathway and continued propagation of the impulse in the long pathway.

impulse spreads progressively around the circle until it returns to the 12-o'clock position. If the originally stimulated muscle fibers are still in a refractory state, the impulse then dies out because refractory muscle cannot transmit a second impulse. However, three different conditions can cause this impulse to continue to travel around the circle, that is, to cause "reentry" of the impulse into muscle that has already been excited (circus movement).

First, if the *pathway around the circle is much longer than normal*, by the time the impulse returns to the 12-o'clock position, the originally stimulated muscle will no longer be refractory and the impulse will continue around the circle again and again.

Second, if the length of the pathway remains constant but the *velocity of conduction becomes decreased* enough, an increased interval of time will elapse before the impulse returns to the 12-o'clock position. By this time, the originally stimulated muscle might be out of the refractory state, and the impulse can continue around the circle again and again.

Third, *the refractory period of the muscle might become greatly shortened*. In this case, the impulse could also continue around and around the circle.

All these conditions occur in different pathological states of the human heart as follows: (1) a long pathway typically occurs in dilated hearts; (2) decreased rate of conduction frequently results from blockage of the Purkinje system, ischemia of the muscle, high blood potassium levels, or many other factors; (3) a shortened refractory period commonly occurs in response to various drugs, such as epinephrine, or after repetitive electrical stimulation. Thus, in many cardiac disturbances, reentry can cause abnormal patterns of cardiac contraction or abnormal cardiac rhythms that ignore the pace-setting effects of the sinus node.

ELECTROCARDIOGRAM IN VENTRICULAR FIBRILLATION

In ventricular fibrillation, the ECG is bizarre (Figure 34-14) and ordinarily shows no tendency toward a regular rhythm of any type. During the first few seconds of ventricular fibrillation, relatively large masses of muscle contract simultaneously, which causes coarse, irregular waves in the ECG. After another few seconds, the coarse contractions of the ventricles disappear and the ECG changes into a new pattern of low-voltage, very irregular waves. Thus, no repetitive electrocardiographic pattern can be ascribed to ventricular fibrillation. Instead, the ventricular muscle contracts at as many as 30–50 small patches of muscle at a time, and electrocardiographic potentials change constantly and spasmodically because the electrical currents in the heart flow first in one direction and then in another and seldom repeat any specific cycle.

The voltages of the waves in the ECG in ventricular fibrillation are usually about 0.5 mV when ventricular fibrillation first begins, but they decay rapidly and thus after 20–30 seconds, they are usually only 0.2–0.3 mV. Minute voltages of 0.1 mV or less may be recorded for 10 minutes or longer after ventricular fibrillation begins. As already pointed out, because no pumping of blood occurs during ventricular fibrillation, this

state is lethal unless stopped by some heroic therapy, such as immediate electroshock through the heart, as explained in the next section.

ELECTROSHOCK DEFIBRILLATION OF THE VENTRICLES

Although a moderate alternating-current voltage applied directly to the ventricles almost invariably throws the ventricles into fibrillation, a strong high-voltage electrical current passed through the ventricles for a fraction of a second can stop fibrillation by throwing all the ventricular muscle into refractoriness simultaneously. This feat is accomplished by passing intense current through large electrodes placed on two sides of the heart. The current penetrates most of the fibers of the ventricles at the same time, thus stimulating essentially all parts of the ventricles simultaneously and causing them all to become refractory. All action potentials stop, and the heart remains quiescent for 3–5 seconds after which it begins to beat again, usually with the sinus node or some other part of the heart becoming the pacemaker. However, if the same reentrant focus that had originally thrown the ventricles into fibrillation is still present, fibrillation may begin again immediately.

When electrodes are applied directly to the two sides of the heart, fibrillation can usually be stopped using 1000 V of direct current applied for a few thousandths of a second. When applied through two electrodes on the chest wall, as shown in Figure 34-15, the usual procedure is to charge a large electrical capacitor up to several thousand volts and then to cause the capacitor to discharge for a few thousandths of a second through the electrodes and through the heart.

In patients with high risk for ventricular fibrillation, a small battery-powered implantable cardioverter-defibrillator (ICD) with electrode wires lodged in the right ventricle may be implanted in the patient. The device is programmed to detect ventricular fibrillation and revert it by delivering a brief electrical

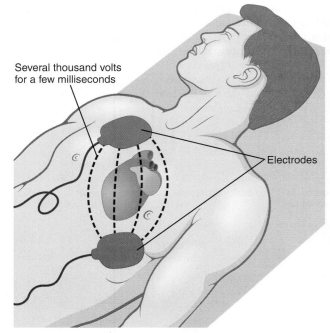

Figure 34-15 Application of electrical current to the chest to stop ventricular fibrillation.

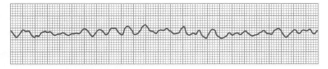

Figure 34-14 Ventricular fibrillation (lead II).

impulse to the heart. Recent advances in electronics and batteries have permitted development of ICDs that can deliver enough electrical current to defibrillate the heart through electrode wires implanted subcutaneously, outside the rib cage near the heart rather than in or on the heart itself. These devices can be implanted with a minor surgical procedure.

HAND PUMPING OF THE HEART (CARDIOPULMONARY RESUSCITATION) AS AN AID TO DEFIBRILLATION

Unless defibrillated within 1 minute after fibrillation begins, the heart is usually too weak to be revived by defibrillation because of the lack of nutrition from coronary blood flow. However, it is still possible to revive the heart by preliminarily pumping the heart by hand (intermittent hand squeezing) and then defibrillating the heart later. In this way, small quantities of blood are delivered into the aorta and a renewed coronary blood supply develops. Then, after a few minutes of hand pumping, electrical defibrillation often becomes possible. Indeed, fibrillating hearts have been pumped by hand for as long as 90 minutes followed by successful defibrillation.

A technique for pumping the heart without opening the chest consists of intermittent thrusts of pressure on the chest wall along with artificial respiration. This process plus defibrillation is called *cardiopulmonary resuscitation*, or CPR.

Lack of blood flow to the brain for more than 5–8 minutes usually causes permanent mental impairment or even destruction of brain tissue. Even if the heart is revived, the person may die from the effects of brain damage or may live with permanent mental impairment.

Atrial Fibrillation

Remember that except for the conducting pathway through the A-V bundle, the atrial muscle mass is separated from the ventricular muscle mass by fibrous tissue. Therefore, ventricular fibrillation often occurs without atrial fibrillation. Likewise, fibrillation often occurs in the atria without ventricular fibrillation (shown to the right in Figure 34-17).

The mechanism of atrial fibrillation is identical to that of ventricular fibrillation, except that the process occurs only in the atrial muscle mass instead of the ventricular mass. A frequent cause of atrial fibrillation is atrial enlargement that can result, for example, from heart valve lesions that prevent the atria from emptying adequately into the ventricles, or from ventricular failure with excess damming of blood in the atria. The dilated atrial walls provide ideal conditions of a long conductive pathway as well as slow conduction, both of which predispose to atrial fibrillation.

Impaired Pumping of the Atria During Atrial Fibrillation. For the same reasons that the ventricles will not pump blood during ventricular fibrillation, neither do the atria pump blood in atrial fibrillation. Therefore, the atria become useless as primer pumps for the ventricles. Even so, blood flows passively through the atria into the ventricles and the efficiency of ventricular pumping is decreased only 20–30%. Therefore, in contrast to the lethality of ventricular fibrillation, a person can live for years with atrial fibrillation, although at reduced efficiency of overall heart pumping.

Electrocardiogram in Atrial Fibrillation. Figure 34-16 shows the ECG during atrial fibrillation. Numerous small depolarization

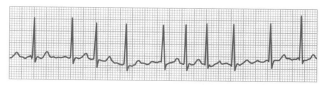

Figure 34-16 Atrial fibrillation (lead II). The waves that can be seen are ventricular QRS and T waves.

waves spread in all directions through the atria during atrial fibrillation. Because the waves are weak and many of them are of opposite polarity at any given time, they usually almost completely electrically neutralize one another. Therefore, in the ECG, one can see either no P waves from the atria or only a fine, high-frequency, very low-voltage wavy record. Conversely, the QRS–T complexes are normal unless there is some pathology of the ventricles, but their timing is irregular, as explained next.

Irregularity of Ventricular Rhythm During Atrial Fibrillation. When the atria are fibrillating, impulses arrive from the atrial muscle at the A-V node rapidly but also irregularly. Because the A-V node will not pass a second impulse for about 0.35 second after a previous one, at least 0.35 second must elapse between one ventricular contraction and the next. Then an additional but variable interval of 0–0.6 second occurs before one of the irregular atrial fibrillatory impulses happens to arrive at the A-V node. Thus, the interval between successive ventricular contractions varies from a minimum of about 0.35 second to a maximum of about 0.95 second causing a very irregular heartbeat. In fact, this irregularity, demonstrated by the variable spacing of the heartbeats in the ECG of Figure 34-16, is one of the clinical findings used to diagnose the condition. Also, because of the rapid rate of the fibrillatory impulses in the atria, the ventricle is driven at a fast heart rate, usually between 125 and 150 beats/minute.

Electroshock Treatment of Atrial Fibrillation. In the same manner that ventricular fibrillation can be converted back to a normal rhythm by electroshock, so too can atrial fibrillation be converted by electroshock. The procedure is essentially the same as for ventricular fibrillation conversion—passage of a single strong electric shock through the heart, which throws the entire heart into refractoriness for a few seconds; a normal rhythm often follows *if the heart is capable of generating a normal rhythm.*

Atrial Flutter

Atrial flutter is another condition caused by a circus movement in the atria. Atrial flutter is different from atrial fibrillation, in that the electrical signal travels as a single large wave always in one direction around and around the atrial muscle mass, as shown to the left in Figure 34-17. Atrial flutter causes a rapid rate of contraction of the atria, usually between 200 and 350 beats/minute. However, because one side of the atria is contracting while the other side is relaxing, the amount of blood pumped by the atria is slight. Furthermore, the signals reach the A-V node too rapidly for all of them to be passed into the ventricles because the refractory periods of the A-V node and A-V bundle are too long to pass more than a fraction of the atrial signals. Therefore, there are usually two to three beats of the atria for every single beat of the ventricles.

Figure 34-18 shows a typical ECG in atrial flutter. The P waves are strong because of contraction of semicoordinate

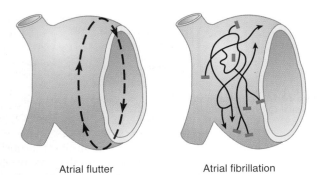

Figure 34-17 Pathways of impulses in atrial flutter and atrial fibrillation.

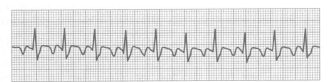

Figure 34-18 Atrial flutter—2:1 and 3:1 atrial to ventricle rhythm (lead II).

masses of muscle. However, note in the record that a QRS–T complex follows an atrial P wave only once for every two to three beats of the atria, giving a 2:1 or 3:1 rhythm.

Cardiac Arrest

A final serious abnormality of the cardiac rhythmicity–conduction system is *cardiac arrest*, which results from cessation of all electrical control signals in the heart. That is, no spontaneous rhythm remains.

Cardiac arrest may occur *during deep anesthesia*, when severe hypoxia may develop because of inadequate respiration. The hypoxia prevents the muscle fibers and conductive fibers from maintaining normal electrolyte concentration differentials across their membranes, and their excitability may be so affected that the automatic rhythmicity disappears.

In many instances of cardiac arrest from anesthesia, CPR (for many minutes or even hours) is quite successful in reestablishing a normal heart rhythm. In some patients, severe myocardial disease can cause permanent or semipermanent cardiac arrest, which can cause death. To treat the condition, rhythmical electrical impulses from an *implanted electronic cardiac pacemaker* have been used successfully to keep patients alive for months to years.

Vectorial Analysis of the ECG and its Application to Ventricular Hypertrophy

From the discussion in Chapter 32 on impulse transmission through the heart, it is obvious that any change in the pattern of this transmission can cause abnormal electrical potentials around the heart and, consequently, alter the shapes of the waves in the ECG. For this reason, most serious abnormalities of the heart muscle can be diagnosed by analyzing the contours of the waves in the different electrocardiographic leads.

PRINCIPLES OF VECTORIAL ANALYSIS OF ELECTROCARDIOGRAMS

To understand how cardiac abnormalities affect the contours of the ECG, one must first become familiar with the concept of

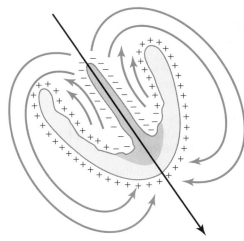

Figure 34-19 Mean vector through the partially depolarized ventricles.

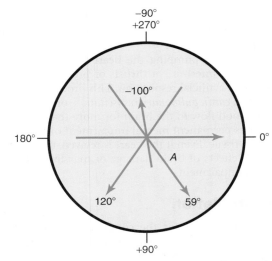

Figure 34-20 Vectors drawn to represent potentials for several different hearts, and the axis of the potential (expressed in degrees) for each heart.

vectors and *vectorial analysis* as applied to electrical potentials in and around the heart.

A vector is an arrow that points in the direction of the electrical potential generated by the current flow, *with the arrowhead in the positive direction*. Also, by convention, the length of the arrow is drawn *proportional to the voltage of the potential*.

"Resultant" Vector in the Heart at Any Given Instant. Figure 34-19 shows, by the shaded area and the minus signs, depolarization of the ventricular septum and of parts of the apical endocardial walls of the two ventricles. Although the electrical current flows in different directions, considerably more current flows downward from the base of the ventricles toward the apex than in the upward direction. Therefore, the summated vector of the generated potential at this particular instant, called the *instantaneous mean vector*, is represented by the long *black* arrow drawn through the center of the ventricles in a direction from the base toward the apex. Furthermore, because the summated current is considerable in quantity, the potential is large and the vector is long.

When a vector is exactly horizontal and directed toward the person's left side, the vector is said to extend in the direction of 0 degree, as shown in Figure 34-20. From this zero reference point, the scale of vectors rotates clockwise: when the vector extends from above and straight downward, it has a direction of

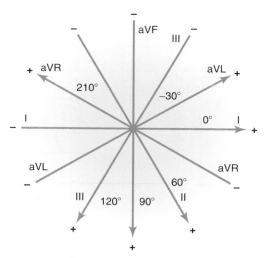

Figure 34-21 Axes of the three bipolar and three unipolar leads.

+90 degrees; when it extends from the person's left to right, it has a direction of +180 degrees; and when it extends straight upward, it has a direction of −90 (or +270) degrees.

In a normal heart, the average direction of the vector during spread of the depolarization wave through the ventricles, called the *mean QRS vector*, is about +59 degrees, which is shown by vector *A* drawn through the center of Figure 34-20 in the +59-degree direction. This means that during most of the depolarization wave, the apex of the heart remains positive with respect to the base of the heart.

The Hexagonal Reference System

In Chapter 33, the three standard bipolar and the three unipolar limb leads are described. Each lead is actually a pair of electrodes connected to the body on opposite sides of the heart, and the direction from negative electrode to positive electrode is called the "axis" of the lead. Lead I is recorded from two electrodes placed, respectively, on the two arms. Because the electrodes lie exactly in the horizontal direction, with the positive electrode to the left, the axis of lead I is 0 degree.

In recording lead II, electrodes are placed on the right arm and left leg. The right arm connects to the torso in the upper right-hand corner and the left leg connects in the lower left-hand corner. Therefore, the direction of this lead is about +60 degrees.

By similar analysis, it can be seen that lead III has an axis of about +120 degrees; lead aVR, +210 degrees; aVF, +90 degrees; and aVL, −30 degrees. The directions of the axes of all these leads are shown in Figure 34-21, which is known as the *hexagonal reference system*. The polarities of the electrodes are shown by the plus and minus signs in the figure. *The reader must learn these axes and their polarities, particularly for the bipolar limb leads I, II, and III, to understand the remainder of this chapter.*

Vectorial Analysis of the Normal Electrocardiogram

VECTORS THAT OCCUR AT SUCCESSIVE INTERVALS DURING DEPOLARIZATION OF THE VENTRICLES—THE QRS COMPLEX

When the cardiac impulse enters the ventricles through the A-V bundle, the first part of the ventricles to become depolarized is the left endocardial surface of the septum. Then depolarization spreads rapidly to involve both endocardial surfaces of the septum, as demonstrated by the darker shaded portion of the ventricle in Figure 34-22A. Next, depolarization spreads along the endocardial surfaces of the remainder of the two ventricles, as shown in Figure 34-22B and C. Finally, it spreads through the ventricular muscle to the outside of the heart, as shown progressively in Figure 34-22C–E.

At each stage in Figure 34-22, parts A–E, the instantaneous mean electrical potential of the ventricles is represented by a red vector superimposed on the ventricle and in relation to the axes of the three bipolar leads. To the right in each figure is shown progressive development of the electrocardiographic QRS complex. *Keep in mind that a positive vector (one that points in the positive direction of a lead) will cause recording in the ECG above the zero line, whereas a negative vector will cause recording below the zero line.*

ELECTROCARDIOGRAM DURING REPOLARIZATION—THE T WAVE

After the ventricular muscle has become depolarized, about 0.15 second later, repolarization begins and proceeds until complete at about 0.35 second. This repolarization causes the T wave in the ECG.

Because the septum and endocardial areas of the ventricular muscle depolarize first, it seems logical that these areas should repolarize first as well. However, this is not the usual case because the septum and other endocardial areas have a longer period of contraction than do most of the external surfaces of the heart. Therefore, *the greatest portion of ventricular muscle mass to repolarize first is the entire outer surface of the ventricles, especially near the apex of the heart.* The endocardial areas, conversely, normally repolarize last. This sequence of repolarization is postulated to be caused by the high blood pressure inside the ventricles during contraction, which greatly reduces coronary blood flow to the endocardium, thereby slowing repolarization in the endocardial areas.

Because the outer apical surfaces of the ventricles repolarize before the inner surfaces, the positive end of the overall ventricular vector during repolarization is toward the apex of the heart. *As a result, the normal T wave in all three bipolar limb leads is positive, which is also the polarity of most of the normal QRS complex.*

DEPOLARIZATION OF THE ATRIA—THE P WAVE

Depolarization of the atria begins in the sinus node and spreads in all directions over the atria. Therefore, the point of original electronegativity in the atria is about at the point of entry of the superior vena cava where the sinus node lies, and the direction of initial depolarization is denoted by the black vector in Figure 34-23. Furthermore, the vector remains generally in this direction throughout the process of normal atrial depolarization. Because this direction is generally in the positive directions of the axes of the three standard bipolar limb leads I, II, and III, the ECGs recorded from the atria during depolarization are also usually positive in all three of these leads, as shown in Figure 34-23. This record of atrial depolarization is known as the atrial P wave.

Mean Electrical Axis of the Ventricular QRS—And its Significance

The vectorcardiogram during ventricular depolarization (the QRS vectorcardiogram) shown in Figure 34-24 is that of a normal heart. Note from this vectorcardiogram that the

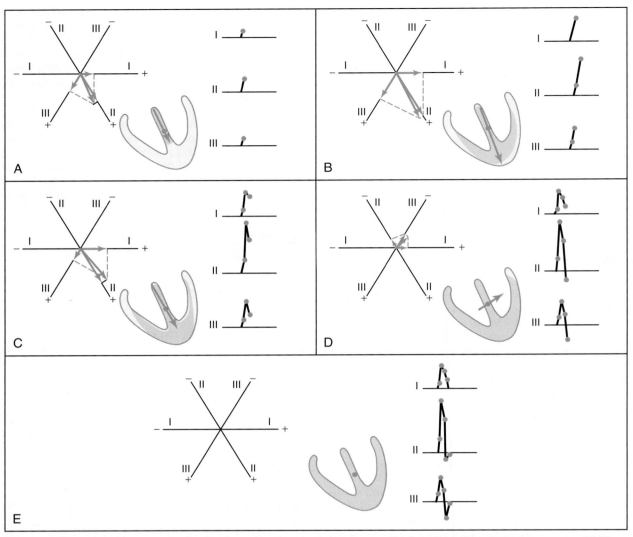

Figure 34-22   Shaded areas of the ventricles are depolarized (−); nonshaded areas are still polarized (+). The ventricular vectors and QRS complexes 0.01 second after onset of ventricular depolarization (*A*); 0.02 second after onset of depolarization (*B*); 0.035 second after onset of depolarization (*C*); 0.05 second after onset of depolarization (*D*); and after depolarization of the ventricles is complete, 0.06 second after onset (*E*).

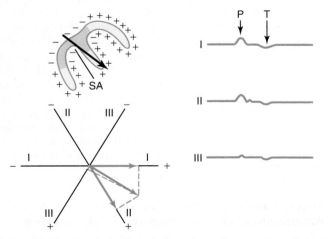

Figure 34-23   Depolarization of the atria and generation of the P wave, showing the maximum vector through the atria and the resultant vectors in the three standard leads. At the right are the atrial P and T waves. *SA*, sinoatrial node.

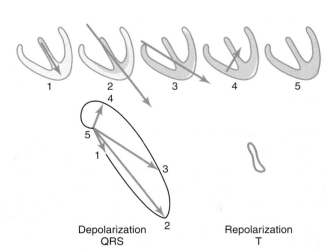

Depolarization
QRS

Repolarization
T

Figure 34-24   QRS and T vectorcardiograms.

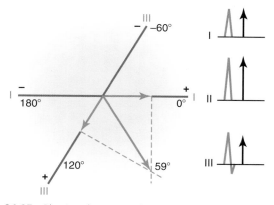

Figure 34-25 Plotting the mean electrical axis of the ventricles from two electrocardiographic leads (leads I and III).

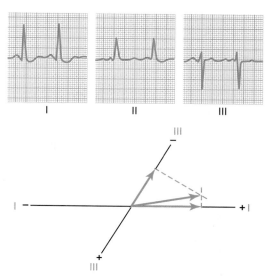

Figure 34-26 Left axis deviation in a *hypertensive heart (hypertrophic left ventricle)*. Note the slightly prolonged QRS complex as well.

preponderant direction of the vectors of the ventricles during depolarization is mainly toward the apex of the heart. That is, during most of the cycle of ventricular depolarization, the direction of the electrical potential (negative to positive) is from the base of the ventricles toward the apex. This preponderant direction of the potential during depolarization is called the *mean electrical axis of the ventricles*. The mean electrical axis of the normal ventricles is 59 degrees. In many pathological conditions of the heart, this direction changes markedly, sometimes even to opposite poles of the heart.

DETERMINING THE ELECTRICAL AXIS FROM STANDARD LEAD ELECTROCARDIOGRAMS

Clinically, the electrical axis of the heart is usually estimated from the standard bipolar limb lead ECGs rather than from the vectorcardiogram. Figure 34-25 shows a method for performing this estimation. After recording the standard leads, one determines the net potential and polarity of the recordings in leads I and III. In lead I of Figure 34-25, the recording is positive, and in lead III, the recording is mainly positive but negative during part of the cycle. If any part of a recording is negative, *this negative potential is subtracted from the positive part of the potential* to determine the *net potential* for that lead, as shown by the arrow to the right of the QRS complex for lead III. Then each net potential for leads I and III is plotted on the axes of the respective leads, with the base of the potential at the point of intersection of the axes, as shown in Figure 34-25.

If the net potential of lead I is positive, it is plotted in a positive direction along the line depicting lead I. Conversely, if this potential is negative, it is plotted in a negative direction. Also, for lead III, the net potential is placed with its base at the point of intersection, and, if positive, it is plotted in the positive direction along the line depicting lead III. If it is negative, it is plotted in the negative direction.

To determine the vector of the total QRS ventricular mean electrical potential, one draws perpendicular lines (the dashed lines in the figure) from the apices of leads I and III, respectively. The point of intersection of these two perpendicular lines represents, by vectorial analysis, the apex of the *mean* QRS vector in the ventricles, and the point of intersection of the lead I and lead III axes represents the negative end of the mean vector. Therefore, the *mean QRS vector* is drawn between these two points. The approximate average potential generated by the ventricles during depolarization is represented by the length of this mean QRS

vector, and the mean electrical axis is represented by the direction of the mean vector. Thus, the orientation of the mean electrical axis of the normal ventricles, as determined in Figure 34-25, is 59 degrees positive (+59 degrees).

Ventricular Hypertrophy and Axis Deviation

Hypertrophy of One Ventricle. When one ventricle greatly hypertrophies, *the axis of the heart shifts toward the hypertrophied ventricle* for two reasons. First, a greater quantity of muscle exists on the hypertrophied side of the heart than on the other side, which allows generation of greater electrical potential on that side. Second, more time is required for the depolarization wave to travel through the hypertrophied ventricle than through the normal ventricle. Consequently, the *normal* ventricle becomes depolarized considerably in advance of the *hypertrophied* ventricle, and this situation causes a strong vector from the normal side of the heart toward the hypertrophied side, which remains strongly positively charged. Thus, the axis deviates toward the hypertrophied ventricle.

Vectorial Analysis of Left Axis Deviation Resulting from Hypertrophy of the Left Ventricle. Figure 34-26 shows the three standard bipolar limb lead ECGs. Vectorial analysis demonstrates left axis deviation with mean electrical axis pointing in the −15-degree direction. This is a typical ECG caused by increased muscle mass of the left ventricle. In this instance, the axis deviation was caused by *hypertension* (high arterial blood pressure), which caused the left ventricle to hypertrophy so that it could pump blood against elevated systemic arterial pressure. A similar picture of left axis deviation occurs when the left ventricle hypertrophies as a result of *aortic valvular stenosis*, *aortic valvular regurgitation*, or any number of *congenital heart conditions* in which the left ventricle enlarges while the right ventricle remains relatively normal in size.

Vectorial Analysis of Right Axis Deviation Resulting from Hypertrophy of the Right Ventricle. The ECG of Figure 34-27 shows intense right axis deviation, to an electrical axis of 170 degrees, which is 111 degrees to the right of the normal 59-degree mean ventricular QRS axis. The right axis deviation demonstrated in this figure was caused by hypertrophy of the

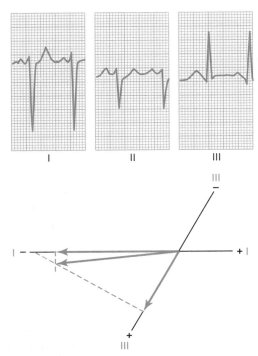

Figure 34-27 High-voltage electrocardiogram in *congenital pulmonary valve stenosis with right ventricular hypertrophy*. Intense right axis deviation and a slightly prolonged QRS complex also are seen.

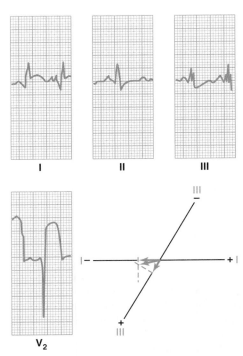

Figure 34-28 Current of injury in *acute anterior wall infarction*. Note the intense injury potential in lead V_2.

right ventricle as a result of *congenital pulmonary valve stenosis*. Right axis deviation also can occur in other congenital heart conditions that cause hypertrophy of the right ventricle, such as *tetralogy of Fallot* and *interventricular septal defect*.

Coronary Ischemia

CURRENT OF INJURY

Many different cardiac abnormalities, especially those that damage the heart muscle, often cause part of the heart to remain partially or totally *depolarized all the time*. When this condition occurs, current flows between the pathologically depolarized and the normally polarized areas, even between heartbeats. This condition is called a *current of injury*. Note especially that *the injured part of the heart is negative, because this is the part that is depolarized and emits negative charges into the surrounding fluids, whereas the remainder of the heart is neutral or in positive polarity.* When the uninjured part of the heart is completely depolarized, all the ventricular muscle is in a negative state. Therefore, at this instant in the ECG, no current flows from the ventricles to the ECG electrodes. This instant, where the wave of depolarization just completes its passage through the heart, occurs at the end of the QRS complex. The potential of the ECG at this instant is at zero voltage and this point on the ECG is known as the "J point."

Insufficient blood flow to the cardiac muscle depresses the metabolism of the muscle for three reasons: (1) lack of oxygen, (2) excess accumulation of carbon dioxide, and (3) lack of sufficient food nutrients. Consequently, repolarization of the muscle membrane cannot occur in areas of severe myocardial ischemia. Often the heart muscle does not die because the blood flow is sufficient to maintain life of the muscle even though it is not sufficient to cause normal repolarization of the membranes. As long as this state exists, an injury potential continues to flow during the diastolic portion (the T–P portion) of each heart cycle.

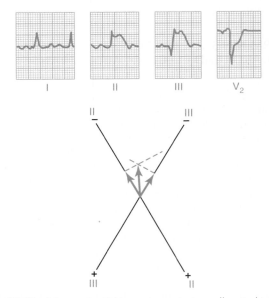

Figure 34-29 Injury potential in *acute posterior wall, apical infarction*.

Extreme ischemia of the cardiac muscle occurs after coronary occlusion, and a strong current of injury flows from the infarcted area of the ventricles during the T–P interval between heartbeats, as shown in Figures 34-28 and 34-29. Therefore, one of the most important diagnostic features of ECGs recorded after acute coronary thrombosis is the current of injury.

ACUTE ANTERIOR WALL INFARCTION

Figure 34-28 shows the ECG in the three standard bipolar limb leads and in one chest lead (lead V_2) recorded from a patient with acute anterior wall cardiac infarction. The most important diagnostic feature of this ECG is the intense injury potential in chest

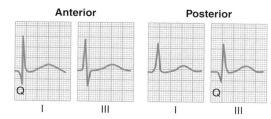

Anterior **Posterior**

I III I III

Figure 34-30 Electrocardiograms of anterior and posterior wall infarctions that occurred about 1 year previously, showing a Q wave in lead I in anterior wall infarction and a Q wave in lead III in *posterior wall infarction.*

lead V$_2$. If one draws a zero horizontal potential line through the J point of this ECG, a strong *negative* injury potential during the T–P interval is found, which means that the chest electrode over the front of the heart is in an area of strongly negative potential. In other words, the negative end of the injury potential vector in this heart is against the anterior chest wall. This means that the current of injury is emanating from the anterior wall of the ventricles, which diagnoses this condition as *anterior wall infarction.*

When analyzing the injury potentials in leads I and III, one finds a negative potential in lead I and a positive potential in lead III. This finding means that the resultant vector of the injury potential in the heart is about +150 degrees, with the negative end pointing toward the left ventricle and the positive pointing toward the right ventricle. Thus, in this ECG, the current of injury is coming mainly from the left ventricle, as well as from the anterior wall of the heart. Therefore, one would conclude that this anterior wall infarction almost certainly is caused by thrombosis of the anterior descending branch of the left coronary artery.

POSTERIOR WALL INFARCTION

Figure 34-29 shows the three standard bipolar limb leads and one chest lead (lead V$_2$) from a patient with posterior wall infarction. The major diagnostic feature of this ECG is also in the chest lead. If a zero potential reference line is drawn through the J point of this lead, it is readily apparent that during the T–P interval, the potential of the current of injury is positive. This means that the positive end of the vector is in the direction of the anterior chest wall and the negative end (the injured end of the vector) points away from the chest wall. In other words, the current of injury is coming from the back of the heart opposite

to the anterior chest wall, which is the reason this type of ECG is the basis for diagnosing posterior wall infarction.

If one analyzes the injury potentials from leads II and III of Figure 34-29, it is readily apparent that the injury potential is negative in both leads. By vectorial analysis, as shown in the figure, one finds that the resultant vector of the injury potential is about −95 degrees, with the negative end pointing downward and the positive end pointing upward. Thus, because the infarct, as indicated by the chest lead, is on the posterior wall of the heart and, as indicated by the injury potentials in leads II and III, is in the apical portion of the heart, one would suspect that this infarct is near the apex on the posterior wall of the left ventricle.

OLD RECOVERED MYOCARDIAL INFARCTION

Figure 34-30 shows leads I and III after *anterior infarction* and leads I and III after *posterior infarction* about 1 year after the acute heart attack. The records show what might be called the "ideal" configurations of the QRS complex in these types of recovered myocardial infarction. Usually a Q wave has developed at the beginning of the QRS complex in lead I in anterior infarction because of loss of muscle mass in the anterior wall of the left ventricle, but in posterior infarction, a Q wave has developed at the beginning of the QRS complex in lead III because of loss of muscle in the posterior apical part of the ventricle.

These configurations are certainly not found in all cases of old cardiac infarction. Local loss of muscle and local points of cardiac signal conduction block can cause very bizarre QRS patterns (especially prominent Q waves, eg), decreased voltage, and QRS prolongation.

CURRENT OF INJURY IN ANGINA PECTORIS

"Angina pectoris" means pain from the heart felt in the pectoral regions of the upper chest. This pain usually also radiates into the left neck area and down the left arm. The pain is typically caused by moderate ischemia of the heart. Usually, no pain is felt as long as the person is quiet, but as soon as he or she overworks the heart, the pain appears.

An injury potential sometimes appears in the ECG during an attack of severe angina pectoris because the coronary insufficiency becomes great enough to prevent adequate repolarization of some areas of the heart during diastole.

BIBLIOGRAPHY

Adler A, Rosso R, Viskin D, et al: What do we know about the "malignant form" of early repolarization? *J. Am. Coll. Cardiol.* 62:863, 2013.

Darby AE, DiMarco JP: Management of atrial fibrillation in patients with structural heart disease, *Circulation* 125:945, 2012.

Dobrzynski H, Boyett MR, Anderson RH: New insights into pacemaker activity: promoting understanding of sick sinus syndrome, *Circulation* 115:1921, 2007.

Jalife J: Ventricular fibrillation: mechanisms of initiation and maintenance, *Annu. Rev. Physiol.* 62:25, 2000.

Lampert R: Managing with pacemakers and implantable cardioverter defibrillators, *Circulation* 128:1576, 2013.

Olshansky B, Sullivan RM: Inappropriate sinus tachycardia, *J. Am. Coll. Cardiol.* 61:793, 2013.

Park DS, Fishman GI: The cardiac conduction system, *Circulation* 123:904, 2011.

Schwartz PJ, Ackerman MJ, George AL Jr, Wilde AA: Impact of genetics on the clinical management of channelopathies, *J. Am. Coll. Cardiol.* 62:169, 2013.

Shen MJ, Zipes DP: Role of the autonomic nervous system in modulating cardiac arrhythmias, *Circ. Res.* 114:1004, 2014.

Zimetbaum PJ, Josephson ME: Use of the electrocardiogram in acute myocardial infarction, *N. Engl. J. Med.* 348:933, 2003.

35

Cardiac Cycle

LEARNING OBJECTIVES

- List the phases of the cardiac cycle.
- Describe the pressure and volume changes in each phase of the cardiac cycle.
- Describe the genesis of the heart sounds.
- Diagrammatically summarize events during a single cardiac cycle (Wiggers diagram).
- List the determinants of myocardial oxygen consumption.

GLOSSARY OF TERMS

- **Cardiac cycle:** The electrical and mechanical cardiac events that occur from the beginning of one heartbeat to the beginning of the next

- **Diastole:** Period of relaxation, during which the heart fills with blood

- **Isovolumetric contraction:** The early phase of systole during which the ventricular volume does not change (the pressure in the ventricles rises rapidly, but not enough to overcome the aortic and pulmonary end-diastolic pressures and open the aortic and pulmonary valves)

- **Isovolumetric relaxation:** The phase of diastole following closure of the semilunar valves during which the ventricular pressures fall rapidly but ventricular volumes do not change

- **Protodiastole:** The early part of ventricular relaxation, terminating when the semilunar (aortic and pulmonary) valves close

- **Systole:** Period of contraction

The heart, shown in Figure 35-1, is actually two separate pumps: a *right heart* that pumps blood through the lungs and a *left heart* that pumps blood through the systemic circulation that provides blood flow to the other organs and tissues of the body. In turn, each of these hearts is a pulsatile two-chamber pump composed of an *atrium* and a *ventricle*. The ventricles supply the main pumping force that propels the blood either (1) through the pulmonary circulation by the right ventricle or (2) through the systemic circulation by the left ventricle.

The cardiac events that occur from the beginning of one heartbeat to the beginning of the next are called the *cardiac cycle*. Each cycle is initiated by spontaneous generation of an action potential in the *sinus node*, as explained in Chapter 32. The action potential travels from here rapidly through both atria and then through the atrioventricular (A-V) bundle into the ventricles. Because of this special arrangement of the conducting system from the atria into the ventricles, there is a delay of more than 0.1 second during passage of the cardiac impulse from the

atria into the ventricles. This delay allows the atria to contract ahead of ventricular contraction, thereby pumping blood into the ventricles before the strong ventricular contraction begins. Thus, the atria act as *primer pumps* for the ventricles, and the ventricles in turn provide the major source of power for moving blood through the body's vascular system.

Diastole and Systole

The cardiac cycle consists of a period of relaxation called *diastole*, during which the heart fills with blood, followed by a period of contraction called *systole*.

The total *duration of the cardiac cycle*, including systole and diastole, is the reciprocal of the heart rate. For example, if heart rate is 72 beats/minute, the duration of the cardiac cycle is 0.833 second/beat.

Figure 35-2 (often called Wiggers diagram) shows the different events during the cardiac cycle for the left side of the heart. The top three curves show the pressure changes in the aorta, left ventricle, and left atrium, respectively. The fourth curve depicts the changes in left ventricular volume, the fifth depicts the electrocardiogram, and the sixth depicts a phonocardiogram, which is a recording of the sounds produced by the heart—mainly by the heart valves—as it pumps. It is especially important that the reader study in detail this figure and understand the causes of all the events shown. In order to simplify things, this diagram is broken up to show individual events in subsequent sections.

Increasing Heart Rate Decreases the Duration of Cardiac Cycle. When heart rate increases, the duration of each cardiac cycle decreases, including the contraction and relaxation phases. The duration of the action potential and the period of contraction (systole) also decrease, but not by as great a percentage as does the relaxation phase (diastole). At a normal heart rate of 72 beats/minute, systole comprises about 0.4 of the entire cardiac cycle. At 3 times the normal heart rate, systole is about 0.65 of the entire cardiac cycle. This means that the heart beating at a very fast rate does not remain relaxed long enough to allow complete filling of the cardiac chambers before the next contraction.

MECHANICAL EVENTS IN THE HEART

The Ventricles Fill with Blood During Diastole

During ventricular systole, large amounts of blood accumulate in the right and left atria because of the closed A-V valves. Therefore, as soon as systole is over and the ventricular pressures fall again to their low diastolic values, the moderately increased pressures that have developed in the atria during ventricular systole immediately push the A-V valves open and allow blood to flow rapidly into the ventricles, as shown by the rise of the left *ventricular volume curve* in Figure 35-2. This period is called the *period of rapid filling of the ventricles*.

The period of rapid filling lasts for about the first third of diastole. During the middle third of diastole, only a small amount

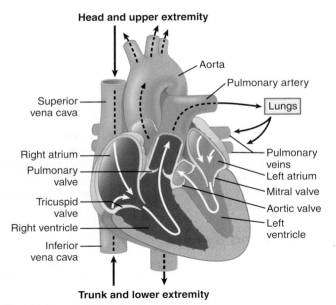

Head and upper extremity

Aorta

Pulmonary artery

Lungs

Superior vena cava

Right atrium

Pulmonary valve

Tricuspid valve

Right ventricle

Inferior vena cava

Pulmonary veins

Left atrium

Mitral valve

Aortic valve

Left ventricle

Trunk and lower extremity

Figure 35-1   Structure of the heart and course of blood flow through the heart chambers and heart valves.

of blood normally flows into the ventricles; this is blood that continues to empty into the atria from the veins and passes through the atria directly into the ventricles.

During the last third of diastole, the atria contract and give an additional thrust to the inflow of blood into the ventricles. This mechanism accounts for about 20% of the filling of the ventricles during each heart cycle. Since about 80% of the blood flows directly through the atria into the ventricles even before the atria contract, the atria simply function as primer pumps that increase the ventricular pumping effectiveness. However, the heart can continue to operate under most conditions even without this extra 20% effectiveness because it normally has the capability of pumping 300–400% more blood than is required by the resting body. Therefore, when the atria fail to function, the difference is unlikely to be noticed unless a person exercises; then acute signs of heart failure occasionally develop, especially shortness of breath.

Outflow of Blood from the Ventricles During Systole

Period of Isovolumic (Isometric) Contraction. Immediately after ventricular contraction begins, the ventricular pressure rises abruptly, as shown in Figure 35-2, causing the A-V valves to close. Then an additional 0.02–0.03 second is required for the ventricle to build up sufficient pressure to push the semilunar (aortic and pulmonary) valves open against the pressures in the aorta and pulmonary artery. Therefore, during this period, contraction is occurring in the ventricles, but no emptying occurs. This period is called the period of *isovolumic* or *isometric contraction* meaning that cardiac muscle tension is increasing but little or no shortening of the muscle fibers is occurring.

Period of Ejection. When the left ventricular pressure rises slightly above 80 mmHg (and the right ventricular pressure rises slightly above 8 mmHg), the ventricular pressures push the semilunar valves open. Immediately, blood begins to pour out of the ventricles. Approximately 60% of the blood in the ventricle at the end of diastole is ejected during systole; 70% of this portion flows out during the first third of the ejection period with the remaining 30% emptying during the next two thirds.

Therefore, the first third is called the *period of rapid ejection* and the last two thirds are called the *period of slow ejection*.

Period of Isovolumic (Isometric) Relaxation. At the end of systole, ventricular relaxation begins suddenly allowing both the right and left *intraventricular pressures* to decrease rapidly. The elevated pressures in the distended large arteries that have just been filled with blood from the contracted ventricles immediately push blood back toward the ventricles, which snaps the aortic and pulmonary valves closed. This brief period during which there is a backflow of blood associated with closure of the aortic and pulmonary valves is called *protodiastole*. For another 0.03–0.06 second, the ventricular muscle continues to relax, even though the ventricular volume does not change, giving rise to the period of *isovolumic* or *isometric relaxation*. During this period, the intraventricular pressures rapidly decrease back to their low diastolic levels. Then the A-V valves open to begin a new cycle of ventricular pumping. The ventricular pressure–volume changes are depicted separately in Figure 35-3.

Thus the phases of the cardiac cycle are as follows:
1. rapid filling of the ventricles
2. slow filling of the ventricles
3. atrial systole
4. isovolumetric contraction
5. rapid ejection
6. slow ejection
7. protodiastole
8. isovolumetric relaxation

ELECTRICAL EVENTS OF THE CARDIAC CYCLE

The electrocardiogram in Figure 35-2 shows the *P, Q, R, S,* and *T waves*, which are discussed in Chapter 33. They are electrical voltages generated by the heart and recorded by the electrocardiograph from the surface of the body.

The *P wave* is caused by *spread of depolarization* through the atria, and is followed by atrial contraction, which causes a slight rise in the atrial pressure curve immediately after the electrocardiographic P wave.

About 0.16 second after the onset of the P wave, the *QRS waves* appear as a result of electrical depolarization of the ventricles, which initiates contraction of the ventricles and causes the ventricular pressure to begin rising, as also shown in the figure. Therefore, the QRS complex begins slightly before the onset of ventricular systole.

Finally the *ventricular T wave* represents the stage of repolarization of the ventricles when the ventricular muscle fibers begin to relax. Therefore, the T wave occurs slightly before the end of ventricular contraction. The ECG changes are depicted separately in Figure 35-4.

Pressure Changes in the Atria—A, C, and V Waves

In the atrial pressure curve of Figure 35-2, three minor pressure elevations, called the *a, c,* and *v atrial pressure waves*, are shown.

The *a wave* is caused by atrial contraction. Ordinarily, the *right* atrial pressure increases 4–6 mmHg during atrial contraction, and the *left* atrial pressure increases about 7–8 mmHg.

The *c wave* occurs when the ventricles begin to contract; it is caused partly by slight backflow of blood into the atria at the onset of ventricular contraction but mainly by bulging of the A-V valves backward toward the atria because of increasing pressure in the ventricles.

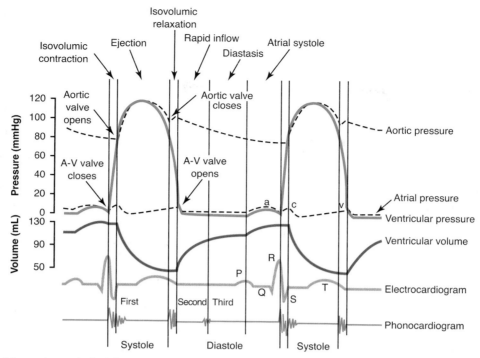

Figure 35-2 Events of the cardiac cycle for left ventricular function showing changes in left atrial pressure, left ventricular pressure, aortic pressure, ventricular volume, the electrocardiogram, and the phonocardiogram. *A-V,* atrioventricular.

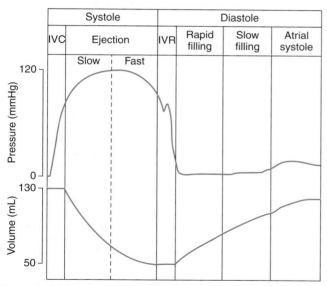

Figure 35-3 Left ventricular volume and pressure changes during the different phases of the cardiac cycle. The brief period of backflow resulting in closure of the aortic valve is called *protodiastole. IVC,* isovolumetric contraction; *IVR,* isovolumetric relaxation.

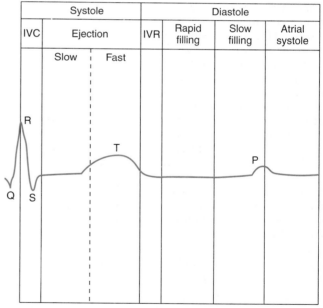

Figure 35-4 ECG changes during the different phases of the cardiac cycle. *IVC,* isovolumetric contraction; *IVR,* isovolumetric relaxation; *P,* atrial depolarization; *QRS complex,* ventricular depolarization; *T,* ventricular repolarization.

The *v wave* occurs toward the end of ventricular contraction; it results from slow flow of blood into the atria from the veins while the A-V valves are closed during ventricular contraction. Then, when ventricular contraction is over, the A-V valves open, allowing this stored atrial blood to flow rapidly into the ventricles and causing the *v wave* to disappear. These right atrial pressure changes that are also reflected in the jugular venous pressure trace are depicted separately in Figure 35-5.

Aortic Pressure Curve

When the left ventricle contracts, the ventricular pressure increases rapidly until the aortic valve opens. Then, after the valve opens, the pressure in the ventricle rises much less rapidly, as shown in Figure 35-2, because blood immediately flows out of the ventricle into the aorta and then into the systemic distribution arteries.

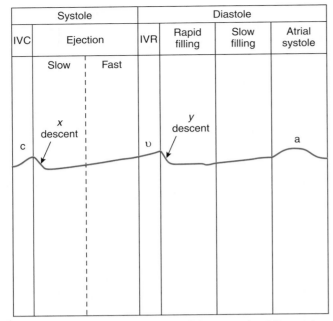

Figure 35-5   Right atrial pressure changes during the different phases of the cardiac cycle. *v*, buildup of pressure during atrial filling; *a*, atrial systole; A-V, atrioventricular; *c*, bulging of A-V valve into the atrium; *IVC*, isovolumetric contraction; *IVR*, isovolumetric relaxation.

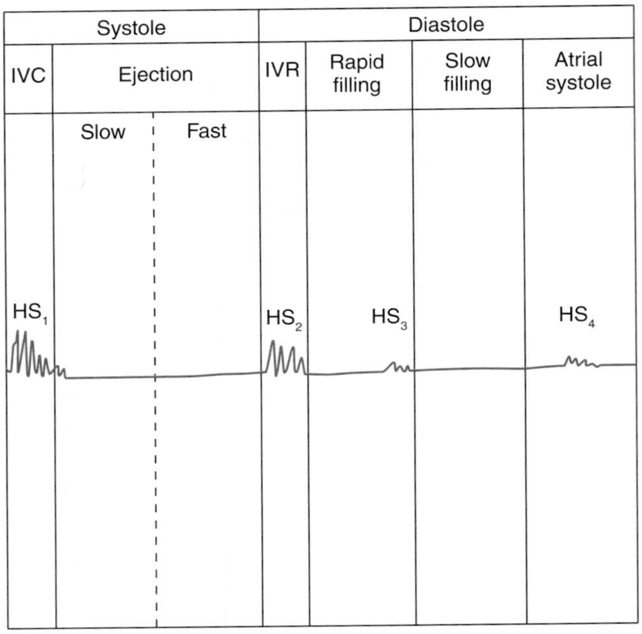

Figure 35-6   Location of the heart sounds in relation to the different phases of the cardiac cycle. A-V, atrioventricular; HS_1, closure of A-V valves; HS_2, closure of semilunar valves; HS_3, rapid filling; HS_3, atrial systole; *IVC*, isovolumetric contraction; *IVR*, isovolumetric relaxation.

The entry of blood into the arteries during systole causes the walls of these arteries to stretch and the pressure to increase to about 120 mmHg.

Next, at the end of systole, after the left ventricle stops ejecting blood and the aortic valve closes, the elastic walls of the arteries maintain a high pressure in the arteries even during diastole.

An *incisura* occurs in the aortic pressure curve when the aortic valve closes. This is caused by a short period of backward flow of blood (*protodiastole*) immediately before closure of the valve followed by sudden cessation of the backflow.

After the aortic valve has closed, the pressure in the aorta decreases slowly throughout diastole because the blood stored in the distended elastic arteries flows continually through the peripheral vessels back to the veins. Before the ventricle contracts again, the aortic pressure usually has fallen to about 80 mmHg (diastolic pressure), which is two-thirds the maximal pressure of 120 mmHg (systolic pressure) that occurs in the aorta during ventricular contraction.

The pressure curves in the *right ventricle* and *pulmonary artery* are similar to those in the aorta, except that the pressures are only about one-sixth as great as discussed in Chapter 29.

Heart Sounds During the Cardiac Cycle

When listening to the heart with a stethoscope, one does not hear the opening of the valves because this is a relatively slow process that normally makes no noise. However, when the valves close, the vanes of the valves and the surrounding fluids vibrate under the influence of sudden pressure changes, giving off sound that travels in all directions through the chest.

When the ventricles contract, one first hears a sound caused by closure of the A-V valves. The vibration pitch is low and relatively long-lasting and is known as the *first heart sound*. When the aortic and pulmonary valves close at the end of systole, one hears a rapid snap because these valves close rapidly and the surroundings vibrate for a short period. This sound is called the *second heart sound*. There are two additional heart sounds:

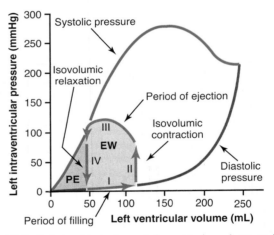

Figure 35-7   Relationship between left ventricular volume and intraventricular pressure during diastole and systole. Also shown by the red lines is the "volume–pressure diagram," demonstrating changes in intraventricular volume and pressure during the normal cardiac cycle. *EW*, net external work; *PE*, potential energy.

the *third heart sound* related to the turbulence of blood in the rapid filling phase and the *fourth heart sound* related to the turbulence of blood during atrial systole, which may not always be heard. *The location of these heart sounds in relation to the cardiac cycle is depicted in Figure 35-6.*

Graphical Analysis of Ventricular Pumping

Figure 35-7 shows a diagram that is especially useful in explaining the pumping mechanics of the *left* ventricle. The most important components of the diagram are the two curves labeled "diastolic pressure" and "systolic pressure." These curves are volume–pressure curves.

The diastolic pressure curve is determined by filling the heart with progressively greater volumes of blood and then measuring

Figure 35-8 The "volume–pressure diagram" demonstrating changes in intraventricular volume and pressure during a single cardiac cycle (*red line*). The shaded area represents the net external work (*EW*) output by the left ventricle during the cardiac cycle.

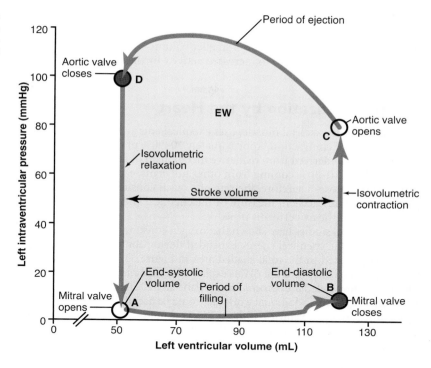

the diastolic pressure immediately before ventricular contraction occurs, which is the *end-diastolic pressure* of the ventricle.

The systolic pressure curve is determined by recording the systolic pressure achieved during ventricular contraction at each volume of filling.

Until the volume of the noncontracting ventricle rises above about 150 mL, the "diastolic" pressure does not increase greatly. Therefore, up to this volume, blood can flow easily into the ventricle from the atrium. Above 150 mL, the ventricular diastolic pressure increases rapidly, partly because of fibrous tissue in the heart that will stretch no more and partly because the pericardium that surrounds the heart becomes filled nearly to its limit.

During ventricular contraction, the "systolic" pressure increases even at low ventricular volumes and reaches a maximum at a ventricular volume of 150–170 mL. Then, as the volume increases still further, the systolic pressure actually decreases under some conditions, as demonstrated by the falling systolic pressure curve in Figure 35-7, because at these great volumes, the actin and myosin filaments of the cardiac muscle fibers are pulled apart far enough that the strength of each cardiac fiber contraction becomes less than optimal.

Note especially in the figure that the maximum systolic pressure for the normal *left* ventricle is between 250 and 300 mmHg, but this varies widely with each person's heart strength and degree of heart stimulation by cardiac nerves. For the normal *right* ventricle, the maximum systolic pressure is between 60 and 80 mmHg.

"Volume–Pressure Diagram" During the Cardiac Cycle; Cardiac Work Output

The red lines in Figure 35-7 form a loop called the *volume–pressure diagram* of the cardiac cycle for normal function of the *left* ventricle. A more detailed version of this loop is shown in Figure 35-8. It is divided into four phases:

Phase I: period of filling. Phase I in the volume–pressure diagram begins at a ventricular volume of about 50 mL and a diastolic pressure of 2–3 mmHg. The amount of blood that remains in the ventricle after the previous heartbeat,

50 mL, is called the *end-systolic volume*. As venous blood flows into the ventricle from the left atrium, the ventricular volume normally increases to about 120 mL, called the *end-diastolic volume*, an increase of 70 mL. Therefore, the volume–pressure diagram during phase I extends along the line labeled "I," and from point A to point B, with the volume increasing to 120 mL and the diastolic pressure rising to about 5–7 mmHg.

Phase II: period of isovolumic contraction. During isovolumic contraction, the volume of the ventricle does not change because all valves are closed. However, the pressure inside the ventricle increases to equal the pressure in the aorta, at a pressure value of about 80 mmHg, as depicted by point C.

Phase III: period of ejection. During ejection, the systolic pressure rises even higher because of still more contraction of the ventricle. At the same time, the volume of the ventricle decreases because the aortic valve has now opened and blood flows out of the ventricle into the aorta. Therefore, the curve labeled "III," or "period of ejection," traces the changes in volume and systolic pressure during this period of ejection.

Phase IV: period of isovolumic relaxation. At the end of the period of ejection (point D), the aortic valve closes and the ventricular pressure falls back to the diastolic pressure level. The line labeled "IV" traces this decrease in intraventricular pressure without any change in volume. Thus, the ventricle returns to its starting point with about 50 mL of blood left in the ventricle and at an atrial pressure of 2–3 mmHg.

The area subtended by this functional volume–pressure diagram (the shaded area, labeled EW) represents the *net external work (EW) output* of the ventricle during its contraction cycle. In experimental studies of cardiac contraction, this diagram is used for calculating cardiac work output.

When the heart pumps large quantities of blood, the area of the work diagram becomes much larger. That is, it extends far to the right because the ventricle fills with more blood during diastole, it rises much higher because the ventricle contracts with greater pressure, and it usually extends farther to the left because the ventricle contracts to a smaller volume—especially if the ventricle is stimulated to increased activity by the sympathetic nervous system.

Oxygen Utilization by the Heart

Heart muscle, like skeletal muscle, uses chemical energy to provide the work of contraction. Approximately 70–90% of this energy is normally derived from oxidative metabolism of fatty acids with about 10–30% coming from other nutrients, especially lactate and glucose. Therefore, the rate of oxygen consumption by the heart is an excellent measure of the chemical energy liberated while the heart performs its work.

Experimental studies have shown that oxygen consumption of the heart and the chemical energy expended during contraction are directly related to the total shaded area in Figure 35-7. This shaded portion consists of the *EW* as explained earlier and an additional portion called the *potential energy*, labeled PE. The potential energy represents additional work that could be accomplished by contraction of the ventricle if the ventricle should completely empty all the blood in its chamber with each contraction.

Oxygen consumption has also been shown to be nearly proportional to the *tension* that occurs in the heart muscle during contraction multiplied by the *duration of time* that the contraction persists, called the *tension–time index*. Because tension is high when systolic pressure is high, correspondingly more oxygen is used. Also, much more chemical energy is expended even at normal systolic pressures when the ventricle is abnormally dilated because the heart muscle tension during contraction is proportional to pressure times the diameter of the ventricle. This becomes especially important in heart failure when the heart ventricle is dilated and, paradoxically, the amount of chemical energy required for a given amount of work output is greater than normal even though the heart is already failing.

Efficiency of Cardiac Contraction

During heart muscle contraction, most of the expended chemical energy is converted into *heat* and a much smaller portion is converted into *work output*. The ratio of work output to total chemical energy expenditure is called the *efficiency of cardiac contraction*, or simply *efficiency of the heart*. Maximum efficiency of the normal heart is between 20 and 25%. In persons with heart failure, this efficiency can decrease to as low as 5–10%.

BIBLIOGRAPHY

Guyton AC: Determination of cardiac output by equating venous return curves with cardiac response curves, *Physiol. Rev.* 35:123, 1955.

Knaapen P, Germans T, Knuuti J, et al: Myocardial energetic and efficiency: current status of the noninvasive approach, *Circulation* 115:918, 2007.

Olson EN: A decade of discoveries in cardiac biology, *Nat. Med.* 10:467, 2004.

Rudy Y, Ackerman MJ, Bers DM, et al: Systems approach to understanding electromechanical activity in the human heart: a National Heart, Lung, and Blood Institute workshop summary, *Circulation* 118:1202, 2008.

Sarnoff SJ: Myocardial contractility as described by ventricular function curves, *Physiol. Rev.* 35:107, 1955.

Starling EH: *The Linacre Lecture on the Law of the Heart*, London, 1918, Longmans Green.

36

Cardiac Output and Venous Return

LEARNING OBJECTIVES

- Define cardiac output and state its resting value.
- Describe the determinants of cardiac output and venous return, and their control.
- Describe different methods that can be used to measure cardiac output.

GLOSSARY OF TERMS

- **Cardiac index:** Cardiac output per unit body surface area
- **Cardiac output:** The amount of blood ejected per ventricle per minute, normal ~5 L/minute
- **Mean systemic filling pressure:** The pressure at which (7 mmHg) all flow in the systemic circulation ceases and both the arterial and the venous pressures come to equilibrium
- **Stroke volume:** The amount of blood ejected per ventricle per contraction, normal ~70 mL
- **Venous return:** Quantity of blood flowing into the right atrium per minute

Cardiac output is the quantity of blood pumped into the aorta each minute by the heart. This is also the quantity of blood that flows through the circulation. Cardiac output is one of the most important factors in relation to the circulation because it is the sum of the blood flows to all the tissues of the body.

Venous return is the quantity of blood flowing from the veins into the right atrium each minute. The venous return and the cardiac output must equal each other except for a few heartbeats at a time when blood is temporarily stored in or removed from the heart and lungs.

Normal Values for Cardiac Output at Rest and During Activity

Cardiac output varies widely with the level of activity of the body. The following factors, among others, directly affect cardiac output: (1) the basic level of body metabolism, (2) whether the person is exercising, (3) the person's age, and (4) the size of the body.

For *young, healthy men*, resting cardiac output averages about 5.6 L/minute. For *women*, this value is about 4.9 L/minute. When one considers the factor of age as well—because with increasing age, body activity and mass of some tissues (eg, skeletal muscle) diminish—the average cardiac output for the resting adult, in round numbers, is often stated to be about 5 L/minute.

CARDIAC INDEX

Experiments have shown that the cardiac output increases approximately in proportion to the surface area of the body.

Therefore, cardiac output is frequently stated in terms of the *cardiac index*, which is the *cardiac output per square meter of body surface area*. The average human being who weighs 70 kg has a body surface area of about 1.7 m², which means that the normal average cardiac index for adults is about 3 L/minute per square meter of body surface area.

Effect of Age on Cardiac Output. Figure 36-1 shows the cardiac output, expressed as cardiac index, at different ages. The cardiac index rises rapidly to a level greater than 4 L/minute per square meter at age 10 years, and declines to about 2.4 L/minute per square meter at age 80 years. We explain later in the chapter that the cardiac output is regulated throughout life almost directly in proportion to overall metabolic activity. Therefore, the declining cardiac index is indicative of declining activity or declining muscle mass with age.

Control of Cardiac Output by Venous Return—The Frank–Starling Mechanism of the Heart

When one states that cardiac output is controlled by venous return, this means that it is not the heart itself that is normally the primary controller of cardiac output. Instead, it is the various factors of the peripheral circulation that affect flow of blood into the heart from the veins, called *venous return*, that are the primary controllers.

The main reason peripheral factors are usually so important in controlling cardiac output is that the heart has a built-in mechanism that normally allows it to pump automatically whatever amount of blood that flows into the right atrium from the veins. This mechanism, called the *Frank–Starling law of the heart*, was discussed in Chapter 30. Basically, this law states that when increased quantities of blood flow into the heart, the increased blood stretches the walls of the heart chambers. As a result of the stretch, the cardiac muscle contracts with increased force and this action empties the extra blood that has entered from the systemic circulation.

Another important factor is that stretching the heart causes the heart to pump faster—resulting in an increased heart rate. That is, stretch of the *sinus node* in the wall of the right atrium has a direct effect on the rhythmicity of the node to increase the heart rate as much as 10–15%. In addition, the stretched right atrium initiates a nervous reflex called the *Bainbridge reflex*, passing first to the vasomotor center of the brain and then back to the heart by way of the sympathetic nerves and vagi, also to increase the heart rate.

Under most normal unstressed conditions, the cardiac output is controlled mainly by peripheral factors that determine venous return. However, as will be discussed later in the chapter, if the returning blood does become more than the heart can pump, then the heart becomes the limiting factor that determines cardiac output.

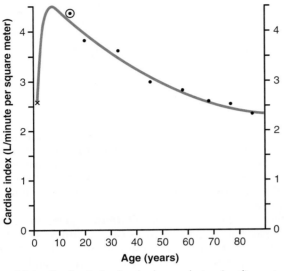

Figure 36-1 *Cardiac index* for the human being (cardiac output per square meter of surface area) at different ages. *Modified from Guyton, A.C., Jones, C.E., Coleman, T.B., 1973. Circulatory Physiology: Cardiac Output and its Regulation, second ed. W.B. Saunders, Philadelphia.*

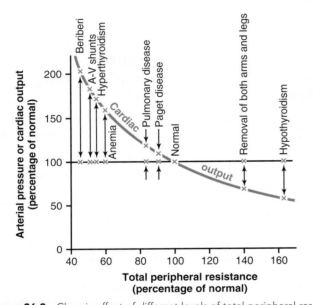

Figure 36-2 Chronic effect of different levels of total peripheral resistance on cardiac output, showing a reciprocal relationship between total peripheral resistance and cardiac output. *A-V, atrioventricular. Modified from Guyton, A.C., 1980. Arterial Pressure and Hypertension. W.B. Saunders, Philadelphia.*

Long-Term Cardiac Output Varies Inversely with Total Peripheral Resistance when Arterial Pressure Is Unchanged. Figure 36-2 illustrates an extremely important principle in cardiac output control. Under many conditions, the long-term cardiac output level varies reciprocally with changes in total peripheral vascular resistance, as long as the arterial pressure is unchanged. Note in Figure 36-2 that when the total peripheral resistance is exactly normal (at the 100% mark in the figure), the cardiac output is also normal. Then, when the total peripheral resistance increases above normal, the cardiac output falls; conversely, when the total peripheral resistance decreases, the cardiac output increases. One can easily understand this phenomenon by reconsidering one of the forms of Ohm's law, as expressed in Chapter 38:

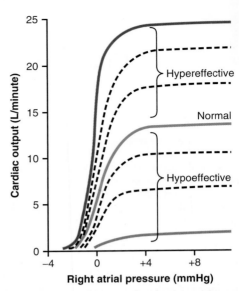

Figure 36-3 Cardiac output curves for the normal heart and for hypoeffective and hypereffective hearts. *Modified from Guyton, A.C., Jones, C.E., Coleman, T.B., 1973. Circulatory Physiology: Cardiac Output and its Regulation, second ed. W.B. Saunders, Philadelphia.*

$$Cardiac\ output = \frac{arterial\ pressure}{total\ peripheral\ resistance}$$

Thus, anytime the long-term level of total peripheral resistance changes (but no other functions of the circulation change), the cardiac output changes quantitatively in exactly the opposite direction.

FACTORS THAT CAUSE A HYPEREFFECTIVE HEART

There are definite limits to the amount of blood that the heart can pump, which can be expressed quantitatively in the form of *cardiac output curves* (Figure 36-3).

Two types of factors that can make the heart a better pump than normal are as follows: (1) nervous stimulation and (2) hypertrophy of the heart muscle.

Nervous Excitation Can Increase Heart Pumping

In Chapter 30 we saw that a combination of (1) sympathetic *stimulation* and (2) parasympathetic *inhibition* does two things to increase the pumping effectiveness of the heart: (1) it greatly increases the heart rate—sometimes, in young people, from the normal level of 72 up to 180–200 beats/minute—and (2) it increases the strength of heart contraction (which is called increased "contractility") to twice its normal strength. Combining these two effects, maximal nervous excitation of the heart can raise the plateau level of the cardiac output curve to almost twice the plateau of the normal curve, as shown by the 25-L/minute level of the uppermost curve in Figure 36-3.

Heart Hypertrophy Can Increase Pumping Effectiveness

A long-term increased workload, but not so much excess load that it damages the heart, causes the heart muscle to increase in mass and contractile strength in the same way that heavy exercise causes skeletal muscles to hypertrophy. For instance, it is common for the hearts of marathon runners to be increased in mass by

50–75%. This factor increases the plateau level of the cardiac output curve, sometimes 60–100%, and therefore allows the heart to pump much greater than usual amounts of cardiac output.

When one combines nervous excitation of the heart and hypertrophy, as occurs in marathon runners, the total effect can allow the heart to pump as much as 30–40 L/minute, about 2.5 times the level that can be achieved in the average person; this increased level of pumping is one of the most important factors in determining the runner's running time.

FACTORS THAT CAUSE A HYPOEFFECTIVE HEART

Any factor that decreases the heart's ability to pump blood causes hypoeffectivity. Some of the factors that can decrease the heart's ability to pump blood are the following:

- increased arterial pressure against which the heart must pump, such as in severe hypertension;
- inhibition of nervous excitation of the heart;
- pathological factors that cause abnormal heart rhythm or rate of heartbeat;
- coronary artery blockage causing a "heart attack";
- valvular heart disease;
- congenital heart disease;
- myocarditis, an inflammation of the heart muscle;
- cardiac hypoxia.

ROLE OF THE NERVOUS SYSTEM IN CONTROLLING CARDIAC OUTPUT

Importance of the Nervous System in Maintaining Arterial Pressure when Peripheral Blood Vessels Are Dilated and Venous Return and Cardiac Output Increase

Figure 36-4 shows an important difference in cardiac output control with and without a functioning autonomic nervous system. The solid curves demonstrate the effect in the normal dog of intense dilation of the peripheral blood vessels caused by administering the drug dinitrophenol, which increased the metabolism of virtually all tissues of the body about fourfold. With nervous

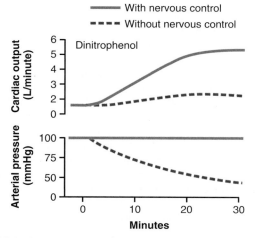

Figure 36-4 Experiment in a dog to demonstrate the importance of nervous maintenance of the arterial pressure as a prerequisite for cardiac output control. Note that with pressure control, the metabolic stimulant *dinitrophenol* increases cardiac output greatly; without pressure control, the arterial pressure falls and the cardiac output rises very little. *Drawn from experiments by Dr. M. Banet.*

control mechanisms intact dilating all the peripheral blood vessels caused almost no change in arterial pressure but increased the cardiac output almost fourfold. However, after autonomic control of the nervous system had been blocked, vasodilation of the vessels with dinitrophenol (dashed curves) then caused a profound fall in arterial pressure to about one-half normal, and the cardiac output rose only 1.6-fold instead of 4-fold.

Thus, maintenance of a normal arterial pressure by the nervous reflexes, by mechanisms explained in Chapter 43, is essential to achieve high cardiac outputs when the peripheral tissues dilate their vessels to increase the venous return.

Effect of the Nervous System to Increase the Arterial Pressure During Exercise. During exercise, intense increase in metabolism in active skeletal muscles acts directly on the muscle arterioles to relax them and to allow adequate oxygen and other nutrients needed to sustain muscle contraction. Obviously, this greatly decreases the total peripheral resistance, which normally would decrease the arterial pressure as well. However, the nervous system immediately compensates. The same brain activity that sends motor signals to the muscles sends simultaneous signals into the autonomic nervous centers of the brain to excite circulatory activity, causing large vein constriction, increased heart rate, and increased contractility of the heart. All these changes acting together increase the arterial pressure above normal, which in turn forces still more blood flow through the active muscles.

In summary, when local tissue blood vessels dilate and increase venous return and cardiac output above normal, the nervous system plays a key role in preventing the arterial pressure from falling to disastrously low levels. In fact, during exercise, the nervous system goes further, providing additional signals to raise the arterial pressure even above normal, which serves to increase the cardiac output an extra 30–100%.

Venous Return Curves

The venous return to the heart is the sum of all the local blood flows through all the individual tissue segments of the peripheral circulation (Figure 36-5). All the local blood flows summate to form the venous return, and the heart automatically pumps this returning blood back into the arteries to flow around the system again.

The entire systemic circulation must be considered before total analysis of cardiac regulation can be achieved. To analyze the function of the systemic circulation, we first remove the heart and lungs from the circulation of an animal and replace them with a pump and artificial oxygenator system. Then, different factors, such as blood volume, vascular resistances, and central venous pressure in the right atrium, are altered to determine how the systemic circulation operates in different circulatory states. In these studies, one finds the following three principal factors that affect venous return to the heart from the systemic circulation:

1. *right atrial pressure*, which exerts a backward force on the veins to impede flow of blood from the veins into the right atrium;
2. degree of filling of the systemic circulation [measured by the *mean systemic filling pressure* (Psf)], which forces the systemic blood toward the heart (this is the pressure measured everywhere in the systemic circulation when all flow of blood is stopped and is discussed in detail later);
3. *resistance to blood flow* between the peripheral vessels and the right atrium.

These factors can all be expressed quantitatively by the *venous return curve*, as we explain in the next sections.

Cardiac output = total tissue blood flow

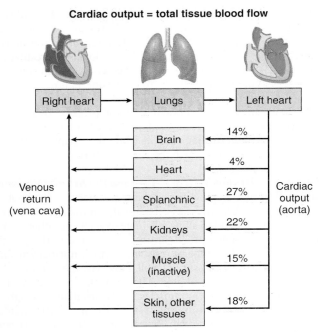

Figure 36-5   Cardiac output is equal to venous return and is the sum of tissue and organ blood flows. Except when the heart is severely weakened and unable to adequately pump the venous return, cardiac output (total tissue blood flow) is determined mainly by the metabolic needs of the tissues and organs of the body.

NORMAL VENOUS RETURN CURVE

In the same way that the cardiac output curve relates pumping of blood by the heart to right atrial pressure, the *venous return curve relates venous return also to right atrial pressure*—that is, the venous flow of blood into the heart from the systemic circulation at different levels of right atrial pressure.

The curve in Figure 36-6 is the *normal* venous return curve. This curve shows that when heart pumping capability becomes diminished and causes the right atrial pressure to rise, the backward force of the rising atrial pressure on the veins of the systemic circulation decreases venous return of blood to the heart. *If all nervous circulatory reflexes are prevented from acting*, venous return decreases to zero when the right atrial pressure rises to about +7 mmHg. Such a slight rise in right atrial pressure causes a drastic decrease in venous return because any increase in back pressure causes blood to dam up in the systemic circulation instead of returning to the heart.

At the same time that the right atrial pressure is rising and causing venous stasis, pumping by the heart also approaches zero because of decreasing venous return. Both the arterial and the venous pressures come to equilibrium when all flow in the systemic circulation ceases at a pressure of 7 mmHg, which, by definition, is the *Psf*.

Plateau in the Venous Return Curve at Negative Atrial Pressures Caused by Collapse of the Large Veins. When the right atrial pressure falls *below* zero—that is, below atmospheric pressure—further increase in venous return almost ceases and by the time the right atrial pressure has fallen to about −2 mmHg, the venous return reaches a plateau. It remains at this plateau level even though the right atrial pressure falls to −20 or −50 mmHg, or even further. This plateau is caused by *collapse of the veins* entering the chest. Negative pressure in the

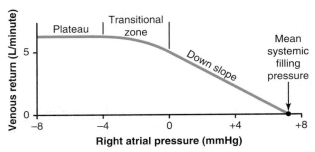

Figure 36-6   Normal *venous return curve.* The plateau is caused by *collapse* of the large veins entering the chest when the right atrial pressure falls below atmospheric pressure. Note also that venous return becomes zero when the right atrial pressure rises to equal the mean systemic filling pressure.

right atrium sucks the walls of the veins together where they enter the chest, which prevents any additional flow of blood from the peripheral veins. Consequently, even very negative pressures in the right atrium cannot increase venous return significantly above that which exists at a normal atrial pressure of 0 mmHg.

MEAN CIRCULATORY FILLING PRESSURE, MEAN SYSTEMIC FILLING PRESSURE, AND THEIR EFFECT ON VENOUS RETURN

When heart pumping is stopped by shocking the heart with electricity to cause ventricular fibrillation or is stopped in any other way, flow of blood everywhere in the circulation ceases a few seconds later. Without blood flow, the pressures everywhere in the circulation become equal. This equilibrated pressure level is called the *mean circulatory filling pressure.*

Effect of Blood Volume on Mean Circulatory Filling Pressure. The greater the volume of blood in the circulation, the greater is the mean circulatory filling pressure because extra blood volume stretches the walls of the vasculature. The *red curve* in Figure 36-7 shows the approximate normal effect of different levels of blood volume on the mean circulatory filling pressure. Note that at a blood volume of about 4000 mL, the mean circulatory filling pressure is close to zero because this is the "unstressed volume" of the circulation, but at a volume of 5000 mL, the filling pressure is the normal value of 7 mmHg. Similarly, at still higher volumes, the mean circulatory filling pressure increases almost linearly.

Sympathetic Nervous Stimulation Increases Mean Circulatory Filling Pressure. The *green curve* and *blue curve* in Figure 36-7 show the effects, respectively, of high and low levels of sympathetic nervous activity on the mean circulatory filling pressure. Strong sympathetic stimulation constricts all the systemic blood vessels, as well as the larger pulmonary blood vessels and even the chambers of the heart. Therefore, the capacity of the system decreases so that at each level of blood volume, the mean circulatory filling pressure is increased. At normal blood volume, maximal sympathetic stimulation increases the mean circulatory filling pressure from 7 mmHg to about 2.5 times that value, or about 17 mmHg.

Conversely, complete inhibition of the sympathetic nervous system relaxes both the blood vessels and the heart, decreasing the mean circulatory filling pressure from the normal value of 7 mmHg down to about 4 mmHg. Note in Figure 36-7 how steep the curves are, which means that even slight changes in

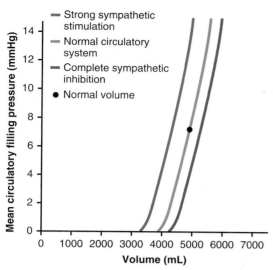

Figure 36-7 Effect of changes in total blood volume on the *mean circulatory filling pressure* (ie, "volume–pressure curves" for the entire circulatory system). These curves also show the effects of strong sympathetic stimulation and complete sympathetic inhibition.

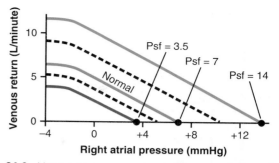

Figure 36-8 Venous return curves showing the normal curve when the mean systemic filling pressure (Psf) is 7 mmHg and the effect of altering the Psf to either 3.5 or 14 mmHg. *Modified from Guyton, A.C., Jones, C.E., Coleman, T.B., 1973. Circulatory Physiology: Cardiac Output and its Regulation, second ed. W.B. Saunders, Philadelphia.*

blood volume or capacity of the system caused by various levels of sympathetic activity can have large effects on the mean circulatory filling pressure.

Mean Systemic Filling Pressure and its Relation to Mean Circulatory Filling Pressure. The *Psf* is slightly different from the mean circulatory filling pressure. It is the pressure measured everywhere *in the systemic circulation* after blood flow has been stopped by clamping the large blood vessels at the heart, so the pressures in the systemic circulation can be measured independently from those in the pulmonary circulation. The Psf, although almost impossible to measure in the living animal, *is almost always nearly equal to the mean circulatory filling pressure* because the pulmonary circulation has less than one-eighth as much capacitance as the systemic circulation and only about one-tenth as much blood volume.

Effect on the Venous Return Curve of Changes in Mean Systemic Filling Pressure. Figure 36-8 shows the effects on the venous return curve caused by increasing or decreasing Psf. Note that the normal Psf is 7 mmHg. Then, for the uppermost curve in the figure, the Psf has been increased to 14 mmHg, and for the lowermost curve, it has been decreased to 3.5 mmHg. These curves demonstrate that the greater the Psf (which also means the greater the "tightness" with which the circulatory system is filled with blood), the more the venous return curve shifts *upward* and *to the right*. Conversely, the lower the Psf, the more the curve shifts *downward* and *to the left*.

Expressing this another way, the greater the degree to which the system is filled, the easier it is for blood to flow into the heart. The lesser the degree to which the system is filled, the more difficult it is for blood to flow into the heart.

When the "Pressure Gradient for Venous Return" Is Zero, There Is No Venous Return. When the right atrial pressure rises to equal the Psf, there is no longer any pressure difference between the peripheral vessels and the right atrium. Consequently, there can no longer be any blood flow from peripheral vessels back to the right atrium. However, when the right atrial pressure

falls progressively lower than the Psf, the flow to the heart increases proportionately, as one can see by studying any of the venous return curves in Figure 36-8. That is, *the greater the difference between the Psf and the right atrial pressure, the greater becomes the venous return.* Therefore, the difference between these two pressures is called the *pressure gradient for venous return*.

RESISTANCE TO VENOUS RETURN

In the same way that Psf represents a pressure pushing venous blood from the periphery toward the heart, there is also resistance to this venous flow of blood. It is called the *resistance to venous return*. Most of the resistance to venous return occurs in the veins, although some occurs in the arterioles and small arteries as well.

Why is venous resistance so important in determining the resistance to venous return? The answer is that when the resistance in the veins increases, blood begins to be dammed up, mainly in the veins themselves. However, the venous pressure rises very little because the veins are highly distensible. Therefore, this rise in venous pressure is not very effective in overcoming the resistance, and blood flow into the right atrium decreases drastically. Conversely, when arteriolar and small artery resistances increase, blood accumulates in the arteries, which have a capacitance only one-thirtieth as great as that of the veins. Therefore, even slight accumulation of blood in the arteries raises the pressure greatly—30 times as much as in the veins—and this high pressure overcomes much of the increased resistance. Mathematically, it turns out that about two-thirds of the so-called "resistance to venous return" is determined by venous resistance, and about one-third is determined by the arteriolar and small artery resistance.

Venous return can be calculated by the following formula:

$$VR = \frac{Psf - PRA}{RVR}$$

where VR is venous return, Psf is mean systemic filling pressure, PRA is right atrial pressure, and RVR is resistance to venous return. In the healthy human adult, the values for these are as follows: VR equals 5 L/minute, Psf equals 7 mmHg, PRA equals 0 mmHg, and RVR equals 1.4 mmHg/L per minute of blood flow.

Effect of Resistance to Venous Return on the Venous Return Curve. Figure 36-9 demonstrates the effect of different levels of resistance to venous return on the venous return curve, showing

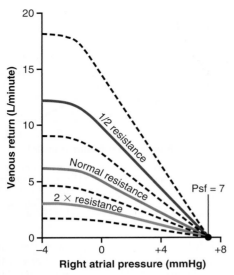

Figure 36-9 Venous return curves depicting the effect of altering the "resistance to venous return." Psf, mean systemic filling pressure. *Modified from Guyton, A.C., Jones, C.E., Coleman, T.B., 1973. Circulatory Physiology: Cardiac Output and its Regulation, second ed. W.B. Saunders, Philadelphia.*

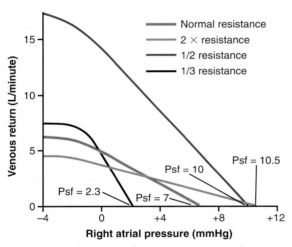

Figure 36-10 Combinations of the major patterns of venous return curves, showing the effects of simultaneous changes in mean systemic filling pressure (Psf) and in "resistance to venous return." *Modified from Guyton, A.C., Jones, C.E., Coleman, T.B., 1973. Circulatory Physiology: Cardiac Output and its Regulation, second ed. W.B. Saunders, Philadelphia.*

that a *decrease* in this resistance to one-half normal allows twice as much flow of blood and, therefore, *rotates the curve upward* to twice as great a slope. Conversely, an *increase* in resistance to twice normal *rotates the curve downward* to one-half as great a slope.

Note also that when the right atrial pressure rises to equal the Psf, venous return becomes zero at all levels of resistance to venous return because then there is no pressure gradient to cause flow of blood. Therefore, *the highest level to which the right atrial pressure can rise*, regardless of how much the heart might fail, is equal to the Psf.

Combinations of Venous Return Curve Patterns. Figure 36-10 shows the effects on the venous return curve caused by simultaneous changes in Psf and resistance to venous return, demonstrating that both these factors can operate simultaneously.

Summary of Factors Affecting Venous Return

It is useful here to summarize the factors that affect venous return. Some of these factors are merely listed since the preceding discussion is quite comprehensive and include the following:

1. the muscle pump: where muscle contraction forces venous return to the heart, aided by the unidirectional venous valves;
2. changes in the intrathoracic pressure including right atrial pressure (the respiratory pump) [during inspiration abdominal pressure increases due to the downward movement of the diaphragm while intrathoracic pressure simultaneously decreases (because of the increased thoracic volume); the pressure gradient from the abdomen to the thorax favors a return of venous blood to the heart; the changes are reversed during expiration];
3. resistance to blood flow between the peripheral veins and the right atrium;
4. blood volume;
5. posture;
6. Psf;
7. sympathetic nervous activation.

Analysis of Cardiac Output and Right Atrial Pressure Using Simultaneous Cardiac Output and Venous Return Curves

In the complete circulation, the heart and the systemic circulation must operate together. This requirement means that (1) the venous return from the systemic circulation must equal the cardiac output from the heart and (2) the right atrial pressure is the same for both the heart and the systemic circulation.

Therefore, one can predict the cardiac output and right atrial pressure in the following way: (1) determine the momentary pumping ability of the heart and depict this ability in the form of a cardiac output curve; (2) determine the momentary state of flow from the systemic circulation into the heart and depict this state of flow in the form of a venous return curve; and (3) "equate" these curves against each other, as shown in Figure 36-11.

Two curves in the figure depict the *normal cardiac output curve* (red line) and the *normal venous return curve* (blue line). There is only one point on the graph, point A, at which the venous return equals the cardiac output and at which the right atrial pressure is the same for both the heart and the systemic circulation. Therefore, in the normal circulation, the right atrial pressure, cardiac output, and venous return are all depicted by point A, called the *equilibrium point*, giving a normal value for cardiac output of 5 L/minute and a right atrial pressure of 0 mmHg.

Effect of Increased Blood Volume on Cardiac Output. A sudden increase in blood volume of about 20% increases the cardiac output to about 2.5–3 times normal. An analysis of this effect is shown in Figure 36-11. Immediately on infusing the large quantity of extra blood, the increased filling of the system causes the Psf to increase to 16 mmHg, which shifts the venous return curve to the right. At the same time, the increased blood volume distends the blood vessels, thus reducing their resistance and thereby reducing the resistance to venous return, which rotates the curve upward. As a result of these two effects, the venous return curve of Figure 36-11 is shifted to the right. This new curve

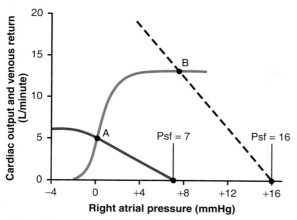

Figure 36-11 The two *solid curves* demonstrate an analysis of cardiac output and right atrial pressure when the cardiac output (*red line*) and venous return (*blue line*) curves are normal. Transfusion of blood equal to 20% of the blood volume causes the venous return curve to become the *dashed curve*; as a result, the cardiac output and right atrial pressure shift from point A to point B. Psf, mean systemic filling pressure.

equates with the cardiac output curve at point B, showing that the cardiac output and venous return increase 2.5–3 times and that the right atrial pressure rises to about +8 mmHg.

Compensatory Effects Initiated in Response to Increased Blood Volume. The greatly increased cardiac output caused by increased blood volume lasts for only a few minutes because several compensatory effects immediately begin to occur: (1) the increased cardiac output *increases the capillary pressure* so that fluid begins to transude out of the capillaries into the tissues, thereby returning the blood volume toward normal; (2) the increased pressure in the veins causes the veins to continue distending gradually by the mechanism called *stress relaxation*, especially causing the venous blood reservoirs, such as the liver and spleen, to distend, thus *reducing the Psf*; (3) the excess blood flow through the peripheral tissues causes autoregulatory increase in the peripheral vascular resistance, thus increasing the *resistance to venous return*. These factors cause the Psf to return toward normal and the resistance vessels of the systemic circulation to constrict. Therefore, gradually, over a period of 10–40 minutes, the cardiac output returns almost to normal.

Effect of Sympathetic Stimulation on Cardiac Output. Sympathetic stimulation affects both the heart and the systemic circulation: (1) it *makes the heart a stronger pump* and (2) in the systemic circulation, it *increases the* Psf because of contraction of the peripheral vessels, especially the veins, and it *increases the resistance to venous return*.

In Figure 36-12, the *normal* cardiac output and venous return curves are depicted; these equate with each other at point A, which represents a normal venous return and cardiac output of 5 L/minute and a right atrial pressure of 0 mmHg. Note in the figure that maximal sympathetic stimulation (green curves) increases the Psf to 17 mmHg (depicted by the point at which the venous return curve reaches the zero venous return level). Sympathetic stimulation also increases pumping effectiveness of the heart by nearly 100%. As a result, the cardiac output rises from the normal value at equilibrium point A to about double normal at equilibrium point D—and yet *the right atrial pressure hardly changes*. Thus, different degrees of sympathetic stimulation can increase the cardiac output progressively to about twice

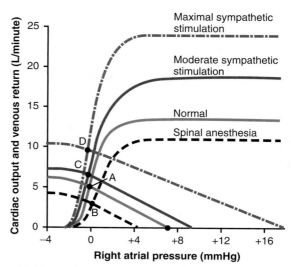

Figure 36-12 Analysis of the effect on cardiac output of (1) moderate sympathetic stimulation (from point A to point C), (2) maximal sympathetic stimulation (point D), and (3) sympathetic inhibition caused by total spinal anesthesia (point B). *Modified from Guyton, A.C., Jones, C.E., Coleman, T.B., 1973. Circulatory Physiology: Cardiac Output and its Regulation, second ed. W.B. Saunders, Philadelphia.*

normal *for short periods*, until other compensatory effects occur within seconds or minutes to return cardiac output to nearly normal.

Effect of Sympathetic Inhibition on Cardiac Output. The sympathetic nervous system can be blocked by inducing *total spinal anesthesia* or by using a drug, such as *hexamethonium*, that blocks transmission of nerve signals through the autonomic ganglia. The lowermost curves in Figure 36-12 show the effect of sympathetic inhibition caused by total spinal anesthesia demonstrating that (1) the *Psf falls to about 4 mmHg* and (2) the *effectiveness of the heart as a pump decreases to about 80% of normal*. The cardiac output falls from point A to point B, which is a decrease to about 60% of normal.

Methods for Measuring Cardiac Output

In animal experiments, one can cannulate the aorta, pulmonary artery, or great veins entering the heart and measure the cardiac output using a flowmeter. An electromagnetic or ultrasonic flowmeter can also be placed on the aorta or pulmonary artery to measure cardiac output.

In humans, except in rare instances, cardiac output is measured by indirect methods that do not require surgery. Two of the methods that have been used for experimental studies are the *oxygen Fick method* and the *indicator dilution method*.

Cardiac output can also be estimated by *echocardiography*, a method that uses ultrasound waves from a transducer placed on the chest wall or passed into the patient's esophagus to measure the size of the heart's chambers, as well as the velocity of blood flowing from the left ventricle into the aorta. Stroke volume is calculated from the velocity of blood flowing into the aorta and the aorta cross-sectional area determined from the aorta diameter that is measured by ultrasound imaging. Cardiac output is then calculated from the product of the stroke volume and the heart rate.

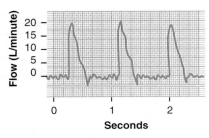

Figure 36-13 Pulsatile blood flow in the root of the aorta recorded using an electromagnetic flowmeter.

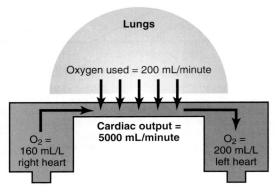

Figure 36-14 Fick principle for determining cardiac output.

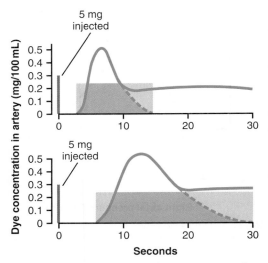

Figure 36-15 *Extrapolated dye concentration curves* used to calculate two separate cardiac outputs by the dilution method. (The rectangular areas are the calculated average concentrations of dye in the arterial blood for the durations of the respective extrapolated curves.)

PULSATILE OUTPUT OF THE HEART MEASURED BY AN ELECTROMAGNETIC OR ULTRASONIC FLOWMETER

Figure 36-13 shows a recording in a dog of blood flow in the root of the aorta; this recording was made using an electromagnetic flowmeter. It demonstrates that the blood flow rises rapidly to a peak during systole, and then at the end of systole it reverses for a fraction of a second. This reverse flow causes the aortic valve to close and the flow to return to zero.

MEASUREMENT OF CARDIAC OUTPUT USING THE OXYGEN FICK PRINCIPLE

The Fick principle is explained by Figure 36-14. This figure shows that 200 mL of oxygen is being absorbed from the lungs into the pulmonary blood each minute. It also shows that the blood entering the right heart has an oxygen concentration of 160 mL/L of blood, whereas that leaving the left heart has an oxygen concentration of 200 mL/L of blood. From these data, one can calculate that each liter of blood passing through the lungs absorbs 40 mL of oxygen.

Because the total quantity of oxygen absorbed into the blood from the lungs each minute is 200 mL, dividing 200 by 40 calculates a total of five 1-L portions of blood that must pass through the pulmonary circulation each minute to absorb this amount of oxygen. Therefore, the quantity of blood flowing through the lungs each minute is 5 L, which is also a measure of the cardiac output. Thus, the cardiac output can be calculated by the following formula:

$$\text{Cardiac output (L/min)} = \frac{\text{O}_2 \text{ absorbed per minute by the lungs (mL/min)}}{\text{arteriovenous O}_2 \text{ difference (mL/L of blood)}}$$

By applying this Fick procedure for measuring cardiac output in humans, *mixed venous blood* is usually obtained through a catheter inserted up the brachial vein of the forearm, through the subclavian vein, down to the right atrium, and, finally, into the right ventricle or pulmonary artery. *Systemic arterial blood* can then be obtained from any systemic artery in the body. The *rate of oxygen absorption* by the lungs is measured by the rate of disappearance of oxygen from the respired air, using any type of oxygen meter.

INDICATOR DILUTION METHOD FOR MEASURING CARDIAC OUTPUT

To measure cardiac output by the "indicator dilution method," a small amount of *indicator*, such as a dye, is injected into a large systemic vein or, preferably, into the right atrium. This indicator passes rapidly through the right side of the heart, then through the blood vessels of the lungs, through the left side of the heart, and, finally, into the systemic arterial system. The concentration of the dye is recorded as the dye passes through one of the peripheral arteries, giving a curve as shown in Figure 36-15. In each of these instances, 5 mg of Cardiogreen dye was injected at zero time. In the top recording, none of the dye passed into the arterial tree until about 3 seconds after the injection, but then the arterial concentration of the dye rose rapidly to a maximum in about 6–7 seconds. After that, the concentration fell rapidly, but before the concentration reached zero, some of the dye had already circulated all the way through some of the peripheral systemic vessels and returned through the heart for a second time. Consequently, the dye concentration in the artery began to rise again. For the purpose of calculation, it is necessary to *extrapolate* the early downslope of the curve to the zero point, as shown by the dashed portion of each curve. In this way, the *extrapolated time–concentration curve* of the dye in the systemic artery without recirculation can be measured in its first portion and estimated reasonably accurately in its latter portion.

Once the extrapolated time–concentration curve has been determined, one then calculates the mean concentration of dye in the arterial blood for the duration of the curve. For instance, in the top example of Figure 36-15, this calculation was done by measuring the area under the entire initial and extrapolated curves and then averaging the concentration of dye for the duration of the curve; one can see from the shaded rectangle straddling the curve in the upper figure that the average concentration of dye was 0.25 mg/dL of blood and that the duration of this average value was 12 seconds. A total of 5 mg of dye had been injected at the beginning of the experiment. For blood carrying only 0.25 mg of dye in each 100 mL to carry the entire 5 mg of dye through the heart and lungs in 12 seconds, a total of 20 portions each with 100 mL of blood would have passed through the heart during the 12 seconds, which would be the same as a cardiac output of 2 L/12 seconds, or 10 L/minute. We leave it to the reader to calculate the cardiac output from the bottom *extrapolated* curve of Figure 36-15. To summarize, the cardiac output can be determined using the following formula:

$$\text{Cardiac output (mL/min)} = \frac{\text{milligrams of dye injected} \times 60}{\substack{\text{(average concentration of dye in each milliliter} \\ \text{of blood for the duration of the curve)} \times \\ \text{(duration of the curve in seconds)}}}$$

BIBLIOGRAPHY

Guyton AC: Determination of cardiac output by equating venous return curves with cardiac response curves, *Physiol. Rev.* 35:123, 1955.

Guyton AC: Venous return, Hamilton WF, editor: *Handbook of Physiology, Section 2*, vol. 2, Baltimore, 1963, Williams & Wilkins, p. 1099.

Guyton AC, Lindsey AW, Kaufmann BN: Effect of mean circulatory filling pressure and other peripheral circulatory factors on cardiac output, *Am. J. Physiol.* 180:463-468, 1955.

Guyton AC, Jones CE, Coleman TG: *Circulatory Physiology: Cardiac Output and its Regulation*, Philadelphia, 1973, W.B. Saunders.

Hall JE: Integration and regulation of cardiovascular function, *Am. J. Physiol.* 277:S174, 1999.

Hall JE: The pioneering use of systems analysis to study cardiac output regulation, *Am. J. Physiol. Regul. Integr. Comp. Physiol.* 287:R1009, 2004.

Hollenberg SM: Hemodynamic monitoring, *Chest* 143:1480, 2013.

Koch WJ, Lefkowitz RJ, Rockman HA: Functional consequences of altering myocardial adrenergic receptor signaling, *Annu. Rev. Physiol.* 62:237, 2000.

Rothe CF: Reflex control of veins and vascular capacitance, *Physiol. Rev.* 63:1281, 1983.

Sarnoff SJ, Berglund E: Ventricular function. 1. Starling's law of the heart, studied by means of simultaneous right and left ventricular function curves in the dog, *Circulation* 9:706, 1953.

Uemura K, Sugimachi M, Kawada T, et al: A novel framework of circulatory equilibrium, *Am. J. Physiol. Heart Circ. Physiol.* 286:H2376, 2004.

Vatner SF, Braunwald E: Cardiovascular control mechanisms in the conscious state, *N. Engl. J. Med.* 293:970, 1975.

Regulation of Cardiac Output

When a person is at rest, the heart pumps only 4–6 L of blood each minute. During severe exercise, the heart may be required to pump four to seven times this amount. The basic means by which the volume pumped by the heart is regulated are (1) intrinsic cardiac regulation of pumping in response to changes in volume of blood flowing into the heart and (2) control of heart rate and strength of heart pumping by the autonomic nervous system.

Intrinsic Regulation of Heart Pumping—The Frank–Starling Mechanism

Under most conditions, the amount of blood pumped by the heart each minute is normally determined almost entirely by the rate of blood flow into the heart from the veins, which is called *venous return*. That is, each peripheral tissue of the body controls its own local blood flow, and all the local tissue flows combine and return by way of the veins to the right atrium. The heart, in turn, automatically pumps this incoming blood into the arteries so that it can flow around the circuit again.

This intrinsic ability of the heart to adapt to increasing volumes of inflowing blood is called the *Frank–Starling mechanism of the heart*, in honor of Otto Frank and Ernest Starling, two great physiologists of a century ago. Basically, the Frank–Starling mechanism means that the greater the heart muscle is stretched during filling, the greater is the force of contraction and the greater the quantity of blood pumped into the aorta.

Since this regulation of stroke volume is based on changing length of the muscle fiber, it is often referred to as *heterometric regulation*. Stated another way: *Within physiological limits, the heart pumps all the blood that returns to it by the way of the veins.*

What Is the Explanation of the Frank–Starling Mechanism?

When an extra amount of blood flows into the ventricles, the cardiac muscle is stretched to a greater length. This stretching in turn causes the muscle to contract with increased force because the actin and myosin filaments are brought to a more nearly optimal degree of overlap for force generation. Therefore, the ventricle, because of its increased pumping, automatically pumps the extra blood into the arteries.

This ability of stretched muscle, up to an optimal length, to contract with increased work output is characteristic of all striated muscle and is not simply a characteristic of cardiac muscle.

In addition to the important effect of lengthening the heart muscle, still another factor increases heart pumping when its volume is increased. Stretch of the right atrial wall directly increases the heart rate by 10–20% through the Bainbridge reflex, which also helps increase the amount of blood pumped each minute, although its contribution is much less than that of the Frank–Starling mechanism.

VENTRICULAR FUNCTION CURVES

One of the best ways to express the functional ability of the ventricles to pump blood is by *ventricular function curves*. Figure 37-1 shows a type of ventricular function curve called the *stroke work output curve*. Note that as the atrial pressure for each side of the heart increases, the stroke work output for that side increases until it reaches the limit of the ventricle's pumping ability.

Figure 37-2 shows another type of ventricular function curve called the *ventricular volume output curve*. The two curves of this figure represent function of the two ventricles of the human heart based on data extrapolated from experimental animal studies. As the right and left atrial pressures increase, the respective ventricular volume outputs per minute also increase.

Thus, *ventricular function curves* are another way of expressing the Frank–Starling mechanism of the heart. That is, as the ventricles fill in response to higher atrial pressures, each ventricular volume and strength of cardiac muscle contraction increases causing the heart to pump increased quantities of blood into the arteries.

CONTROL OF THE HEART BY THE SYMPATHETIC AND PARASYMPATHETIC NERVES

The pumping effectiveness of the heart also is controlled by the *sympathetic* and *parasympathetic (vagus)* nerves, which

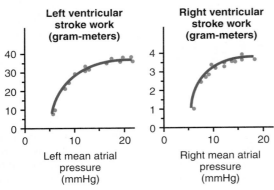

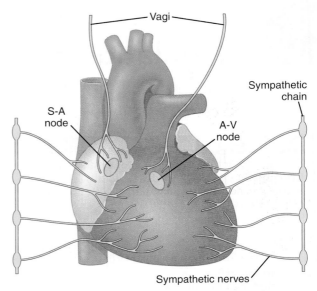

Figure 37-1 Left and right ventricular function curves recorded from dogs, depicting *ventricular stroke work output* as a function of left and right mean atrial pressures. *Data from Sarnoff, S.J., 1955. Myocardial contractility as described by ventricular function curves. Physiol. Rev. 35, 107.*

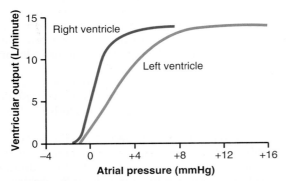

Figure 37-2 Approximate normal right and left *ventricular volume output curves* for the normal resting human heart as extrapolated from data obtained in dogs and data from human beings.

Figure 37-3 Cardiac *sympathetic* and *parasympathetic* nerves. (The vagus nerves to the heart are parasympathetic nerves.) *A-V*, atrioventricular; *S-A*, sinoatrial.

decreasing the level of cardiac pumping as much as 30% below normal.

Parasympathetic (Vagal) Stimulation Reduces Heart Rate and Strength of Contraction

Strong stimulation of the parasympathetic nerve fibers in the vagus nerves to the heart can stop the heartbeat for a few seconds, but then the heart usually "escapes" and beats at a rate of 20–40 beats/minute as long as the parasympathetic stimulation continues. In addition, strong vagal stimulation can decrease the strength of heart muscle contraction by 20–30%.

The vagal fibers are distributed mainly to the atria and not much to the ventricles, where the power contraction of the heart occurs. This distribution explains why the effect of vagal stimulation is mainly to decrease the heart rate rather than to decrease greatly the strength of heart contraction. Nevertheless, the great decrease in heart rate combined with a slight decrease in heart contraction strength can decrease ventricular pumping 50% or more.

Effect of Sympathetic or Parasympathetic Stimulation on the Cardiac Function Curve

Figure 37-4 shows four cardiac function curves. These curves are similar to the ventricular function curves of Figure 37-2. However, they represent function of the entire heart rather than of a single ventricle. They show the relation between right atrial pressure at the input of the right heart and cardiac output from the left ventricle into the aorta.

The curves of Figure 37-4 demonstrate that at any given right atrial pressure, the cardiac output increases during increased sympathetic stimulation and decreases during increased parasympathetic stimulation. These changes in output caused by autonomic nervous system stimulation result both from *changes in heart rate* and from *changes in contractile strength of the heart*.

It is clear that the Frank–Starling mechanism of regulation of stroke volume can be modulated by the autonomic

abundantly supply the heart, as shown in Figure 37-3. For given levels of atrial pressure, the amount of blood pumped each minute (*cardiac output*) often can be increased more than 100% by sympathetic stimulation.

Mechanisms of Excitation of the Heart by the Sympathetic Nerves

Strong sympathetic stimulation can increase the heart rate in young adult humans from the normal rate of 70 up to 180–200 beats/minute and, rarely, even 250 beats/minute. Also, sympathetic stimulation increases the force of heart contraction (positive inotropy) to as much as double the normal rate, thereby increasing the volume of blood pumped and increasing the ejection pressure. Thus, sympathetic stimulation often can increase the maximum cardiac output as much as twofold to threefold, in addition to the increased output caused by the Frank–Starling mechanism already discussed.

Conversely, *inhibition* of the sympathetic nerves to the heart can decrease cardiac pumping to a moderate extent. Under normal conditions, the sympathetic nerve fibers to the heart discharge continuously at a slow rate that maintains pumping at about 30% above that with no sympathetic stimulation. Therefore, when the activity of the sympathetic nervous system is depressed below normal, both the heart rate and the strength of ventricular muscle contraction decrease, thereby

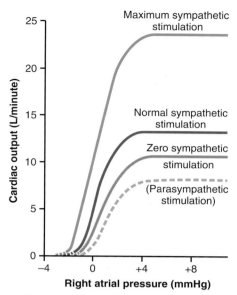

Figure 37-4 Effect on the cardiac output curve of different degrees of sympathetic or parasympathetic stimulation.

nervous system such that for a given degree of muscle stretch, the sympathetic nervous system increases contractility while the parasympathetic nervous system decreases contractility. Factors such as the autonomic nervous system and ions (discussed later) that alter stroke volume independent of the initial muscle length constitute the *homeometric regulation* of cardiac output.

Effect of Potassium and Calcium Ions on Heart Function

In the discussion of membrane potentials (see Chapters 7 and 31), it was pointed out that potassium ions have a marked effect on membrane potentials. Calcium ions (see Chapters 14 and 30) also play an especially important role in activating the muscle contractile process. Therefore, it is to be expected that the concentrations of each of these two ions in the extracellular fluids also have important effects on cardiac pumping.

Effect of Potassium Ions

Excess potassium in the extracellular fluids causes the heart to become dilated and flaccid, and also slows the heart rate. Large quantities of potassium can also block conduction of the cardiac impulse from the atria to the ventricles through the atrioventricular (A-V) bundle. Elevation of potassium concentration to only 8–12 mEq/L—two to three times the normal value—can cause severe weakness of the heart, abnormal rhythm, and death.

These effects result partially from the fact that a high potassium concentration in the extracellular fluids decreases the resting membrane potential in the cardiac muscle fibers. That is, high extracellular fluid potassium concentration partially depolarizes the cell membrane causing the membrane potential to be less negative. As the membrane potential decreases, the intensity of the action potential also decreases, which makes contraction of the heart progressively weaker.

Effect of Calcium Ions

Excess calcium ions have effects almost exactly opposite to those of potassium ions causing the heart to move toward spastic contraction. This effect is caused by a direct effect of calcium ions on the cardiac contractile process.

Conversely, deficiency of calcium ions causes cardiac *weakness*, similar to the effect of high potassium. Fortunately, calcium ion levels in the blood normally are regulated within a very narrow range. Therefore, cardiac effects of abnormal calcium concentrations are seldom of clinical concern.

Effect of Temperature on Heart Function

Increased body temperature, such as that which occurs when one has a fever, increases the heart rate, sometimes to double the normal rate. Decreased temperature greatly decreases the heart rate, which may fall to as low as a few beats per minute when a person is near death from hypothermia in the body temperature range of 60–70°F. These effects presumably result from the fact that heat increases the permeability of the cardiac muscle membrane to ions that control heart rate resulting in acceleration of the self-excitation process.

Contractile strength of the heart often is enhanced temporarily by a moderate increase in temperature, such as that which occurs during body exercise, but prolonged elevation of temperature exhausts the metabolic systems of the heart and eventually causes weakness. Therefore, optimal function of the heart depends greatly on proper control of body temperature by the temperature control mechanisms explained in Chapter 128.

Increasing the Arterial Pressure Load (Up to a Limit) Does Not Decrease the Cardiac Output

Note in Figure 37-5 that increasing the arterial pressure in the aorta does not decrease the cardiac output until the mean arterial pressure rises above about 160 mmHg. In other words, during normal function of the heart at normal systolic arterial pressures (80–140 mmHg), the cardiac output is determined almost entirely by the ease of blood flow through the body's tissues, which in turn controls *venous return* of blood to the heart.

The factors that affect cardiac output are summarized in Figure 37-6.

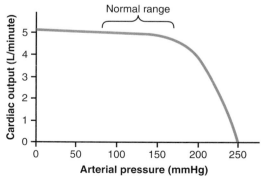

Figure 37-5 Constancy of cardiac output up to a pressure level of 160 mmHg. Only when the arterial pressure rises above this normal limit does the increasing pressure load cause the cardiac output to fall significantly.

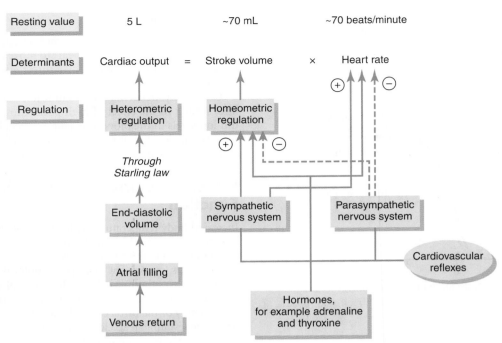

Figure 37-6 Summary of factors affecting cardiac output. Solid lines are stimulatory (ie, increase stroke volume or heart rate) while dotted lines are inhibitory.

BIBLIOGRAPHY

Chantler PD, Lakatta EG, Najjar SS: Arterial–ventricular coupling: mechanistic insights into cardiovascular performance at rest and during exercise, *J. Appl. Physiol.* 105:1342, 2008.

Fuchs F, Smith SH: Calcium, cross-bridges, and the Frank–Starling relationship, *News Physiol. Sci.* 16:5, 2001.

Guyton AC: Determination of cardiac output by equating venous return curves with cardiac response curves, *Physiol. Rev.* 35:123, 1955.

Guyton AC, Jones CE, Coleman TG: *Circulatory Physiology: Cardiac Output and its Regulation*, second ed., Philadelphia, 1973, W.B. Saunders.

Saks V, Dzeja P, Schlattner U, et al: Cardiac system bioenergetics: metabolic basis of the Frank–Starling law, *J. Physiol.* 571:253, 2006.

Sarnoff SJ: Myocardial contractility as described by ventricular function curves, *Physiol. Rev.* 35:107, 1955.

Starling EH: *The Linacre Lecture on the Law of the Heart*, London, 1918, Longmans Green.

Hemodynamics

Interrelationships of Pressure, Flow, and Resistance

Blood flow through a blood vessel is determined by two factors: (1) *pressure difference* of the blood between the two ends of the vessel, also sometimes called "pressure gradient" along the vessel, which pushes the blood through the vessel, and (2) the impediment to blood flow through the vessel, which is called *vascular resistance*. Figure 38-1 demonstrates these relationships showing a blood vessel segment located anywhere in the circulatory system.

P_1 represents the pressure at the origin of the vessel; at the other end, the pressure is P_2. Resistance occurs as a result of friction between the flowing blood and the intravascular endothelium all along the inside of the vessel. The flow through the vessel can be calculated by the following formula, which is called *Ohm's law*:

$$F = \frac{\Delta P}{R}$$

where F is blood flow, ΔP is the pressure difference ($P_1 - P_2$) between the two ends of the vessel, and R is the resistance. This formula states that the blood flow is directly proportional to the pressure difference but inversely proportional to the resistance.

Note that it is the *difference* in pressure between the two ends of the vessel, not the absolute pressure in the vessel, which determines rate of flow. For example, if the pressure at both ends of a vessel is 100 mmHg and yet no difference exists between the two ends, there will be no flow despite the presence of 100 mmHg pressure.

Ohm's law, illustrated in the preceding formula, expresses the most important of all the relations that the reader needs to understand to comprehend the hemodynamics of the circulation. Because of the extreme importance of this formula, the reader should also become familiar with its other algebraic forms:

$$\Delta P = F \times R$$

$$R = \frac{\Delta P}{F}$$

BLOOD FLOW

Blood flow means the quantity of blood that passes a given point in the circulation in a given period of time. Ordinarily, blood flow is expressed in *milliliters per minute* or *liters per minute*, but it can be expressed in milliliters per second or in any other units of flow and time.

The overall blood flow in the total circulation of an adult person at rest is about 5000 mL/minute. This is called the *cardiac output* because it is the amount of blood pumped into the aorta by the heart each minute.

Laminar Flow of Blood in Vessels. When blood flows at a steady rate through a long, smooth blood vessel, it flows in *streamlines*, with each layer of blood remaining the same distance from the vessel wall. Also, the central-most portion of the blood stays in the center of the vessel. This type of flow is called *laminar flow* or *streamline flow* and it is the opposite of *turbulent flow*, which is blood flowing in all directions in the vessel and continually mixing within the vessel, as discussed subsequently.

Parabolic Velocity Profile During Laminar Flow. When laminar flow occurs, the velocity of flow in the center of the vessel is far greater than that toward the outer edges. This phenomenon is demonstrated in Figure 38-2. In Figure 38-2A, a vessel contains two fluids, the one at the left colored by a dye and the one at the right a clear fluid, but there is no flow in the vessel. When the fluids are made to flow, a parabolic interface develops between them, as shown 1 second later in Figure 38-2B; the portion of fluid adjacent to the vessel wall has hardly moved, the portion slightly away from the wall has moved a small distance, and the portion in the center of the vessel has moved a long distance. This effect is called the "parabolic profile for velocity of blood flow."

The cause of the parabolic profile is the following: The fluid molecules touching the wall move slowly because of adherence to the vessel wall. The next layer of molecules slips over these, the third layer over the second, the fourth layer over the third, and so forth. Therefore, the fluid in the middle of the vessel can move rapidly because many layers of slipping molecules exist

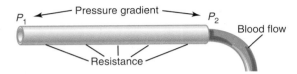

Figure 38-1 Interrelationships of pressure, resistance, and blood flow. P_1, pressure at the origin of the vessel; P_2, pressure at the other end of the vessel.

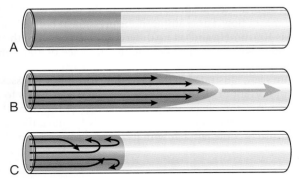

Figure 38-2 (A) Two fluids (one dyed red and the other clear) before flow begins; (B) the same fluids 1 second after flow begins; (C) turbulent flow with elements of the fluid moving in a disorderly pattern.

between the middle of the vessel and the vessel wall; thus, each layer toward the center flows progressively more rapidly than the outer layers.

Turbulent Flow of Blood Under Some Conditions. When the rate of blood flow becomes too great, when it passes by an obstruction in a vessel, when it makes a sharp turn, or when it passes over a rough surface, the flow may become *turbulent*, or disorderly, rather than streamlined (see Figure 38-2C). Turbulent flow means that the blood flows crosswise in the vessel and along the vessel, usually forming whorls in the blood, called *eddy currents*. These eddy currents are similar to the whirlpools that one frequently sees in a rapidly flowing river at a point of obstruction.

When eddy currents are present, the blood flows with much greater resistance than when the flow is streamlined because eddies add tremendously to the overall friction of flow in the vessel.

The tendency for turbulent flow increases in direct proportion to the velocity of blood flow, the diameter of the blood vessel, and the density of the blood and is inversely proportional to the viscosity of the blood, in accordance with the following equation:

$$Re = \frac{v \cdot d \cdot \rho}{\eta}$$

where Re is "*Reynolds*" *number* and is the measure of the tendency for turbulence to occur, v is the mean velocity of blood flow (in centimeters per second), d is the vessel diameter (in centimeters), ρ is density, and η is the viscosity (in poise). The viscosity of blood is normally about 1/30 P, and the density is only slightly greater than 1. When "Reynolds" number rises above 200–400, turbulent flow will occur at some branches of vessels but will die out along the smooth portions of the vessels. However, when "Reynolds" number rises above approximately 2000, turbulence will usually occur even in a straight, smooth vessel.

"Reynolds" number for flow in the vascular system normally rises to 200–400 even in large arteries; as a result there is almost always some turbulence of flow at the branches of these vessels. In the proximal portions of the aorta and pulmonary artery, "Reynolds" number can rise to several thousand during the rapid phase of ejection by the ventricles, which causes considerable turbulence in the proximal aorta and pulmonary artery where many conditions are appropriate for turbulence: (1) high velocity of blood flow, (2) pulsatile nature of the flow, (3) sudden change in vessel diameter, and (4) large vessel diameter. However, in small vessels, "Reynolds" number is almost never high enough to cause turbulence.

BLOOD PRESSURE

Standard Units of Pressure. Blood pressure almost always is measured in millimeters of mercury because the mercury manometer has been used as the standard reference for measuring pressure since its invention in 1846 by Poiseuille. Actually, blood pressure means the *force exerted by the blood against any unit area of the vessel wall*. When one says that the pressure in a vessel is 50 mmHg, this means that the force exerted is sufficient to push a column of mercury against gravity up to a level 50 mm high. If the pressure is 100 mmHg, it will push the column of mercury up to 100 mm.

Occasionally, pressure is measured in *centimeters of water*. A pressure of 10 cm H$_2$O means a pressure sufficient to raise a column of water against gravity to a height of 10 cm. *One millimeter of mercury pressure equals 1.36 cm water pressure* because the specific gravity of mercury is 13.6 times that of water and 1 cm is 10 times as great as 1 mm.

RESISTANCE TO BLOOD FLOW

Units of Resistance. Resistance is the impediment to blood flow in a vessel, but it cannot be measured by any direct means. Instead, resistance must be calculated from measurements of blood flow and pressure difference between two points in the vessel. If the pressure difference between two points is 1 mmHg and the flow is 1 mL/second, the resistance is said to be 1 *peripheral resistance unit*, usually abbreviated PRU.

Expression of Resistance in CGS Units. Occasionally, a basic physical unit called the CGS (centimeters, grams, seconds) unit is used to express resistance. This unit is dyne seconds/cm^5. Resistance in these units can be calculated by the following formula:

$$R \left(\text{in } \frac{\text{dyne second}}{\text{cm}^5} \right) = \frac{1333 \times \text{millimeters of mercury}}{\text{milliliter per second}}$$

Total Peripheral Vascular Resistance and Total Pulmonary Vascular Resistance. The rate of blood flow through the entire circulatory system is equal to the rate of blood pumping by the heart—that is, it is equal to the cardiac output. In the adult human being, this is approximately 100 mL/second. The pressure difference from the systemic arteries to the systemic veins is about 100 mmHg. Therefore, the resistance of the entire systemic circulation, called the *total peripheral resistance*, is about 100/100, or 1 PRU.

In conditions in which all the blood vessels throughout the body become strongly constricted, the total peripheral resistance occasionally rises to as high as 4 PRU. Conversely, when the vessels become greatly dilated, the resistance can fall to as little as 0.2 PRU.

In the pulmonary system, the mean pulmonary arterial pressure averages 16 mmHg and the mean left atrial pressure

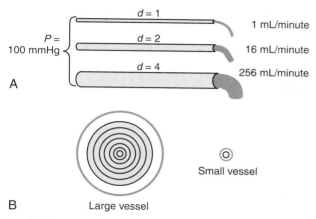

Figure 38-3 (A) Demonstration of the effect of vessel diameter on blood flow; (B) concentric rings of blood flowing at different velocities; the farther away from the vessel wall, the faster is the flow. *d*, diameter; *P*, pressure difference between the two ends of the vessels.

averages 2 mmHg, giving a net pressure difference of 14 mm. Therefore, when the cardiac output is normal at about 100 mL/second, the *total pulmonary vascular resistance* calculates to be about 0.14 PRU (about one-seventh that in the systemic circulation).

"Conductance" of Blood in a Vessel Is the Reciprocal of Resistance. Conductance is a measure of the blood flow through a vessel for a given pressure difference. This measurement is generally expressed in terms of milliliters per second per millimeter of mercury pressure, but it can also be expressed in terms of liters per second per millimeter of mercury or in any other units of blood flow and pressure.

It is evident that conductance is the exact reciprocal of resistance in accord with the following equation:

$$\text{Conductance} = \frac{1}{\text{resistance}}$$

Small Changes in Vessel Diameter Markedly Change its Conductance. Small changes in the diameter of a vessel cause tremendous changes in the vessel's ability to conduct blood when the blood flow is streamlined. This phenomenon is demonstrated by the experiment illustrated in Figure 38-3A, which shows three vessels with relative diameters of 1, 2, and 4 but with the same pressure difference of 100 mmHg between the two ends of the vessels. Although the diameters of these vessels increase only 4-fold, the respective flows are 1, 16, and 256 mL/minute, which is a 256-fold increase in flow. Thus, the conductance of the vessel increases in proportion to the *fourth power of the diameter*, in accordance with the following formula:

$$\text{Conductance} \propto \text{diameter}^4$$

Poiseuille's Law. The cause of this great increase in conductance when the diameter increases can be explained by referring to Figure 38-3B, which shows cross-sections of a large and a small vessel. The concentric rings inside the vessels indicate that the velocity of flow in each ring is different from that in the adjacent rings because of *laminar* flow, which was discussed earlier in the chapter. That is, the blood in the ring touching the wall

of the vessel is barely flowing because of its adherence to the vascular endothelium. The next ring of blood toward the center of the vessel slips past the first ring and, therefore, flows more rapidly. The third, fourth, fifth, and sixth rings likewise flow at progressively increasing velocities. Thus, the blood that is near the wall of the vessel flows slowly, whereas that in the middle of the vessel flows much more rapidly.

In the small vessel, essentially all the blood is near the wall, so the extremely rapidly flowing central stream of blood simply does not exist. By integrating the velocities of all the concentric rings of flowing blood and multiplying them by the areas of the rings, one can derive the following formula, known as Poiseuille's law:

$$F \to \frac{\pi \Delta P r^4}{8 \eta l}$$

where F is the rate of blood flow, ΔP is the pressure difference between the ends of the vessel, r is the radius of the vessel, l is length of the vessel, and η is viscosity of the blood.

Note particularly in this equation that the rate of blood flow is directly proportional to the *fourth power of the radius* of the vessel, which demonstrates once again that the diameter of a blood vessel (which is equal to twice the radius) plays by far the greatest role of all factors in determining the rate of blood flow through a vessel.

Importance of the Vessel Diameter "Fourth Power Law" in Determining Arteriolar Resistance. In the systemic circulation, about two-thirds of the total systemic resistance to blood flow is arteriolar resistance in the small arterioles. The internal diameters of the arterioles range from as little as 4 μm to as great as 25 μm. However, their strong vascular walls allow the internal diameters to change tremendously, often as much as fourfold. From the fourth power law discussed earlier that relates blood flow to diameter of the vessel, one can see that a 4-fold increase in vessel diameter can increase the flow as much as 256-fold. Thus, this fourth power law makes it possible for the arterioles, responding with only small changes in diameter to nervous signals or local tissue chemical signals, either to turn off almost completely the blood flow to the tissue or at the other extreme to cause a vast increase in flow. Indeed, ranges of blood flow of more than 100-fold in separate tissue areas have been recorded between the limits of maximum arteriolar constriction and maximum arteriolar dilation.

Resistance to Blood Flow in Series and Parallel Vascular Circuits. Blood pumped by the heart flows from the high-pressure part of the systemic circulation (ie, aorta) to the low-pressure side (ie, vena cava) through many miles of blood vessels arranged in series and in parallel. The arteries, arterioles, capillaries, venules, and veins are collectively arranged in series. When blood vessels are arranged in series, flow through each blood vessel is the same and the total resistance to blood flow (R_{total}) is equal to the sum of the resistances of each vessel:

$$R_{\text{total}} = R_1 + R_2 + R_3 + R_4 \cdots$$

The total peripheral vascular resistance is therefore equal to the sum of resistances of the arteries, arterioles, capillaries, venules, and veins. In the example shown in Figure 38-4A, the total vascular resistance is equal to the sum of R_1 and R_2.

Blood vessels branch extensively to form parallel circuits that supply blood to the many organs and tissues of the body. This

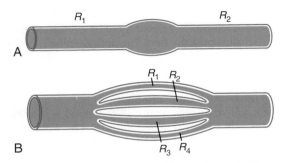

Figure 38-4 Vascular resistances (R): (A) in series and (B) in parallel.

parallel arrangement permits each tissue to regulate its own blood flow, to a great extent, independently of flow to other tissues.

For blood vessels arranged in parallel (Figure 38-4B), the total resistance to blood flow is expressed as follows:

$$\frac{1}{R_{total}} = \frac{1}{R_1} + \frac{1}{R_2} + \frac{1}{R_3} + \frac{1}{R_4} \cdots$$

It is obvious that for a given pressure gradient, far greater amounts of blood will flow through this parallel system than through any of the individual blood vessels. Therefore, the total resistance is far less than the resistance of any single blood vessel. Flow through each of the parallel vessels in Figure 38-4B is determined by the pressure gradient and its own resistance, not the resistance of the other parallel blood vessels. However, increasing the resistance of any of the blood vessels increases the total vascular resistance.

It may seem paradoxical that adding more blood vessels to a circuit reduces the total vascular resistance. Many parallel blood vessels, however, make it easier for blood to flow through the circuit because each parallel vessel provides another pathway, or *conductance*, for blood flow. The total conductance (C_{total}) for blood flow is the sum of the conductance of each parallel pathway:

$$C_{total} = C_1 + C_2 + C_3 + C_4 \cdots$$

For example, brain, kidney, muscle, gastrointestinal, skin, and coronary circulations are arranged in parallel, and each tissue contributes to the overall conductance of the systemic circulation. Blood flow through each tissue is a fraction of the total blood flow (cardiac output) and is determined by the resistance (the reciprocal of conductance) for blood flow in the tissue, as well as the pressure gradient. Therefore, amputation of a limb or surgical removal of a kidney also removes a parallel circuit and reduces the total vascular conductance and total blood flow (ie, cardiac output) while increasing total peripheral vascular resistance.

Effect of Blood Hematocrit and Blood Viscosity on Vascular Resistance and Blood Flow

Note that another important factor in Poiseuille's equation is the viscosity of the blood. The greater the viscosity, the lower is the flow in a vessel if all other factors are constant. Furthermore, *the viscosity of normal blood is about three times as great as the viscosity of water.*

What makes the blood so viscous? It is mainly the large numbers of suspended red cells in the blood, each of which exerts frictional drag against adjacent cells and against the wall of the blood vessel.

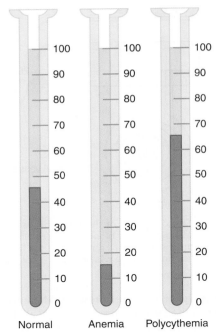

Figure 38-5 Hematocrits in a healthy (normal) person and in patients with anemia and polycythemia. The numbers refer to percentage of the blood composed of red blood cells.

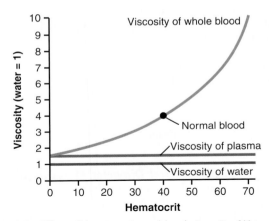

Figure 38-6 Effect of hematocrit on blood viscosity. (Water viscosity = 1.)

Hematocrit—The Proportion of Blood that Is Red Blood Cells.
If a person has a hematocrit of 40, this means that 40% of the blood volume is cells and the remainder is plasma. The hematocrit of adult men averages about 42, whereas that of women averages about 38. These values vary tremendously depending on whether the person has anemia, the degree of bodily activity, and the altitude at which the person resides. These changes in hematocrit are discussed in relation to the red blood cells and their oxygen transport function in Chapter 59.

Hematocrit is determined by centrifuging blood in a calibrated tube, as shown in Figure 38-5. The calibration allows direct reading of the percentage of cells.

Increasing Hematocrit Markedly Increases Blood Viscosity.
The viscosity of blood increases drastically as the hematocrit increases, as shown in Figure 38-6. The viscosity of whole blood at normal hematocrit is about 3–4, which means that three to four

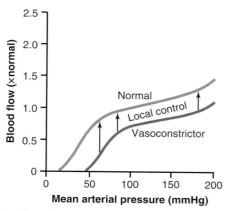

Figure 38-7 Effect of changes in arterial pressure over a period of several minutes on blood flow in a tissue such as skeletal muscle. Note that between pressure of 70 and 175 mmHg blood flow is "autoregulated." The *blue line* shows the effect of sympathetic nerve stimulation or vasoconstriction by hormones such as norepinephrine, angiotensin II, vasopressin, or endothelin on this relationship. Reduced tissue blood flow is rarely maintained for more than a few hours because of the activation of local autoregulatory mechanisms that eventually return blood flow toward normal.

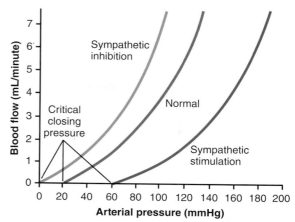

Figure 38-8 Effect of arterial pressure on blood flow through a *passive* blood vessel at different degrees of vascular tone caused by increased or decreased sympathetic stimulation of the vessel.

times as much pressure is required to force whole blood as to force water through the same blood vessel. When the hematocrit rises to 60–70, which it often does in persons with polycythemia, the blood viscosity can become as great as 10 times that of water and its flow through blood vessels is greatly retarded.

Other factors that affect blood viscosity are the plasma protein concentration and types of proteins in the plasma, but these effects are so much less than the effect of hematocrit that they are not significant considerations in most hemodynamic studies. The viscosity of blood plasma is about 1.5 times that of water.

EFFECTS OF PRESSURE ON VASCULAR RESISTANCE AND TISSUE BLOOD FLOW

"Autoregulation" Attenuates the Effect of Arterial Pressure on Tissue Blood Flow. From the discussion thus far, one might expect an increase in arterial pressure to cause a proportionate increase in blood flow through the various tissues of the body. However, the effect of arterial pressure on blood flow in many tissues is usually far less than one might expect, as shown in Figure 38-7. The reason for this is that an increase in arterial pressure not only increases the force that pushes blood through the vessels but also initiates compensatory increases in vascular resistance within a few seconds through activation of the local control mechanisms. Conversely, with reductions in arterial pressure vascular resistance is promptly reduced in most tissues and blood flow is maintained at a relatively constant rate. The ability of each tissue to adjust its vascular resistance and to maintain normal blood flow during changes in arterial pressure between approximately 70 and 175 mmHg is called blood flow autoregulation.

Note in Figure 38-7 that changes in blood flow can be caused by strong sympathetic stimulation, which *constricts* the blood vessels. Likewise, hormonal vasoconstrictors, such as *norepinephrine, angiotensin II, vasopressin,* or *endothelin,* can also reduce blood flow, at least transiently.

Blood flow changes in tissue blood flow rarely last for more than a few hours in most tissues even when increases in arterial pressure or increased levels of vasoconstrictors are sustained. The reason for the relative constancy of blood flow is that each tissue's local autoregulatory mechanisms eventually override most of the effects of vasoconstrictors to provide a blood flow that is appropriate for the needs of the tissue.

Pressure–Flow Relationship in Passive Vascular Beds. In isolated blood vessels or in tissues that do not exhibit autoregulation, changes in arterial pressure may have important effects on blood flow. In fact, the effect of pressure on blood flow may be greater than predicted by Poiseuille's equation, as shown by the upward curving lines in Figure 38-8. The reason for this is that increased arterial pressure not only increases the force that pushes blood through the vessels but also distends the elastic vessels, actually *decreasing* vascular resistance. Conversely, decreased arterial pressure in passive blood vessels increases resistance as the elastic vessels gradually collapse due to reduced distending pressure. When pressure falls below a critical level, called the *critical closing pressure,* flow ceases as the blood vessels are completely collapsed.

Sympathetic stimulation and other vasoconstrictors can alter the passive pressure–flow relationship shown in Figure 38-8. Thus, *inhibition of* sympathetic activity *greatly dilates* the vessels and can increase the blood flow twofold or more. Conversely, very strong sympathetic stimulation *can constrict* the vessels so much that blood flow occasionally decreases to as low as zero for a few seconds despite high arterial pressure.

In reality, there are few physiological conditions in which tissues display the passive pressure–flow relationship shown in Figure 38-8. Even in tissues that do not effectively autoregulate blood flow during acute changes in arterial pressure, blood flow is regulated according to the needs of the tissue when the pressure changes are sustained.

BIBLIOGRAPHY

See bibliography for Chapter 42.

39

Microcirculation

LEARNING OBJECTIVES

- Describe the structure of the microcirculation.
- List the functions of the microcirculation.
- Describe how blood flow through the microcirculation is controlled.
- List Starling forces and their role in capillary fluid exchange.
- List the factors that affect the exchange of nutrients in the capillaries.

GLOSSARY OF TERMS

- **Filtration coefficient:** A measure of a membrane's permeability to water (a higher coefficient indicates greater water permeability)

- **Hydrostatic pressure:** Force exerted by the blood volume on the vessel wall

- **Osmotic pressure:** The pressure exerted by a solution to prevent osmosis into that solution [it is a colligative property (depends on the molar concentration of the solute)]

- **Starling forces:** Those pressures that regulate the flow of fluid across the capillary membrane and include the hydrostatic pressures in the capillary and interstitial fluid, and the osmotic pressures in the capillary and interstitial fluid

The most purposeful function of the microcirculation is *transport of nutrients to the tissues and removal of cell excreta*. The small arterioles control blood flow to each tissue and local conditions in the tissues in turn control the diameters of the arterioles. The walls of the capillaries are thin and constructed of single-layer, highly permeable endothelial cells. Therefore, water, cell nutrients, and cell excreta can all interchange quickly and easily between the tissues and the circulating blood.

The peripheral circulation of the entire body has about 10 billion capillaries with a total surface area estimated to be 500–700 m^2 (about one-eighth the surface area of a football field). Indeed, it is rare that any single functional cell of the body is more than 20–30 μm away from a capillary.

Structure of the Microcirculation and Capillary System

The microcirculation of each organ is organized to serve that organ's specific needs. In general, each nutrient artery entering an organ branches six to eight times before the arteries become small enough to be called *arterioles*, which generally have internal diameters of only 10–15 μm. Then the arterioles themselves branch two to five times, reaching diameters of 5–9 μm at their ends where they supply blood to the capillaries.

The arterioles are highly muscular and their diameters can change manyfold. The metarterioles (the terminal arterioles) do not have a continuous muscular coat, but smooth muscle fibers encircle the vessel at intermittent points, as shown in Figure 39-1.

At the point where each true capillary originates from a metarteriole, a smooth muscle fiber usually encircles the capillary. This structure is called the *precapillary sphincter*. This sphincter can open and close the entrance to the capillary.

The venules are larger than the arterioles and have a much weaker muscular coat. Yet the pressure in the venules is much less than that in the arterioles, so the venules can still contract considerably despite the weak muscle.

This typical arrangement of the capillary bed is not found in all parts of the body, although a similar arrangement may serve the same purposes. Most important, the metarterioles and the precapillary sphincters are in close contact with the tissues they serve. Therefore, the local conditions of the tissues—the concentrations of nutrients, end products of metabolism, hydrogen ions, and so forth—can cause direct effects on the vessels to control local blood flow in each small tissue area.

Structure of the Capillary Wall. Figure 39-2 shows the ultramicroscopic structure of typical endothelial cells in the capillary wall as found in most organs of the body, especially in

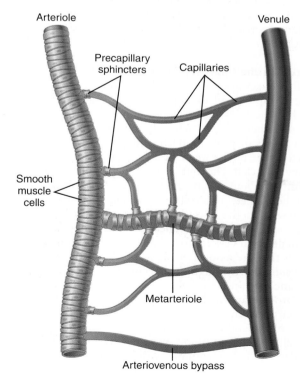

Figure 39-1 Structure of the mesenteric capillary bed.

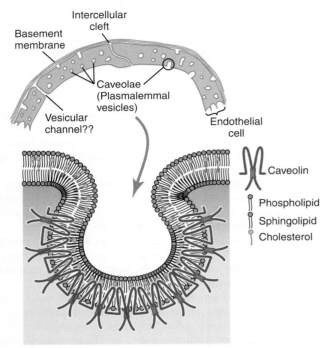

Figure 39-2 Structure of the capillary wall. Note especially the *intercellular cleft* at the junction between adjacent endothelial cells; it is believed that most water-soluble substances diffuse through the capillary membrane along the clefts. Small membrane invaginations, called *caveolae*, are believed to play a role in transporting macromolecules across the cell membrane. Caveolae contain caveolins, which are proteins that interact with cholesterol and polymerize to form the caveolae.

muscles and connective tissue. Note that the wall is composed of a unicellular layer of endothelial cells and is surrounded by a thin basement membrane on the outside of the capillary. The total thickness of the capillary wall is only about 0.5 μm. The internal diameter of the capillary is 4–9 μm, barely large enough for red blood cells and other blood cells to squeeze through.

"Pores" in the Capillary Membrane. Figure 39-2 shows two small passageways connecting the interior of the capillary with the exterior. One of these passageways is an *intercellular cleft*, which is the thin-slit, curving channel that lies between adjacent endothelial cells. Each cleft is interrupted periodically by short ridges of protein attachments that hold the endothelial cells together, but between these ridges fluid can percolate freely through the cleft. The cleft normally has a uniform spacing with a width of about 6–7 nm (60–70 Å), which is slightly smaller than the diameter of an albumin protein molecule.

Present in the endothelial cells are many minute *plasmalemmal vesicles*, also called *caveolae (small caves)*. These plasmalemmal vesicles form oligomers of proteins called *caveolins* that are associated with molecules of *cholesterol* and *sphingolipids*. Although the precise functions of caveolae are still unclear, they are believed to play a role in *endocytosis* (the process by which the cell engulfs material from outside the cell) and *transcytosis* of macromolecules across the interior of the endothelial cells. The caveolae at the surface of the cell appear to imbibe small packets of plasma or extracellular fluid that contain plasma proteins. These vesicles can then move slowly through the endothelial cell. Some of these vesicles may coalesce to form *vesicular channels* all the

way through the endothelial cell, which is demonstrated in Figure 39-2.

Special Types of "Pores" Occur in the Capillaries of Certain Organs. The "pores" in the capillaries of some organs have special characteristics to meet the peculiar needs of the organs. Some of these characteristics are as follows:

1. In the *brain*, the junctions between the capillary endothelial cells are mainly "tight" junctions that allow only extremely small molecules such as water, oxygen, and carbon dioxide to pass into or out of the brain tissues.
2. In the *liver*, the opposite is true. The clefts between the capillary endothelial cells are wide open so that almost all dissolved substances of the plasma, including the plasma proteins, can pass from the blood into the liver tissues.
3. The pores of the *gastrointestinal capillary membranes* are midway in size between those of the muscles and those of the liver.
4. In the *glomerular capillaries of the kidney*, numerous small oval windows called *fenestrae* penetrate all the way through the middle of the endothelial cells so that tremendous amounts of small molecular and ionic substances (but not the large molecules of the plasma proteins) can filter through the glomeruli without having to pass through the clefts between the endothelial cells.

Flow of Blood in the Capillaries— Vasomotion

Blood usually does not flow continuously through the capillaries. Instead, it flows intermittently, turning on and off every few seconds or minutes. The cause of this intermittency is the phenomenon called *vasomotion*, which means intermittent contraction of the metarterioles and precapillary sphincters (and sometimes even the very small arterioles).

Regulation of Vasomotion. The most important factor affecting the degree of opening and closing of the metarterioles and precapillary sphincters that has been found thus far is the concentration of *oxygen* in the tissues. When the rate of oxygen usage by the tissue is high so that tissue oxygen concentration decreases below normal, the intermittent periods of capillary blood flow occur more often, and the duration of each period of flow lasts longer, thereby allowing the capillary blood to carry increased quantities of oxygen (as well as other nutrients) to the tissues.

AVERAGE FUNCTION OF THE CAPILLARY SYSTEM

Despite the fact that blood flow through each capillary is intermittent, so many capillaries are present in the tissues that their overall function becomes averaged. That is, there is an *average rate of blood flow* through each tissue capillary bed, an *average capillary pressure* within the capillaries, and an *average rate of transfer of substances* between the blood of the capillaries and the surrounding interstitial fluid. In the remainder of this chapter, we are concerned with these averages, although one should remember that the average functions are, in reality, the functions of literally billions of individual capillaries, each operating intermittently in response to local conditions in the tissues.

Exchange of Water, Nutrients, and Other Substances Between the Blood and Interstitial Fluid

DIFFUSION THROUGH THE CAPILLARY MEMBRANE

By far the most important means by which substances are transferred between the plasma and the interstitial fluid is *diffusion*. Figure 39-3 illustrates this process, showing that as the blood flows along the lumen of the capillary, large numbers of water molecules and dissolved particles diffuse back and forth through the capillary wall providing continual mixing between the interstitial fluid and the plasma. *Diffusion results from thermal motion of the water molecules and dissolved substances in the fluid*, with the different molecules and ions moving first in one direction and then another, bouncing randomly in every direction.

Lipid-Soluble Substances Diffuse Directly Through the Cell Membranes of the Capillary Endothelium. If a substance is lipid soluble, it can diffuse directly through the cell membranes of the capillary without having to go through the pores. Such substances include *oxygen* and *carbon dioxide*. Because these substances can permeate all areas of the capillary membrane, their rates of transport through the capillary membrane are many times faster than the rates for lipid-insoluble substances, such as sodium ions and glucose that can go only through the pores.

Water-Soluble, Nonlipid-Soluble Substances Diffuse Through Intercellular "Pores" in the Capillary Membrane. Many substances needed by the tissues are soluble in water but cannot pass through the lipid membranes of the endothelial cells; such substances include *water molecules, sodium ions, chloride ions,* and *glucose*. Although only 1/1000 of the surface area of the capillaries is represented by the intercellular clefts between the endothelial cells, the velocity of thermal molecular motion in the clefts is so great that even this small area is sufficient to allow tremendous diffusion of water and water-soluble substances through these cleft pores. To give one an idea of the rapidity with which these substances diffuse, *the rate at which*

TABLE 39-1	Relative Permeability of Skeletal Muscle Capillary Pores to Different-Sized Molecules	
Substance	**Molecular Weight**	**Permeability**
Water	18	1
NaCl	58.5	0.96
Urea	60	0.8
Glucose	180	0.6
Sucrose	342	0.4
Inulin	5,000	0.2
Myoglobin	17,600	0.03
Hemoglobin	68,000	0.01
Albumin	69,000	0.001

Data from Pappenheimer, J.R., 1953. Passage of molecules through capillary walls. Physiol. Rev. 33, 387.

water molecules diffuse through the capillary membrane is about 80 times as high as the rate at which plasma itself flows linearly along the capillary. That is, the water of the plasma is exchanged with the water of the interstitial fluid 80 times before the plasma can flow the entire distance through the capillary.

Effect of Molecular Size on Passage Through the Pores. The width of the capillary intercellular cleft pores, 6–7 nm, is about 20 times the diameter of the water molecule, which is the smallest molecule that normally passes through the capillary pores. The diameters of plasma protein molecules, however, are slightly greater than the width of the pores. Other substances, such as sodium ions, chloride ions, glucose, and urea, have intermediate diameters. Therefore, the permeability of the capillary pores for different substances varies according to their molecular diameters.

Table 39-1 lists the relative permeabilities of the capillary pores in skeletal muscle for substances commonly encountered, demonstrating, for instance, that the permeability for glucose molecules is 0.6 times that for water molecules, whereas the permeability for albumin molecules is very slight, only 1/1000 that for water molecules.

A word of caution must be issued at this point. The capillaries in various tissues have extreme differences in their permeabilities.

Effect of Concentration Difference on Net Rate of Diffusion Through the Capillary Membrane. The "net" rate of diffusion of a substance through any membrane is proportional to the *concentration difference of the substance* between the two sides of the membrane. That is, the greater the difference between the concentrations of any given substance on the two sides of the capillary membrane, the greater is the net movement of the substance in one direction through the membrane. The rates of diffusion through the capillary membranes of most nutritionally important substances are so high that only slight concentration differences suffice to cause more than adequate transport between the plasma and interstitial fluid. For instance, the concentration of oxygen in the interstitial fluid immediately outside the capillary is not more than a few percent less than its concentration in the plasma of the blood, yet this slight difference causes enough oxygen to move from the blood into the interstitial spaces to provide all the oxygen required for tissue metabolism, often as much as several liters of oxygen per minute during very active states of the body.

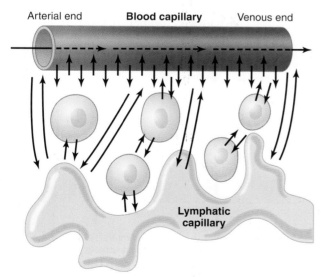

Arterial end   **Blood capillary**   Venous end

Lymphatic capillary

Figure 39-3 Diffusion of fluid molecules and dissolved substances between the capillary and interstitial fluid spaces.

Interstitium and Interstitial Fluid

About one-sixth of the total volume of the body consists of spaces between cells, which collectively are called the *interstitium*. The fluid in these spaces is called the *interstitial fluid*.

The structure of the interstitium is shown in Figure 39-4. It contains two major types of solid structures: (1) *collagen fiber bundles* and (2) *proteoglycan filaments*. The collagen fiber bundles extend long distances in the interstitium. They are extremely strong and therefore provide most of the tensional strength of the tissues. The proteoglycan filaments, however, are extremely thin-coiled or twisted molecules composed of about 98% *hyaluronic acid* and 2% protein. These molecules are so thin that they cannot be seen with a light microscope and are difficult to demonstrate even with the electron microscope. Nevertheless, they form a mat of very fine reticular filaments aptly described as a "brush pile."

"Gel" in the Interstitium. The fluid in the interstitium is derived by filtration and diffusion from the capillaries. It contains almost the same constituents as plasma except for much lower concentrations of proteins because proteins do not easily pass outward through the pores of the capillaries. The interstitial fluid is entrapped mainly in the minute spaces among the proteoglycan filaments. This combination of proteoglycan filaments and fluid entrapped within them has the characteristics of a *gel* and therefore is called *tissue gel*.

"Free" Fluid in the Interstitium. Although almost all the fluid in the interstitium normally is entrapped within the tissue gel, occasionally small *rivulets of "free" fluid* and *small free fluid vesicles* are also present, which means fluid that is free of the proteoglycan molecules and therefore can flow freely. The amount of "free" fluid present in *normal* tissues is slight, usually less than 1%. Conversely, when the tissues develop edema, *these small pockets and rivulets of free fluid expand tremendously* until one-half or more of the edema fluid becomes freely flowing fluid independent of the proteoglycan filaments.

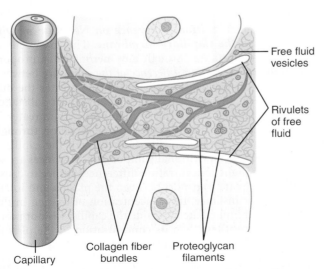

Figure 39-4 Structure of the interstitium. Proteoglycan filaments are everywhere in the spaces between the collagen fiber bundles. Free fluid vesicles and small amounts of free fluid in the form of rivulets occasionally also occur.

Fluid Filtration Across Capillaries Is Determined by Hydrostatic and Colloid Osmotic Pressures and the Capillary Filtration Coefficient

The hydrostatic pressure in the capillaries tends to force fluid and its dissolved substances through the capillary pores into the interstitial spaces. Conversely, osmotic pressure caused by the plasma proteins (called *colloid osmotic pressure*) tends to cause fluid movement by osmosis from the interstitial spaces into the blood. This osmotic pressure exerted by the plasma proteins normally prevents significant loss of fluid volume from the blood into the interstitial spaces.

HYDROSTATIC AND COLLOID OSMOTIC FORCES DETERMINE FLUID MOVEMENT THROUGH THE CAPILLARY MEMBRANE

Figure 39-5 shows the four primary forces that determine whether fluid will move out of the blood into the interstitial fluid or in the opposite direction. These forces, called "Starling forces" in honor of the physiologist Ernst Starling who first demonstrated their importance, are as follows:

1. the *capillary pressure* (Pc), which tends to force fluid *outward* through the capillary membrane;
2. the *interstitial fluid pressure* (Pif), which tends to force fluid *inward* through the capillary membrane when Pif is positive but outward when Pif is negative;
3. the capillary *plasma colloid osmotic pressure* (Πp), which tends to cause osmosis of fluid *inward* through the capillary membrane;
4. the *interstitial fluid colloid osmotic pressure* (Πif), which tends to cause osmosis of fluid *outward* through the capillary membrane.

If the sum of these forces—the *net filtration pressure* (NFP)—is positive, there will be a net *fluid filtration* across the capillaries. If the sum of the Starling forces is negative, there will be a net *fluid absorption* from the interstitial spaces into the capillaries. The NFP is calculated as follows:

$$NFP = Pc - Pif - \Pi p - \Pi if$$

As discussed later, the NFP is slightly positive under normal conditions, resulting in a net filtration of fluid across the capillaries into the interstitial space in most organs. The rate of fluid filtration in a tissue is also determined by the number and size of the pores in each capillary, as well as the number of capillaries in which blood is flowing. These factors are usually expressed

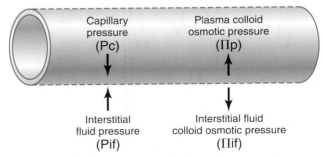

Figure 39-5 Fluid pressure and colloid osmotic pressure forces operate at the capillary membrane, and tend to move fluid either outward or inward through the membrane pores.

together as the *capillary filtration coefficient* (K_f). The K_f is therefore a measure of the capacity of the capillary membranes to filter water for a given NFP and is usually expressed as milliliter per minute per millimeter of mercury NFP.

The rate of capillary fluid filtration is therefore determined as follows:

$$Filtration = K_f \times NFP$$

In the following sections we discuss each of the forces that determine the rate of capillary fluid filtration.

CAPILLARY HYDROSTATIC PRESSURE

Various methods have been used to estimate the capillary hydrostatic pressure: (1) *direct micropipette cannulation of the capillaries*, which has given an average mean capillary pressure of about 25 mmHg in some tissues, such as the skeletal muscle and the gut, and (2) *indirect functional measurement of the capillary pressure*, which has given a capillary pressure averaging about 17 mmHg in these tissues.

INTERSTITIAL FLUID HYDROSTATIC PRESSURE

There are several methods for measuring interstitial fluid hydrostatic pressure and each of these gives slightly different values, depending on the method used and the tissue in which the pressure is measured. In loose subcutaneous tissue, interstitial fluid pressure measured by the different methods is usually a few millimeters of mercury less than atmospheric pressure; that is, the values are called *negative interstitial fluid pressure*. In other tissues that are surrounded by capsules, such as the kidneys, the interstitial pressure is generally *positive* (greater than atmospheric pressure). The methods most widely used have been (1) direct cannulation of the tissues with a micropipette, (2) measurement of the pressure from implanted perforated capsules, and (3) measurement of the pressure from a cotton wick inserted into the tissue.

PLASMA COLLOID OSMOTIC PRESSURE

Plasma Proteins Cause Colloid Osmotic Pressure. In the basic discussion of osmotic pressure in Chapter 4, we pointed out that only the molecules or ions that fail to pass through the pores of a semipermeable membrane exert osmotic pressure. Because the proteins are the only dissolved constituents in the plasma and interstitial fluids that do not readily pass through the capillary pores, it is the proteins of the plasma and interstitial fluids that are responsible for the osmotic pressures on the two sides of the capillary membrane. To distinguish this osmotic pressure from that which occurs at the cell membrane, it is called either *colloid osmotic pressure* or *oncotic pressure*. The term "colloid" osmotic pressure is derived from the fact that a protein solution resembles a colloidal solution despite the fact that it is actually a true molecular solution.

Normal Values for Plasma Colloid Osmotic Pressure. The colloid osmotic pressure of normal human plasma averages about 28 mmHg; 19 mmHg of this pressure is caused by molecular effects of the dissolved protein and 9 mmHg is caused by the *Donnan effect*—that is, extraosmotic pressure caused by sodium, potassium, and the other cations held in the plasma by the proteins.

Effect of the Different Plasma Proteins on Colloid Osmotic Pressure. The plasma proteins are a mixture that contains albumin, globulins, and fibrinogen with an average molecular weight of 69,000, 140,000, and 400,000, respectively. Thus, 1 g of globulin contains only half as many molecules as 1 g of albumin, and 1 g of fibrinogen contains only one-sixth as many molecules as 1 g of albumin. It should be recalled from the discussion of osmotic pressure in Chapter 4 that osmotic pressure is determined by the number of molecules dissolved in a fluid rather than by the mass of these molecules. Therefore, when corrected for number of molecules rather than mass, the following table gives both the relative mass concentrations (gram per deciliter) of the different types of proteins in normal plasma and their respective contributions to the total plasma colloid osmotic pressure (Πp):

	Gram Per Deciliter	Πp (mmHg)
Albumin	4.5	21.8
Globulins	2.5	6.0
Fibrinogen	0.3	0.2
Total	7.3	28.0

Thus, about 80% of the total colloid osmotic pressure of the plasma results from the albumin, 20% from the globulins, and almost none from fibrinogen. Therefore, from the point of view of capillary and tissue fluid dynamics, it is mainly albumin that is important.

INTERSTITIAL FLUID COLLOID OSMOTIC PRESSURE

Although the size of the usual capillary pore is smaller than the molecular sizes of the plasma proteins, this is not true of all the pores. Therefore, small amounts of plasma proteins do leak into the interstitial spaces through pores and by transcytosis in small vesicles.

The total quantity of protein in the entire 12 L of interstitial fluid of the body is slightly greater than the total quantity of protein in the plasma itself, but because this volume is four times the volume of plasma, the average protein *concentration* of the interstitial fluid of most tissues is usually only 40% of that in plasma, or about 3 g/dL. Quantitatively, one finds that the average interstitial fluid colloid osmotic pressure for this concentration of proteins is about 8 mmHg.

EXCHANGE OF FLUID VOLUME THROUGH THE CAPILLARY MEMBRANE

Now that the different factors affecting fluid movement through the capillary membrane have been discussed, we can put all these factors together to see how the capillary system maintains normal fluid volume distribution between the plasma and the interstitial fluid.

The average capillary pressure at the arterial ends of the capillaries is 15–25 mmHg greater than at the venous ends. Because of this difference, fluid "filters" out of the capillaries at their arterial ends, but at their venous ends fluid is reabsorbed back into the capillaries. Thus, a small amount of fluid actually "flows" through the tissues from the arterial ends of the capillaries to the venous ends. The dynamics of this flow are as follows.

Analysis of the Forces Causing Filtration at the Arterial End of the Capillary. The approximate average forces operative at the *arterial end* of the capillary that cause movement through the capillary membrane are shown as follows:

	Millimeter of Mercury
Forces tending to move fluid outward	
Capillary pressure (arterial end of capillary)	30
Negative interstitial free fluid pressure	3
Interstitial fluid colloid osmotic pressure	8
Total outward force	41
Forces tending to move fluid inward	
Plasma colloid osmotic pressure	28
Total inward force	28
Summation of forces	
Outward	41
Inward	28
Net outward force (at arterial end)	13

Thus, the summation of forces at the arterial end of the capillary shows a NFP of 13 mmHg, tending to move fluid outward through the capillary pores.

This 13 mmHg filtration pressure causes, on average, about 1/200 of the plasma in the flowing blood to filter out of the arterial ends of the capillaries into the interstitial spaces each time the blood passes through the capillaries.

Analysis of Reabsorption at the Venous End of the Capillary. The low blood pressure at the venous end of the capillary changes the balance of forces in favor of absorption as follows:

	Millimeter of Mercury
Forces tending to move fluid inward	
Plasma colloid osmotic pressure	28
Total inward force	28
Forces tending to move fluid outward	
Capillary pressure (venous end of capillary)	10
Negative interstitial free fluid pressure	3
Interstitial fluid colloid osmotic pressure	8
Total outward force	21
Summation of forces	
Inward	28
Outward	21
Net inward force	7

Thus, the force that causes fluid to move into the capillary, 28 mmHg, is greater than that opposing reabsorption, 21 mmHg. The difference, 7 mmHg, is the *net reabsorption pressure* at the venous ends of the capillaries. This reabsorption pressure is considerably less than the filtration pressure at the capillary arterial ends, but remember that the venous capillaries are more numerous and more permeable than the arterial capillaries, and thus less reabsorption pressure is required to cause inward movement of fluid.

The reabsorption pressure causes about nine-tenths of the fluid that has filtered out of the arterial ends of the capillaries to be reabsorbed at the venous ends. The remaining one-tenth flows into the lymph vessels and returns to the circulating blood.

STARLING EQUILIBRIUM FOR CAPILLARY EXCHANGE

Ernest Starling pointed out more than a century ago that under normal conditions, a state of near-equilibrium exists in most capillaries. That is, the amount of fluid filtering outward from the arterial ends of capillaries equals almost exactly the fluid returned to the circulation by absorption. The slight disequilibrium that does occur accounts for the fluid that is eventually returned to the circulation by way of the lymphatics.

The following table shows the principles of the Starling equilibrium. For this table, the pressures in the arterial and venous capillaries are averaged to calculate mean *functional* capillary pressure for the entire length of the capillary. This mean functional capillary pressure calculates to be 17.3 mmHg.

	Millimeter of Mercury
Mean forces tending to move fluid outward	
Mean capillary pressure	17.3
Negative interstitial free fluid pressure	3.0
Interstitial fluid colloid osmotic pressure	8.0
Total outward force	28.3
Mean force tending to move fluid inward	
Plasma colloid osmotic pressure	28.0
Total inward force	28.0
Summation of mean forces	
Outward	28.3
Inward	28.0
Net outward force	0.3

Thus, for the total capillary circulation, we find a near-equilibrium between the total outward forces, 28.3 mmHg, and the total inward force, 28.0 mmHg. This slight imbalance of forces, 0.3 mmHg, causes slightly more filtration of fluid into the interstitial spaces than reabsorption. This slight excess of filtration is called *net filtration*, and it is the fluid that must be returned to the circulation through the lymphatics. The normal rate of net filtration *in the entire body*, not including the kidneys, is only about 2 mL/minute.

Capillary Filtration Coefficient. In the previous example, an average net imbalance of forces at the capillary membranes of 0.3 mmHg causes net fluid filtration in the entire body of 2 mL/minute. Expressing the net fluid filtration rate for each millimeter of mercury imbalance, one finds a net filtration rate of 6.67 mL/minute of fluid per millimeter of mercury for the entire body. This value is called the whole-body capillary *filtration coefficient*.

The filtration coefficient can also be expressed for separate parts of the body in terms of rate of filtration per minute per millimeter of mercury per 100 g of tissue. On this basis, the capillary filtration coefficient of the average tissue is about 0.01 mL/minute per millimeter of mercury per 100 g of tissue. However, because of extreme differences in permeabilities of the capillary systems in different tissues, this coefficient varies more than 100-fold among the different tissues. It is very small in brain and muscle, moderately large in subcutaneous tissue, large in the intestine, and extremely large in the liver and glomerulus of the kidney where the pores are either numerous or wide open. By the same token, the permeation of proteins through the capillary membranes varies greatly as well. The concentration of protein in the interstitial fluid of muscles is about 1.5 g/dL; in subcutaneous tissue, 2 g/dL; in intestine, 4 g/dL; and in liver, 6 g/dL.

Effect of Abnormal Imbalance of Forces at the Capillary Membrane

If the mean capillary pressure rises above 17 mmHg, the net force tending to cause filtration of fluid into the tissue spaces rises. Thus, a 20 mmHg rise in mean capillary pressure causes an increase in NFP from 0.3 to 20.3 mmHg, which results in 68 times as much net filtration of fluid into the interstitial spaces as normally occurs. To prevent accumulation of excess fluid in these spaces would require 68 times the normal flow of fluid into the lymphatic system, an amount that is 2–5 times too much for the lymphatics to carry away. As a result, fluid will begin to accumulate in the interstitial spaces and edema will result.

Conversely, if the capillary pressure falls very low, net reabsorption of fluid into the capillaries will occur instead of net filtration and the blood volume will increase at the expense of the interstitial fluid volume.

BIBLIOGRAPHY

Chidlow JH Jr, Sessa WC: Caveolae, caveolins, and cavins: complex control of cellular signalling and inflammation, *Cardiovasc. Res.* 86:219, 2010.

Dejana E: Endothelial cell–cell junctions: happy together, *Nat. Rev. Mol. Cell Biol.* 5:261, 2004.

Guyton AC: Concept of negative interstitial pressure based on pressures in implanted perforated capsules, *Circ. Res.* 12:399, 1963.

Guyton AC: Interstitial fluid pressure: II. Pressure–volume curves of interstitial space, *Circ. Res.* 16:452, 1965.

Guyton AC, Granger HJ, Taylor AE: Interstitial fluid pressure, *Physiol. Rev.* 51:527, 1971.

Kolka CM, Bergman RN: The barrier within: endothelial transport of hormones, *Physiology (Bethesda)* 27:237, 2012.

Mehta D, Malik AB: Signaling mechanisms regulating endothelial permeability, *Physiol. Rev.* 86:279, 2006.

Parker JC: Hydraulic conductance of lung endothelial phenotypes and Starling safety factors against edema, *Am. J. Physiol. Lung Cell. Mol. Physiol.* 292:L378, 2007.

Parker JC, Townsley MI: Physiological determinants of the pulmonary filtration coefficient, *Am. J. Physiol. Lung Cell. Mol. Physiol.* 295:L235, 2008.

Predescu SA, Predescu DN, Malik AB: Molecular determinants of endothelial transcytosis and their role in endothelial permeability, *Am. J. Physiol. Lung Cell. Mol. Physiol.* 293:L823, 2007.

40

The Lymphatic System

Formation of Lymph

Lymph is derived from interstitial fluid that flows into the lymphatics. Therefore, lymph as it first enters the terminal lymphatics has almost the same composition as the interstitial fluid.

The protein concentration in the interstitial fluid of most tissues averages about 2 g/dL and the protein concentration of lymph flowing from these tissues is near this value. Lymph formed in the liver has a protein concentration as high as 6 g/dL and lymph formed in the intestines has a protein concentration as high as 3–4 g/dL. Because about two-thirds of all lymph normally is derived from the liver and intestines, the thoracic duct lymph, which is a mixture of lymph from all areas of the body, usually has a protein concentration of 3–5 g/dL.

The lymphatic system is also one of the major routes for absorption of nutrients from the gastrointestinal tract, especially for absorption of virtually all fats in food, as discussed in Chapter 72. Indeed, after a fatty meal, thoracic duct lymph sometimes contains as much as 1–2% fat.

Finally, even large particles, such as bacteria, can push their way between the endothelial cells of the lymphatic capillaries and in this way enter the lymph. As the lymph passes through the lymph nodes, these particles are almost entirely removed and destroyed.

Rate of Lymph Flow

About 100 mL/hour of lymph flows through the *thoracic duct* of a resting human, and approximately another 20 mL flows into the circulation each hour through other channels, making a total estimated lymph flow of about 120 mL/hour or 2–3 L/day.

Effect of Interstitial Fluid Pressure on Lymph Flow. Figure 40-1 shows the effect of different levels of interstitial fluid pressure on lymph flow as measured in animals. Note that

normal lymph flow is very little at interstitial fluid pressures more negative than the normal value of −6 mmHg. Then, as the pressure rises to 0 mmHg (atmospheric pressure), flow increases more than 20-fold. Therefore, any factor that increases interstitial fluid pressure also increases lymph flow if the lymph vessels are functioning normally. Such factors include the following:

- elevated capillary hydrostatic pressure
- decreased plasma colloid osmotic pressure
- increased interstitial fluid colloid osmotic pressure
- increased permeability of the capillaries

All of these factors cause a balance of fluid exchange at the blood capillary membrane to favor fluid movement into the interstitium, thus increasing interstitial fluid volume, interstitial fluid pressure, and lymph flow all at the same time.

However, note in Figure 40-1 that when the interstitial fluid pressure becomes 1 or 2 mmHg greater than atmospheric pressure (>0 mmHg), lymph flow fails to rise any further at still higher pressures. This results from the fact that the increasing tissue pressure not only increases entry of fluid into the lymphatic capillaries but also compresses the outside surfaces of the larger lymphatics, thus impeding lymph flow. At the higher pressures, these two factors balance each other almost exactly, so lymph flow reaches a "maximum lymph flow rate." This is illustrated by the upper-level plateau in Figure 40-1.

Lymphatic Pump Increases Lymph Flow. Valves exist in all lymph channels. Figure 40-2 shows typical valves in collecting lymphatics into which the lymphatic capillaries empty.

When a collecting lymphatic or larger lymph vessel becomes stretched with fluid, the smooth muscle in the wall of the vessel automatically contracts. Furthermore, each segment of the

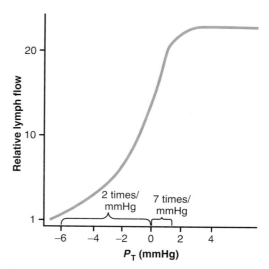

Figure 40-1 Relation between interstitial fluid pressure and lymph flow in the leg of a dog. Note that lymph flow reaches a maximum when the interstitial pressure, P_T, rises slightly above atmospheric pressure (0 mmHg). *Courtesy Drs. Harry Gibson and Aubrey Taylor.*

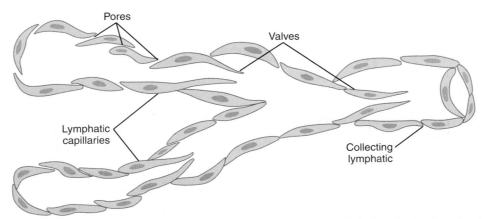

Figure 40-2 Structure of lymphatic capillaries and a collecting lymphatic, with the lymphatic valves also shown.

lymph vessel between successive valves functions as a separate automatic pump. That is, even slight filling of a segment causes it to contract and the fluid is pumped through the next valve into the next lymphatic segment. This fluid fills the subsequent segment and a few seconds later it, too, contracts, the process continuing all along the lymph vessel until the fluid is finally emptied into the blood circulation. In a very large lymph vessel such as the thoracic duct, this lymphatic pump can generate pressures as great as 50–100 mmHg.

Pumping Caused by External Intermittent Compression of the Lymphatics

In addition to the pumping caused by intrinsic intermittent contraction of the lymph vessel walls, any external factor that intermittently compresses the lymph vessel also can cause pumping. In order of their importance, such factors are as follows:
- contraction of surrounding skeletal muscles
- movement of the parts of the body
- pulsations of arteries adjacent to the lymphatics
- compression of the tissues by objects outside the body

The lymphatic pump becomes very active during exercise, often increasing lymph flow 10- to 30-fold. Conversely, during periods of rest, lymph flow is sluggish, almost zero.

Lymphatic Capillary Pump. The terminal lymphatic capillary is also capable of pumping lymph, in addition to the pumping by the larger lymph vessels. The walls of the lymphatic capillaries are tightly adherent to the surrounding tissue cells by means of their anchoring filaments. Therefore, each time excess fluid enters the tissue and causes the tissue to swell, the anchoring filaments pull on the wall of the lymphatic capillary and fluid flows into the terminal lymphatic capillary through the junctions between the endothelial cells. Then, when the tissue is compressed, the pressure inside the capillary increases and causes the overlapping edges of the endothelial cells to close like valves. Therefore, the pressure pushes the lymph forward into the collecting lymphatic instead of backward through the cell junctions.

The lymphatic capillary endothelial cells also contain a few contractile actomyosin filaments.

Summary of Factors that Determine Lymph Flow. From the previous discussion, one can see that the two primary factors that determine lymph flow are (1) the interstitial fluid pressure and (2) the activity of the lymphatic pump. Therefore, one can state that, roughly, *the rate of lymph flow is determined by the product of interstitial fluid pressure times the activity of the lymphatic pump.*

The Lymphatic System Plays a Key Role in Controlling Interstitial Fluid Protein Concentration, Volume, and Pressure

It is already clear that the lymphatic system functions as an "overflow mechanism" to return excess proteins and excess fluid volume from the tissue spaces to the circulation. Therefore, the lymphatic system also plays a central role in controlling (1) the concentration of proteins in the interstitial fluids, (2) the volume of interstitial fluid, and (3) the interstitial fluid pressure. Let us explain how these factors interact.

First, remember that small amounts of proteins leak continuously out of the blood capillaries into the interstitium. Only minute amounts, if any, of the leaked proteins return to the circulation by way of the venous ends of the blood capillaries. Therefore, these proteins tend to accumulate in the interstitial fluid, which in turn increases the colloid osmotic pressure of the interstitial fluids.

Second, the increasing colloid osmotic pressure in the interstitial fluid shifts the balance of forces at the blood capillary membranes in favor of fluid filtration into the interstitium. Therefore, in effect, fluid is translocated osmotically outward through the capillary wall by the proteins and into the interstitium, thus increasing both interstitial fluid volume and interstitial fluid pressure.

Third, the increasing interstitial fluid pressure greatly increases the rate of lymph flow, which in turn carries away the excess interstitial fluid volume and excess protein that has accumulated in the spaces.

Thus, once the interstitial fluid protein concentration reaches a certain level and causes comparable increases in interstitial fluid volume and pressure, the return of protein and fluid by way of the lymphatic system becomes great enough to balance the rate of leakage of these into the interstitium from the blood capillaries. Therefore, the quantitative values of all these factors

BOX 40-1 LYMPHATIC SYSTEM: SUMMARY OF FUNCTIONS

- Route of absorption of nutrients, especially fats, from the gastrointestinal tract (GIT)
- Role in immunity
- Regulation of interstitial fluid protein concentration
- Regulation of interstitial fluid volume
- Regulation of interstitial fluid pressure

reach a steady state and they will remain balanced at these steady-state levels until something changes the rate of leakage of proteins and fluid from the blood capillaries. The functions of the lymphatic system are surmised in Box 40-1.

SIGNIFICANCE OF NEGATIVE INTERSTITIAL FLUID PRESSURE AS A MEANS FOR HOLDING THE BODY TISSUES TOGETHER

Traditionally, it has been assumed that the different tissues of the body are held together entirely by connective tissue fibers. However, connective tissue fibers are very weak or even absent at many places in the body, particularly at points where tissues slide over one another (eg, the skin sliding over the back of the hand or over the face). Yet, even at these places, the tissues are held together by the negative interstitial fluid pressure, which is actually a partial vacuum. When the tissues lose their negative pressure, fluid accumulates in the spaces and the condition known as *edema* occurs.

BIBLIOGRAPHY

Gashev AA: Physiologic aspects of lymphatic contractile function: current perspectives, *Ann. N. Y. Acad. Sci.* 979:178, 2002.

Gashev AA: Basic mechanisms controlling lymph transport in the mesenteric lymphatic net, *Ann. N. Y. Acad. Sci.* 1207(Suppl. 1):E16, 2010.

Oliver G: Lymphatic vasculature development, *Nat. Rev. Immunol.* 4:35, 2004.

Predescu SA, Predescu DN, Malik AB: Molecular determinants of endothelial transcytosis and their role in endothelial permeability, *Am. J. Physiol. Lung Cell. Mol. Physiol.* 293:L823, 2007.

41

Vascular Distensibility of the Venous System

LEARNING OBJECTIVES

- Describe the factors that regulate right atrial pressure.
- List and briefly describe the determinants of peripheral venous pressure.
- Describe the mechanism and treatment of varicose veins.
- Describe how venous pressure is estimated.
- List the various blood reservoirs in the body and their relative importance.

GLOSSARY OF TERMS

- **Central venous pressure:** The pressure measured at the right atrium by inserting a catheter through the median cubital vein into the superior vena cava
- **Varicose veins:** Enlarged and tortuous veins that are most commonly seen in the lower limbs, although they may occur elsewhere

The veins provide passageways for flow but they also perform other special functions that are necessary for operation of the circulation. Of special importance is that they are capable of constricting and enlarging, and thereby storing either small or large quantities of blood and making this blood available when it is required by the remainder of the circulation. The peripheral veins can also propel blood forward by means of a so-called *venous pump*, and they even help to regulate cardiac output, an exceedingly important function that is described in detail in Chapter 36.

Right Atrial Pressure (Central Venous Pressure) and its Regulation

To understand the various functions of the veins, it is first necessary to know something about pressure in the veins and what determines the pressure.

Blood from all the systemic veins flows into the right atrium of the heart; therefore, the pressure in the right atrium is called the *central venous pressure*.

Right atrial pressure is regulated by a balance between (1) the ability of the heart to pump blood out of the right atrium and ventricle into the lungs and (2) the tendency for blood to flow from the peripheral veins into the right atrium. If the right heart is pumping strongly, the right atrial pressure decreases. Conversely, weakness of the heart elevates the right atrial pressure. Also, any effect that causes rapid inflow of blood into the right atrium from the peripheral veins elevates the right atrial pressure. Some of the factors that can increase this venous return and thereby increase the right atrial pressure are (1) increased blood volume,

(2) increased large vessel tone throughout the body with resultant increased peripheral venous pressures, and (3) dilation of the arterioles, which decreases the peripheral resistance and allows rapid flow of blood from the arteries into the veins.

The same factors that regulate right atrial pressure also contribute to regulation of cardiac output because the amount of blood pumped by the heart depends on both the ability of the heart to pump and the tendency for blood to flow into the heart from the peripheral vessels. Therefore, we discuss the regulation of right atrial pressure in much more depth in Chapter 36 in connection with regulation of cardiac output.

The *normal right atrial pressure* is about 0 mmHg, which is equal to the atmospheric pressure around the body. It can increase to 20–30 mmHg under very abnormal conditions, such as (1) serious heart failure or (2) after massive transfusion of blood, which greatly increases the total blood volume and causes excessive quantities of blood to attempt to flow into the heart from the peripheral vessels.

The lower limit to the right atrial pressure is usually about −3 to −5 mmHg below atmospheric pressure, which is also the pressure in the chest cavity that surrounds the heart. The right atrial pressure approaches these low values when the heart pumps with exceptional vigor or when blood flow into the heart from the peripheral vessels is greatly depressed, such as after severe hemorrhage.

Peripheral Venous Pressure and its Determinants

VENOUS RESISTANCE AND PERIPHERAL VENOUS PRESSURE

Large veins have so little resistance to blood flow *when they are distended* that the resistance then is almost zero and is of almost no importance. However, as shown in Figure 41-1, most of the large veins that enter the thorax are compressed at many points by the surrounding tissues so that blood flow is impeded at these points. For instance, the veins from the arms are compressed by their sharp angulations over the first rib. Also, the pressure in the neck veins often falls so low that the atmospheric pressure on the outside of the neck causes these veins to collapse. Finally, veins coursing through the abdomen are often compressed by different organs and by the intraabdominal pressure, so they usually are at least partially collapsed to an ovoid or slit-like state. For these reasons, the *large veins do usually offer some resistance to blood flow*, and, thus, the pressure in the more peripheral small veins in a person lying down is usually +4 to +6 mmHg greater than the right atrial pressure.

Effect of High Right Atrial Pressure on Peripheral Venous Pressure

When the right atrial pressure rises above its normal value of 0 mmHg, blood begins to back up in the large veins. This

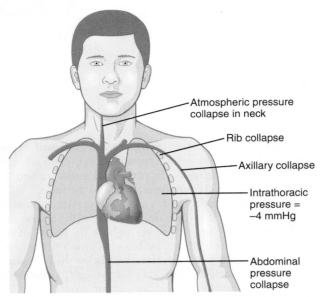

Figure 41-1   Compression points that tend to collapse the veins entering the thorax.

Labels on Figure 41-1:
- Atmospheric pressure collapse in neck
- Rib collapse
- Axillary collapse
- Intrathoracic pressure = –4 mmHg
- Abdominal pressure collapse

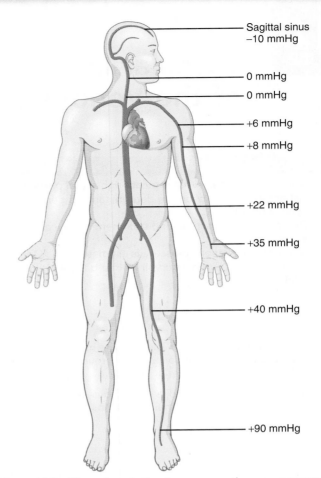

Figure 41-2   Effect of gravitational pressure on the venous pressures throughout the body in the standing person.

Labels on Figure 41-2:
- Sagittal sinus –10 mmHg
- 0 mmHg
- 0 mmHg
- +6 mmHg
- +8 mmHg
- +22 mmHg
- +35 mmHg
- +40 mmHg
- +90 mmHg

backup of blood enlarges the veins and even the collapse points in the veins open up when the right atrial pressure rises above +4 to +6 mmHg. Then, as the right atrial pressure rises still further, the additional increase causes a corresponding rise in peripheral venous pressure in the limbs and elsewhere. Because the heart must be weakened significantly to cause a rise in right atrial pressure as high as +4 to +6 mmHg, the peripheral venous pressure is not noticeably elevated even in the early stages of heart failure as long as the person is at rest.

Effect of Intraabdominal Pressure on Venous Pressures of the Leg

The pressure in the abdominal cavity of a recumbent person normally averages about +6 mmHg, but it can rise to +15 to +30 mmHg as a result of pregnancy, large tumors, abdominal obesity, or excessive fluid (called "ascites") in the abdominal cavity. When the intraabdominal pressure rises, the pressure in the veins of the legs must rise *above* the abdominal pressure before the abdominal veins open and allow the blood to flow from the legs to the heart. Thus, if the intraabdominal pressure is +20 mmHg, the lowest possible pressure in the femoral veins is also about +20 mmHg.

EFFECT OF GRAVITATIONAL PRESSURE ON VENOUS PRESSURE

In any body of water that is exposed to air, the pressure at the surface of the water is equal to atmospheric pressure, but the pressure rises 1 mmHg for each 13.6 mm of distance below the surface. This pressure results from the weight of the water and therefore is called *gravitational pressure* or *hydrostatic pressure.*

Gravitational pressure also occurs in the vascular system of the human being because of weight of the blood in the vessels, as shown in Figure 41-2. When a person is standing, the pressure in the right atrium remains about 0 mmHg because the heart pumps into the arteries any excess blood that attempts to accumulate at this point. However, in an adult *who is standing absolutely still*, the pressure in the veins of the feet is about +90 mmHg simply because of the gravitational weight of the

blood in the veins between the heart and the feet. The venous pressures at other levels of the body are proportionately between 0 and 90 mmHg.

In the arm veins, the pressure at the level of the top rib is usually about +6 mmHg because of compression of the subclavian vein as it passes over this rib. The gravitational pressure down the length of the arm then is determined by the distance below the level of this rib. Thus, if the gravitational difference between the level of the rib and the hand is +29 mmHg, this gravitational pressure is added to the +6 mmHg pressure caused by compression of the vein as it crosses the rib, making a total of +35 mmHg pressure in the veins of the hand.

The neck veins of a person standing upright collapse almost completely all the way to the skull because of atmospheric pressure on the outside of the neck. This collapse causes the pressure in these veins to remain at zero along their entire extent. Any tendency for the pressure to rise above this level opens the veins and allows the pressure to fall back to zero because of flow of the blood. Conversely, any tendency for the neck vein pressure to fall below zero collapses the veins still more, which further increases their resistance and again returns the pressure back to zero.

The veins inside the skull, on the other hand, are in a non-collapsible chamber (the skull cavity) and thus they cannot collapse. Consequently, *negative pressure can exist in the dural sinuses of the head*; in the standing position, the venous pressure in the sagittal sinus at the top of the brain is about −10 mmHg

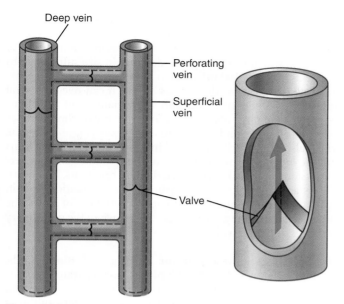

Figure 41-3   Venous valves of the leg.

because of the hydrostatic "suction" between the top of the skull and the base of the skull. Therefore, if the sagittal sinus is opened during surgery, air can be sucked immediately into the venous system; the air may even pass downward to cause air embolism in the heart, and death.

Effect of the Gravitational Factor on Arterial and Other Pressures

The gravitational factor also affects pressures in the peripheral arteries and capillaries. For instance, a standing person who has a mean arterial pressure of 100 mmHg at the level of the heart has an arterial pressure in the feet of about 190 mmHg. Therefore, when one states that the arterial pressure is 100 mmHg, this statement generally means that 100 mmHg is the pressure at the gravitational level of the heart but not necessarily elsewhere in the arterial vessels.

VENOUS VALVES AND THE "VENOUS PUMP": THEIR EFFECTS ON VENOUS PRESSURE

Were it not for valves in the veins, the gravitational pressure effect would cause the venous pressure in the feet always to be about +90 mmHg in a standing adult. However, every time one moves the legs, one tightens the muscles and compresses the veins in or adjacent to the muscles, which squeezes the blood out of the veins. However, the valves in the veins, shown in Figure 41-3, are arranged so that the direction of venous blood flow can be only toward the heart. Consequently, every time a person moves the legs or even tenses the leg muscles, a certain amount of venous blood is propelled toward the heart. This pumping system is known as the "venous pump" or "muscle pump," and it is efficient enough that under ordinary circumstances, the venous pressure in the feet of a walking adult remains less than +20 mmHg.

If a person stands perfectly still, the venous pump does not work, and the venous pressures in the lower legs increase to the full gravitational value of 90 mmHg in about 30 seconds. The pressures in the capillaries also increase greatly causing fluid to leak from the circulatory system into the tissue spaces. As a result, the legs swell and the blood volume diminishes. Indeed,

10–20% of the blood volume can be lost from the circulatory system within the 15–30 minutes of standing absolutely still, which may lead to fainting as sometimes occurs when a soldier is made to stand at rigid attention. This situation can be avoided by simply flexing the leg muscles periodically and slightly bending the knees, thus permitting the venous pump to work.

Varicose Veins

The valves of the venous system may become "incompetent" or even be destroyed when the veins have been overstretched by excess venous pressure lasting weeks or months. This can occur in pregnancy or when one stands most of the time. Stretching the veins increases their cross-sectional areas, but the leaflets of the valves do not increase in size. Therefore, the leaflets of the valves no longer close completely. When this lack of complete closure occurs, the pressure in the veins of the legs increases greatly because of failure of the venous pump, which further increases the sizes of the veins and finally destroys the function of the valves entirely. Thus, the person develops "varicose veins," which are characterized by large, bulbous protrusions of the veins beneath the skin of the entire leg, particularly the lower leg.

Whenever people with varicose veins stand for more than a few minutes, the venous and capillary pressures become very high and leakage of fluid from the capillaries causes constant edema in the legs. The edema in turn prevents adequate diffusion of nutritional materials from the capillaries to the muscle and skin cells, so the muscles become painful and weak and the skin may even become gangrenous and ulcerate. The best treatment for such a condition is continual elevation of the legs to a level at least as high as the heart. Tight binders or long "compression" stockings on the legs also can be of considerable assistance in preventing the edema and its sequelae.

CLINICAL ESTIMATION OF VENOUS PRESSURE

Venous pressure often can be estimated by simply observing the degree of distention of the peripheral veins—especially of the neck veins. For instance, in the sitting position, the neck veins are never distended in the normal quietly resting person. However, when the right atrial pressure becomes increased to as much as +10 mmHg, the lower veins of the neck begin to protrude, and at +15 mmHg atrial pressure essentially all the veins in the neck become distended.

Direct Measurement of Venous Pressure and Right Atrial Pressure

Venous pressure can also be measured with ease by inserting a needle directly into a vein and connecting it to a pressure recorder. The only means by which *right atrial pressure* can be measured accurately is by inserting a catheter through the peripheral veins and into the right atrium. Pressures measured through such *central venous catheters* are often used in some types of hospitalized cardiac patients to provide constant assessment of heart's pumping ability.

Pressure Reference Level for Measuring Venous and Other Circulatory Pressures

In discussions up to this point, we often have spoken of right atrial pressure as being 0 mmHg and arterial pressure as being 100 mmHg, but we have not stated the gravitational level in the circulatory system to which this pressure is referred. There is one point in the circulatory system at which gravitational pressure factors caused by changes in body position of a healthy

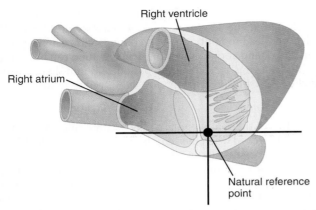

Figure 41-4   Reference point for circulatory pressure measurement (located near the tricuspid valve).

person usually do not affect the pressure measurement by more than 1–2 mmHg. This is at or near the level of the tricuspid valve, as shown by the crossed axes in Figure 41-4. Therefore, all circulatory pressure measurements discussed in this text are referred to this level, which is called the *reference level for pressure measurement*.

The reason for lack of gravitational effects at the tricuspid valve is that the heart automatically prevents significant gravitational changes in pressure at this point in the following way.

If the pressure at the tricuspid valve rises slightly above normal, the right ventricle fills to a greater extent than usual, causing the heart to pump blood more rapidly and therefore to decrease the pressure at the tricuspid valve back toward the normal mean value. Conversely, if the pressure falls, the right ventricle fails to fill adequately, its pumping decreases, and blood dams up in the venous system until the pressure at the tricuspid level again rises to the normal value. In other words, *the heart acts as a feedback regulator of pressure* at the tricuspid valve.

When a person is lying on his or her back, the tricuspid valve is located at almost exactly 60% of the chest thickness in front of the back. This is the *zero pressure reference level* for a person lying down.

Blood Reservoir Function of the Veins

As pointed out in Chapter 29, more than 60% of all the blood in the circulatory system is usually in the veins. For this reason and also because the veins are so compliant, it is said that the venous system serves as a *blood reservoir* for the circulation.

When blood is lost from the body and the arterial pressure begins to fall, nervous signals are elicited from the carotid sinuses and other pressure-sensitive areas of the circulation, as discussed in Chapter 43. These signals in turn elicit nerve signals from the brain and spinal cord mainly through sympathetic nerves to the veins, causing them to constrict. This process takes up much of the slack in the circulatory system caused by the lost blood. Indeed, even after as much as 20% of the total blood volume has been lost, the circulatory system often functions almost normally because of this variable reservoir function of the veins.

Specific Blood Reservoirs. Certain portions of the circulatory system are so extensive and/or so compliant that they are called "specific blood reservoirs." These reservoirs include (1) the *spleen*, which sometimes can decrease in size sufficiently to release as much as 100 mL of blood into other areas of the circulation; (2) the *liver*, the sinuses of which can release several hundred milliliters of blood into the remainder of the circulation; (3) the *large abdominal veins*, which can contribute as much as 300 mL; and (4) the *venous plexus beneath the skin*, which also can contribute several hundred milliliters. The *heart* and the *lungs*, although not parts of the systemic venous reservoir system, may also be considered blood reservoirs. The heart, for instance, shrinks during sympathetic stimulation and in this way can contribute approximately 50–100 mL of blood; the lungs can contribute another 100–200 mL when the pulmonary pressures decrease to low values.

The Spleen as a Reservoir for Storing Red Blood Cells. Figure 41-5 shows that the spleen has two separate areas for storing blood: the *venous sinuses* and the *pulp*. The sinuses can swell the same as any other part of the venous system and store whole blood.

In the splenic pulp, the capillaries are so permeable that whole blood, including the red blood cells, oozes through the capillary walls into a trabecular mesh, forming the *red pulp*. The red cells are trapped by the trabeculae, while the plasma flows on into the venous sinuses and then into the general circulation. As a consequence, the red pulp of the spleen is a *special reservoir that contains large quantities of concentrated red blood cells*. These concentrated red blood cells can then be expelled into the general circulation whenever the sympathetic nervous system becomes excited and causes the spleen and its vessels to contract. As much as 50 mL of concentrated red blood cells can be released into the circulation, raising the hematocrit 1–2%.

In other areas of the splenic pulp are islands of white blood cells, which collectively are called the *white pulp*. Here lymphoid cells are manufactured that are similar to those manufactured in the lymph nodes. They are part of the body's immune system, described in Chapter 25.

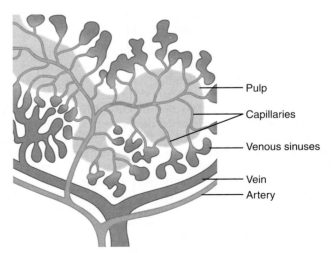

Figure 41-5   Functional structures of the spleen.

BIBLIOGRAPHY

Badeer HS: Hemodynamics for medical students, *Am. J. Physiol. (Adv. Physiol. Educ)* 25:44, 2001.

Bazigou E, Makinen T: Flow control in our vessels: vascular valves make sure there is no way back, *Cell. Mol. Life Sci.* 70:1055, 2013.

Guyton AC, Jones CE: Central venous pressure: physiological significance and clinical implications, *Am. Heart J.* 86:431, 1973.

Guyton AC, Jones CE, Coleman TG: *Circulatory Physiology: Cardiac Output and its Regulation*, Philadelphia, 1973, W.B. Saunders.

Hall JE: Integration and regulation of cardiovascular function, *Am. J. Physiol. (Adv. Physiol. Educ.)* 22:S174, 1999.

Hicks JW, Badeer HS: Gravity and the circulation: "open" vs. "closed" systems, *Am. J. Physiol.* 262:R725-R732, 1992.

Determinants of Arterial Blood Pressure

Blood pressure is usually measured in millimeters of mercury and is defined as the *force exerted by the blood against any unit area of the vessel wall.*

Blood pressure, unless otherwise specified, refers to the systemic arterial pressure. This pressure is not constant but is pulsatile, as described later. The highest pressure is achieved during systole and is referred to as the systolic pressure while the lowest pressure occurs in diastole and is referred to as the diastolic pressure. Systolic and diastolic blood pressures have different determinants; this is illustrated by the fact that they alter differentially. For example, with strenuous whole-body isotonic exercise, the diastolic blood pressure may fall while the systolic blood pressure rises. Systolic blood pressure is determined, in part, by cardiac output that increases during strenuous exercise. In contrast, diastolic blood pressure is determined by the total peripheral resistance (TPR). TPR falls during strenuous exercise because of vasodilation in the skeletal muscles and in the

skin (for thermoregulation), as a result, the diastolic pressure falls. A more detailed discussion of TPR has been presented in Chapter 38. Vascular pressures, including arterial blood pressure, are influenced by posture and gravity and this has been discussed in Chapter 41.

Arterial Pressure Pulsations

With each beat of the heart a new surge of blood fills the arteries. The aorta at the outlet of the left ventricle is highly elastic. The ejection of the blood from the ventricle distends the aorta and subsequent elastic recoil (Windkessel effect) maintains the pressure head and allows for steady blood flow to the peripheral arteries.

Were it not for distensibility of the arterial system, all the ejected blood would have to flow through the peripheral blood vessels almost instantaneously, only during cardiac systole, and no flow would occur during diastole. However, the compliance of the arterial tree normally reduces the pressure pulsations to almost no pulsations by the time the blood reaches the capillaries; therefore, tissue blood flow is mainly continuous with very little pulsation.

The *pressure pulsations* at the root of the aorta are illustrated in Figure 42-1. In the healthy young adult, the pressure at the top of each pulse, called the *systolic pressure*, is about 120 mmHg. At the lowest point of each pulse, called the *diastolic pressure*, it is about 80 mmHg. The difference between these two pressures, about 40 mmHg, is called the *pulse pressure*.

Two major factors affect the pulse pressure: (1) the *stroke volume output* of the heart and (2) the *compliance (total distensibility)* of the arterial tree. A third, less important, factor is the character of ejection from the heart during systole.

In general, the greater the stroke volume output, the greater is the amount of blood that must be accommodated in the

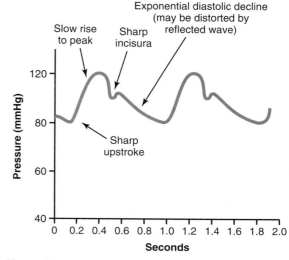

Figure 42-1 Pressure pulse contour in the ascending aorta.

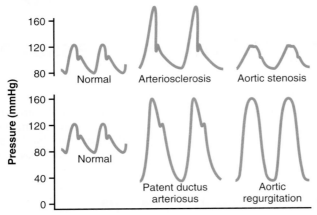

Figure 42-2 Aortic pressure pulse contours in arteriosclerosis, aortic stenosis, patent ductus arteriosus, and aortic regurgitation.

arterial tree with each heartbeat, and, therefore, the greater the pressure rise and fall during systole and diastole, thus causing a greater pulse pressure. Conversely, the less the compliance of the arterial system, the greater is the rise in pressure for a given stroke volume of blood pumped into the arteries. For instance, as demonstrated by the middle top curves in Figure 42-2, the pulse pressure in old age sometimes rises to twice normal because the arteries have become hardened with *arteriosclerosis* and therefore are relatively noncompliant.

In effect, pulse pressure is determined approximately by the *ratio of stroke volume output to compliance of the arterial tree*. Any condition of the circulation that affects either of these two factors also affects the pulse pressure:

$$\text{Pulse pressure} \approx \frac{\text{stroke volume}}{\text{arterial compliance}}$$

TRANSMISSION OF PRESSURE PULSES TO THE PERIPHERAL ARTERIES

When the heart ejects blood into the aorta during systole, at first only the proximal portion of the aorta becomes distended because the inertia of the blood prevents sudden blood movement all the way to the periphery. However, the rising pressure in the proximal aorta rapidly overcomes this inertia, and the wave front of distention spreads farther and farther along the aorta, as shown in Figure 42-3. This phenomenon is called *transmission of the pressure pulse* in the arteries.

The velocity of pressure pulse transmission is 3–5 m/second in the normal aorta, 7–10 m/second in the large arterial branches, and 15–35 m/second in the small arteries. In general, the greater the compliance of each vascular segment, the slower is the velocity, which explains the slow transmission in the aorta and the much faster transmission in the much less compliant small distal arteries. In the aorta, the velocity of transmission of the pressure pulse is 15 or more times the velocity of blood flow because the pressure pulse is simply a moving wave of *pressure* that involves little forward total movement of blood volume.

Pressure Pulses Are Damped in the Smaller Arteries, Arterioles, and Capillaries. Figure 42-4 shows typical changes in the contours of the pressure pulse as the pulse travels into the peripheral vessels. Note especially in the three lower curves that the intensity of pulsation becomes progressively less in the smaller arteries, the arterioles, and, especially, the capillaries. In fact, only

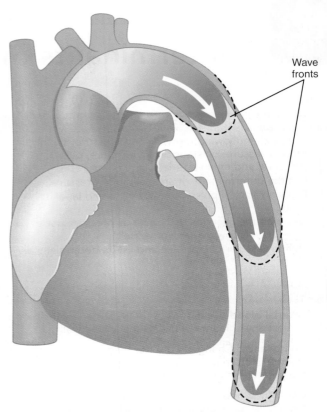

Figure 42-3 Progressive stages in transmission of the pressure pulse along the aorta.

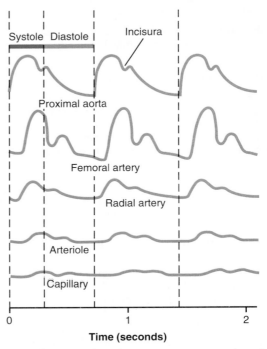

Figure 42-4 Changes in the pulse pressure contour as the pulse wave travels toward the smaller vessels.

when the aortic pulsations are extremely large or the arterioles are greatly dilated can pulsations be observed in the capillaries.

This progressive diminution of the pulsations in the periphery is called *damping* of the pressure pulses. The cause of this damping is twofold: (1) resistance to blood movement in the vessels and (2) compliance of the vessels. The resistance damps the pulsations because a small amount of blood must flow forward at the pulse wave front to distend the next segment of the vessel; the greater the resistance, the more difficult it is for this to occur. The compliance damps the pulsations because the more compliant a vessel, the greater is the quantity of blood required at the pulse wave front to cause an increase in pressure. Therefore, *the degree of damping is almost directly proportional to the product of resistance times compliance.*

Vascular Distensibility

A valuable characteristic of the vascular system is that all blood vessels are *distensible*. The distensible nature of the arteries allows them to accommodate the pulsatile output of the heart and to average out the pressure pulsations. This capability provides smooth, continuous flow of blood through the very small blood vessels of the tissues.

The most distensible by far of all the vessels are the veins. Venous distensibility has been discussed in greater detail in Chapter 41. Even slight increases in venous pressure cause the veins to store 0.5–1.0 L of extra blood. Therefore, the veins provide a *reservoir* for storing large quantities of extra blood that can be called into use whenever blood is required elsewhere in the circulation.

Units of Vascular Distensibility. Vascular distensibility normally is expressed as the fractional increase in volume for each millimeter of mercury rise in pressure, in accordance with the following formula:

$$\text{Vascular distensibility} = \frac{\text{increase in volume}}{\text{increase in pressure} \times \text{original volume}}$$

That is, if 1 mmHg causes a vessel that originally contained 10 mm of blood to increase its volume by 1 mL, the distensibility would be 0.1 mmHg^{-1}, or 10%/mmHg.

The Veins Are More Distensible than the Arteries. The walls of the arteries are thicker and far stronger than those of the veins. Consequently, the veins, on average, are about eight times more distensible than the arteries. That is, a given increase in pressure causes about eight times as much increase in blood in a vein as in an artery of comparable size.

In the pulmonary circulation, the pulmonary vein distensibilities are similar to those of the systemic circulation. However, the pulmonary arteries normally operate under pressures about one-sixth of those in the systemic arterial system, and their distensibilities are correspondingly greater, about six times the distensibility of systemic arteries.

VASCULAR COMPLIANCE (OR VASCULAR CAPACITANCE)

In hemodynamic studies, it usually is much more important to know the *total quantity of blood* that can be stored in a given portion of the circulation for each millimeter of mercury pressure rise than to know the distensibilities of the individual vessels. This value is called the *compliance* or *capacitance* of the respective vascular bed, that is:

$$\text{Vascular compliance} = \frac{\text{increase in volume}}{\text{increase in pressure}}$$

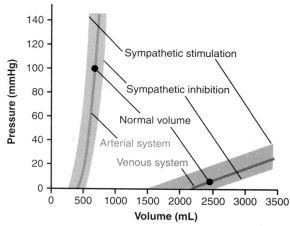

Figure 42-5 "Volume–pressure curves" of the systemic arterial and venous systems, showing the effects of stimulation or inhibition of the sympathetic nerves to the circulatory system.

Compliance and distensibility are quite different. A highly distensible vessel that has a small volume may have far less compliance than a much less distensible vessel that has a large volume because *compliance is equal to distensibility times volume.*

The compliance of a systemic vein is about 24 times that of its corresponding artery because it is about 8 times as distensible and has a volume about 3 times as great ($8 \times 3 = 24$).

VOLUME–PRESSURE CURVES OF THE ARTERIAL AND VENOUS CIRCULATIONS

A convenient method for expressing the relation of pressure to volume in a vessel or in any portion of the circulation is to use a *volume–pressure curve*. The red and blue solid curves in Figure 42-5 represent, respectively, the volume–pressure curves of the normal systemic arterial system and venous system, showing that when the arterial system of the average adult person (including all the large arteries, small arteries, and arterioles) is filled with about 700 mL of blood, the mean arterial pressure is 100 mmHg, but when it is filled with only 400 mL of blood, the pressure falls to zero.

In the entire systemic venous system, the volume normally ranges from 2000 to 3500 mL, and a change of several hundred millimeters in this volume is required to change the venous pressure only 3–5 mmHg. This requirement mainly explains why as much as 0.5 L of blood can be transfused into a healthy person in only a few minutes without greatly altering the function of the circulation.

Effect of Sympathetic Stimulation or Sympathetic Inhibition on the Volume–Pressure Relations of the Arterial and Venous Systems. Also shown in Figure 42-5 are the effects on the volume–pressure curves when the vascular sympathetic nerves are excited or inhibited. It is evident that an increase in vascular smooth muscle tone caused by sympathetic stimulation increases the pressure at each volume of the arteries or veins, whereas sympathetic inhibition decreases the pressure at each volume. Control of the vessels in this manner by the sympathetics is a valuable means for diminishing the dimensions of one segment of the circulation, thus transferring blood to other segments. For instance, an increase in vascular tone throughout the systemic circulation can cause large volumes of blood to shift into the heart, which is one of the principal methods that the body uses to rapidly increase heart pumping.

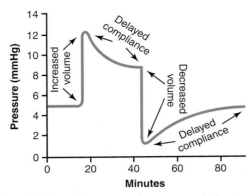

Figure 42-6 Effect on the intravascular pressure of injecting a volume of blood into a venous segment and later removing the excess blood, demonstrating the principle of delayed compliance.

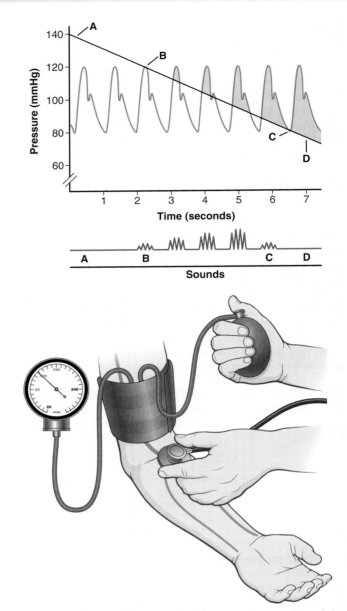

Figure 42-7 The auscultatory method for measuring systolic and diastolic arterial pressures.

Sympathetic control of vascular capacitance is also highly important during hemorrhage. Enhancement of sympathetic tone, especially to the veins, reduces the vessel sizes enough that the circulation continues to operate almost normally even when as much as 25% of the total blood volume has been lost.

Delayed Compliance (Stress Relaxation) of Vessels. The term "delayed compliance" means that a vessel exposed to increased volume at first exhibits a large increase in pressure, but progressive delayed stretching of smooth muscle in the vessel wall allows the pressure to return toward normal over a period of minutes to hours. This effect is shown in Figure 42-6. In this figure, the pressure is recorded in a small segment of a vein that is occluded at both ends. An extra volume of blood is suddenly injected until the pressure rises from 5 to 12 mmHg. Even though none of the blood is removed after it is injected, the pressure begins to decrease immediately and approaches about 9 mmHg after several minutes. In other words, the volume of blood injected causes immediate *elastic* distention of the vein, but then the smooth muscle fibers of the vein begin to "creep" to longer lengths, and their tensions correspondingly decrease. This effect is a characteristic of all smooth muscle tissues and is called *stress relaxation.*

Delayed compliance is a valuable mechanism by which the circulation can accommodate extra blood when necessary, such as after too large a transfusion. Delayed compliance in the reverse direction is one of the ways in which the circulation automatically adjusts itself over a period of minutes or hours to diminished blood volume after serious hemorrhage.

Clinical Methods for Measuring Systolic and Diastolic Pressures

It is not practical to use pressure recorders that require needle insertion into an artery for making routine arterial pressure measurements in human patients, although these types of recorders are used on occasion when special studies are necessary. Instead, the clinician determines systolic and diastolic pressures through indirect means, usually by the *auscultatory method.*

Auscultatory Method. Figure 42-7 shows the auscultatory method for determining systolic and diastolic arterial pressures. A stethoscope is placed over the antecubital artery and a blood pressure cuff is inflated around the upper arm. As long as the cuff continues to compress the arm with too little pressure to close the brachial artery, no sounds are heard from the

antecubital artery with the stethoscope. However, when the cuff pressure is great enough to close the artery during part of the arterial pressure cycle, a sound then is heard with each pulsation. These sounds are called *Korotkoff sounds,* named after *Nikolai Korotkoff,* a Russian physician who described them in 1905.

The Korotkoff sounds are believed to be caused mainly by blood jetting through the partly occluded vessel and by vibrations of the vessel wall. The jet causes turbulence in the vessel beyond the cuff, and this turbulence sets up the vibrations heard through the stethoscope.

In determining blood pressure by the auscultatory method, the pressure in the cuff is first elevated well above arterial systolic pressure. As long as this cuff pressure is higher than systolic pressure, the brachial artery remains collapsed so that no blood jets into the lower artery during any part of the pressure cycle. Therefore, no Korotkoff sounds are heard in the lower artery. But then the cuff pressure gradually is reduced. Just as soon as the pressure in the cuff falls below systolic pressure (point B, Figure 42-7), blood begins to flow through the artery beneath the cuff during the peak of systolic pressure, and one begins to hear *tapping* sounds from the antecubital artery in synchrony with the heartbeat. As soon as these sounds begin to be heard, the pressure level indicated by the manometer connected to the cuff is about equal to the systolic pressure.

As the pressure in the cuff is lowered still more, the Korotkoff sounds change in quality, having less of the tapping quality and more of a rhythmical and harsher quality. Then, finally, when the pressure in the cuff falls near diastolic pressure, the sounds suddenly change to a muffled quality (point C, Figure 42-7). One notes the manometer pressure when the Korotkoff sounds change to the muffled quality and this pressure is about equal to the diastolic pressure, although it slightly overestimates the diastolic pressure determined by direct intraarterial catheter. As the cuff pressure falls a few millimeters of mercury further, the artery no longer closes during diastole, which means that the basic factor causing the sounds (the jetting of blood through a squeezed artery) is no longer present. Therefore, the sounds disappear entirely. Many clinicians believe that the pressure at which the Korotkoff sounds completely disappear should be used as the diastolic pressure, except in situations in which the disappearance of sounds cannot reliably be determined because sounds are audible even after complete deflation of the cuff. For example, in patients with arteriovenous fistulas for hemodialysis or with aortic insufficiency, Korotkoff sounds may be heard after complete deflation of the cuff.

The auscultatory method for determining systolic and diastolic pressures is not entirely accurate, but it usually gives values within 10% of those determined by direct catheter measurement from inside the arteries.

Normal Arterial Pressures as Measured by the Auscultatory Method. Figure 42-8 shows the approximate normal systolic and diastolic arterial pressures at different ages. The progressive increase in pressure with age results from the effects of aging on the blood pressure control mechanisms. We shall see in Chapter 44 that the kidneys are primarily responsible for this long-term regulation of arterial pressure; it is well known that

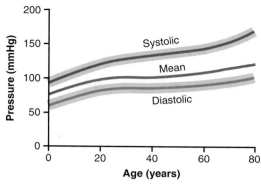

Figure 42-8   Changes in systolic, diastolic, and mean arterial pressures with age. The shaded areas show the approximate normal ranges.

the kidneys exhibit definitive changes with age, especially after the age of 50 years.

A slight extra increase in *systolic* pressure usually occurs beyond the age of 60 years. This results from decreasing distensibility, or "hardening," of the arteries, which is often a result of *atherosclerosis*. The final effect is a higher systolic pressure with considerable increase in pulse pressure, as previously explained.

Mean Arterial Pressure. The mean arterial pressure is the average of the arterial pressures measured millisecond by millisecond over a period of time. It is not equal to the average of systolic and diastolic pressures because at normal heart rates, a greater fraction of the cardiac cycle is spent in diastole than in systole; thus, the arterial pressure remains nearer to diastolic pressure than to systolic pressure during the greater part of the cardiac cycle. The mean arterial pressure is therefore determined about 60% by the diastolic pressure and 40% by the systolic pressure. Mean arterial pressure can be calculated as diastolic pressure + 1/3 pulse pressure. Note in Figure 42-8 that the mean pressure (solid green line) at all ages is nearer to the diastolic pressure than to the systolic pressure. However, at very high heart rates diastole comprises a smaller fraction of the cardiac cycle and the mean arterial pressure is more closely approximated as the average of systolic and diastolic pressures.

BIBLIOGRAPHY

Badeer HS: Hemodynamics for medical students, *Am. J. Physiol. (Adv. Physiol. Educ)* 25:44, 2001.

Chirinos JA: Arterial stiffness: basic concepts and measurement techniques, *J. Cardiovasc. Transl. Res.* 5:255, 2012.

Guyton AC: *Arterial Pressure and Hypertension*, Philadelphia, 1980, W.B. Saunders.

Hall JE: Integration and regulation of cardiovascular function, *Am. J. Physiol. (Adv. Physiol. Educ.)* 22:s174, 1999.

Hicks JW, Badeer HS: Gravity and the circulation: "open" vs. "closed" systems, *Am. J. Physiol.* 262:R725, 1992.

Kass DA: Ventricular arterial stiffening: integrating the pathophysiology, *Hypertension* 46:185, 2005.

Kurtz TW, Griffin KA, Bidani AK, et al: Recommendations for blood pressure measurement in humans and experimental animals. Part 2: blood pressure measurement in experimental animals: a statement for professionals from the Subcommittee of Professional and Public Education of the American Heart Association Council on High Blood pressure Research, *Hypertension* 45:299, 2005.

Laurent S, Boutouyrie P, Lacolley P: Structural and genetic bases of arterial stiffness, *Hypertension* 45:1050, 2005.

O'Rourke MF, Adji A: Noninvasive studies of central aortic pressure, *Curr. Hypertens. Rep.* 14:8, 2012.

Pickering TG, Hall JE, Appel LJ, et al: Recommendations for blood pressure measurement in humans and experimental animals: part 1: blood pressure measurement in humans: a statement for professionals from the Subcommittee of Professional and Public Education of the American Heart Association Council on High Blood Pressure Research, *Hypertension* 45:142, 2005.

Short-Term Regulation of Arterial Blood Pressure

GLOSSARY OF TERMS

- **Bainbridge reflex:** An increase in heart rate following direct stretch of the atrial wall, mediated by the vagus nerve

- **Cushing's CNS ischemic response:** Intense sympathetic stimulation and increase in arterial blood pressure following cerebral ischemia

- **Vasovagal syncope:** Vagally mediated bradycardia resulting in a fall in blood pressure and fainting

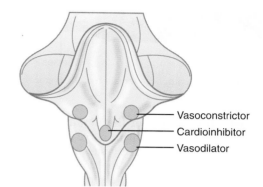

The nervous system controls the circulation almost entirely through the *autonomic nervous system*. The total function of this system is presented in Chapter 119. In this chapter we consider additional specific anatomical and functional characteristics.

Autonomic Nervous System

By far the most important part of the autonomic nervous system for regulating the circulation is the *sympathetic nervous system*. The *parasympathetic nervous system*, however, contributes importantly to regulation of heart function, as described later in the chapter.

Sympathetic Nervous System. Figure 43-1 shows the anatomy of sympathetic nervous control of the circulation. Sympathetic vasomotor nerve fibers leave the spinal cord through all the thoracic spinal nerves and through the first one or two lumbar spinal nerves. They then pass immediately into a *sympathetic chain*, one of which lies on each side of the vertebral column. Next, they pass by two routes to the circulation: (1) through specific *sympathetic nerves* that innervate mainly the vasculature of the internal viscera and the heart, as shown on the right side of Figure 43-1, and (2) almost immediately into peripheral portions of the *spinal nerves* distributed to the vasculature of the peripheral areas. The precise pathways of these fibers in the spinal cord and in the sympathetic chains are discussed in Chapter 119.

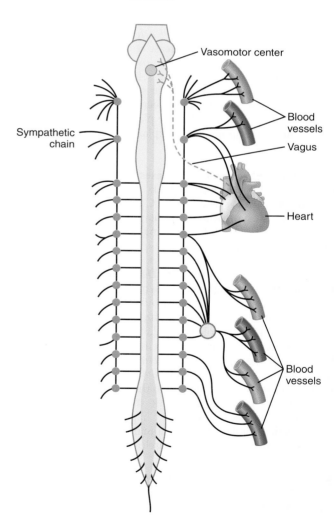

Figure 43-1 Anatomy of *sympathetic nervous control* of the circulation. Also shown by the *dashed red line*, a vagus nerve that carries *parasympathetic signals* to the heart.

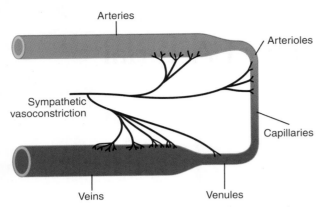

Figure 43-2 Sympathetic innervation of the systemic circulation.

Sympathetic Innervation of the Blood Vessels. Figure 43-2 shows distribution of sympathetic nerve fibers to the blood vessels demonstrating that in most tissues all the vessels *except* the capillaries are innervated. Precapillary sphincters and metarterioles are innervated in some tissues, such as the mesenteric blood vessels, although their sympathetic innervation is usually not as dense as in the small arteries, arterioles, and veins.

The innervation of the *small arteries* and *arterioles* allows sympathetic stimulation to increase *resistance* to blood flow and thereby *decrease* the rate of blood flow through the tissues.

The innervation of the large vessels, particularly of the *veins*, makes it possible for sympathetic stimulation to *decrease* the volume of these vessels. This decrease in volume can push blood into the heart and thereby plays a major role in regulation of heart pumping, as we explain later in this and subsequent chapters.

Sympathetic Stimulation Increases Heart Rate and Contractility. Sympathetic fibers also go directly to the heart, as shown in Figure 43-1 and as discussed in Chapters 30 and 32. It should be recalled that sympathetic stimulation markedly increases the activity of the heart, both increasing the heart rate and enhancing its strength and volume of pumping.

Parasympathetic Stimulation Decreases Heart Rate and Contractility. Although the parasympathetic nervous system is exceedingly important for many other autonomic functions of the body, such as control of multiple gastrointestinal actions, it plays only a minor role in regulation of vascular function in most tissues. Its most important circulatory effect is to control heart rate by way of *parasympathetic nerve fibers* to the heart in the *vagus nerves*, shown in Figure 43-1 by the dashed red line from the brain medulla directly to the heart.

The effects of parasympathetic stimulation on heart function were discussed in detail in Chapter 32. Principally, parasympathetic stimulation causes a marked *decrease* in heart rate and a slight decrease in heart muscle contractility.

SYMPATHETIC VASOCONSTRICTOR SYSTEM AND ITS CONTROL BY THE CENTRAL NERVOUS SYSTEM

The sympathetic nerves carry tremendous numbers of *vasoconstrictor nerve fibers* and only a few vasodilator fibers. The vasoconstrictor fibers are distributed to essentially all segments of the circulation, but more to some tissues than to others. This

sympathetic vasoconstrictor effect is especially powerful in the kidneys, intestines, spleen, and skin but much less potent in skeletal muscle and the brain.

Vasomotor Center in the Brain and its Control of the Vasoconstrictor System

Located bilaterally mainly in the reticular substance of the medulla and of the lower third of the pons is an area called the *vasomotor center*, shown in Figures 43-1 and 43-3. This center transmits parasympathetic impulses through the vagus nerves to the heart and sympathetic impulses through the spinal cord and peripheral sympathetic nerves to virtually all arteries, arterioles, and veins of the body.

Although the total organization of the vasomotor center is still unclear, experiments have made it possible to identify certain important areas in this center:

1. A *vasoconstrictor area* located bilaterally in the anterolateral portions of the upper medulla. The neurons originating in this area distribute their fibers to all levels of the spinal cord, where they excite preganglionic vasoconstrictor neurons of the sympathetic nervous system.

2. A *vasodilator area* located bilaterally in the anterolateral portions of the lower half of the medulla. The fibers from these neurons project upward to the vasoconstrictor area just described; they inhibit the vasoconstrictor activity of this area, thus causing vasodilation.

3. A *sensory area* located bilaterally in the *nucleus tractus solitarius* in the posterolateral portions of the medulla and lower pons. The neurons of this area receive sensory nerve signals from the circulatory system mainly through the *vagus* and *glossopharyngeal nerves*, and output signals from this sensory area then help to control activities of both the vasoconstrictor and vasodilator areas of the vasomotor center, thus providing "reflex" control of many circulatory functions. An example is the baroreceptor reflex for controlling arterial pressure, described later in this chapter.

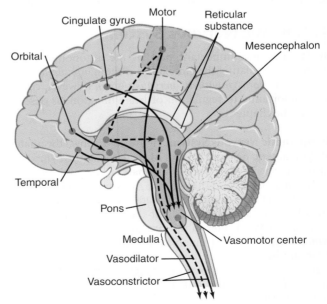

Figure 43-3 Areas of the brain that play important roles in the nervous regulation of the circulation. The *dashed lines* represent inhibitory pathways.

Continuous Partial Constriction of the Blood Vessels Is Normally Caused by Sympathetic Vasoconstrictor Tone

Under normal conditions, the vasoconstrictor area of the vasomotor center transmits signals continuously to the sympathetic vasoconstrictor nerve fibers over the entire body, causing slow firing of these fibers at a rate of about one-half to two impulses per second. This continual firing is called *sympathetic vasoconstrictor tone*. These impulses normally maintain a partial state of contraction in the blood vessels called *vasomotor tone*.

Figure 43-4 demonstrates the significance of vasoconstrictor tone. In the experiment of this figure, a total spinal anesthetic was administered to an animal. This anesthetic blocked all transmission of sympathetic nerve impulses from the spinal cord to the periphery. As a result, the arterial pressure fell from 100 to 50 mmHg, demonstrating the effect of the loss of vasoconstrictor tone throughout the body. A few minutes later, a small amount of the hormone norepinephrine was injected into the blood (norepinephrine is the principal vasoconstrictor hormonal substance secreted at the endings of the sympathetic vasoconstrictor nerve fibers). As this injected hormone was transported in the blood to blood vessels, the vessels once again became constricted and the arterial pressure rose to a level even greater than normal for 1–3 minutes, until the norepinephrine was destroyed.

Control of Heart Activity by the Vasomotor Center

At the same time that the vasomotor center regulates the amount of vascular constriction, it also controls heart activity. The *lateral* portions of the vasomotor center transmit excitatory impulses through the sympathetic nerve fibers to the heart when there is a need to increase heart rate and contractility. Conversely, when there is a need to decrease heart pumping, the *medial* portion of the vasomotor center sends signals to the adjacent *dorsal motor nuclei of the vagus nerves*, which then transmit parasympathetic impulses through the vagus nerves to the heart to decrease heart rate and heart contractility. Therefore, the vasomotor center can either increase or decrease heart activity. Heart rate and strength of heart contraction ordinarily increase when vasoconstriction occurs and ordinarily decrease when vasoconstriction is inhibited.

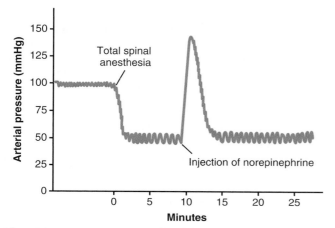

Figure 43-4 Effect of total spinal anesthesia on the arterial pressure showing marked decrease in pressure resulting from loss of "vasomotor tone."

Control of the Vasomotor Center by Higher Nervous Centers

Large numbers of small neurons located throughout the *reticular substance* of the *pons, mesencephalon,* and *diencephalon* can either excite or inhibit the vasomotor center. This reticular substance is shown in Figure 43-3. In general, the neurons in the more lateral and superior portions of the reticular substance cause excitation, whereas the more medial and inferior portions cause inhibition.

The *hypothalamus* plays a special role in controlling the vasoconstrictor system because it can exert powerful excitatory or inhibitory effects on the vasomotor center. The *posterolateral portions* of the hypothalamus cause mainly excitation, whereas the *anterior portion* can cause either mild excitation or inhibition, depending on the precise part of the anterior hypothalamus that is stimulated.

Many parts of the *cerebral cortex* can also excite or inhibit the vasomotor center. Stimulation of the *motor cortex*, for instance, excites the vasomotor center because of impulses transmitted downward into the hypothalamus and then to the vasomotor center. Also, stimulation of the *anterior temporal lobe*, the *orbital areas of the frontal cortex*, the *anterior part of the cingulate gyrus*, the *amygdala*, the *septum*, and the *hippocampus* can all either excite or inhibit the vasomotor center, depending on the precise portions of these areas that are stimulated and the intensity of the stimulus. Thus, widespread basal areas of the brain can have profound effects on cardiovascular function.

Norepinephrine Is the Sympathetic Vasoconstrictor Neurotransmitter

The substance secreted at the endings of the vasoconstrictor nerves is almost entirely norepinephrine, which acts directly on the *alpha adrenergic receptors* of the vascular smooth muscle to cause vasoconstriction, as discussed in Chapter 119.

Adrenal Medullae and their Relation to the Sympathetic Vasoconstrictor System

Sympathetic impulses are transmitted to the adrenal medullae at the same time that they are transmitted to the blood vessels. These impulses cause the medullae to *secrete both epinephrine and norepinephrine into the circulating blood*. These two hormones are carried in the bloodstream to all parts of the body, where they act directly on all blood vessels, usually to cause vasoconstriction. In a few tissues, epinephrine causes vasodilation because it also has a "beta" adrenergic receptor stimulatory effect, which dilates rather than constricts certain vessels, as discussed in Chapter 119.

Emotional Fainting—Vasovagal Syncope

An interesting vasodilatory reaction occurs in people who experience intense emotional disturbances that cause fainting. In this case, the muscle vasodilator system becomes activated, and at the same time, the vagal cardioinhibitory center transmits strong signals to the heart to slow the heart rate markedly. The arterial pressure falls rapidly, which reduces blood flow to the brain and causes the person to lose consciousness. This overall effect is called *vasovagal syncope*. Emotional fainting begins with disturbing thoughts in the cerebral cortex. The pathway probably then goes to the vasodilatory center of the anterior hypothalamus next to the vagal centers of the medulla, to the heart through the vagus nerves, and also through the spinal cord to the *sympathetic vasodilator* nerves of the muscles.

Role of the Nervous System in Rapid Control of Arterial Pressure

One of the most important functions of nervous control of the circulation is its capability to cause rapid increases in arterial pressure. For this purpose, the entire vasoconstrictor and cardioaccelerator functions of the sympathetic nervous system are stimulated together. At the same time, there is reciprocal inhibition of parasympathetic vagal inhibitory signals to the heart. Thus, the following three major changes occur simultaneously, each of which helps to increase arterial pressure. They are as follows:

1. *Most arterioles of the systemic circulation are constricted,* which greatly increases the total peripheral resistance, thereby increasing the arterial pressure.
2. *The veins especially (but the other large vessels of the circulation as well) are strongly constricted.* This constriction displaces blood out of the large peripheral blood vessels toward the heart, thus increasing the volume of blood in the heart chambers. The stretch of the heart then causes the heart to beat with far greater force and therefore to pump increased quantities of blood. This also increases the arterial pressure.
3. Finally, *the heart is directly stimulated by the autonomic nervous system, further enhancing cardiac pumping.* Much of this enhanced cardiac pumping is caused by an increase in the heart rate, which sometimes increases to as much as three times normal. In addition, sympathetic nervous signals have a significant direct effect to increase contractile force of the heart muscle, increasing the capability of the heart to pump larger volumes of blood. During strong sympathetic stimulation, the heart can pump about two times as much blood as under normal conditions, which contributes still more to the acute rise in arterial pressure.

Nervous Control of Arterial Pressure Is Rapid. An especially important characteristic of nervous control of arterial pressure is its rapidity of response, beginning within seconds and often increasing the pressure to two times normal within 5–10 seconds. Conversely, sudden inhibition of nervous cardiovascular stimulation can decrease the arterial pressure to as little as one-half normal within 10–40 seconds. Therefore, nervous control is by far the most rapid mechanism for arterial blood pressure regulation.

REFLEX MECHANISMS FOR MAINTAINING NORMAL ARTERIAL PRESSURE

Aside from the exercise and stress functions of the autonomic nervous system to increase arterial pressure, multiple subconscious special nervous control mechanisms operate all the time to maintain the arterial pressure at or near normal. Almost all of these are *negative feedback reflex mechanisms,* which we describe in the following sections.

Baroreceptor Arterial Pressure Control System— Baroreceptor Reflexes

By far the best known of the nervous mechanisms for arterial pressure control is the *baroreceptor reflex.* Basically, this reflex is initiated by stretch receptors, called either *baroreceptors* or *pressoreceptors,* located at specific points in the walls of several large systemic arteries. A rise in arterial pressure stretches the baroreceptors and causes them to transmit signals into the central nervous system (CNS). "Feedback" signals are then sent back through the autonomic nervous system to the circulation to reduce arterial pressure downward toward the normal level.

Physiological Anatomy of the Baroreceptors and their Innervation. Baroreceptors are spray-type nerve endings that lie in the walls of the arteries and are stimulated when stretched. A few baroreceptors are located in the wall of almost every large artery of the thoracic and neck regions, but, as shown in Figure 43-5, baroreceptors are extremely abundant in (1) the wall of each internal carotid artery slightly above the carotid bifurcation, an area known as the *carotid sinus,* and (2) the wall of the aortic arch.

Figure 43-5 shows that signals from the "carotid baroreceptors" are transmitted through small *Hering nerves* to the *glossopharyngeal nerves* in the high neck, and then to the *nucleus tractus solitarius* in the medullary area of the brainstem. Signals from the "aortic baroreceptors" in the arch of the aorta are transmitted through the *vagus nerves* to the same nucleus tractus solitarius of the medulla.

Response of the Baroreceptors to Arterial Pressure. Figure 43-6 shows the effect of different arterial pressure levels on the rate of impulse transmission in a Hering carotid sinus nerve. Note that the carotid sinus baroreceptors are not stimulated at all by pressures between 0 and 50–60 mmHg, but above these levels, they respond progressively more rapidly and reach a maximum at about 180 mmHg. The responses of the aortic baroreceptors are similar to those of the carotid receptors except that they operate, in general, at arterial pressure levels about 30 mmHg higher.

Note especially that in the normal operating range of arterial pressure, around 100 mmHg, even a slight change in pressure causes a strong change in the baroreflex signal to readjust arterial pressure back toward normal. Thus, the baroreceptor feedback mechanism functions most effectively in the pressure range where it is most needed.

The baroreceptors respond rapidly to changes in arterial pressure; in fact, the rate of impulse firing increases in the fraction of a second during each systole and decreases again during diastole. Furthermore, the baroreceptors *respond much more to a rapidly changing pressure* than to a stationary pressure. That is, if the mean arterial pressure is 150 mmHg but at that moment is rising rapidly, the rate of impulse transmission may be as much as twice that when the pressure is stationary at 150 mmHg.

Circulatory Reflex Initiated by the Baroreceptors. After the baroreceptor signals have entered the tractus solitarius of the medulla, secondary signals *inhibit the vasoconstrictor center* of the medulla and *excite the vagal parasympathetic center.* The net effects are (1) *vasodilation* of the veins and arterioles throughout the peripheral circulatory system and (2) *decreased heart rate* and *strength of heart contraction.* Therefore, excitation of the baroreceptors by high pressure in the arteries reflexly *causes the arterial pressure to decrease* because of both a decrease in peripheral resistance and a decrease in cardiac output. Conversely, low pressure has opposite effects, reflexly causing the pressure to rise back toward normal.

Table 43-1 summarizes the working of the baroreflex.

The Baroreceptors Attenuate Blood Pressure Changes During Changes in Body Posture. The ability of the baroreceptors to maintain relatively constant arterial pressure in the upper body

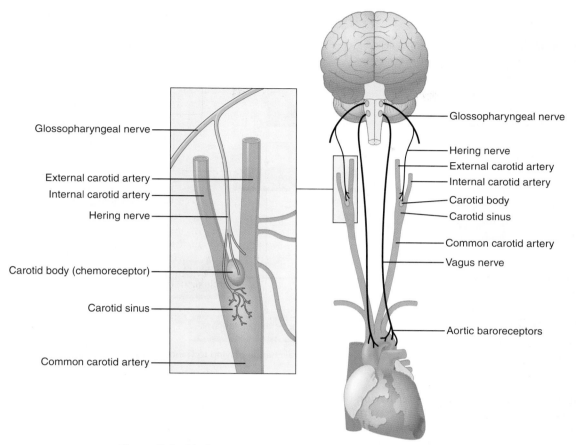

Figure 43-5 The baroreceptor system for controlling arterial pressure.

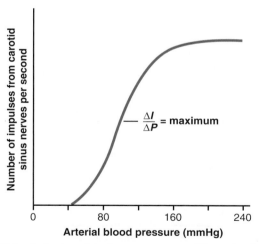

Figure 43-6 Activation of the baroreceptors at different levels of arterial pressure. ΔI, change in carotid sinus nerve impulses per second; ΔP, change in arterial blood pressure in millimeters of mercury.

TABLE 43-1	Working of the Baroreflex
Components of a Typical Reflex	**Components of the Baroreflex**
Stimulus	Increased arterial blood pressure
Receptor	Baroreceptors: carotid sinus, aortic arch baroreceptors
Afferent nerve	Hering nerve (IX cranial nerve) from carotid sinus
	Depressor nerve (X cranial nerve) from arch of the aorta
Integrating center	Nucleus tractus solitarius—vasomotor center
Efferent nerve	Vagus: increased activity
	Sympathetic: decreased activity
Effector organs	Heart, blood vessels
Physiological effects	Decreased heart rate, decreased cardiac contractility
	Vasodilation resulting in decreased cardiac output and decreased resistance

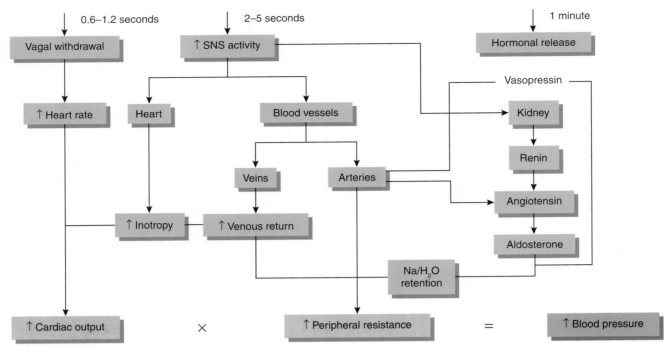

Figure 43-7   Maintenance of blood pressure during a postural change of lying to standing. *SNS,* sympathetic nervous system.

is important when a person stands up after having been lying down. Immediately on standing, the arterial pressure in the head and upper part of the body tends to fall, and marked reduction of this pressure could cause loss of consciousness. However, the falling pressure at the baroreceptors elicits an immediate reflex, resulting in strong sympathetic discharge throughout the body that minimizes the decrease in pressure in the head and upper body. These changes are summarized in Figure 43-7.

Pressure "Buffer" Function of the Baroreceptor Control System. Because the baroreceptor system opposes either increases or decreases in arterial pressure, it is called a *pressure buffer system* and the nerves from the baroreceptors are called *buffer nerves.*

Figure 43-8 shows the importance of this buffer function of the baroreceptors. The upper record in this figure shows an arterial pressure recording for 2 hours from a normal dog, and the lower record shows an arterial pressure recording from a dog whose baroreceptor nerves from both the carotid sinuses and the aorta had been removed. Note the extreme variability of pressure in the denervated dog caused by simple events of the day, such as lying down, standing, excitement, eating, defecation, and noises.

Figure 43-9 shows the frequency distributions of the mean arterial pressures recorded for a 24-hour day in both the normal dog and the denervated dog. Note that when the baroreceptors were functioning normally, the mean arterial pressure remained within a narrow range of between 85 and 115 mmHg throughout the day and for most of the day it remained at about 100 mmHg. After denervation of the baroreceptors, however, the frequency distribution curve became the broad, low curve of the figure, showing that the pressure range increased 2.5-fold, frequently falling to as low as 50 mmHg or rising to more than 160 mmHg. Thus, one can see the extreme variability of pressure in the absence of the arterial baroreceptor system.

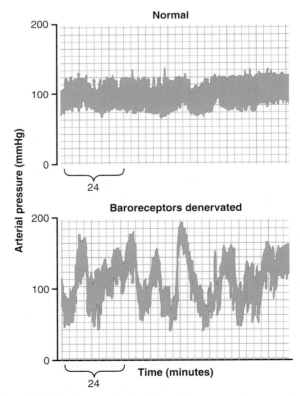

Figure 43-8   Two-hour records of arterial pressure in a normal dog (*top*) and in the same dog (*bottom*) several weeks after the baroreceptors had been denervated. *Modified from Cowley Jr., A.W., Liard, J.F., Guyton, A.C., 1973. Role of baroreceptor reflex in daily control of arterial blood pressure and other variables in dogs. Circ. Res. 32, 564. By permission of the American Heart Association, Inc.*

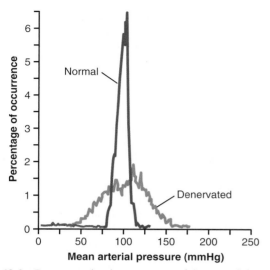

Figure 43-9 Frequency distribution curves of the arterial pressure for a 24-hour period in a normal dog and in the same dog several weeks after the baroreceptors had been denervated. *Modified from Cowley Jr., A.W., Liard, J.P., Guyton, A.C., 1973. Role of baroreceptor reflex in daily control of arterial blood pressure and other variables in dogs. Circ. Res. 32, 564. By permission of the American Heart Association, Inc.*

Thus, a primary purpose of the arterial baroreceptor system is to reduce the minute-by-minute variation in arterial pressure to about one-third that which would occur if the baroreceptor system was not present.

Are the Baroreceptors Important in Long-Term Regulation of Arterial Pressure?

Although the arterial baroreceptors provide powerful moment-to-moment control of arterial pressure, their importance in long-term blood pressure regulation has been controversial. One reason that the baroreceptors have been considered by some physiologists to be relatively unimportant in chronic regulation of arterial pressure is that they tend to *reset* in 1–2 days to the pressure level to which they are exposed. That is, if the arterial pressure rises from the normal value of 100 to 160 mmHg, a very high rate of baroreceptor impulses are at first transmitted. During the next few minutes, the rate of firing diminishes considerably; then it diminishes much more slowly during the next 1–2 days, at the end of which time the rate of firing will have returned to nearly normal despite the fact that the mean arterial pressure still remains at 160 mmHg. Conversely, when the arterial pressure falls to a very low level, the baroreceptors at first transmit no impulses, but gradually, over 1–2 days, the rate of baroreceptor firing returns toward the control level.

This "resetting" of the baroreceptors may attenuate their potency as a control system for correcting disturbances that tend to change arterial pressure for longer than a few days at a time. Experimental studies, however, have suggested that the baroreceptors do not completely reset and may therefore contribute to long-term blood pressure regulation, especially by influencing sympathetic nerve activity of the kidneys. For example, with prolonged increases in arterial pressure, the baroreceptor reflexes may mediate decreases in renal sympathetic nerve activity that promote increased excretion of sodium and water by the kidneys. This action, in turn, causes a gradual decrease in blood volume, which helps to restore arterial pressure toward normal. Thus, long-term regulation of mean arterial pressure by the baroreceptors requires interaction with additional systems, principally the renal–body fluid–pressure control system (along with its associated nervous and hormonal mechanisms), discussed in Chapter 44.

Control of Arterial Pressure by the Carotid and Aortic Chemoreceptors—Effect of Low Oxygen on Arterial Pressure.

Closely associated with the baroreceptor pressure control system is a *chemoreceptor reflex* that operates in much the same way as the baroreceptor reflex except that *chemoreceptors*, instead of stretch receptors, initiate the response.

The chemoreceptors are chemosensitive to low oxygen, carbon dioxide excess, and hydrogen ion excess. They are located in several small *chemoreceptor organs* about 2 mm in size (two *carotid bodies*, one of which lies in the bifurcation of each common carotid artery, and usually one to three *aortic bodies* adjacent to the aorta). The chemoreceptors excite nerve fibers that, along with the baroreceptor fibers, pass through Hering nerves and the vagus nerves into the vasomotor center of the brainstem.

Each carotid or aortic body is supplied with an abundant blood flow through a small nutrient artery, so the chemoreceptors are always in close contact with arterial blood. Whenever the arterial pressure falls below a critical level, the chemoreceptors become stimulated because diminished blood flow causes decreased oxygen, as well as excess buildup of carbon dioxide and hydrogen ions that are not removed by the slowly flowing blood.

The signals transmitted from the chemoreceptors *excite* the vasomotor center, and this response elevates the arterial pressure back toward normal. However, this chemoreceptor reflex is not a powerful arterial pressure controller until the arterial pressure falls below 80 mmHg. Therefore, it is at the lower pressures that this reflex becomes important to help prevent further decreases in arterial pressure.

The chemoreceptors are discussed in much more detail in Chapter 61 in relation to *respiratory control*, in which they play a far more important role than in blood pressure control.

Atrial and Pulmonary Artery Reflexes Regulate Arterial Pressure.

Both the atria and the pulmonary arteries have in their walls stretch receptors called *low-pressure receptors*. Low-pressure receptors are similar to the baroreceptor stretch receptors of the large systemic arteries. These low-pressure receptors play an important role, especially in minimizing arterial pressure changes in response to changes in blood volume. For example, if 300 mL of blood suddenly is infused into a dog with all receptors intact, the arterial pressure rises only about 15 mmHg. With the *arterial baroreceptors* denervated, the pressure rises about 40 mmHg. If the *low-pressure receptors* also are denervated, the arterial pressure rises about 100 mmHg.

Thus, one can see that even though the low-pressure receptors in the pulmonary artery and in the atria cannot detect the systemic arterial pressure, they do detect simultaneous increases in pressure in the low-pressure areas of the circulation caused by increase in volume, and they elicit reflexes parallel to the baroreceptor reflexes to make the total reflex system more potent for control of arterial pressure.

Atrial Reflexes that Activate the Kidneys—The "Volume Reflex".

Stretch of the atria also causes significant reflex dilation of the afferent arterioles in the kidneys. Signals are also transmitted simultaneously from the atria to the hypothalamus to decrease secretion of antidiuretic hormone (ADH). The decreased afferent arteriolar resistance in the kidneys causes the glomerular capillary pressure to rise, with resultant increase in filtration of fluid into the kidney tubules. The diminution of ADH diminishes the reabsorption of water from the tubules. The combination of these two effects—an increase in glomerular filtration and a decrease in reabsorption of the fluid—increases fluid loss by the kidneys and reduces an increased blood volume back toward normal. Atrial stretch caused by increased blood volume also elicits a hormonal effect on the kidneys—release of *atrial natriuretic peptide*—that adds still further to the excretion of fluid in the urine and return of blood volume toward normal.

All these mechanisms that tend to return the blood volume back toward normal after a volume overload act indirectly as pressure controllers, as well as blood volume controllers, because excess volume drives the heart to greater cardiac output and leads to greater arterial pressure. This volume reflex mechanism is discussed again in Chapter 44, along with other mechanisms of blood volume control.

Atrial Reflex Control of Heart Rate (the Bainbridge Reflex). An increase in atrial pressure also causes an increase in heart rate, sometimes increasing the heart rate as much as 75%. A small part of this increase is caused by a direct effect of the increased atrial volume to stretch the sinus node; such direct stretch can increase the heart rate as much as 15%. An additional 40–60% increase in rate is caused by a nervous reflex called the *Bainbridge reflex*. The stretch receptors of the atria that elicit the Bainbridge reflex transmit their afferent signals through the vagus nerves to the medulla of the brain. Then efferent signals are transmitted back through vagal and sympathetic nerves to increase heart rate and strength of heart contraction. Thus, this reflex helps prevent damming of blood in the veins, atria, and pulmonary circulation.

CNS ISCHEMIC RESPONSE—CONTROL OF ARTERIAL PRESSURE BY THE BRAIN'S VASOMOTOR CENTER IN RESPONSE TO DIMINISHED BRAIN BLOOD FLOW

Most nervous control of blood pressure is achieved by reflexes that originate in the baroreceptors, the chemoreceptors, and the low-pressure receptors, all of which are located in the peripheral circulation outside the brain. However, when blood flow to the vasomotor center in the lower brainstem becomes decreased severely enough to cause nutritional deficiency—that is, to cause *cerebral ischemia*—the vasoconstrictor and cardioaccelerator neurons in the vasomotor center respond directly to the ischemia and become strongly excited. When this excitation occurs, the systemic arterial pressure often rises to a level as high as the heart can possibly pump. This effect is believed to be caused by failure of the slowly flowing blood to carry carbon dioxide away from the brainstem vasomotor center: At low levels of blood flow to the vasomotor center, the local concentration of carbon dioxide increases greatly and has an extremely potent effect in stimulating the sympathetic vasomotor nervous control areas in the brain's medulla.

It is possible that other factors, such as buildup of lactic acid and other acidic substances in the vasomotor center, also contribute to the marked stimulation and elevation in arterial pressure. This arterial pressure elevation in response to cerebral ischemia is known as the *CNS ischemic response*.

The ischemic effect on vasomotor activity can elevate the mean arterial pressure dramatically, sometimes to as high as 250 mmHg for as long as 10 minutes. *The degree of sympathetic vasoconstriction caused by intense cerebral ischemia is often so great that some of the peripheral vessels become totally or almost totally occluded.* The kidneys, for instance, often entirely cease their production of urine because of renal arteriolar constriction in response to the sympathetic discharge. Therefore, *the CNS ischemic response is one of the most powerful of all the activators of the sympathetic vasoconstrictor system.*

Importance of the CNS Ischemic Response as a Regulator of Arterial Pressure. Despite the powerful nature of the CNS ischemic response, it does not become significant until the arterial pressure falls far below normal, down to 60 mmHg and below, reaching its greatest degree of stimulation at a pressure of 15–20 mmHg. Therefore, the CNS ischemic response is not one of the normal mechanisms for regulating arterial pressure. Instead, it operates principally as an *emergency pressure control system* that acts rapidly and powerfully to prevent further decrease in arterial pressure whenever blood flow to the brain decreases dangerously close to the lethal level. It is sometimes called the "last ditch stand" pressure control mechanism.

Cushing Reaction to Increased Pressure Around the Brain. The so-called *Cushing reaction* is a special type of CNS ischemic response that results from increased pressure of the cerebrospinal fluid around the brain in the cranial vault. For instance, when the cerebrospinal fluid pressure rises to equal the arterial pressure, it compresses the whole brain, as well as the arteries in the brain, and cuts off the blood supply to the brain. This action initiates a CNS ischemic response that causes the arterial pressure to rise. When the arterial pressure has risen to a level higher than the cerebrospinal fluid pressure, blood will flow once again into the vessels of the brain to relieve the brain ischemia. Ordinarily, the blood pressure comes to a new equilibrium level slightly higher than the cerebrospinal fluid pressure, thus allowing blood to begin to flow through the brain again. The Cushing reaction helps protect vital centers of the brain from loss of nutrition if the cerebrospinal fluid pressure ever rises high enough to compress the cerebral arteries.

Special Features of Nervous Control of Arterial Pressure

ROLE OF THE SKELETAL NERVES AND SKELETAL MUSCLES IN INCREASING CARDIAC OUTPUT AND ARTERIAL PRESSURE

Increased Cardiac Output and Arterial Pressure Caused by Skeletal Muscle Contraction During Exercise. When the skeletal muscles contract during exercise, they compress blood vessels throughout the body. Even anticipation of exercise tightens the muscles, thereby compressing the vessels in the muscles and in the abdomen. This compression translocates blood from the peripheral vessels into the heart and lungs and, therefore, increases cardiac output. This effect is essential in helping to cause the fivefold to sevenfold increase in cardiac output that sometimes occurs during heavy exercise. The rise in cardiac output in turn is an essential ingredient in increasing the arterial pressure during exercise, an increase usually from a normal mean of 100 up to 130–160 mmHg.

RESPIRATORY WAVES IN THE ARTERIAL PRESSURE

With each cycle of respiration, the arterial pressure usually rises and falls 4–6 mmHg in a wave-like manner, causing *respiratory waves* in the arterial pressure. The waves result from several different effects, some of which are reflex in nature, as follows:

1. Many of the "breathing signals" that arise in the respiratory center of the medulla "spill over" into the vasomotor center with each respiratory cycle.
2. Every time a person inspires, the pressure in the thoracic cavity becomes more negative than usual, causing the blood vessels in the chest to expand. This reduces the quantity of blood returning to the left side of the heart and thereby momentarily decreases the cardiac output and arterial pressure.
3. The pressure changes caused in the thoracic vessels by respiration can excite vascular and atrial stretch receptors.

Although it is difficult to analyze the exact relations of all these factors in causing the respiratory pressure waves, the net result during normal respiration is usually an increase in arterial pressure during the early part of expiration and a decrease in pressure during the remainder of the respiratory cycle. During deep respiration, the blood pressure can rise and fall as much as 20 mmHg with each respiratory cycle.

ARTERIAL PRESSURE "VASOMOTOR" WAVES—OSCILLATION OF PRESSURE REFLEX CONTROL SYSTEMS

Often while recording arterial pressure, in addition to the small pressure waves caused by respiration, some much larger waves are also noted—as great as 10–40 mmHg at times—that rise and fall more slowly than the respiratory waves. The duration of each cycle varies from 26 seconds in the anesthetized dog to 7–10 seconds in the unanesthetized human. These waves are called *vasomotor waves* or "*Mayer waves*." Such records are demonstrated in Figure 43-10, showing the cyclical rise and fall in arterial pressure.

The cause of vasomotor waves is "reflex oscillation" of one or more nervous pressure control mechanisms.

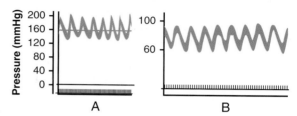

Figure 43-10 (A) Vasomotor waves caused by oscillation of the CNS ischemic response; (B) vasomotor waves caused by baroreceptor reflex oscillation.

BIBLIOGRAPHY

DiBona GF: Physiology in perspective: the wisdom of the body. Neural control of the kidney, *Am. J. Physiol. Regul. Integr. Comp. Physiol.* 289:R633, 2005.

Fadel PJ, Raven PB: Human investigations into the arterial and cardiopulmonary baroreflexes during exercise, *Exp. Physiol.* 97:39, 2012.

Freeman R: Clinical practice. Neurogenic orthostatic hypotension, *N. Engl. J. Med.* 358:615, 2008.

Guyenet PG: The sympathetic control of blood pressure, *Nat. Rev. Neurosci.* 7:335, 2006.

Guyenet PG, Abbott SB, Stornetta RL: The respiratory chemoreception conundrum: light at the end of the tunnel? *Brain Res.* 1511:126, 2013.

Guyton AC: *Arterial Pressure and Hypertension*, Philadelphia, 1980, W.B. Saunders.

Hall JE, da Silva AA, do Carmo JM, et al: Obesity-induced hypertension: role of sympathetic nervous system, leptin, and melanocortins, *J. Biol. Chem.* 285:17271, 2010.

Jardine DL: Vasovagal syncope: new physiologic insights, *Cardiol. Clin.* 31:75, 2013.

Joyner MJ: Baroreceptor function during exercise: resetting the record, *Exp. Physiol.* 91:27, 2006.

Kaufman MP: The exercise pressor reflex in animals, *Exp. Physiol.* 97:51, 2012.

Ketch T, Biaggioni I, Robertson R, Robertson D: Four faces of baroreflex failure: hypertensive crisis, volatile hypertension, orthostatic tachycardia, and malignant vagotonia, *Circulation* 105:2518, 2002.

Lohmeier TE, Iliescu R: Chronic lowering of blood pressure by carotid baroreflex activation: mechanisms and potential for hypertension therapy, *Hypertension* 57:880, 2011.

Parati G, Esler M: The human sympathetic nervous system: its relevance in hypertension and heart failure, *Eur. Heart J.* 33:1058, 2012.

Paton JF, Sobotka PA, Fudim M, et al: The carotid body as a therapeutic target for the treatment of sympathetically mediated diseases, *Hypertension* 61:5, 2013.

Schultz HD, Li YL, Ding Y: Arterial chemoreceptors and sympathetic nerve activity: implications for hypertension and heart failure, *Hypertension* 50:6, 2007.

Seifer C: Carotid sinus syndrome, *Cardiol. Clin.* 31:111, 2013.

Stewart JM: Common syndromes of orthostatic intolerance, *Pediatrics* 131:968, 2013.

Zucker IH: Novel mechanisms of sympathetic regulation in chronic heart failure, *Hypertension* 48:1005, 2006.

Long-Term Regulation of Arterial Blood Pressure

GLOSSARY OF TERMS

- **Pressure diuresis:** The increase in renal output of water following an increase in arterial blood pressure
- **Pressure natriuresis:** The increase in renal output of sodium following an increase in arterial blood pressure

The sympathetic nervous system plays a major role in the short-term control of arterial pressure primarily through the effects of the nervous system on total peripheral vascular resistance and capacitance, as well as on cardiac pumping ability as discussed in Chapter 43.

The body, however, also has powerful mechanisms for regulating arterial pressure week after week and month after month. This long-term control of arterial pressure is closely intertwined with homeostasis of body fluid volume; for long-term survival, fluid intake and output must be precisely balanced. In this chapter we discuss these renal–body fluid systems that play a major role in long-term blood pressure regulation.

The renal–body fluid system for arterial pressure control acts slowly but powerfully as follows: If blood volume increases and vascular capacitance is not altered, arterial pressure will also increase. The rising pressure in turn causes the kidneys to excrete the excess volume, thus returning the pressure back toward normal. Indeed, an increase in arterial pressure in the human of only a few millimeters of mercury can double renal output of water, which is called *pressure diuresis*, as well as double the output of salt, which is called *pressure natriuresis*.

Quantification of Pressure Diuresis as a Basis for Arterial Pressure Control

Figure 44-1 shows the approximate average effect of different arterial pressure levels on urinary volume output by an isolated kidney, demonstrating markedly increased urine volume output as the pressure rises. This increased urinary output is the phenomenon of *pressure diuresis*. The curve in this figure is called a *renal urinary output curve* or a *renal function curve*. In the human being, at an arterial pressure of 50 mmHg, the urine output is essentially zero. At 100 mmHg it is normal, and at 200 mmHg

it is about six to eight times normal. Furthermore, not only does increasing the arterial pressure increase urine volume output, but it also causes an approximately equal increase in sodium output, which is the phenomenon of *pressure natriuresis*.

THE RENAL–BODY FLUID MECHANISM PROVIDES "NEARLY INFINITE FEEDBACK GAIN" FOR LONG-TERM ARTERIAL PRESSURE CONTROL

Figure 44-2 shows a graphical method that can be used for analyzing arterial pressure control by the renal–body fluid system. This analysis is based on two separate curves that intersect each other: (1) the renal output curve for water and salt in response to rising arterial pressure, which is the same renal output curve as that shown in Figure 44-1, and (2) the line that represents the net water and salt intake.

Over a long period, the water and salt output must equal the intake. Furthermore, the only place on the graph in Figure 44-2 at which output equals intake is where the two curves intersect, called the *equilibrium point*. Now, let us see what happens if the arterial pressure increases above, or decreases below, the equilibrium point.

First, assume that the arterial pressure rises to 150 mmHg. At this level, the renal output of water and salt is about three times as great as intake. Therefore, the body loses fluid, the blood volume decreases, and the arterial pressure decreases. Furthermore, this "negative balance" of fluid will not cease until the pressure falls *all the way* back exactly to the equilibrium level. Indeed, even when the arterial pressure is only a few millimeters of mercury greater than the equilibrium level, there still is slightly more loss of water and salt than intake, so the pressure continues to fall that last few millimeters of mercury *until the pressure eventually returns to the equilibrium point*.

If the arterial pressure falls below the equilibrium point, the intake of water and salt is greater than the output. Therefore, body fluid volume increases, blood volume increases, and the arterial pressure rises until once again it returns *exactly* to the equilibrium point. This return of the arterial pressure *always back to the equilibrium point* is the *near infinite feedback gain principle* for control of arterial pressure by the renal–body fluid mechanism.

TWO KEY DETERMINANTS OF LONG-TERM ARTERIAL PRESSURE

In Figure 44-2, one can also see that two basic long-term factors determine the long-term arterial pressure level. As long as the two curves representing (1) renal output of salt and water, and (2) intake of salt and water remain exactly as they are shown in Figure 44-2, the mean arterial pressure level will eventually readjust to 100 mmHg, which is the pressure level depicted by the equilibrium point of this figure. Furthermore, there are only

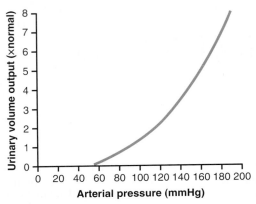

Figure 44-1   A typical renal urinary output curve measured in a per-fused isolated kidney, showing pressure diuresis when the arterial pressure rises above normal.

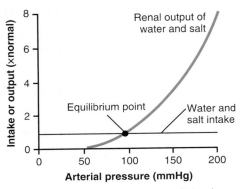

Figure 44-2   Analysis of arterial pressure regulation by equating the "renal output curve" with the "salt and water intake curve." The equilibrium point describes the level to which the arterial pressure will be regulated. (The small portion of the salt and water intake that is lost from the body through nonrenal routes is ignored in this and similar figures in this chapter.)

two ways in which the pressure of this equilibrium point can be changed from the 100 mmHg level. One way is by shifting the pressure level of the renal output curve for salt and water, and the other is by changing the level of the water and salt intake line. Therefore, expressed simply, the two primary determinants of the long-term arterial pressure level are as follows:

1. the degree of pressure shift of the renal output curve for water and salt;
2. the level of the water and salt intake.

Operation of these two determinants in the control of arterial pressure is demonstrated in Figure 44-3. In Figure 44-3A, some abnormality of the kidneys has caused the renal output curve to shift 50 mmHg in the high-pressure direction (to the right). Note that the equilibrium point has also shifted to 50 mmHg higher than normal. Therefore, one can state that if the renal output curve shifts to a new pressure level, the arterial pressure will follow to this new pressure level within a few days.

Figure 44-3B shows how a change in the level of salt and water intake also can change the arterial pressure. In this case, the intake level has increased fourfold and the equilibrium point has shifted to a pressure level of 160 mmHg, 60 mmHg above the normal level. Conversely, a decrease in the intake level would reduce the arterial pressure.

Thus, it is *impossible to change the long-term mean arterial pressure level* to a new value without changing one or both of the

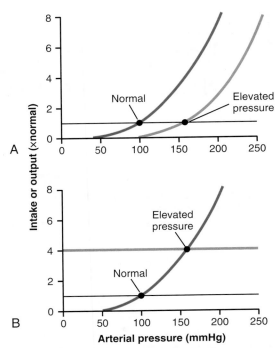

Figure 44-3   Two ways in which the arterial pressure can be increased: (A) by shifting the renal output curve in the right-hand direction toward a higher pressure level or (B) by increasing the intake level of salt and water.

two basic determinants of long-term arterial pressure—either (1) the level of salt and water intake or (2) the degree of shift of the renal function curve along the pressure axis. However, if either of these is changed, one finds the arterial pressure thereafter to be regulated at a new pressure level, the arterial pressure at which the two new curves intersect.

In most people, however, the renal function curve is much steeper than shown in Figure 44-3 and changes in salt intake have only a modest effect on arterial pressure, as discussed in the next section.

The Renin–Angiotensin System: Its Role in Arterial Pressure Control

Aside from the capability of the kidneys to control arterial pressure through changes in extracellular fluid volume, the kidneys also have another powerful mechanism for controlling pressure: the renin–angiotensin system.

Renin is a protein enzyme released by the kidneys when the arterial pressure falls too low. In turn, it raises the arterial pressure in several ways, thus helping to correct the initial fall in pressure.

COMPONENTS OF THE RENIN–ANGIOTENSIN SYSTEM

Figure 44-4 shows the functional steps by which the renin–angiotensin system helps to regulate arterial pressure.

Renin is synthesized and stored in an inactive form called *prorenin* in the *juxtaglomerular cells* (JG cells) of the kidneys. The JG cells are modified smooth muscle cells located mainly *in the walls of the afferent arterioles immediately proximal to the glomeruli*. When the arterial pressure falls, intrinsic reactions in the kidneys cause many of the prorenin molecules in the JG

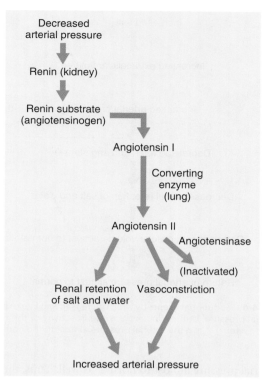

Decreased
arterial pressure

↓

Renin (kidney)

↓

Renin substrate
(angiotensinogen)

↓

Angiotensin I

Converting
enzyme
(lung)

↓

Angiotensin II

Angiotensinase

(Inactivated)

Renal retention   Vasoconstriction
of salt and water

↓

Increased arterial pressure

Figure 44-4 The renin–angiotensin vasoconstrictor mechanism for arterial pressure control.

cells to split and release renin. Most of the renin enters the renal blood and then passes out of the kidneys to circulate throughout the entire body. However, small amounts of the renin do remain in the local fluids of the kidney and initiate several intrarenal functions.

Renin itself is an enzyme, not a vasoactive substance. As shown in the schema of Figure 44-4, renin acts enzymatically on another plasma protein, a globulin called *renin substrate* (or *angiotensinogen*), to release a 10–amino acid peptide, *angiotensin I*. Angiotensin I has mild vasoconstrictor properties but not enough to cause significant changes in circulatory function. The renin persists in the blood for 30 minutes to 1 hour and continues to cause formation of still more angiotensin I during this entire time.

Within a few seconds to minutes after formation of angiotensin I, two additional amino acids are split from the angiotensin I to form the 8–amino acid peptide *angiotensin II*. This conversion occurs to a great extent in the lungs while the blood flows through the small vessels of the lungs, catalyzed by an enzyme called *angiotensin-converting enzyme* that is present in the endothelium of the lung vessels. Other tissues such as the kidneys and blood vessels also contain converting enzyme and therefore form angiotensin II locally.

Angiotensin II is an extremely powerful vasoconstrictor and it affects circulatory function in other ways as well. However, it persists in the blood only for 1 or 2 minutes because it is rapidly inactivated by multiple blood and tissue enzymes collectively called *angiotensinases.*

Angiotensin II has two principal effects that can elevate arterial pressure. The first of these, *vasoconstriction in many areas of the body*, occurs rapidly. Vasoconstriction occurs intensely in the arterioles and much less in the veins. Constriction of the arterioles increases the total peripheral resistance, thereby raising the

arterial pressure, as demonstrated at the bottom of the schema in Figure 44-4. Also, the mild constriction of the veins promotes increased venous return of blood to the heart, thereby helping the heart pump against the increasing pressure.

The second principal means by which angiotensin II increases the arterial pressure is to *decrease excretion of both salt and water* by the kidneys. This action slowly increases the extracellular fluid volume, which then increases the arterial pressure during subsequent hours and days. This long-term effect, acting through the extracellular fluid volume mechanism, is even more powerful than the acute vasoconstrictor mechanism in eventually raising the arterial pressure.

Angiotensin II Causes Renal Retention of Salt and Water—An Important Means for Long-Term Control of Arterial Pressure

Angiotensin II causes the kidneys to retain both salt and water in two major ways:

1. Angiotensin II acts directly on the kidneys to cause salt and water retention.
2. Angiotensin II causes the adrenal glands to secrete aldosterone, and the aldosterone in turn increases salt and water reabsorption by the kidney tubules.

Thus, whenever excess amounts of angiotensin II circulate in the blood, the entire long-term renal–body fluid mechanism for arterial pressure control automatically becomes set to a higher arterial pressure level than normal.

Mechanisms of the Direct Renal Effects of Angiotensin II to Cause Renal Retention of Salt and Water. Angiotensin has several direct renal effects that make the kidneys retain salt and water. One major effect is to constrict the renal arterioles, thereby diminishing blood flow through the kidneys. The slow flow of blood reduces the pressure in the peritubular capillaries, which causes rapid reabsorption of fluid from the tubules. Angiotensin II also has important direct actions on the tubular cells to increase tubular reabsorption of sodium and water. The combined result of all these effects is that angiotensin II can sometimes decrease urine output to less than one-fifth of normal.

Angiotensin II Increases Salt and Water Retention by the Kidneys by Stimulating Aldosterone. Angiotensin II is also one of the most powerful stimulators of aldosterone secretion by the adrenal glands, as we shall discuss in relation to body fluid regulation in Chapter 80 and in relation to adrenal gland function in Chapter 91. Therefore, when the renin–angiotensin system becomes activated, the rate of aldosterone secretion usually also increases, and an important subsequent function of aldosterone is to cause marked increase in sodium reabsorption by the kidney tubules, thus increasing the total body extracellular fluid sodium. This increased sodium then causes water retention, as already explained, increasing the extracellular fluid volume and leading secondarily to still more long-term elevation of the arterial pressure.

Thus both the direct effect of angiotensin on the kidney and its effect acting through aldosterone are important in long-term arterial pressure control. However, research in our laboratory has suggested that the direct effect of angiotensin on the kidneys is perhaps three or more times as potent as the indirect effect acting through aldosterone—even though the indirect effect is the one most widely known.

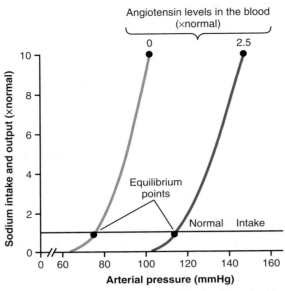

Figure 44-5 The effect of two angiotensin II levels in the blood on the renal output curve, showing regulation of the arterial pressure at an equilibrium point of 75 mmHg when the angiotensin II level is low and at 115 mmHg when the angiotensin II level is high.

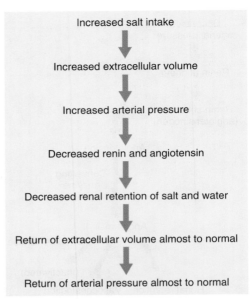

Figure 44-6 Sequential events by which increased salt intake increases the arterial pressure, but feedback decrease in activity of the renin–angiotensin system returns the arterial pressure almost to the normal level.

Quantitative Analysis of Arterial Pressure Changes Caused by Angiotensin II. Figure 44-5 shows a quantitative analysis of the effect of angiotensin in arterial pressure control. This figure shows two renal function curves, as well as a line depicting a normal level of sodium intake. The left-hand renal function curve is that measured in dogs whose renin–angiotensin system had been blocked by an angiotensin-converting enzyme inhibitor drug that blocks the conversion of angiotensin I to angiotensin II. The right-hand curve was measured in dogs infused continuously with angiotensin II at a level about 2.5 times the normal rate of angiotensin formation in the blood. Note the shift of the renal output curve toward higher pressure levels under the influence of angiotensin II. This shift is caused by both the direct effects of angiotensin II on the kidney and the indirect effect acting through aldosterone secretion, as explained earlier.

Finally, note the two equilibrium points, one for zero angiotensin showing an arterial pressure level of 75 mmHg and one for elevated angiotensin showing a pressure level of 115 mmHg. Therefore, the action of angiotensin to cause renal retention of salt and water can have a powerful effect in promoting chronic elevation of the arterial pressure.

Role of the Renin–Angiotensin System in Maintaining a Normal Arterial Pressure Despite Large Variations in Salt Intake

One of the most important functions of the renin–angiotensin system is to allow a person to eat either very small or very large amounts of salt without causing great changes in either extracellular fluid volume or arterial pressure. This function is explained by the schema in Figure 44-6, which shows that the initial effect of increased salt intake is to elevate the extracellular fluid volume, in turn elevating the arterial pressure. Then, the increased arterial pressure causes increased blood flow through the kidneys, as well as other effects, which reduce the rate of secretion of renin to a much lower level and lead sequentially to decreased renal retention of salt and water, return of the extracellular fluid volume almost to normal, and, finally, return of

the arterial pressure almost to normal as well. Thus, the renin–angiotensin system is an automatic feedback mechanism that helps maintain the arterial pressure at or near the normal level even when salt intake is increased. When salt intake is decreased below normal, exactly opposite effects take place.

To emphasize the efficacy of the renin–angiotensin system in controlling arterial pressure, when the system functions normally, the pressure rises no more than 4–6 mmHg in response to as much as a 100-fold increase in salt intake. Conversely, when the renin–angiotensin system is blocked and the usual suppression of angiotensin is prevented, the same increase in salt intake sometimes causes the pressure to rise 50–60 mmHg, as much as 10 times the normal increase.

Hypertension

About 90–95% of all people who have hypertension are said to have "primary hypertension," also widely known as "essential hypertension" by many clinicians. These terms mean simply that *the hypertension is of unknown origin*, in contrast to the forms of hypertension that are *secondary* to known causes, such as renal artery stenosis or monogenic forms of hypertension.

In most patients, *excess weight gain* and *a sedentary lifestyle* appear to play a major role in causing hypertension. The majority of patients with hypertension are overweight, and studies of different populations suggest that excess weight gain and obesity may account for as much as 65–75% of the risk for developing primary hypertension.

The following characteristics of primary hypertension, among others, are caused by excess weight gain and obesity:

1. *Cardiac output is increased.*
2. *Sympathetic nerve activity, especially in the kidneys, is increased in overweight patients.*
3. *Angiotensin II and aldosterone levels are increased twofold to threefold in many obese patients.*
4. *The renal-pressure natriuresis mechanism is impaired, and the kidneys will not excrete adequate amounts of salt and water unless the arterial pressure is high or kidney function is somehow improved.*

BIBLIOGRAPHY

Brands MW: Chronic blood pressure control, *Compr. Physiol.* 2:2481, 2012.

Chobanian AV, Bakris GL, Black HR, Joint National Committee on Prevention, Detection, Evaluation, and Treatment of High Blood Pressure, National High Blood Pressure Education Program Coordinating Committee: et al: Seventh report of the Joint National Committee on Prevention, Detection, Evaluation, and Treatment of High Blood Pressure, *Hypertension* 42:1206, 2003.

Coffman TM: Under pressure: the search for the essential mechanisms of hypertension, *Nat. Med.* 17:1402, 2011.

Cowley AW: Long-term control of arterial blood pressure, *Physiol. Rev.* 72:231, 1992.

Guyton AC: *Arterial Pressure and Hypertension*, Philadelphia, 1980, W.B. Saunders.

Hall JE: The kidney, hypertension, and obesity, *Hypertension* 41:625, 2003.

Hall JE, daSilva AA, doCarmo JM, et al: Obesity-induced hypertension: role of sympathetic nervous system, leptin and melanocortins, *J. Biol. Chem.* 285:17271, 2010.

Hall JE, Granger JP, do Carmo JM, et al: Hypertension: physiology and pathophysiology, *Compr. Physiol.* 2:2393, 2012.

Lohmeier TE, Iliescu R: Chronic lowering of blood pressure by carotid baroreflex activation: mechanisms and potential for hypertension therapy, *Hypertension* 57:880, 2011.

Maranon R, Reckelhoff JF: Sex and gender differences in control of blood pressure, *Clin. Sci. (Lond.)* 125:311, 2013.

45

Regional Circulation: An Overview

A fundamental principle of circulatory function is that most tissues have the ability to control their own local blood flow in proportion to their specific metabolic needs.

The specific needs of the tissues for blood flow are many, and include the following:

1. delivery of oxygen to the tissues;
2. delivery of other nutrients, such as glucose, amino acids, and fatty acids;
3. removal of carbon dioxide from the tissues;
4. removal of hydrogen ions from the tissues;
5. maintenance of proper concentrations of ions in the tissues;
6. transport of various hormones and other substances to the different tissues.

Certain organs have special requirements. For instance, blood flow to the skin determines heat loss from the body and in this way helps to control body temperature. Also, delivery of adequate quantities of blood plasma to the kidneys allows the kidneys to filter and excrete the waste products of the body and to regulate body fluid volumes and electrolytes.

Variations in Blood Flow in Different Tissues and Organs

Note the very large blood flows in some organs listed in Table 45-1—for example, several hundred milliliters per minute per 100 g of thyroid or adrenal gland tissue and a total blood flow of 1350 mL/minute in the liver, which is 95 mL/minute per 100 g of liver tissue.

Also note the extremely large blood flow through the kidneys—1100 mL/minute. This extreme amount of flow is required for the kidneys to perform their function of cleansing the blood of waste products and precisely regulating the composition of body fluids.

Conversely, most surprising is the low blood flow to all the *inactive* muscles of the body, only a total of 750 mL/minute, even though the muscles constitute between 30 and 40% of the total body mass. In the resting state, the metabolic activity of the muscles is low, as is the blood flow, only 4 mL/minute per 100 g. Yet, during heavy exercise, muscle metabolic activity can increase more than 60-fold and the blood flow as much as 20-fold, increasing to as high as 16,000 mL/minute in the body's total muscle vascular bed (or 80 mL/minute per 100 g of muscle).

Mechanisms of Blood Flow Control

Local blood flow control can be divided into two phases: (1) acute control and (2) long-term control.

Acute control is achieved by rapid changes in local vasodilation or vasoconstriction of the arterioles, metarterioles, and precapillary sphincters that occurs within seconds to minutes to provide very rapid maintenance of appropriate local tissue blood flow.

Long-term control means slow, controlled changes in flow over a period of days, weeks, or even months. In general, these long-term changes provide even better control of the flow in proportion to the needs of the tissues. These changes come about as a result of an increase or decrease in the physical sizes and numbers of blood vessels supplying the tissues.

ACUTE CONTROL OF LOCAL BLOOD FLOW

Increases in Tissue Metabolism Increase Tissue Blood Flow. Figure 45-1 shows the approximate acute effect on blood flow of increasing the rate of metabolism in a local tissue, such as in a skeletal muscle. Note that an increase in metabolism up to eight times normal increases the blood flow acutely about fourfold.

Reduced Increases Tissue Blood Flow. One of the most necessary of the metabolic nutrients is oxygen. Whenever the availability of oxygen to the tissues decreases, such as (1) at a high altitude at the top of a high mountain, (2) in pneumonia, (3) in carbon monoxide poisoning (which poisons the ability of hemoglobin to transport oxygen), or (4) in cyanide poisoning (which poisons the ability of the tissues to use oxygen), the blood flow through the tissues increases markedly. Figure 45-2 shows that as the arterial oxygen saturation decreases to about 25% of normal, the blood flow through an isolated leg increases about threefold; that is, the blood flow increases almost enough, but not quite enough, to make up for the decreased amount of oxygen in the blood, thus almost maintaining a relatively constant supply of oxygen to the tissues.

TABLE 45-1	Blood Flow to Different Organs and Tissues Under Basal Conditions		
	Percent of Cardiac Output	Milliliters Per Minute	Milliliters Per Minute Per 100 g of Tissue Weight
Brain	14	700	50
Heart	4	200	70
Bronchi	2	100	25
Kidneys	22	1100	360
Liver	27	1350	95
Portal	(21)	1050	
Arterial	(6)	300	
Muscle (inactive state)	15	750	4
Bone	5	250	3
Skin (cool weather)	6	300	3
Thyroid gland	1	50	160
Adrenal glands	0.5	25	300
Other tissues	3.5	175	1.3
Total	100	5000	

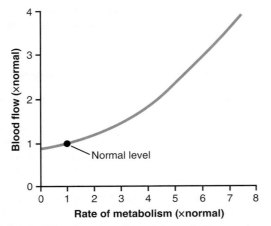

Figure 45-1 Effect of increasing rate of metabolism on tissue blood flow.

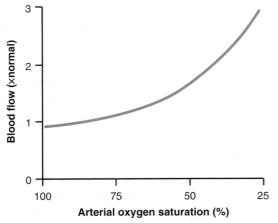

Figure 45-2 Effect of decreasing arterial oxygen saturation on blood flow through an isolated dog leg.

Vasodilator Theory for Acute Local Blood Flow Regulation—Possible Special Role of Adenosine. According to the vasodilator theory, the greater the rate of metabolism or the lesser the availability of oxygen or some other nutrients to a tissue, the greater is the rate of formation of *vasodilator substances* in the tissue cells. The vasodilator substances then are believed to diffuse through the tissues to the precapillary sphincters, metarterioles, and arterioles to cause dilation. Some of the different vasodilator substances that have been suggested are *adenosine, carbon dioxide, adenosine phosphate compounds, histamine, potassium ions,* and *hydrogen ions.*

Many physiologists believe that *adenosine* is an important local vasodilator for controlling local blood flow. For example, minute quantities of adenosine are released from heart muscle cells when coronary blood flow becomes too little and this causes enough local vasodilation in the heart to return coronary blood flow back to normal. Also, whenever the heart becomes more active than normal and the heart's metabolism increases an extra amount, this, too, causes increased utilization of oxygen, followed by (1) decreased oxygen concentration in the heart muscle cells with (2) consequent degradation of adenosine triphosphate (ATP), which (3) increases the release of adenosine. It is believed that much of this adenosine leaks out of the heart muscle cells to cause coronary vasodilation, providing increased coronary blood flow to supply the increased nutrient demands of the active heart.

Oxygen Demand Theory for Local Blood Flow Control. Although the vasodilator theory is widely accepted, several critical facts have made other physiologists favor another theory, which can be called either the *oxygen demand theory* or, more accurately, the *nutrient demand theory* (because other nutrients besides oxygen are involved). Oxygen is one of the metabolic nutrients required to cause vascular muscle contraction (together with other nutrients as well). Therefore, in the absence of adequate oxygen, it is reasonable to believe that the blood vessels would relax and therefore dilate. Also, increased utilization of oxygen in the tissues as a result of increased metabolism theoretically could decrease the availability of oxygen to the smooth muscle fibers in the local blood vessels, and this decreased availability, too, would cause local vasodilation.

Possible Role of Other Nutrients Besides Oxygen in Control of Local Blood Flow. Under special conditions, it has been shown that lack of glucose in the perfusing blood can cause local tissue vasodilation. It also is possible that this same effect occurs when other nutrients, such as amino acids or fatty acids, are deficient, although this issue has not been studied adequately. In addition, vasodilation occurs in the vitamin deficiency disease *beriberi*, in which the patient has deficiencies of the vitamin B substances *thiamine*, *niacin*, and *riboflavin*. In this disease, the peripheral vascular blood flow almost everywhere in the body often increases twofold to threefold. Because all these vitamins are necessary for oxygen-induced phosphorylation, which is required to produce ATP in the tissue cells, one can well understand how deficiency of these vitamins might lead to diminished smooth muscle contractile ability and therefore local vasodilation as well.

Special Examples of Acute "Metabolic" Control of Local Blood Flow

The mechanisms we have described thus far for local blood flow control are called "metabolic mechanisms" because all of them function in response to the metabolic needs of the tissues. Two additional special examples of metabolic control of local blood flow are *reactive hyperemia* and *active hyperemia*.

"Reactive Hyperemia" Occurs After the Tissue Blood Supply Is Blocked for a Short Time. When the blood supply to a tissue is blocked for a few seconds to as long as an hour or more and then is unblocked, blood flow through the tissue usually increases immediately to four to seven times normal; this increased flow will continue for a few seconds if the block has lasted only a few seconds but sometimes continues for as long as many hours if the blood flow has been stopped for an hour or more. This phenomenon is called reactive hyperemia.

Reactive hyperemia is another manifestation of the local "metabolic" blood flow regulation mechanism; that is, lack of flow sets into motion all of the factors that cause vasodilation. After short periods of vascular occlusion, the extra blood flow during the reactive hyperemia phase lasts long enough to repay almost exactly the tissue oxygen deficit that has accrued during the period of occlusion. This mechanism emphasizes the close connection between local blood flow regulation and delivery of oxygen and other nutrients to the tissues.

"Active Hyperemia" Occurs When Tissue Metabolic Rate Increases. When any tissue becomes highly active, such as an exercising muscle, a gastrointestinal gland during a hypersecretory period, or even the brain during increased mental activity, the rate of blood flow through the tissue increases. The increase in local metabolism causes the cells to devour tissue fluid nutrients rapidly and also to release large quantities of vasodilator substances. The result is dilation of local blood vessels and increased local blood flow. In this way, the active tissue receives the additional nutrients required to sustain its new level of function. As pointed out earlier, active hyperemia in skeletal muscle can increase local muscle blood flow as much as 20-fold during intense exercise.

"Autoregulation" of Blood Flow During Changes in Arterial Pressure—"Metabolic" and "Myogenic" Mechanisms

In any tissue of the body, a rapid increase in arterial pressure causes an immediate rise in blood flow. However, within less

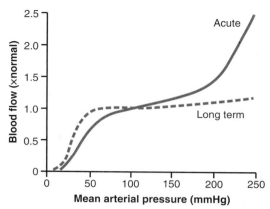

Figure 45-3 Effect of different levels of arterial pressure on blood flow through a muscle. The *solid red curve* shows the effect if the arterial pressure is raised over a period of a few minutes. The *dashed green curve* shows the effect if the arterial pressure is raised slowly over a period of many weeks.

than a minute, the blood flow in most tissues returns almost to the normal level, even though the arterial pressure is kept elevated. This return of flow toward normal is called "*autoregulation*." After autoregulation has occurred, the local blood flow in most body tissues will be related to arterial pressure approximately in accord with the solid "acute" curve in Figure 45-3. Note that between arterial pressures of about 70 and 175 mmHg the blood flow increases only 20–30% even though the arterial pressure increases 150%. In some tissues, such as the brain and the heart, this autoregulation is even more precise.

For almost a century, two views have been proposed to explain this acute autoregulation mechanism. They have been called (1) the metabolic theory and (2) the myogenic theory.

The *metabolic theory* can be understood easily by applying the basic principles of local blood flow regulation discussed in previous sections. Thus, when the arterial pressure becomes too high, the excess flow provides too much oxygen and too many other nutrients to the tissues and "washes out" the vasodilators released by the tissues. These nutrients (especially oxygen) and decreased tissue levels of vasodilators then cause the blood vessels to constrict and return flow to nearly normal despite the increased pressure.

The *myogenic theory*, however, suggests that still another mechanism not related to tissue metabolism explains the phenomenon of autoregulation. This theory is based on the observation that sudden stretch of small blood vessels causes the smooth muscle of the vessel wall to contract. Therefore, it has been proposed that when high arterial pressure stretches the vessel, this in turn causes reactive vascular constriction that reduces blood flow nearly back to normal. Conversely, at low pressures, the degree of stretch of the vessel is less, so that the smooth muscle relaxes, reducing vascular resistance and helping to return flow toward normal.

The myogenic response is inherent to vascular smooth muscle and can occur in the absence of neural or hormonal influences. It is most pronounced in arterioles but can also be observed in arteries, venules, veins, and even lymphatic vessels. Myogenic contraction is initiated by stretch-induced vascular depolarization, which then rapidly increases calcium ion entry from the extracellular fluid into the cells, causing them to contract. Changes in vascular pressure may also open or close

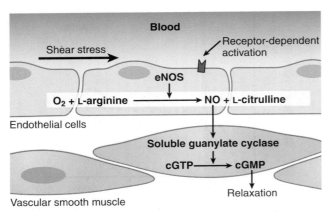

Figure 45-4 Nitric oxide synthase (eNOS) enzyme in endothelial cells synthesizes nitric oxide (NO) from arginine and oxygen. NO activates soluble guanylate cyclases in vascular smooth muscle cells resulting in conversion of cyclic guanosine triphosphate (cGTP) to cyclic guanosine monophosphate (cGMP), which ultimately causes the blood vessels to relax.

other ion channels that influence vascular contraction. The precise mechanisms by which changes in pressure cause opening or closing of vascular ion channels are still uncertain but likely involve mechanical effects of pressure on extracellular proteins that are tethered to cytoskeleton elements of the vascular wall or to the ion channels themselves.

The myogenic mechanism appears to be important in preventing excessive stretching of blood vessel when blood pressure is increased. However, the role of the myogenic mechanism in blood flow regulation is unclear because this pressure-sensing mechanism cannot directly detect changes in blood flow in the tissue. Indeed, metabolic factors appear to override the myogenic mechanism in circumstances in which the metabolic demands of the tissues are significantly increased, such as during vigorous muscle exercise, which can cause dramatic increases in skeletal muscle blood flow.

Control of Tissue Blood Flow by Endothelial-Derived Relaxing or Constricting Factors

The endothelial cells lining the blood vessels synthesize several substances that, when released, can affect the degree of relaxation or contraction of the arterial wall. For many of these endothelial-derived relaxing or constrictor factors, the physiological roles are just beginning to be understood and clinical applications have, in most cases, not yet been developed.

Nitric Oxide—A Vasodilator Released from Healthy Endothelial Cells. The most important of the endothelial-derived relaxing factors is nitric oxide (NO), a lipophilic gas that is released from endothelial cells in response to a variety of chemical and physical stimuli. Endothelial-derived nitric oxide synthase (NOS) enzymes synthesize NO from arginine and oxygen and by reduction of inorganic nitrate. After diffusing out of the endothelial cell, NO has a half-life in the blood of only about 6 seconds and acts mainly in the local tissues where it is released. NO activates soluble guanylate cyclases in vascular smooth muscle cells (Figure 45-4), resulting in conversion of cyclic guanosine triphosphate (cGTP) to cyclic guanosine monophosphate (cGMP) and activation of cGMP-dependent protein kinase (PKG), which has several actions that cause the blood vessels to relax.

The flow of blood through the arteries and arterioles causes *shear stress* on the endothelial cells because of viscous drag of the blood against the vascular walls. This stress contorts the endothelial cells in the direction of flow and causes significant NO release. The NO then relaxes the blood vessels, which is fortunate because the local metabolic mechanisms for controlling tissue blood flow dilate the very small arteries and arterioles in each tissue. Yet, when blood flow through a microvascular portion of the circulation increases, this action secondarily stimulates the release of NO from larger vessels as a result of increased flow and shear stress in these vessels. The released NO increases the diameters of the larger upstream blood vessels whenever microvascular blood flow increases downstream. Without such a response, the effectiveness of local blood flow control would be decreased because a significant part of the resistance to blood flow is in the upstream small arteries.

NO synthesis and release from endothelial cells are also stimulated by some vasoconstrictors, such as *angiotensin II*, which bind to specific receptors on endothelial cells. The increased NO release protects against excessive vasoconstriction.

When endothelial cells are damaged by chronic hypertension or atherosclerosis, impaired NO synthesis may contribute to excessive vasoconstriction and worsening of the hypertension and endothelial damage, which, if untreated, may eventually cause vascular injury and damage to vulnerable tissues such as the heart, kidneys, and brain.

Even before NO was discovered, clinicians used nitroglycerin, amyl nitrates, and other nitrate derivatives to treat patients who had *angina pectoris*, that is, severe chest pain caused by ischemia of the heart muscle. These drugs, when broken down chemically, release NO and evoke dilation of blood vessels throughout the body, including the coronary blood vessels.

Other important applications of NO physiology and pharmacology are the development and clinical use of drugs (eg, sildenafil) that inhibit *cGMP-specific phosphodiesterase-5 (PDE-5)*, an enzyme that degrades cGMP. By preventing the degradation of cGMP, the PDE-5 inhibitors effectively prolong the actions of NO to cause vasodilation. The primary clinical use of the PDE-5 inhibitors is to treat erectile dysfunction. Penile erection is caused by parasympathetic nerve impulses through the pelvic nerves to the penis, where the neurotransmitters acetylcholine and NO are released. By preventing the degradation of NO, the PDE-5 inhibitors enhance the dilation of the blood vessels in the penis and aid in erection, as discussed in Chapter 97.

Endothelin—A Powerful Vasoconstrictor Released from Damaged Endothelium. Endothelial cells also release vasoconstrictor substances. The most important of these is endothelin, a large 21–amino acid peptide that requires only minute amounts (nanogram) to cause powerful vasoconstriction. This substance is present in the endothelial cells of all or most blood vessels but greatly increases when the vessels are injured. The usual stimulus for release is damage to the endothelium, such as that caused by crushing the tissues or injecting a traumatizing chemical into the blood vessel. After severe blood vessel damage, release of local endothelin and subsequent vasoconstriction helps to prevent extensive bleeding from arteries as large as 5 mm in diameter that might have been torn open by crushing injury.

Increased endothelin release is also believed to contribute to vasoconstriction when the endothelium is damaged by hypertension. Drugs that block endothelin receptors have been used to treat *pulmonary hypertension* but generally have not been used for lowering blood pressure in patients with systemic arterial hypertension.

LONG-TERM BLOOD FLOW REGULATION

Thus far, most of the mechanisms for local blood flow regulation that we have discussed act within a few seconds to a few minutes after the local tissue conditions have changed. Yet, even after full activation of these acute mechanisms, the blood flow usually is adjusted only about three-quarters of the way to the exact additional requirements of the tissues. However, over a period of hours, days, and weeks, a long-term type of local blood flow regulation develops in addition to the acute control. This long-term regulation gives far more complete control of blood flow. For instance, in the aforementioned example, if the arterial pressure remains at 150 mmHg indefinitely, within a few weeks the blood flow through the tissues gradually approaches almost exactly the normal flow level. Figure 45-3 shows by the dashed green curve the extreme effectiveness of this long-term local blood flow regulation. Note that once the long-term regulation has had time to occur, long-term changes in arterial pressure between 50 and 250 mmHg have little effect on the rate of local blood flow.

Long-term regulation of blood flow is especially important when the metabolic demands of a tissue change. Thus, if a tissue becomes chronically overactive and therefore requires increased quantities of oxygen and other nutrients, the arterioles and capillary vessels usually increase in both number and size within a few weeks to match the needs of the tissue—unless the circulatory system has become pathological or too old to respond.

Blood Flow Regulation by Changes in "Tissue Vascularity"

A key mechanism for long-term local blood flow regulation is to change the amount of vascularity of the tissues. For instance, if the metabolism in a tissue is increased for a prolonged period, vascularity increases, a process generally called *angiogenesis*; if the metabolism is decreased, vascularity decreases. Figure 45-5 shows the large increase in the number of capillaries in a rat anterior tibialis muscle that was stimulated electrically to contract for short periods each day for 30 days, compared with the unstimulated muscle in the other leg of the animal.

Thus, actual physical reconstruction of the tissue vasculature occurs to meet the needs of the tissues. This reconstruction occurs rapidly (within days) in young animals. It also occurs rapidly in new growth tissue, such as in scar tissue and cancerous tissue, but it occurs much more slowly in old, well-established tissues. Therefore, the time required for long-term regulation to take place may be only a few days in the neonate or as long as months in the elderly person. Furthermore, the final degree of response is much better in younger than in older tissues; thus in the neonate, the vascularity will adjust to match almost exactly the needs of the tissue for blood flow, whereas in older tissues, vascularity frequently lags far behind the needs of the tissues.

Role of Oxygen in Long-Term Regulation. Oxygen is important not only for acute control of local blood flow but also for long-term control. One example of this is increased vascularity in tissues of animals that live at high altitudes, where the atmospheric oxygen is low. In premature human babies who are put into oxygen tents for therapeutic purposes, the excess oxygen causes almost immediate cessation of new vascular growth in the retina of the premature baby's eyes and even causes degeneration of some of the small vessels that already have formed. When the infant is taken out of the oxygen tent, explosive

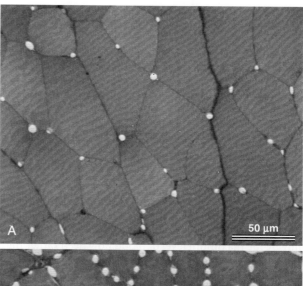
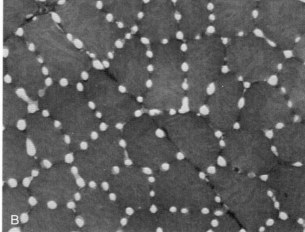

Figure 45-5 A large increase in the number of capillaries (*white dots*) in a rat anterior tibialis muscle that was stimulated electrically to contract for short periods each day for 30 days (B), compared with the unstimulated muscle (A). The 30 days of intermittent electrical stimulation converted the predominantly fast twitch, glycolytic anterior tibialis muscle to a predominantly slow twitch, oxidative muscle with increased numbers of capillaries and decreased fiber diameter as shown. *Photo courtesy Dr. Thomas Adair.*

overgrowth of new vessels then occurs to make up for the sudden decrease in available oxygen. Indeed, often so much overgrowth occurs that the retinal vessels grow out from the retina into the eye's vitreous humor, eventually causing blindness, a condition called *retrolental fibroplasia*.

Importance of Vascular Growth Factors in Formation of New Blood Vessels

A dozen or more factors that increase growth of new blood vessels have been found, almost all of which are small peptides. The four that have been best characterized are *vascular endothelial growth factor (VEGF)*, *fibroblast growth factor*, *platelet-derived growth factor (PDGF)*, and *angiogenin*, each of which has been isolated from tissues that have inadequate blood supply. Presumably, it is deficiency of tissue oxygen or other nutrients, or both, that leads to formation of the vascular growth factors (also called "angiogenic factors").

Certain other substances, such as some steroid hormones, have exactly the opposite effect on small blood vessels, occasionally even causing dissolution of vascular cells and disappearance of vessels. Therefore, blood vessels can also be made to disappear when they are not needed. Peptides produced in the tissues can also block the growth of new blood vessels. For example, *angiostatin*, a fragment of the protein plasminogen, is a naturally occurring inhibitor of angiogenesis. *Endostatin* is another anti-angiogenic peptide that is derived from the breakdown of collagen type XVII. Although the precise physiological functions of these antiangiogenic substances are still unknown, there is great interest in their potential use in arresting blood vessel growth in cancerous tumors and therefore preventing the large increases in blood flow needed to sustain the nutrient supply of rapidly growing tumors.

Vascularity Is Determined by Maximum Blood Flow Need, Not by Average Need. An especially valuable characteristic of long-term vascular control is that vascularity is determined mainly by the maximum level of blood flow need rather than by average need. For instance, during heavy exercise the need for whole-body blood flow often increases to six to eight times the resting blood flow. This great excess of flow may not be required for more than a few minutes each day. Nevertheless, even this short need can cause enough angiogenic factors to be formed by the muscles to increase their vascularity as required. Were it not for this capability, every time that a person attempted heavy exercise, the muscles would fail to receive the required nutrients, especially the required oxygen, so that the muscles simply would fail to contract.

However, after extravascularity does develop, the extra blood vessels normally remain mainly vasoconstricted, opening to allow extra flow only when appropriate local stimuli such as lack of oxygen, nerve vasodilatory stimuli, or other stimuli call forth the required extra flow.

BLOOD FLOW DEVELOPMENT BY DEVELOPMENT OF COLLATERAL CIRCULATION

In most tissues of the body, when an artery or a vein is blocked, a new vascular channel usually develops around the blockage and allows at least partial resupply of blood to the affected tissue. Within 1 day as much as half the tissue needs may be met, and within a few days the blood flow is usually sufficient to meet the tissue needs. The collateral vessels continue to grow for many months thereafter, usually forming multiple small collateral channels rather than one single large vessel. Under resting conditions, the blood flow may return to nearly normal, but the new channels seldom become large enough to supply the blood flow needed during strenuous tissue activity. Thus, development of collateral vessels follows the usual principles of both acute and long-term local blood flow control, the acute control being rapid metabolic dilation, followed chronically by growth and enlargement of new vessels over a period of weeks and months.

An important example of the development of collateral blood vessels occurs after thrombosis of one of the coronary arteries. By the age of 60 years most people have experienced closure or partial closure of at least one of the smaller branches of the coronary vessels, but may be unaware of it because collaterals have developed rapidly enough to prevent myocardial damage. When collateral blood vessels are unable to develop quickly enough to maintain blood flow because of the rapidity or severity of the coronary insufficiency, serious heart attacks occur.

Humoral Control of the Circulation

Humoral control of the circulation means control by substances secreted or absorbed into the body fluids—such as hormones and locally produced factors. Some of these substances are formed by special glands and transported in the blood throughout the entire body. Others are formed in local tissue areas and cause only local circulatory effects. Among the most important of the humoral factors that affect circulatory function are those that are described in the following sections.

VASOCONSTRICTOR AGENTS

Norepinephrine and Epinephrine. *Norepinephrine* is an especially powerful vasoconstrictor hormone; *epinephrine* is less so and in some tissues even causes mild vasodilation. (A special example of vasodilation is that which is caused by epinephrine to dilate the coronary arteries during increased heart activity.)

When the sympathetic nervous system is stimulated in most parts of the body during stress or exercise, the sympathetic nerve endings in the individual tissues release norepinephrine, which excites the heart and contracts the veins and arterioles. In addition, the sympathetic nerves to the adrenal medullae cause these glands to secrete both norepinephrine and epinephrine into the blood. These hormones then circulate to all areas of the body and cause almost the same effects on the circulation as direct sympathetic stimulation, thus providing a dual system of control: (1) direct nerve stimulation and (2) indirect effects of norepinephrine and/or epinephrine in the circulating blood.

Angiotensin II. Angiotensin II is another powerful vasoconstrictor substance. As little as *one-millionth* of a gram can increase the arterial pressure of a human being by 50 mmHg or more.

The effect of angiotensin II is to powerfully constrict the small arterioles. If this constriction occurs in an isolated tissue area, the blood flow to that area can be severely depressed. However, the real importance of angiotensin II is that it normally acts on many of the arterioles of the body at the same time to increase the *total peripheral resistance* and to decrease sodium and water excretion by the kidneys, thereby increasing the arterial pressure. Thus, this hormone plays an integral role in the regulation of arterial pressure, as is discussed in detail in Chapter 44.

Vasopressin. *Vasopressin*, also called *antidiuretic hormone*, is even more powerful than angiotensin II as a vasoconstrictor, thus making it one of the body's most potent vascular constrictor substances. It is formed in nerve cells in the hypothalamus of the brain (see Chapter 88) but is then transported downward by nerve axons to the posterior pituitary gland, where it is finally secreted into the blood.

It is clear that vasopressin could have enormous effects on circulatory function. Yet, because only minute amounts of vasopressin are secreted in most physiological conditions, most physiologists have thought that vasopressin plays little role in vascular control. However, experiments have shown that the concentration of circulating blood vasopressin after severe hemorrhage can increase enough to raise the arterial pressure as much as 60 mmHg. In many instances, this action can, by itself, bring the arterial pressure almost back up to normal.

Vasopressin has the major function of greatly increasing water reabsorption from the renal tubules back into the blood (discussed in Chapter 88), and therefore helps to control body fluid volume. That is why this hormone is also called *antidiuretic hormone*.

VASODILATOR AGENTS

Bradykinin. Several substances called *kinins* cause powerful vasodilation when formed in the blood and tissue fluids of some organs.

The kinins are small polypeptides that are split away by proteolytic enzymes from α_2-globulins in the plasma or tissue fluids. A proteolytic enzyme of particular importance for this purpose is *kallikrein*, which is present in the blood and tissue fluids in an inactive form. This inactive kallikrein is activated by maceration of the blood, tissue inflammation, or other similar chemical or physical effects on the blood or tissues. As kallikrein becomes activated, it acts immediately on α_2-globulin to release a kinin called *kallidin* that is then converted by tissue enzymes into *bradykinin*. Once formed, bradykinin persists for only a few minutes because it is inactivated by the enzyme *carboxypeptidase* or by *converting enzyme*, the same enzyme that also plays an essential role in activating angiotensin. The activated kallikrein enzyme is destroyed by a *kallikrein inhibitor* also present in the body fluids.

Bradykinin causes both powerful *arteriolar dilation* and *increased capillary permeability*. For instance, injection of *1 mcg* of bradykinin into the brachial artery of a person increases blood flow through the arm as much as sixfold, and even smaller amounts injected locally into tissues can cause marked local edema resulting from increase in capillary pore size.

Kinins appear to play special roles in regulating blood flow and capillary leakage of fluids in inflamed tissues. It also is believed that bradykinin plays a normal role to help regulate blood flow in the skin, as well as in the salivary and gastrointestinal glands.

Histamine. Histamine is released in essentially every tissue of the body if the tissue becomes damaged or inflamed or is the subject of an allergic reaction. Most of the histamine is derived from *mast cells* in the damaged tissues and from *basophils* in the blood.

Histamine has a powerful vasodilator effect on the arterioles and, like bradykinin, has the ability to increase greatly capillary porosity, allowing leakage of both fluid and plasma protein into the tissues. In many pathological conditions, the intense arteriolar dilation and increased capillary porosity produced by histamine cause tremendous quantities of fluid to leak out of the circulation into the tissues, inducing edema. The local vasodilatory and edema-producing effects of histamine are especially prominent during allergic reactions and are discussed in Chapter 25.

VASCULAR CONTROL BY IONS AND OTHER CHEMICAL FACTORS

Many different ions and other chemical factors can either dilate or constrict local blood vessels. The following list details some of their specific effects:

1. An increase in *calcium ion* concentration causes *vasoconstriction* because of the general effect of calcium to stimulate smooth muscle contraction.
2. An increase in *potassium ion* concentration, within the physiological range, causes *vasodilation*. This effect results from the ability of potassium ions to inhibit smooth muscle contraction.
3. An increase in *magnesium* ion concentration causes *powerful vasodilation* because magnesium ions inhibit smooth muscle contraction.
4. An *increase in hydrogen ion* concentration (decrease in pH) causes dilation of the arterioles. Conversely, a *slight decrease in hydrogen ion* concentration causes arteriolar constriction.
5. *Anions* that have significant effects on blood vessels are *acetate* and *citrate*, both of which cause mild degrees of vasodilation.
6. An *increase in carbon dioxide concentration* causes moderate vasodilation in most tissues but marked vasodilation in the brain. Also, carbon dioxide in the blood, acting on the brain vasomotor center, has an extremely powerful indirect effect, transmitted through the sympathetic nervous vasoconstrictor system, to cause widespread vasoconstriction throughout the body.

BIBLIOGRAPHY

Adair TH: Growth regulation of the vascular system: an emerging role for adenosine, *Am. J. Physiol. Regul. Integr. Comp. Physiol.* 289:R283, 2005.

Bolduc V, Thorin-Trescases N, Thorin E: Endothelium-dependent control of cerebrovascular functions through age: exercise for healthy cerebrovascular aging, *Am. J. Physiol. Heart Circ. Physiol.* 305:H620, 2013.

Campbell WB, Falck JR: Arachidonic acid metabolites as endothelium-derived hyperpolarizing factors, *Hypertension* 49:590, 2007.

Casey DP, Joyner MJ: Compensatory vasodilatation during hypoxic exercise: mechanisms responsible for matching oxygen supply to demand, *J. Physiol.* 590:6321, 2012.

Dhaun N, Goddard J, Kohan DE, et al: Role of endothelin-1 in clinical hypertension: 20 years on, *Hypertension* 52:452, 2008.

Drummond HA, Grifoni SC, Jernigan NL: A new trick for an old dogma: ENaC proteins as mechanotransducers in vascular smooth muscle, *Physiology (Bethesda)* 23:23, 2008.

Ferrara N, Gerber HP, LeCouter J: The biology of VEGF and its receptors, *Nat. Med.* 9:669, 2003.

Folkman J: Angiogenesis: an organizing principle for drug discovery? *Nat. Rev. Drug Discov.* 6:273, 2007.

Hall JE, Brands MW, Henegar JR: Angiotensin II and long-term arterial pressure regulation: the overriding dominance of the kidney, *J. Am. Soc. Nephrol.* 10(Suppl. 12):S258, 1999.

Heerkens EH, Izzard AS, Heagerty AM: Integrins, vascular remodeling, and hypertension, *Hypertension* 49:1, 2007.

Hellsten Y, Nyberg M, Jensen LG, Mortensen SP: Vasodilator interactions in skeletal muscle blood flow regulation, *J. Physiol.* 590:6297, 2012.

Keeley EC, Mehrad B, Strieter RM: Chemokines as mediators of neovascularization, *Arterioscler. Thromb. Vasc. Biol.* 28:2008, 1928.

Marshall JM, Ray CJ: Contribution of non-endothelium-dependent substances to exercise hyperaemia: are they O(2) dependent? *J. Physiol.* 590:6307, 2012.

Renkin EM: Control of microcirculation and blood-tissue exchange, Renkin EM, Michel CC, editors: *Handbook of Physiology, Section 2,* vol. IV, Bethesda, 1984, American Physiological Society, pp 627.

Silvestre JS, Smadja DM, Lévy BI: Postischemic revascularization: from cellular and molecular mechanisms to clinical applications, *Physiol. Rev.* 93:1743, 2013.

Simons M: An inside view: VEGF receptor trafficking and signaling, *Physiology (Bethesda)* 27:213, 2012.

Speed JS, Pollock DM: Endothelin, kidney disease, and hypertension, *Hypertension* 61:1142, 2013.

Coronary Circulation

About one-third of all deaths in industrialized countries of the Western world result from coronary artery disease. However, this has become an increasing problem in developing countries as life spans increase and lifestyle behaviors change. For this reason, understanding normal and pathological physiology of the coronary circulation is one of the most important subjects in medicine.

Physiological Anatomy of the Coronary Blood Supply

Figure 46-1 shows the heart and its coronary blood supply. Note that the main coronary arteries lie on the surface of the heart and smaller arteries then penetrate from the surface into the cardiac muscle mass. It is almost entirely through these arteries that the heart receives its nutritive blood supply. Only the inner 1/10 mm of the endocardial surface can obtain significant nutrition directly from the blood inside the cardiac chambers, so this source of muscle nutrition is minuscule.

The *left coronary artery* supplies mainly the anterior and left lateral portions of the left ventricle, whereas the *right coronary artery* supplies most of the right ventricle, as well as the posterior part of the left ventricle in 80–90% of people.

Most of the coronary venous blood flow from the left ventricular muscle returns to the right atrium of the heart by way of the *coronary sinus*, which is about 75% of the total coronary blood flow. On the other hand, most of the coronary venous blood from the right ventricular muscle returns through small anterior cardiac veins that flow directly into the right atrium, not by way of the coronary sinus. A very small amount of coronary venous blood also flows back into the heart through very minute *Thebesian veins*, which empty directly into all chambers of the heart.

Normal Coronary Blood Flow— Averages 5% of Cardiac Output

The normal coronary blood flow in the resting human being averages 70 mL/minute per 100 g of heart weight, or about 225 mL/minute, which is about 4–5% of the total cardiac output (Box 46-1).

During strenuous exercise, the heart in the young adult increases its cardiac output fourfold to sevenfold, and it pumps this blood against a higher than normal arterial pressure. Consequently, the work output of the heart under severe conditions may increase sixfold to ninefold. At the same time, the coronary blood flow increases threefold to fourfold to supply the extra nutrients needed by the heart.

Phasic Changes in Coronary Blood Flow During Systole and Diastole—Effect of Cardiac Muscle Compression. Figure 46-2 shows the changes in blood flow through the nutrient capillaries of the left ventricular coronary system in milliliters per minute in the human heart during systole and diastole, as extrapolated from studies in experimental animals. Note from this diagram that the coronary capillary blood flow in the left ventricle muscle falls to a low value during systole. The reason for this phenomenon is strong compression of the intramuscular blood vessels by the left ventricular muscle during systolic contraction.

During diastole, the cardiac muscle relaxes and no longer obstructs blood flow through the left ventricular muscle capillaries, so blood flows rapidly during all of diastole.

Blood flow through the coronary capillaries of the right ventricle also undergoes phasic changes during the cardiac cycle, but because the force of contraction of the right ventricular muscle is far less than that of the left ventricular muscle, the inverse phasic changes are only partial, in contrast to those in the left ventricular muscle.

Epicardial Versus Subendocardial Coronary Blood Flow— Effect of Intramyocardial Pressure. Figure 46-3 demonstrates the special arrangement of the coronary vessels at different depths in the heart muscle, showing on the outer surface *epicardial coronary arteries* that supply most of the muscle. Smaller, intramuscular arteries derived from the epicardial arteries penetrate the muscle, supplying the needed nutrients. Lying immediately beneath the endocardium is a plexus of

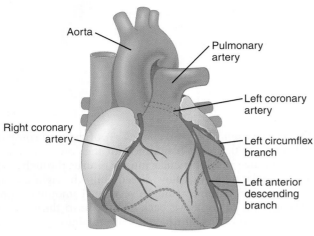

Figure 46-1   The coronary arteries.

BOX 46-1   SALIENT FEATURES OF THE CORONARY CIRCULATION

1. Four to 5% of cardiac output, that is, 225 mL/minute, is received
2. Distribution of blood flow in right and left coronary arteries varies; some individuals are left coronary artery dominant, others right coronary artery dominant
3. Extraction of oxygen from coronary arteries at rest is high
4. Coronary blood flow is closely coupled to cardiac metabolism
5. Coronary circulation shows "autoregulation" of blood flow
6. Coronary blood flow is phasic: more during diastole, and minimal during systole. This phasic nature is more pronounced in the left ventricle
7. Coronary blood vessels have "collaterals"

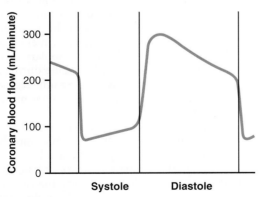

Figure 46-2   Phasic flow of blood through the coronary capillaries of the human left ventricle during cardiac systole and diastole (as extrapolated from measured flows in dogs).

subendocardial arteries. During systole, blood flow through the subendocardial plexus of the left ventricle, where the intramuscular coronary vessels are compressed greatly by ventricular muscle contraction, tends to be reduced. However, the extra vessels of the subendocardial plexus normally compensate for this reduction. Later in the chapter, we explain how this peculiar difference between blood flow in the epicardial and subendocardial arteries plays an important role in certain types of coronary ischemia.

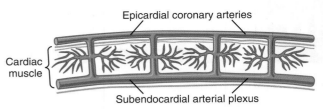

Figure 46-3   Diagram of the epicardial, intramuscular, and subendocardial coronary vasculature.

Control of Coronary Blood Flow

LOCAL MUSCLE METABOLISM IS THE PRIMARY CONTROLLER OF CORONARY FLOW

Blood flow through the coronary system is regulated mostly by local arteriolar vasodilation in response to the nutritional needs of cardiac muscle. That is, whenever the vigor of cardiac contraction is increased, the rate of coronary blood flow also increases. This local regulation of coronary blood flow is similar to that occurring in many other tissues of the body, especially in the skeletal muscles.

Oxygen Demand as a Major Factor in Local Coronary Blood Flow Regulation

Blood flow in the coronary arteries usually is regulated almost exactly in proportion to the need of the cardiac musculature for oxygen. Normally, about 70% of the oxygen in the coronary arterial blood is removed as the blood flows through the heart muscle. Because not much oxygen is left, little additional oxygen can be supplied to the heart musculature unless the coronary blood flow increases. Fortunately, the coronary blood flow increases almost in direct proportion to any additional metabolic consumption of oxygen by the heart.

The exact means by which increased oxygen consumption causes coronary dilation has not been determined. A substance with great vasodilator propensity is adenosine. In the presence of very low concentrations of oxygen in the muscle cells, a large proportion of the cell's adenosine triphosphate (ATP) degrades to adenosine monophosphate. Small portions of this substance are then further degraded and release adenosine into the tissue fluids of the heart muscle, with a resultant increase in local coronary blood flow. After the adenosine causes vasodilation, much of it is reabsorbed into the cardiac cells to be reused for the production of ATP.

Other vasodilators include adenosine phosphate compounds, potassium ions, hydrogen ions, carbon dioxide, prostaglandins, and nitric oxide. The mechanisms of coronary vasodilation during increased cardiac activity are not fully explained by adenosine. Pharmacological agents that block or partially block the vasodilator effect of adenosine do not prevent coronary vasodilation caused by increased heart muscle activity.

NERVOUS CONTROL OF CORONARY BLOOD FLOW

Stimulation of the autonomic nerves to the heart can affect coronary blood flow both directly and indirectly. The direct effects result from action of the nervous transmitter substances acetylcholine from the vagus nerves and norepinephrine from the sympathetic nerves on the coronary vessels. The indirect effects result from secondary changes in coronary blood flow caused by increased or decreased activity of the heart.

The indirect effects, which are mostly opposite to the direct effects, play a far more important role in normal control of coronary blood flow. Thus, sympathetic stimulation, which releases norepinephrine from the sympathetic nerves and norepinephrine and epinephrine from the adrenal medullae, increases both heart rate and heart contractility and increases the rate of metabolism of the heart. In turn, the increased metabolism of the heart sets off local blood flow regulatory mechanisms for dilating the coronary vessels, and the blood flow increases approximately in proportion to the metabolic needs of the heart muscle. In contrast, vagal stimulation, with its release of acetylcholine, slows the heart and has a slight depressive effect on heart contractility. These effects decrease cardiac oxygen consumption and, therefore, indirectly constrict the coronary arteries.

Direct Effects of Nervous Stimuli on the Coronary Vasculature

The distribution of parasympathetic (vagal) nerve fibers to the ventricular coronary system is not very great. However, the acetylcholine released by parasympathetic stimulation has a direct effect to dilate the coronary arteries.

More extensive sympathetic innervation of the coronary vessels occurs. In Chapter 119, we see that the sympathetic transmitter substances, norepinephrine and epinephrine, can have either vascular constrictor or vascular dilator effects, depending on the presence or absence of constrictor or dilator receptors in the blood vessel walls. The constrictor receptors are called *alpha receptors* and the dilator receptors are called *beta receptors*. Both alpha and beta receptors exist in the coronary vessels. In general, the epicardial coronary vessels have a preponderance of alpha receptors, whereas the intramuscular arteries may have a preponderance of beta receptors. Therefore, sympathetic stimulation can, at least theoretically, cause slight overall coronary constriction or dilation, but usually constriction. In some people, the alpha vasoconstrictor effects seem to be disproportionately severe, and these people can have vasospastic myocardial ischemia during periods of excess sympathetic drive, often with resultant anginal pain.

Metabolic factors, especially myocardial oxygen consumption, are the major controllers of myocardial blood flow. Whenever the direct effects of nervous stimulation reduce the coronary blood flow, the metabolic control of coronary flow usually overrides the direct coronary nervous effects within seconds.

Special Features of Cardiac Muscle Metabolism

The basic principles of cellular metabolism apply to cardiac muscle the same as for other tissues, but some quantitative differences exist. Most important, under resting conditions, cardiac muscle normally consumes fatty acids instead of carbohydrates to supply most of its energy (about 70% of the energy is derived from fatty acids). However, as is also true of other tissues, under anaerobic or ischemic conditions, cardiac metabolism must call on anaerobic glycolysis mechanisms for energy. However, glycolysis consumes large quantities of the blood glucose and at the same time forms large amounts of lactic acid in the cardiac tissue, which is probably one of the causes of cardiac pain in cardiac ischemic conditions, as discussed later in this chapter.

As is true in other tissues, more than 95% of the metabolic energy liberated from foods is used to form ATP in the mitochondria. This ATP in turn acts as the conveyer of energy for cardiac muscular contraction and other cellular functions. In severe coronary ischemia, the ATP degrades first to adenosine diphosphate, and then to adenosine monophosphate and adenosine. Because the cardiac muscle cell membrane is slightly permeable to adenosine, much of this agent can diffuse from the muscle cells into the circulating blood.

The released adenosine is believed to be one of the substances that causes dilation of the coronary arterioles during coronary hypoxia, as discussed earlier. However, loss of adenosine also has a serious cellular consequence. Within as little as 30 minutes of severe coronary ischemia, as occurs after a myocardial infarct, about one-half of the adenine base can be lost from the affected cardiac muscle cells. Furthermore, this loss can be replaced by new synthesis of adenine at a rate of only 2%/hour. Therefore, once a serious bout of coronary ischemia has persisted for 30 or more minutes, relief of the ischemia may be too late to prevent injury and death of the cardiac cells. This occurrence almost certainly is one of the major causes of cardiac cellular death during myocardial ischemia.

Ischemic Heart Disease

Atherosclerosis as a Cause of Ischemic Heart Disease. A frequent cause of diminished coronary blood flow is atherosclerosis. In people who have a genetic predisposition to atherosclerosis, who are overweight or obese and have a sedentary lifestyle, or who have high blood pressure and damage to the endothelial cells of the coronary blood vessels, large quantities of cholesterol gradually become deposited beneath the endothelium at many points in arteries throughout the body. Gradually, these areas of deposit are invaded by fibrous tissue and frequently become calcified. The net result is the development of atherosclerotic plaques that actually protrude into the vessel lumens and either block or partially block blood flow. A common site for development of atherosclerotic plaques is the first few centimeters of the major coronary arteries.

ACUTE CORONARY OCCLUSION

Acute occlusion of a coronary artery most frequently occurs in a person who already has underlying atherosclerotic coronary heart disease but almost never in a person with a normal coronary circulation.

Lifesaving Value of Collateral Circulation in the Heart

The degree of damage to the heart muscle caused either by slowly developing atherosclerotic constriction of the coronary arteries or by sudden coronary occlusion is determined to a great extent by the degree of collateral circulation that has already developed or that can open within minutes after the occlusion.

In a normal heart, almost no large communications exist among the larger coronary arteries. However, many anastomoses do exist among the smaller arteries sized 20–250 μm in diameter, as shown in Figure 46-4.

When a sudden occlusion occurs in one of the larger coronary arteries, the small anastomoses begin to dilate within seconds. However, the blood flow through these minute collaterals is usually less than one-half that needed to keep alive most of the cardiac muscle that they now supply; the diameters of the collateral vessels do not enlarge much more for the next 8–24 hours. But then collateral flow begins to increase, doubling by the second or third day and often reaching normal or almost normal coronary flow within about 1 month. Because of these developing collateral channels, many patients recover almost completely from various degrees of coronary occlusion when the area of muscle involved is not too great.

MYOCARDIAL INFARCTION

Immediately after an acute coronary occlusion, blood flow ceases in the coronary vessels beyond the occlusion except for small amounts of collateral flow from surrounding vessels. The area of muscle that has either zero flow or so little flow that it cannot sustain cardiac muscle function is said to be *infarcted*. The overall process is called a *myocardial infarction*.

Soon after the onset of the infarction, small amounts of collateral blood begin to seep into the infarcted area, which, combined with progressive dilation of local blood vessels, causes the area to become overfilled with stagnant blood. Simultaneously the muscle fibers use the last vestiges of the oxygen in the blood causing the hemoglobin to become totally deoxygenated. Therefore, the infarcted area takes on a bluish-brown hue and the blood vessels of the area appear to be engorged despite lack of blood flow. Within a few hours of almost no blood supply, the cardiac muscle cells die.

Cardiac muscle requires about 1.3 mL of oxygen per 100 g of muscle tissue per minute just to remain alive. In comparison, about 8 mL of oxygen per 100 g is delivered to the normal resting left ventricle each minute. Therefore, if there is even 15–30% of normal resting coronary blood flow, the muscle will not die. In the central portion of a large infarct, however, where there is almost no collateral blood flow, the muscle does die.

Subendocardial Infarction

The subendocardial muscle frequently becomes infarcted even when there is no evidence of infarction in the outer surface portions of the heart. The reason for this is that the subendocardial muscle has a higher oxygen consumption and extra difficulty obtaining adequate blood flow because the blood vessels in the

subendocardium are intensely compressed by systolic contraction of the heart, as explained earlier. Therefore, any condition that compromises blood flow to any area of the heart usually causes damage first in the subendocardial regions, and the damage then spreads outward toward the epicardium.

Causes of Death After Acute Coronary Occlusion

The most common causes of death after acute myocardial infarction are (1) decreased cardiac output; (2) damming of blood in the pulmonary blood vessels and then death resulting from pulmonary edema; (3) fibrillation of the heart; and, occasionally, (4) rupture of the heart.

Stages of Recovery from Acute Myocardial Infarction

The upper left part of Figure 46-5 shows the effects of acute coronary occlusion in a patient with a small area of muscle ischemia; to the right is shown a heart with a large area of ischemia. When the area of ischemia is small, little or no death of the muscle cells may occur, but part of the muscle often does become temporarily nonfunctional because of inadequate nutrition to support muscle contraction.

When the area of ischemia is large, some of the muscle fibers in the center of the area die rapidly, within 1–3 hours where there is total cessation of coronary blood supply. Immediately around the dead area is a nonfunctional area, with failure of contraction and usually failure of impulse conduction. Then, extending circumferentially around the nonfunctional area is an area that is still contracting but only weakly because of mild ischemia.

Replacement of Dead Muscle by Scar Tissue. In the lower part of Figure 46-5, the various stages of recovery after a large myocardial infarction are shown. Shortly after the occlusion, the muscle fibers in the center of the ischemic area die. Then, during the ensuing days, this area of dead fibers becomes bigger because many of the marginal fibers finally succumb to the prolonged ischemia. At the same time, because of enlargement of collateral arterial channels supplying the outer rim of the infarcted area, much of the nonfunctional muscle recovers. After a few days to 3 weeks, most of the nonfunctional muscle becomes functional again or dies—one or the other. In the meantime, fibrous tissue begins developing among the dead fibers because ischemia can stimulate growth of fibroblasts and promote development

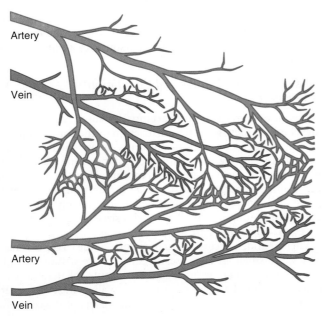

Figure 46-4 Minute anastomoses in the normal coronary arterial system.

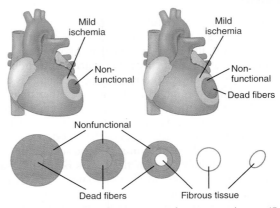

Figure 46-5 (*Top*) Small and large areas of coronary ischemia. (*Bottom*) Stages of recovery from myocardial infarction.

of greater than normal quantities of fibrous tissue. Therefore, the dead muscle tissue is gradually replaced by fibrous tissue. Then, because it is a general property of fibrous tissue to undergo progressive contraction and dissolution, the fibrous scar may grow smaller over a period of several months to a year.

Finally, the normal areas of the heart gradually hypertrophy to compensate at least partially for the lost dead cardiac musculature. By these means, the heart recovers either partially or almost completely within a few months.

Value of Rest in Treating Myocardial Infarction. The degree of cardiac cellular death is determined by the degree of ischemia and the workload on the heart muscle. When the workload is greatly increased, such as during exercise, in severe emotional strain, or as a result of fatigue, the heart needs increased oxygen and other nutrients for sustaining its life. Furthermore, anastomotic blood vessels that supply blood to ischemic areas of the heart must also still supply the areas of the heart that they normally supply. When the heart becomes excessively active, the vessels of the normal musculature become greatly dilated. This dilation allows most of the blood flowing into the coronary vessels to flow through the normal muscle tissue, thus leaving little blood to flow through the small anastomotic channels into the ischemic area; as a result the ischemic condition worsens. This condition is called the *"coronary steal" syndrome.* Consequently, one of the most important factors in the treatment of a patient with myocardial infarction is observance of absolute body rest during the recovery process.

Function of the Heart After Recovery from Myocardial Infarction

Occasionally, a heart that has recovered from a large myocardial infarction returns almost to full functional capability, but more frequently its pumping capability is permanently decreased below that of a healthy heart. This does not mean that the person is necessarily a cardiac invalid or that the resting cardiac output is depressed below normal, because the normal heart is capable of pumping 300–400% more blood per minute than the body requires during rest—that is, a normal person has a "cardiac reserve" of 300–400%. Even when the cardiac reserve is reduced to as little as 100%, the person can still perform most normal daily activities but not strenuous exercise that would overload the heart.

Pain in Coronary Heart Disease

Normally, a person cannot "feel" his or her heart, but ischemic cardiac muscle often does cause pain sensation that is sometimes severe. Exactly what causes this pain is not known, but it is believed that ischemia causes the muscle to release acidic substances, such as lactic acid, or other pain-promoting products, such as histamine, kinins, or cellular proteolytic enzymes, that are not removed rapidly enough by the slowly moving coronary blood flow. The high concentrations of these abnormal products then stimulate pain nerve endings in the cardiac muscle, sending pain impulses through sensory afferent nerve fibers into the central nervous system.

ANGINA PECTORIS (CARDIAC PAIN)

In most people who sustain progressive constriction of their coronary arteries, cardiac pain, called *angina pectoris*, begins to appear whenever the load on the heart becomes too great in relation to the available coronary blood flow. This pain is usually felt beneath the upper sternum over the heart, and in addition it is often referred to distant surface areas of the body, most commonly to the left arm and left shoulder but also frequently to the neck and even to the side of the face. The reason for this distribution of pain is that during embryonic life the heart originates in the neck, as do the arms. Therefore, both the heart and these surface areas of the body receive pain nerve fibers from the same spinal cord segments.

Most people who have chronic angina pectoris feel pain when they exercise or when they experience emotions that increase metabolism of the heart or temporarily constrict the coronary vessels because of sympathetic vasoconstrictor nerve signals. Anginal pain is also exacerbated by cold temperatures or by having a full stomach, both of which increase the workload of the heart. The pain usually lasts for only a few minutes. However, some patients have such severe and lasting ischemia that the pain is present all the time. The pain is frequently described as hot, pressing, and constricting and is of such quality that it usually makes the patient stop all unnecessary body activity.

Treatment with Drugs

Several vasodilator drugs, when administered during an acute anginal attack, can often provide immediate relief from the pain. Commonly used short-acting vasodilators are nitroglycerin and other nitrate drugs. Other vasodilators, such as angiotensin-converting enzyme inhibitors, angiotensin receptor blockers, calcium channel blockers, and ranolazine, may be beneficial in treating chronic stable angina pectoris.

Another class of drugs used for prolonged treatment of angina pectoris is the *beta-blockers,* such as propranolol. These drugs block sympathetic beta-adrenergic receptors, which prevents sympathetic enhancement of heart rate and cardiac metabolism during exercise or emotional episodes. Therefore, therapy with a beta-blocker decreases the need of the heart for extra metabolic oxygen during stressful conditions. For obvious reasons, this therapy can also reduce the number of anginal attacks, as well as their severity.

Surgical Treatment of Coronary Artery Disease

Aortic–Coronary Bypass Surgery. In many patients with coronary ischemia, the constricted areas of the coronary arteries are located at only a few discrete points blocked by atherosclerotic disease and the coronary vessels elsewhere are normal or almost normal. In the 1960s a surgical procedure called *aortic–coronary bypass* was developed in which a section of a subcutaneous vein from an arm or leg was removed and then grafted from the root of the aorta to the side of a peripheral coronary artery beyond the atherosclerotic blockage point.

Coronary Angioplasty. Since the 1980s, a procedure has been used to open partially blocked coronary vessels before they become totally occluded. This procedure, called *coronary artery angioplasty*, is as follows: A small balloon-tipped catheter, about 1 mm in diameter, is passed under radiographic guidance into the coronary system and pushed through the partially occluded artery until the balloon portion of the catheter straddles the partially occluded point. The balloon is then inflated with high pressure, which markedly stretches the diseased artery. After this procedure is performed, the blood flow through the vessel often increases threefold to fourfold, and more than 75% of the patients who undergo the procedure are relieved of the coronary ischemic symptoms for at least several years, although many of the patients still eventually require coronary bypass surgery.

Small stainless steel mesh tubes called "stents" are sometimes placed inside a coronary artery dilated by angioplasty to hold the artery open, thus preventing its restenosis. Within a few weeks after the stent is placed in the coronary artery, the endothelium usually grows over the metal surface of the stent, allowing blood to flow smoothly through the stent. However, reclosure (restenosis) of the blocked coronary artery occurs in about 25–40% of patients treated with angioplasty, often within 6 months of the initial procedure. Restenosis is usually due to excessive formation of scar tissue that develops underneath the healthy new endothelium that has grown over the stent. Stents that slowly release drugs (drug-eluting stents) may help prevent the excessive growth of scar tissue.

Newer procedures for opening atherosclerotic coronary arteries are constantly in experimental development. One of these procedures employs a laser beam from the tip of a coronary artery catheter aimed at the atherosclerotic lesion. The laser literally dissolves the lesion without substantially damaging the rest of the arterial wall.

BIBLIOGRAPHY

Armstrong EJ, Rutledge JC, Rogers JH: Coronary artery revascularization in patients with diabetes mellitus, *Circulation* 128:1675, 2013.

Beyer AM, Gutterman DD: Regulation of the human coronary microcirculation, *J. Mol. Cell. Cardiol.* 52:814, 2012.

Crea F, Liuzzo G: Pathogenesis of acute coronary syndromes, *J. Am. Coll. Cardiol.* 61:1, 2013.

Deussen A, Ohanyan V, Jannasch A, et al: Mechanisms of metabolic coronary flow regulation, *J. Mol. Cell. Cardiol.* 52:794, 2012.

Duncker DJ, Bache RJ: Regulation of coronary blood flow during exercise, *Physiol. Rev.* 88:1009, 2008.

Guyton AC, Jones CE, Coleman TG: *Circulatory Pathology: Cardiac Output and its Regulation*, Philadelphia, 1973, W.B. Saunders.

Khand A, Fisher M, Jones J, et al: The collateral circulation of the heart in coronary total arterial occlusions in man: systematic review of assessment and pathophysiology, *Am. Heart J.* 166:941, 2013.

Koerselman J, van der Graaf Y, de Jaegere PP, et al: Coronary collaterals: an important and underexposed aspect of coronary artery disease, *Circulation* 107:2507, 2003.

Levine BD: VO2max: what do we know, and what do we still need to know? *J. Physiol.* 586:25, 2008.

Meier P, Schirmer SH, Lansky AJ, et al: The collateral circulation of the heart, *BMC Med.* 11:143, 2013.

Renault MA, Losordo DW: Therapeutic myocardial angiogenesis, *Microvasc. Res.* 74:159, 2007.

Reynolds HR, Hochman J: Cardiogenic shock: current concepts and improving outcomes, *Circulation* 117:686, 2008.

Yellon DM, Downey JM: Preconditioning the myocardium: from cellular physiology to clinical cardiology, *Physiol. Rev.* 83:1113, 2003.

Cerebral Circulation

Abnormalities of cerebral blood flow can profoundly affect brain function. For instance, total cessation of blood flow to the brain causes unconsciousness within 5–10 seconds because lack of oxygen delivery to the brain cells nearly shuts down metabolism in these cells.

Anatomy of Cerebral Blood Flow

Blood flow of the brain is supplied by four large arteries—two carotid and two vertebral arteries—that merge to form the *circle of Willis* at the base of the brain. The arteries arising from the circle of Willis travel along the brain surface and give rise to *pial* arteries, which branch out into smaller vessels called *penetrating arteries and arterioles* (Figure 47-1). The penetrating vessels are separated slightly from the brain tissue by an extension of the subarachnoid space called the *Virchow–Robin space*. The penetrating vessels dive down into the brain tissue, giving rise to intracerebral arterioles, which eventually branch into capillaries where exchange among the blood and the tissues of oxygen, nutrients, carbon dioxide, and metabolites occurs.

Regulation of Cerebral Blood Flow

Normal blood flow through the brain of the adult person averages 50–65 mL per 100 g of brain tissue per minute. For the entire brain, this amounts to 750–900 mL/minute. Thus, the brain constitutes only about 2% of the body weight but receives 15% of the resting cardiac output.

As in most other tissues, cerebral blood flow is highly related to the tissue metabolism. Several metabolic factors are believed to contribute to cerebral blood flow regulation: (1) carbon dioxide concentration, (2) hydrogen ion concentration, (3) oxygen concentration, and (4) substances released from *astrocytes*, which are specialized, nonneuronal cells that appear to couple neuronal activity with local blood flow regulation.

Excesses of Carbon Dioxide or Hydrogen Ion Concentration Increase of Cerebral Blood Flow. An increase in carbon dioxide concentration in the arterial blood perfusing the brain greatly increases cerebral blood flow. This is demonstrated in Figure 47-2, which shows that a 70% increase in arterial partial pressure of carbon dioxide (PCO_2) approximately doubles cerebral blood flow.

Carbon dioxide is believed to increase cerebral blood flow by combining first with water in the body fluids to form carbonic acid, with subsequent dissociation of this acid to form hydrogen ions. The hydrogen ions then cause vasodilation of the cerebral vessels—with the dilation being almost directly proportional to the increase in hydrogen ion concentration up to a blood flow limit of about twice normal.

Other substances that increase the acidity of the brain tissue and therefore increase hydrogen ion concentration will likewise increase cerebral blood flow. Such substances include lactic acid, pyruvic acid, and any other acidic material formed during the course of tissue metabolism.

Importance of Cerebral Blood Flow Control by Carbon Dioxide and Hydrogen Ions. Increased hydrogen ion concentration greatly depresses neuronal activity. Therefore, it is fortunate that increased hydrogen ion concentration also causes increased blood flow, which in turn carries hydrogen ions, carbon dioxide, and other acid-forming substances away from the brain tissues. Loss of carbon dioxide removes carbonic acid from the tissues; this action, along with removal of other acids, reduces the hydrogen ion concentration back toward normal. Thus, this mechanism helps maintain a constant hydrogen ion concentration in the cerebral fluids and thereby helps to maintain a normal, constant level of neuronal activity.

Oxygen Deficiency as a Regulator of Cerebral Blood Flow. Except during periods of intense brain activity, the rate of oxygen utilization by the brain tissue remains within narrow limits—almost exactly 3.5 (±0.2) mL of oxygen per 100 g of brain tissue per minute. If blood flow to the brain ever becomes insufficient to supply this needed amount of oxygen, the oxygen deficiency almost immediately causes vasodilation, returning the brain blood flow and transport of oxygen to the cerebral tissues to near normal. Thus, this local blood flow regulatory mechanism is almost exactly the same in the brain as in coronary blood vessels, in skeletal muscle, and in most other circulatory areas of the body.

Substances Released from Astrocytes Regulate Cerebral Blood Flow. Increasing evidence suggests that the close coupling between neuronal activity and cerebral blood flow is due, in part, to substances released from *astrocytes* (also called *astroglial cells*)

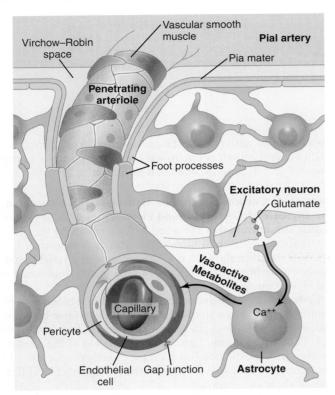

Figure 47-1 Architecture of cerebral blood vessels and potential mechanism for blood flow regulation by astrocytes. The pial arteries lie on the glia limitans and the penetrating arteries are surrounded by astrocyte foot processes. Note that the astrocytes also have fine processes that are closely associated with synapses.

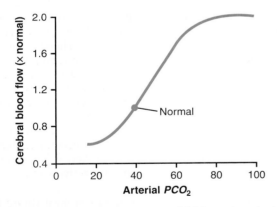

Figure 47-2 Relationship between arterial PCO_2 and cerebral blood flow.

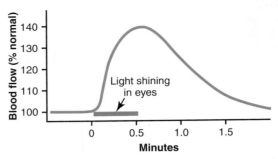

Figure 47-3 Increase in blood flow to the occipital regions of a cat's brain when light is shined into its eyes.

suggested that the vasodilation is mediated by several vasoactive metabolites released from astrocytes. Although the precise mediators are still unclear, nitric oxide, metabolites of arachidonic acid, potassium ions, adenosine, and other substances generated by astrocytes in response to stimulation of adjacent excitatory neurons have all been suggested to be important in mediating local vasodilation.

Measurement of Cerebral Blood Flow and Effect of Brain Activity on Flow. Cerebral blood flow was originally measured using Fick principle, based on the inhalation of nitrous oxide. This method was originally developed by Kety and is often referred to as Kety method.

A method has been developed to record blood flow in as many as 256 isolated segments of the human cerebral cortex simultaneously. To record blood flow in these segments, *a radioactive substance, such as radioactive xenon, is injected into the carotid artery; then the radioactivity of each segment of the cortex is recorded as the radioactive substance passes through the brain tissue. For this purpose, 256 small radioactive scintillation detectors are pressed against the surface of the cortex.* The rapidity of rise and decay of radioactivity in each tissue segment is a direct measure of the rate of blood flow through that segment.

Using this technique, it has become clear that blood flow in each individual segment of the brain changes as much as 100–150% within seconds in response to changes in local neuronal activity. For instance, simply making a fist of the hand causes an immediate increase in blood flow in the motor cortex of the opposite side of the brain. Reading a book increases the blood flow, especially in the visual areas of the occipital cortex and in the language perception areas of the temporal cortex. This measuring procedure can also be used for localizing the origin of epileptic attacks because local brain blood flow increases acutely and markedly at the focal point of each attack.

Demonstrating the effect of local neuronal activity on cerebral blood flow, Figure 47-3 shows a typical increase in occipital blood flow recorded in a cat's brain when intense light is shined into its eyes for 0.5 minute.

Blood flow and neural activity in different regions of the brain can also be assessed indirectly by *functional magnetic resonance imaging (fMRI)*. This method is based on the observation that oxygen-rich hemoglobin (oxyhemoglobin) and oxygen-poor hemoglobin (deoxyhemoglobin) in the blood behave differently in a magnetic field.

An alternative MRI method called *arterial spin labeling (ASL)* can be used to provide a more quantitative assessment of regional blood flow. ASL works by manipulating the MR signal of arterial blood before it is delivered to different areas of the brain. By subtracting two images in which the arterial blood is

that surround blood vessels of the central nervous system. Astrocytes are star-shaped *nonneuronal cells* that support and protect neurons, as well as provide nutrition. They have numerous projections that make contact with neurons and the surrounding blood vessels, providing a potential mechanism for neurovascular communication. Gray matter astrocytes (*protoplasmic astrocytes*) extend fine processes that cover most synapses and large *foot processes* that are closely apposed to the vascular wall (see Figure 47-1).

Experimental studies have shown that electrical stimulation of excitatory glutaminergic neurons leads to increases in intracellular calcium ion concentration in astrocyte foot processes and vasodilation of nearby arterioles. Additional studies have

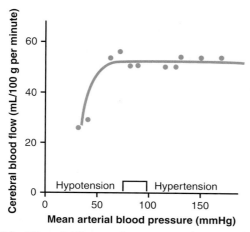

Figure 47-4 Effect of differences in mean arterial pressure, from hypotensive to hypertensive level, on cerebral blood flow in different human beings. *Modified from Lassen, N.A., 1959. Cerebral blood flow and oxygen consumption in man. Physiol. Rev. 39, 183.*

BOX 47-1   SALIENT FEATURES OF THE CEREBRAL CIRCULATION

1. Fifteen percent of cardiac output, that is, 750 mL/minute, is received
2. There are two separate circulations: internal carotid and vertebrobasilar, which anastomose at the circle of Willis
3. Cerebral blood flow is closely coupled to metabolism
4. Cerebral blood flow shows wide regional variations—dependent on the area of the brain that is metabolically active
5. Cerebral circulation shows "autoregulation" of blood flow

Refer to Box 47-1 for the salient features of cerebral circulation.

Cerebral Microcirculation

As is true for almost all other tissues of the body, the number of blood capillaries in the brain is greatest where the metabolic needs are greatest. The overall metabolic rate of the brain gray matter where the neuronal cell bodies lie is about four times as great as that of white matter; correspondingly, the number of capillaries and rate of blood flow are also about four times as great in the gray matter.

An important structural characteristic of the brain capillaries is that most of them are much less "leaky" than the blood capillaries in almost any other tissue of the body. One reason for this phenomenon is that the capillaries are supported on all sides by "glial feet," which are small projections from the surrounding glial cells (eg, astroglial cells) that abut against all surfaces of the capillaries and provide physical support to prevent overstretching of the capillaries in case of high capillary blood pressure.

The walls of the small arterioles leading to the brain capillaries become greatly thickened in people in whom high blood pressure develops and these arterioles remain significantly constricted all the time to prevent transmission of the high pressure to the capillaries. We shall see later in the chapter that whenever these systems for protecting against transudation of fluid into the brain break down, serious brain edema ensues, which can lead rapidly to coma and death.

"Cerebral Stroke" Occurs when Cerebral Blood Vessels Are Blocked

Almost all elderly people have blockage of some small arteries in the brain and up to 10% eventually have enough blockage to cause serious disturbance of brain function, a condition called a "stroke."

Most strokes are caused by arteriosclerotic plaques that occur in one or more of the feeder arteries to the brain. The plaques can activate the clotting mechanism of the blood causing a blood clot to occur and block blood flow in the artery, thereby leading to acute loss of brain function in a localized area.

In about one-quarter of people in whom strokes develop, high blood pressure makes one of the blood vessels burst; hemorrhage then occurs, compressing the local brain tissue and further compromising its functions. The neurological effects of a stroke are determined by the affected brain area. One of the most common types of stroke is blockage of the *middle cerebral artery* that supplies the midportion of one brain hemisphere. For instance, if the middle cerebral artery is blocked on the left side of the brain, the person is likely to become almost totally demented because of lost function in Wernicke's speech comprehension area in the left cerebral hemisphere, and he or she also becomes

manipulated differently, the static proton signal in the rest of the tissue subtracts out, leaving only the signal arising from the delivered arterial blood.

Cerebral Blood Flow Autoregulation Protects the Brain from Fluctuations in Arterial Pressure Changes. During normal daily activities, arterial pressure can fluctuate widely, rising to high levels during states of excitement or strenuous activity and falling to low levels during sleep. However, cerebral blood flow is "autoregulated" extremely well between arterial pressure limits of 60 and 140 mmHg. That is, mean arterial pressure can be decreased acutely to as low as 60 mmHg or increased to as high as 140 mmHg without significant change in cerebral blood flow. In addition, in people who have hypertension, autoregulation of cerebral blood flow occurs even when the mean arterial pressure rises to as high as 160–180 mmHg. This is demonstrated in Figure 47-4, which shows cerebral blood flow measured in both persons with normal blood pressure, and hypertensive and hypotensive patients. Note the extreme constancy of cerebral blood flow between the limits of 60 and 180 mmHg mean arterial pressure. Therefore, if the arterial pressure falls below 60 mmHg, cerebral blood flow becomes severely decreased.

Role of the Sympathetic Nervous System in Controlling Cerebral Blood Flow. The cerebral circulatory system has strong sympathetic innervation that passes upward from the superior cervical sympathetic ganglia in the neck and then into the brain along with the cerebral arteries. This innervation supplies both the large brain arteries and the arteries that penetrate into the substance of the brain. However, transection of the sympathetic nerves or mild to moderate stimulation of them usually causes little change in cerebral blood flow because the blood flow autoregulation mechanism can override the nervous effects.

When mean arterial pressure rises acutely to an exceptionally high level, such as during strenuous exercise or during other states of excessive circulatory activity, the sympathetic nervous system normally constricts the large- and intermediate-sized brain arteries enough to prevent the high pressure from reaching the smaller brain blood vessels. This mechanism is important in preventing vascular hemorrhages into the brain—that is, for preventing the occurrence of "cerebral stroke."

unable to speak words because of loss of Broca's motor area for word formation. In addition, loss of function of neural motor control areas of the left hemisphere can create spastic paralysis of most muscles on the opposite side of the body.

In a similar manner, blockage of a *posterior cerebral artery* will cause infarction of the occipital pole of the hemisphere on the same side as the blockage, which causes loss of vision in both eyes in the half of the retina on the same side as the stroke lesion. Especially devastating are strokes that involve the blood supply to the midbrain because this effect can block nerve conduction in major pathways between the brain and spinal cord causing *both sensory and motor abnormalities.*

BIBLIOGRAPHY

Ainslie PN, Duffin J: Integration of cerebrovascular CO2 reactivity and chemoreflex control of breathing: mechanisms of regulation, measurement, and interpretation, *Am. J. Physiol. Regul. Integr. Comp. Physiol.* 296:R1473, 2009.

Barres BA: The mystery and magic of glia: a perspective on their roles in health and disease, *Neuron* 60:430, 2008.

Chesler M: Regulation and modulation of pH in the brain, *Physiol. Rev.* 83:1183, 2003.

Damkier HH, Brown PD, Praetorius J: Cerebrospinal fluid secretion by the choroid plexus, *Physiol. Rev.* 93:1847, 2013.

Dunn KM, Nelson MT: Neurovascular signaling in the brain and the pathological consequences of hypertension, *Am. J. Physiol. Heart Circ. Physiol.* 306:H1, 2014.

Filosa JA, Iddings JA: Astrocyte regulation of cerebral vascular tone, *Am. J. Physiol. Heart Circ. Physiol.* 305:H609, 2013.

Gore JC: Principles and practice of functional MRI of the human brain, *J. Clin. Invest.* 112:4, 2003.

Haydon PG, Carmignoto G: Astrocyte control of synaptic transmission and neurovascular coupling, *Physiol. Rev.* 86:1009, 2006.

Iadecola C, Nedergaard M: Glial regulation of the cerebral microvasculature, *Nat. Neurosci.* 10:1369, 2007.

Iliff JJ, Nedergaard M: Is there a cerebral lymphatic system? *Stroke* 44(6 Suppl. 1):S93, 2013.

Kahle KT, Simard JM, Staley KJ, et al: Molecular mechanisms of ischemic cerebral edema: role of electroneutral ion transport, *Physiology (Bethesda)* 24:257, 2009.

Pires PW, Dams Ramos CM, Matin N, Dorrance AM: The effects of hypertension on the cerebral circulation, *Am. J. Physiol. Heart Circ. Physiol.* 304:H1598, 2013.

Schönfeld P, Reiser G: Why does brain metabolism not favor burning of fatty acids to provide energy? Reflections on disadvantages of the use of free fatty acids as fuel for brain, *J. Cereb. Blood Flow Metab.* 33:1493, 2013.

Sloan SA, Barres BA: Mechanisms of astrocyte development and their contributions to neurodevelopmental disorders, *Curr. Opin. Neurobiol.* 27C:75, 2014.

Syková E, Nicholson C: Diffusion in brain extracellular space, *Physiol. Rev.* 88(1277), 2008.

Splanchnic Circulation

- Describe the anatomy of the splanchnic circulation.
- Describe the countercurrent blood flow mechanism in villi.
- List the factors that regulate gastrointestinal blood flow.

GLOSSARY OF TERMS

- **Portal circulation:** Two capillary beds in series [in this case, blood flow from the gut (the first capillary bed) flows through the portal vein into the liver (the second capillary bed)]

- **Splanchnic circulation:** Blood flow through the gut plus blood flow through the liver, spleen, and pancreas

The blood vessels of the gastrointestinal system are part of a more extensive system called the *splanchnic circulation* shown in Figure 48-1. It includes the blood flow through the gut plus blood flows through the spleen, pancreas, and liver. The design of this system is such that all the blood that courses through the gut, spleen, and pancreas then flows immediately into the liver by way of the *portal vein*. In the liver, the blood passes through millions of minute *liver sinusoids* and finally leaves the liver by way of *hepatic veins* that empty into the vena cava of the general circulation. This flow of blood through the liver, before it empties into the vena cava, allows the *reticuloendothelial cells* that line the liver sinusoids to remove bacteria and other particulate matter that might enter the blood from the gastrointestinal tract, thus preventing direct transport of potentially harmful agents into the remainder of the body.

The *nonfat, water-soluble nutrients* absorbed from the gut (eg, carbohydrates and proteins) are transported in the portal venous blood to the same liver sinusoids. Here, both the reticuloendothelial cells and the principal parenchymal cells of the liver, the *hepatic cells*, absorb and store temporarily from one-half to three-quarters of the nutrients. Also, much chemical intermediary processing of these nutrients occurs in the liver cells. Almost all of the *fats* absorbed from the intestinal tract *are not carried in the portal blood* but instead are absorbed into the intestinal lymphatics and then conducted to the systemic circulating blood by way of the *thoracic duct* bypassing the liver.

Anatomy of the Gastrointestinal Blood Supply

Figure 48-2 shows the general features of the arterial blood supply to the gut, including the superior mesenteric and inferior mesenteric arteries supplying the walls of the small and large intestines by way of an arching arterial system. Not shown in the figure is the celiac artery, which provides a similar blood supply to the stomach.

On entering the wall of the gut, the arteries branch and send smaller arteries circling in both directions around the gut, with the tips of these arteries meeting on the side of the gut wall opposite the mesenteric attachment. From the circling arteries, still much smaller arteries penetrate into the intestinal wall and spread (1) along the muscle bundles, (2) into the intestinal villi, and (3) into submucosal vessels beneath the epithelium to serve the secretory and absorptive functions of the gut.

Figure 48-3 shows the special organization of the blood flow through an intestinal villus, including a small arteriole and venule that interconnect with a system of multiple looping capillaries. The walls of the arterioles are highly muscular and highly active in controlling villus blood flow.

Effect of Gut Activity and Metabolic Factors on Gastrointestinal Blood Flow

Under normal conditions, the blood flow in each area of the gastrointestinal tract, as well as in each layer of the gut wall, is directly related to the level of local activity. For instance, during active absorption of nutrients, blood flow in the villi and adjacent regions of the submucosa increases as much as eightfold. Likewise, blood flow in the muscle layers of the intestinal wall increases with increased motor activity in the gut. For instance, after a meal, the motor activity, secretory activity, and absorptive activity all increase; likewise, the blood flow increases greatly but then decreases back to the resting level over another 2–4 hours.

Possible Causes of the Increased Blood Flow During Gastrointestinal Activity. Although the precise causes of the increased blood flow during increased gastrointestinal activity are still unclear, some facts are known.

First, several vasodilator substances are released from the mucosa of the intestinal tract during the digestive process. Most of these substances are peptide hormones, including *cholecystokinin, vasoactive intestinal peptide, gastrin,* and *secretin*. These same hormones control specific motor and secretory activities of the gut, as discussed in Chapters 67–69.

Second, some of the gastrointestinal glands also release into the gut wall two kinins, *kallidin* and *bradykinin*, at the same time that they secrete other substances into the lumen. These kinins are powerful vasodilators that are believed to cause much of the increased mucosal vasodilation that occurs along with secretion.

Third, *decreased oxygen concentration* in the gut wall can increase intestinal blood flow at least 50–100%; therefore, the increased mucosal and gut wall metabolic rate during gut activity probably lowers the oxygen concentration enough to cause much of the vasodilation. The decrease in oxygen can also lead to as much as a fourfold increase of *adenosine*, a well-known vasodilator that could be responsible for much of the increased flow.

Thus, the increased blood flow during increased gastrointestinal activity is probably a combination of many of the aforementioned factors plus still others yet undiscovered.

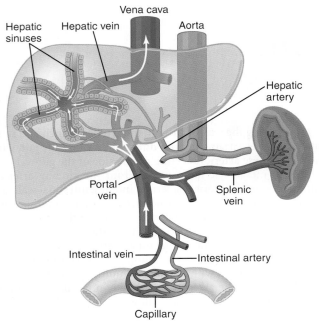

Figure 48-1 Splanchnic circulation.

"Countercurrent" Blood Flow in the Villi. Note in Figure 48-3 that the arterial flow into the villus and the venous flow out of the villus are in directions opposite to each other and that the vessels lie in close apposition to each other. Because of this vascular arrangement, much of the blood oxygen diffuses out of the arterioles directly into the adjacent venules without ever being carried in the blood to the tips of the villi. As much as 80% of the oxygen may take this short-circuit route and is therefore not available for local metabolic functions of the villi. The reader will recognize that this type of countercurrent mechanism in the villi is analogous to the countercurrent mechanism in the vasa recta of the kidney medulla, which is discussed in detail in Chapter 79.

Under normal conditions, this shunting of oxygen from the arterioles to the venules is not harmful to the villi, but in disease conditions in which blood flow to the gut becomes greatly curtailed, such as in circulatory shock, the oxygen deficit in the tips of the villi can become so great that the villus tip or even the whole villus undergoes ischemic death and disintegrates. For this reason and other reasons, villi become seriously blunted in many gastrointestinal diseases, leading to greatly diminished intestinal absorptive capacity.

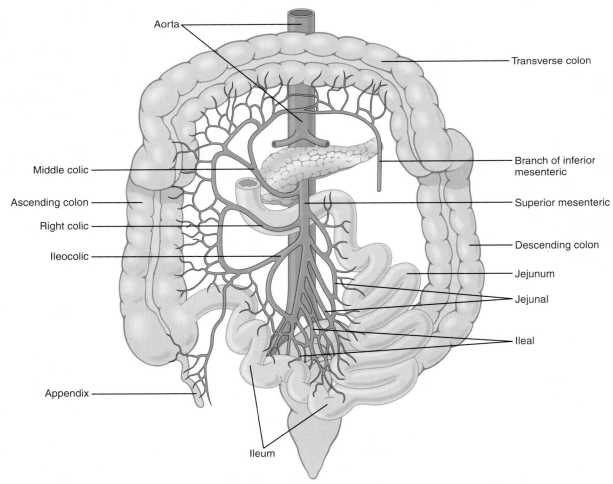

Figure 48-2 Arterial blood supply to the intestines through the mesenteric web.

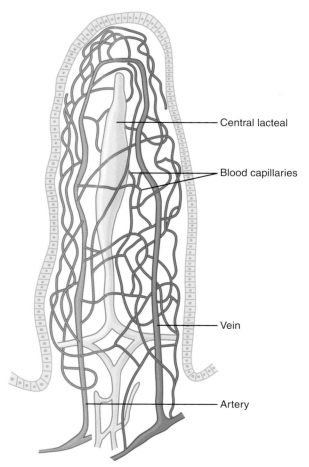

Figure 48-3 Microvasculature of the villus showing a countercurrent arrangement of blood flow in the arterioles and venules.

Labels: Central lacteal; Blood capillaries; Vein; Artery

Sympathetic stimulation, by contrast, has a direct effect on essentially all the gastrointestinal tract to cause intense vasoconstriction of the arterioles with greatly decreased blood flow. After a few minutes of this vasoconstriction, the flow often returns to near normal by means of a mechanism called "autoregulatory escape." That is, the local metabolic vasodilator mechanisms that are elicited by ischemia override the sympathetic vasoconstriction, returning toward normal the necessary nutrient blood flow to the gastrointestinal glands and muscles.

Importance of Nervous Depression of Gastrointestinal Blood Flow when Other Parts of the Body Need Extra Blood Flow. A major value of sympathetic vasoconstriction in the gut is that it allows shutoff of gastrointestinal and other splanchnic blood flow for short periods during heavy exercise, when the skeletal muscle and heart need increased flow. Also, in circulatory shock, when all the body's vital tissues are in danger of cellular death for lack of blood flow—especially the brain and the heart—sympathetic stimulation can decrease splanchnic blood flow to very little for many hours.

Sympathetic stimulation also causes strong vasoconstriction of the large-volume *intestinal* and *mesenteric* veins. This vasoconstriction decreases the volume of these veins, thereby displacing large amounts of blood into other parts of the circulation. In hemorrhagic shock or other states of low blood volume, this mechanism can provide as much as 200–400 mL of extra blood to sustain the general circulation. Box 48-1 summarizes the salient features of the splanchnic circulation.

Nervous Control of Gastrointestinal Blood Flow

Stimulation of the parasympathetic nerves going to the *stomach* and *lower colon* increases local blood flow at the same time that it increases glandular secretion. This increased flow probably results secondarily from the increased glandular activity, not as a direct effect of the nervous stimulation.

BIBLIOGRAPHY

Jeays AD, Lawford PV, Gillott R, et al: A framework for the modeling of gut blood flow regulation and postprandial hyperaemia, *World J. Gastroenterol.* 13:1393, 2007.

Kolkman JJ, Bargeman M, Huisman AB, Geelkerken RH: Diagnosis and management of splanchnic ischemia, *World J. Gastroenterol.* 14:7309, 2008.

49 Fetal and Neonatal Circulation

LEARNING OBJECTIVES

- Describe the anatomical organization of the fetal circulation.
- Describe the changes in the fetal circulation at birth.
- Describe the circulatory adjustments that occur with:
  - patent ductus arteriosus (left-to-right shunt);
  - tetralogy of Fallot (right-to-left shunt).

GLOSSARY OF TERMS

- **Congenital heart disease:** Heart disease present at birth due to abnormal development of the heart in utero
- **Left-to-right shunt:** Abnormal flow of blood either from the left heart to the right or from the systemic to the pulmonary circulation
- **Right-to-left shunt:** Abnormal flow of blood from the right heart to the left heart or from the pulmonary circulation to the systemic circulation

The human heart begins beating during the fourth week after fertilization, contracting at a rate of about 65 beats/minute. This rate increases steadily to about 140 beats/minute immediately before birth.

Circulatory Readjustments at Birth

Equally essential as the onset of breathing at birth are immediate circulatory adjustments that allow adequate blood flow through the lungs. In addition, circulatory adjustments during the first few hours of life cause more and more blood flow through the baby's liver, which up to this point has had little blood flow. To describe these readjustments, we first consider the anatomical structure of the fetal circulation.

Specific Anatomical Structure of the Fetal Circulation. Because the lungs are mainly nonfunctional during fetal life and because the liver is only partially functional, it is not necessary for the fetal heart to pump much blood through either the lungs or the liver. However, the fetal heart must pump large quantities of blood through the placenta. Therefore, special anatomical arrangements cause the fetal circulatory system to operate much differently from that of the newborn baby.

First, as shown in Figure 49-1, blood returning from the placenta through the umbilical vein passes through the *ductus venosus*, mainly bypassing the liver. Then most of the blood entering the right atrium from the inferior vena cava is directed in a straight pathway across the posterior aspect of the right atrium and through the *foramen ovale* directly into the left atrium. Thus, the well-oxygenated blood from the placenta enters mainly the left side of the heart, rather than the right side, and is pumped by the left ventricle mainly into the arteries of the head and forelimbs.

The blood entering the right atrium from the superior vena cava is directed downward through the tricuspid valve into the right ventricle. This blood is mainly deoxygenated blood from the head region of the fetus. It is pumped by the right ventricle into the pulmonary artery and then mainly through the *ductus arteriosus* into the descending aorta, and then through the two umbilical arteries into the placenta, where the deoxygenated blood becomes oxygenated.

Figure 49-2 shows the relative percentages of the total blood pumped by the heart that pass through the different vascular circuits of the fetus. Approximately 55% of all the blood goes through the placenta, leaving only 45% to pass through all the tissues of the fetus. Furthermore, during fetal life, only 12% of the blood flows through the lungs, whereas immediately after birth, virtually all the blood flows through the lungs.

Changes in the Fetal Circulation at Birth. Briefly, these changes are given in the following subsections.

Decreased Pulmonary and Increased Systemic Vascular Resistances at Birth. The primary changes in the circulation at birth are, first, loss of the tremendous blood flow through the

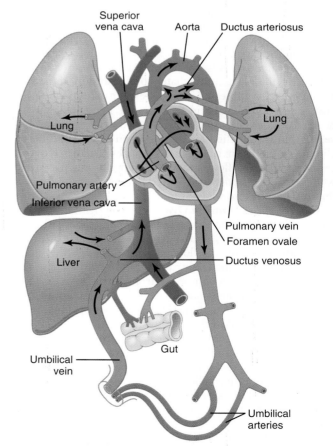

Figure 49-1 Organization of the fetal circulation.

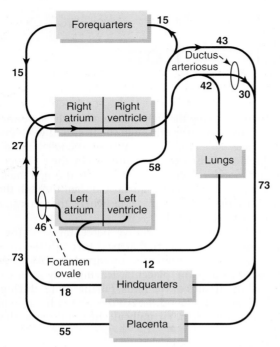

Figure 49-2 Diagram of the fetal circulatory system, showing relative distribution of blood flow to the different vascular areas. The numerals represent the percentage of the total output from both sides of the heart flowing through each particular area.

placenta, which approximately doubles the systemic vascular resistance at birth. This doubling of the systemic vascular resistance increases the aortic pressure, as well as the pressures in the left ventricle and left atrium.

Second, the *pulmonary vascular resistance greatly decreases* as a result of expansion of the lungs. In the unexpanded fetal lungs, the blood vessels are compressed because of the small volume of the lungs. Immediately on expansion, these vessels are no longer compressed and the resistance to blood flow decreases severalfold. Also, in fetal life, the hypoxia of the lungs causes considerable tonic vasoconstriction of the lung blood vessels, but vasodilation takes place when aeration of the lungs eliminates the hypoxia. All these changes together reduce the resistance to blood flow through the lungs as much as fivefold, which *reduces the pulmonary arterial pressure*, *right ventricular pressure*, and *right atrial pressure*.

Closure of the Foramen Ovale. The *low right atrial pressure* and the *high left atrial pressure* that occur secondarily to the changes in pulmonary and systemic resistances at birth cause blood now to attempt to flow backward through the foramen ovale, that is, from the left atrium into the right atrium, rather than in the other direction, as occurred during fetal life. Consequently, the small valve that lies over the foramen ovale on the left side of the atrial septum closes over this opening, thereby preventing further flow through the foramen ovale.

In two-thirds of all people, the valve becomes adherent over the foramen ovale within a few months to a few years and forms a permanent closure. However, even if permanent closure does not occur (a condition called *patent foramen ovale*), throughout life the left atrial pressure normally remains 2–4 mmHg greater than the right atrial pressure and the backpressure keeps the valve closed.

Closure of the Ductus Arteriosus. The ductus arteriosus also closes, but for different reasons. First, the increased systemic resistance elevates the aortic pressure while the decreased pulmonary resistance reduces the pulmonary arterial pressure. As a consequence, after birth, blood begins to flow backward from the aorta into the pulmonary artery through the ductus arteriosus rather than in the other direction, as in fetal life. However, after only a few hours, the muscle wall of the ductus arteriosus constricts markedly and within 1–8 days, the constriction is usually sufficient to stop all blood flow. This is called *functional closure* of the ductus arteriosus. Then, during the next 1–4 months, the ductus arteriosus ordinarily becomes anatomically occluded by growth of fibrous tissue into its lumen.

The cause of ductus arteriosus closure relates to the increased oxygenation of the blood flowing through the ductus as well as loss of the vascular relaxing effects of *prostaglandin E₂ (PGE₂)*. In fetal life, the partial pressure of oxygen (PO_2) of the ductus blood is only 15–20 mmHg, but it increases to about 100 mmHg within a few hours after birth. Furthermore, many experiments have shown that the degree of contraction of the smooth muscle in the ductus wall is highly related to this availability of oxygen.

In one of several thousand infants, the ductus fails to close resulting in a *patent ductus arteriosus*. The failure of closure has been postulated to result from excessive ductus dilation caused by vasodilating prostaglandins, especially PGE_2, in the ductus wall. In fact, administration of the drug *indomethacin*, which blocks synthesis of prostaglandins, often leads to closure.

Closure of the Ductus Venosus. In fetal life, the portal blood from the fetus's abdomen joins the blood from the umbilical vein, and these together pass by way of the *ductus venosus* directly into the vena cava immediately below the heart but above the liver, thus bypassing the liver.

Immediately after birth, blood flow through the umbilical vein ceases, but most of the portal blood still flows through the ductus venosus, with only a small amount passing through the channels of the liver. However, within 1–3 hours the muscle wall of the ductus venosus contracts strongly and closes this avenue of flow. As a consequence, the portal venous pressure rises from near 0 to 6–10 mmHg, which is enough to force portal venous blood flow through the liver sinuses. Although the ductus venosus rarely fails to close, we know little about what causes the closure.

Special Functional Problems in the Circulation of the Neonate

Blood Volume. The blood volume of a neonate immediately after birth averages about 300 mL, but if the infant is left attached to the placenta for a few minutes after birth or if the umbilical cord is stripped to force blood out of its vessels into the baby, an additional 75 mL of blood enters the infant, to make a total of 375 mL. Then, during the ensuing few hours, fluid is lost into the neonate's tissue spaces from this blood, which increases the hematocrit but returns the blood volume once again to the normal value of about 300 mL. Some pediatricians believe that this extra blood volume that results from stripping the umbilical cord can lead to mild pulmonary edema with some degree of respiratory distress, but the extra red blood cells are often valuable to the infant.

Cardiac Output. The cardiac output of the neonate averages 500 mL/minute, which, like respiration and body metabolism, is about twice as much in relation to body weight as in the adult. Occasionally, a child is born with an especially low cardiac output caused by hemorrhage of much of its blood volume from the placenta at birth.

Arterial Pressure. The arterial pressure during the first day after birth averages about 70 mmHg systolic and 50 mmHg diastolic and increases slowly during the next several months to about 90/60. A much slower rise then occurs during the subsequent years until the adult pressure of 115/70 is attained at adolescence.

Abnormal Circulatory Dynamics in Congenital Heart Defects

Occasionally, the heart or its associated blood vessels are malformed during fetal life; the defect is called a *congenital anomaly*. There are three major types of congenital anomalies of the heart and its associated vessels: (1) *stenosis* of the channel of blood flow at some point in the heart or in a closely allied major blood vessel; (2) an anomaly that allows blood to flow backward from the left side of the heart or aorta to the right side of the heart or pulmonary artery, thus failing to flow through the systemic circulation, which is called a *left-to-right shunt*; and (3) an anomaly that allows blood to flow directly from the right side of the heart into the left side of the heart, thus failing to flow through the lungs—called a *right-to-left shunt*.

PATENT DUCTUS ARTERIOSUS IS A LEFT-TO-RIGHT SHUNT

As described earlier, during fetal life, the lungs are collapsed and almost all the pulmonary arterial blood to flow occurs through a special artery present in the fetus that connects the pulmonary artery with the aorta (Figure 49-3) called the *ductus arteriosus*,

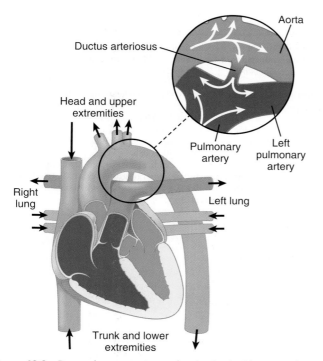

Figure 49-3 Patent ductus arteriosus, showing by the blue color that venous blood changes into oxygenated blood at different points in the circulation. The right-hand diagram shows backflow of blood from the aorta into the pulmonary artery and then through the lungs for a second time.

thus bypassing the lungs. This allows immediate recirculation of the blood through the systemic arteries of the fetus without the blood going through the lungs. This lack of blood flow through the lungs is not detrimental to the fetus because the blood is oxygenated by the placenta. Most often, the ductus arteriosus closes within a few hours to a few days after birth. Unfortunately, in about 1 of every 5500 babies, the ductus does not close, causing the condition known as *patent ductus arteriosus*, which is shown in Figure 49-3.

Dynamics of the Circulation with a Persistent Patent Ductus. During the early months of an infant's life, a patent ductus usually does not cause severely abnormal function. However, as the child grows older, the differential between the high pressure in the aorta and the lower pressure in the pulmonary artery progressively increases with corresponding increase in backward flow of blood from the aorta into the pulmonary artery. Also, the high aortic blood pressure usually causes the diameter of the partially open ductus to increase with time, making the condition even worse.

Recirculation Through the lungs. In an older child with a patent ductus, one-half to two-thirds of the aortic blood flows backward through the ductus into the pulmonary artery, then through the lungs, and finally back into the left ventricle and aorta, passing through the lungs and left side of the heart two or more times for every one time that it passes through the systemic circulation. People with this condition do not show cyanosis until later in life, when the heart fails or the lungs become congested. Indeed, early in life, the arterial blood is often better oxygenated than normal because of the extra times it passes through the lungs.

Diminished Cardiac and Respiratory Reserve. The major effects of patent ductus arteriosus on the patient are decreased cardiac and respiratory reserve. The left ventricle is pumping about two or more times the normal cardiac output, and the maximum that it can pump after hypertrophy of the heart has occurred is about four to seven times normal. Therefore, during exercise, the net blood flow through the remainder of the body can never increase to the levels required for strenuous activity. With even moderately strenuous exercise, the person is likely to become weak and may even faint from momentary heart failure.

The high pressures in the pulmonary vessels caused by excess flow through the lungs may also lead to pulmonary congestion and pulmonary edema. As a result of the excessive load on the heart, and especially because the pulmonary congestion becomes progressively more severe with age, most patients with uncorrected patent ductus die from heart disease between ages 20 and 40 years.

Heart Sounds: Machinery Murmur. In a newborn infant with patent ductus arteriosus, occasionally no abnormal heart sounds are heard because the quantity of reverse blood flow through the ductus may be insufficient to cause a heart murmur. But as the baby grows older, reaching age 1–3 years, a harsh, blowing murmur begins to be heard in the pulmonary artery area of the chest, as shown in recording F (Figure 50-2). This sound is much more intense during systole when the aortic pressure is high and much less intense during diastole when the aortic pressure falls low, so that the murmur waxes and wanes with each beat of the heart, creating the so-called *machinery murmur*.

Surgical Treatment. Surgical treatment of patent ductus arteriosus is simple; one need to only ligate the patent ductus or divide it and then close the two ends. In fact, this procedure was one of the first successful heart surgeries ever performed.

TETRALOGY OF FALLOT IS A RIGHT-TO-LEFT SHUNT

Tetralogy of Fallot is shown in Figure 49-4; it is the most common cause of "blue baby." Most of the blood bypasses the lungs, so the aortic blood is mainly unoxygenated venous blood. In this condition, four abnormalities of the heart occur simultaneously:

1. The aorta originates from the right ventricle rather than the left, or it overrides a hole in the septum, as shown in Figure 49-4, receiving blood from both ventricles.
2. Because the pulmonary artery is stenosed, much lower than normal amounts of blood pass from the right ventricle into the lungs; instead, most of the blood passes directly into the aorta, thus bypassing the lungs.
3. Blood from the left ventricle flows either through a ventricular septal hole into the right ventricle and then into the aorta or directly into the aorta that overrides this hole.
4. Because the right side of the heart must pump large quantities of blood against the high pressure in the aorta, its musculature is highly developed, causing an enlarged right ventricle.

Abnormal Circulatory Dynamics. It is readily apparent that the major physiological difficulty caused by tetralogy of Fallot is the shunting of blood past the lungs without becoming oxygenated. As much as 75% of the venous blood returning to the heart passes directly from the right ventricle into the aorta without becoming oxygenated.

A diagnosis of tetralogy of Fallot is usually based on (1) the fact that the baby's skin is *cyanotic* (blue); (2) measurement of high systolic pressure in the right ventricle, recorded through a catheter; (3) characteristic changes in the radiological silhouette of the heart, showing an enlarged right ventricle; and (4) angiograms (X-ray pictures) showing abnormal blood flow through

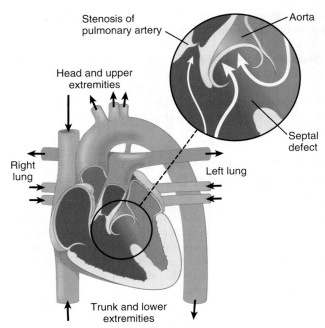

Figure 49-4 Tetralogy of Fallot, showing by the blue color that most of the venous blood is shunted from the right ventricle into the aorta without passing through the lungs.

the interventricular septal hole and into the overriding aorta, but much less flow through the stenosed pulmonary artery.

Surgical Treatment. Tetralogy of Fallot can usually be treated successfully with surgery. The usual operation is to open the pulmonary stenosis, close the septal defect, and reconstruct the flow pathway into the aorta. When surgery is successful, the average life expectancy increases from only 3–4 to 50 or more years.

BIBLIOGRAPHY

Crean A: Cardiovascular MR and CT in congenital heart disease, *Heart* 93(12):1637, 2007.

Fahed AC, Gelb BD, Seidman JG, Seidman CE: Genetics of congenital heart disease glass half empty, *Circ. Res.* 112(4):707, 2013.

Gao Y, Raj JU: Regulation of the pulmonary circulation in the fetus and newborn, *Physiol. Rev.* 90(4):1291, 2010.

Hoffman JI, Kaplan S: The incidence of congenital heart disease, *J. Am. Coll. Cardiol.* 39:1890, 2002.

Jenkins KJ, Correa A, Feinstein JA, et al: Noninherited risk factors and congenital cardiovascular defects: current knowledge: a scientific statement from

the American Heart Association Council on Cardiovascular Disease in the Young: endorsed by the American Academy of Pediatrics, *Circulation* 115:2995, 2007.

Osol G, Mandala M: Maternal uterine vascular remodeling during pregnancy, *Physiology (Bethesda)* 24:58, 2009.

Rhodes JF, Hijazi ZM, Sommer RJ: Pathophysiology of congenital heart disease in the adult, part II. Simple obstructive lesions, *Circulation* 117:1228, 2008.

Saigal S, Doyle LW: An overview of mortality and sequelae of preterm birth from infancy to adulthood, *Lancet* 371:261, 2008.

Schneider DJ: The patent ductus arteriosus in term infants, children, and adults, *Semin. Perinatol* 36:146, 2012.

Sommer RJ, Hijazi ZM, Rhodes JF Jr: Pathophysiology of congenital heart disease in the adult: part I: shunt lesions, *Circulation* 117:1090, 2008a.

Sommer RJ, Hijazi ZM, Rhodes JF: Pathophysiology of congenital heart disease in the adult: part III: complex congenital heart disease, *Circulation* 117:1340, 2008b.

Yuan S, Zaidi S, Brueckner M: Congenital heart disease: emerging themes linking genetics and development, *Curr. Opin. Genet. Dev.* 23:352, 2013.

Valvular Heart Disease

LEARNING OBJECTIVES

- Describe the causes of the heart sounds.
- Identify the auscultatory areas on the chest wall.
- Describe the murmurs caused by common valvular lesions.
- Describe the circulatory dynamics associated with common valvular lesions.

GLOSSARY OF TERMS

- **Phonocardiogram:** The recording of the heart sounds from a microphone specially designed to detect low-frequency sound when applied to the chest wall

- **Rheumatic heart disease:** An autoimmune disease affecting the valves of the heart and that follows a sore throat with group A hemolytic streptococci

- **Valvular "incompetence":** Valves that are "leaky" following disease, and that allow the backflow of blood when the valve should normally be closed

- **Valvular "stenosis":** Valves that are extra tight following disease, and that open with difficulty and increased pressure

When listening to a normal heart with a stethoscope, one hears a sound usually described as "lub, dub, lub, dub." The "lub" is associated with closure of the atrioventricular (A-V) valves at the beginning of systole, and the "dub" is associated with closure of the semilunar (aortic and pulmonary) valves at the end of systole. The "lub" sound is called the *first heart sound* and the "dub" is called the *second heart sound* because the normal pumping cycle of the heart is considered to start when the A-V valves close at the onset of ventricular systole.

Causes of Heart Sounds

The First Sound Is Associated with Closure of the A-V Valves.
The cause of the heart sound is the *vibration of the taut valves immediately after closure* along with *vibration of the adjacent walls of the heart and major vessels around the heart*. That is, in generating the first heart sound, contraction of the ventricles first causes sudden backflow of blood against the A-V valves (the tricuspid and mitral valves) causing them to close and bulge toward the atria until the chordae tendineae abruptly stop the back bulging. The elastic tautness of the chordae tendineae and of the valves then causes the back-surging blood to bounce forward again into each respective ventricle. This mechanism causes the blood and the ventricular walls, as well as the taut valves, to vibrate and causes vibrating turbulence in the blood. The vibrations travel through the adjacent tissues to the chest wall, where they can be heard as sound by using the stethoscope.

The Second Heart Sound Is Associated with Closure of the Aortic and Pulmonary Valves.
The second heart sound results from sudden closure of the semilunar (ie, the aortic and pulmonary) valves at the end of systole. When the semilunar valves close, they bulge backward toward the ventricles and their elastic stretch recoils the blood back into the arteries, which causes a short period of reverberation of blood back and forth between the walls of the arteries and the semilunar valves, as well as between these valves and the ventricular walls. The vibrations occurring in the arterial walls are then transmitted mainly along the arteries. When the vibrations of the vessels or ventricles come into contact with a "sounding board," such as the chest wall, they create sound that can be heard.

Duration and Pitch of the First and Second Heart Sounds.
The duration of each of the heart sounds is slightly more than 0.10 second with the first sound about 0.14 second and the second about 0.11 second. The reason for the shorter second sound is that the semilunar valves are more taut than the A-V valves, so they vibrate for a shorter time than do the A-V valves.

The second heart sound normally has a higher frequency than the first heart sound for two reasons: (1) the tautness of the semilunar valves in comparison with the much less taut A-V valves and (2) the greater elastic coefficient of the taut arterial walls that provide the principal vibrating chambers for the second sound, in comparison with the much looser, less elastic ventricular chambers that provide the vibrating system for the first heart sound. The clinician uses these differences to distinguish special characteristics of the two respective sounds and these are summarized as follows:

	First Heart Sound	Second Heart Sound
Cause	Closure of A-V valves	Closure of semilunar valves
Duration (second)	0.14	0.11
Frequency	Lower	Higher

A-V, atrioventricular.

The Third Heart Sound Occurs at the Beginning of the Middle Third of Diastole.
Occasionally a weak, rumbling third heart sound is heard at the beginning of the *middle third of diastole*. A logical but unproved explanation of this sound is oscillation of blood back and forth between the walls of the ventricles initiated by inrushing blood from the atria. The reason the third heart sound does not occur until the middle third of diastole is believed to be that in the early part of diastole, the ventricles are not filled sufficiently to create even the small amount of elastic tension necessary for reverberation. The frequency of this sound is usually so low that the ear cannot hear it, yet it can often be recorded in the phonocardiogram. The third heart sound may be normally present in children, adolescents, and young adults but generally indicates systolic heart failure in older adults.

Atrial Contraction Sound (Fourth Heart Sound). An atrial heart sound can sometimes be recorded in the phonocardiogram, but it can almost never be heard with a stethoscope because of its weakness and very low frequency—usually 20 cycles/second or less. This sound occurs when the atria contract, and, presumably, it is caused by the inrush of blood into the ventricles, which initiates vibrations similar to those of the third heart sound. A fourth heart sound is common in persons who derive benefit from atrial contraction for ventricular filling as a result of decreased ventricular wall compliance and increased resistance to ventricular filling. For example, a fourth heart sound is often heard in older patients with left ventricular hypertrophy.

CHEST SURFACE AREAS FOR AUSCULTATION OF NORMAL HEART SOUNDS

Listening to the sounds of the body, usually with the aid of a stethoscope, is called *auscultation*. Figure 50-1 shows the areas of the chest wall from which the different heart valvular sounds can best be distinguished. Although the sounds from all the valves can be heard from all these areas, the cardiologist distinguishes the sounds from the different valves by a process of elimination. That is, he or she moves the stethoscope from one area to another, noting the loudness of the sounds in different areas and gradually picking out the sound components from each valve.

The areas for listening to the different heart sounds are not directly over the valves themselves. The aortic area is upward along the aorta because of sound transmission up the aorta and the pulmonic area is upward along the pulmonary artery. The tricuspid area is over the right ventricle, and the mitral area is over the apex of the left ventricle, which is the portion of the heart nearest the surface of the chest; the heart is rotated so that the remainder of the left ventricle lies more posteriorly.

PHONOCARDIOGRAM

If a microphone specially designed to detect low-frequency sound is placed on the chest, the heart sounds can be amplified and recorded by a high-speed recording apparatus. The recording is called a *phonocardiogram*, and the heart sounds appear as

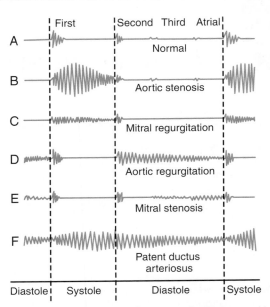

Figure 50-2 Phonocardiograms from normal and abnormal hearts.

waves, as shown schematically in Figure 50-2. Recording A is an example of normal heart sounds showing the vibrations of the first, second, and third heart sounds and even the very weak atrial sound. Note specifically that the third and atrial heart sounds are each a very low rumble. The third heart sound can be recorded in only one-third to one-half of all people and the atrial heart sound can be recorded in perhaps one-fourth of all people.

Valvular Lesions

RHEUMATIC VALVULAR LESIONS

By far the greatest number of valvular lesions results from *rheumatic fever*. Rheumatic fever is an autoimmune disease in which the heart valves are likely to be damaged or destroyed. The disease is usually initiated by streptococcal toxin following a sore throat with group A hemolytic streptococci. The streptococci also release several different proteins against which the person's reticuloendothelial system produces *antibodies*. The antibodies react not only with the streptococcal protein but also with other protein tissues of the body, often causing severe immunologic damage. These reactions continue to take place as long as the antibodies persist in the blood—1 year or more.

Rheumatic fever particularly causes damage in certain susceptible areas, such as the heart valves. In rheumatic fever, large hemorrhagic, fibrinous, bulbous lesions grow along the inflamed edges of the heart valves. Because the mitral valve receives more trauma during valvular action than any of the other valves, it is the one most often seriously damaged and the aortic valve is the second most frequently damaged. The right heart valves, the tricuspid and pulmonary valves, are usually affected much less severely, probably because the low-pressure stresses that act on these valves are slight compared with the high-pressure stresses that act on the left heart valves.

Scarring of the Valves

The lesions of acute rheumatic fever frequently occur on adjacent valve leaflets simultaneously, so the edges of the leaflets become stuck together. Then, weeks, months, or years later, the

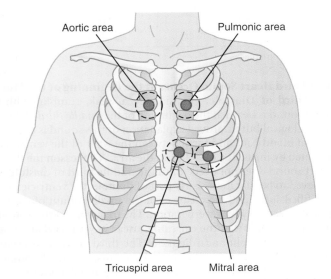

Figure 50-1 Chest areas from which sound from each valve is best heard.

lesions become scar tissue, permanently fusing portions of adjacent valve leaflets. Also, the free edges of the leaflets, which are normally filmy and free-flapping, often become solid, scarred masses.

A valve in which the leaflets adhere to one another so extensively that blood cannot flow through it normally is said to be *stenosed*. Conversely, when the valve edges are so destroyed by scar tissue that they cannot close as the ventricles contract, *regurgitation* (backflow) of blood occurs when the valve should be closed. Stenosis usually does not occur without the coexistence of at least some degree of regurgitation and vice versa.

Other Causes of Valvular Lesions

Stenosis or lack of one or more leaflets of a valve also occurs occasionally as a *congenital defect*. Complete lack of leaflets is rare; *congenital stenosis* is more common, as is discussed later in this chapter.

HEART MURMURS ARE CAUSED BY VALVULAR LESIONS

As shown by the phonocardiograms in Figure 50-2, many abnormal heart sounds, known as "heart murmurs," occur when abnormalities of the valves are present.

Systolic Murmur of Aortic Stenosis

In persons with aortic stenosis, blood is ejected from the left ventricle through only a small fibrous opening of the aortic valve. Because of the resistance to ejection, sometimes the blood pressure in the left ventricle rises as high as 300 mmHg, while the pressure in the aorta is still normal. Thus, a nozzle effect is created *during systole*, with blood jetting at tremendous velocity through the small opening of the valve. This phenomenon causes *severe turbulence* of the blood in the root of the aorta. The turbulent blood impinging against the aortic walls causes intense vibration, and a loud murmur (see recording B, Figure 50-2) occurs during systole and is transmitted throughout the superior thoracic aorta and even into the large arteries of the neck. This sound is harsh and in persons with severe stenosis it may be so loud that it can be heard several feet away from the patient. Also, the sound vibrations can often be felt with the hand on the upper chest and lower neck, a phenomenon known as a "*thrill*."

Diastolic Murmur of Aortic Regurgitation

In aortic regurgitation, no abnormal sound is heard during systole, but *during diastole*, blood flows backward from the high-pressure aorta into the left ventricle, causing a "blowing" murmur of relatively high pitch with a swishing quality heard maximally over the left ventricle (see recording D, Figure 50-2). This murmur results from *turbulence* of blood jetting backward into the blood already in the low-pressure diastolic left ventricle.

Systolic Murmur of Mitral Regurgitation

In persons with mitral regurgitation, blood flows backward through the mitral valve into the left atrium *during systole*. This backward flow also causes a high-frequency "blowing," swishing sound (see recording C, Figure 50-2) similar to that of aortic regurgitation but occurring during systole rather than diastole. It is transmitted most strongly into the left atrium. However, the left atrium is so deep within the chest that it is difficult to hear this sound directly over the atrium. As a result, the sound of mitral regurgitation is transmitted to the chest wall mainly through the left ventricle to the apex of the heart.

Diastolic Murmur of Mitral Stenosis

In persons with mitral stenosis, blood passes with difficulty through the stenosed mitral valve from the left atrium into the left ventricle, and because the pressure in the left atrium seldom rises above 30 mmHg, a large pressure differential forcing blood from the left atrium into the left ventricle does not develop. Consequently, the abnormal sounds heard in mitral stenosis (see recording E, Figure 50-2) are usually weak and of very low frequency, so most of the sound spectrum is below the low-frequency end of human hearing.

During the early part of diastole, a left ventricle with a stenotic mitral valve has so little blood in it and its walls are so flabby that blood does not reverberate back and forth between the walls of the ventricle. For this reason, even in persons with severe mitral stenosis, no murmur may be heard during the first third of diastole. Then, after partial filling, the ventricle has stretched enough for blood to reverberate and a low rumbling murmur begins.

Phonocardiograms of Valvular Murmurs

Phonocardiograms B, C, D, and E of Figure 50-2 show, respectively, idealized records obtained from patients with aortic stenosis, mitral regurgitation, aortic regurgitation, and mitral stenosis. It is obvious from these phonocardiograms that the aortic stenotic lesion causes the loudest murmur and the mitral stenotic lesion causes the weakest murmur. The phonocardiograms show how the intensity of the murmurs varies during different portions of systole and diastole, and the relative timing of each murmur is also evident. Note especially that the murmurs of aortic stenosis and mitral regurgitation occur only during systole, whereas the murmurs of aortic regurgitation and mitral stenosis occur only during diastole.

Abnormal Circulatory Dynamics in Valvular Heart Disease

DYNAMICS OF THE CIRCULATION IN AORTIC STENOSIS AND AORTIC REGURGITATION

In *aortic stenosis*, the contracting left ventricle fails to empty adequately, whereas in *aortic regurgitation*, blood flows backward into the ventricle from the aorta after the ventricle has just pumped the blood into the aorta. Therefore, in either case, the *net stroke volume output* of the heart is reduced.

Several important compensations take place that can ameliorate the severity of the circulatory defects. Some of these compensations are described in the following sections.

Hypertrophy of the Left Ventricle. In both aortic stenosis and aortic regurgitation, the left ventricular musculature hypertrophies because of the increased ventricular workload.

In *regurgitation*, the left ventricular chamber also enlarges to hold all the regurgitant blood from the aorta. Sometimes the left ventricular muscle mass increases fourfold to fivefold, creating a tremendously large left side of the heart.

When the aortic valve is seriously *stenosed*, the hypertrophied muscle allows the left ventricle to develop as much as 400 mmHg of intraventricular pressure at systolic peak.

In persons with severe aortic regurgitation, sometimes the hypertrophied muscle allows the left ventricle to pump a stroke volume output as great as 250 mL, although as much as three-fourths of this blood returns to the ventricle during diastole and only one-fourth flows through the aorta to the body.

Increase in Blood Volume. Another effect that helps compensate for the diminished net pumping by the left ventricle is increased blood volume. This increased volume results from (1) an initial slight decrease in arterial pressure plus (2) peripheral circulatory reflexes induced by the decrease in pressure. These mechanisms together diminish renal output of urine causing the blood volume to increase and the mean arterial pressure to return to normal. Also, red blood cell mass eventually increases because of a slight degree of tissue hypoxia.

The increase in blood volume tends to increase venous return to the heart, which, in turn, causes the left ventricle to pump with the extra power required to overcome the abnormal pumping dynamics.

Aortic Valvular Lesions May Be Associated with Inadequate Coronary Blood Flow. When a person has stenosis of the aortic valve, the ventricular muscle must develop a high tension to create the high intraventricular pressure needed to force blood through the stenosed valve. This action increases workload and oxygen consumption of the ventricle, necessitating increased coronary blood flow to deliver this oxygen. The high wall tension of the ventricle, however, causes marked decreases in coronary flow during systole, particularly in the subendocardial vessels. Intraventricular diastolic pressure is also increased when there is aortic valve stenosis, and this increased pressure may cause compression of the inner layers of the heart muscle and reduced coronary blood flow. Thus, severe aortic valve stenosis often causes ischemia of the heart muscle.

With aortic regurgitation the intraventricular diastolic pressure also increases, compressing the inner layer of the heart muscle and decreasing coronary blood flow. Aortic diastolic pressure decreases during aortic regurgitation, which can also decrease coronary blood flow and cause ischemia of the heart muscle.

Eventual Failure of the Left Ventricle and Development of Pulmonary Edema

In the early stages of aortic stenosis or aortic regurgitation, the intrinsic ability of the left ventricle to adapt to increasing loads prevents significant abnormalities in circulatory function in the person during rest, other than increased work output required of the left ventricle. Therefore, considerable degrees of aortic stenosis or aortic regurgitation often occur before the person knows that he or she has serious heart disease (eg, a resting left ventricular systolic pressure as high as 200 mmHg in persons with aortic stenosis or a left ventricular stroke volume output as high as double normal in persons with aortic regurgitation).

Beyond a critical stage in these aortic valve lesions, the left ventricle finally cannot keep up with the work demand. As a consequence, the left ventricle dilates and cardiac output begins to fall; blood simultaneously dams up in the left atrium and in the lungs behind the failing left ventricle. The left atrial pressure rises progressively and at mean left atrial pressures above 25–40 mmHg, serious edema appears in the lungs, as discussed in Chapter 51.

DYNAMICS OF MITRAL STENOSIS AND MITRAL REGURGITATION

In persons with mitral stenosis, blood flow from the left atrium into the left ventricle is impeded and in persons with mitral regurgitation, much of the blood that has flowed into the left ventricle during diastole leaks back into the left atrium during systole rather than being pumped into the aorta. Therefore, either of these conditions reduces net movement of blood from the left atrium into the left ventricle.

Pulmonary Edema in Mitral Valvular Disease. The buildup of blood in the left atrium causes progressive increase in left atrial pressure, eventually resulting in the development of serious pulmonary edema. Ordinarily, lethal edema does not occur until the mean left atrial pressure rises above 25 mmHg and sometimes as high as 40 mmHg because the lung lymphatic vessels enlarge manyfold and can rapidly carry fluid away from the lung tissues.

Enlarged Left Atrium and Atrial Fibrillation. The high left atrial pressure in mitral valvular disease also causes progressive enlargement of the left atrium, which increases the distance that the cardiac electrical excitatory impulse must travel in the atrial wall. This pathway may eventually become so long that it predisposes to the development of excitatory signal *circus movements*, as discussed in Chapter 34. Therefore, in late stages of mitral valvular disease, especially in mitral stenosis, atrial fibrillation often occurs. This development further reduces the pumping effectiveness of the heart and causes further cardiac debility.

Compensation in Early Mitral Valvular Disease. As also occurs in aortic valvular disease and in many types of congenital heart disease, the blood volume increases in mitral valvular disease principally because of diminished excretion of water and salt by the kidneys. This increased blood volume increases venous return to the heart, thereby helping to overcome the effect of the cardiac debility. Therefore, after compensation, cardiac output may fall only minimally until the late stages of mitral valvular disease, even though the left atrial pressure is rising.

As the left atrial pressure rises, blood begins to dam up in the lungs, eventually all the way back to the pulmonary artery. In addition, incipient edema of the lungs causes pulmonary arteriolar constriction. These two effects together increase systolic pulmonary arterial pressure and also right ventricular pressure, sometimes to as high as 60 mmHg, which is more than double normal. This increased pressure, in turn, causes hypertrophy of the right side of the heart, which partially compensates for its increased workload.

CIRCULATORY DYNAMICS DURING EXERCISE IN PATIENTS WITH VALVULAR LESIONS

During exercise, large quantities of venous blood are returned to the heart from the peripheral circulation. Therefore, all the dynamic abnormalities that occur in the different types of valvular heart disease become tremendously exacerbated. Even in persons with mild valvular heart disease, in which the symptoms may be unrecognizable at rest, severe symptoms often develop during heavy exercise. For instance, in patients with aortic valvular lesions, exercise can cause acute left ventricular failure followed by *acute pulmonary edema*. Also, in patients with mitral disease, exercise can cause so much damming of blood in the lungs that serious or even lethal pulmonary edema may ensue in as little as 10 minutes.

Even in mild to moderate cases of valvular disease, the patient's *cardiac reserve* diminishes in proportion to the severity of the valvular dysfunction. That is, the cardiac output does not increase as much as it should during exercise. Therefore, the muscles of the body fatigue rapidly because of too little increase in muscle blood flow.

Hypertrophy of the Heart in Valvular Heart Disease

Hypertrophy of cardiac muscle is one of the most important mechanisms by which the heart adapts to increased workloads, whether these loads are caused by increased pressure against which the heart muscle must contract or by increased cardiac output that must be pumped. Some physicians believe that the increased strength of contraction of the heart muscle causes the hypertrophy; others believe that the increased metabolic rate of the muscle is the primary stimulus. Regardless of which of these is correct, one can calculate approximately how much hypertrophy will occur in each chamber of the heart by multiplying ventricular output by the pressure against which the ventricle must work, with emphasis on pressure. Thus, hypertrophy occurs in most types of valvular and congenital disease, sometimes causing heart weights as great as 800 g instead of the normal 300 g.

Detrimental Effects of Late Stages of Cardiac Hypertrophy. Although the most common cause of cardiac hypertrophy is hypertension, almost all forms of cardiac diseases including valvular and congenital disease can stimulate enlargement of the heart.

"Physiological" cardiac hypertrophy is generally considered to be a compensatory response of the heart to increased workload and is usually beneficial for maintaining cardiac output in the face of abnormalities that impair the heart's effectiveness as a pump. However, extreme degrees of hypertrophy can lead to heart failure. One of the reasons for this is that the coronary vasculature typically does not increase to the same extent as the mass of cardiac muscle increases. The second reason is that fibrosis often develops in the muscle, especially in the subendocardial muscle where the coronary blood flow is poor, with fibrous tissue replacing degenerating muscle fibers. Because of the disproportionate increase in muscle mass relative to coronary blood flow, relative ischemia may develop as the cardiac muscle hypertrophies and coronary blood flow insufficiency may ensue. Anginal pain is therefore a frequent accompaniment of cardiac hypertrophy associated with valvular and congenital heart diseases. Enlargement of the heart is also associated with greater risk for developing arrhythmias, which in turn can lead to further impairment of cardiac function and sudden death because of fibrillation.

BIBLIOGRAPHY

Burchfield JS, Xie M, Hill JA: Pathological ventricular remodeling: mechanisms: part 1 of 2, *Circulation* 128:388, 2013.

Gould ST, Srigunapalan S, Simmons CA, Anseth KS: Hemodynamic and cellular response feedback in calcific aortic valve disease, *Circ. Res.* 113:186, 2013.

Kari FA, Siepe M, Sievers HH, Beyersdorf F: Repair of the regurgitant bicuspid or tricuspid aortic valve: background, principles, and outcomes, *Circulation* 128:854, 2013.

Lindman BR, Bonow RO, Otto CM: Current management of calcific aortic stenosis, *Circ. Res.* 113:223, 2013.

Manning WJ: Asymptomatic aortic stenosis in the elderly: a clinical review, *JAMA* 310:1490, 2013.

Marijon E, Mirabel M, Celermajer DS, Jouven X: Rheumatic heart disease, *Lancet* 379:953, 2012.

Maron BJ, Maron MS: Hypertrophic cardiomyopathy, *Lancet* 381:242, 2013.

Towler DA: Molecular and cellular aspects of calcific aortic valve disease, *Circ. Res.* 113:198, 2013.

Zaid RR, Barker CM, Little SH, Nagueh SF: Pre- and post-operative diastolic dysfunction in patients with valvular heart disease: diagnosis and therapeutic implications, *J. Am. Coll. Cardiol.* 62:1922, 2013.

51

Cardiac Failure

LEARNING OBJECTIVES

- Describe the circulatory dynamics in heart failure.
- Distinguish between left and right heart failure.
- Distinguish between compensated and decompensated heart failure.
- Describe the principles of treatment of heart failure.
- Explain the concept of "cardiac reserve."

GLOSSARY OF TERMS

- **Cardiac failure:** Failure of the heart to pump enough blood to satisfy the needs of the body

- **Cardiac reserve:** The maximum percentage that the cardiac output can increase above normal (typically 400–500%, ie, four to five times)

- **Left heart failure:** Impaired functioning of the left side of the heart resulting in elevated pulmonary pressures and pulmonary congestion

- **Pulmonary edema:** Buildup of fluid in the tissues of the lung following an increase in pulmonary vascular pressures and associated with shortness in breath and dyspnea

- **Right heart failure:** Impaired functioning of the right ventricle, which results in back pressure and is manifested clinically by an elevated jugular venous pulse, hepatomegaly, and peripheral edema

One of the most important ailments treated by the physician is cardiac failure (heart failure). This ailment can result from any heart condition that reduces the ability of the heart to pump enough blood to meet the body's needs. The cause is usually decreased contractility of the myocardium resulting from diminished coronary blood flow. However, failure can also be caused by damaged heart valves, external pressure around the heart, vitamin B deficiency, primary cardiac muscle disease, or any other abnormality that makes the heart a hypoeffective pump.

In this chapter, we will discuss mainly cardiac failure caused by ischemic heart disease resulting from partial blockage of the coronary blood vessels, which is the most common cause of heart failure.

Circulatory Dynamics in Cardiac Failure

ACUTE EFFECTS OF MODERATE CARDIAC FAILURE

If a heart suddenly becomes severely damaged, such as by myocardial infarction, the pumping ability of the heart is immediately depressed. As a result, two main effects occur: (1) reduced cardiac output and (2) damming of blood in the veins resulting in increased venous pressure.

The progressive changes in heart's pumping effectiveness at different times after an acute myocardial infarction are shown graphically in Figure 51-1. The top curve of this figure shows a normal cardiac output curve. Point A on this curve is the normal operating point showing a normal cardiac output under resting conditions of 5 L/minute and a right atrial pressure of 0 mmHg.

Immediately after the heart becomes damaged, the cardiac output curve becomes greatly depressed, falling to the lowest curve at the bottom of the graph. Within a few seconds, a new circulatory state is established at point B illustrating that the cardiac output has fallen to 2 L/minute, about two-fifths normal, whereas the right atrial pressure has risen to +4 mmHg because venous blood returning to the heart from the body is dammed up in the right atrium. This low cardiac output is still sufficient to sustain life for perhaps a few hours, but it is likely to be associated with fainting. Fortunately, this acute stage usually lasts for only a few seconds because sympathetic nervous reflexes occur almost immediately and compensate, to a great extent, for the damaged heart as follows.

Compensation for Acute Cardiac Failure by Sympathetic Nervous Reflexes. When the cardiac output falls precariously low, many of the circulatory reflexes discussed in Chapter 43 are rapidly activated. The best known of these is the *baroreceptor reflex*, which is activated by diminished arterial pressure. The *chemoreceptor reflex*, the *central nervous system ischemic response*, and even *reflexes that originate in the damaged heart* also likely contribute to activation of the sympathetic nervous system. The sympathetics therefore become strongly stimulated within a few seconds and the parasympathetic nervous signals to the heart become reciprocally inhibited at the same time.

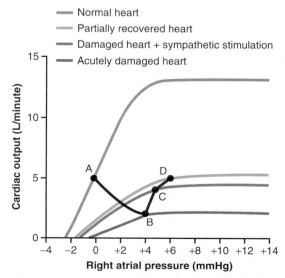

Figure 51-1 Progressive changes in the cardiac output curve after acute myocardial infarction. Both the cardiac output and right atrial pressure change progressively from point A to point D (illustrated by the *black line*) over a period of seconds, minutes, days, and weeks.

Strong sympathetic stimulation has major effects on the heart and on the peripheral vasculature. If all the ventricular musculature is diffusely damaged but is still functional, sympathetic stimulation strengthens this damaged musculature. If part of the muscle is nonfunctional and part of it is still normal, the normal muscle is strongly stimulated by the sympathetic stimulation, in this way partially compensating for the nonfunctional muscle. Thus, *the heart becomes a stronger pump* as a result of sympathetic stimulation. This effect is illustrated in Figure 51-1, which shows about twofold elevation of the very low cardiac output curve after sympathetic compensation.

Sympathetic stimulation also increases venous return because it increases the tone of most of the blood vessels of the circulation, especially the veins, *raising the mean systemic filling* pressure to 12–14 mmHg, almost 100% above normal. As discussed in Chapter 36, this increased filling pressure greatly increases the tendency for blood to flow from the veins back into the heart. Therefore, the damaged heart becomes primed with more inflowing blood than usual and the right atrial pressure rises still further, which helps the heart to pump still larger quantities of blood. Thus, in Figure 51-1, the new circulatory state is depicted by point C showing a cardiac output of 4.2 L/minute and a right atrial pressure of 5 mmHg.

The sympathetic reflexes become maximally developed in about 30 seconds. Therefore, a person who has a sudden, moderate heart attack might experience nothing more than cardiac pain and a few seconds of fainting. Shortly thereafter, with the aid of the sympathetic reflex compensations, the cardiac output may return to a level adequate to sustain the person if he or she remains quiet, although the pain might persist.

CHRONIC STAGE OF FAILURE—FLUID RETENTION AND COMPENSATED CARDIAC OUTPUT

After the first few minutes of an acute heart attack, a prolonged semichronic state begins characterized mainly by two events: (1) retention of fluid by the kidneys and (2) varying degrees of recovery of the heart itself over a period of weeks to months as illustrated by the light green curve in Figure 51-1.

Renal Retention of Fluid and Increase in Blood Volume Occur for Hours to Days

A low cardiac output has a profound effect on renal function, sometimes causing anuria when the cardiac output falls to 50–60% of normal. In general, the urine output remains below normal as long as the cardiac output and arterial pressure remain significantly less than normal; urine output usually does not return all the way to normal after an acute heart attack until the cardiac output and arterial pressure rise almost to normal levels.

Moderate Fluid Retention in Cardiac Failure Can Be Beneficial. Many cardiologists have considered fluid retention to always have a detrimental effect in cardiac failure. However, a moderate increase in body fluid and blood volume is an important factor in helping to compensate for the diminished pumping ability of the heart by increasing the venous return. The increased blood volume increases venous return in two ways: First, it increases the mean systemic filling pressure, which increases the pressure gradient for causing venous flow of blood toward the heart. Second, it distends the veins, which reduces the venous resistance and allows even more ease of flow of blood to the heart.

If the heart is not too greatly damaged, this increased venous return can almost fully compensate for the heart's diminished pumping ability—enough so that even when the heart's pumping ability is reduced to as low as 40–50% of normal, the increased venous return can often cause nearly normal cardiac output as long as the person remains in a quiet resting state.

When the heart's pumping capability is reduced further, blood flow to the kidneys finally becomes too low for the kidneys to excrete enough salt and water to equal salt and water intake. Therefore, fluid retention begins and continues indefinitely, unless major therapeutic procedures are used to prevent this outcome. Furthermore, because the heart is already pumping at its maximum capacity, *this excess fluid no longer has a beneficial effect* on the circulation. Instead, the fluid retention increases the workload on the already damaged heart and severe edema develops throughout the body, which can be very detrimental and can lead to death.

Detrimental Effects of Excess Fluid Retention in Severe Cardiac Failure. In contrast to the beneficial effects of moderate fluid retention in cardiac failure, in severe cardiac failure extreme excesses of fluid can have serious physiological consequences. These consequences include (1) increasing the workload on the damaged heart; (2) overstretching of the heart, which further weakens the heart; (3) filtration of fluid into the lungs causing pulmonary edema and consequent deoxygenation of the blood; and (4) development of extensive edema in most parts of the body. These detrimental effects of excessive fluid are discussed in later sections of this chapter.

Recovery of the Heart After Myocardial Infarction

After a heart becomes suddenly damaged as a result of myocardial infarction, the natural reparative processes of the body begin to help restore normal cardiac function. For instance, a new collateral blood supply begins to penetrate the peripheral portions of the infarcted area of the heart, often causing much of the heart muscle in the fringe areas to become functional again. Also, the undamaged portion of the heart musculature hypertrophies, offsetting much of the cardiac damage.

The degree and extent of recovery depends on the type of cardiac damage. After acute myocardial infarction, the heart ordinarily recovers rapidly during the first few days and weeks and achieves most of its final state of recovery within 5–7 weeks, although mild degrees of additional recovery can continue for months.

Cardiac Output Curve After Partial Recovery. Figure 51-1 shows function of the partially recovered heart a week or so after acute myocardial infarction. By this time, considerable fluid has been retained in the body and the tendency for venous return has increased markedly as well; therefore, the right atrial pressure has risen even more. As a result, the state of the circulation is now changed from point C to point D, which shows a normal cardiac output of 5 L/minute but right atrial pressure increased to 6 mmHg.

Because the cardiac output has returned to normal, renal output of fluid also returns to normal and no further fluid retention occurs, except that *the retention of fluid that has already occurred continues to maintain moderate excesses of fluid.* Therefore, except for the high right atrial pressure represented by point D in this figure, the person now has essentially normal cardiovascular dynamics *as long as he or she remains at rest.*

If the heart recovers to a significant extent and if adequate fluid volume has been retained, the sympathetic stimulation gradually abates toward normal for the following reasons: Just as with sympathetic stimulation the partial recovery of the heart can elevate the cardiac output curve. Therefore, as the heart recovers even slightly, the fast pulse rate, cold skin, and pallor resulting from sympathetic stimulation in the acute stage of cardiac failure gradually disappear.

SUMMARY OF THE CHANGES THAT OCCUR AFTER ACUTE CARDIAC FAILURE—"COMPENSATED HEART FAILURE"

To summarize the events discussed in the past few sections describing the dynamics of circulatory changes after an acute, moderate heart attack, we can divide the stages into (1) the instantaneous effect of the cardiac damage; (2) compensation by the sympathetic nervous system, which occurs mainly within the first 30 seconds to 1 minute; and (3) chronic compensations resulting from partial heart recovery and renal retention of fluid. All these changes are shown graphically by the black line in Figure 51-1. The progression of this line shows the normal state of the circulation (point A), the state a few seconds after the heart attack but before sympathetic reflexes have occurred (point B), the rise in cardiac output toward normal caused by sympathetic stimulation (point C), and final return of the cardiac output to almost normal after several days to several weeks of partial cardiac recovery and fluid retention (point D). This final state is called *compensated heart failure*.

Compensated Heart Failure. Note especially in Figure 51-1 that the maximum pumping ability of the partly recovered heart, as depicted by the plateau level of the light green curve, is still depressed to less than one-half normal. This demonstrates that an increase in right atrial pressure can maintain the cardiac output at a normal level despite continued weakness of the heart. Thus, many people, especially older people, have normal resting cardiac outputs but mildly to moderately elevated right atrial pressures because of various degrees of "compensated heart failure." These persons may not know that they have cardiac damage because the damage often has occurred a little at a time and the compensation has occurred concurrently with the progressive stages of damage.

When a person is in a state of compensated heart failure, any attempt to perform heavy exercise usually causes immediate return of the symptoms of acute heart failure because the heart is not able to increase its pumping capacity to the levels required for the exercise. Therefore, it is said that the *cardiac reserve* is reduced in compensated heart failure. This concept of cardiac reserve is discussed more fully later in the chapter.

DYNAMICS OF SEVERE CARDIAC FAILURE—DECOMPENSATED HEART FAILURE

If the heart becomes severely damaged, no amount of compensation, either by sympathetic nervous reflexes or by fluid retention, can make the excessively weakened heart pump a normal cardiac output. As a consequence, the cardiac output cannot rise high enough to make the kidneys excrete normal quantities of fluid. Therefore, fluid continues to be retained, the person develops more and more edema, and this state of events eventually leads to death. This condition is called *decompensated heart failure*. Thus, a major cause of decompensated heart failure is failure of the heart to pump sufficient

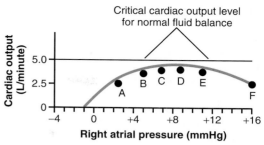

Figure 51-2 Greatly depressed cardiac output that indicates decompensated heart disease. Progressive fluid retention raises the right atrial pressure over a period of days, and the cardiac output progresses from point A to point F, until death occurs.

blood to make the kidneys excrete the necessary amounts of fluid every day.

Graphical Analysis of Decompensated Heart Failure. Figure 51-2 shows greatly depressed cardiac output at different times (points A–F) after the heart has become severely weakened. Point A on this curve represents the approximate state of the circulation before any compensation has occurred, and point B the state a few minutes later after sympathetic stimulation has compensated as much as it can but before fluid retention has begun. At this time, the cardiac output has risen to 4 L/minute and the right atrial pressure has risen to 5 mmHg. The person appears to be in reasonably good condition, but this state will not remain stable because the cardiac output has not risen high enough to cause adequate kidney excretion of fluid; therefore, fluid retention continues and can eventually be the cause of death. These events can be explained quantitatively in the following way.

Note the straight line in Figure 51-2, at a cardiac output level of 5 L/minute. This level is approximately the critical cardiac output level that is required in the normal adult person to make the kidneys reestablish normal fluid balance—that is, for the output of salt and water to be as great as the intake of these substances. At cardiac outputs below this level, the fluid-retaining mechanisms discussed in the earlier section remain in play and the body fluid volume increases progressively. Because of this progressive increase in fluid volume, the mean systemic filling pressure of the circulation continues to rise, which forces progressively increasing quantities of blood from the person's peripheral veins into the right atrium, thus increasing the right atrial pressure. After 1 day or so, the state of the circulation changes in Figure 51-2 from point B to point C with the right atrial pressure rising to 7 mmHg and the cardiac output rising to 4.2 L/minute. Note again that the cardiac output is still not high enough to cause normal renal output of fluid; therefore, fluid continues to be retained. After another day or so, the right atrial pressure rises to 9 mmHg, and the circulatory state becomes that depicted by point D. Still, the cardiac output is not enough to establish normal fluid balance.

After another few days of fluid retention, the right atrial pressure has risen still further, but by now, cardiac function is beginning to decline toward a lower level. This decline is caused by overstretch of the heart, edema of the heart muscle, and other factors that diminish the heart's pumping performance. It is now clear that further retention of fluid will be more detrimental than beneficial to the circulation. Yet the cardiac output still is not high enough to bring about normal renal function, so fluid retention not only continues but also accelerates because of the falling cardiac output (and falling arterial pressure that also occurs). Consequently, within a few days, the state of the circulation has reached point F on the curve with the cardiac output now less than 2.5 L/minute and the right atrial pressure 16 mmHg. This state has approached or reached incompatibility with life and the patient will die unless this chain of events can be reversed. This state of heart failure in which the failure continues to worsen is called *decompensated heart failure.*

Thus, one can see from this analysis that failure of the cardiac output (and arterial pressure) to rise to the critical level required for normal renal function results in (1) progressive retention of more and more fluid, which causes (2) progressive elevation of the mean systemic filling pressure, and (3) progressive elevation of the right atrial pressure until finally the heart is so overstretched or so edematous that it cannot pump even moderate quantities of blood and, therefore, fails completely. Clinically, one detects this serious condition of decompensation principally by the progressing edema, especially edema of the lungs, which leads to bubbling *rales* (a crackling sound) in the lungs and to *dyspnea* (air hunger). Lack of appropriate therapy at this stage rapidly leads to death.

Treatment of Decompensation. The decompensation process can often be stopped by (1) *strengthening the heart* in any one of several ways, especially by administering a cardiotonic drug, such as *digitalis*, so that the heart becomes strong enough to pump adequate quantities of blood required to make the kidneys function normally again, or (2) *administering diuretic drugs to increase kidney excretion* while at the same time reducing water and salt intake, which brings about a balance between fluid intake and output despite low cardiac output.

Both methods stop the decompensation process by reestablishing normal fluid balance so that at least as much fluid leaves the body as enters it.

Mechanism of Action of the Cardiotonic Drugs Such as Digitalis. Cardiotonic drugs, such as digitalis, when administered to a person with a healthy heart have little effect on increasing the contractile strength of the cardiac muscle. However, when administered to a person with a chronically failing heart, the same drugs can sometimes increase the strength of the failing myocardium as much as 50–100%. Therefore, they are one of the mainstays of therapy in persons with chronic heart failure.

Digitalis and other cardiotonic glycosides are believed to strengthen heart contractions by increasing the quantity of calcium ions in muscle fibers. This effect is likely due to inhibition of sodium–potassium ATPase in cardiac cell membranes. Inhibition of the sodium–potassium pump increases intracellular sodium concentration and slows the sodium–calcium exchange pump, which extrudes calcium from the cell in exchange for sodium. Because the sodium–calcium exchange pump relies on a high sodium gradient across the cell membrane, accumulation of sodium inside the cell reduces its activity.

In the failing heart muscle, the sarcoplasmic reticulum fails to accumulate normal quantities of calcium and, therefore, cannot release enough calcium ions into the free-fluid compartment of the muscle fibers to cause full contraction of the muscle. The effect of digitalis to depress the sodium–calcium exchange pump and raise calcium ion concentration in cardiac muscle provides the extra calcium needed to increase the muscle contractile force. Therefore, it is usually beneficial to depress the calcium pumping mechanism to a moderate amount using digitalis, allowing the muscle fiber intracellular calcium level to rise slightly.

Unilateral Left Heart Failure

In the discussions thus far, we have considered failure of the heart as a whole. Yet, in a large number of patients, especially those with early acute heart failure, left-sided failure predominates over right-sided failure, and, in rare instances, the right side fails without significant failure of the left side.

When the left side of the heart fails without concomitant failure of the right side, blood continues to be pumped into the lungs with usual right heart vigor, whereas it is not pumped adequately out of the lungs by the left heart into the systemic circulation. As a result, the *mean pulmonary filling pressure* rises because of the shift of large volumes of blood from the systemic circulation into the pulmonary circulation.

As the volume of blood in the lungs increases, the pulmonary capillary pressure increases, and if this pressure rises above a value approximately equal to the colloid osmotic pressure of the plasma, about 28 mmHg, fluid begins to filter out of the capillaries into the lung interstitial spaces and alveoli, resulting in pulmonary edema.

Thus, among the most important problems of left heart failure are *pulmonary vascular congestion* and *pulmonary edema.* In severe, acute left heart failure, pulmonary edema occasionally occurs so rapidly that it can cause death by suffocation in 20–30 minutes.

Low-Output Cardiac Failure—Cardiogenic Shock

In many instances after acute heart attacks and often after prolonged periods of slow progressive cardiac deterioration, the heart becomes incapable of pumping even the minimal amount of blood flow required to keep the body alive. Consequently, the body tissues, including the heart, begin to suffer and even to deteriorate, often leading to death within a few hours to a few days. This circulatory shock syndrome caused by inadequate cardiac pumping is called *cardiogenic shock* or simply *cardiac shock.* Once a person develops cardiogenic shock, the survival rate is often less than 30% even with appropriate medical care.

Vicious Cycle of Cardiac Deterioration in Cardiogenic Shock. The discussion of circulatory shock in Chapter 52 emphasizes the tendency for the heart to become progressively more damaged when its coronary blood supply is reduced during the course of the shock. That is, the low arterial pressure that occurs during shock reduces the coronary blood supply even more. This reduction further weakens the heart, due to which the arterial pressure falls still more, which makes the shock progressively worse; the process eventually becomes a vicious cycle of cardiac deterioration. In cardiogenic shock caused by myocardial infarction, this problem is greatly compounded by already existing coronary vessel blockage. For instance, in a healthy heart, the arterial pressure usually must be reduced below about 45 mmHg before cardiac deterioration sets in. However, in a heart that already has a blocked major coronary vessel, deterioration begins when the coronary arterial pressure falls below 80–90 mmHg. In other words, even a small decrease in arterial pressure can now set off a vicious cycle of cardiac deterioration. For this reason, in treating myocardial infarction, it is extremely important to prevent even short periods of hypotension.

Physiology of Treatment. Often a patient dies of cardiogenic shock before the various compensatory processes can return the cardiac output (and arterial pressure) to a life-sustaining level. Therefore, treatment of this condition is one of the most important problems in the management of acute heart attacks.

Digitalis is often administered to strengthen the heart if the ventricular muscle shows signs of deterioration. Also, infusion of whole blood, plasma, or a blood pressure–raising drug is used to sustain the arterial pressure. If the arterial pressure can be elevated to a high enough level, the coronary blood flow often will increase enough to prevent the vicious cycle of deterioration. This process allows enough time for appropriate compensatory mechanisms in the circulatory system to correct the shock.

Some success has also been achieved in saving the lives of patients in cardiogenic shock by using one of the following procedures: (1) surgically removing the clot in the coronary artery, often in combination with a coronary bypass graft, or (2) catheterizing the blocked coronary artery and infusing either *streptokinase* or *tissue-type plasminogen activator* enzymes that cause dissolution of the clot. The results are occasionally astounding when one of these procedures is instituted within the first hour of cardiogenic shock but of little, if any, benefit after 3 hours.

Edema in Patients with Cardiac Failure

Acute Cardiac Failure Does Not Cause Immediate Peripheral Edema. Acute *left* heart failure can cause rapid congestion of the lungs with development of *pulmonary edema* and even death within minutes to hours.

However, either left or right heart failure is very slow to cause *peripheral edema*. This situation can best be explained by referring to Figure 51-3. When a previously healthy heart acutely

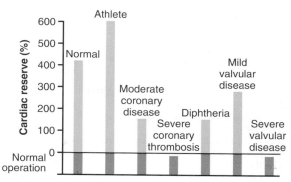

Figure 51-4 Cardiac reserve in different conditions, showing less than zero reserve for two of the conditions.

fails as a pump, the aortic pressure falls and the right atrial pressure rises. As the cardiac output approaches zero, these two pressures approach each other at an equilibrium value of about 13 mmHg. Capillary pressure also falls from its normal value of 17 mmHg to the new equilibrium pressure of 13 mmHg. Thus, *severe acute cardiac failure often causes a fall in peripheral capillary pressure rather than a rise*. Therefore, animal experiments, as well as experience in humans, show that acute cardiac failure almost never causes immediate development of peripheral edema.

Cardiac Reserve

The maximum percentage that the cardiac output can increase above normal is called the *cardiac reserve*. Thus, in the healthy young adult, the cardiac reserve is 300–400%. In athletically trained persons, it is 500–600% or more. However, in persons with severe heart failure, there is no cardiac reserve. As an example of normal reserve, during vigorous exercise the cardiac output of a healthy young adult can rise to about five times normal, which is an increase above normal of 400%—that is, *a cardiac reserve of 400%*.

Any factor that prevents the heart from pumping blood satisfactorily will decrease the cardiac reserve. A decrease in cardiac reserve can result from ischemic heart disease, primary myocardial disease, vitamin deficiency that affects cardiac muscle, physical damage to the myocardium, valvular heart disease, and many other factors, some of which are shown in Figure 51-4.

DIAGNOSIS OF LOW CARDIAC RESERVE— EXERCISE TEST

As long as persons with low cardiac reserve remain in a state of rest, they usually will not experience major symptoms of heart disease. However, a diagnosis of low cardiac reserve usually can be made by requiring the person to exercise either on a treadmill or by walking up and down steps, either of which requires greatly increased cardiac output. The increased load on the heart rapidly uses up the small amount of reserve that is available and the cardiac output soon fails to rise high enough to sustain the body's new level of activity. Exercise tests are part of the armamentarium of the cardiologist. These tests take the place of cardiac output measurements that cannot be made with ease in most clinical settings.

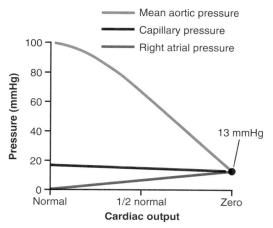

Figure 51-3 Progressive changes in mean aortic pressure, peripheral tissue capillary pressure, and right atrial pressure as the cardiac output falls from normal to zero.

BIBLIOGRAPHY

Andrew P: Diastolic heart failure demystified, *Chest* 124:744, 2003.

Bayeva M, Gheorghiade M, Ardehali H: Mitochondria as a therapeutic target in heart failure, *J. Am. Coll. Cardiol.* 61:599, 2013.

Bers DM: Altered cardiac myocyte Ca regulation in heart failure, *Physiology (Bethesda)* 21:380, 2006.

Braunwald E: Biomarkers in heart failure, *N. Engl. J. Med.* 358:2148, 2008.

Burchfield JS, Xie M, Hill JA: Pathological ventricular remodeling: mechanisms: part 1 of 2, *Circulation* 128:388, 2013.

Cahill TJ, Ashrafian H, Watkins H: Genetic cardiomyopathies causing heart failure, *Circ. Res.* 113:660, 2013.

Despa S, Bers DM: Na$^+$ transport in the normal and failing heart—remember the balance, *J. Mol. Cell. Cardiol.* 61:2, 2013.

Doenst T, Nguyen TD, Abel ED: Cardiac metabolism in heart failure: implications beyond ATP production, *Circ. Res.* 113:709, 2013.

Guyton AC, Jones CE, Coleman TG: *Circulatory Physiology: Cardiac Output and its Regulation*, Philadelphia, 1973, W.B. Saunders.

Kirk JA, Kass DA: Electromechanical dyssynchrony and resynchronization of the failing heart, *Circ. Res.* 113:765, 2013.

Luo M, Anderson ME: Mechanisms of altered Ca^{2+} handling in heart failure, *Circ. Res.* 113:690, 2013.

Lymperopoulos A, Rengo G, Koch WJ: Adrenergic nervous system in heart failure: pathophysiology and therapy, *Circ. Res.* 113:739, 2013.

Morita H, Seidman J, Seidman CE: Genetic causes of human heart failure, *J. Clin. Invest.* 115:518, 2005.

Nickel A, Löffler J, Maack C: Myocardial energetics in heart failure, *Basic Res. Cardiol.* 108:358, 2013.

Zile MR, Brutsaert DL: New concepts in diastolic dysfunction and diastolic heart failure: part I: diagnosis, prognosis, and measurements of diastolic function, *Circulation* 105:1387, 2002.

52

Circulatory Shock

LEARNING OBJECTIVES

- Define shock.
- Describe the physiological pathways operative in shock.
- Describe the stages of shock.
- List the causes of shock and briefly describe them.
- Discuss the principles of treatment of shock.

GLOSSARY OF TERMS

- **Anaphylactic shock:** Shock resulting from a severe generalized allergic reaction with the resultant release of histamine (this causes vasodilation and loss of fluid into the tissues)

- **Circulatory shock:** Reduced tissue perfusion resulting in inadequate oxygen and nutrient supply, and leading to tissue damage, if untreated

- **Compensated shock:** An early stage of shock where cardiovascular compensatory mechanisms overcome shock without external treatment

- **Hypovolemic shock:** Shock resulting from reduced blood volume resulting in reduced venous return and inadequate cardiac output

- **Irreversible shock:** A late stage of shock where the patient is still alive but where treatment is ineffective in stopping the further progression of shock

- **Neurogenic shock:** Shock often resulting from brain damage and the subsequent widespread loss of vascular tone resulting in increased vascular capacity

- **Septic shock:** Shock resulting from severe disseminated bacterial infection and widespread vasodilation

Circulatory shock means generalized inadequate blood flow through the body to the extent that the body tissues are damaged, especially because too little oxygen and other nutrients are delivered to the tissue cells. Even the cardiovascular system itself—the heart musculature, walls of the blood vessels, vasomotor system, and other circulatory parts—begins to deteriorate, so the shock, once begun, is prone to become progressively worse.

Physiological Causes of Shock

CIRCULATORY SHOCK CAUSED BY DECREASED CARDIAC OUTPUT

Shock usually results from an inadequate cardiac output. Therefore, any condition that reduces the cardiac output far below

normal may lead to circulatory shock. Two types of factors can severely reduce cardiac output:

1. *Cardiac abnormalities that decrease the ability of the heart to pump blood.* These abnormalities include, in particular, myocardial infarction but also toxic states of the heart, severe heart valve dysfunction, heart arrhythmias, and other conditions. The circulatory shock that results from diminished cardiac pumping ability is called *cardiogenic shock.*

2. *Factors that decrease venous return* also decrease cardiac output because the heart cannot pump blood that does not flow into it. The most common cause of decreased venous return is *diminished blood volume,* but venous return can also be reduced as a result of *decreased vascular tone,* especially of the venous blood reservoirs, or *obstruction to blood flow* at some point in the circulation, especially in the venous return pathway to the heart.

CIRCULATORY SHOCK WITHOUT DIMINISHED CARDIAC OUTPUT

Occasionally, cardiac output is normal or even greater than normal, yet the person is in a state of circulatory shock. This situation can result from (1) *excessive metabolic rate, so even a normal cardiac output is inadequate,* or (2) *abnormal tissue perfusion patterns, so most of the cardiac output is passing through blood vessels other than those that supply the local tissues with nutrition.*

WHAT HAPPENS TO THE ARTERIAL PRESSURE IN CIRCULATORY SHOCK?

In the minds of many physicians, the arterial pressure level is the principal measure of adequacy of circulatory function. However, the arterial pressure can often be seriously misleading. At times, a person may be in severe shock and still have an almost normal arterial pressure because of powerful nervous reflexes that keep the pressure from falling. At other times, the arterial pressure can fall to half of normal, but the person still has normal tissue perfusion and is not in shock.

In most types of shock, especially shock caused by severe blood loss, the arterial blood pressure decreases at the same time the cardiac output decreases, although usually not as much.

TISSUE DETERIORATION IS THE END RESULT OF CIRCULATORY SHOCK

Once circulatory shock reaches a critical state of severity, regardless of its initiating cause, *the shock itself leads to more shock.* That is, the inadequate blood flow causes the body tissues to begin deteriorating including the heart and circulatory system. This deterioration causes an even greater decrease in cardiac output and a vicious cycle ensues, with progressively increasing circulatory shock, less adequate tissue perfusion, more shock, and so forth until death occurs.

STAGES OF SHOCK

Because the characteristics of circulatory shock change with different degrees of severity, shock is often divided into the following three major stages:

1. a *nonprogressive stage* (sometimes called the *compensated stage*), in which the normal circulatory compensatory mechanisms eventually cause full recovery without help from outside therapy;
2. a *progressive stage*, in which, without therapy, the shock becomes steadily worse until death occurs;
3. an *irreversible stage*, in which the shock has progressed to such an extent that all forms of known therapy are inadequate to save the person's life, even though, for the moment, the person is still alive.

We will now discuss the stages of circulatory shock caused by decreased blood volume, which illustrate the basic principles. Then we will consider special characteristics of shock initiated by other causes.

Causes of Shock

HYPOVOLEMIA—HEMORRHAGIC SHOCK

Hypovolemia means diminished blood volume. Hemorrhage is the most common cause of hypovolemic shock. Hemorrhage *decreases the filling pressure of the circulation* and, as a consequence, decreases venous return. As a result, the cardiac output falls below normal and shock may ensue.

Relationship of Bleeding Volume to Cardiac Output and Arterial Pressure

Figure 52-1 shows the approximate effects on cardiac output and arterial pressure of removing blood from the circulatory system over a period of about 30 minutes. About 10% of the total blood volume can be removed with almost no effect on either arterial pressure or cardiac output, but greater blood loss usually diminishes the cardiac output first and later the arterial pressure, both of which fall to zero when about 40–45% of the total blood volume has been removed.

Sympathetic Reflex Compensations in Shock—Their Special Value to Maintain Arterial Pressure. The decrease in arterial pressure after hemorrhage as well as decreases in pressures in the pulmonary arteries and veins in the thorax causes

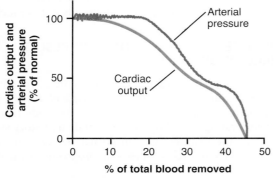

Figure 52-1 Effect of hemorrhage on cardiac output and arterial pressure.

powerful sympathetic reflexes (as explained in Chapter 43). These reflexes stimulate the sympathetic vasoconstrictor system in most tissues of the body resulting in three important effects: (1) the arterioles constrict in most parts of the systemic circulation, thereby increasing the total peripheral resistance; (2) the veins and venous reservoirs constrict, thereby helping to maintain adequate venous return despite diminished blood volume; (3) heart rate increases markedly, sometimes from the normal value of 72 beats/minute to as high as 160–180 beats/minute.

Value of the Sympathetic Nervous Reflexes. In the absence of the sympathetic reflexes, only 15–20% of the blood volume can be removed over a period of 30 minutes before a person dies; in contrast a person can sustain a 30–40% loss of blood volume when the reflexes are intact.

Greater Effect of the Sympathetic Nervous Reflexes in Maintaining Arterial Pressure than in Maintaining Cardiac Output. Referring again to Figure 52-1, note that the arterial pressure is maintained at or near normal levels in the hemorrhaging person longer than in maintaining the cardiac output. The reason for this difference is that the sympathetic reflexes are geared more for maintaining arterial pressure than for maintaining cardiac output. They increase the arterial pressure mainly by increasing the total peripheral resistance, which has no beneficial effect on cardiac output; however, the *sympathetic constriction of the veins is important to keep venous return and cardiac output from falling too much*, in addition to their role in maintaining arterial pressure.

Especially interesting is the second plateau occurring at about 50 mmHg in the arterial pressure curve of Figure 52-1. This second plateau results from activation of the central nervous system ischemic response, which causes extreme stimulation of the sympathetic nervous system when the brain begins to experience lack of oxygen or excess buildup of carbon dioxide as discussed in Chapter 43. This effect of the central nervous system ischemic response can be called the "last-ditch stand" of the sympathetic reflexes in their attempt to keep the arterial pressure from falling too low.

Protection of Coronary and Cerebral Blood Flow by the Reflexes. A special value of the maintenance of normal arterial pressure even in the presence of decreasing cardiac output is protection of blood flow through the coronary and cerebral circulations. The sympathetic stimulation does not cause significant constriction of either the cerebral or the cardiac vessels. In addition, in both vascular beds, local blood flow autoregulation is excellent, which prevents moderate decreases in arterial pressure from significantly decreasing their blood flows. Therefore, blood flow through the heart and brain is maintained essentially at normal levels as long as the arterial pressure does not fall below about 70 mmHg, despite the fact that blood flow in some other areas of the body might be decreased to as little as one-third to one-quarter normal by this time because of vasoconstriction.

Nonprogressive Shock—Compensated Shock. If shock is not severe enough to cause its own progression, the person eventually recovers. Therefore, shock of this lesser degree is called *nonprogressive shock* or *compensated shock*, meaning that the sympathetic reflexes and other factors compensate enough to prevent further deterioration of the circulation.

The factors that cause a person to recover from moderate degrees of shock are all the negative feedback control mechanisms of the circulation that attempt to return cardiac output and arterial pressure back to normal levels. They include the following:

1. *baroreceptor reflexes*, which elicit powerful sympathetic stimulation of the circulation;
2. *central nervous system ischemic response*, which elicits even more powerful sympathetic stimulation throughout the body but is not activated significantly until the arterial pressure falls below 50 mmHg;
3. *reverse stress relaxation of the circulatory system*, which causes the blood vessels to contract around the diminished blood volume so that the blood volume that is available more adequately fills the circulation;
4. *increased secretion of renin by the kidneys and formation of angiotensin II*, which constricts the peripheral arterioles and also causes decreased output of water and salt by the kidneys, both of which help prevent progression of shock;
5. *increased secretion by the posterior pituitary gland of vasopressin (antidiuretic hormone)*, which constricts the peripheral arterioles and veins, and greatly increases water retention by the kidneys;
6. *increased secretion by the adrenal medullae of epinephrine and norepinephrine*, which constricts the peripheral arterioles and veins, and increases the heart rate;
7. *compensatory mechanisms that return the blood volume back toward normal*, including absorption of large quantities of fluid from the intestinal tract, absorption of fluid into the blood capillaries from the interstitial spaces of the body, conservation of water and salt by the kidneys, and increased thirst and increased appetite for salt, which make the person drink water and eat salty foods if they are able to do so.

The sympathetic reflexes and increased secretion of catecholamines by the adrenal medullae provide rapid help toward bringing about recovery because they become maximally activated within 30 seconds to a few minutes after hemorrhage.

The angiotensin and vasopressin mechanisms, as well as the reverse stress relaxation that causes contraction of the blood vessels and venous reservoirs, all require 10 minutes to 1 hour to respond completely, but they aid greatly in increasing the arterial pressure or increasing the circulatory filling pressure, thereby increasing the return of blood to the heart.

Finally, readjustment of blood volume by absorption of fluid from the interstitial spaces and intestinal tract, as well as oral ingestion and absorption of additional quantities of water and salt, may require from 1 to 48 hours, but recovery eventually takes place, provided the shock does not become severe enough to enter the progressive stage.

"Progressive Shock" Is Caused by a Vicious Cycle of Cardiovascular Deterioration. Figure 52-2 shows some of the positive feedbacks that further depress cardiac output in shock, thus causing the shock to become progressive. Some of the more important feedbacks are described in the following sections.

Cardiac Depression. When the arterial pressure falls low enough, coronary blood flow decreases below that required for adequate nutrition of the myocardium. This occurrence weakens the heart muscle and thereby decreases the cardiac output more. Thus, a positive feedback cycle has developed, whereby the shock becomes more and more severe.

Thus, one of the important features of progressive shock, whether it is hemorrhagic in origin or caused in another way, is eventual progressive deterioration of the heart. In the early stages of shock, this deterioration plays very little role in the

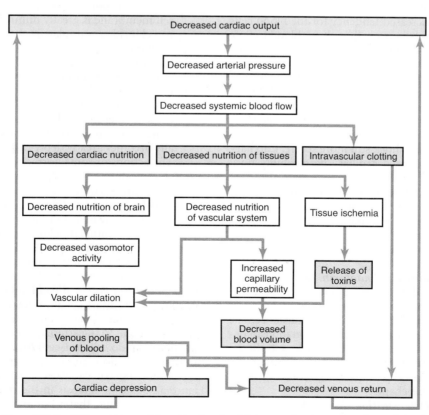

Figure 52-2 Different types of "positive feedback" that can lead to progression of shock.

condition of the person, partly because deterioration of the heart is not severe during the first hour or so of shock, but mainly because the heart has tremendous reserve capability that normally allows it to pump 300–400% more blood than is required by the body for adequate tissue nutrition. In the latest stages of shock, however, deterioration of the heart is probably the most important factor in the final lethal progression of the shock.

Vasomotor Failure. In the early stages of shock, various circulatory reflexes cause intense activity of the sympathetic nervous system. This activity, as discussed earlier, helps delay depression of the cardiac output and especially helps prevent decreased arterial pressure. However, there comes a point when diminished blood flow to the brain's vasomotor center depresses the center so much that it, too, becomes progressively less active and finally totally inactive. For instance, during the first 4–8 minutes, complete circulatory arrest to the brain causes the most intense of all sympathetic discharges, but by the end of 10–15 minutes, the vasomotor center becomes so depressed that no further evidence of sympathetic discharge can be demonstrated. Fortunately, the vasomotor center usually does not fail in the early stages of shock if the arterial pressure remains above 30 mmHg.

Blockage of Very Small Vessels by "Sludged Blood". In time, blockage occurs in many of the very small blood vessels in the circulatory system and this blockage also causes the shock to progress. The initiating cause of this blockage is sluggish blood flow in the microvessels. Because tissue metabolism continues despite the low flow, large amounts of acid, both carbonic acid and lactic acid, continue to empty into the local blood vessels and greatly increase the local acidity of the blood. This acid, plus other deterioration products from the ischemic tissues, causes local blood agglutination, resulting in minute blood clots, leading to very small plugs in the small vessels. Even if the vessels do not become plugged, an increased tendency for the blood cells to stick to one another makes it more difficult for blood to flow through the microvasculature giving rise to the term sludged blood.

Increased Capillary Permeability. After many hours of capillary hypoxia and lack of other nutrients, the permeability of the capillaries gradually increases and large quantities of fluid begin to transude into the tissues. This phenomenon decreases the blood volume even more, with a resultant further decrease in cardiac output, making the shock still more severe. Capillary hypoxia does not cause increased capillary permeability until the late stages of prolonged shock.

Release of Toxins by Ischemic Tissue. Shock has been suggested to cause tissues to release toxic substances, such as histamine, serotonin, and tissue enzymes, that cause further deterioration of the circulatory system. Experimental studies have proved the significance of at least one toxin, endotoxin, in some types of shock.

Cardiac Depression Caused by Endotoxin. Endotoxin is released from the bodies of dead gram-negative bacteria in the intestines. Diminished blood flow to the intestines often causes enhanced formation and absorption of this toxic substance. The circulating toxin then causes increased cellular metabolism despite inadequate nutrition of the cells, which has a specific effect on the heart muscle causing cardiac depression. Endotoxin can play a major role in some types of shock, especially "septic shock," discussed later in this chapter.

Generalized Cellular Deterioration. As shock becomes severe, many signs of generalized cellular deterioration occur

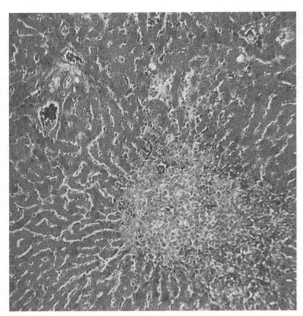

Figure 52-3 Necrosis of the central portion of a liver lobule during severe circulatory shock. *Courtesy Dr. J.W. Crowell.*

throughout the body. One organ especially affected is the liver as illustrated in Figure 52-3. The liver is especially affected mainly because of lack of enough nutrients to support the normally high rate of metabolism in liver cells, but also partly because of the exposure of the liver cells to any vascular toxin or other abnormal metabolic factor occurring in shock.

Among the damaging cellular effects that are known to occur in most body tissues are the following:

1. Active transport of sodium and potassium through the cell membrane is greatly diminished. As a result, sodium and chloride accumulate in the cells and potassium is lost from the cells. In addition, the cells begin to swell.
2. Mitochondrial activity in the liver cells, as well as in many other tissues of the body, becomes severely depressed.
3. Lysosomes in the cells in widespread tissue areas begin to break open with intracellular release of *hydrolases* that cause further intracellular deterioration.
4. Cellular metabolism of nutrients, such as glucose, eventually becomes greatly depressed in the last stages of shock. The actions of some hormones are depressed as well, including almost 100% depression of the actions of insulin.

All these effects contribute to further deterioration of many organs of the body, including especially (1) the *liver*, with depression of its many metabolic and detoxification functions; (2) the *lungs*, with eventual development of pulmonary edema and poor ability to oxygenate the blood; and (3) the *heart*, thereby further depressing its contractility.

Tissue Necrosis in Severe Shock—Patchy Areas of Necrosis Occur Because of Patchy Blood Flows in Different Organs. Not all cells of the body are equally damaged by shock because some tissues have better blood supplies than do others. For instance, the cells adjacent to the arterial ends of capillaries receive better nutrition than do cells adjacent to the venous ends of the same capillaries. Therefore, more nutritive deficiency occurs around the venous ends of capillaries than elsewhere. For instance, Figure 52-3 shows necrosis in the center of a liver lobule, the portion of the lobule that is last to be exposed to the blood as it passes through the liver sinusoids.

Similar punctate lesions occur in heart muscle, although here a definite repetitive pattern, such as occurs in the liver, cannot be demonstrated. Nevertheless, the cardiac lesions play an important role in leading to the final irreversible stage of shock. Deteriorative lesions also occur in the kidneys, especially in the epithelium of the kidney tubules, leading to kidney failure and occasionally uremic death several days later. Deterioration of the lungs also often leads to respiratory distress and death several days later—called the *shock lung syndrome.*

Acidosis in Shock. Metabolic derangements that occur in shocked tissue can lead to acidosis all through the body. This results from poor delivery of oxygen to the tissues, which greatly diminishes oxidative metabolism of the foodstuffs. When this occurs, the cells obtain most of their energy by the anaerobic process of glycolysis, which leads to tremendous quantities of excess lactic acid in the blood. In addition, poor blood flow through tissues prevents normal removal of carbon dioxide. The carbon dioxide reacts locally in the cells with water to form high concentrations of intracellular carbonic acid, which, in turn, reacts with various tissue chemicals to form additional intracellular acidic substances. Thus, another deteriorative effect of shock is both generalized and local tissue acidosis leading to further progression of the shock.

Positive Feedback Deterioration of Tissues in Shock and the Vicious Circle of Progressive Shock. All the factors just discussed that can lead to further progression of shock are types of *positive feedback.* Each increase in the degree of shock causes a further increase in the shock.

However, positive feedback does not necessarily lead to a vicious cycle. A vicious cycle develops depending on the intensity of the positive feedback. In mild degrees of shock, the negative feedback mechanisms of the circulation—sympathetic reflexes, reverse stress-relaxation mechanism of the blood reservoirs, absorption of fluid into the blood from the interstitial spaces, and others—can easily overcome the positive feedback influences and, therefore, cause recovery. In severe degrees of shock, however, the deteriorative feedback mechanisms become more and more powerful leading to such rapid deterioration of the circulation that all the normal negative feedback systems of circulatory control acting together cannot return the cardiac output to normal.

Considering once again the principles of positive feedback and vicious circle discussed in Chapter 1, one can readily understand why there is a critical cardiac output level above which a person in shock recovers and below which a person enters a vicious cycle of circulatory deterioration that proceeds until death.

Irreversible Shock

After shock has progressed to a certain stage, transfusion or any other type of therapy becomes incapable of saving the person's life. The person is then said to be in the *irreversible stage of shock.* Ironically, even in this irreversible stage, therapy can, on rare occasions, return the arterial pressure and even the cardiac output to normal or near normal for short periods, but the circulatory system nevertheless continues to deteriorate and death ensues in another few minutes to few hours.

Figure 52-4 demonstrates this effect showing that transfusion during the irreversible stage can sometimes cause the cardiac output (as well as the arterial pressure) to return to nearly normal. However, the cardiac output soon begins to fall again, and subsequent transfusions have less and less effect. By this time, multiple deteriorative changes have occurred in the muscle

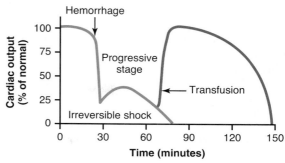

Figure 52-4   Failure of transfusion to prevent death in irreversible shock.

cells of the heart that may not necessarily affect the heart's *immediate* ability to pump blood but, over a long period, depress heart's pumping enough to cause death. Beyond a certain point, so much tissue damage has occurred, so many destructive enzymes have been released into the body fluids, so much acidosis has developed, and so many other destructive factors are now in progress that even a normal cardiac output for a few minutes cannot reverse the continuing deterioration. Therefore, in severe shock, a stage is eventually reached at which the person will die even though vigorous therapy might still return the cardiac output to normal for short periods.

Depletion of Cellular High-Energy Phosphate Reserves in Irreversible Shock. The high-energy phosphate reserves in the tissues of the body, especially in the liver and the heart, are greatly diminished in severe shock. Essentially all the *creatine phosphate* has been degraded and almost all the *adenosine triphosphate* has downgraded to *adenosine diphosphate, adenosine monophosphate,* and, eventually, *adenosine.* Much of this adenosine then diffuses out of the cells into the circulating blood and is converted into uric acid, a substance that cannot reenter the cells to reconstitute the adenosine phosphate system. New adenosine can be synthesized at a rate of only about 2% of the normal cellular amount an hour, meaning that once the high-energy phosphate stores of the cells are depleted, they are difficult to replenish.

Thus, one of the most devastating end results in shock, and the one that is perhaps most significant for development of the final state of irreversibility, is this cellular depletion of these high-energy compounds.

Hypovolemic Shock Caused by Plasma Loss

Loss of plasma from the circulatory system, even without loss of red blood cells, can sometimes be severe enough to reduce the total blood volume markedly, causing typical hypovolemic shock similar in almost all details to that caused by hemorrhage. Severe plasma loss occurs in the following conditions:

1. *Intestinal obstruction* may cause severely reduced plasma volume. Distention of the intestine in intestinal obstruction partly blocks venous blood flow in the intestinal walls, which increases intestinal capillary pressure. This pressure increase in turn causes fluid to leak from the capillaries into the intestinal walls and also into the intestinal lumen. Because the lost fluid has high protein content, the result is reduced total blood plasma protein as well as reduced plasma volume.

2. *Severe burns* or other denuding conditions of the skin cause loss of plasma through the denuded skin areas so that the plasma volume becomes markedly reduced.

The hypovolemic shock that results from plasma loss has almost the same characteristics as the shock caused by hemorrhage, except for one additional complicating factor: the blood viscosity increases greatly as a result of increased red blood cell concentration in the remaining blood, and this increase in blood viscosity exacerbates the sluggishness of blood flow.

Loss of fluid from all fluid compartments of the body is called *dehydration*; this condition, too, can reduce the blood volume and cause hypovolemic shock similar to that resulting from hemorrhage. Some of the causes of this type of shock are (1) excessive sweating, (2) fluid loss in severe diarrhea or vomiting, (3) excess loss of fluid by the kidneys, (4) inadequate intake of fluid and electrolytes, or (5) destruction of the adrenal cortices with loss of aldosterone secretion and consequent failure of the kidneys to reabsorb sodium, chloride, and water, which occurs in the absence of the adrenocortical hormone aldosterone.

Hypovolemic Shock Caused by Trauma

One of the most common causes of circulatory shock is trauma to the body. Often the shock results simply from hemorrhage caused by the trauma, but it can also occur even without hemorrhage because extensive contusion of the body can damage the capillaries sufficiently to allow excessive loss of plasma into the tissues. This phenomenon results in greatly reduced plasma volume with resultant hypovolemic shock.

Various attempts have been made to implicate toxic factors released by the traumatized tissues as one of the causes of shock after trauma. However, cross-transfusion experiments with normal animals have failed to show significant toxic elements.

Traumatic shock, therefore, seems to result mainly from hypovolemia, although there might also be a moderate degree of concomitant neurogenic shock caused by loss of vasomotor tone, as discussed next.

NEUROGENIC SHOCK—INCREASED VASCULAR CAPACITY

Shock occasionally results without any loss of blood volume. Instead, the *vascular capacity* increases so much that even the normal amount of blood is incapable of filling the circulatory system adequately. One of the major causes of this condition is *sudden loss of vasomotor tone* throughout the body resulting especially in massive dilation of the veins. The resulting condition is known as *neurogenic shock*.

The role of vascular capacity in helping to regulate circulatory function was discussed in Chapters 36 and 41, where it was pointed out that either an increase in vascular capacity or a decrease in blood volume *reduces the mean systemic filling pressure*, which reduces venous return to the heart. Diminished venous return caused by vascular dilation is called *venous pooling* of blood.

Causes of Neurogenic Shock

Some neurogenic factors that can cause loss of vasomotor tone include the following:
1. *Deep general anesthesia* often depresses the vasomotor center enough to cause vasomotor paralysis with resulting neurogenic shock.
2. *Spinal anesthesia*, especially when this extends all the way up the spinal cord, blocks the sympathetic nervous outflow from the nervous system and can be a potent cause of neurogenic shock.

3. *Brain damage* is often a cause of vasomotor paralysis. Many patients who have had brain concussion or contusion of the basal regions of the brain experience profound neurogenic shock. Also, even though brain ischemia for a few minutes almost always causes extreme vasomotor stimulation and increased blood pressure, prolonged ischemia (lasting longer than 5–10 minutes) can cause the opposite effect—total inactivation of the vasomotor neurons in the brainstem with consequent decrease in arterial blood pressure and the development of severe neurogenic shock.

ANAPHYLACTIC SHOCK AND HISTAMINE SHOCK

Anaphylaxis is an allergic condition in which the cardiac output and arterial pressure often decrease drastically. It results primarily from an antigen–antibody reaction that rapidly occurs after an antigen to which the person is sensitive enters the circulation. One of the principal effects is to cause the *basophils* in the blood and *mast* cells in the pericapillary tissues to release *histamine* or a *histamine-like substance*. The histamine causes (1) an increase in vascular capacity because of venous dilation, thus causing a marked decrease in venous return; (2) dilation of the arterioles, resulting in greatly reduced arterial pressure; and (3) greatly increased capillary permeability with rapid loss of fluid and protein into the tissue spaces. The net effect is a great reduction in venous return and sometimes such serious shock that the person may die within minutes.

Intravenous injection of large amounts of histamine causes "histamine shock," which has characteristics almost identical to those of anaphylactic shock.

SEPTIC SHOCK

A condition that was formerly known by the popular name "blood poisoning" is now called *septic shock* by most clinicians. This term refers to a bacterial infection widely disseminated to many areas of the body with the infection being borne through the blood from one tissue to another and causing extensive damage. There are many varieties of septic shock because of the many types of bacterial infections that can cause it and because infection in different parts of the body produces different effects. Most cases of septic shock, however, are caused by gram-positive bacteria, followed by endotoxin-producing gram-negative bacteria.

Septic shock is extremely important to the clinician because other than cardiogenic shock, septic shock is the most frequent cause of shock-related death in the modern hospital.

Some of the typical causes of septic shock include the following:
1. peritonitis caused by spread of infection from the uterus and fallopian tubes, sometimes resulting from instrumental abortion performed under unsterile conditions;
2. peritonitis resulting from rupture of the gastrointestinal system, sometimes caused by intestinal disease and sometimes by wounds;
3. generalized bodily infection resulting from spread of a skin infection such as streptococcal or staphylococcal infection;
4. generalized gangrenous infection resulting specifically from gas gangrene bacilli, spreading first through peripheral tissues and finally by way of the blood to the internal organs, especially the liver;
5. infection spreading into the blood from the kidney or urinary tract, often caused by colon bacilli.

Special Features of Septic Shock

Because of the multiple types of septic shock, it is difficult to categorize this condition. The following features are often observed:

1. high fever;
2. often marked vasodilation throughout the body, especially in the infected tissues;
3. high cardiac output in perhaps half of patients, caused by arteriolar dilation in the infected tissues and by high metabolic rate and vasodilation elsewhere in the body resulting from bacterial toxin stimulation of cellular metabolism and from high body temperature;
4. sludging of the blood, caused by red cell agglutination in response to degenerating tissues;
5. development of microblood clots in widespread areas of the body, a condition called *disseminated intravascular coagulation*; also, this causes the blood clotting factors to be used up, so hemorrhaging occurs in many tissues, especially in the gut wall of the intestinal tract.

In early stages of septic shock, the patient usually does not have signs of circulatory collapse but only signs of the bacterial infection. As the infection becomes more severe, the circulatory system usually becomes involved either because of direct extension of the infection or secondarily as a result of toxins from the bacteria with resultant loss of plasma into the infected tissues through deteriorating blood capillary walls. There finally comes a point at which deterioration of the circulation becomes progressive in the same way that progression occurs in all other types of shock. The end stages of septic shock are not greatly different from the end stages of hemorrhagic shock, even though the initiating factors are markedly different in the two conditions.

Physiology of Treatment in Shock

REPLACEMENT THERAPY

Blood and Plasma Transfusion. If a person is in shock caused by hemorrhage, the best possible therapy is usually transfusion of whole blood. If the shock is caused by plasma loss, the best therapy is administration of plasma. When dehydration is the cause, administration of an appropriate electrolyte solution can correct the shock.

Whole blood is not always available, such as under battlefield conditions. Plasma can usually substitute adequately for whole blood because it increases the blood volume and restores normal hemodynamics. Plasma cannot restore a normal hematocrit, but the human body can usually stand a decrease in hematocrit to about half of normal before serious consequences result, if cardiac output is adequate. Therefore, in emergency conditions, it is reasonable to use plasma in place of whole blood for treatment of hemorrhagic or most other types of hypovolemic shock.

Sometimes plasma is unavailable. In these instances, various *plasma substitutes* have been developed that perform almost exactly the same hemodynamic functions as plasma. One of these is dextran solution.

Dextran Solution as a Plasma Substitute. The principal requirement of a truly effective plasma substitute is that it remain in the circulatory system—that is, it does not filter through the capillary pores into the tissue spaces. In addition, the solution must be nontoxic and must contain appropriate electrolytes to prevent derangement of the body's extracellular fluid electrolytes on administration.

To remain in the circulation, the plasma substitute must contain some substance that has a large enough molecular size to exert colloid osmotic pressure. One substance developed for this purpose is *dextran*, a large polysaccharide polymer of glucose. Certain bacteria secrete dextran as a by-product of their growth, and commercial dextran can be manufactured using a bacterial culture procedure. By varying the growth conditions of the bacteria, the molecular weight of the dextran can be controlled to the desired value. Dextrans of appropriate molecular size do not pass through the capillary pores and, therefore, can replace plasma proteins as colloid osmotic agents.

Few toxic reactions have been observed when using purified dextran to provide colloid osmotic pressure; therefore, solutions containing this substance have been used as substitute for plasma in fluid replacement therapy.

TREATMENT OF NEUROGENIC AND ANAPHYLACTIC SHOCK WITH SYMPATHOMIMETIC DRUGS

A *sympathomimetic drug* is a drug that mimics sympathetic stimulation. These drugs include *norepinephrine*, *epinephrine*, and a large number of long-acting drugs that have the same effect as epinephrine and norepinephrine.

In two types of shock, sympathomimetic drugs have proved to be especially beneficial. The first of these is *neurogenic shock*, in which the sympathetic nervous system is severely depressed. Administering a sympathomimetic drug takes the place of the diminished sympathetic actions and can often restore full circulatory function.

The second type of shock in which sympathomimetic drugs are valuable is *anaphylactic shock*, in which excess histamine plays a prominent role. The sympathomimetic drugs have a vasoconstrictor effect that opposes the vasodilating effect of histamine. Therefore, epinephrine, norepinephrine, or other sympathomimetic drugs are often lifesaving.

Sympathomimetic drugs have not proved to be very valuable in hemorrhagic shock. The reason is that in this type of shock, the sympathetic nervous system is almost always maximally activated by the circulatory reflexes already; so much norepinephrine and epinephrine are already circulating in the blood that sympathomimetic drugs have essentially no additional beneficial effect.

OTHER THERAPY

Treatment by the Head-Down Position. When the pressure falls too low in most types of shock, especially in hemorrhagic and neurogenic shock, placing the patient with the head at least 12 in. lower than the feet helps in promoting venous return, thereby also increasing cardiac output. This head-down position is the first essential step in the treatment of many types of shock.

Oxygen Therapy. Because a major deleterious effect of most types of shock is too little delivery of oxygen to the tissues, giving the patient oxygen to breathe can be of benefit in some instances. However, this intervention is frequently far less beneficial than one might expect because the problem in most types of shock is not inadequate oxygenation of the blood by the lungs but inadequate transport of the blood after it is oxygenated.

Treatment with Glucocorticoids. Glucocorticoids—adrenal cortex hormones that control glucose metabolism— are frequently given to patients in severe shock for several reasons: (1) experiments have shown empirically that glucocorticoids frequently increase the strength of the heart in the late stages of shock; (2) glucocorticoids stabilize lysosomes in tissue cells and thereby prevent release of lysosomal enzymes into the cytoplasm of the cells, thus preventing deterioration from this source; and

(3) glucocorticoids might aid in the metabolism of glucose by the severely damaged cells.

Circulatory Arrest

A condition closely allied to circulatory shock is circulatory arrest, in which all blood flow stops. This condition can occur, for example, as a result of *cardiac arrest* or *ventricular fibrillation*.

Ventricular fibrillation can usually be stopped by strong electroshock of the heart, the basic principles of which are described in Chapter 34.

In the case of a cardiac arrest a normal cardiac rhythm can be restored by immediately applying cardiopulmonary resuscitation procedures, while at the same time supplying the patient's lungs with adequate quantities of ventilatory oxygen.

EFFECT OF CIRCULATORY ARREST ON THE BRAIN

A special problem in circulatory arrest is to prevent detrimental effects in the brain as a result of the arrest. In general, more than 5–8 minutes of total circulatory arrest can cause at least some degree of permanent brain damage in more than half of patients. Circulatory arrest for as long as 10–15 minutes almost always permanently destroys significant amounts of mental power.

For many years, it was taught that this detrimental effect on the brain was caused by the acute cerebral hypoxia that occurs during circulatory arrest. However, experiments have shown that if blood clots are prevented from occurring in the blood vessels of the brain, this will also prevent much of the early deterioration of the brain during circulatory arrest. For instance, in animal experiments, all the blood was removed from the animal's blood vessels at the beginning of circulatory arrest and then replaced at the end of circulatory arrest so that no intravascular blood clotting could occur. In this experiment, the brain was usually able to withstand up to 30 minutes of circulatory arrest without permanent brain damage. Also, administration of heparin or streptokinase (to prevent blood coagulation) before cardiac arrest was shown to increase the survivability of the brain up to two to four times longer than usual.

Figure 52-5 outlines the stages of shock and the pathophysiological mechanisms at each stage.

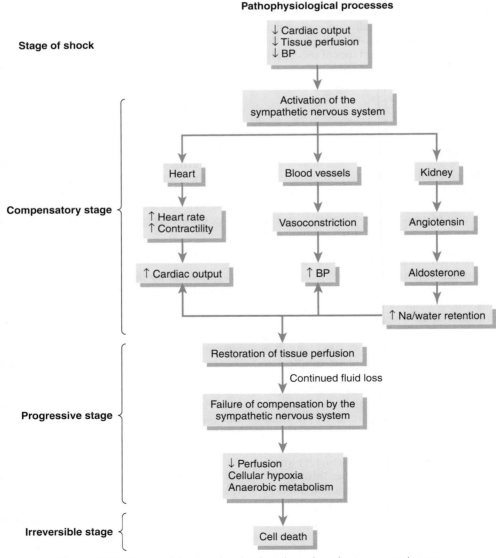

Figure 52-5 Stages of shock and pathophysiological mechanisms at each stage.

BIBLIOGRAPHY

Angus DC, van der Poll T: Severe sepsis and septic shock, *N. Engl. J. Med.* 369:840, 2013.

Annane D, Sebille V, Charpentier C, et al: Effect of treatment with low doses of hydrocortisone and fludrocortisone on mortality in patients with septic shock, *JAMA* 288:862, 2002.

Burry LD, Wax RS: Role of corticosteroids in septic shock, *Ann. Pharmacother.* 38:464, 2004.

Crowell JW, Smith EE: Oxygen deficit and irreversible hemorrhagic shock, *Am. J. Physiol.* 206:313, 1964.

Galli SJ, Tsai M, Piliponsky AM: The development of allergic inflammation, *Nature* 454:445, 2008.

Goodnough LT, Shander A: Evolution in alternatives to blood transfusion, *Hematol. J.* 4:87, 2003.

Guyton AC, Jones CE, Coleman TG: *Circulatory Physiology: Cardiac Output and its Regulation*, Philadelphia, 1973, W.B. Saunders.

Huet O, Chin-Dusting JP: Septic shock: desperately seeking treatment, *Clin. Sci. (Lond.)* 126:31, 2014.

Kar B, Basra SS, Shah NR, Loyalka P: Percutaneous circulatory support in cardiogenic shock: interventional bridge to recovery, *Circulation* 125:1809, 2012.

Kobayashi L, Costantini TW, Coimbra R: Hypovolemic shock resuscitation, *Surg. Clin. North Am.* 92:1403, 2012.

Lam SW, Bauer SR, Guzman JA: Septic shock: the initial moments and beyond, *Cleve. Clin. J. Med.* 80:175, 2013.

Lieberman PL: Recognition and first-line treatment of anaphylaxis, *Am. J. Med.* 127(1 Suppl.):S6, 2014.

McNeer RR, Varon AJ: Pitfalls of hemodynamic monitoring in patients with trauma, *Anesthesiol. Clin.* 31:179, 2013.

Myburgh JA, Mythen MG: Resuscitation fluids, *N. Engl. J. Med.* 369:1243, 2013.

Neligan PJ, Baranov D: Trauma and aggressive homeostasis management, *Anesthesiol. Clin.* 31:21, 2013.

Reynolds HR, Hochman J: Cardiogenic shock: current concepts and improving outcomes, *Circulation* 117:686, 2008.

Rushing GD, Britt LD: Reperfusion injury after hemorrhage: a collective review, *Ann. Surg.* 247:929, 2008.

Toh CH, Dennis M: Disseminated intravascular coagulation: old disease, new hope, *BMJ* 327:974, 2003.

Wilson M, Davis DP, Coimbra R: Diagnosis and monitoring of hemorrhagic shock during the initial resuscitation of multiple trauma patients: a review, *J. Emerg. Med.* 24:413, 2003.

SECTION V

Respiratory Physiology

TONY RAJ

53

Organization of the Respiratory System

The main functions of respiration are to provide oxygen to the tissues and remove carbon dioxide. As most tissues in the body survive on oxygen to produce energy, there is a requirement for a continuous supply of oxygen and removal of carbon dioxide. The four major components of respiration are as follows:

1. *pulmonary ventilation*, which means the inflow and outflow of air between the atmosphere and the lung alveoli;
2. *diffusion of oxygen (O_2) and carbon dioxide (CO_2) between the alveoli and the blood*;
3. *transport of oxygen and carbon dioxide in the blood and body fluids* to and from the body's tissue cells;
4. *regulation of ventilation* and other facets of respiration.

The respiratory system also performs several "nonrespiratory" functions, which are described later in this chapter.

The respiratory system in humans has evolved to include the following structures:

1. the lungs;
2. the conducting airways, including the oral and nasal cavities;
3. the nerves that control respiration and the respiratory centers in the central nervous system;
4. the structures involved in moving air in and out of the lungs such as:
   a. rib cage
   b. intercostal muscles
   c. diaphragm
   d. abdominal muscles

Anatomical Organization of the Lungs and Airways

THE LUNGS

The lungs are the organs for respiration and are two in number, the left and the right lung. Each lung is further divided into lobes. The right lung is divided into three lobes (upper, middle, and lower lobes) and the left lung is divided into two lobes (upper and lower lobes) (Figure 53-1). The lungs are covered by thin membranous layers called the pleura. The visceral pleura lines the lungs and is separated from the parietal pleura by a pleural space or cavity, which is filled by pleural fluid. This interface helps the lungs to glide smoothly during inspiration and expiration (Figure 53-2).

THE TRACHEA, BRONCHI, BRONCHIOLES, AND RESPIRATORY UNIT

Figure 53-3 shows the respiratory system, demonstrating especially the respiratory passageways, and Figure 53-4 demonstrates the organization of the airways. The air is distributed to the lungs by way of the trachea, bronchi, and bronchioles.

The trachea branches out into two main bronchi, which further branch out into lobar bronchi that connect each lobe (see Figure 53-2). These lobar bronchi further branch out into segmental bronchi and into smaller branches until they reach the terminal bronchioles, which are the smallest airways without any alveoli attached. All these airways do not participate in any gas exchange and are referred to as the "conducting zone."

The terminal bronchioles are further divided into respiratory bronchioles. These bronchioles differ from the terminal bronchioles because they have alveoli occasionally attached to their walls.

The respiratory bronchioles lead to the alveolar ducts and finally to the alveoli. This region where alveoli are present in the lungs and where gas exchange takes place is called the "respiratory zone."

RESPIRATORY UNIT

Figure 53-5 shows the *respiratory unit* (also called "respiratory lobule"), which is composed of a *respiratory bronchiole*, *alveolar ducts*, and *alveoli*. There are about 300 million alveoli in the two lungs, and each alveolus has an average diameter of about 0.2 mm. The alveolar walls are extremely thin and between the alveoli is an almost solid network of interconnecting capillaries, shown in Figure 53-6. Indeed, because of the extensiveness of the capillary plexus, the flow of blood in the alveolar wall has been described as a "sheet" of flowing blood. Thus, it is obvious that the alveolar gases are in very close proximity to the blood, gas exchange between the alveolar air and the pulmonary blood occurs through the membranes of all the terminal portions of

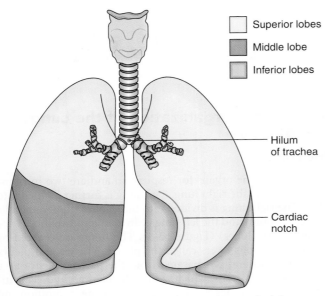

Figure 53-1   Anatomy of the lungs indicating the lobes.

Superior lobes

Middle lobe

Inferior lobes

Hilum
of trachea

Cardiac
notch

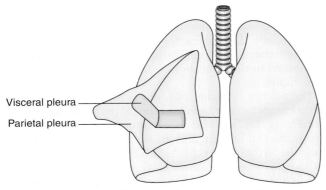

Figure 53-2   The pleural membranes covering the lungs.

Visceral pleura

Parietal pleura

the lungs, not merely in the alveoli. All these membranes are collectively known as the *respiratory membrane*, also called the *pulmonary membrane* which is described later.

RESPIRATORY MEMBRANE

Figure 53-7 shows the ultrastructure of the respiratory membrane drawn in cross-section on the left and a red blood cell on the right. It also shows the diffusion of O_2 from the alveolus into the red blood cell and diffusion of CO_2 in the opposite direction.

Box 53-1 lists the different layers of the respiratory membrane.

Despite the large number of layers, the overall thickness of the respiratory membrane in some areas is as little as 0.2 μm, and averages about 0.6 μm, except where there are cell nuclei. From histological studies, it has been estimated that the total surface area of the respiratory membrane is about 70 m^2 in the healthy adult human male, which is equivalent to the floor area of a 25 × 30–ft. room. The total quantity of blood in the capillaries of the lungs at any given instant is 60–140 mL. Now

imagine this small amount of blood spread over the entire surface of a 25 × 30–ft. floor, and it is easy to understand the rapidity of the respiratory exchange of O_2 and CO_2.

The average diameter of the pulmonary capillaries is only about 5 μm, which means that red blood cells must squeeze through them. The red blood cell membrane usually touches the capillary wall, so O_2 and CO_2 need not pass through significant amounts of plasma as they diffuse between the alveolus and the red blood cell. This, too, increases the rapidity of diffusion.

Physical Laws Applicable in Respiratory Physiology

For a student to understand the various concepts in respiratory physiology, it is important to understand the various physical gas laws and their applicability to respiratory physiology (Table 53-1).

BOYLE'S LAW

Boyle's law states that under constant temperature, the volume of a fixed mass of dry gas is inversely proportional to the pressure exerted on it.

It is denoted by an equation: $P_1V_1 = P_2V_2$ (at constant temperature), where P_1 is the original pressure, P_2 is the new pressure, V_1 is the original volume, and V_2 is the new volume.

CHARLES' LAW

Charles' law states that the volume occupied by a fixed mass of gas at a constant pressure is directly proportional to the absolute temperature:

$$V/T = \text{constant}$$

where V is the volume and T is the absolute temperature (measured in kelvin).

IDEAL GAS LAW

Boyle's and Charles' laws can be combined to form a single generalization of the behavior of gases known as an equation of state, which is given by the following equation:

$$PV = nRT,$$

where P is the pressure in atmospheres, V is the volume in liters, n is the number of gram-moles of a gas, R is called the universal gas constant, and T is the temperature in kelvin. Although this law describes the behavior of an ideal gas, it closely approximates the behavior of real gases.

AVOGADRO'S LAW

It states that under the same conditions of temperature and pressure, equal volumes of different gases contain an equal number of molecules.

The volume occupied by 1 mol of gas is about 22.4 L [0.791 (ft.)^3] at standard temperature and pressure (0°C, 1 atm) and is the same for all gases, according to Avogadro's law.

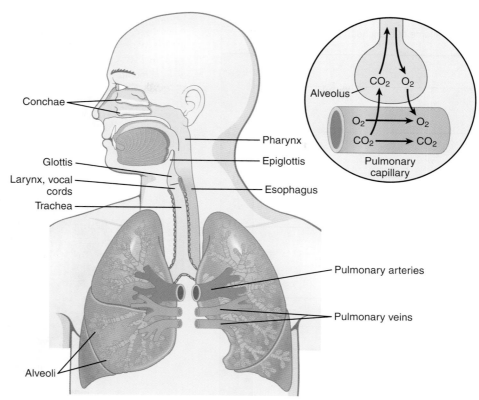

Figure 53-3 Respiratory passages.

DALTON'S LAW

Dalton's law states that in a mixture of gases, the total pressure exerted is equal to the sum of the partial pressures of the individual component gases.

The partial pressure is the pressure that each gas would exert if it alone occupied the volume of the mixture at the same temperature.

HENRY'S LAW

Henry's law states that at constant temperature, the amount of gas dissolved in a liquid will be directly proportional to the partial pressure of the gas with which the liquid is in equilibrium.

GRAHAM'S LAW

In a gas phase, Graham's law states that the rate of diffusion of a gas is inversely proportional to its molecular weight.

FICK'S LAW

Fick's law of diffusion states that the net diffusion rate of a gas through a membrane is proportional to the tissue area (A) and the difference in partial pressure ($P_1 - P_2$) between the two sides, and is inversely proportional to the thickness (T):

$$V_{gas} = A \times D \times (P_1 - P_2) / T,$$

where D is a constant that depends on the solubility of the gas and inversely to the molecular weight and is given by

$$D \propto \text{Solubility} / \text{Square root of molecular weight}$$

Nonrespiratory Functions of the Lungs

Although the lungs function primarily for respiration, they also perform several other functions that are not directly related to respiration and these are listed in Box 53-2.

FILTRATION FUNCTION

The hairs at the entrance to the nostrils are important for filtering out large particles. Much more important, though, is the removal of particles by *turbulent precipitation*. That is, the air passing through the nasal passageways hits many obstructing vanes: the *conchae* (also called *turbinates*, because they cause turbulence of the air), the septum, and the pharyngeal wall. Each time air hits one of these obstructions, it must change its direction of movement. The particles suspended in the air, having far more mass and momentum than air, cannot change their direction of travel as rapidly as the air can. Therefore, they continue forward, striking the surfaces of the obstructions, and are entrapped in the mucous coating and transported by the cilia to the pharynx to be swallowed.

Size of Particles Entrapped in the Respiratory Passages. The nasal turbulence mechanism for removing particles from air is so effective that almost no particles larger than 6 μm in diameter enter the lungs through the nose. This size is smaller than the size of red blood cells.

Of the remaining particles, many that are between 1 and 5 μm *settle* in the smaller bronchioles as a result of *gravitational*

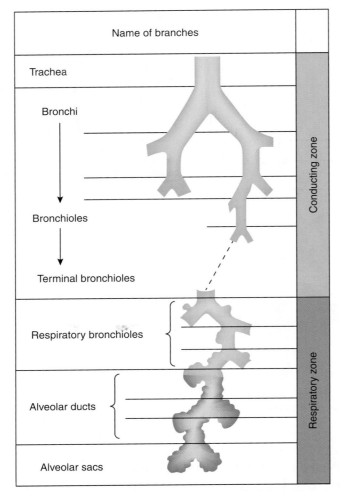

Figure 53-4 Organization of the airways. *Modified from Widmaier, E.P., Raff, H., Strang, K.T., 2005. Vander's Human Physiology: The Mechanisms of Body Function, 10th ed. McGraw-Hill, New York.*

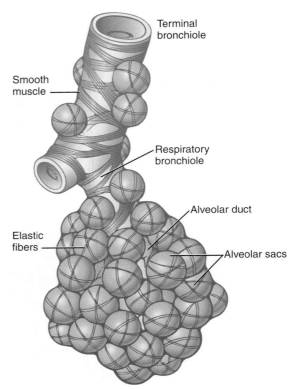

Figure 53-5 Respiratory unit.

precipitation. For instance, terminal bronchiolar disease is common in coal miners because of settled dust particles. Some of the still smaller particles (smaller than 1 μm in diameter) *diffuse* against the walls of the alveoli and adhere to the alveolar fluid. However, many particles smaller than 0.5 μm in diameter remain suspended in the alveolar air and are expelled by expiration. For instance, the particles of cigarette smoke are about 0.3 μm. Almost none of these particles are precipitated in the respiratory passageways before they reach the alveoli. Unfortunately, up to one-third of them do precipitate in the alveoli by the diffusion process, with the balance remaining suspended and expelled in the expired air.

IMMUNE FUNCTIONS

Another route by which invading organisms frequently enter the body is through the lungs. Large numbers of tissue macrophages are present as integral components of the alveolar walls. They can phagocytize particles that become entrapped in the alveoli. Many of the particles that become entrapped in the alveoli are removed by *alveolar macrophages* and others are carried away by the lung lymphatics. If the particles are digestible,

the macrophages can also digest them and release the digestive products into the lymph. If the particle is not digestible, the macrophages often form a "giant cell" capsule around the particle until such time—if ever—that it can be slowly dissolved. Such capsules are frequently formed around tuberculosis bacilli, silica dust particles, and even carbon particles. An excess of particles can cause growth of fibrous tissue in the alveolar septa leading to permanent debility.

METABOLIC FUNCTIONS

The cells of the lungs, especially the endothelial cells of the capillary beds that line the alveoli, have developed the capacity to metabolize various metabolic and vasoactive substances. Some of these substances include proteins, lipids, cytokines, and vasoactive amines.

Other notable examples are as follows:
1. Angiotensin I is activated to angiotensin II by angiotensin-converting enzyme present on the surface of the endothelial cells.
2. Serotonin is metabolized by the endothelial cells after being internalized into the cell.

Some of the substances that are synthesized and secreted by the endothelial cells include cytokines, prostaglandins, prostacyclin, nitric oxide, and clotting factors.

VOCALIZATION AND PHONATION

Speech involves not only the respiratory system but also (1) specific speech nervous control centers in the cerebral cortex; (2) respiratory control centers of the brain; and (3) the articulation

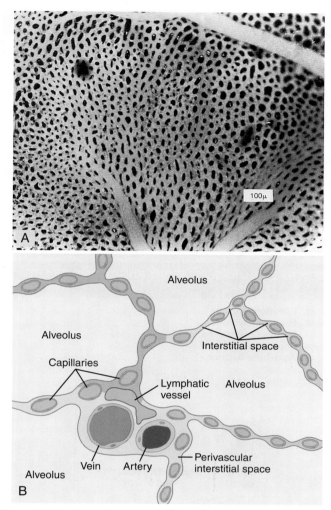

Figure 53-6 (A) Surface view of capillaries in an alveolar wall; (B) cross-sectional view of alveolar walls and their vascular supply. *(A) From Maloney, J.E., Castle, B.L., 1969. Pressure–diameter relations of capillaries and small blood vessels in frog lung. Respir. Physiol. 7, 150. Reproduced by permission of ASP Biological and Medical Press, North-Holland Division.*

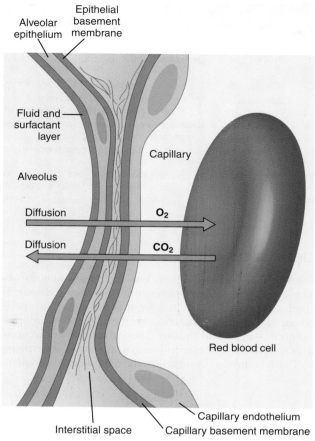

Figure 53-7 Ultrastructure of the alveolar respiratory membrane, shown in cross-section.

---

and resonance structures of the mouth and nasal cavities. Speech is composed of two mechanical functions: (1) *phonation*, which is achieved by the larynx, and (2) *articulation*, which is achieved by the structures of the mouth.

Phonation. The larynx, shown in Figure 53-8A, is especially adapted to act as a vibrator. The vibrating elements are the *vocal folds*, commonly called the *vocal cords*.

Figure 53-8B shows the vocal cords as they are seen when looking into the glottis with a laryngoscope. During phonation, the cords move together so that passage of air between them will cause vibration. The pitch of the vibration is determined mainly by the degree of stretch of the cords, but also by how tightly the cords are approximated to one another and by the mass of their edges. Figure 53-8A shows a dissected view of the vocal folds after removal of the mucous epithelial lining.

BOX 53-1 DIFFERENT LAYERS OF THE RESPIRATORY MEMBRANE

1. A layer of fluid containing surfactant that lines the alveolus and reduces the surface tension of the alveolar fluid
2. The alveolar epithelium, which is composed of thin epithelial cells
3. An epithelial basement membrane
4. A thin interstitial space between the alveolar epithelium and the capillary membrane
5. A capillary basement membrane that in many places fuses with the alveolar epithelial basement membrane
6. The capillary endothelial membrane

Also, slips of muscles *within* the vocal cords can change the *shapes and masses of the vocal cord edges*, sharpening them to emit high-pitched sounds and blunting them for the more bass sounds.

Articulation and Resonance. The resonators include the *mouth*, the *nose* and *associated nasal sinuses*, the *pharynx*, and even the *chest cavity*. Again, we are all familiar with the resonating qualities of these structures. For instance, the function of the nasal resonators is demonstrated by the change in voice quality when a person has a severe cold that blocks the air passages to these resonators.

TABLE 53-1		Physical Gas Laws Applicable in Respiratory Physiology
	Law	**Description**
01	Boyle's law	Under constant temperature, the volume of a fixed mass of dry gas is inversely proportional to the pressure exerted on it
02	Charles' law	The volume occupied by a fixed mass of gas at a constant pressure is directly proportional to the absolute temperature
03	Ideal gas law	$PV = nRT$, where P is the pressure in atmospheres, V is the volume in liters, n is the number of gram-moles of a gas, R is called the universal gas constant, and T is the temperature in kelvin
04	Avogadro's law	Under the same conditions of temperature and pressure, equal volumes of different gases contain an equal number of molecules
05	Dalton's law	In a mixture of gases, the total pressure exerted is equal to the sum of the partial pressures of the individual component gases
06	Henry's law	At constant temperature, the amount of gas dissolved in a liquid will be directly proportional to the partial pressure of the gas with which the liquid is in equilibrium
07	Graham's law	In a gas phase, Graham's law states that the rate of diffusion of a gas is inversely proportional to its molecular weight

ACID–BASE BALANCE

The respiratory system also participates in maintaining the acid–base balance of the body by eliminating CO_2 from the body. This is discussed later in detail; however, it is important to note that there are chemosensors that monitor the CO_2 and hydrogen ion concentrations in blood and any change that indicates accumulation of CO_2 in the arterial blood leads to alterations in respiratory rate. This is controlled by centers in the central nervous system.

> **BOX 53-2   NONRESPIRATORY FUNCTIONS OF THE LUNG**
>
> 1. Filtration function
> 2. Immune functions
> 3. Metabolic functions
> 4. Phonation
> 5. Acid–base balance

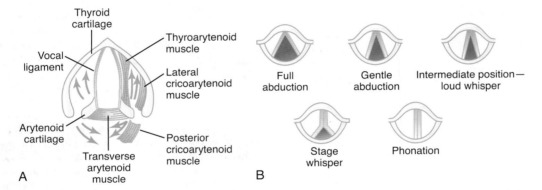

Figure 53-8   (A) Anatomy of the larynx; (B) laryngeal function in phonation, showing the positions of the vocal cords during different types of phonation. *Modified from Greene, M.C., 1980. The Voice and its Disorders, fourth ed. J.B. Lippincott, Philadelphia.*

BIBLIOGRAPHY

Encyclopædia Britannica, 2012. Avogadro's law. Encyclopædia Britannica Online. Encyclopædia Britannica Inc., May 11. <http://www.britannica.com/EBchecked/topic/45902/Avogadros-law>.

Encyclopædia Britannica, 2012. Dalton's law. Encyclopædia Britannica Online. Encyclopædia Britannica Inc., May 11. <http://www.britannica.com/EBchecked/topic/150311/Daltons-law>.

Fahy JV, Dickey BF: Airway mucus function and dysfunction, *N. Engl. J. Med.* 363:2233, 2010.

Hilaire G, Duron B: Maturation of the mammalian respiratory system, *Physiol. Rev.* 79:325, 1999.

Lai-Fook SJ: Pleural mechanics and fluid exchange, *Physiol. Rev.* 84:385, 2004.

Lalley PM: The aging respiratory system—pulmonary structure, function and neural control, *Respir. Physiol. Neurobiol.* 187:199, 2013.

Lopez-Rodriguez E, Pérez-Gil J: Structure–function relationships in pulmonary surfactant membranes: from biophysics to therapy, *Biochim. Biophys. Acta* 1838:1568, 2014.

Mason RJ, Broaddus CV, Martin T, et al: Gas exchange. *Murray and Nadel's Textbook of Respiratory Medicine*, sixth ed., Philadelphia, 2015, Saunders Elsevier.

Paton JF, Dutschmann M: Central control of upper airway resistance regulating respiratory airflow in mammals, *J. Anat.* 201:319, 2002.

Powell FL, Hopkins SR: Comparative physiology of lung complexity: implications for gas exchange, *News Physiol. Sci.* 19:55, 2004.

Sant'Ambrogio G, Widdicombe J: Reflexes from airway rapidly adapting receptors, *Respir. Physiol.* 125:33, 2001.

Strohl KP, Butler JP, Malhotra A: Mechanical properties of the upper airway, *Compr. Physiol.* 2:1853, 2012.

Suki B, Sato S, Parameswaran H, et al: Emphysema and mechanical stress-induced lung remodeling, *Physiology (Bethesda)* 28:404, 2013.

Uhlig S, Taylor AE: *Methods in Pulmonary Research*, Basel, 1998, Springer Basel AG.

Voynow JA, Rubin BK: Mucins, mucus, and sputum, *Chest* 135:505, 2009.

West JB: Why doesn't the elephant have a pleural space? *News Physiol. Sci.* 17:47, 2002.

West JB: *Respiratory Physiology*, ninth ed., Philadelphia, 2012, Lippincott Williams & Wilkins, Wolters Kluwers.

Widdicombe J: Reflexes from the lungs and airways: historical perspective, *J. Appl. Physiol.* 101:628, 2006.

Widdicombe J: Lung afferent activity: implications for respiratory sensation, *Respir. Physiol. Neurobiol.* 167:2, 2009.

Wright JR: Pulmonary surfactant: a front line of lung host defense, *J. Clin. Invest.* 111:1453, 2003.

Zeitels SM, Healy GB: Laryngology and phonosurgery, *N. Engl. J. Med.* 349:882, 2003.

54 Mechanics of Breathing

GLOSSARY OF TERMS

- **Alveolar pressure:** The pressure of the air inside the lung alveoli
- **Alveolar ventilation:** The rate at which new air reaches the alveoli, alveolar sacs, alveolar ducts, and respiratory bronchioles
- **Compliance:** Stretchability of the lung tissue
- **Intrapleural pressure:** The pressure of the fluid in the thin space between the lung pleura and the chest wall pleura
- **Mediastinum:** The region in the thoracic cavity between the two pleural sacs containing the heart, trachea, and other viscera other than the lungs
- **Surfactant:** A complex mixture of several phospholipids, proteins, and ions that is present on the inner surface of the alveoli and helps in reducing surface tension
- **Transpulmonary pressure:** The difference between the alveolar pressure and the intrapleural pressure

Mechanics of Pulmonary Ventilation

MUSCLES THAT CAUSE LUNG EXPANSION AND CONTRACTION

The lungs can be expanded and contracted in two ways:

1. by downward and upward movement of the diaphragm to lengthen or shorten the chest cavity;
2. by elevation and depression of the ribs to increase and decrease the anteroposterior diameter of the chest cavity using the intercostal muscles. Figure 54-1 shows these two methods and Figure 54-2 shows the actions of the intercostal muscles.

Normal quiet breathing is accomplished almost entirely by the first method, that is, by movement of the diaphragm. During inspiration, contraction of the diaphragm pulls the lower surfaces of the lungs downward. Then, during expiration, the diaphragm simply relaxes and the *elastic recoil* of the lungs, chest wall, and abdominal structures compresses the lungs and expels the air. During heavy breathing, however, the elastic forces are not powerful enough to cause the necessary rapid expiration, so extra force is achieved mainly by contraction of the *abdominal muscles*, which pushes the abdominal contents upward against the bottom of the diaphragm, thereby compressing the lungs.

The second method for expanding the lungs is to raise the rib cage. Raising the rib cage expands the lungs because, in the natural resting position, the ribs slant downward, as shown on the left side of Figure 54-1, thus allowing the sternum to fall backward toward the vertebral column. When the rib cage is elevated, however, the ribs project almost directly forward, so the sternum also moves forward, away from the spine, making the anteroposterior thickness of the chest about 20% greater during maximum inspiration than during expiration. Therefore, all the muscles that elevate the chest cage are classified as muscles of inspiration and the muscles that depress the chest cage are classified as muscles of expiration. The most important muscles that raise the rib cage are the *external intercostals*, but others that help are the (1) *sternocleidomastoid* muscles, which lift upward on the sternum; (2) *anterior serrati*, which lift many of the ribs; (3) *scaleni*, which lift the first two ribs; and (4) *alae nasi*, which cause flaring of the nostrils.

The muscles that pull the rib cage downward during expiration are mainly the (1) *abdominal recti*, which have the powerful effect of pulling downward on the lower ribs at the same time that these and other abdominal muscles also compress the abdominal contents upward against the diaphragm, and (2) the *internal intercostals*.

Figure 54-1 also shows the mechanism by which the external and internal intercostals act to cause inspiration and expiration. To the left, the ribs during expiration are angled downward and the external intercostals are elongated forward and downward. As they contract, they pull the upper ribs forward in relation to the lower ribs, which causes leverage on the ribs to raise them upward, thereby causing inspiration. The internal intercostals function exactly in the opposite manner, functioning as expiratory muscles because they angle between the ribs in the opposite direction and cause opposite leverage. The actions of the intercostal muscles are shown in Figure 54-2, summary of events during inspiration and expiration is shown in Figure 54-3, and a list of muscles acting during inspiration and expiration is given in Box 54-1.

PRESSURES THAT CAUSE THE MOVEMENT OF AIR IN AND OUT OF THE LUNGS

The lung is an elastic structure that collapses like a balloon and expels all its air through the trachea whenever there is no force

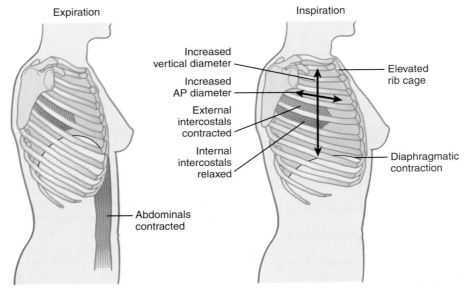

Figure 54-1 Contraction and expansion of the thoracic cage during expiration and inspiration, demonstrating diaphragmatic contraction, function of the intercostal muscles, and elevation and depression of the rib cage. *AP*, anteroposterior.

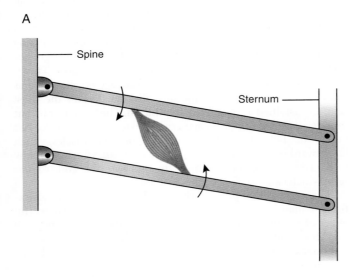

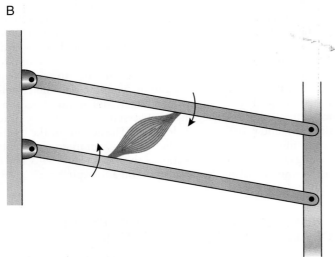

Figure 54-2 Actions of the intercostal muscles. (A) External intercostal; (B) internal intercostal.

to keep it inflated. Also, there are no attachments between the lung and the walls of the chest cage, except where it is suspended at its hilum from the *mediastinum*, the middle section of the chest cavity. Instead, the lung "floats" in the thoracic cavity, surrounded by a thin layer of *pleural fluid* that lubricates movement of the lungs within the cavity. Further, continual suction of excess fluid into lymphatic channels maintains a slight suction between the visceral surface of the lung pleura and the parietal pleural surface of the thoracic cavity. Therefore, the lungs are held to the thoracic wall as if glued there, except that they are well lubricated and can slide freely as the chest expands and contracts.

Pleural Pressure and its Changes During Respiration

Pleural pressure is the pressure of the fluid in the thin space between the lung pleura and the chest wall pleura. As noted earlier, this pressure is normally a slight suction, which means a slightly *negative* pressure. The normal pleural pressure at the beginning of inspiration is about −5 cm H_2O, which is the amount of suction required to hold the lungs open to their resting level. During normal inspiration, expansion of the chest cage pulls outward on the lungs with greater force and creates more negative pressure, to an average of about −7.5 cm H_2O.

These relationships between pleural pressure and changing lung volume are demonstrated in Figure 54-4, showing in the lower panel the increasing negativity of the pleural pressure from −5 to −7.5 during inspiration and in the upper panel an increase in lung volume of 0.5 L. Then, during expiration, the events are essentially reversed.

Alveolar Pressure—The Air Pressure Inside the Lung Alveoli

When the glottis is open and no air is flowing into or out of the lungs, the pressures in all parts of the respiratory tree, all the way to the alveoli, are equal to atmospheric pressure, which is considered to be zero reference pressure in the airways—that is, 0 cm H_2O pressure. To cause inward flow of air into the alveoli during inspiration, the pressure in the alveoli must fall to a value

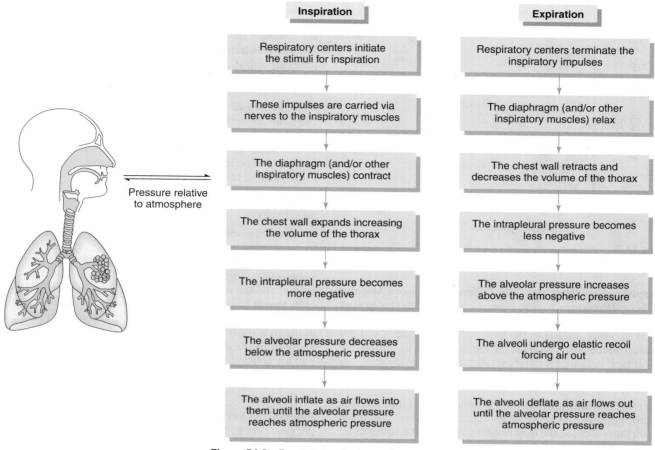

Figure 54-3 Events in inspiration and expiration.

BOX 54-1 SUMMARY OF MUSCLES ACTING DURING INSPIRATION AND EXPIRATION

INSPIRATORY MUSCLES

1. Diaphragm
2. External intercostal muscles

ACCESSORY INSPIRATORY MUSCLES

1. Sternocleidomastoid muscles
2. Anterior serrati
3. Scaleni
4. Alae nasi

EXPIRATORY MUSCLES (HYPERVENTILATION)

1. Rectus abdominis
2. Internal intercostal muscles
3. Internal and external obliques
4. Transversus abdominis

slightly below atmospheric pressure (below 0). The second curve (labeled "alveolar pressure") of Figure 54-4 demonstrates that during normal inspiration, alveolar pressure decreases to about −1 cm H_2O. This slight negative pressure is enough to pull 0.5 L of air into the lungs in the 2 seconds required for normal quiet inspiration.

During expiration, alveolar pressure rises to about +1 cm H_2O, which forces the 0.5 L of inspired air out of the lungs during the 2–3 seconds of expiration.

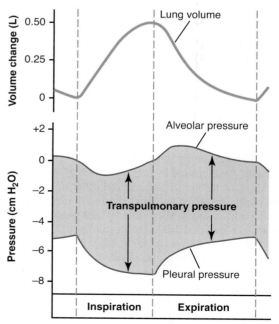

Figure 54-4 Changes in lung volume, alveolar pressure, pleural pressure, and transpulmonary pressure during normal breathing.

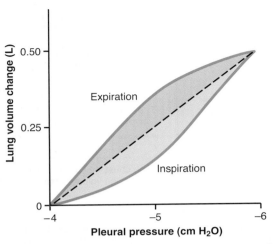

Figure 54-5 Compliance diagram in a healthy person. This diagram shows compliance of the lungs alone.

Transpulmonary Pressure—The Difference Between Alveolar and Pleural Pressures. Note in Figure 54-4 that the *transpulmonary pressure* is the pressure difference between that in the alveoli and that on the outer surfaces of the lungs (pleural pressure), and it is a measure of the elastic forces in the lungs that tend to collapse the lungs at each instant of respiration called the *recoil pressure*.

Compliance of the Lungs

The extent to which the lungs will expand for each unit increase in transpulmonary pressure (if enough time is allowed to reach equilibrium) is called the *lung compliance*. The total compliance of both lungs together in the normal adult human averages about 200 mL of air per centimeter of water transpulmonary pressure. That is, every time the transpulmonary pressure increases 1 cm H_2O, the lung volume, after 10–20 seconds, will expand 200 mL.

Compliance Diagram of the Lungs. Figure 54-5 is a diagram relating lung volume changes to changes in pleural pressure, which, in turn, alters transpulmonary pressure. Note that the relation is different for inspiration and expiration. Each curve is recorded by changing the pleural pressure in small steps and allowing the lung volume to come to a steady level between successive steps. The two curves are called, respectively, the *inspiratory compliance curve* and the *expiratory compliance curve*, and the entire diagram is called the *compliance diagram of the lungs*.

The characteristics of the compliance diagram are determined by the elastic forces of the lungs. These forces can be divided into two parts:
1. *elastic forces of the lung tissue*;
2. *elastic forces caused by surface tension of the fluid that lines the inside walls of the alveoli* and other lung air spaces.

The elastic forces of the lung tissue are determined mainly by *elastin* and *collagen* fibers interwoven among the lung parenchyma. In deflated lungs, these fibers are in an elastically contracted and kinked state; then, when the lungs expand, the fibers become stretched and unkinked, thereby elongating and exerting even more elastic force.

The elastic forces caused by surface tension are much more complex. The significance of surface tension is shown in Figure 54-6, which compares the compliance diagram of the lungs when filled with saline solution and when filled with air. When the lungs are filled with air, there is an interface between the alveolar fluid and the air in the alveoli. In lungs filled with saline solution, there is no air–fluid interface, and, therefore, the surface tension effect is not present—only tissue elastic forces are operative in the lung filled with saline solution (Box 54-2).

Note that transpleural pressures required to expand air-filled lungs are about three times as high as those required to expand lungs filled with saline solution. Thus, one can conclude that *the tissue elastic forces tending to cause collapse of the air-filled lung represent only about one-third of the total lung elasticity, whereas the fluid–air surface tension forces in the alveoli represent about two-thirds.*

The fluid–air surface tension elastic forces of the lungs also increase tremendously when the substance called *surfactant* is *not* present in the alveolar fluid.

Regional Variation of Compliance and Effect of Gravity

The basal regions of the lungs are gravity-dependent and receive more ventilation as compared to the upper regions of the lungs. The basal regions of the lungs have less negative intrapleural pressure as compared to the upper regions of the lungs due to gravity and the weight of the lungs. This results in the upper region alveoli having larger volumes as compared to those in the basal and more dependent regions. The alveoli in the upper regions are already filled with air and are less compliant compared to those in the dependent regions, which are more compliant and are able to increase their volume with each breath.

Surfactant, Surface Tension, and Collapse of the Alveoli

Principle of Surface Tension. When water forms a surface with air, the water molecules on the surface of the water have an especially strong attraction for one another. As a result, the water surface is always attempting to contract. This is what holds raindrops together—a tight contractile membrane of water molecules around the entire surface of the raindrop. Now let us reverse these principles and see what happens on the inner surfaces of the alveoli. Here, the water surface is also attempting to contract. This tends to force air out of the alveoli through the bronchi and, in doing so, causes the alveoli to try to collapse. The net effect is to cause an elastic contractile force of the entire lungs, which is called the *surface tension elastic force*.

Surfactant and its Effect on Surface Tension. Surfactant is a *surface active agent in water*, which means that it greatly reduces the surface tension of water. It is secreted by special surfactant-secreting epithelial cells called *type II alveolar epithelial cells*, which constitute about 10% of the surface area of the alveoli. These cells are granular, containing lipid inclusions that are secreted in the surfactant into the alveoli.

Surfactant (Box 54-3) is a complex mixture of several phospholipids, proteins, and ions. The most important components are the phospholipid *dipalmitoyl phosphatidylcholine, surfactant apoproteins*, and *calcium ions*. The *dipalmitoyl phosphatidylcholine* and several less important phospholipids are responsible for reducing the surface tension. They perform this function by not dissolving uniformly in the fluid lining the alveolar surface. Instead, part of the molecule dissolves while the remainder spreads over the surface of the water in the alveolus. This surface has from one-twelfth to one-half the surface tension of a pure water surface.

In quantitative terms, the surface tension of different water fluids is approximately the following: pure water, 72 dynes/cm; normal fluids lining the alveoli but without surfactant, 50 dynes/cm; normal fluids lining the alveoli and *with* normal amounts of surfactant included, between 5 and 30 dynes/cm.

Figure 54-6 Comparison of the compliance diagrams of saline-filled and air-filled lungs and explanation of Laplace's law. *Netter illustration from www.netterimages.com.* © Elsevier Inc. All rights reserved.

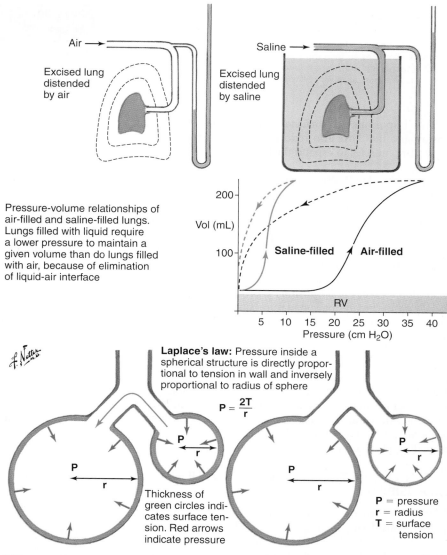

Pressure-volume relationships of air-filled and saline-filled lungs. Lungs filled with liquid require a lower pressure to maintain a given volume than do lungs filled with air, because of elimination of liquid-air interface

Laplace's law: Pressure inside a spherical structure is directly proportional to tension in wall and inversely proportional to radius of sphere

$$P = \frac{2T}{r}$$

Thickness of green circles indicates surface tension. Red arrows indicate pressure

P = pressure
r = radius
T = surface tension

Without surfactant. Surface tension in both alveoli is the same. A greater pressure is required to keep small alveolus open. Small alveolus tends to empty into larger one

With surfactant. Surface tension reduced in small alveolus. Pressure distending both alveoli is approximately the same. Alveoli are stabilized, and the tendency for small alveolus to empty into larger one is reduced

---

BOX 54-2 SUMMARY OF FACTORS THAT DETERMINE LUNG COMPLIANCE

1. Elastic forces of the lung tissue:
   a. Elastin fibers woven in the lung parenchyma
   b. Collagen fibers woven in the lung parenchyma
2. Elastic forces inside walls of the alveoli:
   a. Surface tension of the fluid that lines the inside walls of the alveoli (surfactant helps reduce this surface tension)

BOX 54-3 PULMONARY SURFACTANT

- Surfactant is a complex mixture of several phospholipids, proteins, and ions
- It contains *dipalmitoylphosphatidylcholine*
- It is responsible for reducing the surface tension within the alveoli
- It is produced by the *type II alveolar epithelial cells*

Pressure in Occluded Alveoli Caused by Surface Tension. If the air passages leading from the alveoli of the lungs are blocked, the surface tension in the alveoli tends to collapse the alveoli. This collapse creates positive pressure in the alveoli, attempting to push the air out. The amount of pressure generated in this way in an alveolus can be calculated using Laplace's law (Figure 54-6), which describes the relationship between surface tension (T), radius of the alveoli (r), and pressure (P) from the following formula:

$$\text{Pressure} = \frac{2 \times \text{surface tension}}{\text{radius of alveolus}}$$

For the average-sized alveolus with a radius of about 100 μm and lined with *normal surfactant*, this calculates to be about 4 cm H_2O pressure (3 mmHg). If the alveoli were lined with pure water without any surfactant, the pressure would calculate to be about 18 cm H_2O pressure, 4.5 times higher. Thus, one

TABLE 54-1	**Conditions of Increased or Decreased Compliance**
Conditions of Increased Compliance	**Conditions of Decreased Compliance**
• Normal aging • Bronchial asthma • Emphysema	• Fibrosis • Pulmonary hypertension • Alveolar atelectasis • Reduced surfactant • Premature infants

sees the importance of surfactant in reducing alveolar surface tension and therefore also reducing the effort required by the respiratory muscles to expand the lungs.

Effect of Alveolar Radius on the Pressure Caused by Surface Tension. Note from the preceding formula that the pressure generated as a result of surface tension in the alveoli is *inversely* affected by the radius of the alveolus, which means that the smaller the alveolus, the greater is the alveolar pressure caused by the surface tension. Thus, when the alveoli have half the normal radius (50 instead of 100 μm), the pressures noted earlier are doubled. To summarize, the factors that stabilize the alveoli are listed in Box 54-4.

Pathophysiology of Respiratory Distress Syndrome. This is especially significant in small premature babies, many of whom have alveoli with radii less than one-quarter that of an adult person. Further, surfactant does not normally begin to be secreted into the alveoli until between the sixth and seventh months of gestation, and in some cases, even later. Therefore, many premature babies have little or no surfactant in the alveoli when they are born, and their lungs have an extreme tendency to collapse, sometimes as high as six to eight times that in a normal adult person. This situation causes the condition called *respiratory distress syndrome of the newborn.* It is fatal if not treated with strong measures, especially properly applied continuous positive pressure breathing.

EFFECT OF THE THORACIC CAGE ON LUNG EXPANSIBILITY

Thus far, we have discussed the expansibility of the lungs alone, without considering the thoracic cage. The thoracic cage has its own elastic and viscous characteristics, similar to those of the lungs; even if the lungs were not present in the thorax, muscular effort would still be required to expand the thoracic cage.

Compliance of the Thorax and the Lungs Together

The compliance of the entire pulmonary system (the lungs and thoracic cage together) is measured while expanding the lungs of a totally relaxed or paralyzed subject. To measure compliance, air is forced into the lungs a little at a time while recording lung pressures and volumes. To inflate this total pulmonary system, almost twice as much pressure as is required to inflate the same lungs after removal from the chest cage is necessary. Therefore, the compliance of the combined lung–thorax system is almost exactly one-half that of the lungs alone—110 mL of volume per centimeter of water pressure for the combined system, compared with 200 mL/cm for the lungs alone. Furthermore, when the lungs are expanded to high volumes or compressed to low volumes, the limitations of the chest become extreme. When near these limits, the compliance of the combined lung–thorax system can be less than one-fifth that of the lungs alone. Conditions of increased or decreased compliance are shown in Table 54-1.

"WORK" OF BREATHING

We have already pointed out that during normal quiet breathing, all respiratory muscle contraction occurs during inspiration; expiration is almost entirely a passive process caused by elastic recoil of the lungs and chest cage. Thus, under resting conditions, the respiratory muscles normally perform "work" to cause inspiration but not to cause expiration.

The work of inspiration can be divided into three fractions: (1) that required to expand the lungs against the lung and chest elastic forces, called *compliance work* or *elastic work*; (2) that required to overcome the viscosity of the lung and chest wall structures, called *tissue resistance work*; and (3) that required to overcome airway resistance to movement of air into the lungs, called *airway resistance work.* Figure 54-7 compares work of breathing in normal individuals with obstructive disease and restrictive disease.

Energy Required for Respiration. During normal quiet respiration, only 3–5% of the total energy expended by the body is required for pulmonary ventilation. However, during heavy exercise, the amount of energy required can increase as much as 50-fold, especially if the person has any degree of increased airway resistance or decreased pulmonary compliance. Therefore, one of the major limitations on the intensity of exercise that can be performed is the person's ability to provide enough muscle energy for the respiratory process alone.

Minute Respiratory Volume

The *minute respiratory volume* is the total amount of new air moved into the respiratory passages each minute, and is equal to the *tidal volume* times the *respiratory rate per minute.* The normal tidal volume is about 500 mL and the normal respiratory rate is about 12 breaths/minute. Therefore, the *minute respiratory volume averages about 6 L/minute.*

Alveolar Ventilation

The rate at which new air reaches the alveoli, alveolar sacs, alveolar ducts, and respiratory bronchioles is called *alveolar ventilation.* The ultimate importance of pulmonary ventilation is to continually renew the air in the gas exchange areas of the lungs, where air is in proximity to the pulmonary blood.

"DEAD SPACE"

Definition. Some of the air a person breathes never reaches the gas exchange areas but simply fills respiratory passages where gas exchange does not occur, such as the nose, pharynx, and trachea. This air is called *dead space air* because it is not useful for gas exchange.

On expiration, the air in the dead space is expired first, before any of the air from the alveoli reaches the atmosphere. Therefore, the dead space is very disadvantageous for removing the expiratory gases from the lungs.

Work of Breathing

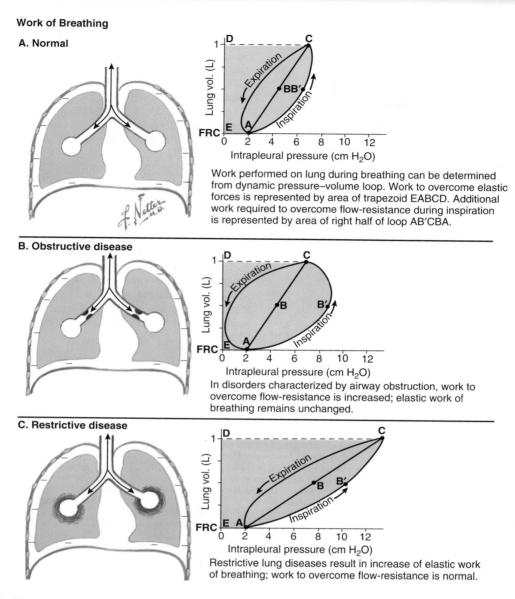

A. Normal

Work performed on lung during breathing can be determined from dynamic pressure–volume loop. Work to overcome elastic forces is represented by area of trapezoid EABCD. Additional work required to overcome flow-resistance during inspiration is represented by area of right half of loop AB'CBA.

B. Obstructive disease

In disorders characterized by airway obstruction, work to overcome flow-resistance is increased; elastic work of breathing remains unchanged.

C. Restrictive disease

Restrictive lung diseases result in increase of elastic work of breathing; work to overcome flow-resistance is normal.

Figure 54-7 Work of breathing in obstructive and restrictive lung disease compared to work performed in normal breathing (A). Work performed on lung during breathing can be determined from dynamic pressure–volume loop. Work required to overcome elastic forces is represented by area of trapezoid EABCD. Additional work required to overcome flow resistance during inspiration is represented by area of right half of loop AB'CBA. In obstructive disease, while compliance may be unchanged, the work of breathing is increased by the elevated airway resistance (B). While the elastic work of breathing remains unchanged. In restrictive lung diseases, lung compliance is low, and the elastic work of breathing is increased (C). Work required to overcome flow resistance is normal. *FRC*, functional residual capacity. *Netter illustration from www.netterimages.com. © Elsevier Inc. All rights reserved.*

Measurement of the Dead Space Volume. A simple method for measuring dead space volume is demonstrated by the graph in Figure 54-8. In making this measurement, the subject suddenly takes a deep breath of 100% O_2 which fills the entire dead space with pure O_2. Some oxygen also mixes with the alveolar air but does not completely replace this air. Then the person expires through a rapidly recording nitrogen meter, which makes the record shown in the figure. The first portion of the expired air comes from the dead space regions of the respiratory passageways, where the air has been completely replaced by O_2. Therefore, in the early part of the record, only O_2 appears and the nitrogen concentration is zero. Then, when alveolar air begins to reach the nitrogen meter, the nitrogen concentration rises rapidly because alveolar air containing large amounts of nitrogen begins to mix with the dead space air. After still more air has been expired, all the dead

space air has been washed from the passages and only alveolar air remains. Therefore, the recorded nitrogen concentration reaches a plateau level equal to its concentration in the alveoli, as shown to the right in the figure. With a little thought, the student can see that the gray area represents the air that has no nitrogen in it; this area is a measure of the volume of dead space air. For exact quantification, the following equation is used:

$$V_D = \frac{\text{gray area} \times V_E}{\text{pink area} + \text{gray area}}$$

where V_D is dead space air and V_E is the total volume of expired air.

Let us assume, for instance, that the gray area on the graph is 30 cm^2, the pink area is 70 cm^2, and the total volume expired is 500 mL. The dead space would be

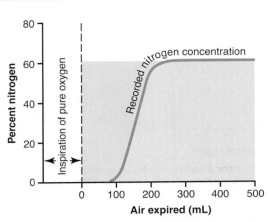

Figure 54-8   Record of the changes in nitrogen concentration in the expired air after a single previous inspiration of pure oxygen. This record can be used to calculate dead space, as discussed in the text.

$$\frac{30}{30+70} \times 500 = 150\,\text{mL}$$

Normal Dead Space Volume. The normal dead space air in a young adult man is about 150 mL. Dead space air increases slightly with age.

Anatomical Versus Physiological Dead Space

Anatomical Dead Space. The method just described for measuring the dead space measures the volume of all the space of the respiratory system other than the alveoli and their other closely related gas exchange areas; this space is called the *anatomical dead space.*

Physiological Dead Space. On occasion, some of the alveoli themselves are nonfunctional or only partially functional because of absent or poor blood flow through the adjacent pulmonary capillaries. Therefore, from a functional point of view, these alveoli must also be considered dead space. When the alveolar dead space is included in the total measurement of dead space, this is called the *physiological dead space,* in contradistinction to the anatomical dead space.

In a normal person, the anatomical and physiological dead spaces are nearly equal because all alveoli are functional in the normal lung, but in a person with partially functional or nonfunctional alveoli in some parts of the lungs, the physiological dead space may be as much as 10 times the volume of the anatomical dead space, or 1–2 L. These problems are discussed further in Chapter 56 in relation to pulmonary gaseous exchange and in Chapter 64 in relation to certain pulmonary diseases.

BIBLIOGRAPHY

Ayas NT, Zakynthinos S, Roussos C, Par PA: Respiratory system mechanics and energetics. In Murray, Nadel's, editors: *Textbook of Respiratory Medicine,* sixth ed., Philadelphia, 2015, Saunders Elsevier.

Daniels CB, Orgeig S: Pulmonary surfactant: the key to the evolution of air breathing, *News Physiol. Sci.* 18:151, 2003.

Fahy JV, Dickey BF: Airway mucus function and dysfunction, *N. Engl. J. Med.* 363:2233, 2010.

Henderson WR, Sheel AW: Pulmonary mechanics during mechanical ventilation, *Respir. Physiol. Neurobiol.* 180:162, 2012.

Lai-Fook SJ: Pleural mechanics and fluid exchange, *Physiol. Rev.* 84:385, 2004.

Lalley PM: The aging respiratory system—pulmonary structure, function and neural control, *Respir. Physiol. Neurobiol.* 187:199, 2013.

Lopez-Rodriguez E, Pérez-Gil J: Structure–function relationships in pulmonary surfactant membranes: from biophysics to therapy, *Biochim. Biophys. Acta* 1838:1568, 2014.

Powell FL, Hopkins SR: Comparative physiology of lung complexity: implications for gas exchange, *News Physiol. Sci.* 19:55, 2004.

Suki B, Sato S, Parameswaran H, et al: Emphysema and mechanical stress-induced lung remodeling, *Physiology (Bethesda)* 28:404, 2013.

Wagner PD, Powell FL, West JB: Ventilation, blood flow, and gas exchange. In Murray, Nadel's, editors: *Textbook of Respiratory Medicine,* sixth ed., Philadelphia, 2015, Saunders Elsevier.

West JB: *Respiratory Physiology,* ninth ed., Philadelphia, 2012, Lippincott Williams & Wilkins, Wolters Kluwers.

Widdicombe J: Reflexes from the lungs and airways: historical perspective, *J. Appl. Physiol.* 101:628, 2006.

Widdicombe J: Lung afferent activity: implications for respiratory sensation, *Respir. Physiol. Neurobiol.* 167:2, 2009.

Wright JR: Pulmonary surfactant: a front line of lung host defense, *J. Clin. Invest.* 111:1453, 2003.

55

Lung Volumes and Capacities

GLOSSARY OF TERMS

- **Anaphylaxis:** A type of allergic reaction that is rapidly progressive and could be fatal
- **Asthenic:** Pertaining to a condition of weakness or an individual who is very slim and feeble
- **Functional residual capacity:** The volume of air that remains in the lungs at the end of each normal expiration
- **Kyphosis:** The forward deformity of the spine also known as "hunchback"
- **Microemboli:** Small emboli or blood clots that travel in the blood stream
- **Peak expiratory flow rate:** The maximum flow rate that is attained during a forceful expiratory effort
- **Scoliosis:** A condition where there is a lateral deviation deformity in the curvature of the spine
- **Silicosis:** A progressive lung disease that results from the exposure to particles of silica from sand, rocks, or similar substances
- **Spirometry:** A lung function test to measure the lung volumes and capacities using an instrument called a spirometer
- **Tuberculosis:** An infectious disease caused by *Mycobacterium tuberculosis* that primarily affects the lungs and could be potentially fatal

Pulmonary Volumes and Capacities

RECORDING CHANGES IN PULMONARY VOLUME—SPIROMETRY

Pulmonary ventilation can be studied by recording the volume movement of air into and out of the lungs by a method called *spirometry*. A typical basic spirometer is shown in Figure 55-1. It consists of a drum inverted over a chamber of water, with the drum counterbalanced by a weight. In the drum is a breathing gas, usually air or oxygen; a tube connects the mouth with the gas chamber. When one breathes into and out of the chamber, the drum rises and falls, and an appropriate recording is made on a moving sheet of paper.

Figure 55-2 shows a spirogram indicating changes in lung volume under different conditions of breathing. For ease in describing the events of pulmonary ventilation, the air in the lungs has been subdivided in this diagram into four *volumes* and four *capacities*, which are the average for a *young adult man*. Table 55-1 summarizes the volumes and capacities.

Pulmonary Volumes

To the left in Figure 55-2 are listed four pulmonary lung volumes that, when added together, equal the maximum volume to which the lungs can be expanded. The significance of each of these volumes is the following:

1. The *tidal volume* is the volume of air inspired or expired with each normal breath; it amounts to about 500 mL in the adult male.
2. The *inspiratory reserve volume* is the extra volume of air that can be inspired over and above the normal tidal volume when the person inspires with full force; it is usually equal to about 3000 mL.
3. The *expiratory reserve volume* (ERV) is the maximum extra volume of air that can be expired by forceful expiration after the end of a normal tidal expiration; this volume normally amounts to about 1100 mL.
4. The *residual volume* (RV) is the volume of air remaining in the lungs after the most forceful expiration; this volume averages about 1200 mL.

Pulmonary Capacities

In describing events in the pulmonary cycle, it is sometimes desirable to consider two or more of the volumes together. Such combinations are called *pulmonary capacities*. To the right in Figure 55-2 are listed the important pulmonary capacities, which can be described as follows:

1. The *inspiratory capacity* (IC) equals the *tidal volume* plus the *inspiratory reserve volume*. This capacity is the amount of air (about 3500 mL) a person can breathe in, beginning at the normal expiratory level and distending the lungs to the maximum amount.
2. The *functional residual capacity* (FRC) equals the *ERV* plus the *RV*. This capacity is the amount of air that remains in the lungs at the end of normal expiration (about 2300 mL).
3. The *vital capacity* equals the *inspiratory reserve volume* plus the *tidal volume* plus the *ERV*. This capacity is the maximum amount of air a person can expel from the lungs after first filling the lungs to their maximum extent and then expiring to the maximum extent (about 4600 mL).
4. The *total lung capacity* (TLC) is the maximum volume to which the lungs can be expanded with the greatest possible effort (about 5800 mL); it is equal to the *vital capacity* plus the *RV*.

All pulmonary volumes and capacities are usually about 20–25% less in women than in men, and they are greater in large and athletic people than in small and asthenic people.

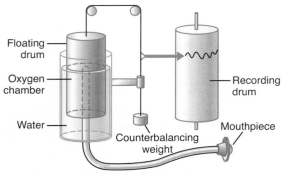

Floating drum

Oxygen chamber

Water

Counterbalancing weight

Recording drum

Mouthpiece

Figure 55-1 Spirometer.

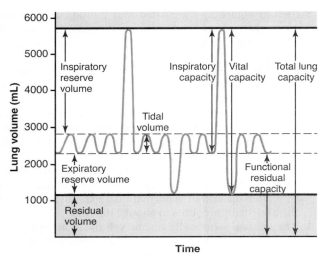

Figure 55-2 Diagram showing respiratory excursions during normal breathing and during maximal inspiration and maximal expiration.

TABLE 55-1	**Lung Volumes and Capacities**	
	Pulmonary Volumes	**Normal Values (mL)**
01	Tidal volume	~500
02	Inspiratory reserve volume	~3000
03	Expiratory reserve volume	~1100
04	Residual volume	~1200
	Pulmonary Capacities	**Normal Values (mL)**
01	Inspiratory capacity	~3500
02	Functional residual capacity	~2300
03	Vital capacity	~4600
04	Total lung capacity	~5800

ABBREVIATIONS AND SYMBOLS USED IN PULMONARY FUNCTION STUDIES

Spirometry is only one of many measurement procedures that the pulmonary physician uses daily. Many of these measurement procedures depend heavily on mathematical computations. To simplify these calculations, as well as the presentation of pulmonary function data, several abbreviations and symbols have become standardized. The more important

of these are given in Table 55-2. Using these symbols, we present here a few simple algebraic exercises showing some of the interrelations among the pulmonary volumes and capacities; the student should think through and verify these interrelations.

$$VC = IRV + V_T + ERV$$

$$VC = IC + ERV$$

$$TLC = VC + RV$$

$$TLC = IC + FRC$$

$$FRC = ERV + RV$$

DETERMINATION OF FUNCTIONAL RESIDUAL CAPACITY, RESIDUAL VOLUME, AND TOTAL LUNG CAPACITY—HELIUM DILUTION METHOD

Definition. The FRC, which is the volume of air that remains in the lungs at the end of each normal expiration, is important to lung function.

Because its value changes markedly in some types of pulmonary disease, it is often desirable to measure this capacity. The spirometer cannot be used in a direct way to measure the FRC because the air in the RV of the lungs cannot be expired into the spirometer and this volume constitutes about one-half of the FRC. To measure FRC, the spirometer must be used in an indirect manner, usually by means of a helium dilution method, as given in the next section (Figure 55-3).

Method.

1. A spirometer of known volume is filled with air mixed with helium at a known concentration.
2. Before breathing from the spirometer, the person expires normally. At the end of this expiration, the remaining volume in the lungs is equal to the FRC.
3. At this point, the subject immediately begins to breathe from the spirometer, and the gases of the spirometer mix with the gases of the lungs.
4. As a result, the helium becomes diluted by the FRC of gases and the volume of the FRC can be calculated from the degree of dilution of the helium, using the following formula:

$$FRC = \left(\frac{Ci_{He}}{Cf_{He}} - 1 \right) Vi_{Spir}$$

where FRC is functional residual capacity, Ci_{He} is initial concentration of helium in the spirometer, Cf_{He} is final concentration of helium in the spirometer, and Vi_{Spir} is initial volume of the spirometer.

Once the FRC has been determined, the RV can be determined by subtracting ERV, as measured by normal spirometry, from the FRC. Also, the TLC can be determined by adding the IC to the FRC. That is,

$$RV = FRC - ERV$$

and

$$TLC = FRC + IC$$

TABLE 55-2	Abbreviations and Symbols for Pulmonary Function		
V_T	Tidal volume	P_B	Atmospheric pressure
FRC	Functional residual capacity	Palv	Alveolar pressure
ERV	Expiratory reserve volume	Ppl	Pleural pressure
RV	Residual volume	P_{O_2}	Partial pressure of oxygen
IC	Inspiratory capacity	P_{CO_2}	Partial pressure of carbon dioxide
IRV	Inspiratory reserve volume	P_{N_2}	Partial pressure of nitrogen
TLC	Total lung capacity	Pa_{O_2}	Partial pressure of oxygen in arterial blood
VC	Vital capacity	Pa_{CO_2}	Partial pressure of carbon dioxide in arterial blood
Raw	Resistance of the airways to flow of air into the lung	PA_{O_2}	Partial pressure of oxygen in alveolar gas
C	Compliance	PA_{CO_2}	Partial pressure of carbon dioxide in alveolar gas
$\dot{V}_D$	Volume of dead space gas	PA_{H_2O}	Partial pressure of water in alveolar gas
$\dot{V}_A$	Volume of alveolar gas	R	Respiratory exchange ratio
$\dot{V}_I$	Inspired volume of ventilation per minute	$\dot{Q}$	Cardiac output
$\dot{V}_E$	Expired volume of ventilation per minute		
$\dot{V}_S$	Shunt flow		
$\dot{V}_A$	Alveolar ventilation per minute	Ca_{O_2}	Concentration of oxygen in arterial blood
$\dot{V}_{O_2}$	Rate of oxygen uptake per minute	$C\bar{v}\text{-}_{O_2}$	Concentration of oxygen in mixed venous blood
$\dot{V}_{CO_2}$	Amount of carbon dioxide eliminated per minute	S_{O_2}	Percentage saturation of hemoglobin with oxygen
$\dot{V}_{CO}$	Rate of carbon monoxide uptake per minute	Sa_{O_2}	Percentage saturation of hemoglobin with oxygen in arterial blood
DL_{O_2}	Diffusing capacity of the lungs for oxygen		
DL_{CO}	Diffusing capacity of the lungs for carbon monoxide		

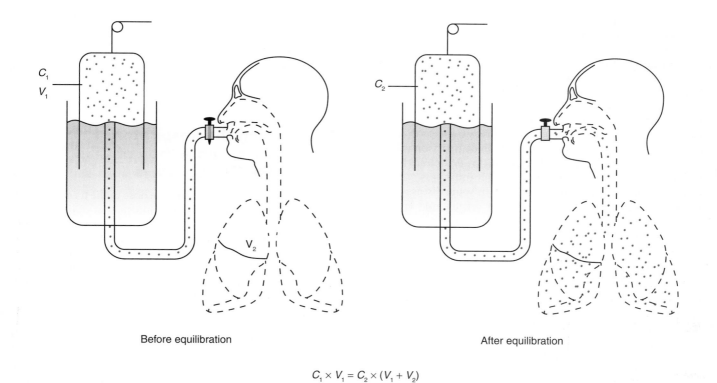

Before equilibration   After equilibration

$$C_1 \times V_1 = C_2 \times (V_1 + V_2)$$

Figure 55-3 Diagram to illustrate measurement of residual volume and functional residual capacity. *Modified from West, J.B., 2008. Respiratory Physiology: The Essentials, eighth ed. Lippincott Williams & Wilkins, Philadelphia.*

Functions of the Respiratory Passageways

TRACHEA, BRONCHI, AND BRONCHIOLES

Figure 55-3 highlights the respiratory passageways. The air is distributed to the lungs by way of the trachea, bronchi, and bronchioles.

One of the most important challenges in the respiratory passageways is to keep them open and allow easy passage of air to and from the alveoli. To keep the trachea from collapsing, multiple cartilage rings extend about five-sixths of the way around the trachea. In the walls of the bronchi, less extensive curved cartilage plates also maintain a reasonable amount of rigidity yet allow sufficient motion for the lungs to expand and contract. These plates become progressively less extensive in the later generations of bronchi and are gone in the bronchioles, which usually have diameters less than 1.5 mm. The bronchioles are not prevented from collapsing by the rigidity of their walls. Instead, they are kept expanded mainly by the same transpulmonary pressures that expand the alveoli. That is, as the alveoli enlarge, the bronchioles also enlarge, but not as much.

Muscular Wall of the Bronchi and Bronchioles and its Control. In all areas of the *trachea* and *bronchi* not occupied by cartilage plates, the walls are composed mainly of smooth muscle. Also, the walls of the *bronchioles* are almost entirely smooth muscle, with the exception of the most terminal bronchiole, called the *respiratory bronchiole*, which is mainly pulmonary epithelium and underlying fibrous tissue plus a few smooth muscle fibers. Many obstructive diseases of the lung result from narrowing of the smaller bronchi and larger bronchioles, often because of excessive contraction of the smooth muscle.

Airway Resistance

Resistance to Airflow in the Bronchial Tree. Under *normal respiratory conditions*, air flows through the respiratory passageways so easily that less than 1 cm H_2O pressure gradient from the alveoli to the atmosphere is sufficient to cause enough airflow for quiet breathing. The greatest amount of resistance to airflow occurs not in the minute air passages of the terminal bronchioles but in some of the larger bronchioles and bronchi near the trachea. The reason for this high resistance is that there are relatively few of these larger bronchi in comparison with the approximately 65,000 parallel terminal bronchioles, through each of which only a minute amount of air must pass.

Determinants of Airway Resistance. In some disease conditions, the smaller bronchioles play a far greater role in determining airflow resistance because of their small size and because they are easily occluded by (Box 55-1):

- muscle contraction in their walls,
- edema occurring in the walls, or
- mucus collecting in the lumens of the bronchioles.

BOX 55-1   DETERMINANTS OF AIRWAY RESISTANCE

- Diameter of airways
- Tone of the smooth muscles lining the airways
- Lung volume
- Gas density and viscosity
- Edema of the airway lining
- Mucus collecting in the lumen

Nervous and Local Control of the Bronchiolar Musculature—"Sympathetic" Dilation of the Bronchioles. Direct control of the bronchioles by sympathetic nerve fibers is relatively weak because few of these fibers penetrate to the central portions of the lung. However, the bronchial tree is very much exposed to *norepinephrine* and *epinephrine* released into the blood by sympathetic stimulation of the adrenal gland medullae. Both these hormones, especially epinephrine because of its greater stimulation of *beta-adrenergic receptors*, cause dilation of the bronchial tree.

Parasympathetic Constriction of the Bronchioles. A few parasympathetic nerve fibers derived from the vagus nerves penetrate the lung parenchyma. These nerves secrete *acetylcholine* and, when activated, cause mild to moderate constriction of the bronchioles. When a disease process such as asthma has already caused some bronchiolar constriction, superimposed parasympathetic nervous stimulation often worsens the condition. When this situation occurs, administration of drugs that block the effects of acetylcholine, such as *atropine*, can sometimes relax the respiratory passages enough to relieve the obstruction.

Sometimes the parasympathetic nerves are also activated by reflexes that originate in the lungs. Most of these reflexes begin with irritation of the epithelial membrane of the respiratory passageways, initiated by noxious gases, dust, cigarette smoke, or bronchial infection. Also, a bronchiolar constrictor reflex often occurs when microemboli occlude small pulmonary arteries.

Local Secretory Factors May Cause Bronchiolar Constriction. Several substances formed in the lungs are often quite active in causing bronchiolar constriction. Two of the most important of these are *histamine* and *slow reactive substance of anaphylaxis*. Both of these substances are released in the lung tissues by *mast cells* during allergic reactions, especially those caused by pollen in the air. Therefore, they play key roles in causing the airway obstruction that occurs in allergic asthma; this is especially true of the slow reactive substance of anaphylaxis.

The same irritants that cause parasympathetic constrictor reflexes of the airways—smoke, dust, sulfur dioxide, and some of the acidic elements in smog—may also act directly on the lung tissues to initiate local, nonnervous reactions that cause obstructive constriction of the airways.

Mucus Lining the Respiratory Passageways, and Action of Cilia to Clear the Passageways

All the respiratory passages, from the nose to the terminal bronchioles, are kept moist by a layer of mucus that coats the entire surface. The mucus is secreted partly by individual mucous goblet cells in the epithelial lining of the passages and partly by small submucosal glands. In addition to keeping the surfaces moist, the mucus traps small particles out of the inspired air and keeps most of these particles from ever reaching the alveoli. The mucus is removed from the passages in the following manner.

The entire surface of the respiratory passages, both in the nose and in the lower passages down as far as the terminal bronchioles, is lined with ciliated epithelium, with about 200 cilia on each epithelial cell. These cilia beat continually at a rate of 10–20 times/second, and the direction of their "power stroke" is always toward the pharynx. That is, the cilia in the lungs beat upward, whereas those in the nose beat downward. This continual beating causes the coat of mucus to flow slowly, at a velocity of a few millimeters per

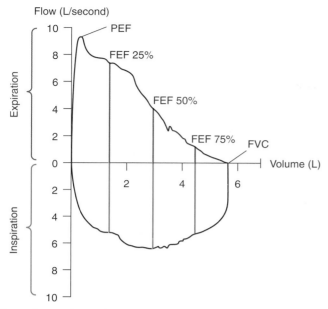

Figure 55-4 Flow–volume loop in a normal individual. *FEF,* forced expiratory flow; *FVC,* forced vital capacity; *PEF,* peak expiratory flow.

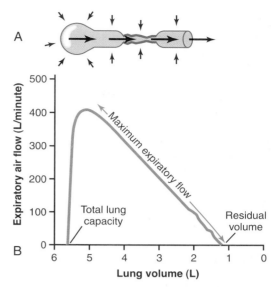

Figure 55-5 (A) Collapse of the respiratory passageway during maximum expiratory effort, an effect that limits expiratory flow rate. (B) Effect of lung volume on the maximum expiratory airflow, showing decreasing maximum expiratory airflow as the lung volume becomes smaller.

minute, toward the pharynx. Then the mucus and its entrapped particles are either swallowed or coughed to the exterior.

Flow–Volume Curves

Lung functions, more recently, are measured clinically using flow–volume curves or loops.

Definition. Flow–volume curves or loops are graphic representations of the relationship between maximal flow rates and volume of gas during a forced maneuver. This can be measured during either inspiration or expiration. In Figure 55-4, expiratory flow rates are shown above the horizontal line while inspiratory flow rates are shown below the horizontal line.

The flow–volume curves can be used to measure the following:
1. flow rates during expiration
2. peak expiratory flow rate (PEFR)
3. forced vital capacity (FVC)

FLOW RATES DURING EXPIRATION

The expiratory flow rates that can be measured include:
1. Forced expiratory flow 25% (FEF_{25}): The flow rate at which time point the vital capacity that has been exhaled is 25%
2. Forced expiratory flow 50% (FEF_{50}): The flow rate at which time point the remaining vital capacity that needs to be exhaled is 50%
3. Forced expiratory flow 75% (FEF_{75}): The flow rate at which time point the vital capacity that has been exhaled is 75%

MAXIMUM EXPIRATORY FLOW

Definition. When a person expires with great force, the expiratory airflow reaches a maximum flow beyond which the flow cannot be increased any more, even with greatly increased additional force. This is the maximal expiratory flow.

Peak Expiratory Flow Rate

The maximum flow rate that is attained during a forceful expiratory effort is called the PEFR.

In many respiratory diseases, and particularly in asthma, the resistance to airflow becomes especially high during expiration, sometimes causing tremendous difficulty in breathing. This condition has led to the concept called *maximal expiratory flow.* The maximal expiratory flow is much greater when the lungs are filled with a large volume of air than when they are almost empty. These principles can be understood by referring to Figure 55-5.

Figure 55-5A shows the effect of increased pressure applied to the outsides of the alveoli and air passageways caused by compressing the chest cage. The arrows indicate that the same pressure compresses the outsides of both the alveoli and the bronchioles. Therefore, not only does this pressure force air from the alveoli toward the bronchioles, but it also tends to collapse the bronchioles at the same time, which will oppose movement of air to the exterior. Once the bronchioles have almost completely collapsed, further expiratory force can still greatly increase the alveolar pressure, but it also increases the degree of bronchiolar collapse and airway resistance by an equal amount, thus preventing further increase in flow. Therefore, beyond a critical degree of expiratory force, a maximum expiratory flow has been reached.

Figure 55-5B shows the effect of different degrees of lung collapse (and therefore of bronchiolar collapse as well) on the maximum expiratory flow. The curve recorded in this section shows the maximum expiratory flow at all levels of lung volume after a healthy person first inhales as much air as possible and then expires with maximum expiratory effort until he or she can expire at no greater rate. Note that the person quickly reaches a *maximum expiratory airflow* of more than 400 L/minute. However, regardless of how much additional expiratory effort the person exerts, this is still the maximum flow rate that he or she can achieve.

Note also that as the lung volume becomes smaller, the maximum expiratory flow rate also becomes less. The main reason for this phenomenon is that in the enlarged lung the bronchi and bronchioles are held open partially by way of elastic pull on their outsides by lung structural elements; however, as the lung becomes smaller, these structures are relaxed so that the bronchi and bronchioles are collapsed more easily by external chest pressure, thus progressively reducing the maximum expiratory flow rate as well.

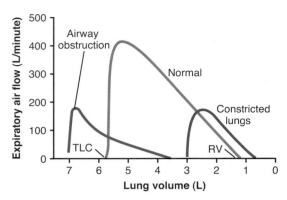

Figure 55-6 Effect of two respiratory abnormalities—constricted lungs and airway obstruction—on the maximum expiratory flow–volume curve. *RV*, residual volume; *TLC*, total lung capacity.

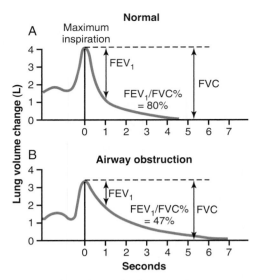

Figure 55-7 Recordings during the forced vital capacity maneuver: (A) in a healthy person and (B) in a person with partial airway obstruction. (The "zero" on the volume scale is residual volume.) *FEV₁*, forced expiratory volume during the first second; *FVC*, forced expiratory vital capacity.

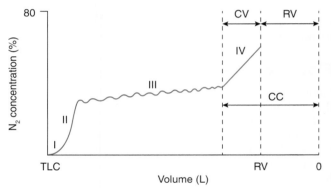

Figure 55-8 Nitrogen concentration in expired air after a single breath inhalation of 100% oxygen to measure closing volume. *CC*, closing capacity; *CV*, closing volume; *RV*, residual volume; *TLC*, total lung capacity. *Redrawn from Yao, F-S.F. (Ed.). Yao and Artusio's Anesthesiology: Problem-Oriented Patient Management, fourth ed. Lippincott Williams & Wilkins, Philadelphia, pp. 3–28, Chapter 1.*

Abnormalities of the Maximum Expiratory Flow–Volume Curve. Figure 55-6 shows the normal maximum expiratory flow–volume curve, along with two additional flow–volume curves recorded in two types of lung diseases: constricted lungs and partial airway obstruction. Note that the *constricted lungs* have both reduced TLC and reduced RV. Furthermore, because the lung cannot expand to a normal maximum volume, even with the greatest possible expiratory effort, the maximal expiratory flow cannot rise equal to that of the normal curve. Constricted lung diseases include fibrotic diseases of the lung, such as *tuberculosis* and *silicosis*, and diseases that constrict the chest cage, such as *kyphosis*, *scoliosis*, and *fibrotic pleurisy*.

In diseases with *airway obstruction*, it is usually much more difficult to expire than to inspire because the closing tendency of the airways is greatly increased by the extra positive pressure required in the chest to cause expiration. By contrast, the extra negative pleural pressure that occurs during inspiration actually "pulls" the airways open at the same time that it expands the alveoli. Therefore, air tends to enter the lung easily but then becomes trapped in the lungs. Over a period of months or years, this effect increases both the TLC and the RV, as shown by the green curve in Figure 55-6. Also, because of the obstruction of the airways and because they collapse more easily than normal airways, the maximum expiratory flow rate is greatly reduced.

The classic disease that causes severe airway obstruction is *asthma*. Serious airway obstruction also occurs in some stages of *emphysema*.

FORCED EXPIRATORY VITAL CAPACITY AND FORCED EXPIRATORY VOLUME

Another useful clinical pulmonary test, and one that is also simple, is to record on a spirometer the *forced expiratory vital capacity* (FVC). Such a recording is shown in Figure 55-7A for a person with normal lungs and in Figure 55-7B for a person with partial airway obstruction. In performing the FVC maneuver, the person first inspires maximally to the TLC and then exhales into the spirometer with maximum expiratory effort as rapidly and as completely as possible. The total distance of the downslope of the lung volume record represents the FVC, as shown in the figure.

Now, study the difference between the two records for (1) normal lungs and (2) *partial* airway obstruction. The total volume changes of the FVCs are not greatly different, indicating only a moderate difference in basic lung volumes in the two persons. There is, however, a *major difference in the amounts of air that these persons can expire each second*, especially during the first second. Therefore, it is customary to compare the recorded

forced expiratory volume during the first second (FEV_1) with the normal. In the normal person (see Figure 55-7A), the percentage of the FVC that is expired in the first second divided by the total FVC ($FEV_1/FVC\%$) is 80%. However, note in Figure 55-7B that, with airway obstruction, this value decreased to only 47%. In persons with serious airway obstruction, as often occurs with acute asthma, this value can decrease to less than 20%.

CLOSING VOLUME

Definition. The closing volume refers to the lung volume that coincides with the beginning of airway closure in the dependent parts of the lungs during expiration. In normal healthy individuals, the closing volume is usually less than the FRC and is above the RV.

The closing volume can be measured by using a similar apparatus as is used to measure anatomical dead space (Fowler method). The person is asked to inhale deeply (100% oxygen) from mid-inspiration and then exhales this steadily into an analyzer that measures nitrogen continuously. The curve is plotted and the closing volume can be determined as shown in Figure 55-8.

BIBLIOGRAPHY

Bel EH: Clinical practice. Mild asthma, *N. Engl. J. Med.* 369:549, 2013.

Booker R: Interpretation and evaluation of pulmonary function tests, *Nurs. Stand.* 23:46, 2009.

Brand PL, de Gooijer A, Postma DS: Changes in peak expiratory flow in healthy subjects and in patients with obstructive lung disease, *Eur. Respir. J. Suppl.* 24:69S, 1997.

Brochard L: What is a pressure–volume curve? *Crit. Care* 10(4):156, 2006.

Decramer M, Janssens W, Miravitlles M: Chronic obstructive pulmonary disease, *Lancet* 379:1341, 2012.

Guarnieri M, Balmes JR: Outdoor air pollution and asthma, *Lancet* 383:1581, 2014.

Heil M, Hazel AL, Smith JA: The mechanics of airway closure, *Respir. Physiol. Neurobiol.* 163:214, 2008.

Hilaire G, Duron B: Maturation of the mammalian respiratory system, *Physiol. Rev.* 79:325, 1999.

Kallet RH: Pressure–volume curves in the management of acute respiratory distress syndrome, *Respir. Care Clin. N. Am.* 9(3):321, 2003.

Lai-Fook SJ: Pleural mechanics and fluid exchange, *Physiol. Rev.* 84:385, 2004.

Lalley PM: The aging respiratory system—pulmonary structure, function and neural control, *Respir. Physiol. Neurobiol.* 187:199, 2013.

Milic-Emili J, Torchio R, D'Angelo E: Closing volume: a reappraisal (1967–2007), *Eur. J. Appl. Physiol.* 99(6):567, 2007.

Paton JF, Dutschmann M: Central control of upper airway resistance regulating respiratory airflow in mammals, *J. Anat.* 201:319, 2002.

Pavord ID, Chung KF: Management of chronic cough, *Lancet* 371:1375, 2008.

Powell FL, Hopkins SR: Comparative physiology of lung complexity: implications for gas exchange, *News Physiol. Sci.* 19:55, 2004.

Sharafkhaneh A, Hanania NA, Kim V: Pathogenesis of emphysema: from the bench to the bedside, *Proc. Am. Thorac. Soc.* 5:475, 2008.

Strohl KP, Butler JP, Malhotra A: Mechanical properties of the upper airway, *Compr. Physiol.* 2:1853, 2012.

Suki B, Sato S, Parameswaran H, et al: Emphysema and mechanical stress-induced lung remodeling, *Physiology (Bethesda)* 28:404, 2013.

Uhlig S, Taylor AE: *Methods in Pulmonary Research*, Basel, 1998, Springer Basel AG.

Voynow JA, Rubin BK: Mucins, mucus, and sputum, *Chest* 135:505, 2009.

West JB: *Respiratory Physiology*, ninth ed., Philadelphia, 2012, Lippincott Williams & Wilkins, Wolters Kluwers.

Widdicombe J: Reflexes from the lungs and airways: historical perspective, *J. Appl. Physiol.* 101:628, 2006.

56

Ventilation

LEARNING OBJECTIVES

- Define minute respiratory volume, alveolar ventilation, maximum voluntary ventilation, and breathing reserve.
- Describe the relation of alveolar ventilation to partial pressures of oxygen and carbon dioxide in blood.
- List the causes of hypoventilation and hyperventilation.

GLOSSARY OF TERMS

- **Alveolar ventilation:** Alveolar ventilation per minute is defined as the total volume of new air entering the alveoli and adjacent gas exchange areas each minute (it does not include dead space air)
- **Breathing reserve:** The difference in maximum voluntary ventilation and the maximal ventilation measured during exercise
- **Maximum voluntary ventilation:** The largest volume of air that an individual can breathe into and out of the lungs in 1 minute with maximum voluntary effort
- **Minute respiratory volume:** The total amount of new air moved into the respiratory passages each minute (it includes the dead space air)
- **Partial pressure:** The total pressure exerted by a mixture of gases being the sum of all the individual pressures exerted by each gas in the mixture (the individual pressures are referred to as "partial pressure" for each gas)

Minute Respiratory Volume (Minute Ventilation)

As discussed earlier in Chapter 54, the *minute respiratory volume* is the total amount of new air moved into the respiratory passages each minute:

Minute respiratory
volume (minute ventilation) = tidal volume × respiratory rate
= 500 mL (tidal volume)
× 12 minute^{-1} (respiratory rate)

Therefore

Minute ventilation = 6000 mL/minute (or 6 L/minute)

It should be understood that not all of this volume of gas is available for gas exchange, as the dead space volume is included in the tidal volume.

A person can live for a short period with a minute respiratory volume as low as 1.5 L/minute and a respiratory rate of only 2–4 breaths/minute.

The respiratory rate occasionally rises to 40–50 minute^{-1}, and the tidal volume can become as great as the vital capacity,

about 4600 mL in a young adult man. This can give a minute respiratory volume greater than 200 L/minute, or more than 30 times normal. Most people cannot sustain more than one-half to two-thirds of these values for longer than 1 minute.

Alveolar Ventilation

The rate at which new air reaches the alveoli, alveolar sacs, alveolar ducts, and respiratory bronchioles is called *alveolar ventilation*. The ultimate importance of pulmonary ventilation is to continually renew the air in the gas exchange areas of the lungs, where air is in proximity to the pulmonary blood.

RATE OF ALVEOLAR VENTILATION

Alveolar ventilation per minute is the total volume of new air entering the alveoli and adjacent gas exchange areas each minute. It is equal to the respiratory rate times the amount of new air that enters these areas with each breath (Figure 56-1):

$$\dot{V}_A = \text{Freq} \times (V_T - V_D)$$

where $\dot{V}_A$ is the volume of alveolar ventilation per minute, "Freq" is the frequency of respiration per minute, V_T is the tidal volume, and V_D is the physiological dead space volume.

Thus, with a normal tidal volume of 500 mL, a normal dead space of 150 mL, and a respiratory rate of 12 breaths/minute, alveolar ventilation equals $12 \times (500 - 150)$, or 4200 mL/minute.

Table 56-1 explains the importance of alveolar ventilation and compares this with minute ventilation and anatomical dead space ventilation in three different subjects with different frequencies and depth of respiration. From Table 56-1, it is clear that alveolar ventilation is one of the major factors determining the concentrations of oxygen and carbon dioxide in the alveoli. Therefore, almost all discussions of gaseous exchange in the following chapters on the respiratory system emphasize alveolar ventilation.

Maximum Voluntary Ventilation

Maximum voluntary ventilation (MVV) is the largest volume of air that an individual can breathe into and out of the lungs in 1 minute with maximum voluntary effort.

The measurement of maximum voluntary ventilation is a nonspecific method to assess the function of ventilation. It is usually measured for about 10–15 seconds and then extrapolated for 1 minute. For example, the MVV can be calculated from the following equation setup for a 10-second maneuver:

$$\text{MVV} = \text{volume measured (in 10 seconds)} \times \frac{60 \text{ seconds}}{10 \text{ seconds}}$$
$$= \text{volume measured (in 10 seconds)} \times 6$$

MVV is usually expressed in liters per minute.

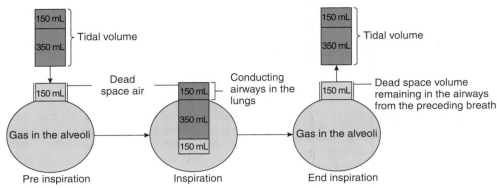

Figure 56-1   Alveolar ventilation. *Modified from Widmaier, E.P., Raff, H., Strang, K.T., 2005. Vander's Human Physiology: The Mechanisms of Body Function, 10th ed. McGraw-Hill, New York.*

TABLE 56-1	Comparison of Alveolar Ventilation with Minute Ventilation and Anatomical Dead Space Ventilation				
Subject	Tidal Volume (mL)	Respiratory Rate (breath/minute)	Anatomical Dead Space Ventilation (mL)	Minute Ventilation (mL)	Alveolar Ventilation (mL)
Subject 1	150	×40	150 × 40 = 6000	6000	0
Subject 2	500	×12	150 × 12 = 1800	6000	4200
Subject 3	1000	×6	150 × 6 = 900	6000	5100

Table 56-1 is a modified version of Table 13-5 from Widmaier, E.P., Raff, H., Strang, K.T., 2005. Vander's Human Physiology: The Mechanisms of Body Function, 10th ed. McGraw-Hill, New York.

Breathing Reserve

Breathing reserve (BR) is the difference in MVV and the maximal ventilation measured during exercise. It can be calculated using the following formulae:

$$BR \; (L/minute) = MVV - maximum \; ventilation \; during \; exercise$$

$$BR = (MVV - maximum \; ventilation)/MVV \times 100$$

The normal BR is between 20 and 50% of the MVV. Individuals with low BR may be limited in their exercise capacity due to limited ventilatory capacity.

Gas Pressures in a Mixture of Gases—"Partial Pressures" of Individual Gases

Pressure is caused by multiple impacts of moving molecules against a surface. Therefore, the pressure of gas acting on the surfaces of the respiratory passages and alveoli is proportional to the summated force of impact of all the molecules of that gas striking the surface at any given instant. This means that *the pressure is directly proportional to the concentration of the gas molecules.*

In respiratory physiology, one deals with mixtures of gases, mainly *oxygen*, *nitrogen*, and *carbon dioxide*. The rate of diffusion of each of these gases is directly proportional to the pressure caused by that gas alone, which is called the *partial pressure* of that gas. The concept of partial pressure can be explained as follows.

Consider air, which has an approximate composition of 79% nitrogen and 21% oxygen. The total pressure of this mixture at sea level averages 760 mmHg. It is clear from the preceding description of the molecular basis of pressure that each gas contributes to the total pressure in direct proportion to its concentration. Therefore, 79% of the 760 mmHg is caused by nitrogen (600 mmHg) and 21% by O_2 (160 mmHg). Thus, the "partial pressure" of nitrogen in the mixture is 600 mmHg and the "partial pressure" of O_2 is 160 mmHg; the total pressure is 760 mmHg, the sum of the individual partial pressures. The partial pressures of individual gases in a mixture are designated by the symbols PO_2, PCO_2, PN_2, PH_2, and so forth.

Pressures of Gases Dissolved in Water and Tissues

Gases dissolved in water or in body tissues also exert pressure because the dissolved gas molecules are moving randomly and have kinetic energy. Further, when the gas dissolved in fluid encounters a surface, such as the membrane of a cell, it exerts its own partial pressure in the same way that a gas in the gas phase does. The partial pressures of the separate dissolved gases are designated the same as the partial pressures in the gas state, that is, PO_2, PCO_2, PN_2, PH_e, and so forth.

Factors that Determine the Partial Pressure of a Gas Dissolved in a Fluid. The partial pressure of a gas in a solution is determined not only by its concentration but also by the *solubility coefficient* of the gas. That is, some types of molecules, especially CO_2, are physically or chemically attracted to water molecules, whereas other types of molecules are repelled. When molecules are attracted, far more of them can be dissolved without building up excess partial pressure within the solution. Conversely, in the case of molecules that are repelled, high partial pressure will develop with fewer dissolved molecules.

These relations are expressed by the following formula, which is *Henry's law*:

$$\text{Partial pressure} = \frac{\text{concentration of dissolved gas}}{\text{solubility coefficient}}$$

When partial pressure is expressed in atmospheres (1 atm pressure equals 760 mmHg) and concentration is expressed in volume of gas dissolved in each volume of water, the solubility coefficients for important respiratory gases at body temperature are the following:

Oxygen	0.024
Carbon dioxide	0.57
Carbon monoxide	0.018
Nitrogen	0.012
Helium	0.008

From this table, one can see that CO_2 is more than 20 times as soluble as O_2. Therefore, the partial pressure of CO_2 (for a given concentration) is less than one-twentieth that exerted by O_2.

Relationship Between Alveolar Ventilation and Partial Pressures of Oxygen and Carbon Dioxide

OXYGEN CONCENTRATION AND PARTIAL PRESSURE IN THE ALVEOLI

Oxygen is continually being absorbed from the alveoli into the blood of the lungs, and new oxygen is continually being breathed into the alveoli from the atmosphere. The more rapidly O_2 is absorbed, the lower its concentration in the alveoli becomes; conversely, the more rapidly new O_2 is breathed into the alveoli from the atmosphere, the higher its concentration becomes. Therefore, O_2 concentration in the alveoli, as well as its partial pressure, is controlled by (1) the rate of absorption of O_2 into the blood and (2) the rate of entry of new O_2 into the lungs by the ventilatory process.

Figure 56-2 shows the effect of alveolar ventilation and rate of O_2 absorption into the blood on the alveolar partial pressure of O_2 (PO_2). One curve represents O_2 absorption at a rate of 250 mL/minute, and the other curve represents a rate of 1000 mL/minute. At a normal ventilatory rate of 4.2 L/minute and an O_2 consumption of 250 mL/minute, the normal operating point in Figure 56-2 is point A. The figure also shows that when 1000 mL of O_2 is being absorbed each minute, as occurs during moderate exercise, the rate of alveolar ventilation must increase fourfold to maintain the alveolar PO_2 at the normal value of 104 mmHg.

Another effect shown in Figure 56-2 is that even an extreme increase in alveolar ventilation can never increase the alveolar PO_2 above 149 mmHg as long as the person is breathing normal atmospheric air at sea level pressure because this 149 mmHg is the maximum PO_2 in humidified air at this pressure. If the person breathes gases that contain partial pressures of O_2 higher than 149 mmHg, the alveolar PO_2 can approach these higher pressures at high rates of ventilation.

CO_2 CONCENTRATION AND PARTIAL PRESSURE IN THE ALVEOLI

Carbon dioxide is continually formed in the body and then carried in the blood to the alveoli, and it is continually removed

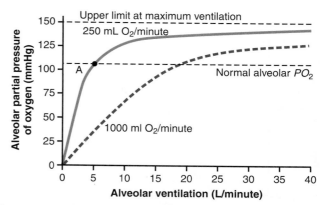

Figure 56-2 Effect of alveolar ventilation on the alveolar PO_2 at two rates of oxygen absorption from the alveoli—250 and 1000 mL/minute. *Point A* is the normal operating point.

from the alveoli by ventilation. Figure 56-3 shows the effects on the alveolar partial pressure of CO_2 (PCO_2) of both alveolar ventilation and two rates of CO_2 excretion, 200 and 800 mL/minute. One curve represents a normal rate of CO_2 excretion of 200 mL/minute. At the normal rate of alveolar ventilation of 4.2 L/minute, the operating point for alveolar PCO_2 is at point A in Figure 56-3 (ie, 40 mmHg).

Two other facts are also evident from Figure 56-3: First, *the alveolar PCO_2 increases directly in proportion to the rate of CO_2 excretion*, as represented by the fourfold elevation of the curve (when 800 mL of CO_2 is excreted per minute). Second, *the alveolar PCO_2 decreases in inverse proportion to alveolar ventilation.* Therefore, the concentrations and partial pressures of both O_2 and CO_2 in the alveoli are determined by the rates of absorption or excretion of the two gases and by the amount of alveolar ventilation.

EXPIRED AIR IS A COMBINATION OF DEAD SPACE AIR AND ALVEOLAR AIR

The overall composition of expired air is determined by (1) the amount of the expired air that is dead space air and (2) the amount that is alveolar air. Figure 56-4 shows the progressive changes in O_2 and CO_2 partial pressures in the expired air during

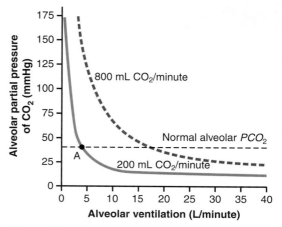

Figure 56-3 Effect of alveolar ventilation on the alveolar PCO_2 at two rates of carbon dioxide excretion from the blood—800 and 200 mL/minute. *Point A* is the normal operating point.

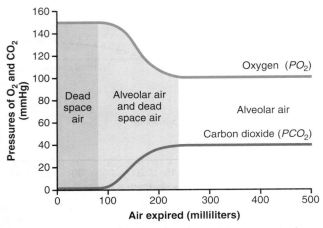

Figure 56-4 Oxygen and carbon dioxide partial pressures in the various portions of normal expired air.

the course of expiration. The first portion of this air, the dead space air from the respiratory passageways, is typical humidified air, as shown in Table 59-1. Then, progressively more and more alveolar air becomes mixed with the dead space air until all the dead space air has finally been washed out and nothing but alveolar air is expired at the end of expiration. Therefore, the method of collecting alveolar air for study is simply to collect a sample of the last portion of the expired air after forceful expiration has removed all the dead space air.

Normal expired air, containing both dead space air and alveolar air, has gas concentrations and partial pressures approximately as shown in Table 59-1 (ie, concentrations between those of alveolar air and humidified atmospheric air).

Causes of Hypoventilation and Hyperventilation

The partial pressure of carbon dioxide is dependent on the ratio of the rate of carbon dioxide production to that of alveolar ventilation:

$$PCO_2 = \frac{\text{carbon dioxide production}}{\text{alveolar ventilation}}$$

Similarly, the partial pressure of oxygen is dependent on ratio of the rate of oxygen consumption to that of alveolar ventilation:

$$PO_2 = \frac{\text{oxygen consumption}}{\text{alveolar ventilation}}$$

HYPOVENTILATION

When there is an increase in the ratio of carbon dioxide production to that of alveolar ventilation, alveolar ventilation cannot keep pace with carbon dioxide production. This state is referred to as "hypoventilation" or "alveolar hypoventilation."

The normal range of arterial PCO_2 is between 37 and 43 mmHg. In clinical states of hypoventilation, the arterial PCO_2 increases beyond 45 mmHg and could increase up to 50–70 mmHg.

Some of the conditions that can cause hypoventilation are listed in Table 56-2.

HYPERVENTILATION

When there is a decrease in the ratio of carbon dioxide production to that of alveolar ventilation, alveolar ventilation is too high for the amount of carbon dioxide production. This state is referred to as "hyperventilation" or "alveolar hypoventilation."

The normal range of arterial PCO_2 is between 37 and 43 mmHg. In clinical states of hyperventilation, the arterial PCO_2 decreases below this normal range of 37–43 mmHg. Dyspnea or difficulty in breathing may be commonly associated with hyperventilation.

Hyperventilation should be differentiated from other conditions, such as tachypnea, where there is just an increase in the respiratory rate, or from hyperpnea where the minute ventilation is increased.

Both these conditions may not be associated with any change in arterial PCO_2.

Some of the conditions that can cause hyperventilation are listed in Table 56-2.

TABLE 56-2	Summary of Causes of Hypoventilation and Hyperventilation	
Hypoventilation	**Hyperventilation**
1. Chronic obstructive lung diseases	1. Acidosis
2. Sleep apnea syndromes	2. Pulmonary disorders such as pneumonia and bronchial asthma
3. Tracheal or laryngeal stenosis	3. Congestive cardiac failure
4. Bulbar poliomyelitis	4. CNS disorders such as infarctions, infections, or tumors
5. Primary alveolar hypoventilation syndrome	5. States of hypoxemia due to high altitude or lung diseases
6. Metabolic alkalosis	6. Hyperthyroidism
7. Prolonged hypoxia	7. Other causes such as sepsis and fever
8. Carotid body trauma and dysfunction	8. Pregnancy
9. Kyphoscoliosis	

BIBLIOGRAPHY

Anthony M: The obesity hypoventilation syndrome, *Respir. Care* 53:1723, 2008.

Glenny RW, Robertson HT: Spatial distribution of ventilation and perfusion: mechanisms and regulation, *Compr. Physiol.* 1:375, 2011.

Hopkins SR, Wielpütz MO, Kauczor HU: Imaging lung perfusion, *J. Appl. Physiol.* 113:328, 2012.

Hughes JM, Pride NB: Examination of the carbon monoxide diffusing capacity (DL(CO)) in relation to its KCO and VA components, *Am. J. Respir. Crit. Care Med.* 186:132, 2012.

Klocke R: Dead space: simplicity to complexity, *J. Appl. Physiol.* 100:1, 2006.

Madama VC: Maximal voluntary ventilation, test for pulmonary mechanics, second revised ed., Pulmonary Function Testing and Cardiopulmonary Stress Testing. Albany, NY, 1998, Delmar Cengage Learning.

Mason RJ, Broaddus CV, Martin T, et al: Hypoventilation and hyperventilation syndromes, sixth ed., Murray and Nadel's Textbook of Respiratory Medicine. Philadelphia, 2015, Saunders Elsevier.

McConnell AK, Romer LM: Dyspnoea in health and obstructive pulmonary disease: the role of respiratory muscle function and training, *Sports Med.* 34:117, 2004.

Powell FL, Hopkins SR: Comparative physiology of lung complexity: implications for gas exchange, *News Physiol. Sci.* 19:55, 2004.

Rahn H, Farhi EE: Ventilation, perfusion, and gas exchange—the Va/Q concept, Fenn WO, Rahn H, editors: *Handbook of Physiology. Section 3*, vol. 1, Baltimore, 1964, Williams & Wilkins, pp 125.

Robertson HT, Buxton RB: Imaging for lung physiology: what do we wish we could measure? *J. Appl. Physiol.* 113:317, 2012.

Uhlig S, Taylor AE: *Methods in Pulmonary Research*, Basel, 1998, Springer Basel AG.

Wasserman K: Breathing reserve, measurements during integrative cardiopulmonary exercise testing, fifth Rev ed., Principles of Exercise Testing and Interpretation: Including Pathophysiology and Clinical Applications. Philadelphia, 2011, Lippincott Williams & Wilkins, Wolters Kluwers.

West JB: *Respiratory Physiology*, ninth ed., Philadelphia, 2012, Lippincott Williams & Wilkins, Wolters Kluwers.

Widdicombe J: Reflexes from the lungs and airways: historical perspective, *J. Appl. Physiol.* 101:628, 2006.

Widmaier EP, Raff H, Strang KT: *Vander's Human Physiology: The Mechanisms of Body Function*, 13th Rev ed., Columbus, 2013, McGraw-Hill Publications.

57 Pulmonary Circulation

The lung has two types of circulations and these are listed as follows:

1. *A high-pressure, low-flow circulation* supplies systemic arterial blood to the trachea, the bronchial tree (including the terminal bronchioles), the supporting tissues of the lung, and the outer coats (adventitia) of the pulmonary arteries and veins.

2. *A low-pressure, high-flow circulation* supplies venous blood from all parts of the body to the alveolar capillaries where oxygen (O_2) is added and carbon dioxide (CO_2) is removed. The *pulmonary artery* (which receives blood from the right ventricle) and its arterial branches carry blood to the alveolar capillaries for gas exchange and the pulmonary veins then return the blood to the left atrium to be pumped by the left ventricle though the systemic circulation.

In this chapter we discuss the special aspects of the pulmonary circulation that are important for gas exchange in the lungs.

Physiological Anatomy of the Pulmonary Circulatory System

Pulmonary Vessels. The pulmonary artery extends only 5 cm beyond the apex of the right ventricle and then divides into right and left main branches that supply blood to the two respective lungs (Figure 57-1).

The pulmonary has a wall thickness one-third that of the aorta. The pulmonary arterial branches are short and all the pulmonary arteries, even the smaller arteries and arterioles, have larger diameters than their counterpart systemic arteries (Figure 57-2). This aspect, combined with the fact that the vessels are thin and distensible, gives the pulmonary arterial tree a *large compliance*, averaging almost 7 mL/mmHg, which is similar to that of the entire systemic arterial tree. This large compliance allows the pulmonary arteries to accommodate the stroke volume output of the right ventricle.

The pulmonary veins, like the pulmonary arteries, are also short. They immediately empty their effluent blood into the left atrium (Figure 57-2).

Bronchial Vessels. Blood also flows to the lungs through small bronchial arteries that originate from the systemic circulation, amounting to 1–2% of the total cardiac output (Figure 57-2). This bronchial arterial blood is *oxygenated* blood, in contrast to the partially deoxygenated blood in the pulmonary arteries. It supplies the supporting tissues of the lungs, including the connective tissue, septa, and large and small bronchi. After this bronchial and arterial blood passes through the supporting tissues, it empties into the pulmonary veins and *enters the left atrium*, rather than passing back to the right atrium. Therefore, the flow into the left atrium and the left ventricular output are about 1–2% greater than that of the right ventricular output.

Lymphatics. Lymph vessels are present in all the supportive tissues of the lung, beginning in the connective tissue spaces that surround the terminal bronchioles, coursing to the hilum of the lung, and then mainly into the *right thoracic lymph duct*. Particulate matter entering the alveoli is partly removed by way of these channels, and plasma protein leaking from the lung capillaries is also removed from the lung tissues, thereby helping to prevent pulmonary edema.

Pressures in the Pulmonary System

Pressures in the Right Ventricle. The pressure pulse curves of the right ventricle and pulmonary artery are shown in the lower portion of Figure 57-3. These curves are contrasted with the much higher aortic pressure curve shown in the upper portion of the figure. The systolic pressure in the right ventricle of the normal human averages about 25 mmHg and the diastolic pressure averages about 0–1 mmHg, values that are only one-fifth those for the left ventricle (Figure 57-4).

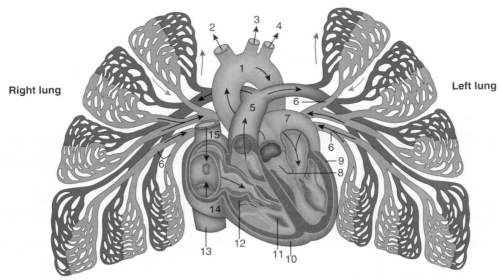

Figure 57-1 Cardiopulmonary circulation. *1*, aorta; *2*, innominate artery; *3*, left common carotid artery; *4*, left subclavian artery; *5*, pulmonary artery; *6*, pulmonary vein; *7*, left auricle; *8*, bicuspid valve; *9*, left ventricle; *10*, right ventricle; *11*, papillary muscle; *12*, tricuspid valve; *13*, inferior vena cava; *14*, right auricle; *15*, superior vena cava.

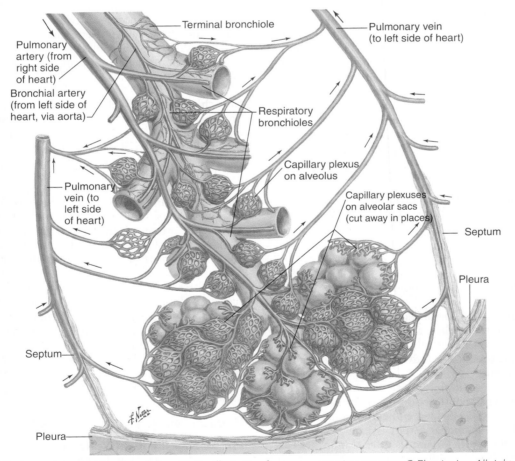

Figure 57-2 Intrapulmonary blood circulation. *Netter illustration from www.netterimages.com. © Elsevier Inc. All rights reserved.*

Pressures in the Pulmonary Artery. As shown in Figures 57-4 and 57-5, the *systolic pulmonary arterial pressure* normally averages about 25 mmHg in the human being, the *diastolic pulmonary arterial pressure* is about 8 mmHg, and the *mean pulmonary arterial pressure* is 15 mmHg.

Pulmonary Capillary Pressure. The mean pulmonary capillary pressure, as diagrammed in Figure 57-5, is about 7 mmHg. The importance of this low capillary pressure is discussed in detail later in the chapter in relation to fluid exchange functions of the pulmonary capillaries.

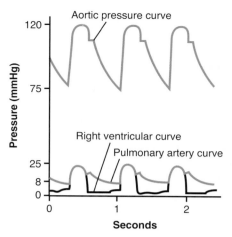

Figure 57-3 Pressure pulse contours in the right ventricle, pulmonary artery, and aorta.

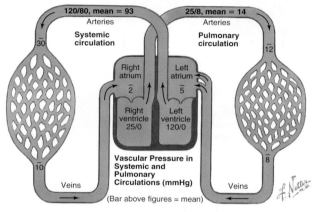

Figure 57-4 Comparison of pressures (mmHg) between the systemic circulation and pulmonary circulation. *RV*, right ventricle; *LV*, left ventricle; *RA*, right atrium; *LA*, left atrium. *Netter illustration from www. netterimages.com. © Elsevier Inc. All rights reserved.*

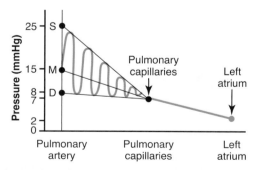

Figure 57-5 Pressures in the different vessels of the lungs. *D*, diastolic; *M*, mean; *red curve*, arterial pulsations; *S*, systolic.

Left Atrial and Pulmonary Venous Pressures. The mean pressure in the left atrium and the major pulmonary veins averages about 2 mmHg in the recumbent human being, varying from as low as 1 mmHg to as high as 5 mmHg. It usually is not feasible to measure a human being's left atrial pressure using a direct measuring device because it is difficult to pass a catheter through the heart chambers into the left atrium. However, the left atrial pressure can be estimated with moderate accuracy by measuring

the so-called *pulmonary wedge pressure.* This measurement is achieved by inserting a catheter first through a peripheral vein to the right atrium, then through the right side of the heart and through the pulmonary artery into one of the small branches of the pulmonary artery, and finally pushing the catheter until it *wedges tightly in the small branch*. The pressure measured through the catheter, called the "wedge pressure," is about 5 mmHg.

Pulmonary Vascular Resistance

As discussed in the earlier section, the pulmonary vascular system has thin walls and less smooth muscle as compared to the systemic vasculature. These vessels offer much lower resistance to blood flow than the systemic arterial vessels and are also more compressible and have more compliance as compared to the systemic arterial vessels.

Since the pulmonary circulation is closely associated with the alveoli, it is influenced by alveolar and intrapleural pressures, which can change dynamically. Therefore, the pulmonary vascular resistance is influenced not only by the smooth muscle tone of the pulmonary vasculature but by other forces as well.

The pulmonary vascular resistance can be calculated using an equation derived from Poiseuille's law detailed as follows:

$$\text{Pulmonary vascular resistance} = \frac{\text{input pressure} - \text{output pressure}}{\text{blood flow}}$$

where input pressure is the mean pulmonary arterial pressure, output pressure is the mean left atrial pressure, and blood flow is the cardiac output.

Although the pulmonary vascular resistance is extremely small under normal circumstances, it can become even lower if the pressure within the pulmonary circulation increases. This is accomplished by two mechanisms (Figure 57-6A):

1. *Recruitment*: Capillaries that are normally closed open up due to the increased pressure, thereby lowering the pulmonary vascular resistance. This is called recruitment.
2. *Distension*: Capillaries distend and accommodate more blood as pulmonary vascular pressures increase. This is called distension.

The effects of lung volume and humoral factors on pulmonary vascular resistance are also detailed in Figure 57-6B and C, respectively.

Blood Volume of the Lungs

The blood volume of the lungs is about 450 mL, about 9% of the total blood volume of the entire circulatory system. Approximately 70 mL of this pulmonary blood volume is in the pulmonary capillaries, and the remainder is divided about equally between the pulmonary arteries and the veins.

The Lungs Serve as a Blood Reservoir. Under various physiological and pathological conditions, the quantity of blood in the lungs can vary from as little as one-half normal up to twice normal. Loss of blood from the systemic circulation by hemorrhage can be partly compensated for by the automatic shift of blood from the lungs into the systemic vessels.

Cardiac Pathology May Shift Blood from the Systemic Circulation to the Pulmonary Circulation. Failure of the left side of the heart or increased resistance to blood flow through

A

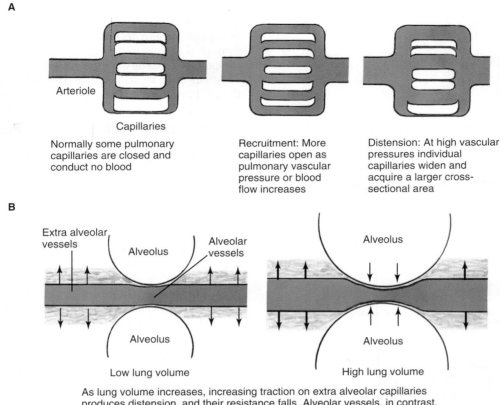

Arteriole

Capillaries

Normally some pulmonary
capillaries are closed and
conduct no blood

Recruitment: More
capillaries open as
pulmonary vascular
pressure or blood
flow increases

Distension: At high vascular
pressures individual
capillaries widen and
acquire a larger cross-
sectional area

B

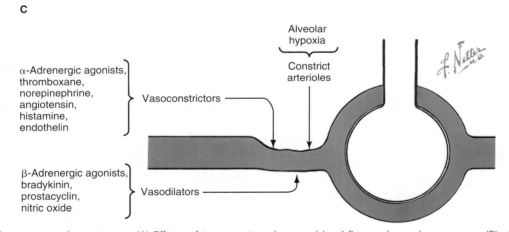

Extra alveolar
vessels

Alveolus

Alveolar
vessels

Alveolus

Alveolus

Alveolus

Low lung volume

High lung volume

As lung volume increases, increasing traction on extra alveolar capillaries
produces distension, and their resistance falls. Alveolar vessels, in contrast,
are compressed by enlarging alveoli, and their resistance increases.

C

Alveolar
hypoxia

Constrict
arterioles

α-Adrenergic agonists,
thromboxane,
norepinephrine,
angiotensin,
histamine,
endothelin

Vasoconstrictors

β-Adrenergic agonists,
bradykinin,
prostacyclin,
nitric oxide

Vasodilators

Figure 57-6   Pulmonary vascular resistance. (A) Effects of increases in pulmonary blood flow and vascular pressures; (B) effects of lung volume; (C) effects of chemical and humoral substances. *Netter illustration from www.netterimages.com.* © Elsevier Inc. All rights reserved.

the mitral valve as a result of mitral stenosis or mitral regurgitation causes blood to dam up in the pulmonary circulation, sometimes increasing the pulmonary blood volume as much as 100% and causing large increases in the pulmonary vascular pressures.

Blood Flow Through the Lungs and its Distribution

The blood flow through the lungs is essentially equal to the cardiac output. Therefore, the factors that control cardiac output also control pulmonary blood flow (Box 57-1). Under most

conditions, the pulmonary vessels act as distensible tubes that enlarge with increasing pressure and narrow with decreasing pressure. For adequate aeration of the blood to occur, the blood must be distributed to the segments of the lungs where the alveoli are best oxygenated. This distribution is achieved by the following mechanism.

Decreased Alveolar Oxygen Reduces Local Alveolar Blood Flow and Regulates Pulmonary Blood Flow Distribution.
When the concentration of O_2 in the air of the alveoli decreases below normal, especially when it falls below 70% of normal (ie, below 73 mmHg PO_2), the adjacent blood vessels constrict with vascular resistance increasing more than fivefold at extremely

low O_2 levels. This effect is *opposite to the effect observed in systemic vessels*, which dilate rather than constrict in response to low O_2 levels. Although the mechanisms that promote pulmonary vasoconstriction during hypoxia are not completely understood, low O_2 concentration may stimulate release of vasoconstrictor substances or decrease release of a vasodilator, such as nitric oxide, from the lung tissue.

Some studies suggest that hypoxia may directly induce vasoconstriction by inhibition of oxygen-sensitive potassium ion channels in pulmonary vascular smooth muscle cell membranes. With low partial pressures of oxygen, these channels are blocked, leading to depolarization of the cell membrane and activation of calcium channels, causing influx of calcium ions. The rise of calcium concentration then causes constriction of small arteries and arterioles.

The increase in pulmonary vascular resistance as a result of low O_2 concentration has the important function of distributing blood flow where it is most effective. That is, if some alveoli are poorly ventilated and have a low O_2 concentration, the local vessels constrict. This constriction causes the blood to flow through other areas of the lungs that are better aerated, thus providing an automatic control system for distributing blood flow to the pulmonary areas in proportion to their alveolar O_2 pressures.

Effect of Hydrostatic Pressure Gradients in the Lungs on Regional Pulmonary Blood Flow

In Chapter 41, we pointed out that the blood pressure in the foot of a standing person can be as much as 90 mmHg greater than the pressure at the level of the heart. This difference is caused by *hydrostatic pressure*—that is, by the weight of the blood itself in the blood vessels. The same effect, but to a lesser degree, occurs in the lungs. In the upright adult, a pressure difference of 23 mmHg exists between the apical regions and the base, about 15 mmHg of which is above the heart and 8 below. That is, the pulmonary arterial pressure in the uppermost portion of the lung of a standing person is about 15 mmHg less than the pulmonary arterial pressure at the level of the heart, and the pressure in the lowest portion of the lungs is about 8 mmHg greater. Such pressure differences have profound effects on blood flow through the different areas of the lungs. This effect is demonstrated by the lower curve in Figure 57-7, which depicts blood flow per unit of lung tissue at different levels of the lung in the upright person. Figure 57-8 also shows the regional differences in pulmonary blood flow. Note that in the standing position at rest, there is little flow in the top of the lung but about five times as much flow in the bottom. To help explain these differences, the lung is often described as being divided into three zones, as shown in Figure 57-9. In each zone, the patterns of blood flow are quite different.

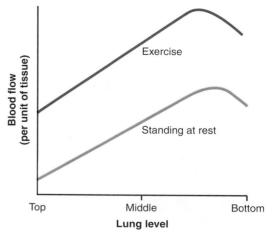

Figure 57-7 Blood flow at different levels in the lung of an upright person *at rest* and *during exercise*. Note that when the person is at rest, the blood flow is very low at the top of the lungs; most of the flow is through the bottom of the lung.

ZONES 1, 2, AND 3 OF PULMONARY BLOOD FLOW

The capillaries in the alveolar walls are distended by the blood pressure inside them, but simultaneously are compressed by the alveolar air pressure on their outsides. Therefore, any time the lung alveolar air pressure becomes greater than the capillary blood pressure, the capillaries close and there is no blood flow. Under different normal and pathological lung conditions, one may find any one of three possible zones (patterns) of pulmonary blood flow, as follows:

Zone 1: *No blood flow during all portions of the cardiac cycle* because the local alveolar capillary pressure in that area of the lung never rises higher than the alveolar air pressure during any part of the cardiac cycle

Zone 2: *Intermittent blood flow* only during the peaks of pulmonary arterial pressure because the systolic pressure is then greater than the alveolar air pressure, but the diastolic pressure is less than the alveolar air pressure

Zone 3: *Continuous blood flow* because the alveolar capillary pressure remains greater than alveolar air pressure during the entire cardiac cycle

Normally, the lungs have only zones 2 and 3 blood flow—zone 2 (intermittent flow) in the apices and zone 3 (continuous flow) in all the lower areas. For example, when a person is in the upright position, the pulmonary arterial pressure at the lung apex is about 15 mmHg less than the pressure at the level of the heart. Therefore, the apical systolic pressure is only 10 mmHg (25 mmHg at heart level minus 15 mmHg hydrostatic pressure difference). This 10 mmHg apical blood pressure is greater than the zero alveolar air pressure, so blood flows through the pulmonary apical capillaries during cardiac systole. Conversely, during diastole, the 8 mmHg diastolic pressure at the level of the heart is not sufficient to push the blood up to the 15 mmHg hydrostatic pressure gradient required to cause diastolic capillary flow. Therefore, blood flow through the apical part of the lung is intermittent with flow during systole but cessation of flow during diastole; this is called *zone 2 blood flow*. Zone 2 blood flow begins in normal lungs about 10 cm above the midlevel of the heart and extends from there to the top of the lungs.

In the lower regions of the lungs, from about 10 cm above the level of the heart all the way to the bottom of the lungs, the pulmonary arterial pressure during both systole and diastole remains greater than the zero alveolar air pressure. Therefore, continuous flow occurs through the alveolar capillaries, or zone

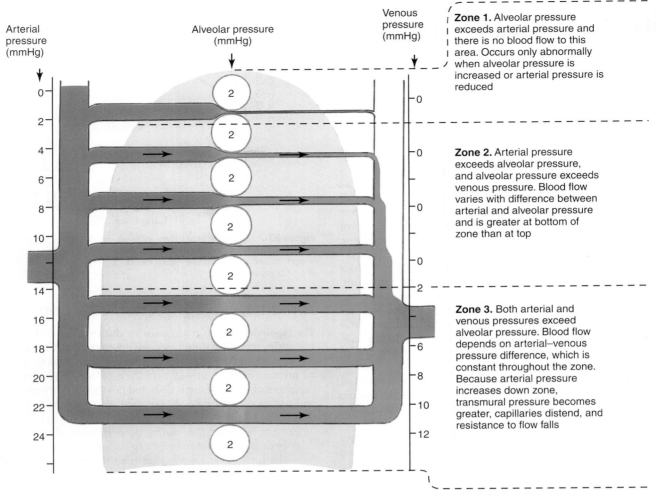

Arterial pressure (mmHg)

Alveolar pressure (mmHg)

Venous pressure (mmHg)

Zone 1. Alveolar pressure exceeds arterial pressure and there is no blood flow to this area. Occurs only abnormally when alveolar pressure is increased or arterial pressure is reduced

Zone 2. Arterial pressure exceeds alveolar pressure, and alveolar pressure exceeds venous pressure. Blood flow varies with difference between arterial and alveolar pressure and is greater at bottom of zone than at top

Zone 3. Both arterial and venous pressures exceed alveolar pressure. Blood flow depends on arterial–venous pressure difference, which is constant throughout the zone. Because arterial pressure increases down zone, transmural pressure becomes greater, capillaries distend, and resistance to flow falls

Figure 57-8   *Distribution of pulmonary blood flow. Netter illustration from www.netterimages.com.* © Elsevier Inc. All rights reserved.

3 blood flow. Also, when a person is lying down, no part of the lung is more than a few centimeters above the level of the heart. In this case, blood flow in a normal person is entirely zone 3 blood flow, including the lung apices.

Zone 1 Blood Flow Occurs Only Under Abnormal Conditions. Zone 1 blood flow, which means no blood flow at any time during the cardiac cycle, occurs when either the pulmonary systolic arterial pressure is too low or the alveolar pressure is too high to allow flow. An instance in which zone 1 blood flow occurs is in an upright person whose pulmonary systolic arterial pressure is exceedingly low, as might occur after severe blood loss.

Exercise Increases Blood Flow Through All Parts of the Lungs. Referring again to Figure 57-7, one sees that the blood flow in all parts of the lung increases during exercise. A major reason for increased blood flow is that the pulmonary vascular pressures rise enough during exercise to convert the lung apices from a zone 2 pattern into a zone 3 pattern of flow.

INCREASED CARDIAC OUTPUT DURING HEAVY EXERCISE IS NORMALLY ACCOMMODATED BY THE PULMONARY CIRCULATION WITHOUT LARGE INCREASES IN PULMONARY ARTERY PRESSURE

During heavy exercise, blood flow through the lungs may increase fourfold to sevenfold. This extra flow is accommodated in the lungs in three ways: (1) by increasing the number of open

capillaries, sometimes as much as threefold; (2) by distending all the capillaries and increasing the rate of flow through each capillary more than twofold (Figure 57-6A); and (3) by increasing the pulmonary arterial pressure. Normally, the first two changes decrease pulmonary vascular resistance so much that the pulmonary arterial pressure rises very little, even during maximum exercise. This effect is shown in Figure 57-10.

The ability of the lungs to accommodate greatly increased blood flow during exercise without increasing the pulmonary arterial pressure conserves the energy of the right side of the heart. This ability also prevents a significant rise in pulmonary capillary pressure, and preventing the development of pulmonary edema.

FUNCTION OF THE PULMONARY CIRCULATION WHEN THE LEFT ATRIAL PRESSURE RISES AS A RESULT OF LEFT-SIDED HEART FAILURE

The left atrial pressure in a healthy person almost never rises above +6 mmHg, even during the most strenuous exercise. These small changes in left atrial pressure have virtually no effect on pulmonary circulatory function because this merely expands the pulmonary venules and opens up more capillaries so that blood continues to flow with almost equal ease from the pulmonary arteries.

When the left side of the heart fails, however, blood begins to dam up in the left atrium. As a result, the left atrial pressure

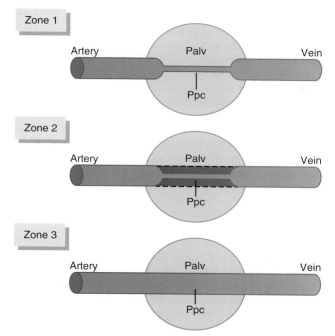

Zone 1

Artery | Palv | Vein

Ppc

Zone 2

Artery | Palv | Vein

Ppc

Zone 3

Artery | Palv | Vein

Ppc

Figure 57-9 Mechanics of blood flow in the three blood flow zones of the lung: *zone 1, no flow*—alveolar air pressure (PALV) is greater than arterial pressure; *zone 2, intermittent flow*—systolic arterial pressure rises higher than alveolar air pressure, but diastolic arterial pressure falls below alveolar air pressure; and *zone 3, continuous flow*—arterial pressure and pulmonary capillary pressure (Ppc) remain greater than alveolar air pressure at all times.

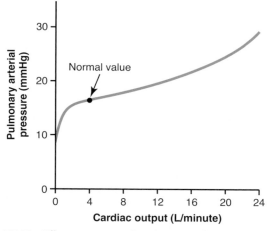

Figure 57-10 Effect on mean pulmonary arterial pressure caused by increasing the cardiac output during exercise.

can rise on occasion from its normal value of 1–5 mmHg all the way up to 40–50 mmHg. The initial rise in atrial pressure, up to about 7 mmHg, has little effect on pulmonary circulatory function. However, when the left atrial pressure rises to greater than 7 or 8 mmHg, further increases in left atrial pressure cause almost equally great increases in pulmonary arterial pressure, thus causing a concomitant increased load on the right heart. Any increase in left atrial pressure above 7 or 8 mmHg increases capillary pressure almost equally as much. When the left atrial pressure rises above 30 mmHg, causing similar increases in capillary pressure, pulmonary edema is likely to develop, as we discuss later in the chapter.

Pulmonary Capillary Dynamics

Exchange of gases between the alveolar air and the pulmonary capillary blood is discussed in Chapter 58. However, it is important to note here that the alveolar walls are lined with so many capillaries that, in most places, the capillaries almost touch one another side by side. Therefore, it is often said that the capillary blood flows in the alveolar walls as a "sheet of flow," rather than in individual capillaries.

Pulmonary Capillary Pressure. No direct measurements of pulmonary capillary pressure have ever been made. However, "isogravimetric" measurement of pulmonary capillary pressure has given a value of 7 mmHg. This measurement is probably nearly correct because the mean left atrial pressure is about 2 mmHg and the mean pulmonary arterial pressure is only 15 mmHg, so the mean pulmonary capillary pressure must lie somewhere between these two values.

Capillary Exchange of Fluid in the Lungs and Pulmonary Interstitial Fluid Dynamics. The dynamics of fluid exchange across the lung capillary membranes are *qualitatively* the same as for peripheral tissues. However, *quantitatively*, there are important differences, as follows:

1. The pulmonary capillary pressure is low, about 7 mmHg, in comparison with a considerably higher functional capillary pressure in the peripheral tissues of about 17 mmHg.
2. The interstitial fluid pressure in the lung is slightly more negative than that in peripheral subcutaneous tissue.
3. The colloid osmotic pressure of the pulmonary interstitial fluid is about 14 mmHg, in comparison with less than half this value in the peripheral tissues.
4. The alveolar walls are extremely thin and the alveolar epithelium covering the alveolar surfaces is so weak that it can be ruptured by any positive pressure in the interstitial spaces greater than alveolar air pressure (>0 mmHg), which allows dumping of fluid from the interstitial spaces into the alveoli. Now let us see how these quantitative differences affect pulmonary fluid dynamics.

Interrelations Between Interstitial Fluid Pressure and Other Pressures in the Lung. Figure 57-11 shows a pulmonary capillary, a pulmonary alveolus, and a lymphatic capillary draining the

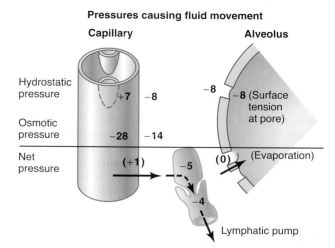

Pressures causing fluid movement

	Capillary		Alveolus
Hydrostatic pressure	+7	−8	−8	−8 (Surface tension at pore)
Osmotic pressure	−28	−14		
Net pressure	(+1)	−5	(0)	(Evaporation)
		−4		
		Lymphatic pump		

Figure 57-11 Hydrostatic and osmotic forces in millimeters of mercury at the capillary (*left*) and alveolar membrane (*right*) of the lungs. Also shown is the tip end of a lymphatic vessel (*center*) that pumps fluid from the pulmonary interstitial spaces.

interstitial space between the blood capillary and the alveolus. Note the balance of forces at the blood capillary membrane, as follows:

	Millimeters of Mercury
Forces tending to cause movement of fluid outward from the capillaries and into the pulmonary interstitium:	
Capillary pressure	7
Interstitial fluid colloid osmotic pressure	14
Negative interstitial fluid pressure	8
TOTAL OUTWARD FORCE	29
Forces tending to cause absorption of fluid into the capillaries:	
Plasma colloid osmotic pressure	28
TOTAL INWARD FORCE	28

Thus, the normal outward forces are slightly greater than the inward forces, providing a *mean filtration pressure* at the pulmonary capillary membrane that can be calculated as follows:

	Millimeters of Mercury
Total outward force	+29
Total inward force	−28
MEAN FILTRATION PRESSURE	+1

This filtration pressure causes a slight continual flow of fluid from the pulmonary capillaries into the interstitial spaces, and except for a small amount that evaporates in the alveoli, this fluid is pumped back to the circulation through the pulmonary lymphatic system.

Negative Pulmonary Interstitial Pressure and the Mechanism for Keeping the Alveoli "Dry". What keeps the alveoli from filling with fluid under normal conditions? If one remembers that the pulmonary capillaries and the pulmonary lymphatic system normally maintain a slight *negative pressure* in the interstitial spaces, it is clear that whenever extra fluid appears in the alveoli, it will simply be sucked mechanically into the lung interstitium through the small openings between the alveolar epithelial cells. The excess fluid is then carried away through the pulmonary lymphatics. Thus, under normal conditions, the alveoli are kept "dry," except for a small amount of fluid that seeps from the epithelium onto the lining surfaces of the alveoli to keep them moist.

PULMONARY EDEMA

Pulmonary edema occurs in the same way that edema occurs elsewhere in the body. Any factor that increases fluid filtration out of the pulmonary capillaries or that impedes pulmonary lymphatic function and causes the pulmonary interstitial fluid pressure to rise from the negative range into the positive range will cause rapid filling of the pulmonary interstitial spaces and alveoli with large amounts of free fluid.

The most common causes of pulmonary edema are as follows:

1. left-sided heart failure or mitral valve disease, with consequent great increases in pulmonary venous pressure and pulmonary capillary pressure and flooding of the interstitial spaces and alveoli;

2. damage to the pulmonary blood capillary membranes caused by infections such as pneumonia or by breathing noxious substances such as chlorine gas or sulfur dioxide gas.

Each of the aforementioned mechanisms causes rapid leakage of both plasma proteins and fluid out of the capillaries and into both the lung interstitial spaces and the alveoli.

"Pulmonary Edema Safety Factor". Experiments in animals have shown that the pulmonary capillary pressure normally must rise to a value at least equal to the colloid osmotic pressure of the plasma inside the capillaries before significant pulmonary edema will occur. Therefore, in the human being, whose normal plasma colloid osmotic pressure is 28 mmHg, one can predict that the pulmonary capillary pressure must rise from the normal level of 7 mmHg to more than 28 mmHg to cause pulmonary edema, giving an *acute safety factor against pulmonary edema* of 21 mmHg.

Safety Factor in Chronic Conditions. When the pulmonary capillary pressure remains elevated chronically (for at least 2 weeks), the lungs become even more resistant to pulmonary edema because the lymph vessels expand greatly, increasing their capability of carrying fluid away from the interstitial spaces perhaps as much as 10-fold. Therefore, in patients with chronic mitral stenosis, pulmonary capillary pressures of 40–45 mmHg have been measured without the development of lethal pulmonary edema.

Rapidity of Death in Persons with Acute Pulmonary Edema. When the pulmonary capillary pressure rises even slightly above the safety factor level, lethal pulmonary edema can occur within hours, or even within 20–30 minutes if the capillary pressure rises 25–30 mmHg above the safety factor level. Thus, in acute left-sided heart failure, in which the pulmonary capillary pressure occasionally does rise to 50 mmHg, death may ensue in less than 30 minutes from acute pulmonary edema.

EFFECT OF THE VENTILATION–PERFUSION RATIO ON ALVEOLAR GAS CONCENTRATION

There are two factors that determine the PO_2 and the PCO_2 in the alveoli: (1) the rate of alveolar ventilation and (2) the rate of transfer of O_2 and CO_2 through the respiratory membrane. The assumption is that all the alveoli are ventilated equally and that blood flow through the alveolar capillaries is the same for each alveolus. However, even normally to some extent, and especially in many lung diseases, some areas of the lungs are well ventilated but have almost no blood flow, whereas other areas may have excellent blood flow but little or no ventilation. In either of these conditions, gas exchange through the respiratory membrane is seriously impaired, and the person may suffer severe respiratory distress despite both normal *total* ventilation and normal *total* pulmonary blood flow, but with the ventilation and blood flow going to different parts of the lungs. Therefore, a highly quantitative concept has been developed to help us understand respiratory exchange when there is imbalance between alveolar ventilation and alveolar blood flow. This concept is called the *ventilation–perfusion ratio.*

In quantitative terms, the ventilation–perfusion ratio is expressed as $\dot{V}_A/\dot{Q}$. When $\dot{V}_A$ (alveolar ventilation) is normal for a given alveolus and $\dot{Q}$ (blood flow) is also normal for the same alveolus, the ventilation–perfusion ratio ($\dot{V}_A/\dot{Q}$) is also said to be normal. When the ventilation ($\dot{V}_A$) is zero, yet there is still perfusion ($\dot{Q}$) of the alveolus, the $\dot{V}_A/\dot{Q}$ is zero. Or, at the other extreme, when there is adequate ventilation ($\dot{V}_A$) but zero perfusion ($\dot{Q}$), the ratio $\dot{V}_A/\dot{Q}$ is infinity. At a ratio of either zero or infinity, there is no exchange of gases through the respiratory membrane

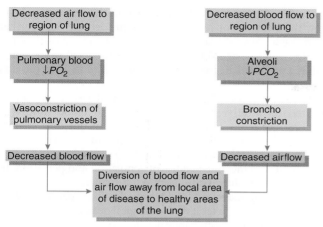

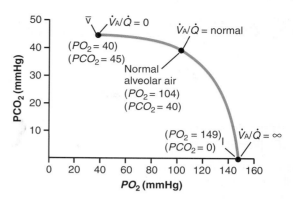

Figure 57-13 Normal $PO_2 - PCO_2$, $\dot{V}_A/\dot{Q}$ diagram.

Figure 57-12 Flow diagram to indicate control of ventilation and perfusion. *Modified from Widmaier, E.P., Raff, H., Strang, K.T., 2005. Vander's Human Physiology: The Mechanisms of Body Function, 10th ed. McGraw-Hill, New York.*

of the affected alveoli, which explains the importance of this concept. Therefore, let us explain the respiratory consequences of these two extremes (Figure 57-12).

ALVEOLAR OXYGEN AND CARBON DIOXIDE PARTIAL PRESSURES WHEN $\dot{V}_A/\dot{Q}$ EQUALS ZERO

When $\dot{V}_A/\dot{Q}$ is equal to zero—that is, without any alveolar ventilation—the air in the alveolus comes to equilibrium with the blood O_2 and CO_2 because these gases diffuse between the blood and the alveolar air. Because the blood that perfuses the capillaries is venous blood returning to the lungs from the systemic circulation, it is the gases in this blood with which the alveolar gases equilibrate. In Chapters 59 and 60, we describe how the normal venous blood ($\overline{v}$) has a PO_2 of 40 mmHg and a PCO_2 of 45 mmHg. Therefore, these are also the normal partial pressures of these two gases in alveoli that have blood flow but no ventilation.

ALVEOLAR OXYGEN AND CARBON DIOXIDE PARTIAL PRESSURES WHEN $\dot{V}_A/\dot{Q}$ EQUALS INFINITY

The effect on the alveolar gas partial pressures when $\dot{V}_A/\dot{Q}$ equals infinity is entirely different from the effect when $\dot{V}_A/\dot{Q}$ equals zero because now there is no capillary blood flow to carry O_2 away or to bring CO_2 to the alveoli. Therefore, instead of the alveolar gases coming to equilibrium with the venous blood, the alveolar air becomes equal to the humidified inspired air. That is, the air that is inspired loses no O_2 to the blood and gains no CO_2 from the blood. Furthermore, because normal inspired and humidified air has a PO_2 of 149 mmHg and a PCO_2 of 0 mmHg, these will be the partial pressures of these two gases in the alveoli.

GAS EXCHANGE AND ALVEOLAR PARTIAL PRESSURES WHEN $\dot{V}_A/\dot{Q}$ IS NORMAL

When there is both normal alveolar ventilation and normal alveolar capillary blood flow (normal alveolar perfusion), exchange of O_2 and CO_2 through the respiratory membrane is nearly optimal, and alveolar PO_2 is normally at a level of 104 mmHg, which lies between that of the inspired air (149 mmHg) and that of venous blood (40 mmHg). Likewise, alveolar PCO_2 lies between two extremes; it is normally 40 mmHg, in contrast to 45 mmHg in venous blood and 0 mmHg in inspired air. Thus, under normal conditions, the alveolar air PO_2 averages 104 mmHg and the PCO_2 averages 40 mmHg.

$PO_2 - PCO_2$, $\dot{V}_A/\dot{Q}$ DIAGRAM

The concepts presented in the preceding sections can be shown in graphical form, as demonstrated in Figure 57-13, called the $PO_2 - PCO_2$, $\dot{V}_A/\dot{Q}$ diagram. The curve in the diagram represents all possible PO_2 and PCO_2 combinations between the limits of $\dot{V}_A/\dot{Q}$ equals zero and $\dot{V}_A/\dot{Q}$ equals infinity when the gas pressures in the venous blood are normal and the person is breathing air at sea-level pressure. Thus, point $\overline{v}$ is the plot of PO_2 and PCO_2 when $\dot{V}_A/\dot{Q}$ equals zero. At this point, the PO_2 is 40 mmHg and the PCO_2 is 45 mmHg, which are the values in normal venous blood.

At the other end of the curve, when $\dot{V}_A/\dot{Q}$ equals infinity, point I represents inspired air, showing PO_2 to be 149 mmHg while PCO_2 is zero. Also plotted on the curve is the point that represents normal alveolar air when is normal. At this point, PO_2 is 104 mmHg and PCO_2 is 40 mmHg.

CONCEPT OF "PHYSIOLOGICAL SHUNT" (WHEN $\dot{V}_A/\dot{Q}$ IS BELOW NORMAL)

Whenever $\dot{V}_A/\dot{Q}$ is below normal, there is inadequate ventilation to provide the O_2 needed to fully oxygenate the blood flowing through the alveolar capillaries. Therefore, a certain fraction of the venous blood passing through the pulmonary capillaries does not become oxygenated. This fraction is called *shunted blood*. Also, some additional blood flows through bronchial vessels rather than through alveolar capillaries, normally about 2% of the cardiac output; this, too, is unoxygenated, shunted blood.

The total quantitative amount of shunted blood per minute is called the *physiological shunt*. This *physiological* shunt is measured in clinical pulmonary function laboratories by analyzing the concentration of O_2 in both mixed venous blood and arterial blood, along with simultaneous measurement of cardiac output. From these values, the physiological shunt can be calculated by the following equation:

$$\frac{\dot{Q}_{PS}}{\dot{Q}_T} = \frac{CiO_2 - CaO_2}{CiO_2 - C\overline{v}O_2}$$

where $\dot{Q}_{PS}$ is the physiological shunt blood flow per minute, $\dot{Q}_T$ is cardiac output per minute, CiO_2 is the concentration of oxygen in the arterial blood if there is an "ideal" ventilation–perfusion ratio, CaO_2 is the measured concentration of oxygen in the arterial blood, and $C\overline{v}O_2$ is the measured concentration of oxygen in the mixed venous blood.

The greater the physiological shunt, the greater is the *amount of blood that fails to be oxygenated* as it passes through the lungs. Refer to Box 57-2 for disorders causing a shunt.

CONCEPT OF THE "PHYSIOLOGICAL DEAD SPACE" (WHEN $\dot{V}_A/\dot{Q}$ IS GREATER THAN NORMAL)

When ventilation of some of the alveoli is great but alveolar blood flow is low, there is far more available oxygen in the alveoli than can be transported away from the alveoli by the flowing blood. Thus, the ventilation of these alveoli is said to be *wasted*. The ventilation of the anatomical dead space areas of the respiratory passageways is also wasted. The sum of these two types of wasted ventilation is called the *physiological dead space*. This space is measured in the clinical pulmonary function laboratory by making appropriate blood and expiratory gas measurements and using the following equation, called the Bohr equation:

$$\frac{\dot{V}_{Dphys}}{\dot{V}_T} = \frac{PaCO_2 - P\overline{e}CO_2}{PaCO_2}$$

where $\dot{V}_{Dphys}$ is the physiological dead space, $\dot{V}_T$ is the tidal volume, $PaCO_2$ is the partial pressure of CO_2 in the arterial blood, and $P\overline{e}CO_2$ is the average partial pressure of carbon dioxide in the entire expired air.

When the physiological dead space is great, much of the *work of ventilation* is wasted effort because so much of the ventilating air never reaches the blood.

ABNORMALITIES OF VENTILATION–PERFUSION RATIO

Abnormal $\dot{V}_A/\dot{Q}$ in the Upper and Lower Normal Lung

In a normal person in the upright position, both pulmonary capillary blood flow and alveolar ventilation are considerably less in the upper part of the lung than in the lower part; however, the decrease of blood flow is considerably greater than the decrease in ventilation is. Therefore, at the top of the lung, $\dot{V}_A/\dot{Q}$ is as much as 2.5 times as great as the ideal value, which causes a moderate degree of *physiological dead space* in this area of the lung.

At the other extreme, in the bottom of the lung, there is slightly too little ventilation in relation to blood flow, with $\dot{V}_A/\dot{Q}$ as low as 0.6 times the ideal value. In this area, a small fraction of the blood fails to become normally oxygenated, and this represents a *physiological shunt*.

In both extremes, inequalities of ventilation and perfusion decrease slightly the lung's effectiveness for exchanging O_2 and CO_2. However, during exercise, blood flow to the upper part of the lung increases markedly, so far less physiological dead space occurs, and the effectiveness of gas exchange now approaches optimum.

Abnormal $\dot{V}_A/\dot{Q}$ in Chronic Obstructive Lung Disease

Most people who smoke for many years develop various degrees of bronchial obstruction; in a large share of these persons, this condition eventually becomes so severe that serious alveolar air trapping develops, with resultant *emphysema*. The emphysema in turn causes many of the alveolar walls to be destroyed. Thus, two abnormalities occur in smokers to cause abnormal $\dot{V}_A/\dot{Q}$. First, because many of the small bronchioles are obstructed, the alveoli beyond the obstructions are unventilated, causing a $\dot{V}_A/\dot{Q}$ that approaches zero. Second, in the areas of the lung where the alveolar walls have been mainly destroyed but there is still alveolar ventilation, most of the ventilation is wasted because of inadequate blood flow to transport the blood gases.

Thus, in chronic obstructive lung disease, some areas of the lung exhibit *serious physiological shunt* and other areas exhibit *serious physiological dead space*. Both conditions tremendously decrease the effectiveness of the lungs as gas exchange organs, sometimes reducing their effectiveness to as little as one-tenth normal. In fact, this condition is the most prevalent cause of pulmonary disability today.

BIBLIOGRAPHY

Bärtsch P, Swenson ER: Clinical practice: acute high-altitude illnesses, *N. Engl. J. Med.* 368:2294, 2013.

Bogaard HJ, Abe K, Vonk Noordegraaf A, Voelkel NF: The right ventricle under pressure: cellular and molecular mechanisms of right-heart failure in pulmonary hypertension, *Chest* 135:794, 2009.

Effros RM, Parker JC: Pulmonary vascular heterogeneity and the Starling hypothesis, *Microvasc. Res.* 78:71, 2009.

Glenny RW, Robertson HT: Spatial distribution of ventilation and perfusion: mechanisms and regulation, *Compr. Physiol.* 1:375, 2011.

Guyton AC, Lindsey AW: Effect of elevated left atrial pressure and decreased plasma protein concentration on the development of pulmonary edema, *Circ. Res.* 7:649, 1959.

Herold S, Gabrielli NM, Vadász I: Novel concepts of acute lung injury and alveolar–capillary barrier dysfunction, *Am. J. Physiol. Lung Cell. Mol. Physiol.* 305:L665, 2013.

Hopkins SR, Wielpütz MO, Kauczor HU: Imaging lung perfusion, *J. Appl. Physiol.* 113:328, 2012.

Hoschele S, Mairbaurl H: Alveolar flooding at high altitude: failure of reabsorption? *News Physiol. Sci.* 18:55, 2003.

Hughes M, West JB: Gravity is the major factor determining the distribution of blood flow in the human lung, *J. Appl. Physiol.* 104:1531, 2008.

Lai-Fook SJ: Pleural mechanics and fluid exchange, *Physiol. Rev.* 84:385, 2004.

Michelakis ED, Wilkins MR, Rabinovitch M: Emerging concepts and translational priorities in pulmonary arterial hypertension, *Circulation* 118:1486, 2008.

Miller RD: The postanesthesia care unit differential diagnosis of arterial hypoxemia in the PACU, eighth ed., Miller's Anesthesia. Philadelphia, 2015, Saunders, Elsevier.

Naeije R, Chesler N: Pulmonary circulation at exercise, *Compr. Physiol.* 2:711, 2012.

Parker JC: Hydraulic conductance of lung endothelial phenotypes and Starling safety factors against edema, *Am. J. Physiol. Lung Cell. Mol. Physiol.* 292:L378, 2007.

Powell FL, Hopkins SR: Comparative physiology of lung complexity: implications for gas exchange, *News Physiol. Sci.* 19:55, 2004.

Rahn H, Farhi EE: Ventilation, perfusion, and gas exchange—the $\dot{V}_A/\dot{Q}$ concept, Fenn WO, Rahn H, editors: *Handbook of Physiology*, vol. 1, Williams & Wilkins, Baltimore, 1964.

Sylvester JT, Shimoda LA, Aaronson PI, Ward JP: Hypoxic pulmonary vasoconstriction, *Physiol. Rev.* 92:367, 2012.

Townsley MI: Structure and composition of pulmonary arteries, capillaries, and veins, *Compr. Physiol.* 2:675, 2012.

Wagner PD: Assessment of gas exchange in lung disease: balancing accuracy against feasibility, *Crit. Care* 11:182, 2007.

Wagner PD: The multiple inert gas elimination technique (MIGET), *Intensive Care Med.* 34:994, 2008.

West JB: *Respiratory Physiology—The Essentials*, ninth ed. Philadelphia, 2012, Lippincott Williams & Wilkins, Wolters Kluwers.

West JB: Role of the fragility of the pulmonary blood–gas barrier in the evolution of the pulmonary circulation, *Am. J. Physiol. Regul. Integr. Comp. Physiol.* 304:R171, 2013.

58

Diffusion of Gases

After the alveoli are ventilated with fresh air, the next step in respiration is *diffusion* of oxygen (O_2) from the alveoli into the pulmonary blood and diffusion of carbon dioxide (CO_2) in the opposite direction, out of the blood into the alveoli. The process of diffusion is simply the random motion of molecules in all directions through the respiratory membrane and adjacent fluids. However, in respiratory physiology, we are concerned not only with the basic mechanism by which diffusion occurs but also with the *rate* at which it occurs, which is a much more complex issue, requiring a deeper understanding of the physics of diffusion and gas exchange.

Physics of Gas Diffusion and Gas Partial Pressures

MOLECULAR BASIS OF GAS DIFFUSION

Definition. All the gases of concern in respiratory physiology are simple molecules that are free to move among one another in a random and spontaneous manner. This process is called "diffusion." This is also true of gases dissolved in the fluids and tissues of the body.

For diffusion to occur there must be a source of energy. This source of energy is provided by the kinetic motion of the molecules. Except at absolute zero temperature, all molecules of all matter are continually undergoing motion. For free molecules that are not physically attached to others, this means linear movement at high velocity until they strike other molecules. They then bounce away in new directions and continue moving until they strike other molecules again. In this way, the molecules move rapidly and randomly among one another.

Net Diffusion of a Gas in One Direction—Effect of a Concentration Gradient. If a gas chamber or a solution has a high concentration of a particular gas at one end of the chamber and a low concentration at the other end, as shown in Figure 58-1, net diffusion of the gas will occur from the high-concentration area toward the low-concentration area. The reason is obvious; there are far more molecules at end A of the chamber to diffuse toward end B than the molecules to diffuse in the opposite direction. Therefore, the rates of diffusion in each of the two directions are proportionately different, as demonstrated by the lengths of the arrows in the figure.

Diffusion of Gases Between the Gas Phase in the Alveoli and the Dissolved Phase in the Pulmonary Blood. The partial pressure of each gas in the alveolar respiratory gas mixture tends to force molecules of that gas into solution in the blood of the alveolar capillaries. Conversely, the molecules of the same gas that are already dissolved in the blood are bouncing randomly in the fluid of the blood, and some of these bouncing molecules escape back into the alveoli. The rate at which they escape is directly proportional to their partial pressure in the blood. This is governed by *Henry's law* as discussed in Chapter 53.

But in which direction will *net diffusion* of the gas occur? The answer is that net diffusion is determined by the difference between the two partial pressures. If the partial pressure is greater in the gas phase in the alveoli, as is normally true for oxygen, then more molecules will diffuse into the blood than in the other direction. Alternatively, if the partial pressure of the gas is greater in the dissolved state in the blood, which is normally true for CO_2, then net diffusion will occur toward the gas phase in the alveoli.

VAPOR PRESSURE OF WATER

When non-humidified air is breathed into the respiratory passageways, water immediately evaporates from the surfaces of these passages and humidifies the air. This results from the fact that water molecules, like the different dissolved gas molecules, are continually escaping from the water surface into the gas phase.

The partial pressure that the water molecules exert to escape through the surface is called the *vapor pressure* of the water. At normal body temperature, 37°C, this vapor pressure is 47 mmHg. Therefore, once the gas mixture has become fully humidified—that is, once it is in "equilibrium" with the water—the partial pressure of the water vapor in the gas mixture is 47 mmHg. This partial pressure, like the other partial pressures, is designated PH_2O.

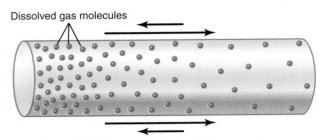

Figure 58-1 Diffusion of oxygen from one end of a chamber to the other. The difference between the lengths of the arrows represents *net diffusion*.

PRESSURE DIFFERENCE CAUSES NET DIFFUSION OF GASES THROUGH FLUIDS

From the preceding discussion, it is clear that when the partial pressure of a gas is greater in one area than in another area, there will be net diffusion from the high-pressure area toward the low-pressure area. Therefore, the *net diffusion* of gas from the area of high pressure to the area of low pressure is equal to the number of molecules bouncing in this forward direction *minus* the number bouncing in the opposite direction, which is proportional to the gas partial pressure difference between the two areas called simply the *pressure difference for causing diffusion*. Diffusion of gases across tissues is governed and described by Fick's law, which is stated in the next section.

Fick's Law. Fick's law of diffusion states that the net diffusion rate of a gas through a membrane is proportional to the tissue area (A) and the difference in partial pressure ($P_1 - P_2$) between the two sides, and is inversely proportional to the thickness (T) (Figure 58-2):

$$V_{\text{gas}} = A \times D \times \frac{P_1 - P_2}{T},$$

where D is a constant that depends on the solubility of the gas and is inversely proportional to the molecular weight (MW) and is given by

$$D \propto \frac{\text{solubility}}{\text{square root of MW}}$$

Quantifying the Net Rate of Diffusion in Fluids. As indicated earlier, in addition to the pressure difference, several other factors affect the rate of gas diffusion in a fluid. They are as follows:
1. the solubility of the gas in the fluid
2. the cross-sectional area of the fluid
3. the distance through which the gas must diffuse
4. the MW of the gas
5. the temperature of the fluid

In the body, the temperature remains reasonably constant and usually need not be considered.

The greater the solubility of the gas, the greater is the number of molecules available to diffuse for any given partial pressure difference. The greater the cross-sectional area of the diffusion pathway, the greater is the total number of molecules that diffuse. Conversely, the greater the distance the molecules must diffuse, the longer it will take the molecules to diffuse the entire distance. Finally, the greater the velocity of kinetic movement of the molecules, which is inversely proportional to the square root of the MW, the greater is the rate of diffusion of the gas.

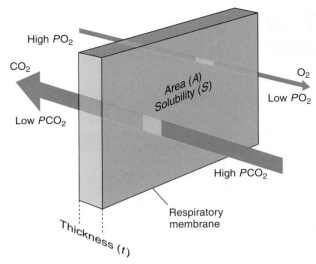

Figure 58-2 Diffusion through the respiratory membrane based on Fick's law. *Modified from Barker, S.J., Tremper, K.K. Physics applied to anesthesia. In: Barash, P.G., Cullen, B.F., Stoelting, R.K. (Eds.), Clinical Anesthesia, 2nd ed. J.B. Lippincott Company, Philadelphia.*

It is obvious from the aforementioned formula that the characteristics of the gas itself determine two factors of the formula: solubility and MW. Together, these two factors determine the *diffusion coefficient of the gas*, which is proportional to $S/\sqrt{MW}$, that is, the relative rates at which different gases at the same partial pressure levels will diffuse are proportional to their diffusion coefficients. Assuming that the diffusion coefficient for oxygen is 1, the *relative* diffusion coefficients for different gases of respiratory importance in the body fluids are as follows:

Oxygen	1.0
Carbon dioxide	20.3
Carbon monoxide	0.81
Nitrogen	0.53
Helium	0.95

DIFFUSION OF GASES THROUGH TISSUES

The gases that are of respiratory importance are all highly soluble in lipids and, consequently, are highly soluble in cell membranes. Because of this, the major limitation to the movement of gases in tissues is the rate at which the gases can diffuse through the tissue water instead of through the cell membranes. Therefore, diffusion of gases through the tissues, including through the respiratory membrane, is almost equal to the diffusion of gases in water, as given in the preceding list.

Diffusion of Gases Through the Respiratory Membrane

RESPIRATORY UNIT

As discussed earlier in Chapter 53, Figure 53-5 shows the *respiratory unit* (also called respiratory lobule). Please refer to Chapter 53 for details.

RESPIRATORY MEMBRANE

The ultrastructure of the respiratory membrane (Figure 53-7) drawn in cross-section on the left and a red blood cell on the right was described in Chapter 53. Please refer to Chapter 53 for details and Box 58-1 for summary of layers of the respiratory membrane.

Diffusion and Perfusion Limitations of Gas Transfer

DIFFUSION LIMITED

If an RBC enters a capillary surrounding an alveolus containing carbon monoxide, the following sequence of events occurs:

1. Carbon monoxide moves rapidly from the alveolus into the RBC via the respiratory membrane.
2. Carbon monoxide forms a strong bond with hemoglobin.
3. Carbon monoxide content increases in the cell but does not cause an increase in partial pressure because it is not dissolved in blood.
4. As the RBC courses through the capillary, no back pressure develops and CO continues to move into the cell from the alveolus.
5. Therefore the partial pressure of CO in the alveoli is always higher than the pulmonary capillary blood, maintaining a gradient that allows diffusion of CO from the alveolus to the RBC for the entire duration that the blood traverses through the pulmonary capillary.
6. It is therefore clear that the quantity of CO that gets into blood is limited by the respiratory membrane and its diffusion properties and not by the quantity of blood available.

This carbon monoxide transfer from the alveolus to the pulmonary capillary is said to be *diffusion limited* (Figure 58-3).

PERFUSION LIMITED

If nitrous oxide (N_2O) is used in lieu of carbon monoxide, the following sequence of events may occur:

1. Nitrous oxide moves rapidly from the alveolus into the RBC via the respiratory membrane.
2. In blood, no bonding of N_2O to hemoglobin occurs.
3. As a result, the partial pressure of N_2O in blood rises rapidly to reach that of the alveolar gas.
4. When the partial pressures are equal, no further nitrous oxide is transferred into the RBC.
5. Therefore the amount of gas that can be transferred into blood from the alveolus is dependent on the blood flow at that point of time and not on the diffusion properties of the respiratory membrane.

The transfer of N_2O is therefore said to be *perfusion limited* (Figure 58-3).

Oxygen—Diffusion or Perfusion Limited

Oxygen's time course through the capillaries around the alveoli is between that of carbon monoxide and that of nitrous oxide.

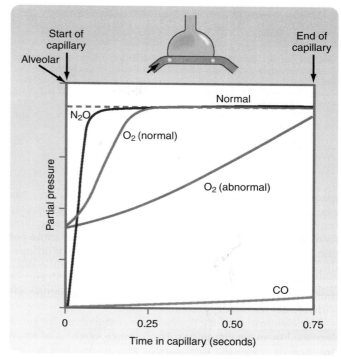

Figure 58-3 Illustration to show perfusion and diffusion limitation. *(Figure 23-3 from Oxygen and carbon dioxide transport. In: Barrett, K.E., Cloutier, M.M., Koeppen, B.M., et al. (Eds.), Berne & Levy Physiology. Elsevier, 2010.)*

1. Oxygen moves from the alveoli into the RBC via the respiratory membrane.
2. Oxygen binds with hemoglobin, but not as strongly as it does with carbon monoxide.
3. The partial pressure of oxygen in the blood rises and is far greater than that of carbon monoxide for the equivalent number of molecules of CO.
4. Under conditions of rest, the partial pressure of oxygen in blood reaches that of alveolar gas, when the red cell has traversed about one-third of its time in the capillary.
5. When the partial pressures are equal, no further oxygen is transferred into the RBC and transfer is perfusion limited just as nitrous oxide.
6. However, in certain disorders of the respiratory membrane, such as thickening of the membrane, the partial pressure of oxygen in blood does not reach the alveolar value even at the end of the capillary and this results in a state of being diffusion limited (Figure 58-3).

FACTORS THAT AFFECT THE RATE OF GAS DIFFUSION THROUGH THE RESPIRATORY MEMBRANE

Referring to the earlier discussion of diffusion of gases in water, one can apply the same principles to diffusion of gases through the respiratory membrane. Thus, the factors that determine how rapidly a gas will pass through the membrane are (1) the *thickness of the membrane*, (2) the *surface area of the membrane*, (3) the *diffusion coefficient* of the gas in the substance of the membrane, and (4) the *partial pressure difference* of the gas between the two sides of the membrane (Box 58-2).

The *thickness of the respiratory membrane* occasionally increases—for instance, as a result of edema fluid in the interstitial space of the membrane and in the alveoli—so the respiratory gases must then diffuse not only through the membrane but also through this fluid. Also, some pulmonary diseases cause fibrosis of the lungs, which can increase the thickness of some portions of the respiratory membrane. Because the rate of diffusion through the membrane is inversely proportional to the thickness of the membrane, any factor that increases the thickness to more than two to three times normal can interfere significantly with normal respiratory exchange of gases.

The *surface area of the respiratory membrane* can be greatly decreased by many conditions. For instance, removal of an entire lung decreases the total surface area to one-half normal. Also, in *emphysema*, many of the alveoli coalesce, with dissolution of many alveolar walls. Therefore, the new alveolar chambers are much larger than the original alveoli, but the total surface area of the respiratory membrane is often decreased as much as fivefold because of loss of the alveolar walls. When the total surface area is decreased to about one-third to one-fourth normal, exchange of gases through the membrane is substantially impeded, *even under resting conditions*, and during competitive sports and other strenuous exercise even the slightest decrease in surface area of the lungs can be a serious detriment to respiratory exchange of gases.

The *diffusion coefficient* for transfer of each gas through the respiratory membrane depends on the gas's *solubility* in the membrane and, inversely, on the *square root* of the gas's *MW*. The rate of diffusion in the respiratory membrane is almost exactly the same as that in water, for reasons explained earlier. Therefore, for a given pressure difference, CO_2 diffuses about 20 times as rapidly as O_2. Oxygen diffuses about twice as rapidly as nitrogen.

The *pressure difference* across the respiratory membrane is the difference between the partial pressure of the gas in the alveoli and the partial pressure of the gas in the pulmonary capillary blood. The partial pressure represents a measure of the total number of molecules of a particular gas striking a unit area of the alveolar surface of the membrane in unit time, and the pressure of the gas in the blood represents the number of molecules that attempt to escape from the blood in the opposite direction. Therefore, the difference between these two pressures is a measure of the *net tendency* for the gas molecules to move through the membrane.

When the partial pressure of a gas in the alveoli is greater than the pressure of the gas in the blood, as is true for O_2, net diffusion from the alveoli into the blood occurs; when the pressure of the gas in the blood is greater than the partial pressure in the alveoli, as is true for CO_2, net diffusion from the blood into the alveoli occurs.

DIFFUSING CAPACITY OF THE RESPIRATORY MEMBRANE

The ability of the respiratory membrane to exchange a gas between the alveoli and the pulmonary blood is expressed in quantitative terms by the *respiratory membrane's diffusing capacity*, which is defined as the *volume of a gas that will diffuse through the membrane each minute for a partial pressure difference of 1 mmHg*.

Diffusing Capacity for Oxygen. In the average young man, the *diffusing capacity for O_2* under resting conditions averages *21 mL/minute per millimeter of mercury*. In functional terms, what does this mean? The mean O_2 pressure difference across the respiratory membrane during normal, quiet breathing is about 11 mmHg. Multiplication of this pressure by the diffusing capacity (11×21) gives a total of about 230 mL of oxygen diffusing through the respiratory membrane each minute, which is equal to the rate at which the resting body uses oxygen.

Increased Oxygen Diffusing Capacity During Exercise. During strenuous exercise or other conditions that greatly increase pulmonary blood flow and alveolar ventilation, the diffusing capacity for O_2 increases in young men to a maximum of about 65 mL/minute per millimeter of mercury, which is three times the diffusing capacity under resting conditions (Box 58-3).

Therefore, during exercise, oxygenation of the blood is increased not only by increased alveolar ventilation but also by greater diffusing capacity of the respiratory membrane for transporting O_2 into the blood.

Diffusing Capacity for Carbon Dioxide. The diffusing capacity for CO_2 has never been measured because CO_2 diffuses through the respiratory membrane so rapidly that the average PCO_2 in the pulmonary blood is not far different from the PCO_2 in the alveoli—the average difference is less than 1 mmHg. With currently available techniques, this difference is too small to be measured.

Nevertheless, measurements of diffusion of other gases have shown that the diffusing capacity varies directly with the diffusion coefficient of the particular gas. Because the diffusion coefficient of CO_2 is slightly more than 20 times that of O_2, one would expect a diffusing capacity for CO_2 under resting conditions of about 400–450 mL/minute per millimeter of mercury and during exercise of about 1200–1300 mL/minute per millimeter of mercury. Figure 58-4 compares the measured or calculated diffusing capacities of carbon monoxide, O_2, and CO_2 at rest and during exercise, showing the extreme diffusing capacity of CO_2 and the effect of exercise on the diffusing capacity of each of these gases.

Measurement of Diffusing Capacity—The Carbon Monoxide Method. The O_2 diffusing capacity can be calculated from measurements of (1) alveolar PO_2, (2) PO_2 in the pulmonary capillary blood, and (3) the rate of O_2 uptake by the blood. However, measuring the PO_2 in the pulmonary capillary blood is so difficult and

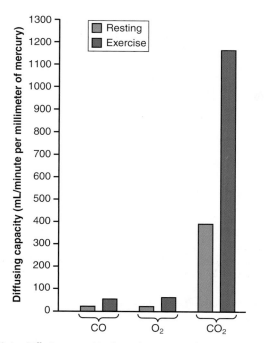

Figure 58-4 *Diffusing capacities* for carbon monoxide, oxygen, and carbon dioxide in the normal lungs under resting conditions and during exercise.

imprecise that it is not practical to measure oxygen diffusing capacity by such a direct procedure, except on an experimental basis.

To obviate the difficulties encountered in measuring oxygen diffusing capacity directly, physiologists usually measure carbon monoxide (CO) diffusing capacity instead and then calculate the O_2 diffusing capacity from this.

The principle of the CO method is the following:

1. A small amount of CO is breathed into the alveoli and the partial pressure of the CO in the alveoli is measured from appropriate alveolar air samples.
2. The CO pressure in the blood is essentially zero because hemoglobin combines with this gas so rapidly that its pressure never has time to build up.
3. Therefore, the pressure difference of CO across the respiratory membrane is equal to its partial pressure in the alveolar air sample.
4. Then, by measuring the volume of CO absorbed in a short period and dividing this by the alveolar CO partial pressure, one can determine accurately the CO diffusing capacity.

To convert CO diffusing capacity to O_2 diffusing capacity, the value is multiplied by a factor of 1.23 because the diffusion coefficient for oxygen is 1.23 times that for CO. Thus, the average diffusing capacity for CO in young men at rest is 17 mL/minute per millimeter of mercury and the diffusing capacity for O_2 is 1.23 times this, or 21 mL/minute per millimeter of mercury.

BIBLIOGRAPHY

Glenny RW, Robertson HT: Spatial distribution of ventilation and perfusion: mechanisms and regulation, *Compr. Physiol.* 1:375, 2011.

Guazzi M: Alveolar–capillary membrane dysfunction in heart failure: evidence of a pathophysiologic role, *Chest* 124:1090, 2003.

Hopkins SR, Wielpütz MO, Kauczor HU: Imaging lung perfusion, *J. Appl. Physiol.* 113:328, 2012.

Hughes JM, Pride NB: Examination of the carbon monoxide diffusing capacity (DL(CO)) in relation to its KCO and VA components, *Am. J. Respir. Crit. Care Med.* 186:132, 2012.

MacIntyre NR: Mechanisms of functional loss in patients with chronic lung disease, *Respir. Care* 53:1177, 2008.

Naeije R, Chesler N: Pulmonary circulation at exercise, *Compr. Physiol.* 2:711, 2012.

O'Donnell DE, Laveneziana P, Webb K, Neder JA: Chronic obstructive pulmonary disease: clinical integrative physiology, *Clin. Chest Med.* 35:51, 2014.

Otis AB: Quantitative relationships in steady-state gas exchange, Fenn WQ, Rahn H, editors: *Handbook of Physiology. Section 3*, vol. 1, Williams & Wilkins, Baltimore, 2000, pp p. 681.

Rahn H, Farhi EE: Ventilation, perfusion, and gas exchange—the $\dot{V}_A/\dot{Q}$ concept, Fenn WO, Rahn H, editors: *Handbook of Physiology. Section 3*, vol. 1, Baltimore, 1964, Williams & Wilkins, pp 125.

Robertson HT, Buxton RB: Imaging for lung physiology: what do we wish we could measure? *J. Appl. Physiol.* 113:317, 2012.

Tuder RM, Petrache I: Pathogenesis of chronic obstructive pulmonary disease, *J. Clin. Invest.* 122:2749, 2012.

Wagner PD: Assessment of gas exchange in lung disease: balancing accuracy against feasibility, *Crit. Care* 11:182, 2007.

Wagner PD: The multiple inert gas elimination technique (MIGET), *Intensive Care Med.* 34:994, 2008.

West JB: Role of the fragility of the pulmonary blood–gas barrier in the evolution of the pulmonary circulation, *Am. J. Physiol. Regul. Integr. Comp. Physiol.* 304:R171, 2013.

59

Oxygen Transport

LEARNING OBJECTIVES

- Compare the composition of the alveolar air, inspired air, and expired air.
- List the methods of transport of oxygen in the blood.
- Draw a diagram to show the oxygen dissociation curve and Bohr effect and explain the curves.
- Define and classify the types of hypoxia with examples.

GLOSSARY OF TERMS

- **2,3-Biphosphoglycerate (BPG):** Also referred to as 2,3-diphosphoglycerate (DPG), is a metabolically important phosphate compound present in the blood in different concentrations under different metabolic conditions

- **Bohr effect:** A shift of the oxygen–hemoglobin dissociation curve to the right in response to increases in blood carbon dioxide and hydrogen ions

- **Hemoglobin:** A complex protein–iron compound present in red blood cells and helps in the transport of oxygen

- **Hypoxia:** Decreased availability of oxygen to the tissues in the body

Compositions of Alveolar Air and Atmospheric Air Are Different

Alveolar air does not have the same concentrations of gases as atmospheric air by any means, which can readily be seen by comparing the alveolar air composition in Table 59-1 with that of atmospheric air. There are several reasons for the differences. First, the alveolar air is only partially replaced by atmospheric air with each breath. Second, oxygen (O_2) is constantly being absorbed into the pulmonary blood from the alveolar air. Third, carbon dioxide is constantly diffusing from the pulmonary blood into the alveoli. And fourth, dry atmospheric air that enters the respiratory passages is humidified even before it reaches the alveoli.

Table 59-1 shows that atmospheric air is composed almost entirely of nitrogen and O_2; it normally contains almost no carbon dioxide and little water vapor. However, as soon as the atmospheric air enters the respiratory passages, it is exposed to the fluids that cover the respiratory surfaces. Even before the air enters the alveoli, it becomes (for all practical purposes) totally humidified. Table 59-1 also shows that humidification of the air dilutes the O_2 partial pressure at sea level from an average of 159 mmHg in atmospheric air to 149 mmHg in the humidified air, and it dilutes the nitrogen partial pressure from 597 to 563 mmHg.

Methods of Oxygen Transport

Once *oxygen (O_2)* has diffused from the alveoli into the pulmonary blood, it is transported to the tissue capillaries in two forms:

1. *Combined with hemoglobin*: Most of the O_2 is transported in this form. The presence of hemoglobin in the red blood cells allows the blood to transport 30–100 times as much O_2 as could be transported in the form of dissolved O_2 in the water of the blood.

2. *Dissolved in the plasma*: The amount of O_2 dissolved obeys Henry's law and is proportional to the partial pressure. However, the amount of O_2 that can be transported in this form is very small and amounts to approximately 0.3 mL of O_2 per 100 mL of blood considering an arterial PO_2 of 100 mmHg.

The purpose of this chapter is to present both qualitatively and quantitatively the physical and chemical principles of O_2 transport in the blood and tissue fluids.

TRANSPORT OF OXYGEN IN THE DISSOLVED STATE

At the normal arterial PO_2 of 95 mmHg, about 0.29 mL of O_2 is dissolved in every 100 mL of water in the blood, and when the PO_2 of the blood falls to the normal 40 mmHg in the tissue capillaries, only 0.12 mL of O_2 remains dissolved. In other words, 0.17 mL of O_2 is normally transported in the dissolved state to the tissues by each 100 mL of arterial blood flow. This compares with almost 5 mL of O_2 transported by the red cell hemoglobin. Therefore, the amount of O_2 transported to the tissues in the dissolved state is normally slight, only about 3% of the total, as compared with 97% transported by the hemoglobin.

During strenuous exercise, when hemoglobin release of O_2 to the tissues increases another threefold, the relative quantity of O_2 transported in the dissolved state falls to as little as 1.5%. But if a person breathes O_2 at very high alveolar PO_2 levels, the amount transported in the dissolved state can become much greater, sometimes so much that a serious excess of O_2 occurs in the tissues, and "oxygen poisoning" ensues. This often leads to brain convulsions and even death, as discussed in detail in Chapter 63 in relation to the high-pressure breathing of O_2 among deep-sea divers.

ROLE OF HEMOGLOBIN IN OXYGEN TRANSPORT

Normally, about 97% of the O_2 transported from the lungs to the tissues is carried in chemical combination with hemoglobin in the red blood cells. The remaining 3% is transported in the dissolved state in the water of the plasma and blood cells. Thus, *under normal conditions*, O_2 is carried to the tissues almost entirely by hemoglobin.

TABLE 59-1	Partial Pressures of Respiratory Gases as they Enter and Leave the Lungs (at Sea Level)			
	Atmospheric Air[a] (mmHg)	Humidified Air (mmHg)	Alveolar Air (mmHg)	Expired Air (mmHg)
N_2	597.0 (78.62%)	563.4 (74.09%)	569.0 (74.9%)	566.0 (74.5%)
O_2	159.0 (20.84%)	149.3 (19.67%)	104.0 (13.6%)	120.0 (15.7%)
CO_2	0.3 (0.04%)	0.3 (0.04%)	40.0 (5.3%)	27.0 (3.6%)
H_2O	3.7 (0.50%)	47.0 (6.20%)	47.0 (6.2%)	47.0 (6.2%)
Total	760.0 (100.0%)	760.0 (100.0%)	760.0 (100.0%)	760.0 (100.0%)

[a]On an average cool, clear day.

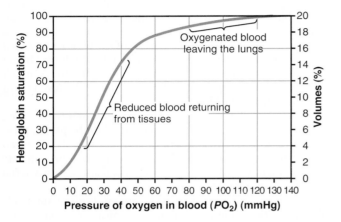

Figure 59-1 Oxygen–hemoglobin dissociation curve.

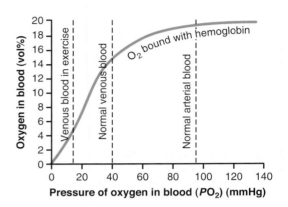

Figure 59-2 Effect of blood PO_2 on the quantity of oxygen bound with hemoglobin in each 100 mL of blood.

REVERSIBLE COMBINATION OF OXYGEN WITH HEMOGLOBIN

The chemistry of hemoglobin is presented in Chapter 21; as described earlier the different types of chains of hemoglobin are designated *alpha chains*, *beta chains*, *gamma chains*, and *delta chains*. The most common form of hemoglobin in the adult human being, *hemoglobin A*, is a combination of *two alpha chains* and *two beta chains*. In the newborn infant, hemoglobin F (fetal) is the predominant form of hemoglobin, which is gradually replaced in the first year of life.

Because each hemoglobin chain has a heme prosthetic group containing an atom of iron, and because there are four hemoglobin chains in each hemoglobin molecule, one finds four iron atoms in each hemoglobin molecule; each of these can bind loosely with one molecule of O_2, making a total of four molecules of O_2 (or eight oxygen atoms) that can be transported by each hemoglobin molecule.

The types of hemoglobin chains in the hemoglobin molecule determine the binding affinity of the hemoglobin for O_2, where it was pointed out that the O_2 molecule combines loosely and reversibly with the heme portion of hemoglobin. When PO_2 is high, as in the pulmonary capillaries, O_2 binds with the hemoglobin, but when PO_2 is low, as in the tissue capillaries, O_2 is released from the hemoglobin. This is the basis for almost all O_2 transport from the lungs to the tissues.

Oxygen–Hemoglobin Dissociation Curve. Figure 59-1 shows the oxygen–hemoglobin dissociation curve, which demonstrates a progressive increase in the percentage of hemoglobin bound with O_2 as blood PO_2 increases, which is called the *percent saturation of hemoglobin*. Because the blood leaving the lungs and entering the systemic arteries usually has a PO_2 of about 95 mmHg, one can see from the dissociation curve that the *usual O_2 saturation of systemic arterial blood averages 97%.*

Conversely, in normal venous blood returning from the peripheral tissues, the PO_2 is about 40 mmHg and *the saturation of hemoglobin averages 75%.*

Maximum Amount of Oxygen that Can Combine with the Hemoglobin of the Blood. The blood of a normal person contains about 15 g of hemoglobin in each 100 mL of blood, and each gram of hemoglobin can bind with a maximum of 1.34 mL of O_2 (1.39 mL when the hemoglobin is chemically pure, but impurities such as methemoglobin reduce this). Therefore, 15 times 1.34 equals 20.1, which means that, on average, the 15 g of hemoglobin in 100 mL of blood can combine with a total of about 20 mL of O_2 if the hemoglobin is 100% saturated. This is usually expressed as *20 vol%*. The O_2–hemoglobin dissociation curve for the normal person can also be expressed in terms of volume percent of O_2, as shown by the far right scale in Figure 59-1, instead of percent saturation of hemoglobin.

Amount of Oxygen Released from the Hemoglobin when Systemic Arterial Blood Flows Through the Tissues. The total quantity of O_2 *bound with hemoglobin* in normal systemic arterial blood, which is 97% saturated, is about 19.4 mL per 100 mL of blood as shown in Figure 59-2. On passing through the tissue capillaries, this amount is reduced, on average, to 14.4 mL (PO_2 of 40 mmHg, 75% saturated hemoglobin). Thus, *under normal conditions, about 5 mL of O_2 is transported from the lungs to the tissues by each 100 mL of blood flow.*

Transport of Oxygen Is Markedly Increased During Strenuous Exercise. During heavy exercise, the muscle cells use O_2 at a rapid rate, which, in extreme cases, can cause the muscle interstitial fluid PO_2 to fall from the normal 40 mmHg to as low as 15 mmHg. At this low pressure, only 4.4 mL of O_2 remains bound with the hemoglobin in each 100 mL of blood, as shown in Figure 59-2. Thus, 19.4 − 4.4, or 15 mL, is the quantity of O_2 actually delivered to the tissues by each 100 mL of blood flow, meaning that three times as much O_2 as normal is delivered in each volume of blood that passes through the tissues.

HEMOGLOBIN "BUFFERS" TISSUE PO_2

Although hemoglobin is necessary for the transport of O_2 to the tissues, it performs another function essential to life. This is its function as a "tissue oxygen buffer" system. That is, the hemoglobin in the blood is mainly responsible for stabilizing the PO_2 in the tissues. This can be explained as follows:

Hemoglobin Helps Maintain Nearly Constant PO_2 ***in the Tissues.*** Under basal conditions, the tissues require about 5 mL of O_2 from each 100 mL of blood passing through the tissue capillaries. Referring to the O_2–hemoglobin dissociation curve in Figure 59-2, one can see that for the normal 5 mL of O_2 to be released per 100 mL of blood flow, the PO_2 must fall to about 40 mmHg. Therefore, the tissue PO_2 normally cannot rise above this 40 mmHg level because, if it did, the amount of O_2 needed by the tissues would not be released from the hemoglobin. In this way, the hemoglobin normally sets an upper limit on the PO_2 in the tissues at about 40 mmHg.

Conversely, during heavy exercise, extra amounts of O_2 (as much as 20 times normal) must be delivered from the hemoglobin to the tissues. However, this delivery of extra O_2 can be achieved with little further decrease in tissue PO_2 because of (1) the steep slope of the dissociation curve and (2) the increase in tissue blood flow caused by the decreased PO_2; that is, a very small fall in PO_2 causes large amounts of extra O_2 to be released from the hemoglobin. It can be seen, then, that the hemoglobin in the blood automatically delivers O_2 to the tissues at a pressure that is held rather tightly between about 15 and 40 mmHg.

When Atmospheric Oxygen Concentration Changes Markedly, the Buffer Effect of Hemoglobin Still Maintains Almost Constant Tissue PO_2. The normal PO_2 in the alveoli is about 104 mmHg, but as one ascends a mountain or ascends in an airplane, the PO_2 can easily fall to less than half this amount. Alternatively, when one enters areas of compressed air, such as deep in the sea or in pressurized chambers, the PO_2 may rise to 10 times this level. Even so, the tissue PO_2 changes little.

It can be seen from the O_2–hemoglobin dissociation curve in Figure 59-1 that when the alveolar PO_2 is decreased to as low as 60 mmHg, the arterial hemoglobin is still 89% saturated with O_2—only 8% below the normal saturation of 97%. Further, the tissues still remove about 5 mL of O_2 from each 100 mL of blood passing through the tissues; to remove this O_2, the PO_2 of the venous blood falls to 35 mmHg—only 5 mmHg below the normal value of 40 mmHg. Thus, the tissue PO_2 hardly changes, despite the marked fall in alveolar PO_2 from 104 to 60 mmHg.

Conversely, when the alveolar PO_2 rises as high as 500 mmHg, the maximum O_2 saturation of hemoglobin can never rise above 100%, which is only 3% above the normal level of 97%. Consequently, the level of alveolar O_2 may vary greatly—from 60 to more than 500 mmHg PO_2—and still the PO_2 in the peripheral tissues does not vary more than a few milliliters from normal, *demonstrating beautifully the tissue "oxygen buffer" function of the blood hemoglobin system.*

FACTORS THAT SHIFT THE OXYGEN–HEMOGLOBIN DISSOCIATION CURVE—THEIR IMPORTANCE FOR OXYGEN TRANSPORT

The O_2–hemoglobin dissociation curves of Figures 59-1 and 59-2 are for normal, average blood. However, several factors can dis-

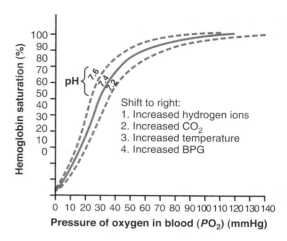

Figure 59-3 Shift of the oxygen–hemoglobin dissociation curve to the right caused by an increase in hydrogen ion concentration (decrease in pH). *BPG*, 2,3-biphosphoglycerate.

BOX 59-1   FACTORS THAT SHIFT THE OXYGEN DISSOCIATION CURVE

Three of these, all of which shift the curve to the *right*, are as follows:
- Increased carbon dioxide concentration
- Increased blood temperature
- Increased 2,3-biphosphoglycerate (BPG), a metabolically important phosphate compound present in the blood in different concentrations under different metabolic conditions

---

place the dissociation curve in one direction or the other in the manner shown in Figure 59-3. This figure shows that when the blood becomes slightly acidic, with the pH decreasing from the normal value of 7.4 to 7.2, the O_2–hemoglobin dissociation curve shifts, on average, about 15% to the right. Conversely, an increase in pH from the normal 7.4 to 7.6 shifts the curve a similar amount to the left.

In addition to pH changes, several other factors are known to shift the curve (Box 59-1).

The Bohr Effect—Increased Delivery of Oxygen to the Tissues when Carbon Dioxide and Hydrogen Ions Shift the Oxygen–Hemoglobin Dissociation Curve. A shift of the O_2–hemoglobin dissociation curve to the right in response to increases in blood CO_2 and hydrogen ions has a significant effect by enhancing the release of O_2 from the blood in the tissues and enhancing oxygenation of the blood in the lungs. This is called the *Bohr effect*, which can be explained as follows: As the blood passes through the tissues, CO_2 diffuses from the tissue cells into the blood. This diffusion increases the blood PO_2, which in turn raises the blood carbonic acid (H_2CO_3) and the hydrogen ion concentration. These effects shift the O_2–hemoglobin dissociation curve to the right and downward, as shown in Figure 59-3, forcing O_2 away from the hemoglobin and therefore delivering increased amounts of O_2 to the tissues.

Exactly the opposite effects occur in the lungs, where CO_2 diffuses from the blood into the alveoli. This reduces the blood PO_2 and decreases the hydrogen ion concentration, shifting the O_2–hemoglobin dissociation curve to the left and upward. Therefore, the quantity of O_2 that binds with the hemoglobin at any given alveolar PO_2 becomes considerably increased, thus allowing greater O_2 transport to the tissues.

Effect of BPG to Cause Rightward Shift of the Oxygen–Hemoglobin Dissociation Curve. The normal 2,3-biphosphoglycerate (BPG) in the blood keeps the O_2–hemoglobin dissociation curve shifted slightly to the right all the time. In hypoxic conditions that last longer than a few hours, the quantity of BPG in the blood increases considerably, thus shifting the O_2–hemoglobin dissociation curve even farther to the right. This causes O_2 to be released to the tissues at as much as 10 mmHg higher tissue O_2 pressure than would be the case without this increased BPG. Therefore, under some conditions, the BPG mechanism can be important for adaptation to hypoxia, especially to hypoxia caused by poor tissue blood flow.

Rightward Shift of the Oxygen–Hemoglobin Dissociation Curve During Exercise. During exercise, several factors shift the dissociation curve considerably to the right, thus delivering extra amounts of O_2 to the active, exercising muscle fibers. The exercising muscles, in turn, release large quantities of CO_2; this and several other acids released by the muscles increase the hydrogen ion concentration in the muscle capillary blood. In addition, the temperature of the muscle often rises 2–3°C, which can increase O_2 delivery to the muscle fibers even more. All these factors act together to shift the O_2–hemoglobin dissociation curve *of the muscle capillary blood* considerably to the right. This rightward shift of the curve forces O_2 to be released from the blood hemoglobin to the muscle at PO_2 levels as high as 40 mmHg, even when 70% of the O_2 has already been removed from the hemoglobin. Then, in the lungs, the shift occurs in the opposite direction allowing the pickup of extra amounts of O_2 from the alveoli.

Hypoxia and Oxygen Therapy

Almost any of the conditions discussed in the past few sections of this chapter can cause serious degrees of cellular hypoxia throughout the body. Sometimes, O_2 therapy is of great value; other times, it is of moderate value, and, at still other times, it is of almost no value. Therefore, it is important to understand the different types of hypoxia; then we can discuss the physiological principles of O_2 therapy. The following is a descriptive classification of the causes of hypoxia (Box 59-2):

1. Inadequate oxygenation of the blood in the lungs because of extrinsic reasons:
   a. Deficiency of O_2 in the atmosphere
   b. Hypoventilation (neuromuscular disorders)

BOX 59-2 CLASSIFICATION OF HYPOXIA

1. Hypoxic hypoxia:
   a. Low atmospheric and alveolar oxygen content
   b. Impairment of diffusion across the respiratory membrane
   c. Venous-to-arterial shunts
   d. Ventilation–perfusion mismatches
2. Anemic hypoxia:
   a. Anemia or abnormal hemoglobin
   b. Poisoning by carbon monoxide
3. Stagnant hypoxia:
   a. General circulatory deficiency
   b. Localized circulatory deficiency (peripheral, cerebral, and coronary vessels)
   c. Tissue edema
4. Histotoxic hypoxia:
   a. Poisoning of cellular oxidation enzymes
   b. Diminished cellular metabolic capacity for using oxygen because of toxicity, vitamin deficiency, or other factors

---

2. Pulmonary disease:
   a. Hypoventilation caused by increased airway resistance or decreased pulmonary compliance
   b. Abnormal alveolar ventilation–perfusion ratio (including either increased physiological dead space or increased physiological shunt)
   c. Diminished respiratory membrane diffusion
3. Venous-to-arterial shunts ("right-to-left" cardiac shunts)
4. Inadequate O_2 transport to the tissues by the blood:
   a. Anemia or abnormal hemoglobin
   b. General circulatory deficiency
   c. Localized circulatory deficiency (peripheral, cerebral, and coronary vessels)
   d. Tissue edema
5. Inadequate tissue capability of using O_2:
   a. Poisoning of cellular oxidation enzymes
   b. Diminished cellular metabolic capacity for using O_2 because of toxicity, vitamin deficiency, or other factors

This classification of the types of hypoxia is mainly self-evident from the discussions earlier in the chapter. Only one type of hypoxia in the classification needs further elaboration: the hypoxia caused by inadequate capability of the body's tissue cells to use oxygen. There is an alternative classification of hypoxia, which is listed in the following.

Inadequate Tissue Capability to Use Oxygen. The classic cause of inability of the tissues to use O_2 is *cyanide poisoning*, in which the action of the enzyme *cytochrome oxidase* is completely blocked by the cyanide—to such an extent that the tissues simply cannot use O_2 even when plenty is available. Also, deficiencies of some of the *tissue cellular oxidative enzymes* or of other elements in the tissue oxidative system can lead to this type of hypoxia. A special example occurs in the disease *beriberi*, in which several important steps in tissue utilization of O_2 and formation of CO_2 are compromised because of *vitamin B deficiency*.

Effects of Hypoxia on the Body. Hypoxia, if severe enough, can cause death of cells throughout the body, but in less severe degrees it causes principally (1) depressed mental activity, sometimes culminating in coma, and (2) reduced work capacity of the muscles. These effects are specifically discussed in Chapter 63 in relation to high-altitude physiology.

Oxygen Therapy in Different Types of Hypoxia. Oxygen can be administered by (1) placing the patient's head in a "tent" that contains air fortified with O_2, (2) allowing the patient to breathe either pure O_2 or high concentrations of O_2 from a mask, or (3) administering O_2 through an intranasal tube.

Recalling the basic physiological principles of the different types of hypoxia, one can readily decide when O_2 therapy will be of value and, if so, how valuable.

In *atmospheric hypoxia*, O_2 therapy can completely correct the depressed O_2 level in the inspired gases and, therefore, provide 100% effective therapy.

In *hypoventilation hypoxia*, a person breathing 100% O_2 can move five times as much O_2 into the alveoli with each breath as when breathing normal air. Therefore, here again O_2 therapy can be extremely beneficial. (However, this provides no benefit for the excess blood CO_2 also caused by the hypoventilation.)

In *hypoxia caused by impaired alveolar membrane diffusion*, essentially the same result occurs as in hypoventilation hypoxia because O_2 therapy can increase the PO_2 in the lung alveoli from the normal value of about 100 mmHg to as high as 600 mmHg. This raises the O_2 pressure gradient for diffusion of O_2 from the alveoli to the blood from the normal value of 60 mmHg to as high as 560 mmHg, an increase of more than 800%. This highly beneficial effect of O_2 therapy in diffusion hypoxia is demonstrated in Figure 59-4, which shows that the pulmonary blood in this patient with pulmonary edema picks up O_2 three to four times as rapidly as would occur with no therapy.

In *hypoxia caused by anemia, abnormal hemoglobin transport of O_2, circulatory deficiency, or physiological shunt*, O_2 therapy is of much less value because normal O_2 is already available in the alveoli. The problem instead is that one or more of the mechanisms for transporting O_2 from the lungs to the tissues are deficient. Even so, a small amount of extra O_2, between 7 and 30%, can be *transported in the dissolved state* in the blood when alveolar O_2 is increased to maximum even though the amount transported by the hemoglobin is hardly altered. This small amount of extra O_2 may be the difference between life and death.

In the different types of *hypoxia caused by inadequate tissue use of O_2*, there is abnormality neither of O_2 pickup by

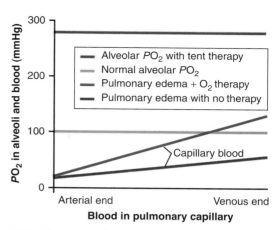

Figure 59-4 Absorption of oxygen into the pulmonary capillary blood in pulmonary edema with and without oxygen tent therapy.

the lungs nor of transport to the tissues. Instead, the tissue metabolic enzyme system is simply incapable of using the O_2 that is delivered. Therefore, O_2 therapy provides no measurable benefit.

BIBLIOGRAPHY

Amann M, Calbet JA: Convective oxygen transport and fatigue, *J. Appl. Physiol.* 104:861, 2008.

Casey DP, Joyner MJ: Compensatory vasodilatation during hypoxic exercise: mechanisms responsible for matching oxygen supply to demand, *J. Physiol.* 590:6321, 2012.

Clanton TL, Hogan MC, Gladden LB: Regulation of cellular gas exchange, oxygen sensing, and metabolic control, *Compr. Physiol.* 3:1135, 2013.

Jensen FB: Red blood cell pH, the Bohr effect, and other oxygenation-linked phenomena in blood O_2 and CO_2 transport, *Acta Physiol. Scand.* 182:215, 2004.

Jensen FB: The dual roles of red blood cells in tissue oxygen delivery: oxygen carriers and regulators of local blood flow, *J. Exp. Biol.* 212:3387, 2009.

Maina JN, West JB: Thin and strong! The bioengineering dilemma in the structural and functional design of the blood–gas barrier, *Physiol. Rev.* 85:811, 2005.

Mairbäurl H: Red blood cells in sports: effects of exercise and training on oxygen supply by red blood cells, *Front. Physiol.* 4:332, 2013.

Mairbäurl H, Weber RE: Oxygen transport by hemoglobin, *Compr. Physiol.* 2:1463, 2012.

Piiper J: Perfusion, diffusion and their heterogeneities limiting blood–tissue O_2 transfer in muscle, *Acta Physiol. Scand.* 168:603, 2000.

Richardson RS: Oxygen transport and utilization: an integration of the muscle systems, *Adv. Physiol. Educ.* 27:183, 2003.

Tsai AG, Johnson PC, Intaglietta M: Oxygen gradients in the microcirculation, *Physiol. Rev.* 83:933, 2003.

Carbon Dioxide Transport

In the body's tissue cells, oxygen (O_2) reacts with various foodstuffs to form large quantities of *carbon dioxide (CO_2)*. This CO_2 enters the tissue capillaries and is transported back to the lungs. Carbon dioxide, like O_2, also combines with chemical substances in the blood that increase CO_2 transport 15- to 20-fold.

The purpose of this chapter is to present both qualitatively and quantitatively the physical and chemical principles of CO_2 transport in the blood and tissue fluids.

Transport of Carbon Dioxide in the Blood

Transport of CO_2 by the blood is not nearly as problematic as transport of O_2 is because even in the most abnormal conditions, CO_2 can usually be transported in far greater quantities than can O_2. However, the amount of CO_2 in the blood has a lot to do with the acid–base balance of the body fluids, which is discussed in Chapter 82. Under normal resting conditions, *an average of 4 mL of CO_2 is transported from the tissues to the lungs in each 100 mL of blood.*

CHEMICAL FORMS IN WHICH CARBON DIOXIDE IS TRANSPORTED

To begin the process of CO_2 transport, CO_2 diffuses out of the tissue cells in the dissolved molecular CO_2 form. On entering the tissue capillaries, the CO_2 initiates a host of almost instantaneous physical and chemical reactions, shown in Figure 60-1, which are essential for CO_2 transport.

Transport of Carbon Dioxide in the Dissolved State

A small portion of the CO_2 is transported in the dissolved state to the lungs. Recall that the PCO_2 of venous blood is 45 mmHg and that of arterial blood is 40 mmHg. The amount of CO_2 dissolved in the fluid of the blood at 45 mmHg is about 2.7 mL/dL (2.7 vol%). The amount dissolved at 40 mmHg is about 2.4 mL, or a difference of 0.3 mL. Therefore, only about 0.3 mL of CO_2 is transported in the dissolved form by each 100 mL of blood flow. This is about 7% of all the CO_2 normally transported.

Transport of Carbon Dioxide in the Form of Bicarbonate Ion

Reaction of Carbon Dioxide with Water in the Red Blood Cells—Effect of Carbonic Anhydrase. The dissolved CO_2 in the blood reacts with water to form carbonic acid. This reaction would occur much too slowly to be of importance, were it not for the fact that inside the red blood cells is a protein enzyme called carbonic anhydrase, which catalyzes the reaction between CO_2 and water, and accelerates its reaction rate about 5000-fold. Therefore, instead of requiring many seconds or minutes to occur, as is true in the plasma, the reaction occurs so rapidly in the red blood cells that it reaches almost complete equilibrium within a small fraction of a second. This phenomenon allows tremendous amounts of CO_2 to react with the red blood cell water even before the blood leaves the tissue capillaries.

Dissociation of Carbonic Acid into Bicarbonate and Hydrogen Ions. In another fraction of a second, the carbonic acid formed in the red cells (H_2CO_3) dissociates into hydrogen and bicarbonate ions (H^+ and HCO_3^-). Most of the H^+ ions then combine with the hemoglobin in the red blood cells because the hemoglobin protein is a powerful acid–base buffer. In turn, many of the HCO_3^- ions diffuse from the red blood cells into the plasma, while chloride ions diffuse into the red blood cells to take their place. This diffusion is made possible by the presence of a special bicarbonate–chloride carrier protein in the red blood cell membrane that shuttles these two ions in opposite directions at rapid velocities. Thus, the chloride content of venous red blood cells is greater than that of arterial red cells, a phenomenon called the chloride shift.

The reversible combination of CO_2 with water in the red blood cells under the influence of carbonic anhydrase accounts for about 70% of the CO_2 transported from the tissues to the lungs. Thus, this means of transporting CO_2 is by far the most important. Indeed, when a carbonic anhydrase inhibitor (acetazolamide) is administered to an animal to block the action of carbonic anhydrase in the red blood cells, CO_2 transport from the tissues becomes so poor that the tissue PCO_2 may rise to 80 mmHg instead of the normal 45 mmHg.

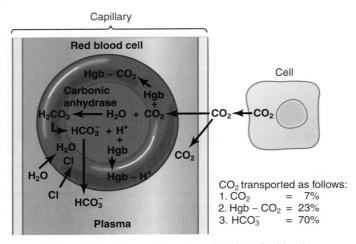

Figure 60-1   Transport of carbon dioxide in the blood.

CO₂ transported as follows:
1. CO_2 = 7%
2. $Hgb - CO_2$ = 23%
3. HCO_3^- = 70%

Transport of Carbon Dioxide in Combination with Hemoglobin and Plasma Proteins—Carbaminohemoglobin. In addition to reacting with water, CO_2 reacts directly with amine radicals of the hemoglobin molecule to form the compound *carbaminohemoglobin* (CO_2Hgb). This combination of CO_2 and hemoglobin is a reversible reaction that occurs with a loose bond, so the CO_2 is easily released into the alveoli, where the PCO_2 is lower than in the pulmonary capillaries.

A small amount of CO_2 also reacts in the same way with the plasma proteins in the tissue capillaries. This reaction is much less significant for the transport of CO_2 because the quantity of these proteins in the blood is only one-fourth as great as the quantity of hemoglobin.

The quantity of CO_2 that can be carried from the peripheral tissues to the lungs by carbamino combination with hemoglobin and plasma proteins is about 30% of the total quantity transported—that is, normally about 1.5 mL of CO_2 in each 100 mL of blood. However, because this reaction is much slower than the reaction of carbon dioxide with water inside the red blood cells, it is doubtful that under normal conditions this carbamino mechanism transports more than 20% of the total CO_2.

DIFFUSION OF CARBON DIOXIDE FROM THE PERIPHERAL TISSUE CELLS INTO THE CAPILLARIES AND FROM THE PULMONARY CAPILLARIES INTO THE ALVEOLI

When O_2 is used by the cells, virtually all of it becomes CO_2 and this increases the intracellular PCO_2; because of this high tissue cell PCO_2, CO_2 diffuses from the cells into the tissue capillaries and is then carried by the blood to the lungs. In the lungs, it diffuses from the pulmonary capillaries into the alveoli and is expired.

Thus, at each point in the gas transport chain, CO_2 diffuses in the direction exactly opposite to the diffusion of O_2. Yet there is one major difference between diffusion of CO_2 and of O_2: CO_2 *can diffuse about 20 times as rapidly as O_2.* Therefore, the pressure differences required to cause CO_2 diffusion are, in each instance, far less than the pressure differences required to cause O_2 diffusion. The CO_2 pressures are approximately the following:

1. Intracellular PCO_2, 46 mmHg; interstitial PCO_2, 45 mmHg. Thus, there is only a 1 mmHg pressure differential, as shown in Figure 60-2.
2. PCO_2 of the arterial blood entering the tissues, 40 mmHg; PCO_2 of the venous blood leaving the tissues, 45 mmHg.

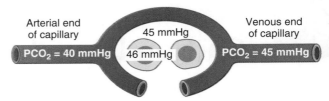

Figure 60-2   Uptake of carbon dioxide by the blood in the tissue capillaries. (PCO_2 in tissue cells = 46 mmHg, and in interstitial fluid = 45 mmHg.)

Thus, as shown in Figure 60-2, the tissue capillary blood comes almost exactly to equilibrium with the interstitial PCO_2 of 45 mmHg.

3. PCO_2 of the blood entering the pulmonary capillaries at the arterial end, 45 mmHg; PCO_2 of the alveolar air, 40 mmHg. Thus, only a 5 mmHg pressure difference causes all the required CO_2 diffusion out of the pulmonary capillaries into the alveoli. Furthermore, as shown in Figure 60-3, the PCO_2 of the pulmonary capillary blood falls to almost exactly equal the alveolar PCO_2 of 40 mmHg before it has passed more than about one-third the distance through the capillaries. This is the same effect that was observed earlier for O_2 diffusion, except that it is in the opposite direction.

Effect of Rate of Tissue Metabolism and Tissue Blood Flow on Interstitial PCO_2. Tissue capillary blood flow and tissue metabolism affect the PCO_2 in ways exactly opposite to their effect on tissue PO_2. Figure 60-4 shows these effects, as follows:

1. A decrease in blood flow from normal (point A) to one-quarter normal (point B) increases peripheral tissue PCO_2 from the normal value of 45 mmHg to an elevated level of 60 mmHg. Conversely, increasing the blood flow to six times normal (point C) decreases the interstitial PCO_2 from the normal value of 45 to 41 mmHg, down to a level almost equal to the PCO_2 in the arterial blood (40 mmHg) entering the tissue capillaries.
2. Note also that a 10-fold increase in tissue metabolic rate greatly elevates the interstitial fluid PCO_2 at all rates of blood flow, whereas decreasing the metabolism to one-quarter normal causes the interstitial fluid PCO_2 to fall to about 41 mmHg, closely approaching that of the arterial blood, 40 mmHg.

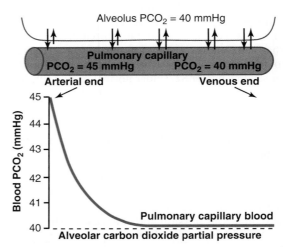

Figure 60-3   Diffusion of carbon dioxide from the pulmonary blood into the alveolus. *Data from Milhorn Jr., H.T., Pulley Jr., P.E., 1968. A theoretical study of pulmonary capillary gas exchange and venous admixture. Biophys. J. 8, 337.*

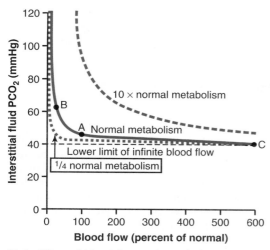

Figure 60-4 Effect of blood flow and metabolic rate on peripheral tissue PCO_2.

CARBON DIOXIDE DISSOCIATION CURVE

The curve shown in Figure 60-5—called the *carbon dioxide dissociation curve*—depicts the dependence of total blood CO_2 in all its forms on PCO_2. Note that the normal blood PCO_2 ranges between a narrow range of 40 mmHg in arterial blood and 45 mmHg in venous blood. Note also that the normal concentration of CO_2 in the blood in all its different forms is about 50 vol%, but only 4 vol% of this is exchanged during normal transport of CO_2 from the tissues to the lungs. That is, the concentration rises to about 52 vol% as the blood passes through the tissues and falls to about 48 vol% as it passes through the lungs.

WHEN OXYGEN BINDS WITH HEMOGLOBIN, CARBON DIOXIDE IS RELEASED (THE HALDANE EFFECT) TO INCREASE CO_2 TRANSPORT

Earlier in the chapter, we pointed out that an increase in CO_2 in the blood causes O_2 to be displaced from the hemoglobin (the Bohr effect), which is an important factor in increasing O_2 transport. The reverse is also true: binding of O_2 with hemoglobin tends to displace CO_2 from the blood. Indeed, this effect, called the *Haldane effect*, is quantitatively far more important in promoting CO_2 transport than is the Bohr effect in promoting O_2 transport (Box 60-1).

Figure 60-6 demonstrates quantitatively the significance of the Haldane effect on the transport of CO_2 from the tissues to the

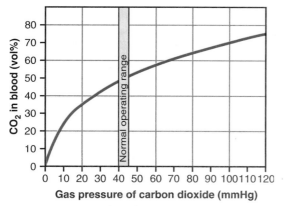

Figure 60-5 Carbon dioxide dissociation curve.

BOX 60-1   HALDANE EFFECT

The Haldane effect results from the simple fact that the combination of oxygen with hemoglobin in the lungs causes the hemoglobin to become a stronger acid. This displaces carbon dioxide from the blood and into the alveoli in two ways:

1. The more highly acidic hemoglobin has less tendency to combine with carbon dioxide to form carbaminohemoglobin, thus displacing much of the carbon dioxide that is present in the carbamino form from the blood.
2. The increased acidity of the hemoglobin also causes it to release an excess of hydrogen ions, and these bind with bicarbonate ions to form carbonic acid; this then dissociates into water and carbon dioxide, and the carbon dioxide is released from the blood into the alveoli and, finally, into the air.

lungs. This figure shows small portions of two CO_2 dissociation curves: (1) when the PO_2 is 100 mmHg, which is the case in the blood capillaries of the lungs, and (2) when the PO_2 is 40 mmHg, which is the case in the tissue capillaries. Point A shows that the normal PCO_2 of 45 mmHg in the tissues causes 52 vol% of CO_2 to combine with the blood. On entering the lungs, the PCO_2 falls to 40 mmHg and the PO_2 rises to 100 mmHg. If the CO_2 dissociation curve did not shift because of the Haldane effect, the CO_2 content of the blood would fall only to 50 vol%, which would be a loss of only 2 vol% of CO_2. However, the increase in PO_2 in the lungs lowers the CO_2 dissociation curve from the top curve to the lower curve of the figure, so the CO_2 content falls to 48 vol% (point B). This represents an additional 2 vol% loss of CO_2. Thus, the Haldane effect approximately doubles the amount of CO_2 released from the blood in the lungs and approximately doubles the pickup of CO_2 in the tissues.

CHANGE IN BLOOD ACIDITY DURING CO_2 TRANSPORT

The carbonic acid formed when CO_2 enters the blood in the peripheral tissues decreases the blood pH. However, reaction of this acid with the acid–base buffers of the blood prevents the H^+ concentration from rising greatly (and the pH from falling greatly). Ordinarily, arterial blood has a pH of about 7.41 and as the blood acquires CO_2 in the tissue capillaries, the pH falls to a venous value of about 7.37. In other words, a pH change of 0.04 U takes place. The reverse occurs when CO_2 is released from the blood in the lungs, with the pH rising to the arterial

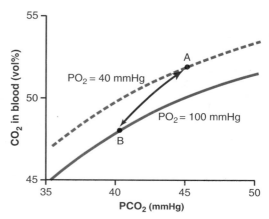

Figure 60-6 Portions of the carbon dioxide dissociation curve when the PO_2 is 100 or 40 mmHg. The arrow represents the Haldane effect on the transport of carbon dioxide.

value of 7.41 once again. In heavy exercise or other conditions of high metabolic activity, or when blood flow through the tissues is sluggish, the decrease in pH in the tissue blood (and in the tissues themselves) can be as much as 0.50, about 12 times normal, thus causing significant tissue acidosis.

CHANGES IN BLOOD GASES DURING HYPOVENTILATION AND HYPERVENTILATION

Blood gas measurements can be monitored either using noninvasive methods or using invasive methods. The invasive methods are described in Chapter 64 and include the measurement of blood PO_2, CO_2, and pH. The arterial blood gas (ABG) measurement is one of the commonly used techniques for measuring PO_2, CO_2, pH, and bicarbonate (HCO_3^-). This measurement technique requires an arterial blood sample of a few milliliters, and is highly reliable and reproducible.

Hypoventilation. Hypoventilation may occur if the respiratory centers are affected by injury or are depressed due to various other reasons. Some of the causes include damage to the nerve supply of the respiratory muscles, spinal cord injuries, conditions such as myasthenia gravis that affect the neuromuscular junction, and dysfunction of the lung mechanics such as chest wall injuries, kyphoscoliosis, and airway obstruction. In those individuals who ascend to high altitudes, alveolar hypoxia may occur due to decreased barometric pressure at higher altitudes. Both hypoventilation and ascent to high altitudes cause alveolar hypoxia, decreased arterial PO_2, and increased CO_2 levels in blood (hypercapnia). Ultimately, hypoventilation will lead to respiratory acidosis (reduced pH with elevated CO_2) and this is compensated by renal HCO_3^- retention and excretion of H^+ ions by the kidneys.

Acid–base nomograms (Figure 82-11) (Davenport diagram) allow simultaneous plotting of pH, CO_2, and HCO_3^-, and help in understanding and interpreting mixed respiratory and metabolic acid–base disturbances.

Hyperventilation. Hyperventilation is a condition where the rate of alveolar ventilation is increased more than the rate of CO_2 production by metabolic processes. This leads to a decrease in arterial PCO_2 levels well below the normal PCO_2 range (37–43 mmHg).

Conditions such as tachypnea (increase in respiratory rate) and hyperpnea (increase in minute ventilation) should be differentiated from hyperventilation. Both tachypnea and hyperpnea do not cause changes in arterial PCO_2 levels.

The causes of alveolar hyperventilation could be due to an *excessive ventilatory drive* caused by either *behavioral* or *metabolic* regulatory *systems*. Some of the causes for hyperventilation include hypoxemia caused by pulmonary diseases, pneumonia, cardiovascular disorders such as congestive cardiac failure, metabolic disorders such as acidosis, hepatic failure, neurological causes such as psychogenic or anxiety, hyperventilation, drugs such as salicylates, beta-adrenergic agonists, and miscellaneous causes such as fever, sepsis, and pregnancy.

In conditions where the arterial PCO_2 is very low due to hyperventilation, it may temporarily cause apnea because of the reduced ventilatory drive. CO_2 that is produced by metabolic processes will then build up and restore the ventilator drive. Chronic hyperventilation leads to respiratory alkalosis and this condition is compensated by renal retention of hydrogen ions and excretion of HCO_3^- by the kidneys.

Respiratory Exchange Ratio

The discerning student will have noted that normal transport of O_2 from the lungs to the tissues by each 100 mL of blood is about 5 mL, whereas normal transport of CO_2 from the tissues to the lungs is about 4 mL. Thus, under normal resting conditions, only about 82% as much CO_2 is expired from the lungs as O_2 is taken up by the lungs. The ratio of CO_2 output to O_2 uptake is called the *respiratory exchange ratio (R)*. That is,

$$R = \frac{\text{rate of carbon dioxide output}}{\text{rate of oxygen uptake}}$$

The value for R changes under different metabolic conditions. When a person is using exclusively carbohydrates for body metabolism, R rises to 1.00. Conversely, when a person is using exclusively fats for metabolic energy, the R level falls to as low as 0.7. The reason for this difference is that when O_2 is metabolized with carbohydrates, one molecule of CO_2 is formed for each molecule of O_2 consumed; when O_2 reacts with fats, a large share of the O_2 combines with hydrogen atoms from the fats to form water instead of CO_2. In other words, when fats are metabolized, the *respiratory quotient of the chemical reactions* in the tissues is about 0.70 instead of 1.00. For a person on a normal diet consuming average amounts of carbohydrates, fats, and proteins, the average value for R is considered to be 0.825.

BIBLIOGRAPHY

Clanton TL, Hogan MC, Gladden LB: Regulation of cellular gas exchange, oxygen sensing, and metabolic control, *Compr. Physiol.* 3:1135, 2013.

Geers C, Gros G: Carbon dioxide transport and carbonic anhydrase in blood and muscle, *Physiol. Rev.* 80:681, 2000.

Jensen FB: Red blood cell pH, the Bohr effect, and other oxygenation-linked phenomena in blood O_2 and CO_2 transport, *Acta Physiol. Scand.* 182:215, 2004.

Levitzky MG: *Pulmonary Physiology*, eight ed., New York, 2013, McGraw-Hill Companies.

Maina JN, West JB: Thin and strong! The bioengineering dilemma in the structural and functional design of the blood–gas barrier, *Physiol. Rev.* 85:811, 2005.

Mason RJ, Broaddus CV, Martin T, et al: Hypoventilation and hyperventilation syndromes. *Murray and Nadel's Textbook of Respiratory Medicine*, sixth ed., Philadelphia, 2015, Saunders Elsevier.

Rakel RE, Rakel DP: *Textbook of Family Medicine*, ninth ed., Philadelphia, 2015, Saunders Elsevier.

West JB: *Respiratory Physiology—The Essentials*, ninth ed., Philadelphia, 2012, Lippincott Williams & Wilkins, Wolters Kluwers.

Chemical Regulation of Respiration

Chemical Control of Respiration

The ultimate goal of respiration is to maintain proper concentrations of O_2, CO_2, and hydrogen ions in the tissues. It is fortunate, therefore, that respiratory activity is highly responsive to changes in each of these substances.

Excess CO_2 or excess hydrogen ions in the blood mainly act directly on the respiratory center itself, causing greatly increased strength of both the inspiratory and the expiratory motor signals to the respiratory muscles.

O_2, in contrast, does not have a significant *direct* effect on the respiratory center of the brain in controlling respiration. Instead, it acts almost entirely on peripheral *chemoreceptors* located in the *carotid* and *aortic bodies*, and these chemoreceptors in turn transmit appropriate nervous signals to the respiratory center for control of respiration (Figure 61-1).

DIRECT CHEMICAL CONTROL OF RESPIRATORY CENTER ACTIVITY BY CO_2 AND HYDROGEN IONS

Chemosensitive Area of the Respiratory Center Beneath the Ventral Surface of the Medulla. There are mainly three areas of the respiratory center: the dorsal respiratory group of neurons, the ventral respiratory group, and the pneumotaxic center. It is believed that none of these is affected directly by changes in blood CO_2 concentration or hydrogen ion concentration. Instead, an additional neuronal area, a *chemosensitive area*, shown in Figure 61-2, is located bilaterally, lying only 0.2 mm beneath the ventral surface of the medulla. This area is highly sensitive to changes in either blood PCO_2 or hydrogen ion concentration, and it in turn excites the other portions of the respiratory center.

Excitation of the Chemosensitive Neurons by Hydrogen Ions Is Likely the Primary Stimulus

The sensor neurons in the chemosensitive area are especially excited by hydrogen ions; in fact, it is believed that hydrogen ions may be the only important direct stimulus for these neurons. However, hydrogen ions do not easily cross the blood–brain barrier. For this reason, changes in hydrogen ion concentration in the blood have considerably less effect in stimulating the chemosensitive neurons than do changes in blood CO_2, even though CO_2 is believed to stimulate these neurons secondarily by changing the hydrogen ion concentration, as explained in the following section.

CO_2 Stimulates the Chemosensitive Area

Although CO_2 has little direct effect in stimulating the neurons in the chemosensitive area, it does have a potent indirect effect. It has this effect by reacting with the water of the tissues to form carbonic acid, which dissociates into hydrogen and bicarbonate ions; the hydrogen ions then have a potent direct stimulatory effect on respiration. These reactions are shown in Figure 61-2.

Why does blood CO_2 have a more potent effect in stimulating the chemosensitive neurons than do blood hydrogen ions? The answer is that the blood–brain barrier is not very permeable to hydrogen ions, but CO_2 passes through this barrier almost as if the barrier did not exist. Consequently, whenever the blood PCO_2 increases, so does the PCO_2 of both the interstitial fluid of the medulla and the cerebrospinal fluid. In both these fluids, the CO_2 immediately reacts with the water to form new hydrogen ions. Thus, paradoxically, more hydrogen ions are released into the respiratory chemosensitive sensory area of the medulla when the blood CO_2 concentration increases than when the blood hydrogen ion concentration increases. For this reason, respiratory center activity is increased very strongly by changes in blood carbon dioxide, a fact that we subsequently discuss quantitatively.

Decreased Stimulatory Effect of CO_2 After the First 1–2 Days. Excitation of the respiratory center by CO_2 is great the first few hours after the blood CO_2 first increases, but then it gradually declines over the next 1–2 days, decreasing to about one-fifth the initial effect. Part of this decline results from renal readjustment of the hydrogen ion concentration in the circulating blood back toward normal after the CO_2 first increases the hydrogen concentration. The kidneys achieve this readjustment by increasing the blood bicarbonate, which binds with the hydrogen ions in the blood and cerebrospinal fluid to reduce their concentrations. But even more important, over a period of hours, the bicarbonate ions also slowly diffuse through the blood–brain and blood–cerebrospinal fluid barriers and combine directly with the hydrogen ions adjacent to the respiratory neurons as well, thus reducing the hydrogen ions back to near normal. A change in blood CO_2 concentration therefore has a potent *acute* effect

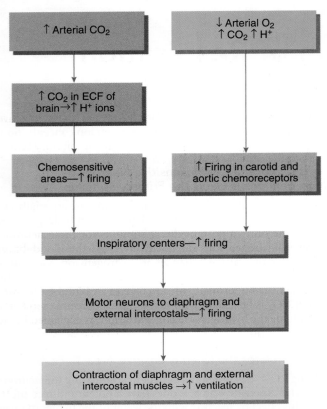

Figure 61-1 Summary of chemical stimuli that regulate ventilation. *ECF*, extracellular fluid.

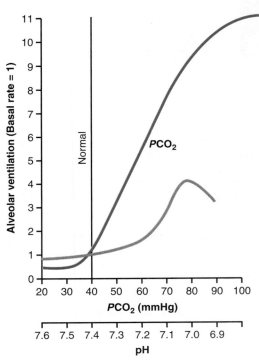

Figure 61-3 Effects of increased arterial blood PCO_2 and decreased arterial pH (increased hydrogen ion concentration) on the rate of alveolar ventilation.

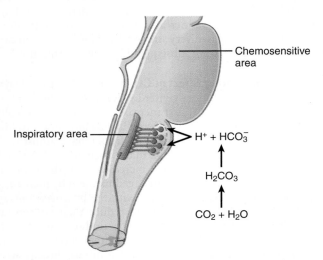

Figure 61-2 Stimulation of the *brainstem inspiratory* area by signals from the *chemosensitive area* located bilaterally in the medulla, lying only a fraction of a millimeter beneath the ventral medullary surface. Note also that hydrogen ions stimulate the chemosensitive area, but carbon dioxide in the fluid gives rise to most of the hydrogen ions.

on controlling respiratory drive but only a weak *chronic* effect after a few days' adaptation.

Quantitative Effects of Blood PCO₂ and Hydrogen Ion Concentration on Alveolar Ventilation

Figure 61-3 shows quantitatively the approximate effects of blood PCO_2 and blood pH (which is an inverse logarithmic measure of hydrogen ion concentration) on alveolar ventilation. Note especially the very marked increase in ventilation caused by an increase in PCO_2 *in the normal range* between 35

and 75 mmHg, which demonstrates the tremendous effect that CO_2 changes have in controlling respiration. By contrast, the change in respiration in the normal blood pH range, which is between 7.3 and 7.5, is less than one-tenth as great.

Changes in O₂ Have Little Direct Effect on Control of the Respiratory Center

Changes in O_2 concentration have virtually no *direct* effect on the respiratory center itself to alter respiratory drive (although O_2 changes do have an indirect effect, acting through the peripheral chemoreceptors, as explained in the next section).

We learned earlier that the hemoglobin–oxygen buffer system delivers almost exactly normal amounts of O_2 to the tissues even when the pulmonary PO_2 changes from a value as low as 60 mmHg up to a value as high as 1000 mmHg. Therefore, except under special conditions, adequate delivery of O_2 can occur despite changes in lung ventilation ranging from slightly below one-half normal to as high as 20 or more times normal. This is not true for CO_2 because both the blood and tissue PCO_2 change inversely with the rate of pulmonary ventilation; thus, the processes of animal evolution have made CO_2 the major controller of respiration, not O_2.

Yet for those special conditions in which the tissues get into trouble for lack of O_2, the body has a special mechanism for respiratory control located in the peripheral chemoreceptors, outside the brain respiratory center; this mechanism responds when the blood O_2 falls too low, mainly below a PO_2 of 70 mmHg, as explained in the next section.

Peripheral Chemoreceptor System for Control of Respiratory Activity—Role of Oxygen in Respiratory Control

In addition to control of respiratory activity by the respiratory center itself, still another mechanism is available for controlling respiration. This mechanism is the *peripheral chemoreceptor*

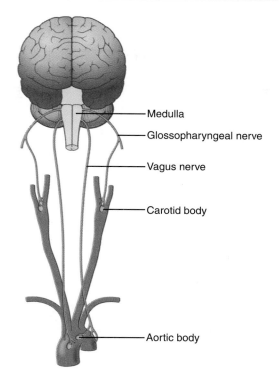

Figure 61-4 Respiratory control by peripheral chemoreceptors in the carotid and aortic bodies.

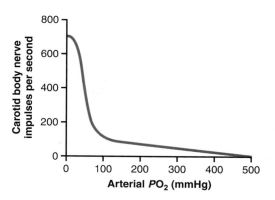

Figure 61-5 Effect of arterial PO_2 on impulse rate from the carotid body.

exposed at all times to arterial blood, not venous blood, and their PO_2 values are arterial PO_2 values.

Decreased Arterial Oxygen Stimulates the Chemoreceptors. When the oxygen concentration in the arterial blood falls below normal, the chemoreceptors become strongly stimulated. This effect is demonstrated in Figure 61-5, which shows the effect of different levels of *arterial PO_2* on the rate of nerve impulse transmission from a carotid body. Note that the impulse rate is particularly sensitive to changes in arterial PO_2 in the range of 60 down to 30 mmHg, a range in which hemoglobin saturation with oxygen decreases rapidly.

Increased Carbon Dioxide and Hydrogen Ion Concentration Stimulates the Chemoreceptors. An increase in either CO_2 concentration or hydrogen ion concentration also excites the chemoreceptors and, in this way, indirectly increases respiratory activity. However, the direct effects of both these factors in the respiratory center are much more powerful than their effects mediated through the chemoreceptors (about seven times as powerful). Yet there is one difference between the peripheral and central effects of CO_2: The stimulation by way of the peripheral chemoreceptors occurs as much as five times as rapidly as central stimulation, so the peripheral chemoreceptors might be especially important in increasing the rapidity of response to CO_2 at the onset of exercise.

Basic Mechanism of Stimulation of the Chemoreceptors by O_2 Deficiency. The exact means by which low PO_2 excites the nerve endings in the carotid and aortic bodies are still not completely understood. However, these bodies have multiple highly characteristic glandular-like cells, called *glomus cells*, that synapse directly or indirectly with the nerve endings. Current evidence suggests that these glomus cells function as the chemoreceptors and then stimulate the nerve endings (Figure 61-6). Glomus cells have O_2-sensitive potassium channels that are

system, shown in Figure 61-4. Special nervous chemical receptors, called *chemoreceptors*, are located in several areas outside the brain. They are especially important for detecting changes in O_2 in the blood, although they also respond to a lesser extent to changes in CO_2 and hydrogen ion concentrations. The chemoreceptors transmit nervous signals to the respiratory center in the brain to help regulate respiratory activity.

Most of the chemoreceptors are in the *carotid bodies*. However, a few are also in the *aortic bodies*, shown in the lower part of Figure 61-4, and a very few are located elsewhere in association with other arteries of the thoracic and abdominal regions.

The *carotid bodies* are located bilaterally in the bifurcations of the common carotid arteries. Their afferent nerve fibers pass through Hering nerves to the *glossopharyngeal nerves* and then to the dorsal respiratory area of the medulla. The *aortic bodies* are located along the arch of the aorta; their afferent nerve fibers pass through the *vagi*, also to the dorsal medullary respiratory area (Table 61-1).

Each of the chemoreceptor bodies receives its own special blood supply through a minute artery directly from the adjacent arterial trunk. Further, blood flow through these bodies is extreme, 20 times the weight of the bodies themselves each minute. Therefore, the percentage of O_2 removed from the flowing blood is virtually zero. This means that *the chemoreceptors are*

TABLE 61-1	**Differences Between the Central and Peripheral Chemoreceptors**	
	Central Chemoreceptors	**Peripheral Chemoreceptors**
Location	Chemosensitive area in the medulla	Carotid and aortic bodies
Stimuli	↑ CO_2 in blood stimulates these receptors indirectly by increasing H^+ ions in the brain extracellular fluids	↓ O_2 arterial concentration primarily stimulates these receptors ↑ CO_2 and H^+ in blood also stimulate these receptors to a lesser extent
Rapidity in response	Slower response as compared to peripheral receptors	Five times as rapid as central stimulation

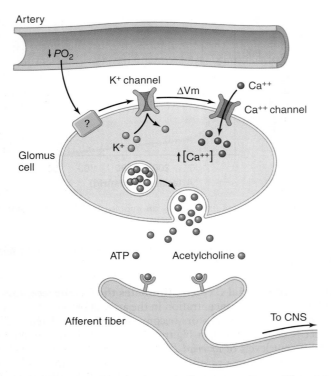

Figure 61-6 Carotid body glomus cell oxygen sensing. When PO_2 decreases below around 60 mmHg, potassium channels close, causing cell depolarization, opening of calcium channels, and increased cytosolic calcium ion concentration. This stimulates transmitter release (ATP is likely the most important), which activates afferent fibers that send signals to the central nervous system (CNS) and stimulate respiration. The mechanisms by which low PO_2 influences potassium channel activity are still unclear. ΔVm, change in membrane voltage. *ATP*, adenosine triphosphate.

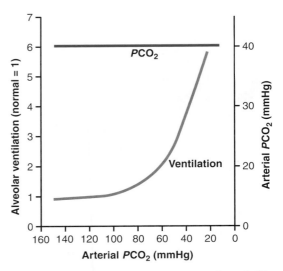

Figure 61-7 The lower curve demonstrates the effect of different levels of arterial PO_2 on alveolar ventilation, showing a sixfold increase in ventilation as the PO_2 decreases from the normal level of 100–20 mmHg. The upper line shows that the arterial PCO_2 was kept at a constant level during the measurements of this study; pH also was kept constant.

inactivated when blood PO_2 decreases markedly. This inactivation causes the cell to depolarize, which, in turn, opens voltage-gated calcium channels and increases intracellular calcium ion concentration. The increased calcium ions stimulate release of a neurotransmitter that activates afferent neurons that send signals to the central nervous system and stimulate respiration. Although early studies suggested that dopamine or acetylcholine might be the main neurotransmitters, more recent studies suggest that during hypoxia, adenosine triphosphate may be the key excitatory neurotransmitter released by carotid body glomus cells.

Effect of Low Arterial PO_2 to Stimulate Alveolar Ventilation when Arterial CO_2 and Hydrogen Ion Concentrations Remain Normal

Figure 61-7 shows the effect of low arterial PO_2 on alveolar ventilation when the PCO_2 and the hydrogen ion concentration are kept constant at their normal levels. In other words, in this figure, only the ventilatory drive, because of the effect of low O_2 on the chemoreceptors, is active. The figure shows almost no effect on ventilation as long as the arterial PO_2 remains greater than 100 mmHg. However, at pressures lower than 100 mmHg, ventilation approximately doubles when the arterial PO_2 falls to 60 mmHg and can increase as much as fivefold at very low PO_2 values. Under these conditions, low arterial PO_2 obviously drives the ventilatory process quite strongly.

Because the effect of hypoxia on ventilation is modest for PO_2 values greater than 60–80 mmHg, the PCO_2 and the hydrogen

ion response are mainly responsible for regulating ventilation in healthy humans at sea level.

Chronic Breathing of Low O_2 Stimulates Respiration Even More—The Phenomenon of "Acclimatization"

Mountain climbers have found that when they ascend a mountain slowly, over a period of days rather than a period of hours, they breathe much more deeply and therefore can withstand far lower atmospheric O_2 concentrations than when they ascend rapidly. This phenomenon is called *acclimatization*.

The reason for acclimatization is that, within 2–3 days, the respiratory center in the brainstem loses about four-fifths of its sensitivity to changes in PCO_2 and hydrogen ions. Therefore, the excess ventilatory blow-off of CO_2 that normally would inhibit an increase in respiration fails to occur, and low O_2 can drive the respiratory system to a much higher level of alveolar ventilation than under acute conditions. Instead of the 70% increase in ventilation that might occur after acute exposure to low O_2, the alveolar ventilation often increases 400–500% after 2–3 days of low O_2, which helps immensely in supplying additional O_2 to the mountain climber.

COMPOSITE EFFECTS OF PCO_2, PH, AND PCO_2 ON ALVEOLAR VENTILATION

Figure 61-8 gives a quick overview of the manner in which the chemical factors PO_2, PCO_2, and pH together affect alveolar ventilation. To understand this diagram, first observe the four red curves. These curves were recorded at different levels of arterial PO_2—40, 50, 60, and 100 mmHg. For each of these curves, the PCO_2 was changed from lower to higher levels. Thus, this "family" of red curves represents the combined effects of alveolar PCO_2 and PO_2 on ventilation.

Now observe the green curves. Whereas the red curves were measured at a blood pH of 7.4, the green curves were measured at a pH of 7.3. We now have two families of curves representing the combined effects of PCO_2 and PO_2 on ventilation at two different pH values. Still other families of curves would be displaced to the right at higher pHs and displaced to the left at

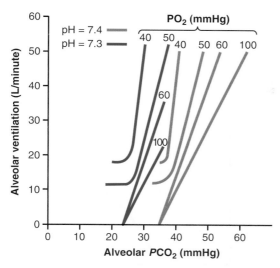

Figure 61-8 Composite diagram showing the interrelated effects of PCO_2, PO_2, and pH on alveolar ventilation. *Data from Cunningham, D.J.C., Lloyd, B.B., 1963. The Regulation of Human Respiration. Blackwell Scientific Publications, Oxford.*

lower pHs. Thus, using this diagram, one can predict the level of alveolar ventilation for most combinations of alveolar PCO_2, alveolar PO_2, and arterial pH.

Regulation of Respiration During Exercise

During strenuous exercise, O_2 consumption and CO_2 formation can increase as much as 20-fold. Yet, in the healthy athlete as illustrated in Figure 61-9, alveolar ventilation ordinarily increases almost exactly in step with the increased level of O_2 metabolism. The arterial PO_2, PCO_2, and pH remain *almost exactly normal*.

In trying to analyze what causes the increased ventilation during exercise, one is tempted to ascribe this increased ventilation to increases in blood CO_2 and hydrogen ions, plus a decrease in blood O_2. However, this attribution is questionable because measurements of arterial PCO_2, pH, and PO_2 show that none of these values changes significantly during exercise, so none of them becomes abnormal enough to stimulate respiration as vigorously as observed during strenuous exercise.

Therefore, what causes intense ventilation during exercise? At least one effect seems to be predominant. The brain, on transmitting motor impulses to the exercising muscles, is believed to transmit collateral impulses into the brainstem at the same time to excite the respiratory center. This action is analogous to the stimulation of the vasomotor center of the brainstem during exercise that causes a simultaneous increase in arterial pressure.

Actually, when a person begins to exercise, a large share of the total increase in ventilation begins immediately on initiation of the exercise, before any blood chemicals have had time to change. It is likely that most of the increase in respiration results from neurogenic signals transmitted directly into the brainstem respiratory center at the same time that signals go to the body muscles to cause muscle contraction.

Interrelation Between Chemical Factors and Nervous Factors in the Control of Respiration During Exercise. When a person exercises, direct nervous signals presumably stimulate the respiratory center *almost* the proper amount to supply the extra O_2 required for exercise and to blow off extra CO_2. Occasionally, however, the nervous respiratory control signals are either too strong or too weak. Chemical factors then play a significant role in bringing about the final adjustment of respiration required to keep the O_2, CO_2, and hydrogen ion concentrations of the body fluids as nearly normal as possible.

This process is demonstrated in Figure 61-10; the lower curve shows changes in alveolar ventilation during a 1-minute period of exercise and the upper curve shows changes in arterial PCO_2. Note that at the onset of exercise, the alveolar ventilation increases almost instantaneously, without an initial increase in arterial PCO_2. In fact, this increase in ventilation is usually great enough so that at first it actually *decreases* arterial PCO_2 below normal, as shown in the figure. The presumed reason that the ventilation forges ahead of the buildup of blood CO_2 is that the brain provides an "anticipatory" stimulation of respiration at the onset of exercise, causing extraalveolar ventilation even before it is necessary. However, after about 30–40 seconds, the amount of CO_2 released into the blood from the active muscles

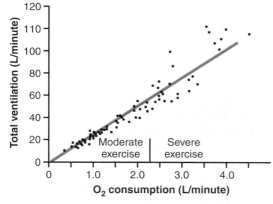

Figure 61-9 Effect of exercise on oxygen consumption and ventilatory rate. *From Gray, J.S., 1950. Pulmonary Ventilation and its Physiological Regulation. Charles C. Thomas, Springfield, IL.*

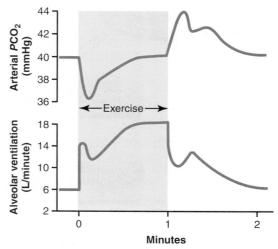

Figure 61-10 Changes in alveolar ventilation (*bottom curve*) and arterial PCO_2 (*top curve*) during a 1-minute period of exercise and also after termination of exercise. *Extrapolated to the human from data in dogs in Bainton, C.R., 1972. Effect of speed versus grade and shivering on ventilation in dogs during active exercise. J. Appl. Physiol. 33, 778.*

approximately matches the increased rate of ventilation, and the arterial PCO_2 returns essentially to normal even as the exercise continues, as shown toward the end of the 1-minute period of exercise in the figure.

Figure 61-11 summarizes the control of respiration during exercise in another way, this time more quantitatively. The lower curve of this figure shows the effect of different levels of arterial PCO_2 on alveolar ventilation when the body is at rest—that is, not exercising. The upper curve shows the approximate shift of this ventilatory curve caused by neurogenic drive from the respiratory center that occurs during heavy exercise. The points indicated on the two curves show the arterial PCO_2 first in the resting state and then in the exercising state. Note in both instances that the PCO_2 is at the normal level of 40 mmHg. In other words, the neurogenic factor shifts the curve about 20-fold in the upward direction, so ventilation almost matches the rate of CO_2 release, thus keeping arterial PCO_2 near its normal value. The upper curve of Figure 61-11 also shows that if, during exercise, the arterial PCO_2 does change from its normal value of 40 mmHg, it has an extra stimulatory effect on ventilation at a PCO_2 value greater than 40 mmHg and a depressant effect at a PCO_2 value less than 40 mmHg. Figure 61-12 summarizes the various factors that regulate ventilation during exercise.

Neurogenic Control of Ventilation During Exercise May Be Partly a Learned Response. Many experiments suggest that the brain's ability to shift the ventilatory response curve during exercise, as shown in Figure 61-11, is at least partly a *learned* response. That is, with repeated periods of exercise, the brain becomes progressively more able to provide the proper signals

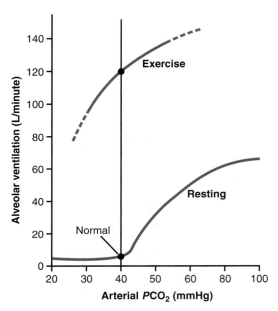

Figure 61-11 Approximate effect of maximum exercise in an athlete to shift the alveolar PCO_2–ventilation response curve to a level much higher than normal. The shift, believed to be caused by neurogenic factors, is almost exactly the right amount to maintain arterial PCO_2 at the normal level of 40 mmHg both in the resting state and during heavy exercise.

required to keep the blood PCO_2 at its normal level. Also, there is reason to believe that even the cerebral cortex is involved in this learning because experiments that block only the cortex also block the learned response.

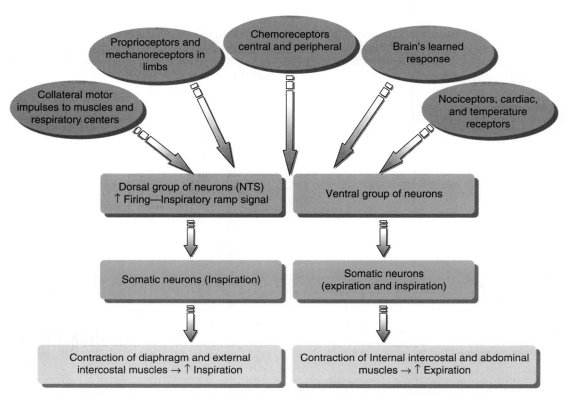

Figure 61-12 Summary of factors that regulate ventilation during exercise. *NTS,* nucleus tractus solitarius.

BIBLIOGRAPHY

Babb TG: Obesity: challenges to ventilatory control during exercise—a brief review, *Respir. Physiol. Neurobiol.* 189:364, 2013.

Guyenet PG: The 2008 Carl Ludwig Lecture: retrotrapezoid nucleus, CO_2 homeostasis, and breathing automaticity, *J. Appl. Physiol.* 105:404, 2008.

Guyenet PG, Abbott SB, Stornetta RL: The respiratory chemoreception conundrum: light at the end of the tunnel? *Brain Res.* 1511:126, 2013.

Guyenet PG, Stornetta RL, Bayliss DA: Central respiratory chemoreception, *J. Comp. Neurol.* 518:3883, 2010.

Jordan AS, McSharry DG, Malhotra A: Adult obstructive sleep apnoea, *Lancet* 383:736, 2014.

Nurse CA, Piskuric NA: Signal processing at mammalian carotid body chemoreceptors, *Semin. Cell Dev. Biol.* 24:22, 2013.

Plataki M, Sands SA, Malhotra A: Clinical consequences of altered chemoreflex control, *Respir. Physiol. Neurobiol.* 189:354, 2013.

Ramirez JM, Doi A, Garcia AJ 3rd, et al: The cellular building blocks of breathing, *Compr. Physiol.* 2:2683, 2012.

Thach BT: Some aspects of clinical relevance in the maturation of respiratory control in infants, *J. Appl. Physiol.* 104:1828, 2008.

West, J.B., Respiratory Physiology—The Essentials. ninth ed., Philadelphia, 2012, Lippincott Williams & Wilkins, Wolters Kluwers.

Neural Regulation of Respiration

LEARNING OBJECTIVES

- List the centers of respiration, and describe their organization.
- Enumerate the peripheral inputs affecting respiration including the peripheral receptors.
- Describe the Hering–Breuer reflex.
- Describe the different types of the abnormal breathing patterns.

GLOSSARY OF TERMS

- **Caudal:** A location that is inferior, underside, or beneath in humans
- **Dyspnea:** Difficulty in breathing
- **Neurogenic:** Originating in or stimulated by the central nervous system or nerve impulses
- **Rostral:** A location that is superior or anteriorly located in humans

The nervous system normally adjusts the rate of alveolar ventilation almost exactly to the demands of the body so that the oxygen partial pressure (PCO_2) and carbon dioxide partial pressure (PO_2) in the arterial blood are hardly altered, even during heavy exercise and most other types of respiratory stress. This chapter describes the function of this neurogenic system for regulation of respiration.

Respiratory Center

The *respiratory center* is composed of several groups of neurons located *bilaterally* in the *medulla oblongata* and pons of the brainstem, as shown in Figure 62-1. It is divided into three major collections of neurons:

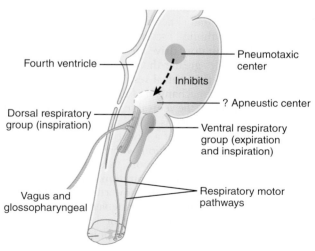

Figure 62-1 Organization of the respiratory center.

1. a *dorsal respiratory group*, located in the dorsal portion of the medulla, which mainly causes inspiration;
2. a *ventral respiratory group*, located in the ventrolateral part of the medulla, which mainly causes expiration;
3. the *pneumotaxic center*, located dorsally in the superior portion of the pons, which mainly controls rate and depth of breathing.

DORSAL RESPIRATORY GROUP OF NEURONS— ITS CONTROL OF INSPIRATION AND OF RESPIRATORY RHYTHM

The dorsal respiratory group of neurons plays a fundamental role in the control of respiration and extends most of the length of the medulla. Most of its neurons are located within the *nucleus of the tractus solitarius (NTS)*, although additional neurons in the adjacent reticular substance of the medulla also play important roles in respiratory control. The NTS is the sensory termination of both the vagal and the glossopharyngeal nerves, which transmit sensory signals into the respiratory center from:

- peripheral chemoreceptors
- baroreceptors
- several types of receptors in the lungs

Figure 62-2 illustrates the schematic organization of the neural regulation of respiration.

Rhythmical Inspiratory Discharges from the Dorsal Respiratory Group. The basic rhythm of respiration is generated mainly in the dorsal respiratory group of neurons. Even when all the peripheral nerves entering the medulla have been sectioned and the brainstem has been transected both above and below the medulla, this group of neurons still emits repetitive bursts of *inspiratory neuronal action potentials*. The basic cause of these repetitive discharges is unknown. In primitive animals, neural networks have been found in which activity of one set of neurons excites a second set, which in turn inhibits the first. Then, after a period, the mechanism repeats itself, continuing throughout the life of the animal. Most respiratory physiologists believe that some similar network of neurons is present in the human being, located entirely within the medulla; it probably involves not only the dorsal respiratory group but adjacent areas of the medulla as well, and it is responsible for the basic rhythm of respiration.

Inspiratory "Ramp" Signal. The nervous signal that is transmitted to the inspiratory muscles, mainly the diaphragm, is not an instantaneous burst of action potentials. Instead, it begins weakly and increases steadily in a ramp manner for about 2 seconds in normal respiration. It then ceases abruptly for approximately the next 3 seconds, which turns off the excitation of the diaphragm and allows elastic recoil of the lungs and the chest wall to cause expiration. Next, the inspiratory signal begins again for another cycle; this cycle repeats again and again, with expiration occurring in between. Thus, the inspiratory signal is a *ramp signal*. The obvious advantage of the ramp is that it causes a steady increase in the volume of the lungs during inspiration, rather than inspiratory gasps.

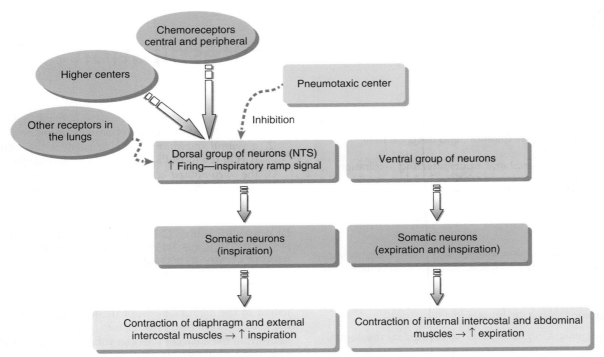

Figure 62-2 Neural control of respiration. *NTS,* nucleus tractus solitarius.

Two qualities of the inspiratory ramp that are controlled are as follows:

1. control of the *rate of increase of the ramp signal* so that during heavy respiration, the ramp increases rapidly and therefore fills the lungs rapidly;
2. control of the *limiting point at which the ramp suddenly ceases,* which is the usual method for controlling the rate of respiration; that is, the earlier the ramp ceases, the shorter is the duration of inspiration. This method also shortens the duration of expiration. Thus, the frequency of respiration is increased.

A PNEUMOTAXIC CENTER LIMITS THE DURATION OF INSPIRATION AND INCREASES THE RESPIRATORY RATE

A *pneumotaxic center,* located dorsally in the *nucleus parabrachialis* of the upper pons, transmits signals to the inspiratory area. The primary effect of this center is to control the "switch-off" point of the inspiratory ramp, thus controlling the duration of the filling phase of the lung cycle. When the pneumotaxic signal is strong, inspiration might last for as little as 0.5 second, thus filling the lungs only slightly; when the pneumotaxic signal is weak, inspiration might continue for 5 or more seconds, thus filling the lungs with a great excess of air.

The function of the pneumotaxic center is primarily to limit inspiration, which has a secondary effect of increasing the rate of breathing because limitation of inspiration also shortens expiration and the entire period of each respiration. A strong pneumotaxic signal can increase the rate of breathing to 30–40 breaths/minute, whereas a weak pneumotaxic signal may reduce the rate to only 3–5 breaths/minute.

VENTRAL RESPIRATORY GROUP OF NEURONS—FUNCTIONS IN BOTH INSPIRATION AND EXPIRATION

Located in each side of the medulla, about 5 mm anterior and lateral to the dorsal respiratory group of neurons, is the *ventral respiratory group of neurons,* found in the *nucleus ambiguus* rostrally and the *nucleus retroambiguus* caudally. The function of this neuronal group differs from that of the dorsal respiratory group in several important ways:

1. The neurons of the ventral respiratory group remain almost totally *inactive* during normal quiet respiration. Therefore, normal quiet breathing is caused only by repetitive inspiratory signals from the dorsal respiratory group transmitted mainly to the diaphragm, and expiration results from elastic recoil of the lungs and thoracic cage.
2. The ventral respiratory neurons do not appear to participate in the basic rhythmical oscillation that controls respiration.
3. When the respiratory drive for increased pulmonary ventilation becomes greater than normal, respiratory signals spill over into the ventral respiratory neurons from the basic oscillating mechanism of the dorsal respiratory area. As a consequence, the ventral respiratory area contributes extra respiratory drive as well.
4. Electrical stimulation of a few of the neurons in the ventral group causes inspiration, whereas stimulation of others causes expiration. Therefore, these neurons contribute to both inspiration and expiration. They are especially important in providing the powerful expiratory signals to the abdominal muscles during very heavy expiration. Thus, this area operates more or less as an overdrive mechanism when high levels of pulmonary ventilation are required, especially during heavy exercise.

THE PERIPHERAL INPUTS AFFECTING THE RESPIRATION INCLUDING THE PERIPHERAL RECEPTORS

There are several peripheral receptors that help in the control of respiration. The levels of oxygen (O_2) and carbon dioxide (CO_2) are detected by central and peripheral chemoreceptors and this is discussed in detail in Chapter 61. The other peripheral receptors that have an influence on respiration are mechanoreceptors and are listed in the following.

THE HERING–BREUER INFLATION REFLEX— LUNG INFLATION SIGNALS LIMIT INSPIRATION

In addition to the central nervous system respiratory control mechanisms operating entirely within the brainstem, sensory nerve signals from the lungs also help control respiration. Most important, located in the muscular portions of the walls of the bronchi and bronchioles throughout the lungs are *stretch receptors* that transmit signals through the *vagi* into the dorsal respiratory group of neurons when the lungs become overstretched. These signals affect inspiration in much the same way as signals from the pneumotaxic center; that is, when the lungs become overly inflated, the stretch receptors activate an appropriate feedback response that "switches off" the inspiratory ramp and thus stops further inspiration. This mechanism is called the *Hering–Breuer inflation reflex*. This reflex also increases the rate of respiration, as is true for signals from the pneumotaxic center.

In humans, the Hering–Breuer reflex probably is not activated until the tidal volume increases to more than three times normal ($> \approx 1.5$ L/breath). Therefore, this reflex appears to be mainly a protective mechanism for preventing excess lung inflation rather than an important ingredient in normal control of ventilation.

CONTROL OF OVERALL RESPIRATORY CENTER ACTIVITY

Up to this point, we have discussed the basic mechanisms for causing inspiration and expiration, but it is also important to know how the intensity of the respiratory control signals is increased or decreased to match the ventilatory needs of the body. For example, during heavy exercise, the rates of O_2 usage and CO_2 formation are often increased to as much as 20 times normal, requiring commensurate increases in pulmonary ventilation. The major purpose of the remainder of this chapter is to discuss this control of ventilation in accord with the respiratory needs of the body.

Other Factors that Affect Respiration

Voluntary Control of Respiration. Thus far, we have discussed the involuntary system for the control of respiration. However, we all know that for short periods, respiration can be controlled voluntarily and that one can hyperventilate or hypoventilate to such an extent that serious derangements in PCO_2, pH, and PCO_2 can occur in the blood.

Effect of Irritant Receptors in the Airways. The epithelium of the trachea, bronchi, and bronchioles is supplied with sensory nerve endings called *pulmonary irritant receptors* that are stimulated by many incidents. These receptors initiate coughing and sneezing. They may also cause bronchial constriction in persons with such diseases as asthma and emphysema.

Function of Lung "J Receptors". A few sensory nerve endings have been described in the alveolar walls in *juxtaposition* to the pulmonary capillaries—hence the name "J receptors." These "J receptors" were first described by an Indian scientist, Autar Singh Paintal, in 1955. They are stimulated especially when the pulmonary capillaries become engorged with blood or when pulmonary edema occurs in such conditions as congestive heart failure. Although the functional role of the J receptors is not clear, their excitation may give the person a feeling of dyspnea.

Brain Edema Depresses the Respiratory Center. The activity of the respiratory center may be depressed or even inactivated by acute brain edema resulting from brain concussion. For instance, the head might be struck against some solid object, after which the damaged brain tissues swell, compressing the cerebral arteries against the cranial vault and thus partially blocking cerebral blood supply.

Occasionally, respiratory depression resulting from brain edema can be relieved temporarily by intravenous injection of hypertonic solutions such as highly concentrated mannitol solution. These solutions osmotically remove some of the fluids of the brain, thus relieving intracranial pressure and sometimes reestablishing respiration within a few minutes.

Anesthesia. Perhaps the most prevalent cause of respiratory depression and respiratory arrest is overdosage with anesthetics or narcotics. For instance, sodium pentobarbital depresses the respiratory center considerably more than many other anesthetics, such as halothane. At one time, morphine was used as an anesthetic, but this drug is now used only as an adjunct to anesthetics because it greatly depresses the respiratory center while having less ability to anesthetize the cerebral cortex.

TYPES OF THE ABNORMAL BREATHING PATTERNS

There are several types of abnormal breathing (Table 62-1). These are listed as follows:
1. Cheyne–Stokes breathing
2. Biot's breathing
3. apneustic breathing
4. Kussmaul's respiration

Periodic Breathing. An abnormality of respiration called *periodic breathing* occurs in several disease conditions. The person breathes deeply for a short interval and then breathes slightly or not at all for an additional interval, with the cycle repeating itself over and over. One type of periodic breathing, *Cheyne–Stokes breathing*, is characterized by slowly waxing and waning respiration occurring about every 40–60 seconds, as illustrated in Figure 62-3. Other types of abnormal or periodic breathing include the following.

Basic Mechanism of Cheyne–Stokes Breathing. The basic cause of Cheyne–Stokes breathing is the following: When a person overbreathes, thus blowing off too much CO_2 from the pulmonary blood while at the same time increasing blood O_2, it takes several seconds before the changed pulmonary blood can be transported to the brain and inhibit the excess ventilation. By this time, the person has already overventilated for

TABLE 62-1	Different Types of Abnormal Breathing	
Type of Abnormal Breathing	**Description**	**Causes**
Cheyne–Stokes breathing	The person breathes deeply for a short interval and then breathes slightly or not at all for an additional interval	Severe cardiac failure, increased negative feedback gain in respiratory control areas
Biot's breathing	Quick bouts of shallow respiration followed by unpredictable periods of apnea	Lesions in the medulla oblongata
Apneustic breathing	Characterized by a prolonged inspiratory gap with a pause at full inspiration	Caused by lesions at the dorsolateral lower half of the pons
Kussmaul's breathing	Characterized by very deep labored regular breathing	Caused by metabolic acidosis or diabetic ketoacidosis

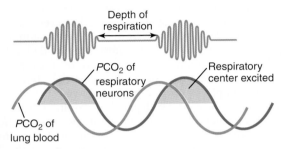

Figure 62-3 Cheyne–Stokes breathing, showing changing PO_2 in the pulmonary blood (*red line*) and delayed changes in the PCO_2 of the fluids of the respiratory center (*blue line*).

an extra few seconds. Therefore, when the overventilated blood finally reaches the brain respiratory center, the center becomes depressed to an excessive amount, at which point the opposite cycle begins, that is, CO_2 increases and O_2 decreases in the alveoli. Again, it takes a few seconds before the brain can respond to these new changes. When the brain does respond, the person breathes hard once again and the cycle repeats.

The basic cause of Cheyne–Stokes breathing occurs in everyone. However, under normal conditions, this mechanism is highly "damped." That is, the fluids of the blood and the respiratory center control areas have large amounts of dissolved and chemically bound CO_2 and O_2. Therefore, normally, the lungs cannot build up enough extra CO_2 or depress the O_2 sufficiently in a few seconds to cause the next cycle of the periodic breathing. But under two separate conditions, the damping factors can be overridden and Cheyne–Stokes breathing does occur:

1. When a *long delay occurs for transport of blood from the lungs to the brain*, changes in CO_2 and O_2 in the alveoli can continue for many more seconds than usual. Under these conditions, the storage capacities of the alveoli and pulmonary blood for these gases are exceeded; then, after a few more seconds, the periodic respiratory drive becomes extreme and Cheyne–Stokes breathing begins. This type of Cheyne–Stokes breathing often occurs in patients with *severe cardiac failure* because blood flow is slow, thus delaying the transport of blood gases from the lungs to the brain. In fact, in patients with chronic heart failure, Cheyne–Stokes breathing can sometimes occur on and off for months.

2. A second cause of Cheyne–Stokes breathing is *increased negative feedback gain* in the respiratory control areas, which means that a change in blood CO_2 or O_2 causes a far greater change in ventilation than normally. For instance, instead of the normal 2- to 3-fold increase in ventilation that occurs when the PCO_2 rises 3 mmHg, the

same 3 mmHg rise might increase ventilation 10- to 20-fold. The brain feedback tendency for periodic breathing is now strong enough to cause Cheyne–Stokes breathing without extra blood flow delay between the lungs and brain. This type of Cheyne–Stokes breathing occurs mainly in patients with *damage to the respiratory centers of the brain*. The brain damage often turns off the respiratory drive entirely for a few seconds; then an extra intense increase in blood CO_2 turns it back on with great force. Cheyne–Stokes breathing of this type is frequently a prelude to death from brain malfunction.

Typical records of changes in pulmonary and respiratory center PCO_2 during Cheyne–Stokes breathing are shown in Figure 62-3. Note that the PCO_2 of the pulmonary blood changes *in advance* of the PCO_2 of the respiratory neurons. However, the depth of respiration corresponds with the PCO_2 in the brain, not with the PCO_2 in the pulmonary blood where the ventilation is occurring.

Biot's Breathing. Biot's breathing (Figure 62-4) is a rare condition where an abnormal breathing pattern occurs in patients with acute neurological disease. This condition is also known as "ataxic breathing" and is characterized by unpredictable

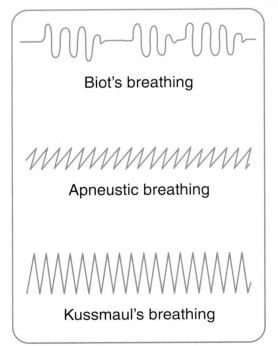

Figure 62-4 Biot's breathing, apneustic breathing, and Kussmaul's breathing patterns.

irregularity. There may be quick bouts of shallow respiration followed by unpredictable periods of apnea.

It may be caused due to lesions in the medulla oblongata. It is named after Camille Biot, a French physician, who characterized this breathing.

Apneustic Breathing. The term "apneuses" is derived from Greek, meaning "breath holding." Apneustic breathing was first described in the year 1888 by Willy Marckwald. This type of breathing (Figure 62-4) is characterized by a prolonged inspiratory gasp with a pause at full inspiration. This type of breathing is usually caused due to lesions at the dorsolateral lower half of the pons.

Kussmaul's Breathing. This type of abnormal breathing (Figure 62-4) is characterized by very deep labored regular breathing, sometimes with increased frequency. It is named after a German physician, Adolf Kussmaul, who first described this in the year 1874. It is seen in patients with metabolic acidosis and more commonly in patients with diabetic ketoacidosis.

BIBLIOGRAPHY

Ainslie PN, Lucas SJ, Burgess KR: Breathing and sleep at high altitude, *Respir. Physiol. Neurobiol.* 188:233, 2013.

Babb TG: Obesity: challenges to ventilatory control during exercise—a brief review, *Respir. Physiol. Neurobiol.* 189:364, 2013.

Hilaire G, Pasaro R: Genesis and control of the respiratory rhythm in adult mammals, *News Physiol. Sci.* 18:23, 2003.

Horner RL, Bradley TD: Update in sleep and control of ventilation 2008, *Am. J. Respir. Crit. Care Med.* 179:528, 2009.

Iggo A: Autar Singh Paintal: 24 September 1925–21 December 2004, *Biogr. Mem. Fellows R. Soc.* 52:251-262, 2006.

Jordan AS, McSharry DG, Malhotra A: Adult obstructive sleep apnoea, *Lancet* 383:736, 2014.

Konecny T, Kara T, Somers VK: Obstructive sleep apnea and hypertension: an update, *Hypertension* 63:203, 2014.

Mador MJ, Tobin MJ: Apneustic breathing. A characteristic feature of brainstem compression in achondroplasia? *Chest* 97:877, 1990.

Prabhakar NR: Sensing hypoxia: physiology, genetics and epigenetics, *J. Physiol.* 591:2245, 2013.

Ramirez JM, Doi A, Garcia AJ 3rd, et al: The cellular building blocks of breathing, *Compr. Physiol.* 2:2683, 2012.

Romero-Corral A, Caples SM, Lopez-Jimenez F, Somers VK: Interactions between obesity and obstructive sleep apnea: implications for treatment, *Chest* 137:711, 2010.

Thach BT: Some aspects of clinical relevance in the maturation of respiratory control in infants, *J. Appl. Physiol.* 104:1828, 2008.

Wijdicks EF: Biot's breathing, *J. Neurol. Neurosurg. Psychiatr.* 78(5):512, 2007.

Respiration in Unusual Environments

GLOSSARY OF TERMS

- **Acclimatization:** Refers to physiological adaptation to a new altitude
- **Angiogenesis:** The process of formation of new blood vessels
- **Euphoria:** A feeling of happiness, great elation, or well-being
- **Hematocrit:** The percentage of packed red cells in a sample of blood after centrifugation (it is also known as "packed cell volume")
- **Hyperbaric:** Refers to pressures that are higher than normal atmospheric pressures
- **Lassitude:** A feeling of weakness, lack of energy, or weariness in an individual
- **SCUBA:** Stands for "self-contained underwater breathing apparatus" and is used by divers during deep-sea diving

As humans have ascended to higher and higher altitudes in aviation, mountain climbing, and space exploration, it has become progressively more important to understand the effects of altitude and low gas pressures on the human body. This chapter deals with these problems, as well as acceleratory forces, weightlessness, and other challenges to body homeostasis that occur at high altitude and in space flight.

Effects of Low Oxygen Pressure on the Body

Barometric Pressures at Different Altitudes. Table 63-1 lists the approximate *barometric* and *oxygen pressures* at different altitudes, showing that at sea level, the barometric pressure is 760 mmHg; at 10,000 ft., it is only 523 mmHg; and at 50,000 ft., it is 87 mmHg. This decrease in barometric pressure is the basic cause of all the hypoxia problems in high-altitude physiology because, as the barometric pressure decreases, the atmospheric oxygen partial pressure (PO_2) decreases proportionately, remaining at all times slightly less than 21% of the total barometric pressure; at sea level PO_2 is about 159 mmHg, but at 50,000 ft. PO_2 is only 18 mmHg.

ALVEOLAR PO_2 AT DIFFERENT ELEVATIONS

Carbon Dioxide and Water Vapor Decrease the Alveolar Oxygen. Even at high altitudes, carbon dioxide (CO_2) is continually excreted from the pulmonary blood into the alveoli. In addition, water vaporizes into the inspired air from the respiratory surfaces. These two gases dilute the O_2 in the alveoli, thus reducing the O_2 concentration. Water vapor pressure in the alveoli remains at 47 mmHg as long as the body temperature is normal, regardless of altitude.

In the case of CO_2, during exposure to very high altitudes, the alveolar partial pressure of CO_2 (PCO_2) falls from the sea-level value of 40 mmHg to lower values. In the *acclimatized* person, who increases ventilation about fivefold, the PCO_2 falls to about 7 mmHg because of increased respiration.

Now let us see how the pressures of these two gases affect the alveolar O_2. For instance, assume that the barometric pressure falls from the normal sea-level value of 760 to 253 mmHg, which is the usual measured value at the top of 29,028-ft. Mount Everest. Forty-seven millimeters of mercury of this must be water vapor, leaving only 206 mmHg for all the other gases. In the *acclimatized* person, 7 mmHg of the 206 mmHg must be CO_2, leaving only 199 mmHg. If there were no use of O_2 by the body, one-fifth of this 199 mmHg would be O_2 and four-fifths would be nitrogen; that is, the PO_2 in the alveoli would be 40 mmHg. However, some of this remaining alveolar O_2 is continually being absorbed into the blood, leaving about 35 mmHg O_2 pressure in the alveoli. At the summit of Mount Everest, only the best of acclimatized people can barely survive when breathing air. However, the effect is very different when the person is breathing pure O_2, as we see in the following discussions.

Alveolar PO_2 at Different Altitudes. The fifth column of Table 63-1 shows the approximate PO_2 values in the alveoli at different altitudes when one is breathing air for both the *unacclimatized* and the *acclimatized* person. At sea level, the alveolar PO_2 is 104 mmHg. At 20,000 ft. altitude, it falls to about 40 mmHg in the unacclimatized person but only to 53 mmHg in the acclimatized person. The reason for the difference between these two is that alveolar ventilation increases much more in the acclimatized person than in the unacclimatized person, as we discuss later.

Saturation of Hemoglobin with Oxygen at Different Altitudes. Figure 63-1 shows arterial blood O_2 saturation at different altitudes while a person is breathing air and while breathing O_2. Up to an altitude of about 10,000 ft., even when air is breathed, the arterial O_2 saturation remains at least as high as 90%. Above 10,000 ft., the arterial O_2 saturation falls rapidly, as shown by the blue curve of the figure, until it is slightly less than 70% at 20,000 ft. and much less at still higher altitudes.

TABLE 63-1	Effects of Acute Exposure to Low Atmospheric Pressures on Alveolar Gas Concentrations and Arterial Oxygen Saturation[a]							
			Breathing Air			**Breathing Pure Oxygen**		
Altitude (ft./m)	Barometric Pressure (mmHg)	PO₂ in Air (mmHg)	PCO₂ in Alveoli (mmHg)	PO₂ in Alveoli (mmHg)	Arterial Oxygen Saturation (%)	PCO₂ in Alveoli (mmHg)	PO₂ in Alveoli (mmHg)	Arterial Oxygen Saturation (%)
0	760	159	40 (40)	104 (104)	97 (97)	40	673	100
10,000/3,048	523	110	36 (23)	67 (77)	90 (92)	40	436	100
20,000/6,096	349	73	24 (10)	40 (53)	73 (85)	40	262	100
30,000/9,144	226	47	24 (7)	18 (30)	24 (38)	40	139	99
40,000/12,192	141	29				36	58	84
50,000/15,240	87	18				24	16	15

[a]Numbers in parentheses are acclimatized values.

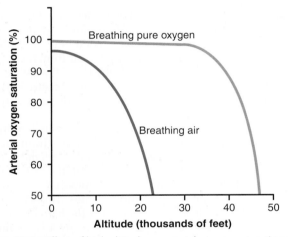

Figure 63-1 Effect of high altitude on arterial oxygen saturation when breathing air and when breathing pure oxygen.

EFFECT OF BREATHING PURE OXYGEN ON ALVEOLAR PO₂ AT DIFFERENT ALTITUDES

When a person breathes pure O_2 instead of air, most of the space in the alveoli formerly occupied by nitrogen becomes occupied by O_2. At 30,000 ft., an aviator could have an alveolar PO_2 as high as 139 mmHg instead of the 18 mmHg when breathing air (see Table 63-1).

The red curve of Figure 63-1 shows arterial blood hemoglobin O_2 saturation at different altitudes when one is breathing pure O_2. Note that the saturation remains above 90% until the aviator ascends to about 39,000 ft.; then it falls rapidly to about 50% at about 47,000 ft.

The "Ceiling" when Breathing Air and when Breathing Oxygen in an Unpressurized Airplane

When comparing the two arterial blood O_2 saturation curves in Figure 63-1, one notes that an aviator breathing pure O_2 in an unpressurized airplane can ascend to far higher altitudes than one breathing air. For instance, the arterial saturation at 47,000 ft. when one is breathing O_2 is about 50% and is equivalent to the arterial O_2 saturation at 23,000 ft. when one is breathing air. In addition, because an unacclimatized person usually can remain conscious until the arterial O_2 saturation falls to 50%, for short exposure times the ceiling for an aviator in an unpressurized airplane when breathing air is about 23,000 ft. and when breathing pure O_2 is about 47,000 ft., provided the equipment supplying the O_2 operates perfectly.

ACUTE EFFECTS OF HYPOXIA

Some of the important acute effects of hypoxia in the unacclimatized person breathing air, beginning at an altitude of about 12,000 ft., are drowsiness, lassitude, mental and muscle fatigue, sometimes headache, occasionally nausea, and sometimes euphoria. These effects progress to a stage of twitchings or seizures above 18,000 ft. and end, above 23,000 ft. in the unacclimatized person, in coma, followed shortly thereafter by death (Box 63-1).

One of the most important effects of hypoxia is decreased mental proficiency, which decreases judgment, memory, and performance of discrete motor movements. For instance, if an unacclimatized aviator stays at 15,000 ft. for 1 hour, mental proficiency ordinarily falls to about 50% of normal, and after 18 hours at this level it falls to about 20% of normal.

PROCESS OF ACCLIMATIZATION TO LOW PO₂

A person remaining at high altitudes for days, weeks, or years becomes more and more *acclimatized* to the low PO_2, so it causes fewer deleterious effects on the body. After acclimatization it becomes possible for the person to work harder without hypoxic effects or to ascend to still higher altitudes (Box 63-2).

Increased Pulmonary Ventilation—Role of Arterial Chemoreceptors. Immediate exposure to low PO_2 stimulates the arterial chemoreceptors, and this stimulation increases alveolar ventilation to a maximum of about 1.65 times normal. Therefore, compensation occurs within seconds for the high altitude, and it alone allows the person to rise several thousand feet higher than would be possible without the increased ventilation. If the person remains at very high altitude for several days, the chemoreceptors increase ventilation still more, up to about five times normal.

The immediate increase in pulmonary ventilation on rising to a high altitude blows off large quantities of CO_2, reducing the PCO_2 and increasing the pH of the body fluids. These changes *inhibit* the brainstem respiratory center and thereby *oppose the effect of low PO_2 to stimulate respiration by way of the peripheral arterial chemoreceptors in the carotid and aortic bodies.* However, this inhibition fades away during the ensuing 2–5 days, allowing the respiratory center to respond with full force to the peripheral chemoreceptor stimulus from hypoxia, and ventilation increases to about five times normal.

The cause of this fading inhibition is believed to be mainly a reduction of bicarbonate ion concentration in the cerebrospinal fluid, as well as in the brain tissues. This reduction in turn decreases the pH in the fluids surrounding the chemosensitive neurons of the respiratory center, thus increasing the respiratory stimulatory activity of the center.

An important mechanism for the gradual decrease in bicarbonate concentration is compensation by the kidneys for the respiratory alkalosis, as discussed in Chapter 82. The kidneys respond to decreased PCO_2 by reducing hydrogen ion secretion and increasing bicarbonate excretion. This metabolic compensation for the respiratory alkalosis gradually reduces plasma and cerebrospinal fluid bicarbonate concentration and pH toward normal and removes part of the inhibitory effect on respiration of low hydrogen ion concentration. Thus, the respiratory centers are much more responsive to the peripheral chemoreceptor stimulus caused by the hypoxia after the kidneys compensate for the alkalosis.

Increase in Red Blood Cells and Hemoglobin Concentration During Acclimatization. As discussed in Chapter 19 hypoxia is the principal stimulus for causing an increase in red blood cell production. Ordinarily, when a person remains exposed to low O_2 for weeks at a time, the hematocrit rises slowly from a normal value of 40–45 to an average of about 60, with an average increase in whole blood hemoglobin concentration from normal of 15 to about 20 g/dL.

In addition, the blood volume also increases, often by 20–30%, and this increase multiplied by the increased blood hemoglobin concentration gives an increase in total body hemoglobin of 50% or more.

Increased Diffusing Capacity After Acclimatization. The normal diffusing capacity for O_2 through the pulmonary membrane is about 21 mL/mmHg per minute, and this diffusing capacity can increase as much as threefold during exercise. A similar increase in diffusing capacity occurs at high altitude.

Part of the increase results from increased pulmonary capillary blood volume, which expands the capillaries and increases the surface area through which O_2 can diffuse into the blood. Another part results from an increase in lung air volume, which expands the surface area of the alveolar–capillary interface still more. A final part results from an increase in pulmonary arterial blood pressure, which forces blood into greater numbers of alveolar capillaries than normally—especially in the upper parts of the lungs, which are poorly perfused under usual conditions.

Peripheral Circulatory System Changes During Acclimatization—Increased Tissue Capillarity. The cardiac output often increases as much as 30% immediately after a person ascends to high altitude but then decreases back toward normal *over a period of weeks as the blood hematocrit increases,* so the amount of O_2 transported to the peripheral body tissues remains about normal.

Another circulatory adaptation is *growth of increased numbers of systemic circulatory capillaries* in the nonpulmonary tissues, which is called *increased tissue capillarity* (or *angiogenesis*). This occurs especially in animals born and bred at high altitudes but less so in animals that later in life become exposed to high altitude.

In active tissues exposed to chronic hypoxia, the increase in capillarity is especially marked. For instance, capillary density in right ventricular muscle increases markedly because of the combined effects of hypoxia and excess workload on the right ventricle caused by pulmonary hypertension at high altitude.

Cellular Acclimatization. In animals native to altitudes of 13,000–17,000 ft., cell mitochondria and cellular oxidative enzyme systems are slightly more plentiful than in sea-level inhabitants. Therefore, it is presumed that the tissue cells of high altitude–acclimatized human beings also can use O_2 more effectively than can their sea-level counterparts.

HYPOXIA-INDUCIBLE FACTORS—A "MASTER SWITCH" FOR THE BODY'S RESPONSE TO HYPOXIA

Hypoxia-inducible factors (HIFs) are DNA-binding transcription factors that respond to decreased oxygen availability and activate several genes that encode proteins needed for adequate oxygen delivery to tissues and energy metabolism. HIFs are found in virtually all oxygen-breathing species, ranging from primitive worms to humans. Some of the genes controlled by HIFs, especially HIF-1, include:

- genes associated with vascular endothelial growth factor, which stimulates angiogenesis;
- erythropoietin genes that stimulate red blood cell production;
- mitochondrial genes involved with energy utilization;
- glycolytic enzyme genes involved with anaerobic metabolism;
- genes that increase availability of nitric oxide, which causes pulmonary vasodilation.

In the presence of adequate oxygen, the subunits of HIF required to activate various genes are downregulated and inactivated by specific HIF hydroxylases. In hypoxia, the HIF hydroxylases are themselves inactive, allowing the formation of a transcriptionally active HIF complex. Thus, the HIFs serve as a "master switch" that permits the body to respond appropriately to hypoxia.

NATURAL ACCLIMATIZATION OF NATIVE HUMAN BEINGS LIVING AT HIGH ALTITUDES

Many native human beings in the Andes and in the Himalayas live at altitudes above 13,000 ft. One group in the Peruvian Andes lives at an altitude of 17,500 ft. and works in a mine at an altitude of 19,000 ft. Many of these natives are born at these altitudes and live there all their lives. The natives are superior to even the best-acclimatized lowlanders in all aspects of acclimatization, even though the lowlanders might have lived at high

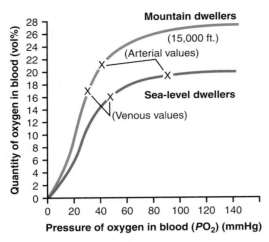

Figure 63-2 Oxygen–hemoglobin dissociation curves for blood of high-altitude residents (*red curve*) and sea-level residents (*blue curve*), showing the respective arterial and venous PO_2 levels and oxygen contents as recorded in their native surroundings. (Data from Oxygendissociation curves for bloods of high-altitude and sea-level residents. PAHO Scientific Publication No. 140, Life at High Altitudes, 1966.)

altitudes for 10 or more years. Acclimatization of the natives begins in infancy. The chest size, especially, is greatly increased, whereas the body size is somewhat decreased, giving a high ratio of ventilatory capacity to body mass. The hearts, of natives, which from birth onward pump extra amount of cardiac output, are also considerably larger than the hearts of lowlanders.

Delivery of O_2 by the blood to the tissues is also highly facilitated in these natives. For instance, Figure 63-2 shows O_2–hemoglobin dissociation curves for natives who live at sea level and for their counterparts who live at 15,000 ft. Note that the arterial PO_2 in the natives at high altitude is only 40 mmHg, but because of the greater quantity of hemoglobin, the quantity of O_2 in their arterial blood is greater than that in the blood of the natives at the lower altitude. Note also that the venous PO_2 in the high-altitude natives is only 15 mmHg less than the venous PO_2 for the lowlanders, despite the very low arterial PO_2, indicating that O_2 transport to the tissues is exceedingly effective in the naturally acclimatized high-altitude natives.

REDUCED WORK CAPACITY AT HIGH ALTITUDES AND POSITIVE EFFECT OF ACCLIMATIZATION

In addition to the mental depression caused by hypoxia, the work capacity of all muscles (not only skeletal muscles but also cardiac muscles) is greatly decreased in a state of hypoxia.

In general, work capacity is reduced in direct proportion to the decrease in maximum rate of O_2 uptake that the body can achieve.

To give an idea of the importance of acclimatization in increasing work capacity, consider the large differences in work capacities as percent of normal for unacclimatized and acclimatized people at an altitude of 17,000 ft.:

	Work Capacity (% of Normal)
Unacclimatized	50
Acclimatized for 2 months	68
Native living at 13,200 ft. but working at 17,000 ft.	87

EFFECTS OF ACUTE MOUNTAIN SICKNESS
1. Acute cerebral edema
2. Acute pulmonary edema

FEATURES OF ACUTE SEVERE MOUNTAIN SICKNESS
1. Dyspnea at rest
2. Inability to walk
3. Cyanosis—bluish discoloration of skin
4. Headache with a sense of confusion
5. Congestion of the chest
6. Cough with blood in the sputum
7. Decreased consciousness
8. Pale appearance

PREVENTION
1. Slow ascent to facilitate acclimatization
2. Breathing oxygen to prevent some of these effects
3. Recognition of the symptoms early
4. Descending to lower altitudes to sleep

Thus, naturally acclimatized native persons can achieve a daily work output even at high altitude almost equal to that of a lowlander at sea level, but even well-acclimatized lowlanders can almost never achieve this result.

ACUTE MOUNTAIN SICKNESS AND HIGH-ALTITUDE PULMONARY EDEMA

A small percentage of people who ascend rapidly to high altitudes become acutely sick and can die if not given O_2 or rapidly moved to a low altitude (Box 63-3). The sickness begins from a few hours up to about 2 days after ascent. Two events frequently occur:

1. *Acute cerebral edema:* This edema is believed to result from local vasodilation of the cerebral blood vessels, which is caused by the hypoxia. Dilation of the arterioles increases blood flow into the capillaries, thus increasing capillary pressure, which in turn causes fluid to leak into the cerebral tissues. The cerebral edema can then lead to severe disorientation and other effects related to cerebral dysfunction.
2. *Acute pulmonary edema:* The cause of acute pulmonary edema is still unknown, but one explanation is the following: The severe hypoxia causes the pulmonary arterioles to constrict potently, but the constriction is much greater in some parts of the lungs than in other parts, so more and more of the pulmonary blood flow is forced through fewer and fewer still unconstricted pulmonary vessels. The postulated result is that the capillary pressure in these areas of the lungs becomes especially high and local edema occurs. Extension of the process to progressively more areas of the lungs leads to spreading pulmonary edema and severe pulmonary dysfunction that can be lethal. Allowing the person to breathe O_2 usually reverses the process within hours.

CHRONIC MOUNTAIN SICKNESS

Occasionally, a person who remains at high altitude too long experiences *chronic mountain sickness* (Box 63-4).

The causes of this sequence of events are probably threefold.

First, the red blood cell mass becomes so great that the blood viscosity increases severalfold; this increased viscosity tends to *decrease* tissue blood flow so that oxygen delivery also begins to decrease.

Second, the pulmonary arterioles become vasoconstricted because of the lung hypoxia. This results from the hypoxic vascular constrictor effect that normally operates to divert blood flow from low-oxygen to high-oxygen alveoli. But because *all* the alveoli are now in the low-O_2 state, all the arterioles become constricted, the pulmonary arterial pressure rises excessively, and the right side of the heart fails.

Third, the alveolar arteriolar spasm diverts much of the blood flow through nonalveolar pulmonary vessels, thus causing an excess of pulmonary shunt blood flow where the blood is poorly oxygenated; this further compounds the problem. Most of these people recover within days or weeks when they are moved to a lower altitude.

Physiology of Deep-Sea Diving and Other Hyperbaric Conditions

When human beings descend beneath the sea, the pressure around them increases tremendously. To keep the lungs from collapsing, air must be supplied at very high pressure to keep them inflated. This maneuver exposes the blood in the lungs to extremely high alveolar gas pressure, a condition called hyperbarism. Beyond certain limits, these high pressures cause major alterations in body physiology and can be lethal.

Relationship of Pressure to Sea Depth. A column of seawater 33 ft. (10.1 m) deep exerts the same pressure at its bottom as the pressure of the atmosphere above the sea. Therefore, a person 33 ft. beneath the ocean surface is exposed to 2 atm pressure, with 1 atm of pressure caused by the weight of the air above the water and 1 atm caused by the weight of the water. At 66 ft. the pressure is 3 atm, and so forth, in accord with the table in Figure 63-3.

Effect of Sea Depth on the Volume of Gases—Boyle's Law. Another important effect of depth is compression of gases to smaller and smaller volumes. The illustration in Figure 63-3 shows a bell jar at sea level containing 1 L of air. At 33 ft. beneath the sea, where the pressure is 2 atm, the volume has been compressed to only one-half liter, and at 8 atm (233 ft.) it has been compressed to one-eighth liter. Thus, the volume to which a given quantity of gas is compressed is inversely proportional to the pressure. This principle of physics is called Boyle's law, and it is extremely important in diving physiology because increased pressure can collapse the air chambers of the diver's body, especially the lungs, and may cause serious damage.

Many times in this chapter it is necessary to refer to actual volume versus sea-level volume. For instance, we might speak of an actual volume of 1 L at a depth of 300 ft.; this is the same quantity of air as a sea-level volume of 10 L.

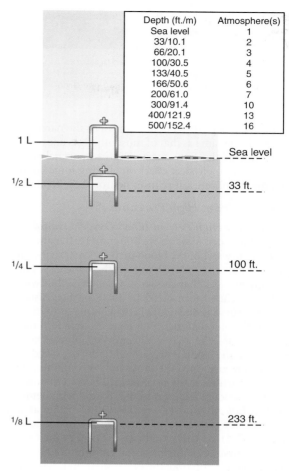

Depth (ft./m)	Atmosphere(s)
Sea level	1
33/10.1	2
66/20.1	3
100/30.5	4
133/40.5	5
166/50.6	6
200/61.0	7
300/91.4	10
400/121.9	13
500/152.4	16

Figure 63-3 Effect of sea depth on pressure (*top table*) and on gas volume (*bottom*).

Changes that Occur with Deep-Sea Diving

EFFECT OF HIGH PARTIAL PRESSURES OF INDIVIDUAL GASES ON THE BODY

The individual gases to which a diver is exposed when breathing air are nitrogen, O_2, and CO_2; each of these at times can cause significant physiological effects at high pressures.

Some of the physiological effects that are seen with deep-sea diving are listed in Box 63-5.

Nitrogen Narcosis at High Nitrogen Pressures

About four-fifths of the air is nitrogen. At sea-level pressure, the nitrogen has no significant effect on bodily function, but at high pressures it can cause varying degrees of narcosis. When the diver remains beneath the sea for an hour or more and is breathing compressed air, the depth at which the first symptoms of mild narcosis appear is about 120 ft. At this level the diver begins to exhibit joviality and loss of many of his or her cares. At 150–200 ft., the diver becomes drowsy. At 200–250 ft., his or her strength wanes considerably, and the diver often becomes too clumsy to perform the work required. Beyond 250 ft. (8.5 atm pressure), the diver usually becomes almost useless as a result of nitrogen narcosis if he or she remains at these depths too long.

Nitrogen narcosis has characteristics similar to those of alcohol intoxication, and for this reason it has frequently been called

BOX 63-5   PHYSIOLOGICAL EFFECTS OF DEEP-SEA DIVING

1. Nitrogen narcosis at high nitrogen pressures
2. Oxygen toxicity at high pressures
3. Carbon dioxide toxicity due to deep-sea diving

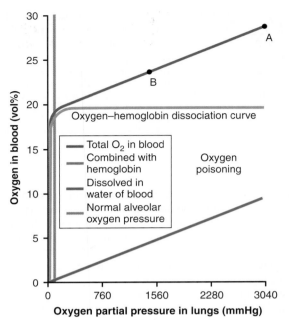

Figure 63-4   Quantity of oxygen dissolved in the fluid of the blood and in combination with hemoglobin at very high PO_2.

"raptures of the depths." The mechanism of the narcotic effect is believed to be the same as that of most other gas anesthetics. That is, it dissolves in the fatty substances in neuronal membranes and, because of its physical effect on altering ionic conductance through the membranes, it reduces neuronal excitability.

Oxygen Toxicity at High Pressures

Effect of Very High PO_2 on Blood Oxygen Transport. When the PO_2 in the blood rises above 100 mmHg, the amount of O_2 dissolved in the water of the blood increases markedly. This effect is shown in Figure 63-4, which depicts the same O_2–hemoglobin dissociation curve as that shown in Chapter 59 but with the alveolar PO_2 extended to more than 3000 mmHg. Also depicted by the lowest curve in the figure is the volume of O_2 dissolved in the fluid of the blood at each PO_2 level. Note that in the normal range of alveolar PO_2 (below 120 mmHg), almost none of the total oxygen in the blood is accounted for by dissolved O_2, but as the O_2 pressure rises into the thousands of millimeters of mercury, a large portion of the total oxygen is then dissolved in the water of the blood, in addition to that bound with hemoglobin.

Effect of High Alveolar PO_2 on Tissue PO_2. Let us assume that the PO_2 in the lungs is about 3000 mmHg (4 atm pressure—point A in Figure 63-4). As this blood passes through the tissue capillaries and the tissues use their normal amount of O_2, about 5 mL from each 100 mL of blood, the O_2 content on leaving the tissue capillaries is still 24 vol% (point B in Figure 63-4). At this point, the PO_2 is approximately 1200 mmHg, which means that O_2 is delivered to the tissues at this extremely high pressure instead of at the normal value of 40 mmHg. Thus, once the alveolar PO_2 rises above a critical level, the hemoglobin–O_2 buffer mechanism (discussed in Chapter 59) is no longer capable of keeping the tissue PO_2 in the normal, safe range between 20 and 60 mmHg.

Acute Oxygen Poisoning. The extremely high tissue PO_2 that occurs when O_2 is breathed at very high alveolar O_2 pressure can be detrimental to many of the body's tissues. For instance, breathing O_2 at 4 atm pressure of O_2 ($P_{O_2} = 3040$ mmHg) will cause brain seizures followed by coma in most people within 30–60 minutes. The seizures often occur without warning and, for obvious reasons, are likely to be lethal to divers submerged beneath the sea.

Other symptoms encountered in acute O_2 poisoning include nausea, muscle twitchings, dizziness, disturbances of vision, irritability, and disorientation. Exercise greatly increases the diver's susceptibility to O_2 toxicity, causing symptoms to appear much earlier and with far greater severity than in the resting person.

Excessive Intracellular Oxidation as a Cause of Nervous System Oxygen Toxicity—"Oxidizing Free Radicals". Molecular O_2 has little capability of oxidizing other chemical compounds. Instead, it must first be converted into an "active" form of O_2. There are several forms of active O_2 called O_2 free radicals. One of the most important of these is the superoxide free radical O_2^-, and another is the peroxide radical in the form of hydrogen peroxide. Even when the tissue PO_2 is normal at the level of 40 mmHg, small amounts of free radicals are continually being formed from the dissolved O_2. Fortunately, the tissues also contain multiple enzymes that rapidly remove these free radicals, including peroxidases, catalases, and superoxide dismutases. Therefore, so long

as the hemoglobin–O_2 buffering mechanism maintains a normal tissue PO_2, the oxidizing free radicals are removed rapidly enough that they have little or no effect in the tissues.

Above a critical alveolar PO_2 (ie, above about 2 atm PO_2), the hemoglobin–O_2 buffering mechanism fails, and the tissue PO_2 can then rise to hundreds or thousands of millimeters of mercury. At these high levels, the amounts of oxidizing free radicals literally swamp the enzyme systems designed to remove them, and now they can have serious destructive and even lethal effects on the cells. One of the principal effects is to oxidize the polyunsaturated fatty acids that are essential components of many of the cell membranes. Another effect is to oxidize some of the cellular enzymes, thus damaging severely the cellular metabolic systems. The nervous tissues are especially susceptible because of their high lipid content. Therefore, most of the acute lethal effects of acute O_2 toxicity are caused by brain dysfunction.

Chronic Oxygen Poisoning Causes Pulmonary Disability. A person can be exposed to only 1 atm pressure of O_2 almost indefinitely without developing the acute O_2 toxicity of the nervous system just described. However, after only about 12 hours of 1 atm O_2 exposure, lung passageway congestion, pulmonary edema, and atelectasis caused by damage to the linings of the bronchi and alveoli begin to develop. The reason for this effect in the lungs but not in other tissues is that the air spaces of the lungs are directly exposed to the high oxygen pressure, but O_2 is delivered to the other body tissues at almost normal PO_2 because of the hemoglobin–O_2 buffer system.

Carbon Dioxide Toxicity at Great Depths in the Sea

If the diving gear is properly designed and functions properly, the diver has no problem due to toxicity because depth alone does not increase the CO_2 partial pressure in the alveoli. This is true because depth does not increase the rate of CO_2 production in the body, and as long as the diver continues to breathe a normal tidal volume and expires the CO_2 as it is formed, alveolar CO_2 pressure will be maintained at a normal value.

In certain types of diving gear, however, such as the diving helmet and some types of rebreathing apparatuses, CO_2 can build up in the dead space air of the apparatus and be rebreathed by the diver. Up to an alveolar CO_2 pressure (PCO_2) of about 80 mmHg, twice that in normal alveoli, the diver usually tolerates this buildup by increasing the minute respiratory volume a maximum of 8- to 11-fold to compensate for the increased CO_2. Beyond 80 mmHg alveolar PCO_2, the situation becomes intolerable, and eventually the respiratory center begins to be depressed, rather than excited, because of the negative tissue metabolic effects of high PCO_2. The diver's respiration then begins to fail rather than to compensate. In addition, the diver experiences severe respiratory acidosis and varying degrees of lethargy, narcosis, and finally even anesthesia, as discussed in Chapter 64.

Decompression of the Diver After Excess Exposure to High Pressure

When a person breathes air under high pressure for a long time, the amount of nitrogen dissolved in the body fluids increases. The reason for this is that blood flowing through the pulmonary capillaries becomes saturated with nitrogen to the same high pressure as that in the alveolar breathing mixture and over several more hours, enough nitrogen is carried to all the tissues of the body to raise their tissue nitrogen partial pressure also to equal the nitrogen pressure in the breathing air.

Because nitrogen is not metabolized by the body, it remains dissolved in all the body tissues until the nitrogen pressure in the lungs is decreased back to some lower level, at which time the nitrogen can be removed by the reverse respiratory process; however, this removal often takes hours to occur and is the source of multiple problems collectively called decompression sickness.

Volume of Nitrogen Dissolved in the Body Fluids at Different Depths. At sea level, almost exactly 1 L of nitrogen is dissolved in the entire body. Slightly less than one-half of this nitrogen is dissolved in the water of the body and a little more than one-half is dissolved in the fat of the body because nitrogen is five times as soluble in fat as in water.

After the diver has become saturated with nitrogen, the sea-level volume of nitrogen dissolved in the body at different depths is as follows:

Feet	Liters
0	1
33	2
100	4
200	7
300	10

Several hours are required for the gas pressures of nitrogen in all the body tissues to come nearly to equilibrium with the gas pressure of nitrogen in the alveoli. The reason for this requirement is that the blood does not flow rapidly enough and the nitrogen does not diffuse rapidly enough to cause instantaneous equilibrium. The nitrogen dissolved in the water of the body comes to almost complete equilibrium in less than 1 hour, but the fat tissue, which requires five times as much transport of nitrogen and has a relatively poor blood supply, reaches equilibrium only after several hours. For this reason, if a person remains under water at deep levels for only a few minutes, not much nitrogen dissolves in the body fluids and tissues, whereas if the person remains at a deep level for several hours, both the body water and body fat become saturated with nitrogen.

Decompression Sickness (Also Known as Bends, Compressed Air Sickness, Caisson Disease, Diver's Paralysis, Dysbarism). If a diver has been beneath the sea long enough that large amounts of

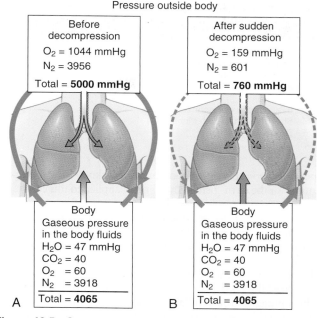

Pressure outside body

Before decompression	After sudden decompression
O_2 = 1044 mmHg	O_2 = 159 mmHg
N_2 = 3956	N_2 = 601
Total = **5000 mmHg**	Total = **760 mmHg**

Body Gaseous pressure in the body fluids	Body Gaseous pressure in the body fluids
H_2O = 47 mmHg	H_2O = 47 mmHg
CO_2 = 40	CO_2 = 40
O_2 = 60	O_2 = 60
N_2 = 3918	N_2 = 3918
Total = **4065**	Total = **4065**

A   B

Figure 63-5 Gaseous pressures both inside and outside the body, showing (A) saturation of the body to high gas pressures when breathing air at a total pressure of 5000 mmHg and (B) the great excesses of intrabody pressures that are responsible for bubble formation in the tissues when the lung intra-alveolar pressure body is suddenly returned from 5000 mmHg to normal pressure of 760 mmHg.

nitrogen have dissolved in his or her body and the diver then suddenly comes back to the surface of the sea, significant quantities of nitrogen bubbles can develop in the body fluids either intracellularly or extracellularly, and can cause minor or serious damage in almost any area of the body, depending on the number and sizes of bubbles formed; this phenomenon is called decompression sickness.

The principles underlying bubble formation are shown in Figure 63-5. In Figure 63-5A, the diver's tissues have become equilibrated to a high dissolved nitrogen pressure (PN_2 = 3918 mmHg), about 6.5 times the normal amount of nitrogen in the tissues. As long as the diver remains deep beneath the sea, the pressure against the outside of his or her body (5000 mmHg) compresses all the body tissues sufficiently to keep the excess nitrogen gas dissolved. However, when the diver suddenly rises to sea level (Figure 63-5B), the pressure on the outside of the body becomes only 1 atm (760 mmHg), while the gas pressure inside the body fluids is the sum of the pressures of water vapor, CO_2, O_2, and nitrogen, or a total of 4065 mmHg, 97% of which is caused by the nitrogen. Obviously, this total value of 4065 mmHg is far greater than the 760 mmHg pressure on the outside of the body. Therefore, the gases can escape from the dissolved state and form bubbles, composed almost entirely of nitrogen, both in the tissues and in the blood where they plug many small blood vessels. The bubbles may not appear for many minutes to hours because sometimes the gases can remain dissolved in the "supersaturated" state for hours before bubbling.

Symptoms of Decompression Sickness ("Bends")

The symptoms of decompression sickness are caused by gas bubbles blocking many blood vessels in different tissues. At first, only the smallest vessels are blocked by minute bubbles, but as the bubbles coalesce, progressively larger vessels are affected. Tissue ischemia and sometimes tissue death result.

In most people with decompression sickness, the symptoms are pain in the joints and muscles of the legs and arms, affecting 85–90%

of persons who experience decompression sickness. The joint pain accounts for the term "bends" that is often applied to this condition.

In 5–10% of people with decompression sickness, nervous system symptoms occur, ranging from dizziness in about 5% to paralysis or collapse and unconsciousness in as many as 3%. The paralysis may be temporary, but in some instances, damage is permanent.

Finally, about 2% of people with decompression sickness experience "the chokes," caused by massive numbers of microbubbles plugging the capillaries of the lungs; this condition is characterized by serious shortness of breath, often followed by severe pulmonary edema and, occasionally, death (Box 63-6).

PHYSIOLOGICAL PRINCIPLES OF PREVENTION AND MANAGEMENT OF DECOMPRESSION SICKNESS

Nitrogen Elimination from the Body; Decompression Tables. If a diver is brought to the surface slowly, enough of the dissolved nitrogen can usually be eliminated by expiration through the lungs to prevent decompression sickness. About two-thirds of the total nitrogen is liberated in 1 hour and about 90% is liberated in 6 hours.

Tables that detail procedures for safe decompression have been prepared by the US Navy. To give the student an idea of the decompression process, a diver who has been breathing air and has been on the sea bottom for 60 minutes at a depth of 190 ft. undergoes decompression according to the following schedule:

10 minutes at 50-ft. depth
17 minutes at 40-ft. depth
19 minutes at 30-ft. depth
50 minutes at 20-ft. depth
84 minutes at 10-ft. depth

Thus, for a work period on the bottom of only 1 hour, the total time for decompression is about 3 hours.

Tank Decompression and Treatment of Decompression Sickness. Another procedure widely used for decompression of professional divers is to put the diver into a pressurized tank and then gradually to lower the pressure back to normal atmospheric pressure, using essentially the same time schedule as noted earlier.

Tank decompression is even more important for treating people in whom symptoms of decompression sickness develop minutes or even hours after they have returned to the surface. In this case, the diver undergoes recompression immediately to a deep level and then decompression is carried out over a period several times as long as the usual decompression period.

"Saturation Diving" and Use of Helium–Oxygen Mixtures in Deep Dives. When divers must work at very deep levels—between 250 and nearly 1000 ft.—they frequently live in a large compression tank for days or weeks at a time, remaining compressed at a pressure level near that at which they will be working. This procedure keeps the tissues and fluids of the body saturated with the gases to which they will be exposed while diving. Then, when they return to the same tank after working, there are no significant changes in pressure, so decompression bubbles do not occur.

In very deep dives, especially during saturation diving, helium is usually used in the gas mixture instead of nitrogen for three reasons: (1) it has only about one-fifth the narcotic effect of nitrogen; (2) only about one-half as much volume of helium dissolves in the body tissues as nitrogen, and the volume that does dissolve diffuses out of the tissues during decompression several times as rapidly as does nitrogen, thus reducing the problem of decompression sickness; and (3) the low density of helium (one-seventh the density of nitrogen) keeps the airway resistance for breathing at a minimum, which is very important because highly compressed nitrogen is so dense that airway resistance can become extreme, sometimes making the work of breathing beyond endurance.

Finally, in very deep dives it is important to reduce the O_2 concentration in the gaseous mixture because otherwise O_2 toxicity would result. For instance, at a depth of 700 ft. (22 atm of pressure), a 1% O_2 mixture will provide all the O_2 required by the diver, whereas a 21% mixture of O_2 (the percentage in air) delivers a PO_2 to the lungs of more than 4 atm, a level very likely to cause seizures in as little as 30 minutes.

Self-Contained Underwater Breathing Apparatus Diving

Before the 1940s, almost all diving was done using a diving helmet connected to a hose through which air was pumped to the diver from the surface. Then, in 1943, French explorer Jacques Cousteau popularized a self-contained underwater breathing apparatus, known as SCUBA. The type of SCUBA used in more than 99% of all sports and commercial diving is the open-circuit demand system shown in Figure 63-6. This system consists

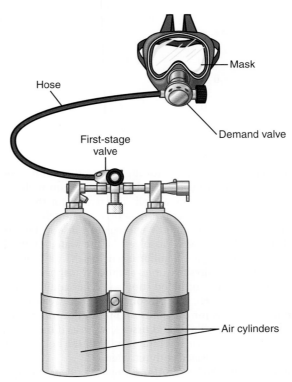

Figure 63-6 Open-circuit demand type of SCUBA.

of the following components: (1) one or more tanks of compressed air or some other breathing mixture, (2) a first-stage "reducing" valve for reducing the very high pressure from the tanks to a low-pressure level, (3) a combination inhalation "demand" valve and exhalation valve that allows air to be pulled into the lungs with slight negative pressure of breathing and then to be exhaled into the sea at a pressure level slightly positive to the surrounding water pressure, and (4) a mask and tube system with small "dead space."

The demand system operates as follows: The first-stage reducing valve reduces the pressure from the tanks so that the air delivered to the mask has a pressure only a few millimeters of mercury greater than the surrounding water pressure. The breathing mixture does not flow continually into the mask. Instead, with each inspiration, slight extra negative pressure in the demand valve of the mask pulls the diaphragm of the valve open, and this action automatically releases air from the tank into the mask and lungs. In this way, only the amount of air needed for inhalation enters the mask. Then, on expiration, the air cannot go back into the tank but instead is expired into the sea.

The most important problem with SCUBA is the limited amount of time one can remain beneath the water surface; for instance, only a few minutes are possible at a 200-ft. depth. The reason for this limitation is that tremendous airflow from the tanks is required to wash CO_2 out of the lungs—the greater the depth, the greater is the airflow in terms of quantity of air per minute that is required, because the volumes have been compressed to small sizes.

BIBLIOGRAPHY

Basnyat B, Murdoch DR: High-altitude illness, *Lancet* 361:1967, 2003.

Butler PJ: Diving beyond the limits, *News Physiol. Sci.* 16:222, 2001.

Hackett PH, Roach RC: High-altitude illness, *N. Engl. J. Med.* 345:107, 2001.

Hainsworth R, Drinkhill MJ: Cardiovascular adjustments for life at high altitude, *Respir. Physiol. Neurobiol.* 158:204, 2007.

Imray C, Wright A, Subudhi A, Roach R: Acute mountain sickness: pathophysiology, prevention, and treatment, *Prog. Cardiovasc. Dis.* 52:467, 2010.

Leach RM, Rees PJ, Wilmshurst P: Hyperbaric oxygen therapy, *BMJ* 317:1140, 1998.

Lindholm P, Lundgren CE: The physiology and pathophysiology of human breath-hold diving, *J. Appl. Physiol.* 106:284, 2009.

Moon RE, Cherry AD, Stolp BW, Camporesi EM: Pulmonary gas exchange in diving, *J. Appl. Physiol.* 106:668, 2009.

Naeije R, Dedobbeleer C: Pulmonary hypertension and the right ventricle in hypoxia, *Exp. Physiol.* 98:1247, 2013.

Neuman TS: Arterial gas embolism and decompression sickness, *News Physiol. Sci.* 17:77, 2002.

Panneton MW: The mammalian diving response: an enigmatic reflex to preserve life? *Physiology (Bethesda)* 28:284, 2013.

Penaloza D, Arias-Stella J: The heart and pulmonary circulation at high altitudes: healthy highlanders and chronic mountain sickness, *Circulation* 115:1132, 2007.

Pendergast DR, Lundgren CE: The underwater environment: cardiopulmonary, thermal, and energetic demands, *J. Appl. Physiol.* 106:276, 2009.

Prabhakar NR, Semenza GL: Adaptive and maladaptive cardiorespiratory responses to continuous and intermittent hypoxia mediated by hypoxia-inducible factors 1 and 2, *Physiol. Rev.* 92:967, 2012.

San T, Polat S, Cingi C, et al: Effects of high altitude on sleep and respiratory system and theirs adaptations, *Sci. World J.* 2013:241569, 2013.

Semenza GL: HIF-1 mediates metabolic responses to intratumoral hypoxia and oncogenic mutations, *J. Clin. Invest.* 123:3664, 2013.

Taylor CT, McElwain JC: Ancient atmospheres and the evolution of oxygen sensing via the hypoxia-inducible factor in metazoans, *Physiology (Bethesda)* 25:272, 2010.

Thom SR: Oxidative stress is fundamental to hyperbaric oxygen therapy, *J. Appl. Physiol.* 106:988, 2008.

Vann RD, Butler FK, Mitchell SJ, Moon RE: Decompression illness, *Lancet* 377:153, 2011.

West JB: High-altitude medicine, *Am. J. Respir. Crit. Care Med.* 186:1229, 2012.

64

Applied Respiratory Physiology

LEARNING OBJECTIVES

- List the various respiratory diseases and describe the pathophysiology.
- Describe the methods of artificial respiration.
- Describe oxygen therapy.

GLOSSARY OF TERMS

- **Atelectasis:** Refers to "collapse of the alveoli" due to various causes
- **Cyanosis:** Bluish discoloration of the skin
- **Hypercapnia:** A condition where there is increased carbon dioxide in blood due to hypoventilation
- **Pneumonia:** Includes any inflammatory or infective condition of the lung in which some or all of the alveoli are filled with fluid and blood cells
- **Polarography:** A technique that is used to measure the concentration of oxygen in a fluid

Respiratory Disorders

Diagnosis and treatment of most respiratory disorders depend heavily on understanding the basic physiological principles of respiration and gas exchange. Some respiratory diseases result from inadequate ventilation. Others result from abnormalities of diffusion through the pulmonary membrane or abnormal blood transport of gases between the lungs and tissues. Therapy is often entirely different for these diseases, so it is no longer satisfactory simply to make a diagnosis of "respiratory insufficiency."

USEFUL METHODS FOR STUDYING RESPIRATORY ABNORMALITIES

In the previous few chapters, we have discussed several methods for studying respiratory abnormalities, including measuring vital capacity, tidal air, functional residual capacity, dead space, physiological shunt, and physiological dead space. This array of measurements is only part of the armamentarium of the clinical pulmonary physiologist. Some other tools are described here.

Study of Blood Gases and Blood pH

Among the most fundamental of all tests of pulmonary performance are determinations of the blood partial pressure of oxygen (PO_2), carbon dioxide (CO_2), and pH. It is often important to make these measurements rapidly as an aid in determining appropriate therapy for acute respiratory distress or acute abnormalities of acid–base balance. The following simple and rapid methods have been developed to make these measurements within minutes, using no more than a few drops of blood.

Determination of Blood pH. Blood pH is measured using a glass pH electrode of the type commonly used in chemical laboratories. However, the electrodes used for this purpose are miniaturized. The voltage generated by the glass electrode is a direct measure of pH, and this is generally read directly from a voltmeter scale, or it is recorded on a chart.

Determination of Blood CO_2. A glass electrode pH meter can also be used to determine blood CO_2: When a weak solution of sodium bicarbonate is exposed to CO_2 gas, the CO_2 dissolves in the solution until an equilibrium state is established. In this equilibrium state, the pH of the solution is a function of the CO_2 and bicarbonate ion concentrations in accordance with the Henderson–Hasselbalch equation that is explained earlier; that is,

$$pH = 6.1 + \log \frac{HCO_3^-}{CO_2}$$

When the glass electrode is used to measure CO_2 in blood, a miniature glass electrode is surrounded by a thin plastic membrane. In the space between the electrode and plastic membrane is a solution of sodium bicarbonate of known concentration. Blood is then superfused onto the outer surface of the plastic membrane, allowing CO_2 to diffuse from the blood into the bicarbonate solution. Only a drop or so of blood is required. Next, the pH is measured by the glass electrode, and the CO_2 is calculated with use of the formula that was previously provided.

Determination of Blood PO_2. The concentration of O_2 in a fluid can be measured by a technique called *polarography*. Electric current is made to flow between a small negative electrode and the solution. If the voltage of the electrode is more than -0.6 V different from the voltage of the solution, O_2 will deposit on the electrode. Furthermore, the rate of current flow through the electrode will be directly proportional to the concentration of O_2 (and therefore to PO_2 as well). In practice, a negative platinum electrode with a surface area of about 1 mm^2 is used, and this electrode is separated from the blood by a thin plastic membrane that allows diffusion of O_2 but not diffusion of proteins or other substances that will "poison" the electrode.

Often all three of the measuring devices for pH, CO_2, and PO_2 are built into the same apparatus, and all these measurements can be made within a minute or so using a single, droplet-size sample of blood. Thus, changes in the blood gases and pH can be followed almost moment by moment at the bedside.

PATHOPHYSIOLOGY OF SPECIFIC PULMONARY ABNORMALITIES

Chronic Pulmonary Emphysema

The term *pulmonary emphysema* literally means excess air in the lungs. However, this term is usually used to describe a complex obstructive and destructive process of the lungs caused by many years of smoking. It results from the following major pathophysiological changes in the lungs:

1. *Chronic infection*, caused by inhaling smoke or other substances that irritate the bronchi and bronchioles. The chronic infection seriously deranges the normal protective mechanisms of the airways, including partial paralysis of the cilia of the respiratory epithelium, an effect caused by nicotine. As a result, mucus cannot be moved easily out of the passageways. Also, stimulation of excess mucus secretion occurs, which further exacerbates the condition. Inhibition of the alveolar macrophages also occurs, so they become less effective in combating infection.
2. The infection, excess mucus, and inflammatory edema of the bronchiolar epithelium together cause *chronic obstruction* of many of the smaller airways.
3. The obstruction of the airways makes it especially difficult to expire, thus causing *entrapment of air in the alveoli* and overstretching them. This effect, combined with the lung infection, causes *marked destruction of as much as 50–80% of the alveolar walls*. Therefore, the final picture of the emphysematous lung is that shown in Figures 64-1 (*top*) and 64-2.

The physiological effects of chronic emphysema are variable, depending on the severity of the disease and the relative degrees of bronchiolar obstruction versus lung parenchymal destruction. Among the different abnormalities are the following:

1. The bronchiolar obstruction *increases airway resistance* and results in greatly increased work of breathing. It is especially difficult for the person to move air through the bronchioles during expiration because the compressive force on the outside of the lung not only compresses the alveoli but also compresses the bronchioles, which further increases their resistance during expiration.
2. The marked loss of alveolar walls greatly *decreases the diffusing capacity* of the lung, which reduces the ability of the lungs to oxygenate the blood and remove CO_2 from the blood.
3. The obstructive process is frequently much worse in some parts of the lungs than in other parts, so some portions of the lungs are well ventilated, whereas other portions are poorly ventilated. This situation often causes *extremely abnormal ventilation–perfusion ratios* leading to very low $\dot{V}_a/\dot{Q}$ in some parts (physiological shunt) and very high $\dot{V}_a/\dot{Q}$ in other parts (physiological dead space), resulting in wasted ventilation, with both effects occurring in the same lungs.
4. Loss of large portions of the alveolar walls also decreases the number of pulmonary capillaries through which blood can pass. As a result, the pulmonary vascular resistance often increases markedly, causing *pulmonary*

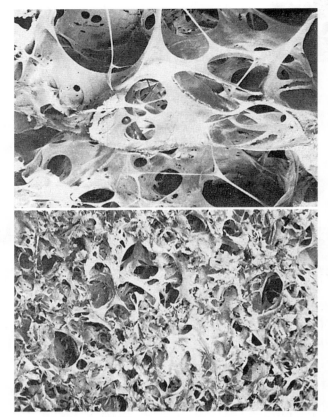

Figure 64-1 Contrast of the emphysematous lung (*top*) with the normal lung (*bottom*) showing extensive alveolar destruction in emphysema. *Courtesy Patricia Delaney and the Department of Anatomy, The Medical College of Wisconsin.*

hypertension which in turn overloads the right side of the heart and frequently causes right-sided heart failure.

Chronic emphysema usually progresses slowly over many years. Both hypoxia and hypercapnia develop because of hypoventilation of many alveoli plus loss of alveolar walls. The net result of all these effects is severe, prolonged, devastating *air hunger* that can last for years until the hypoxia and hypercapnia cause death—a high penalty to pay for smoking.

Pneumonia—Lung Inflammation and Fluid in Alveoli

The term *pneumonia* includes any inflammatory condition of the lung in which some or all of the alveoli are filled with fluid and blood cells, as shown in Figure 64-2. A common type of

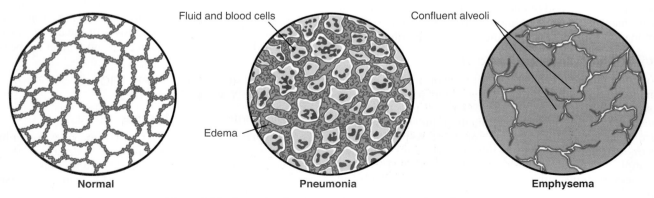

Figure 64-2 Lung alveolar changes in pneumonia and emphysema.

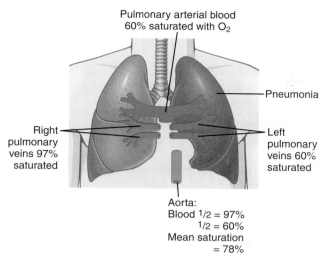

Figure 64-3 Effect of pneumonia on percentage saturation of oxygen (O₂) in the pulmonary artery, the right and left pulmonary veins, and the aorta.

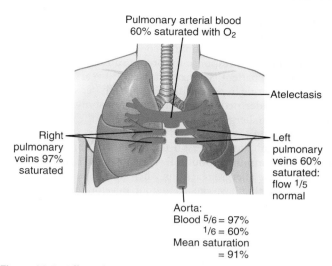

Figure 64-4 Effect of atelectasis on aortic blood oxygen (O₂) saturation.

pneumonia is *bacterial pneumonia*, caused most frequently by *pneumococci*. This disease begins with infection in the alveoli; the pulmonary membrane becomes inflamed and highly porous so that fluid and even red and white blood cells leak out of the blood into the alveoli. Thus, the infected alveoli become progressively filled with fluid and cells, and the infection spreads by extension of bacteria or virus from alveolus to alveolus. Eventually, large areas of the lungs, sometimes whole lobes or even a whole lung, become "consolidated," which means that they are filled with fluid and cellular debris.

In persons with pneumonia, the gas exchange functions of the lungs decline in different stages of the disease. In early stages, the pneumonia process might well be localized to only one lung, with alveolar ventilation reduced while blood flow through the lung continues normally. This condition causes two major pulmonary abnormalities: (1) reduction in the total available surface area of the respiratory membrane and (2) decreased ventilation–perfusion ratio. Both of these effects cause *hypoxemia* (low blood O₂) and *hypercapnia* (high blood CO₂).

Figure 64-3 shows the effect of the decreased ventilation–perfusion ratio in pneumonia. The blood passing through the aerated lung becomes 97% saturated with O₂, whereas that passing through the unaerated lung is about 60% saturated. Therefore, the average saturation of the blood pumped by the left heart into the aorta is only about 78%, which is far below normal.

Atelectasis—Collapse of the Alveoli

Atelectasis means collapse of the alveoli. It can occur in localized areas of a lung or in an entire lung. Common causes of atelectasis are (1) total obstruction of the airway or (2) lack of surfactant in the fluids lining the alveoli.

Airway Obstruction Causes Lung Collapse. The airway obstruction type of atelectasis usually results from (1) blockage of many small bronchi with mucus or (2) obstruction of a major bronchus by either a large mucus plug or some solid object such as a tumor. The air entrapped beyond the block is absorbed within minutes to hours by the blood flowing in the pulmonary capillaries. If the lung tissue is pliable enough, this will lead simply to collapse of the alveoli. However, if the lung is rigid because of fibrotic tissue and cannot collapse, absorption of air from the alveoli creates very negative pressures within the alveoli, which pull

fluid out of the pulmonary capillaries into the alveoli, thus causing the alveoli to fill completely with edema fluid. This process almost always is the effect that occurs when an entire lung becomes atelectatic, a condition called *massive collapse* of the lung.

The effects on overall pulmonary function caused by *massive collapse* (atelectasis) of an entire lung are shown in Figure 64-4. Collapse of the lung tissue not only occludes the alveoli but also almost always increases the *resistance to blood flow* through the pulmonary vessels of the collapsed lung. This resistance increase occurs partially because of the lung collapse, which compresses and folds the vessels as the volume of the lung decreases. In addition, hypoxia in the collapsed alveoli causes additional vasoconstriction, as explained in Chapter 57.

Because of the vascular constriction, blood flow through the atelectatic lung is greatly reduced. Fortunately, most of the blood is routed through the ventilated lung and therefore becomes well aerated. In the situation shown in Figure 64-4, five-sixths of the blood passes through the aerated lung and only one-sixth passes through the unaerated lung. As a result, the overall ventilation–perfusion ratio is only moderately compromised, so the aortic blood has only mild O₂ desaturation despite total loss of ventilation in an entire lung.

Lack of "Surfactant" as a Cause of Lung Collapse. The secretion and function of *surfactant* in the alveoli were discussed in Chapter 54. Surfactant is secreted by special alveolar epithelial cells into the fluids that coat the inside surface of the alveoli. The surfactant in turn decreases the surface tension in the alveoli 2- to 10-fold, which normally plays a major role in preventing alveolar collapse. However, in several conditions, such as in *hyaline membrane disease* (also called *respiratory distress syndrome*), which often occurs in newborn premature babies, the quantity of surfactant secreted by the alveoli is so greatly depressed that the surface tension of the alveolar fluid becomes several times normal. This situation causes a serious tendency for the lungs of these babies to collapse or to become filled with fluid. As explained in Chapter 54, many of these infants die of suffocation when large portions of the lungs become atelectatic.

Asthma—Spasmodic Contraction of Smooth Muscles in Bronchioles

Asthma is characterized by spastic contraction of the smooth muscle in the bronchioles, which partially obstructs the bronchioles and causes extremely difficult breathing. It occurs in 3–5% of all people at some time in life.

The usual cause of asthma is contractile hypersensitivity of the bronchioles in response to foreign substances in the air. In about 70% of patients younger than age 30 years, the asthma is caused by allergic hypersensitivity, especially sensitivity to plant pollens. In older people, the cause is almost always hypersensitivity to nonallergenic types of irritants in the air, such as irritants in smog.

The typical allergic person tends to form abnormally large amounts of immunoglobulin E (IgE) antibodies, and these antibodies cause allergic reactions when they react with the specific antigens that have caused them to develop in the first place. In persons with asthma, these *antibodies are mainly attached to mast cells* that are present in the lung interstitium in close association with the bronchioles and small bronchi. When an asthmatic person breathes in pollen to which he or she is sensitive (ie, to which he or she has developed IgE antibodies), the pollen reacts with the mast cell–attached antibodies and causes the mast cells to release several different substances. Among them are (1) *histamine*, (2) *slow-reacting substance of anaphylaxis* (which is a mixture of leukotrienes), (3) *eosinophilic chemotactic factor*, and (4) *bradykinin*. The combined effects of all these factors, especially the slow-reacting substance of anaphylaxis, are to produce (1) localized edema in the walls of the small bronchioles, as well as secretion of thick mucus into the bronchiolar lumens, and (2) spasm of the bronchiolar smooth muscle. Therefore, the airway resistance increases greatly.

As discussed earlier in this chapter, the bronchiolar diameter becomes more reduced during expiration than during inspiration in persons with asthma, as a result of bronchiolar collapse during expiratory effort that compresses the outsides of the bronchioles. Because the bronchioles of the asthmatic lungs are already partially occluded, further occlusion resulting from the external pressure creates especially severe obstruction during expiration. That is, the asthmatic person often can inspire quite adequately but has great difficulty expiring. Clinical measurements show (1) greatly reduced maximum expiratory rate and (2) reduced timed expiratory volume. Also, all of this altogether results in dyspnea or "air hunger," which is discussed later in this chapter.

The *functional residual capacity* and *residual volume* of the lung become especially increased during an acute asthma attack because of the difficulty in expiring air from the lungs. Also, over a period of years, the chest cage becomes permanently enlarged, causing a "barrel chest," and both the functional residual capacity and lung residual volume become permanently increased.

Tuberculosis

In tuberculosis, the tubercle bacilli cause a peculiar tissue reaction in the lungs, including (1) invasion of the infected tissue by macrophages and (2) "walling off" of the lesion by fibrous tissue to form the so-called *tubercle*. This walling-off process helps to limit further transmission of the tubercle bacilli in the lungs and therefore is part of the protective process against extension of the infection. However, in about 3% of all people in whom tuberculosis develops, if the disease is not treated, the walling-off process fails and tubercle bacilli spread throughout the lungs, often causing extreme destruction of lung tissue with formation of large abscess cavities.

Thus, tuberculosis in its late stages is characterized by many areas of fibrosis throughout the lungs, as well as reduced total amount of functional lung tissue. These effects cause (1)

increased "work" on the part of the respiratory muscles to cause pulmonary ventilation and *reduced vital capacity and breathing capacity*; (2) *reduced total respiratory membrane surface area* and *increased thickness of the respiratory membrane*, causing progressively *diminished pulmonary diffusing capacity*; and (3) *abnormal ventilation–perfusion ratio* in the lungs, further reducing overall pulmonary diffusion of O_2 and CO_2.

Pleural Effusion

Pleural effusion is a condition where there is an abnormal and excessive collection of fluid in the space between the pleural membranes. This results due to either excessive production or reduced absorption of pleural fluid in this space.

Pleural effusion occurs due to an underlying disease process that could be related to the respiratory system or other systems such as the cardiovascular system. Some of the common causes of pleural effusion include pneumonias, malignancies, pulmonary embolism, and congestive heart failure.

The common symptoms of pleural effusion manifest as difficulty in breathing (dyspnea), cough, and chest pain. Other symptoms such as fever, hemoptysis (blood in the sputum), weight loss, and edema may occur and are related to underlying diseases such as pneumonia, malignancy, tuberculosis, or congestive heart failure.

Cyanosis

The term *cyanosis* means blueness of the skin, and its cause is excessive amounts of deoxygenated hemoglobin in the skin blood vessels, especially in the capillaries. This deoxygenated hemoglobin has an intense dark blue–purple color that is transmitted through the skin.

In general, definite cyanosis appears whenever the *arterial blood* contains more than 5 g of deoxygenated hemoglobin in each 100 mL of blood. A person with *anemia* almost never becomes cyanotic because there is not enough hemoglobin for 5 g to be deoxygenated in 100 mL of arterial blood. Conversely, in a person with excess red blood cells, as occurs in *polycythemia vera*, the great excess of available hemoglobin that can become deoxygenated leads frequently to cyanosis, even under otherwise normal conditions.

Hypercapnia—Excess Carbon Dioxide in the Body Fluids

One might suspect, on first thought, that any respiratory condition that causes hypoxia would also cause hypercapnia. However, hypercapnia usually occurs in association with hypoxia only when the hypoxia is caused by *hypoventilation* or *circulatory deficiency* for the following reasons.

Hypoxia caused by *too little O_2 in the air*, *too little hemoglobin*, or *poisoning of the oxidative enzymes* has to do only with the availability of O_2 or use of O_2 by the tissues. Therefore, it is readily understandable that hypercapnia is *not* a concomitant of these types of hypoxia.

In hypoxia resulting from poor diffusion through the pulmonary membrane or through the tissues, serious hypercapnia usually does not occur at the same time because CO_2 diffuses 20 times as rapidly as O_2. If hypercapnia does begin to occur, this immediately stimulates pulmonary ventilation, which corrects the hypercapnia but not necessarily the hypoxia.

Conversely, in hypoxia caused by hypoventilation, CO_2 transfer between the alveoli and the atmosphere is affected as much as is O_2 transfer. Hypercapnia then occurs along with the hypoxia. In circulatory deficiency, diminished flow of blood decreases CO_2 removal from the tissues, resulting in tissue hypercapnia in addition to tissue hypoxia. However, the transport capacity of the blood for CO_2 is more than three times that for O_2, and thus the resulting tissue hypercapnia is much less than the tissue hypoxia.

When the alveolar PCO_2 rises above about 60–75 mmHg, an otherwise normal person by then is breathing about as rapidly and deeply as he or she can, and "air hunger," also called *dyspnea*, becomes severe.

If the PCO_2 rises to 80–100 mmHg, the person becomes lethargic and sometimes even semicomatose. Anesthesia and death can result when the PCO_2 rises to 120–150 mmHg. At these higher levels of PCO_2, the excess CO_2 now begins to depress respiration rather than stimulate it, thus causing a vicious circle: (1) more CO_2, (2) further decrease in respiration, (3) then more CO_2, and so forth—culminating rapidly in a respiratory death.

DYSPNEA

Dyspnea means mental anguish associated with inability to ventilate enough to satisfy the demand for air. A common synonym is *air hunger*.

At least three factors often enter into the development of the sensation of dyspnea. They are (1) abnormality of respiratory gases in the body fluids, especially hypercapnia and, to a much less extent, hypoxia; (2) the amount of work that must be performed by the respiratory muscles to provide adequate ventilation; and (3) state of mind.

A person becomes very dyspneic, especially from excess buildup of CO_2 in the body fluids. At times, however, the levels of both CO_2 and O_2 in the body fluids are normal, but to attain this normality of the respiratory gases, the person has to breathe forcefully. In these instances, the forceful activity of the respiratory muscles frequently gives the person a sensation of dyspnea.

Finally, the person's respiratory functions may be normal and still dyspnea may be experienced because of an abnormal state of mind. This condition is called *neurogenic dyspnea* or *emotional dyspnea*. For instance, almost anyone momentarily thinking about the act of breathing may suddenly start taking breaths a little more deeply than ordinarily because of a feeling of mild dyspnea. This feeling is greatly enhanced in people who have a psychological fear of not being able to receive a sufficient quantity of air, such as on entering small or crowded rooms.

SLEEP APNEA

The term *apnea* means absence of spontaneous breathing. Occasional apneas occur during normal sleep, but in persons with *sleep apnea*, the frequency and duration are greatly increased, with episodes of apnea lasting for 10 seconds or longer and occurring 300–500 times each night. Sleep apneas can be caused by obstruction of the upper airways, especially the pharynx, or by impaired central nervous system respiratory drive.

Obstructive Sleep Apnea Is Caused by Blockage of the Upper Airway. The muscles of the pharynx normally keep this passage open to allow air to flow into the lungs during inspiration. During sleep, these muscles usually relax, but the airway passage remains open enough to permit adequate airflow. Some individuals have an especially narrow passage, and relaxation

---

BOX 64-1 PATHOGENESIS OF OBSTRUCTIVE SLEEP APNEA

1. Blockage of the upper airways during sleep
2. Neural drive to respiratory muscles transiently abolished

---

of these muscles during sleep causes the pharynx to completely close so that air cannot flow into the lungs.

In persons with sleep apnea, loud *snoring* and *labored breathing* occur soon after falling asleep. The snoring proceeds, often becoming louder, and is then interrupted by a long silent period during which no breathing (apnea) occurs. These periods of apnea result in significant decreases in PO_2 and increases in PCO_2, which greatly stimulates respiration. This, in turn, causes sudden attempts to breathe, which result in loud snorts and gasps followed by snoring and repeated episodes of apnea. The periods of apnea and labored breathing are repeated several hundred times during the night, resulting in fragmented, restless sleep. Therefore, patients with sleep apnea usually have excessive daytime *drowsiness*, as well as other disorders, including increased sympathetic activity, high heart rates, pulmonary and systemic hypertension, and a greatly elevated risk for cardiovascular disease (Box 64-1).

Obstructive sleep apnea most commonly occurs in older, obese persons in whom there is increased fat deposition in the soft tissues of the pharynx or compression of the pharynx due to excessive fat masses in the neck. In a few individuals, sleep apnea may be associated with nasal obstruction, a very large tongue, enlarged tonsils, or certain shapes of the palate that greatly increase resistance to the flow of air to the lungs during inspiration. The most common treatments of obstructive sleep apnea include (1) surgery to remove excess fat tissue at the back of the throat (a procedure called *uvulopalatopharyngoplasty*), to remove enlarged tonsils or adenoids, or to create an opening in the trachea (tracheostomy) to bypass the obstructed airway during sleep, and (2) nasal ventilation with *continuous positive airway pressure* (CPAP).

"Central" Sleep Apnea Occurs when the Neural Drive to Respiratory Muscles Is Transiently Abolished. In a few persons with sleep apnea, the central nervous system drive to the ventilatory muscles transiently ceases. Disorders that can cause cessation of the ventilatory drive during sleep include *damage to the central respiratory centers or abnormalities of the respiratory neuromuscular apparatus*. Patients affected by central sleep apnea may have decreased ventilation when they are awake, although they are fully capable of normal voluntary breathing. During sleep, their breathing disorders usually worsen, resulting in more frequent episodes of apnea that decrease PO_2 and increase PCO_2 until a critical level is reached that eventually stimulates respiration. These transient instabilities of respiration cause restless sleep and clinical features similar to those observed in obstructive sleep apnea.

In most patients the cause of central sleep apnea is unknown, although instability of the respiratory drive can result from strokes or other disorders that make the respiratory centers of the brain less responsive to the stimulatory effects of CO_2 and hydrogen ions. Patients with this disease are extremely sensitive to even small doses of sedatives or narcotics, which further reduce the responsiveness of the respiratory centers to the stimulatory effects of CO_2. Medications that stimulate the respiratory centers can sometimes be helpful, but ventilation with CPAP at night is usually necessary.

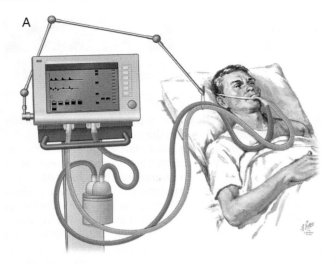

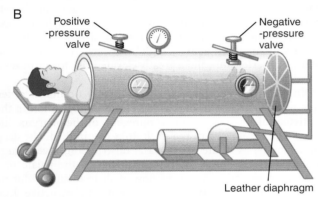

Figure 64-5   (A) Ventilator; (B) tank respirator. *(A) Netter illustration from www.netterimages.com. © Elsevier Inc. All rights reserved.*

Artificial Respiration

Ventilator. Many types of respiratory ventilators are available, and each has its own characteristic principles of operation. The ventilator shown in Figure 64-5A consists of a tank supply of O_2 or air; a mechanism for applying intermittent positive pressure and, with some machines, negative pressure as well; and a mask that fits over the face of the patient or a connector for joining the equipment to an endotracheal tube. This apparatus forces air through the mask or endotracheal tube into the lungs of the patient during the positive-pressure cycle of the ventilator and then usually allows the air to flow passively out of the lungs during the remainder of the cycle.

Earlier ventilators often caused damage to the lungs because of excessive positive pressure. Their usage was at one time greatly decried. However, ventilators now have adjustable positive-pressure limits that are commonly set at 12–15 cm H_2O pressure for normal lungs (but sometimes much higher for noncompliant lungs).

Tank Respirator (the "Iron Lung"). Figure 64-5B shows the tank respirator with a patient's body inside the tank and the head protruding through a flexible but airtight collar. At the end of the tank opposite the patient's head, a motor-driven leather diaphragm moves back and forth with sufficient excursion to raise and lower the pressure inside the tank. As the leather diaphragm moves inward, positive pressure develops around the body and causes expiration; as the diaphragm moves outward, negative pressure causes inspiration. Check valves on the respirator control the positive and negative pressures. Ordinarily these pressures are adjusted so that the negative pressure that causes inspiration falls to −10 to −20 cm H_2O and the positive pressure rises to 0 to +5 cm H_2O.

Effect of the Ventilator and the Tank Respirator on Venous Return. When air is forced into the lungs under positive pressure by a ventilator, or when the pressure around the patient's body is *reduced* by the tank respirator, the pressure inside the lungs becomes greater than pressure everywhere else in the body. Flow of blood into the chest and heart from the peripheral veins becomes impeded. As a result, use of excessive pressures with either the ventilator or the tank respirator can reduce the cardiac output—sometimes to lethal levels. For instance, continuous exposure for more than a few minutes to greater than 30 mmHg positive pressure in the lungs can cause death because of inadequate venous return to the heart.

Oxygen Therapy

O_2 therapy is usually provided to patients with hypoxia and is described in detail in Chapter 59. However, to summarize the different types of O_2 therapy in hypoxic states, the following methods are listed:
1. placing the patient's head in a "tent" that contains air fortified with O_2;
2. providing the patient either pure O_2 or high concentrations of O_2 to breathe from a mask;
3. administering O_2 through an intranasal tube.

Besides O_2 therapy in hypoxic states, there is another method of treating patients with high-pressure O_2 described as follows.

Hyperbaric Oxygen Therapy

The intense oxidizing properties of high-pressure O_2 (hyperbaric oxygen) can have valuable therapeutic effects in several important clinical conditions. Therefore, large pressure tanks are now available in many medical centers into which patients can be placed and treated with hyperbaric O_2. The O_2 is usually administered at PO_2 values of 2–3 atm pressure through a mask or intratracheal tube, whereas the gas around the body is normal air compressed to the same high-pressure level.

It is believed that the same oxidizing free radicals responsible for O_2 toxicity are also responsible for at least some of the therapeutic benefits. Some of the conditions in which hyperbaric O_2 therapy has been especially beneficial are described next.

One successful use of hyperbaric O_2 has been for treatment of gas gangrene. The bacteria that cause this condition, clostridial organisms, grow best under anaerobic conditions and stop growing at O_2 pressures greater than about 70 mmHg. Therefore, hyperbaric oxygenation of the tissues can frequently stop the infectious process entirely and thus convert a condition that formerly was almost 100% fatal into one that is cured in most instances by early treatment with hyperbaric therapy.

Other conditions in which hyperbaric O_2 therapy has been either valuable or possibly valuable include decompression sickness, arterial gas embolism, carbon monoxide poisoning, osteomyelitis, and myocardial infarction.

BIBLIOGRAPHY

Barnes PJ: The cytokine network in asthma and chronic obstructive pulmonary disease, *J. Clin. Invest.* 118:3546, 2008.

Bel EH: Clinical practice. Mild asthma, *N. Engl. J. Med.* 369:549, 2013.

Bradley TD, Floras JS: Obstructive sleep apnoea and its cardiovascular consequences, *Lancet* 373:82, 2009.

Casey KR, Cantillo KO, Brown LK: Sleep-related hypoventilation/hypoxemic syndromes, *Chest* 131:1936, 2007.

Culotta R, Taylor D: Diseases of the pleura. In Ali J, Summer WR, Levitzky MG, editors: *Pulmonary Pathophysiology*, second ed., New York, 2005, Lange Medical Books/McGraw-Hill, pp 194-212.

Decramer M, Janssens W, Miravitlles M: Chronic obstructive pulmonary disease, *Lancet* 379:1341, 2012.

Dempsey JA, McKenzie DC, Haverkamp HC, et al: Update in the understanding of respiratory limitations to exercise performance in fit, active adults, *Chest* 134:613, 2008.

Doolette DJ, Mitchell SJ: Hyperbaric conditions, *Compr. Physiol.* 1:163, 2011.

Eckert DJ, Jordan AS, Merchia P, et al: Central sleep apnea: pathophysiology and treatment, *Chest* 131:595, 2007.

Eder W, Ege MJ, von Mutius E: The asthma epidemic, *N. Engl. J. Med.* 355:2226, 2006.

Fahy JV, Dickey BF: Airway mucus function and dysfunction, *N. Engl. J. Med.* 363:2233, 2010.

Guarnieri M, Balmes JR: Outdoor air pollution and asthma, *Lancet* 383:1581, 2014.

Henderson WR, Sheel AW: Pulmonary mechanics during mechanical ventilation, *Respir. Physiol. Neurobiol.* 180:162, 2012.

Holtzman MJ: Asthma as a chronic disease of the innate and adaptive immune systems responding to viruses and allergens, *J. Clin. Invest.* 122:2741, 2012.

McConnell AK, Romer LM: Dyspnoea in health and obstructive pulmonary disease: the role of respiratory muscle function and training, *Sports Med.* 34:117, 2004.

Mühlfeld C, Rothen-Rutishauser B, Blank F, et al: Interactions of nanoparticles with pulmonary structures and cellular responses, *Am. J. Physiol. Lung Cell. Mol. Physiol.* 294:L817, 2008.

Naureckas ET, Solway J: Clinical practice. Mild asthma, *N. Engl. J. Med.* 345:1257, 2001.

Noble PW, Barkauskas CE, Jiang D: Pulmonary fibrosis: patterns and perpetrators, *J. Clin. Invest.* 122:2756, 2012.

Ramanathan R: Optimal ventilatory strategies and surfactant to protect the preterm lungs, *Neonatology* 93:302, 2008.

Raoof S, Goulet K, Esan A, et al: Severe hypoxemic respiratory failure: part 2: nonventilatory strategies, *Chest* 137:1437, 2010.

Sharafkhaneh A, Hanania NA, Kim V: Pathogenesis of emphysema: from the bench to the bedside, *Proc. Am. Thorac. Soc.* 5:475, 2008.

Sin DD, McAlister FA, Man SF, Anthonisen NR: Contemporary management of chronic obstructive pulmonary disease: scientific review, *JAMA* 290:2301, 2003.

Suki B, Sato S, Parameswaran H, et al: Emphysema and mechanical stress-induced lung remodeling, *Physiology (Bethesda)* 28:404, 2013.

Taraseviciene-Stewart L, Voelkel NF: Molecular pathogenesis of emphysema, *J. Clin. Invest.* 118:394, 2008.

Tarlo SM, Lemiere C: Occupational asthma, *N. Engl. J. Med.* 370:640, 2014.

Tuder RM, Petrache I: Pathogenesis of chronic obstructive pulmonary disease, *J. Clin. Invest.* 122:2749, 2012.

Wilcox ME, Chong CA, Stanbrook MB, Tricco AC, Wong C, Straus SE: Does this patient have an exudative pleural effusion? The Rational Clinical Examination systematic review, *JAMA* 311(23):2422-2431, 2014.

Gastrointestinal Physiology

TONY RAJ

65

Organization of the Gastrointestinal System

LEARNING OBJECTIVES

- List the different types of smooth muscle.
- Outline the process of smooth muscle contraction.
- Compare smooth, skeletal, and cardiac muscles and their functions.
- Illustrate the neural control of the gastrointestinal tract.
- Outline gastrointestinal blood flow.

GLOSSARY OF TERMS

- **Enteric nervous system:** A nervous system that the gastrointestinal tract has for its own functions (it lies entirely in the wall of the gut, beginning in the esophagus and extending all the way to the anus)

- **Slow waves:** Slow, undulating changes in the resting membrane potential and are not action potentials (they determine the rhythmical gastrointestinal contractions)

- **Spike potentials:** True action potentials (they occur automatically when the resting membrane potential of the gastrointestinal smooth muscle becomes more positive than about −40 mV)

- **Syncytium:** Refers to a multinucleated mass of cytoplasm that is not separated into individual cells

The alimentary tract provides the body with a continual supply of water, electrolytes, vitamins, and nutrients, which requires:
- movement of food through the alimentary tract;
- secretion of digestive juices and digestion of the food;
- absorption of water, various electrolytes, vitamins, and digestive products;
- circulation of blood through the gastrointestinal organs to carry away the absorbed substances;
- control of all these functions by local, nervous, and hormonal systems.

Figure 65-1 shows the entire alimentary tract. In this chapter, we discuss the organization and basic principles of function in the entire alimentary tract and in subsequent chapters the specific functions of different segments of the tract will be addressed.

General Principles of Gastrointestinal Motility

PHYSIOLOGICAL ANATOMY OF THE GASTROINTESTINAL WALL

Figure 65-2 shows a typical cross-section of the intestinal wall including the following layers from outer surface inward:
(1) the *serosa*, (2) a *longitudinal smooth muscle layer*, (3) a *circular smooth muscle layer*, (4) the *submucosa*, and (5) the *mucosa*. In addition, sparse bundles of smooth muscle fibers, the *mucosal muscle*, lie in the deeper layers of the mucosa. The motor functions of the gut are performed by the different layers of smooth muscle.

Types of Smooth Muscle. For the sake of simplicity smooth muscle can generally be divided into two major types, which are shown in Figure 65-3:
1. multiunit smooth muscle
2. unitary (or single-unit) smooth muscle

Multiunit smooth muscle. Multiunit smooth muscle is composed of discrete, separate smooth muscle fibers. Each fiber operates independently of the others and often is innervated by a single nerve ending, as occurs for skeletal muscle fibers.

Unitary smooth muscle. Unitary smooth muscle is also called syncytial smooth muscle or visceral smooth muscle. It consists of a mass of hundreds to thousands of smooth muscle fibers that contract together as a single unit.

The specific characteristics of smooth muscle in the gut are the following.

Gastrointestinal Smooth Muscle Functions as a Syncytium. The individual smooth muscle fibers in the gastrointestinal tract are 200–500 μm in length and 2–10 μm in diameter, and they are arranged in bundles of as many as 1000 parallel fibers. In the *longitudinal muscle layer*, the bundles extend longitudinally down the intestinal tract; in the *circular muscle layer*, they extend around the gut.

Within each bundle, the muscle fibers are electrically connected with one another through large numbers of *gap junctions* that allow low-resistance movement of ions from one muscle cell to the next.

Each muscle layer represents a branching latticework of smooth muscle bundles and functions as a *syncytium*; that is, when an action potential is elicited anywhere within the muscle mass, it generally travels in all directions in the muscle. The distance that it travels depends on the excitability of the muscle.

Also, because a few connections exist between the longitudinal and circular muscle layers, excitation of one of these layers often excites the other as well.

Electrical Activity of Gastrointestinal Smooth Muscle

The smooth muscle of the gastrointestinal tract is excited by almost continual slow, intrinsic electrical activity along the membranes of the muscle fibers. This activity has two basic types of electrical waves: (1) *slow waves* and (2) *spikes* (Figure 65-4). In addition, the voltage of the resting membrane potential (RMP) of the gastrointestinal smooth muscle can change to different levels, which can also have important effects in controlling motor activity of the gastrointestinal tract.

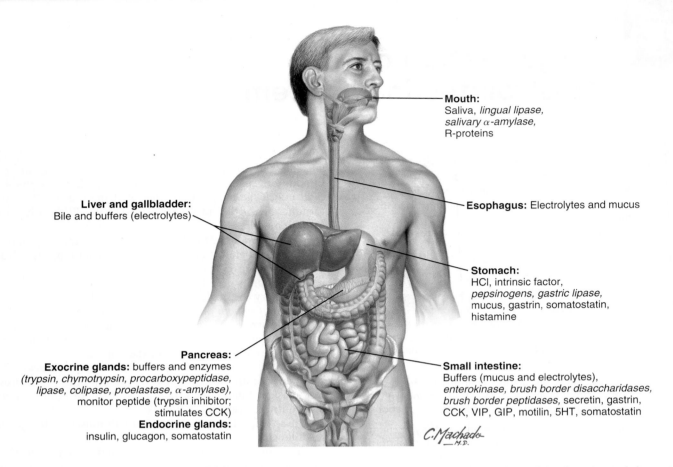

Mouth:
Saliva, *lingual lipase,*
salivary α-amylase,
R-proteins

Esophagus: Electrolytes and mucus

Liver and gallbladder:
Bile and buffers (electrolytes)

Stomach:
HCl, intrinsic factor,
pepsinogens, gastric lipase,
mucus, gastrin, somatostatin,
histamine

Pancreas:
Exocrine glands: buffers and enzymes
(trypsin, chymotrypsin, procarboxypeptidase,
lipase, colipase, proelastase, α-amylase),
monitor peptide (trypsin inhibitor;
stimulates CCK)
Endocrine glands:
insulin, glucagon, somatostatin

Small intestine:
Buffers (mucus and electrolytes),
enterokinase, brush border disaccharidases,
brush border peptidases, secretin, gastrin,
CCK, VIP, GIP, motilin, 5HT, somatostatin

Figure 65-1 Alimentary tract. The alimentary tract begins at the mouth and is made up of discrete areas that aid the digestion and absorption of nutrients. Each area of the tract contributes to the efficient processing of the nutrients. This includes the GI-associated organs (liver, pancreas), which provide important secretions including bile, enzymes, and buffers. GI, gastrointestinal. (*From Netter's Essential Physiology, 2009, Figure 21-1, p. 244*).

Slow Waves. Most gastrointestinal contractions occur rhythmically, and this rhythm is determined mainly by the frequency of so-called "slow waves" of smooth muscle membrane potential. These waves are not action potentials (Figure 65-4). Instead, they are slow, undulating changes in the RMP. Their intensity usually varies between 5 and 15 mV, and their frequency ranges in different parts of the human gastrointestinal tract from 3 to 12 minute^{-1}: about 3 in the body of the stomach, as much as 12 in the duodenum, and about 8 or 9 in the terminal ileum.

The precise cause of the slow waves is not completely understood, although they appear to be caused by complex interactions among the smooth muscle cells and specialized cells, called the *interstitial cells of Cajal*, which are believed to act as *electrical pacemakers* for smooth muscle cells. These interstitial cells form a network with each other and are interposed between the smooth muscle layers, with synaptic-like contacts to smooth muscle cells. The interstitial cells of Cajal undergo cyclic changes in membrane potential due to unique ion channels that periodically open and produce inward (pacemaker) currents that may generate slow wave activity.

The slow waves by themselves usually do not cause muscle contraction in most parts of the gastrointestinal tract, *except*

perhaps in the stomach. Instead, they mainly excite the appearance of intermittent spike potentials, which in turn actually excite the muscle contraction.

Spike Potentials. The spike potentials are true action potentials. They occur automatically when the RMP of the gastrointestinal smooth muscle becomes more positive than about −40 mV (normal RMP in smooth muscle fibers of the gut is between −50 and −60 mV). The higher the slow wave potential rises, the greater the frequency of the spike potentials becomes, usually ranging between 1 and 10 spikes/second. The spike potentials last 10–40 times as long in gastrointestinal muscle as the action potentials in large nerve fibers, with each gastrointestinal spike lasting as long as 10–20 milliseconds.

Another important difference between the action potentials of the gastrointestinal smooth muscle and those of nerve fibers is the manner in which they are generated. In nerve fibers, the action potentials are caused almost entirely by rapid entry of sodium ions through sodium channels to the interior of the fibers. However, in gastrointestinal smooth muscle fibers the channels responsible for the action potentials allow especially large numbers of calcium ions to enter along with smaller numbers of sodium ions and therefore are called *calcium–sodium*

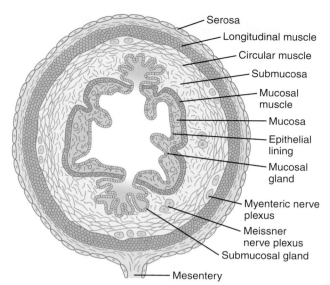

Figure 65-2   Typical cross-section of the gut.

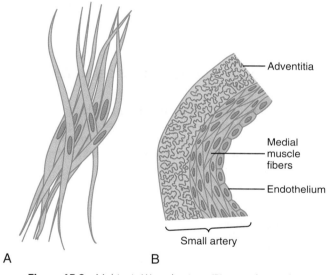

A   B

Figure 65-3   Multiunit (A) and unitary (B) smooth muscle.

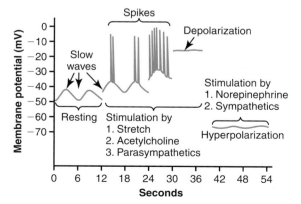

Figure 65-4   Membrane potentials in intestinal smooth muscle. Note the slow waves, the spike potentials, total depolarization, and hyperpolarization, all of which occur under different physiological conditions of the intestine.

channels. These channels are much slower to open and close than are the rapid sodium channels of large nerve fibers, therefore increasing the duration of the action potentials. Also, the movement of large amounts of calcium ions to the interior of the muscle fiber during the action potential plays a special role in causing the intestinal muscle fibers to contract, as we discuss shortly.

Changes in Voltage of the Resting Membrane Potential. In addition to the slow waves and spike potentials, the baseline voltage level of the smooth muscle RMP can also change. Under normal conditions, the RMP averages about -56 mV, but multiple factors can change this level. When the potential becomes less negative, which is called *depolarization* of the membrane, the muscle fibers become more excitable. When the potential becomes more negative, which is called *hyperpolarization*, the fibers become less excitable.

Factors that depolarize the membrane—making it more excitable—are as follows: (1) *stretching* of the muscle, (2) stimulation by *acetylcholine* released from the endings of *parasympathetic nerves*, and (3) stimulation by several *specific gastrointestinal hormones*.

Important factors that make the membrane potential more negative—that is, that hyperpolarize the membrane and make it less excitable—are as follows: (1) the effect of *norepinephrine* or *epinephrine* on the fiber membrane and (2) stimulation of the sympathetic nerves that secrete mainly norepinephrine at their endings.

Entry of Calcium Ions Causes Smooth Muscle Contraction. Smooth muscle contraction occurs in response to entry of calcium ions into the muscle fiber. These calcium ions, acting through a calmodulin control mechanism, activate the myosin filaments in the fiber, causing attractive forces to develop between the myosin filaments and the actin filaments, thereby causing the muscle to contract.

The slow waves do not cause calcium ions to enter the smooth muscle fiber (they cause only entry of sodium ions). Therefore, the slow waves by themselves do not usually cause muscle contraction; however, it is only during the spike potentials that significant quantities of calcium ions do enter the fibers and cause most of the contraction.

Table 65-1 gives the comparison of smooth, skeletal, and cardiac muscles.

Neural Control of Gastrointestinal Function—Enteric Nervous System

The gastrointestinal tract has a nervous system, all its own, called the *enteric nervous system*. It lies entirely in the wall of the gut, beginning in the esophagus and extending all the way to the anus. The number of neurons in this enteric system is about 100 million, nearly equal to the number in the entire spinal cord. This highly developed enteric nervous system is especially important in controlling gastrointestinal movements and secretion.

The enteric nervous system is composed mainly of two plexuses, shown in Figure 65-5:

1. an outer plexus lying between the longitudinal and circular muscle layers, called the *myenteric plexus* or *Auerbach plexus*;

TABLE 65-1	Comparison of Smooth, Skeletal, and Cardiac Muscles		
Features	Smooth Muscle	Skeletal Muscle	Cardiac Muscle
Shape of muscle fiber	Fusiform	Cylindrical	Branched
Attached to bone	No	Yes	No
Mitochondria	Less	Few	Many
Syncytium	Syncytium seen in single-unit smooth muscle	None	Contracts as a syncytium
Sarcotubular system	Poorly developed	Well developed	Moderately developed
Contraction speed	Very slow	Fast	Slow
Electrical spread between fibers	Possible through gap junctions	Absent	Possible through intercalated discs and gap junctions
Resting membrane potential (mV)	−50	−80	−90
Refractory period	Long	Short	Long

2. an inner plexus called the *submucosal plexus* or *Meissner plexus*, which lies in the submucosa.

The nervous connections within and between these two plexuses are also shown in Figure 65-5.

The myenteric plexus controls mainly the gastrointestinal movements, and the submucosal plexus controls mainly gastrointestinal secretion and local blood flow.

In Figure 65-5, note especially the extrinsic sympathetic and parasympathetic fibers that connect to both the myenteric and submucosal plexuses. Although the enteric nervous system can function independently of these extrinsic nerves, stimulation by the parasympathetic and sympathetic systems can greatly enhance or inhibit gastrointestinal functions, as we discuss later.

Also shown in Figure 65-5 are sensory nerve endings that originate in the gastrointestinal epithelium or gut wall and send afferent fibers to both plexuses of the enteric system, as well as

(1) to the prevertebral ganglia of the sympathetic nervous system, (2) to the spinal cord, and (3) in the vagus nerves all the way to the brainstem. These sensory nerves can elicit local reflexes within the gut wall itself and still other reflexes that are relayed to the gut from either the prevertebral ganglia or the basal regions of the brain.

Differences between the myenteric and submucosal plexuses have been given in Table 65-2.

TYPES OF NEUROTRANSMITTERS SECRETED BY ENTERIC NEURONS

In an attempt to understand better the multiple functions of the gastrointestinal enteric nervous system, researchers have identified a dozen or more different neurotransmitter substances that are released by the nerve endings of different types of enteric neurons. These are given in Box 65-1.

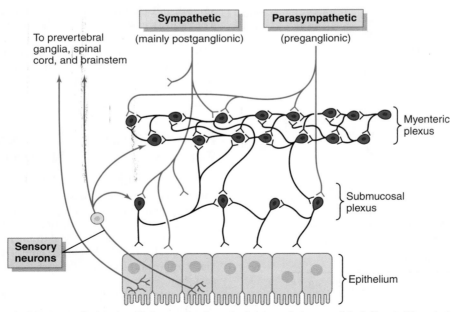

Figure 65-5 Neural control of the gut wall, showing (1) the myenteric and submucosal plexuses (*black fibers*); (2) extrinsic control of these plexuses by the sympathetic and parasympathetic nervous systems (*red fibers*); and (3) sensory fibers passing from the luminal epithelium and gut wall to the enteric plexuses, and then to the prevertebral ganglia of the spinal cord and directly to the spinal cord and brainstem (*green fibers*).

TABLE 65-2	Differences Between the Myenteric and Submucosal Plexuses	
Myenteric Plexus		**Submucosal Plexus**
1	It is concerned mainly with controlling muscle activity along the length of the gut with specific effects: a. Increased "tone" of the gut wall b. Increased intensity of the rhythmic contractions c. Slightly increased rate of the rhythm of contraction d. Increased velocity of conduction of excitatory waves along the gut wall, causing more rapid movement of the gut peristaltic waves	It is mainly concerned with controlling function within the inner wall of each minute segment of the intestine such as: a. Local *intestinal secretion* b. Local *absorption* c. Local *contraction of the submucosal muscle*
2	Composed of excitatory as well as inhibitory neurons Inhibitory neurons are useful for inhibiting some of the intestinal sphincter muscles such as *pyloric sphincter* and the *sphincter of the ileocecal valve*	Composed mainly of excitatory neurons

Autonomic Control of the Gastrointestinal Tract

Parasympathetic Stimulation Increases Activity of the Enteric Nervous System. The parasympathetic supply to the gut is divided into *cranial* and *sacral divisions*, which are discussed in Chapter 119.

Except for a few parasympathetic fibers to the mouth and pharyngeal regions of the alimentary tract, the *cranial parasympathetic* nerve fibers are almost entirely in the *vagus nerves*. These fibers provide extensive innervation to the esophagus, stomach, and pancreas, and somewhat less to the intestines down through the first half of the large intestine.

The *sacral parasympathetics* originate in the second, third, and fourth sacral segments of the spinal cord and pass through the *pelvic nerves* to the distal half of the large intestine and all the way to the anus. The sigmoidal, rectal, and anal regions are considerably better supplied with parasympathetic fibers than are the other intestinal areas. These fibers function especially to execute the defecation reflexes, as discussed in Chapter 74.

The *postganglionic neurons* of the gastrointestinal parasympathetic system are located mainly in the myenteric and submucosal plexuses. Stimulation of these parasympathetic nerves causes general increase in activity of the entire enteric nervous system, which in turn enhances activity of most gastrointestinal functions.

BOX 65-1	DIFFERENT TYPES OF NEUROTRANSMITTERS SECRETED BY ENTERIC NEURONS

1. Acetylcholine
2. Norepinephrine
3. Adenosine triphosphate
4. Serotonin
5. Dopamine
6. Cholecystokinin
7. Substance P
8. Vasoactive intestinal polypeptide
9. Somatostatin
10. Leu-enkephalin
11. Met-enkephalin
12. Bombesin

The specific functions of many of these are not known well enough to justify discussion here, other than to point out the following.

Acetylcholine most often excites gastrointestinal activity. *Norepinephrine* and *epinephrine* almost always inhibit gastrointestinal activity.

Sympathetic Stimulation Usually Inhibits Gastrointestinal Tract Activity. The sympathetic fibers to the gastrointestinal tract originate in the spinal cord between segments T5 and L2. Most of the preganglionic fibers that innervate the gut, after leaving the cord, enter the *sympathetic chains* that lie lateral to the spinal column, and many of these fibers then pass on through the chains to outlying ganglia such as to the *celiac ganglion* and various *mesenteric ganglia*. Most of the *postganglionic sympathetic neuron bodies* are in these ganglia, and postganglionic fibers then spread through postganglionic sympathetic nerves to all parts of the gut. The sympathetics innervate essentially all of the gastrointestinal tract, rather than being more extensive nearest the oral cavity and anus, as is true of the parasympathetics. The sympathetic nerve endings not only secrete mainly *norepinephrine*. In general, stimulation of the sympathetic nervous system *inhibits* activity of the gastrointestinal tract, causing many effects opposite to those of the parasympathetic system. It exerts its effects in two ways: (1) to a slight extent by direct effect of secreted norepinephrine to inhibit intestinal tract smooth muscle (except the mucosal muscle, which it excites) and (2) to a major extent by an inhibitory effect of norepinephrine on the neurons of the entire enteric nervous system.

Strong stimulation of the sympathetic system can inhibit motor movements of the gut so greatly that this can literally block movement of food through the gastrointestinal tract.

Afferent Sensory Nerve Fibers from the Gut

Many afferent sensory nerve fibers innervate the gut. Some of the nerve fibers have their cell bodies in the enteric nervous system and some have them in the dorsal root ganglia of the spinal cord. These sensory nerves can be stimulated by (1) irritation of the gut mucosa, (2) excessive distention of the gut, or (3) the presence of specific chemical substances in the gut. Signals transmitted through the fibers can then cause *excitation* or, under other conditions, *inhibition* of intestinal movements or intestinal secretion.

In addition, other sensory signals from the gut go all the way to multiple areas of the spinal cord and even the brainstem. For example, 80% of the nerve fibers in the vagus nerves are afferent rather than efferent. These afferent fibers transmit sensory signals from the gastrointestinal tract into the brain medulla, which in turn initiates vagal reflex signals that return to the gastrointestinal tract to control many of its functions.

Gastrointestinal Blood Flow— "Splanchnic Circulation"

The blood vessels of the gastrointestinal system are part of a more extensive system called the *splanchnic circulation* (see Figure 48-1). It includes the blood flow through the gut itself plus blood flows through the spleen, pancreas, and liver. This has been explained in Chapter 48; please refer to this chapter for more details.

BIBLIOGRAPHY

Adelson DW, Million M: Tracking the moveable feast: sonomicrometry and gastrointestinal motility, *News Physiol. Sci.* 19:27, 2004.

Brookes SJ, Spencer NJ, Costa M, Zagorodnyuk VP: Extrinsic primary afferent signalling in the gut, *Nat. Rev. Gastroenterol. Hepatol.* 10:286, 2013.

Campbell JE, Drucker DJ: Pharmacology, physiology, and mechanisms of incretin hormone action, *Cell Metab.* 17:819, 2013.

Côté CD, Zadeh-Tahmasebi M, Rasmussen BA, et al: Hormonal signaling in the gut, *J. Biol. Chem.* 289:11642, 2014.

Dimaline R, Varro A: Novel roles of gastrin, *J. Physiol.* 592:2951, 2014.

Furness JB: The enteric nervous system and neurogastroenterology, *Nat. Rev. Gastroenterol. Hepatol.* 9:286, 2012.

Huizinga JD, Lammers WJ: Gut peristalsis is governed by a multitude of cooperating mechanisms, *Am. J. Physiol. Gastrointest. Liver Physiol.* 296:G1, 2009.

Knowles CH, Lindberg G, Panza E, De Giorgio R: New perspectives in the diagnosis and management of enteric neuropathies, *Nat. Rev. Gastroenterol. Hepatol.* 10:206, 2013.

Lake JI, Heuckeroth RO: Enteric nervous system development: migration, differentiation, and disease, *Am. J. Physiol. Gastrointest. Liver Physiol.* 305:G1, 2013.

Lammers WJ, Slack JR: Of slow waves and spike patches, *News Physiol. Sci.* 16:138, 2001.

Neunlist M, Schemann M: Nutrient-induced changes in the phenotype and function of the enteric nervous system, *J. Physiol.* 592:2959, 2014.

Obermayr F, Hotta R, Enomoto H, Young HM: Development and developmental disorders of the enteric nervous system, *Nat. Rev. Gastroenterol. Hepatol.* 10:43, 2013.

Powley TL, Phillips RJ: Musings on the wanderer: what's new in our understanding of vago-vagal reflexes? I. Morphology and topography of vagal afferents innervating the GI tract, *Am. J. Physiol. Gastrointest. Liver Physiol.* 283:G1217, 2002.

Sanders KM, Koh SD, Ro S, Ward SM: Regulation of gastrointestinal motility—insights from smooth muscle biology, *Nat. Rev. Gastroenterol. Hepatol.* 9:633, 2012.

Sanders KM, Ward SM, Koh SD: Interstitial cells: regulators of smooth muscle function, *Physiol. Rev.* 94:859, 2014.

Vanden Berghe P, Tack J, Boesmans W: Highlighting synaptic communication in the enteric nervous system, *Gastroenterology* 135:20, 2008.

66

Salivary Glands and Secretion

LEARNING OBJECTIVES

- List the general principles of alimentary tract secretion.
- List the different salivary glands.
- Describe the composition of saliva.
- Describe the mechanism of secretion of saliva.
- List the functions of saliva.
- Outline the regulatory processes involved in the secretion of saliva.

GLOSSARY OF TERMS

- **Acini:** The plural of "acinus," which refers to small sac-like dilations composing a compound gland

- **Enzymes:** Several complex proteins that are produced by cells and act as catalysts in specific biochemical reactions

- **Mucus:** A thick secretion composed mainly of water, electrolytes, and a mixture of several glycoproteins, which themselves are composed of large polysaccharides bound with much smaller quantities of protein

- **Ptyalin:** A form of amylase (enzyme) found in the saliva of humans and some other animals (this enzyme helps catalyze the hydrolysis of starch into maltose and dextrin)

- **Tactile stimulation:** Stimulation of cells or tissues by the sense of touch

Throughout the gastrointestinal tract, secretory glands subserve two primary functions:

1. *Digestive enzymes* are secreted in most areas of the alimentary tract, from the mouth to the distal end of the ileum.
2. Mucous glands, from the mouth to the anus, provide *mucus* for lubrication and protection of all parts of the alimentary tract.

Most digestive secretions are formed only in response to the presence of food in the alimentary tract, and the quantity secreted in each segment of the tract is usually the precise amount needed for proper digestion. Furthermore, in some portions of the gastrointestinal tract, even the *types of enzymes* and other constituents of the secretions are varied in accordance with the types of food present.

General Principles of Alimentary Tract Secretion

TYPES OF ALIMENTARY TRACT GLANDS

Several types of glands provide the different types of alimentary tract secretions, which are discussed in Table 66-1.

BASIC MECHANISMS OF STIMULATION OF THE ALIMENTARY TRACT GLANDS

Contact of Food with the Epithelium Stimulates Secretion—Function of Enteric Nervous Stimuli. The presence of food in a particular segment of the gastrointestinal tract usually stimulates the glands of that region and adjacent regions to secrete moderate to large quantities of juices. In addition, local epithelial stimulation also activates the *enteric nervous system* of the gut wall. The types of stimuli that activate this system are as follows:

- tactile stimulation;
- chemical irritation;
- distention of the gut wall.

The resulting nervous reflexes stimulate both the mucous cells on the gut epithelial surface and the deep glands in the gut wall to increase their secretion.

Autonomic Stimulation of Secretion

Parasympathetic Stimulation Increases the Alimentary Tract Glandular Secretion Rate. Stimulation of the parasympathetic nerves to the alimentary tract almost invariably increases the rates of alimentary glandular secretion. This increased secretion rate is especially true of the glands such as the salivary glands, esophageal glands, gastric glands, pancreas, and Brunner glands in the duodenum. It is also true of some glands in the distal portion of the large intestine, which are innervated by pelvic parasympathetic nerves.

Sympathetic Stimulation Has a Dual Effect on the Alimentary Tract Glandular Secretion Rate. Sympathetic stimulation can have a dual effect on secretion:

1. Sympathetic stimulation alone usually slightly increases secretion.
2. If parasympathetic or hormonal stimulation is already causing copious secretion by the glands, superimposed sympathetic stimulation usually reduces the secretion, sometimes significantly so, mainly because of vasoconstrictive reduction of the blood supply to the glands.

Regulation of Glandular Secretion by Hormones. In the stomach and intestine, several different *gastrointestinal hormones* help regulate the volume and character of the secretions. These hormones are chemically polypeptides or polypeptide derivatives, and are liberated from the gastrointestinal mucosa in response to the presence of food in the lumen of the gut. The hormones are then absorbed into the blood and carried to the glands, where they stimulate secretion. This type of stimulation is particularly valuable to increase the output of gastric juice and pancreatic juice when food enters the stomach or duodenum.

BASIC MECHANISM OF SECRETION BY GLANDULAR CELLS

Secretion of Organic Substances. Although all the basic mechanisms by which glandular cells function are not known,

TABLE 66-1	Anatomical Types of Glands in the Alimentary Tract and their Functions	
Anatomical Types of Glands		**Description and Functions**
1	*Single-cell mucous glands* called simply *mucous cells* or sometimes *goblet cells*, located on the surface epithelium in most parts of the gastrointestinal tract	They function mainly in response to local irritation of the epithelium. They extrude *mucus* directly onto the epithelial surface to act as a lubricant that also protects the surfaces from excoriation and digestion
2	Invaginations of the epithelium into the submucosa called *pits*, located on many surface areas of the gastrointestinal tract	In the small intestine, these pits, called *crypts of Lieberkühn*, are deep and contain specialized secretory cells (Figure 66-1)
3	Deep *tubular glands* in the stomach and upper duodenum	A typical tubular gland can be seen in Figure 67-1, which shows an acid- and pepsinogen-secreting gland of the stomach (oxyntic gland)
4	Complex glands such as the *salivary glands*, *pancreas*, and *liver*	These glands lie outside the walls of the alimentary tract and, in this, differ from all other alimentary glands. They contain millions of *acini* lined with secreting glandular cells; these acini feed into a system of ducts that finally empty into the alimentary tract itself

experimental evidence points to the following principles of secretion, as shown in Figure 66-1:

1. The nutrient material needed for formation of the secretion must first diffuse or be actively transported by the blood in the capillaries into the base of the glandular cell.
2. Many *mitochondria* located inside the glandular cell near its base use oxidative energy to form adenosine triphosphate (ATP).
3. Energy from the ATP, along with appropriate substrates provided by the nutrients, is then used to synthesize the organic secretory substances; this synthesis occurs almost entirely in the *endoplasmic reticulum* and *Golgi complex* of the glandular cell. *Ribosomes* adherent to the reticulum are specifically responsible for formation of the proteins that are secreted.
4. The secretory materials are transported through the tubules of the endoplasmic reticulum, passing in about 20 minutes all the way to the vesicles of the Golgi complex.
5. In the Golgi complex, the materials are modified, added to, concentrated, and discharged into the cytoplasm in the form of *secretory vesicles*, which are stored in the apical ends of the secretory cells.
6. These vesicles remain stored until nervous or hormonal control signals cause the cells to extrude the vesicular

contents through the cells' surface. This action probably occurs in the following way: The hormone binds to its receptor and, through one of several possible cell signaling mechanisms, *increases the cell membrane permeability to calcium ions*. Calcium enters the cell and causes many of the vesicles to fuse with the apical cell membrane. The apical cell membrane then breaks open, thus emptying the vesicles to the exterior; this process is called *exocytosis*.

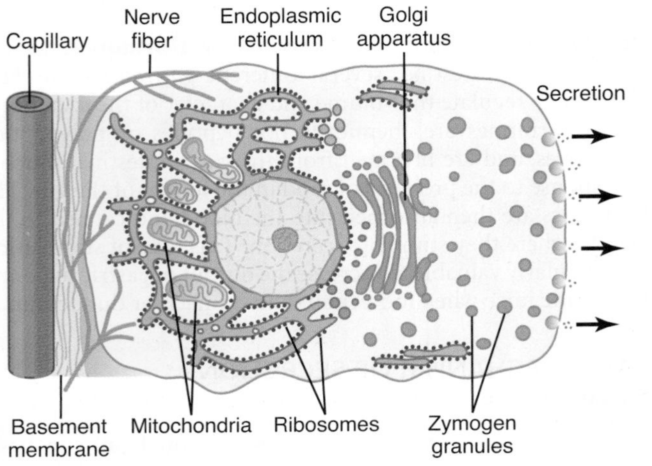

Water and Electrolyte Secretion. A second necessity for glandular secretion is secretion of sufficient water and electrolytes to go along with the organic substances. Secretion by the salivary glands, discussed in more detail later, provides an example of how nervous stimulation causes water and salts to pass through the glandular cells in great profusion, washing the organic substances through the secretory border of the cells at the same time. It is believed that hormones acting on the cell membrane of some glandular cells also cause secretory effects similar to those caused by nervous stimulation.

LUBRICATING AND PROTECTIVE PROPERTIES OF MUCUS, AND THE IMPORTANCE OF MUCUS IN THE GASTROINTESTINAL TRACT

Mucus is a thick secretion composed mainly of water, electrolytes, and a mixture of several glycoproteins that are composed of large polysaccharides bound with much smaller quantities of protein. Mucus is slightly different in different parts of the gastrointestinal tract, but in all locations it has several important characteristics that make it both an excellent lubricant and a protectant for the wall of the gut.

Properties of Mucus in the Gastrointestinal Tract

1. Mucus has adherent qualities that make it adhere tightly to the food or other particles and to spread as a thin film over the surfaces
2. It has sufficient *body* that it coats the wall of the gut and prevents actual contact of most food particles with the mucosa
3. Mucus has a low resistance for slippage, so the particles can slide along the epithelium with great ease
4. Mucus causes fecal particles to adhere to one another to form the feces
5. Mucus is strongly resistant to digestion by the gastrointestinal enzymes

Figure 66-1 Typical function of a glandular cell for formation and secretion of enzymes and other secretory substances.

Properties of Mucus in the Gastrointestinal Tract

6   The glycoproteins of mucus have amphoteric properties, which mean that they are capable of buffering small amounts of either acids or alkalies; also, mucus often contains moderate quantities of bicarbonate ions, which specifically neutralize acids

Thus, mucus has the ability to allow easy slippage of food along the gastrointestinal tract and to prevent excoriative or chemical damage to the epithelium.

Secretion of Saliva

SALIVARY GLANDS AND SECRETIONS

The principal glands of salivation are the *parotid, submandibular,* and *sublingual glands*; in addition, there are many tiny *buccal, labial,* and *glossopalatine* glands (see Figure 66-2).

Daily secretion of saliva normally ranges between 800 and 1500 mL, as shown by the average value of 1000 mL in Table 66-2.

Saliva contains two major types of protein secretion:
1. *serous secretion* that contains *ptyalin* (an α-amylase), which is an enzyme for digesting starches;
2. *mucus secretion* that contains *mucin* for lubricating and for surface protective purposes.

The parotid glands secrete almost entirely the serous type of secretion, whereas the submandibular and sublingual glands secrete both serous secretion and mucus. The buccal, labial, and glossopalatine glands secrete only mucus. Saliva has a pH between 6.0 and 7.0, which is a favorable range for the digestive action of ptyalin.

COMPOSITION OF SALIVA

Saliva contains especially large quantities of potassium and bicarbonate ions. Conversely, the concentrations of both sodium and chloride ions are several times less in saliva than in plasma.

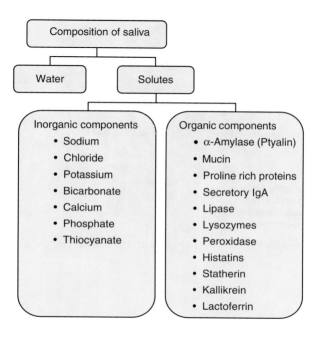

One can understand these special concentrations of ions in the saliva from the following description of the mechanism of secretion of saliva.

MECHANISM OF SECRETION OF SALIVA

Figure 66-3 shows secretion by the submandibular gland, a typical compound gland that contains *acini* and *salivary ducts*. Salivary secretion is a two-stage operation: The first stage involves the acini, and the second stage involves the salivary ducts. The acini secrete a *primary secretion* that contains ptyalin and/or mucin in a solution of ions with concentrations not greatly different from those of typical extracellular fluid. As the primary secretion flows through the ducts, two major active transport processes take place that markedly modify the ionic composition of the fluid in the saliva.

First, *sodium ions* are actively reabsorbed from all the salivary ducts and *potassium ions* are actively secreted in exchange for the sodium. Therefore, the sodium ion concentration of the saliva becomes greatly reduced, whereas the potassium ion concentration becomes increased. However, there is excess sodium reabsorption compared with potassium secretion, which creates electrical negativity of about −70 mV in the salivary ducts; this negativity in turn causes chloride ions to be reabsorbed passively. Therefore, the chloride ion concentration in the salivary fluid falls to a very low level, matching the ductal decrease in sodium ion concentration.

Second, *bicarbonate ions* are secreted by the ductal epithelium into the lumen of the duct. This secretion is at least partly caused by the passive exchange of bicarbonate for chloride ions, but it may also result partly from an active secretory process.

The net result of these transport processes is that *under resting conditions*, the concentrations of sodium and chloride ions in the saliva are only about 15 mEq/L each, about one-seventh to one-tenth their concentrations in plasma. Conversely, the concentration of potassium ions is about 30 mEq/L, seven times as great as in plasma, and the concentration of bicarbonate ions is from 50 to 70 mEq/L, about two to three times that of plasma.

During maximal salivation, the salivary ionic concentrations change considerably because the rate of formation of primary secretion by the acini can increase as much as 20-fold. This acinar secretion then flows through the ducts so rapidly that the ductal reconditioning of the secretion is considerably reduced. Therefore, when copious quantities of saliva are being secreted, the sodium chloride concentration is about one-half or two-thirds that of plasma, and the potassium concentration rises to only four times that of plasma.

FUNCTION OF SALIVA

Under basal awake conditions, about 0.5 mL of saliva, almost entirely of the mucous type, is secreted each minute, but little secretion occurs during sleep (Box 66-1).

Function of Saliva for Oral Hygiene

This secretion plays an exceedingly important role for maintaining healthy oral tissues. The mouth is loaded with pathogenic bacteria that can easily destroy tissues and cause dental caries. Saliva helps prevent the deteriorative processes in several ways:
1. The flow of saliva helps wash away pathogenic bacteria as well as food particles that provide their metabolic support.

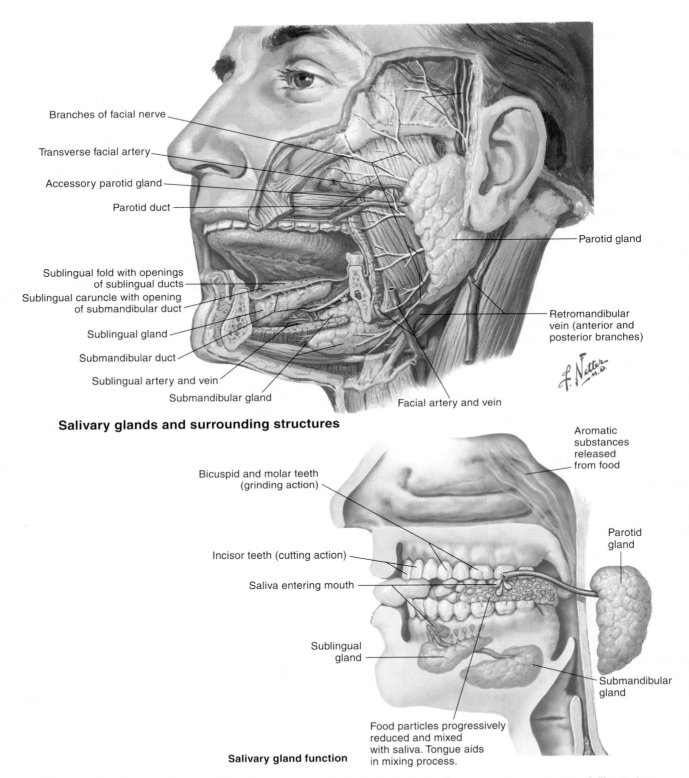

Branches of facial nerve

Transverse facial artery

Accessory parotid gland

Parotid duct

Sublingual fold with openings of sublingual ducts

Sublingual caruncle with opening of submandibular duct

Sublingual gland

Submandibular duct

Sublingual artery and vein

Submandibular gland

Parotid gland

Retromandibular vein (anterior and posterior branches)

Facial artery and vein

Salivary glands and surrounding structures

Bicuspid and molar teeth (grinding action)

Incisor teeth (cutting action)

Saliva entering mouth

Sublingual gland

Aromatic substances released from food

Parotid gland

Submandibular gland

Food particles progressively reduced and mixed with saliva. Tongue aids in mixing process.

Salivary gland function

Figure 66-2 Different salivary glands in relation to the oral cavity. *Netter illustration from www.netterimages.com. © Elsevier Inc. All rights reserved.*

TABLE 66-2	Daily Secretion of Intestinal Juices	
	Daily Volume (mL)	pH
Saliva	1000	6.0–7.0
Gastric secretion	1500	1.0–3.5
Pancreatic secretion	1000	8.0–8.3
Bile	1000	7.8
Small intestine secretion	1800	7.5–8.0
Brunner's gland secretion	200	8.0–8.9
Large intestinal secretion	200	7.5–8.0
Total	6700	

2. Saliva contains several factors that destroy bacteria. One of these is *thiocyanate ions* and another is several *proteolytic enzymes*—most important, *lysozyme*—that (a) attack the bacteria, (b) aid the thiocyanate ions in entering the bacteria where these ions in turn become bactericidal, and (c) digest food particles, thus helping further to remove the bacterial metabolic support.
3. Saliva often contains significant amounts of antibodies that can destroy oral bacteria, including some that cause dental caries. In the absence of salivation, oral tissues often become ulcerated and otherwise infected, and caries of the teeth can become rampant.

NERVOUS REGULATION OF SALIVARY SECRETION

Figure 66-4 shows the parasympathetic nervous pathways for regulating salivation, and demonstrates that the salivary glands are controlled mainly by *parasympathetic nervous signals* all the way from the *superior* and *inferior salivatory nuclei* in the brainstem.

The salivatory nuclei are located approximately at the juncture of the medulla and pons, and are excited by both taste and tactile stimuli from the tongue and other areas of the mouth and pharynx. Many taste stimuli, especially the sour taste (caused by acids), elicit copious secretion of saliva—often 8–20 times the basal rate of secretion. Also, certain tactile stimuli, such as the presence of smooth objects in the mouth (eg, a pebble), cause

marked salivation, whereas rough objects cause less salivation and occasionally even inhibit salivation.

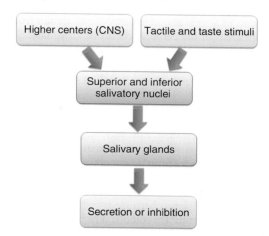

Salivation can also be stimulated or inhibited by nervous signals arriving in the salivatory nuclei from higher centers of the central nervous system. For instance, when a person smells or eats favorite foods, salivation is greater than when food that

BOX 66-1 FUNCTIONS OF SALIVA

1. Defense:
   a. Antibacterial
   b. Antifungal
   c. Antiviral
   d. Immunological
2. Digestive functions:
   a. Digestive enzymes—ptyalin, lipase
   b. Formation of bolus
   c. Taste
3. Protective function:
   a. Protective coating for soft tissues
   b. Protective coating for hard tissues—teeth
4. Lubrication function:
   a. Keeps the oral cavity moist
   b. Facilitates speech
   c. Helps in mastication and swallowing
5. Buffering function

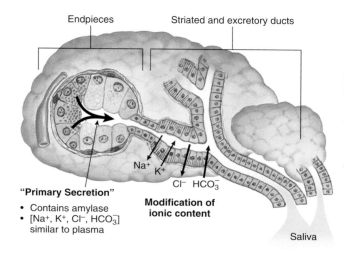

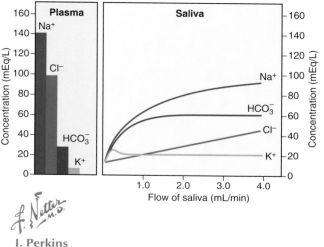

Figure 66-3 Formation and secretion of saliva by a submandibular salivary gland. *From Netter's Essential Physiology, 2009, Figure 23-3, p. 274.*

is disliked is smelled or eaten. The *appetite area* of the brain, which partially regulates these effects, is located in proximity to the parasympathetic centers of the anterior hypothalamus, and it functions to a great extent in response to signals from the taste and smell areas of the cerebral cortex or amygdala.

Salivation also occurs in response to reflexes originating in the stomach and upper small intestines—particularly when irritating foods are swallowed or when a person is nauseated because of some gastrointestinal abnormality. The saliva, when swallowed, helps to remove the irritating factor in the gastrointestinal tract by diluting or neutralizing the irritant substances.

Sympathetic stimulation can also increase salivation a slight amount, much less so than parasympathetic stimulation. The sympathetic nerves originate from the superior cervical ganglia and travel along the surfaces of the blood vessel walls to the salivary glands.

A secondary factor that also affects salivary secretion is the *blood supply to the glands* because secretion always requires adequate nutrients from the blood. The parasympathetic nerve signals that induce copious salivation also moderately dilate the blood vessels. In addition, salivation directly dilates the blood vessels, thus providing increased salivatory gland nutrition as needed by the secreting cells. Part of this additional vasodilator effect is caused by *kallikrein* secreted by the activated salivary cells, which in turn acts as an enzyme to split one of the blood proteins, an alpha-2-globulin, to form *bradykinin*, a strong vasodilator.

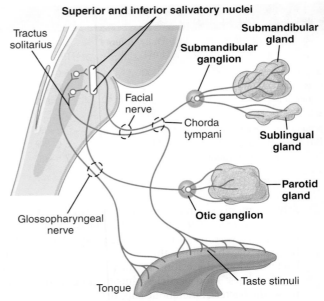

Figure 66-4   Parasympathetic nervous regulation of salivary secretion.

BIBLIOGRAPHY

Bhattacharyya A, Chattopadhyay R, Mitra S, Crowe SE: Oxidative stress: an essential factor in the pathogenesis of gastrointestinal mucosal diseases, *Physiol. Rev.* 94:329, 2014.

de Almeida Pdel V, Grégio AM, Machado MA, et al: Saliva composition and functions: a comprehensive review, *J. Contemp. Dent. Pract.* 9(3):72, 2008.

Dockray GJ: Enteroendocrine cell signalling via the vagus nerve, *Curr. Opin. Pharmacol.* 13:954, 2013.

Heitzmann D, Warth R: Physiology and pathophysiology of potassium channels in gastrointestinal epithelia, *Physiol. Rev.* 88:1119, 2008.

Humphrey SP, Williamson RT: A review of saliva: normal composition, flow, and function, *J. Prosthet. Dent.* 85(2):162, 2001.

Lee MG, Ohana E, Park HW, et al: Molecular mechanism of pancreatic and salivary gland fluid and HCO_3^- secretion, *Physiol. Rev.* 92:39, 2012.

Mandel ID: The functions of saliva, *J. Dent. Res.* 66:623, 1987.

Veerman EC, van den Keybus PA, Vissink A, et al: Human glandular salivas: their separate collection and analysis, *Eur. J. Oral Sci.* 104:346, 1996.

67

Gastric Secretions

LEARNING OBJECTIVES

- List the different types of gastric glands and indicate their secretions.
- List the composition of gastric juice.
- Outline the steps involved in the formation of gastric acid.
- Describe the regulation of gastric acid secretion.
- List the different phases of gastric acid secretion and factors influencing them.
- Outline the basis of the various forms of treatment for acid peptic disease.

GLOSSARY OF TERMS

- **Gastrin:** A hormone secreted by *gastrin cells*, also called *G cells*, and can increase the secretion of gastric acid and influence gastrointestinal motility

- **Histamine:** A substance secreted by *enterochromaffin-like cells* (ECL cells) in the gastric mucosa and increases the secretion of HCl

- **Intrinsic factor:** A substance essential for absorption of vitamin B_{12} in the ileum (it is secreted by the *parietal cells* along with the secretion of hydrochloric acid)

- **Oxyntic glands:** Tubular glands located on the surface of the body and fundus of the stomach [the oxyntic (acid-forming) glands secrete *hydrochloric acid, pepsinogen, intrinsic factor*, and *mucus*]

- **Pepsinogen:** The precursor of the enzyme *pepsin*, causes protein digestion

- **Pyloric glands:** Located in the antral portion of the stomach and mainly secrete mucus and the hormone gastrin

Esophageal Secretion

Esophageal secretions are entirely mucous and mainly provide lubrication for swallowing. The main body of the esophagus is lined with many *simple mucous glands*. At the gastric end, and to a lesser extent in the initial portion of the esophagus, many *compound mucous glands* can also be found. The mucus secreted by the compound glands in the upper esophagus prevents mucosal excoriation by newly entering food, whereas the compound glands located near the esophagogastric junction protect the esophageal wall from digestion by acidic gastric juices that often reflux from the stomach back into the lower esophagus. Despite this protection, a peptic ulcer at times can still occur at the gastric end of the esophagus.

Gastric Secretion

TYPES OF GLANDS AND CHARACTERISTICS OF THEIR SECRETIONS

In addition to mucus-secreting cells that line the entire surface of the stomach, the stomach mucosa has two important types of tubular glands (Figure 67-1):

1. *the oxyntic glands* (also called *gastric* glands)
2. *the pyloric glands*

OXYNTIC GLANDS

The oxyntic (acid-forming) glands secrete *hydrochloric acid, pepsinogen, intrinsic factor*, and *mucus*.

The oxyntic glands are located on the inside surfaces of the body and fundus of the stomach, the proximal 80% of the stomach.

Secretions from the Oxyntic (Gastric) Glands

A typical stomach oxyntic gland is shown in Figure 67-2. It is composed of three types of cells:

1. *mucous neck cells*, which secrete mainly *mucus*;
2. *peptic* (or *chief*) cells, which secrete large quantities of *pepsinogen*;
3. *parietal* (or *oxyntic*) *cells*, which secrete *hydrochloric acid* and *intrinsic factor*.

Secretion of hydrochloric acid by the parietal cells involves special mechanisms, which are described later.

PYLORIC GLANDS

The pyloric glands secrete mainly *mucus* for protection of the pyloric mucosa from the stomach acid. They also secrete the hormone *gastrin*. The pyloric glands are located in the antral portion of the stomach, the distal 20% of the stomach.

Secretions from the Pyloric Glands

The pyloric glands are structurally similar to the oxyntic glands but contain few peptic cells and almost no parietal cells. They are composed of three types of cells:

1. *mucous neck cells* that are identical with the mucous neck cells of the oxyntic glands, which secrete mainly thin *mucus* that helps to lubricate food movement;
2. *peptic* (or *chief*) cells, which secrete *pepsinogen*;
3. *G cells*, which secrete the hormone *gastrin*, which plays a key role in controlling gastric secretion, as we discuss shortly.

SURFACE MUCOUS CELLS

The entire surface of the stomach mucosa between glands has a continuous layer of a special type of mucous cells called simply

Gastric anatomy

Anatomic regions of stomach

Section of gastric wall

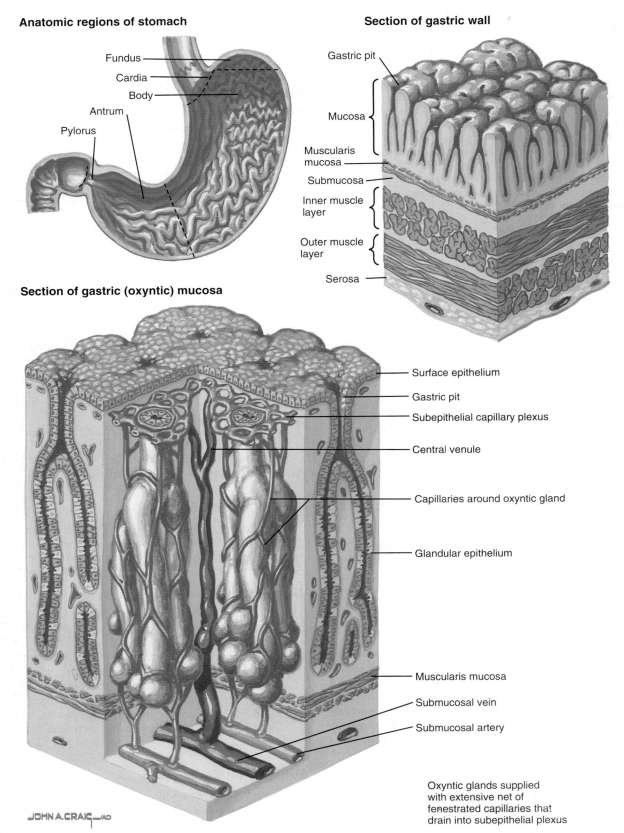

Fundus

Cardia

Body

Antrum

Pylorus

Gastric pit

Mucosa

Muscularis mucosa

Submucosa

Inner muscle layer

Outer muscle layer

Serosa

Section of gastric (oxyntic) mucosa

Surface epithelium

Gastric pit

Subepithelial capillary plexus

Central venule

Capillaries around oxyntic gland

Glandular epithelium

Muscularis mucosa

Submucosal vein

Submucosal artery

Oxyntic glands supplied with extensive net of fenestrated capillaries that drain into subepithelial plexus

JOHN A. CRAIG—AD

Figure 67-1 Functional anatomy of the stomach indicating the different layers of the stomach. *Netter illustration from www.netterimages.com.*

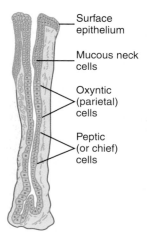

Figure 67-2 Oxyntic gland from the body of the stomach.

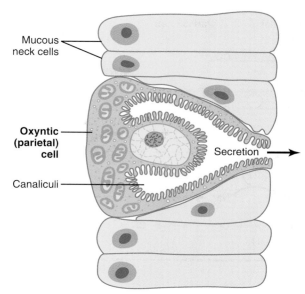

Figure 67-3 Schematic anatomy of the canaliculi in a parietal (oxyntic) cell.

"surface mucous cells." They secrete large quantities of *viscid mucus* that coats the stomach mucosa with a gel layer of mucus often more than 1 mm thick, thus providing a major shell of protection for the stomach wall, as well as contributing to lubrication of food transport.

Another characteristic of this mucus is that *it is alkaline.* Therefore, the *normal* underlying stomach wall is not directly exposed to the highly acidic, proteolytic stomach secretion. Even the slightest contact with food or any irritation of the mucosa directly stimulates the surface mucous cells to secrete additional quantities of this thick, alkaline, viscid mucus.

COMPOSITION OF GASTRIC JUICE

The amount of gastric juice that is secreted by an adult human is approximately about 1.5–2 L.

When a meal is consumed, it stimulates the release of gastric juice from the gastric glands, pyloric glands, and the surface mucous cells.

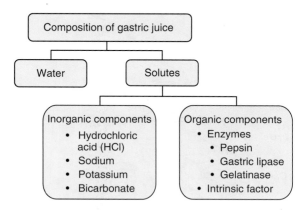

Basic Mechanism of Hydrochloric Acid Secretion. When stimulated, the parietal cells secrete an acid solution that contains about 160 mmol/L of hydrochloric acid, which is nearly isotonic with the body fluids. The pH of this acid is about 0.8, demonstrating its extreme acidity. At this pH, the hydrogen ion concentration is about 3 million times that of the arterial blood. To concentrate the hydrogen ions this tremendous amount requires more than 1500 cal of energy per

liter of gastric juice. At the same time that hydrogen ions are secreted, bicarbonate ions diffuse into the blood so that gastric venous blood has a higher pH than arterial blood when the stomach is secreting acid.

Figure 67-3 shows schematically the functional structure of a parietal cell (also called *oxyntic cell*) demonstrating that it contains large branching intracellular *canaliculi*. The hydrochloric acid is formed at the villus-like projections inside these canaliculi and is then conducted through the canaliculi to the secretory end of the cell.

The main driving force for hydrochloric acid secretion by the parietal cells is a *hydrogen–potassium pump* [H^+–K^+ *adenosine triphosphatase (ATPase)*]. The chemical mechanism of hydrochloric acid formation is shown in Figure 67-4 and consists of the following steps:

1. Water inside the parietal cell becomes dissociated into H^+ and hydroxide (OH^-) in the cell cytoplasm. The H^+ is then actively secreted into the canaliculus in exchange for K^+, an active exchange process that is catalyzed by H^+–K^+ ATPase.

2. Potassium ions transported into the cell by the Na^+–K^+ ATPase pump on the basolateral (extracellular) side of the membrane tend to leak into the lumen but are recycled back into the cell by the H^+–K^+ ATPase.

3. The basolateral Na^+–K^+ ATPase creates low intracellular Na^+, which contributes to Na^+ reabsorption from the lumen of the canaliculus. Thus, most of the K^+ and Na^+ in the canaliculus are reabsorbed into the cell cytoplasm, and hydrogen ions take their place in the canaliculus.

4. The pumping of H^+ out of the cell by the H^+–K^+ ATPase permits OH^- to accumulate and form bicarbonate (HCO_3^-) from CO_2, either formed during metabolism in the cell or while entering the cell from the blood. This reaction is catalyzed by *carbonic anhydrase.*

5. The HCO_3^- is then transported across the basolateral membrane into the extracellular fluid in exchange for chloride ions, which enter the cell and are secreted through chloride channels into the canaliculus, giving a strong solution

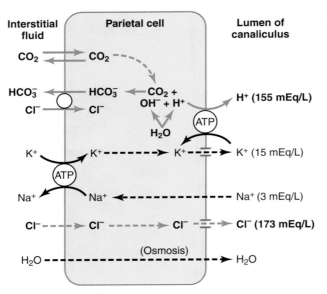

Figure 67-4   Postulated mechanism for secretion of hydrochloric acid. (The points labeled "ATP" indicate active pumps, and the *dashed lines* represent free diffusion and osmosis.)

of hydrochloric acid *in the canaliculus*. The hydrochloric acid is then secreted outward through the open end of the canaliculus into the lumen of the gland.

6. Water passes into the canaliculus by osmosis because of extra ions secreted into the canaliculus. Thus, the final secretion from the canaliculus contains water, hydrochloric acid at a concentration of about 150–160 mEq/L,

potassium chloride at a concentration of 15 mEq/L, and a small amount of sodium chloride.

To produce a concentration of hydrogen ions as great as that found in gastric juice requires minimal backleak into the mucosa of the secreted acid. A major part of the stomach's ability to prevent backleak of acid can be attributed to the *gastric barrier* due to the formation of alkaline mucus and to tight junctions between epithelia cells, as described later. If this barrier is damaged by toxic substances, such as occurs with excessive use of aspirin or alcohol, the secreted acid does leak down an electrochemical gradient into the mucosa, causing stomach mucosal damage.

REGULATION OF GASTRIC ACID SECRETIONS

The Basic Factors that Stimulate Gastric Secretion Are Acetylcholine, Gastrin, and Histamine. As noted earlier in the chapter, the acidity of the fluid secreted by the parietal cells of the oxyntic glands can be great, with pH as low as 0.8. However, secretion of this acid is under continuous control by both endocrine and nervous signals (Figure 67-5).

Stimulation of Acid Secretion by Acetylcholine

Acetylcholine released by parasympathetic stimulation excites secretion of pepsinogen by peptic cells, hydrochloric acid by parietal cells, and mucus by mucous cells. In comparison, both gastrin and histamine strongly stimulate secretion of acid by parietal cells but have little effect on the other cells.

Stimulation of Acid Secretion by Histamine

Furthermore, the parietal cells operate in close association with another type of cell called *enterochromaffin-like cells* (ECL cells), the primary function of which is to secrete *histamine*.

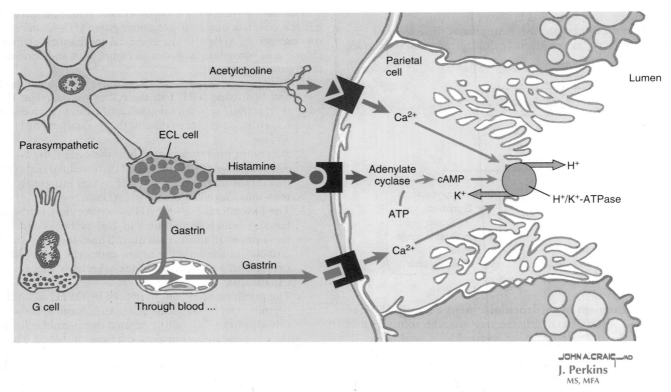

Figure 67-5   Functional summary of factors regulating gastric acid secretion. *ATP*, adenosine triphosphate; *cAMP*, cyclic adenosine monophosphate; *ECL cell*, enterochromaffin-like cell. *Netter illustration from www.netterimages.com.* © Elsevier Inc. All rights reserved.

The ECL cells lie in the deep recesses of the oxyntic glands and therefore release histamine in direct contact with the parietal cells of the glands. The rate of formation and secretion of hydrochloric acid by the parietal cells is directly related to the amount of histamine secreted by the ECL cells. In turn, the ECL cells are stimulated to secrete histamine by the hormone *gastrin*, which is formed almost entirely in the antral portion of the stomach mucosa in response to proteins in the foods being digested. The ECL cells may also be stimulated by hormones secreted by the enteric nervous system of the stomach wall. We will first discuss the gastrin mechanism for control of the ECL cells and their subsequent control of parietal cell secretion of hydrochloric acid.

Stimulation of Acid Secretion by Gastrin

Gastrin is itself a hormone secreted by *gastrin cells*, also called *G cells*. These cells are located in the *pyloric glands* in the distal end of the stomach. Gastrin is a large polypeptide secreted in two forms: a large form called G-34, which contains 34 amino acids, and a smaller form, G-17, which contains 17 amino acids. Although both of these forms are important, the smaller form is more abundant.

When meats or other foods containing protein reach the antral end of the stomach, some of the proteins from these foods have a special stimulatory effect on the *gastrin cells in the pyloric glands* to cause release of *gastrin* into the blood to be transported to the ECL cells of the stomach. The vigorous mixing of the gastric juices transports the gastrin rapidly to the ECL cells in the body of the stomach, causing release of *histamine directly into the deep oxyntic glands*. The histamine then acts quickly to stimulate gastric hydrochloric acid secretion.

PHASES OF GASTRIC SECRETION

Gastric secretion is said to occur in three "phases" (as shown in Figure 67-6 and Table 67-1): a *cephalic phase*, a *gastric phase*, and an *intestinal phase*.

INHIBITION OF GASTRIC SECRETION BY OTHER INTESTINAL FACTORS

Although intestinal chyme slightly stimulates gastric secretion during the early intestinal phase of stomach secretion, it paradoxically inhibits gastric secretion at other times. This inhibition results from at least two influences:

1. The presence of food in the small intestine initiates a *reverse enterogastric reflex*, transmitted through the myenteric nervous system and extrinsic sympathetic and vagus nerves, that inhibits stomach secretion. This reflex can be initiated by:
   a. distending the small bowel;
   b. the presence of acid in the upper intestine;
   c. the presence of protein breakdown products;
   d. irritation of the mucosa.
   This reflex is part of the complex mechanism discussed in Chapter 74 for slowing stomach emptying when the intestines are already filled.
2. The presence of acid, fat, protein breakdown products, hyperosmotic or hypoosmotic fluids, or any irritating factor in the upper small intestine causes release of several intestinal hormones. One of these hormones is *secretin*, which is especially important for control of pancreatic secretion. However, secretin opposes stomach secretion. Three other hormones—*glucose-dependent insulinotropic*

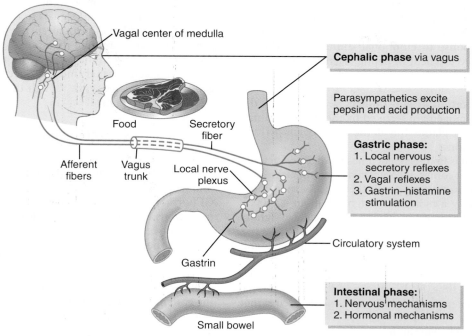

Figure 67-6 Phases of gastric secretion and their regulation.

TABLE 67-1	**Phases of Gastric Secretion**	
Phase	**Description**	**Regulation**
Cephalic phase	Occurs even before food enters the stomach, especially while it is being eaten It results from the sight, smell, thought, or taste of food, and the greater the appetite, the more intense is the stimulation This phase of secretion normally accounts for about 30% of the gastric secretion associated with eating a meal	Neurogenic signals that cause the cephalic phase originate in the cerebral cortex and in the appetite centers of the amygdala and hypothalamus They are transmitted through the dorsal motor nuclei of the vagi and thence through the vagus nerves to the stomach
Gastric phase	Occurs once food enters the stomach, which in turn causes secretion of gastric juice during several hours while food remains in the stomach The gastric phase of secretion accounts for about 60% of the total gastric secretion associated with eating a meal	This phase is regulated by: 1. Long vagovagal reflexes from the stomach to the brain and back to the stomach 2. Local enteric reflexes 3. The gastrin–histamine mechanism
Intestinal phase	When food enters the upper portion of the small intestine, particularly in the duodenum, small amounts of gastric juice continue to be secreted This phase accounts for about 10% of the acid response to a meal	This phase is regulated by: 1. Nervous mechanisms 2. Hormonal mechanisms probably partly because of small amounts of gastrin released by the duodenal mucosa

peptide *(gastric inhibitory peptide)*, *vasoactive intestinal polypeptide*, and *somatostatin*—also have slight to moderate effects in inhibiting gastric secretion.

The purpose of intestinal factors that inhibit gastric secretion is presumably to slow passage of chyme from the stomach when the small intestine is already filled or already overactive. In fact, the enterogastric inhibitory reflexes plus inhibitory hormones usually also reduce stomach motility at the same time that they reduce gastric secretion, as discussed in Chapter 74.

Gastric Secretion During the Interdigestive Period. The stomach secretes a few milliliters of gastric juice each hour during the "interdigestive period," when little or no digestion is occurring anywhere in the gut. The secretion that does occur is usually almost entirely of the nonoxyntic type, composed mainly of *mucus* but little pepsin and almost no acid.

Emotional stimuli may increase interdigestive gastric secretion (which is highly peptic and acidic) to 50 mL or more per hour, in much the same way that the cephalic phase of gastric secretion excites secretion at the onset of a meal. This increase of secretion in response to emotional stimuli is believed to contribute to the development of peptic ulcers, as discussed in Chapter 75.

Secretion and Activation of Pepsinogen. Several slightly different types of pepsinogen are secreted by the peptic and mucous cells of the gastric glands, but all the pepsinogens perform the same basic functions.

When pepsinogen is first secreted, it has no digestive activity. However, as soon as it comes in contact with hydrochloric acid, it is activated to form active *pepsin*. In this process, the pepsinogen molecule, having a molecular weight of about 42,500, is split to form a pepsin molecule, having a molecular weight of about 35,000.

Pepsin functions as an active proteolytic enzyme in a highly acidic medium (optimum pH 1.8–3.5), but above a pH of about 5 it has almost no proteolytic activity and becomes completely inactivated in a short time. Hydrochloric acid is as necessary as pepsin for protein digestion in the stomach, as discussed earlier.

Secretion of Intrinsic Factor by Parietal Cells. The substance *intrinsic factor*, which is essential for absorption of vitamin B_{12} in the ileum, is secreted by the *parietal cells* along with the secretion of hydrochloric acid. When the acid-producing parietal cells of the stomach are destroyed, which frequently occurs in persons with chronic gastritis, not only does *achlorhydria* (lack of stomach acid secretion) develop but *pernicious anemia* also often develops because of failure of maturation of the red blood cells in the absence of vitamin B_{12} stimulation of the bone marrow. This condition is discussed in detail in Chapter 22.

REGULATION OF PEPSINOGEN SECRETION

Stimulation of *pepsinogen* secretion by the peptic cells in the oxyntic glands occurs in response to two main types of signals:
1. *acetylcholine* released from the *vagus nerves* or from the *gastric enteric nervous plexus*;
2. acid in the stomach.

The acid probably does not stimulate the peptic cells directly but instead elicits additional enteric nervous reflexes that support the original nervous signals to the peptic cells. Therefore, the rate of secretion of *pepsinogen*, the precursor of the enzyme *pepsin* that causes protein digestion, is strongly influenced by the amount of acid in the stomach. In people who have lost the ability to secrete normal amounts of acid, secretion of pepsinogen is also decreased, even though the peptic cells may otherwise appear to be normal.

GASTROINTESTINAL HORMONES

The gastrointestinal (GI) tract is considered one of the largest endocrine organs as over 30 peptide hormones genes have been found by researchers and are expressed throughout the GI tract. GI hormones are peptides that are released from various cells or neurons along the GI tract. Table 67-2 lists some of the major GI hormones. Figure 74-6 summarizes the effect of the major GI hormones on GI motility.

Gastrin, *cholecystokinin (CCK)*, and *secretin* are all large polypeptides with approximate molecular weights of 2000, 4200, and 3400, respectively. The terminal five amino acids in the gastrin and CCK molecular chains are the same. The functional activity of gastrin resides in the terminal four amino acids, and the activity for CCK resides in the terminal eight amino acids. All the amino acids in the secretin molecule are essential.

TABLE 67-2	Major GI Hormones		
GI Hormones	**Site of Secretion**	**Primary Stimuli**	**General Actions**
Gastrin	G cells in antrum of stomach and duodenum	Stretch, peptides and amino acids, vagus (through GRP)	↑ *Gastric H⁺* ↑ Gastric mixing ↑ Lower GI tract motility
Secretin	S cells of the duodenum	Acidic chyme	↑ *Pancreatic buffer (HCO_3) secretion* ↑ *Biliary and small intestine buffer secretion* ↓ Gastric H⁺ (by gastrin) ↓ Gastric emptying
CCK	I cells of the duodenum and jejunum	Small peptides and amino acids, fats	↑ *Pancreatic enzyme secretion* contracts gallbladder and relaxes sphincter of Oddi ↑ Pancreatic and biliary buffer secretion ↓ Gastric emptying ↑ Lower GI tract motility
Gastric inhibitory peptide, *aka* GIP	Duodenum and jejunum	Fatty acids, glucose, amino acids	↓ *Gastric H⁺ secretion* ↑ *Pancreatic insulin secretion* ↓ Gastric emptying
Motilin	Mo cells of the duodenum	Fasting	↑ *Phase III contractions of the MMC*
Peptide YY[a]	L cells of the intestine	Fatty acids, glucose, hydrolyzed protein	Inhibition of gastric emptying, pancreatic secretion, gastric acid secretion, intestinal motility, food intake

[a]Cited from Berne & Levy Physiology, sixth ed., Table 26-1, p. 491.
CCK, cholecystokinin; GI, gastrointestinal; GIP, glucose insulinotropic peptide; GRP, gastrin-releasing peptide; MMC, migration myoelectric complex.
Reprinted with permission from Hansen, J., 2002. Netter's Atlas of Human Physiology. Elsevier, Philadelphia.

A synthetic gastrin, composed of the terminal four amino acids of natural gastrin plus the amino acid alanine, has all the same physiological properties as the natural gastrin. This synthetic product is called *pentagastrin*.

Pathophysiology and Treatment Modalities for Acid Peptic Disease

PEPTIC ULCER

A peptic ulcer is an excoriated area of stomach or intestinal mucosa caused principally by the digestive action of gastric juice or upper small intestinal secretions. Figure 67-7 shows the points in the GI tract at which peptic ulcers most frequently occur, demonstrating that the most frequent site is within a few centimeters of the pylorus.

Basic Cause of Peptic Ulceration

The usual cause of peptic ulceration is an *imbalance* between the rate of secretion of gastric juice and the degree of protection

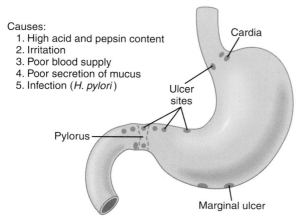

Causes:
1. High acid and pepsin content
2. Irritation
3. Poor blood supply
4. Poor secretion of mucus
5. Infection (*H. pylori*)

Cardia

Ulcer sites

Pylorus

Marginal ulcer

Figure 67-7 Peptic ulcer.

afforded by (1) the gastroduodenal mucosal barrier and (2) the neutralization of the gastric acid by duodenal juices.

In addition to the mucus protection of the mucosa, the duodenum is protected by the *alkalinity of the small intestinal secretions*. Especially important is *pancreatic secretion*, which contains large quantities of sodium bicarbonate that neutralize the hydrochloric acid of the gastric juice, thus also inactivating pepsin and preventing digestion of the mucosa. In addition, large amounts of bicarbonate ions are provided in (1) the secretions of the large Brunner glands in the first few centimeters of the duodenal wall and (2) bile coming from the liver.

Finally, two feedback control mechanisms normally ensure that this neutralization of gastric juices is complete, as follows:

1. When excess acid enters the duodenum, it inhibits gastric secretion and peristalsis in the stomach, both by nervous reflexes and by hormonal feedback from the duodenum, thereby decreasing the rate of gastric emptying.
2. The presence of acid in the small intestine liberates *secretin* from the intestinal mucosa, which then passes by way of the blood to the pancreas to promote rapid secretion of pancreatic juice. This juice also contains a high concentration of sodium bicarbonate, thus making still more sodium bicarbonate available for neutralization of the acid.

Therefore, a peptic ulcer can be caused in either of two ways: (1) excess secretion of acid and pepsin by the gastric mucosa or (2) diminished ability of the gastroduodenal mucosal barrier to protect against the digestive properties of the stomach acid–pepsin secretion.

Specific Causes of Peptic Ulcer

Bacterial Infection by* Helicobacter pylori *Breaks Down the Gastroduodenal Mucosal Barrier and Stimulates Gastric Acid Secretion. At least 75% of persons with peptic ulcer have been found to have chronic infection of the terminal portions of the gastric mucosa and initial portions of the duodenal mucosa, most often caused by the bacterium *Helicobacter* *pylori.* Once this infection begins, it can last a lifetime unless it is eradicated by antibacterial therapy. Furthermore, the bacterium is capable of penetrating the mucosal barrier by virtue of its physical capability to burrow through the barrier and by releasing ammonium that liquefies the barrier and stimulates the secretion of hydrochloric acid. As a result, the strong acidic digestive juices of the stomach secretions can then penetrate into the underlying epithelium and literally digest the GI wall, thus leading to peptic ulceration.

Other Causes of Ulceration. In many people who have peptic ulcers in the initial portion of the duodenum, the rate of gastric acid secretion is greater than normal, sometimes as much as twice normal.

Other factors that predispose to ulcers include (1) *smoking*, presumably because of increased nervous stimulation of the stomach secretory glands; (2) consumption of *alcohol*, because it tends to break down the mucosal barrier; and (3) consumption of *aspirin* and other nonsteroidal anti-inflammatory drugs (NSAIDs) that also have a strong propensity for breaking down this barrier.

Treatment of Peptic Ulcers. Since the discovery that much peptic ulceration has an infectious basis by the bacteria *H. pylori*, therapy has changed immensely. Almost all patients with peptic ulceration can be treated effectively by two measures:

1. use of *antibiotics* along with other agents to kill infectious bacteria;
2. administration of an acid suppressant drug, such as *ranitidine and similar newer molecules*, which are antihistaminic agent that blocks the stimulatory effect of histamine on gastric gland histamine$_2$ receptors, thus reducing gastric acid secretion by 70–80%. More recently, proton pump inhibitors, such as *omeprazole* and *similar newer molecules*, are used to suppress acid production.

Other measures that can be used to treat peptic ulcers include the following:

1. Neutralize the gastric acids with antacids; however, this method is not used often recently.
2. Bismuth compounds are used that probably enhance the mucosal barrier and are antisecretory.
3. Cytoprotective agents such as sucralfate, an aluminum salt of sucrose octasulfate, appear to help with the healing of the ulcer possibly by forming a protective coating.
4. Prostaglandin analogues such as misoprostol can be used to reduce the incidence of peptic ulcers in patients who are on long-term NSAID treatment.
5. Other conservative measures such as quitting smoking, reduction in caffeine and alcohol consumption, and measures to reduce stress can speed up the healing process and prevent ulcers from recurring.

In the past, before these approaches to peptic ulcer therapy were developed, it was often necessary to remove as much as four-fifths of the stomach, thus reducing stomach acid peptic juices enough to cure most patients. Another therapy was to cut the two vagus nerves that supply parasympathetic stimulation to the gastric glands. This procedure blocked almost all secretion of acid and pepsin and often cured the ulcer or ulcers within 1 week after the operation. However, much of the basal stomach secretion returned after a few months and in many patients the ulcer also returned.

The newer physiological approaches to therapy have proven to be much more effective. Even so, in a few instances, the patient's condition is so severe, including massive bleeding from the ulcer, that heroic operative procedures often must still be used.

BIBLIOGRAPHY

Allen A, Flemström G: Gastroduodenal mucus bicarbonate barrier: protection against acid and pepsin, *Am. J. Physiol. Cell Physiol.* 288:C1, 2005.

Bhattacharyya A, Chattopadhyay R, Mitra S, Crowe SE: Oxidative stress: an essential factor in the pathogenesis of gastrointestinal mucosal diseases, *Physiol. Rev.* 94:329, 2014.

Dimaline R, Varro A: Novel roles of gastrin, *J. Physiol.* 592:2951, 2014.

Dockray GJ: Enteroendocrine cell signalling via the vagus nerve, *Curr. Opin. Pharmacol.* 13:954, 2013.

Gareau MG, Barrett KE: Fluid and electrolyte secretion in the inflamed gut: novel targets for treatment of inflammation-induced diarrhea, *Curr. Opin. Pharmacol.* 13:895, 2013.

Heitzmann D, Warth R: Physiology and pathophysiology of potassium channels in gastrointestinal epithelia, *Physiol. Rev.* 88:1119, 2008.

Laine L, Takeuchi K, Tarnawski A: Gastric mucosal defense and cytoprotection: bench to bedside, *Gastroenterology* 135:41, 2008.

Seidler UE: Gastrointestinal HCO$_3^-$ transport and epithelial protection in the gut: new techniques, transport pathways and regulatory pathways, *Curr. Opin. Pharmacol.* 13:900, 2013.

Trauner M, Boyer JL: Bile salt transporters: molecular characterization, function, and regulation, *Physiol. Rev.* 83:633, 2003.

Wallace JL: Prostaglandins, NSAIDs, and gastric mucosal protection: why doesn't the stomach digest itself? *Physiol. Rev.* 88:1547, 2008.

Exocrine Pancreas

GLOSSARY OF TERMS

- **Amylolytic enzymes:** Enzymes that help digest starch, glycogen, and other carbohydrates (except cellulose)
- **Enterokinase:** An enzyme that activates trypsinogen to trypsin (it is secreted by the intestinal mucosa when chyme comes in contact with it)
- **Lipolytic enzymes:** Enzymes that help digest fats to fatty acids and glycerol
- **Pancreatic acini:** Sac-like dilatations within the exocrine pancreas that secrete pancreatic enzymes
- **Pancreatitis:** Inflammation of the pancreas
- **Proteolytic enzymes:** Enzymes that help break down proteins into peptides or amino acids

Pancreatic Secretion

The pancreas, which lies parallel to and beneath the stomach, is a large compound gland and most of its internal structure is similar to that of the salivary glands shown in Figure 66-2. The pancreatic digestive enzymes are secreted by *pancreatic acini*, and large volumes of sodium bicarbonate solution are secreted by the small ductules and larger ducts leading from the acini. The combined product of enzymes and sodium bicarbonate then flows through a long *pancreatic duct* that normally joins the hepatic duct immediately before it empties into the duodenum through the *papilla of Vater*, surrounded by the *sphincter of Oddi*.

COMPOSITION OF PANCREATIC JUICE

Pancreatic juice is secreted most abundantly in response to the presence of chyme in the upper portions of the small intestine, and the characteristics of the pancreatic juice are determined to some extent by the types of food in the chyme. (The pancreas is also an endocrine gland and these are discussed in detail in Chapter 93.)

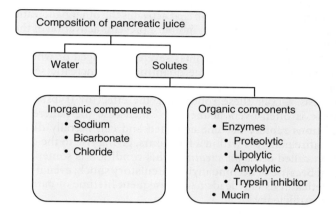

PANCREATIC DIGESTIVE ENZYMES

Pancreatic secretion contains multiple enzymes for digesting all of the three major types of food: proteins, carbohydrates, and fats. It also contains large quantities of bicarbonate ions, which play an important role in neutralizing the acidity of the chyme emptied from the stomach into the duodenum.

The most important pancreatic enzymes for digesting proteins have been discussed in Table 68-1.

When first synthesized in the pancreatic cells, the proteolytic digestive enzymes are in their enzymatically inactive forms *trypsinogen*, *chymotrypsinogen*, and *procarboxypolypeptidase*. They become activated only after they are secreted into the intestinal tract. Trypsinogen is activated by an enzyme called *enterokinase*,

TABLE 68-1	Summary of Pancreatic Enzymes	
Type of Enzymes	**Enzymes**	**Function**
Proteolytic	*Trypsin, chymotrypsin*	Breaks down proteins into peptides
	Carboxypolypeptidase	Splits some peptides into individual amino acids
Amylolytic	*Pancreatic amylase*	Hydrolyzes starches, glycogen, and other carbohydrates (except cellulose) to disaccharides and a few trisaccharides
Lipolytic	*Pancreatic lipase*	Hydrolyzes neutral fat into fatty acids and monoglycerides
	Cholesterol esterase	Hydrolysis of cholesterol esters
	Phospholipase	Splits fatty acids from phospholipids

which is secreted by the intestinal mucosa when chyme comes in contact with the mucosa. Trypsinogen also can be autocatalytically activated by trypsin that has already been formed from previously secreted trypsinogen. Chymotrypsinogen is activated by trypsin to form chymotrypsin, and procarboxypolypeptidase is activated in a similar manner.

Secretion of Trypsin Inhibitor Prevents Digestion of the Pancreas. It is important that the proteolytic enzymes of the pancreatic juice do not become activated until after they have been secreted into the intestine because the trypsin and the other enzymes would digest the pancreas. Fortunately, the same cells that secrete proteolytic enzymes into the acini of the pancreas simultaneously secrete another substance called *trypsin inhibitor*. This substance, which is formed in the cytoplasm of the glandular cells, prevents activation of trypsin both inside the secretory cells and in the acini and ducts of the pancreas. In addition, because it is trypsin that activates the other pancreatic proteolytic enzymes, trypsin inhibitor prevents activation of the other enzymes as well.

When the pancreas becomes severely damaged or when a duct becomes blocked, large quantities of pancreatic secretion sometimes become pooled in the damaged areas of the pancreas. Under these conditions, the effect of trypsin inhibitor is often overwhelmed, in which case the pancreatic secretions rapidly become activated and can literally digest the entire pancreas within a few hours, giving rise to the condition called *acute pancreatitis*. This condition is sometimes lethal because of accompanying circulatory shock; even if it is not lethal, it usually leads to a subsequent lifetime of pancreatic insufficiency.

SECRETION OF BICARBONATE IONS

Although the enzymes of the pancreatic juice are secreted entirely by the acini of the pancreatic glands, the other two important components of pancreatic juice, bicarbonate ions and water, are secreted mainly by the epithelial cells of the ductules and ducts that lead from the acini. When the pancreas is stimulated to secrete copious quantities of pancreatic juice, the bicarbonate ion concentration can rise to as high as 145 mEq/L, a value about five times that of bicarbonate ions in the plasma. This high concentration provides a large quantity of alkali in the pancreatic juice that serves to neutralize the hydrochloric acid emptied into the duodenum from the stomach.

The basic steps in the cellular mechanism for secreting sodium bicarbonate solution into the pancreatic ductules and ducts shown in Figure 68-1 are as follows:

1. Carbon dioxide diffuses to the interior of the cell from the blood and, under the influence of carbonic anhydrase, combines with water to form carbonic acid (H_2CO_3). The carbonic acid dissociates into bicarbonate ions and hydrogen ions (HCO_3^- and H^+). Additional bicarbonate ions enter the cell through the basolateral membrane by cotransport with sodium ions (Na^+). The bicarbonate ions are then exchanged for chloride ions (Cl^-) by secondary active transport through the *luminal border* of the cell into the lumen of the duct. The chloride that enters the cell is recycled back into the lumen by special chloride channels.

2. The hydrogen ions formed by dissociation of carbonic acid inside the cell are *exchanged for sodium ions through the basolateral membrane* of the cell by secondary active

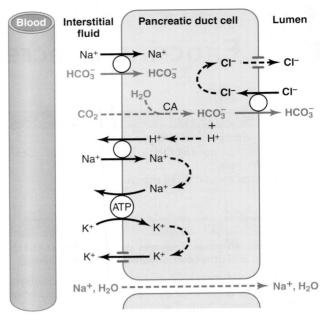

Figure 68-1   Secretion of isosmotic sodium bicarbonate solution by the pancreatic ductules and ducts. CA, carbonic anhydrase.

transport. Sodium ions also enter the cell by cotransport with bicarbonate across the basolateral membrane. Sodium ions are then transported across the *luminal border* into the pancreatic duct lumen. The negative voltage of the lumen also pulls the positively charged sodium ions across the tight junctions between the cells.

3. The overall movement of sodium and bicarbonate ions from the blood into the duct lumen creates an osmotic pressure gradient that causes osmosis of water also into the pancreatic duct, thus forming an almost completely isosmotic bicarbonate solution.

REGULATION OF PANCREATIC SECRETION

Basic Stimuli that Cause Pancreatic Secretion

Three basic stimuli are important in causing pancreatic secretion:

1. *acetylcholine*, which is released from the parasympathetic vagus nerve endings and from other cholinergic nerves in the enteric nervous system;
2. *cholecystokinin* (*CCK*), which is secreted by the duodenal and upper jejunal mucosa when food enters the small intestine;
3. *secretin*, which is also secreted by the duodenal and jejunal mucosa when highly acidic food enters the small intestine.

The first two of these stimuli, acetylcholine and CCK, stimulate the acinar cells of the pancreas, causing production of large quantities of pancreatic digestive enzymes but relatively small quantities of water and electrolytes to go with the enzymes. Without the water most of the enzymes remain temporarily stored in the acini and ducts until more fluid secretion comes along to wash them into the duodenum. Secretin, in contrast to the first two basic stimuli, stimulates secretion of large quantities of water solution of sodium bicarbonate by the pancreatic ductal epithelium.

Multiplicative Effects of Different Stimuli. When all the different stimuli of pancreatic secretion occur at once, the total secretion is far greater than the sum of the secretions caused by each one separately. Therefore, the various stimuli are said to "multiply," or "potentiate," one another. Thus, pancreatic secretion normally results from the combined effects of the multiple basic stimuli, not from one alone.

Phases of Pancreatic Secretion

Pancreatic secretion, as with gastric secretion, occurs in three phases: the *cephalic phase*, the *gastric phase*, and the *intestinal phase*. Their characteristics are described in the following sections.

Cephalic Phase. During the cephalic phase of pancreatic secretion, the same nervous signals from the brain that cause secretion in the stomach also cause acetylcholine release by the vagal nerve endings in the pancreas. This signaling causes moderate amounts of enzymes to be secreted into the pancreatic acini, accounting for about 20% of the total secretion of pancreatic enzymes after a meal. However, little of the secretion flows immediately through the pancreatic ducts into the intestine because only small amounts of water and electrolytes are secreted along with the enzymes.

Gastric Phase. During the gastric phase, the nervous stimulation of enzyme secretion continues, accounting for another 5–10% of pancreatic enzymes secreted after a meal. However, again, only small amounts reach the duodenum because of continued lack of significant fluid secretion.

Intestinal Phase. After chyme leaves the stomach and enters the small intestine, pancreatic secretion becomes copious, mainly in response to the hormone *secretin*.

Secretin Stimulates Copious Secretion of Bicarbonate Ions, which Neutralizes Acidic Stomach Chyme. Secretin is a polypeptide, containing 27 amino acids (with a molecular weight of about 3400). It is present in an inactive form, prosecretin, in so-called S cells in the mucosa of the duodenum and jejunum. When acid chyme with a pH less than 4.5–5.0 enters the duodenum from the stomach, it causes duodenal mucosal release and activation of secretin, which is then absorbed into the blood. The one truly potent constituent of chyme that causes this secretin release is the hydrochloric acid from the stomach.

Secretin in turn causes the pancreas to secrete large quantities of fluid containing a high concentration of bicarbonate ion (up to 145 mEq/L) but a low concentration of chloride ion. The secretin mechanism is especially important for two reasons: First, secretin begins to be released from the mucosa of the small intestine when the pH of the duodenal contents falls below 4.5–5.0, and its release increases greatly as the pH falls to 3.0. This mechanism immediately causes copious secretion of pancreatic juice that contains abundant amounts of sodium bicarbonate. The net result is then the following reaction in the duodenum:

$$HCl + NaHCO_3 \rightarrow NaCl + H_2CO_3$$

The carbonic acid then immediately dissociates into carbon dioxide and water. The carbon dioxide is absorbed into

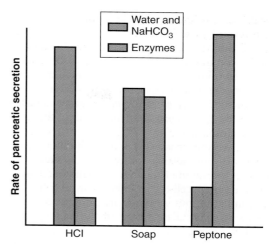

Figure 68-2 Sodium bicarbonate ($NaHCO_3$), water, and enzyme secretion by the pancreas caused by the presence of acid (*HCl*), fat (soap), or peptone solutions in the duodenum.

the blood and expired through the lungs, thus leaving a neutral solution of sodium chloride in the duodenum. In this way, the acid contents that are emptied into the duodenum from the stomach become neutralized, and thus further peptic digestive activity by the gastric juices in the duodenum is immediately blocked. Because the mucosa of the small intestine cannot withstand the digestive action of acid gastric juice, this protective mechanism is essential to prevent the development of duodenal ulcers, as is discussed in further detail in Chapter 75.

Bicarbonate ion secretion by the pancreas provides an appropriate pH for action of the pancreatic digestive enzymes, which function optimally in a slightly alkaline or neutral medium, at a pH of 7.0–8.0. Fortunately, the pH of the sodium bicarbonate secretion averages 8.0.

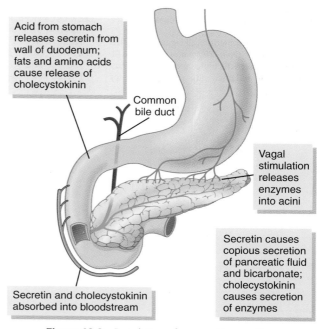

Acid from stomach releases secretin from wall of duodenum; fats and amino acids cause release of cholecystokinin

Common bile duct

Vagal stimulation releases enzymes into acini

Secretin causes copious secretion of pancreatic fluid and bicarbonate; cholecystokinin causes secretion of enzymes

Secretin and cholecystokinin absorbed into bloodstream

Figure 68-3 Regulation of pancreatic secretion.

Cholecystokinin—Contributes to Control of Digestive Enzyme Secretion by the Pancreas. The presence of food in the upper small intestine also causes a second hormone, *CCK*, a polypeptide containing 33 amino acids, to be released from yet another group of cells, *I cells*, in the mucosa of the duodenum and upper jejunum. This release of CCK results especially from the presence of *proteoses* and *peptones* (products of partial protein digestion), and *long-chain fatty acids* in the chyme coming from the stomach.

CCK, like secretin, passes by way of the blood to the pancreas but instead of causing sodium bicarbonate secretion, it mainly causes secretion of much more pancreatic digestive enzymes by the acinar cells. This effect is similar to that caused by vagal stimulation but is even more pronounced, accounting for 70–80% of the total secretion of the pancreatic digestive enzymes after a meal.

The differences between the pancreatic stimulatory effects of secretin and CCK are shown in Figure 68-2 that demonstrates (1) intense sodium bicarbonate secretion in response to acid in the duodenum, stimulated by secretin; (2) a dual effect in response to soap (a fat); and (3) intense digestive enzyme secretion (when peptones enter the duodenum) stimulated by CCK.

Figures 68-3 and 68-4 summarize the more important factors in the regulation of pancreatic secretion. The total amount secreted each day is about 1 L.

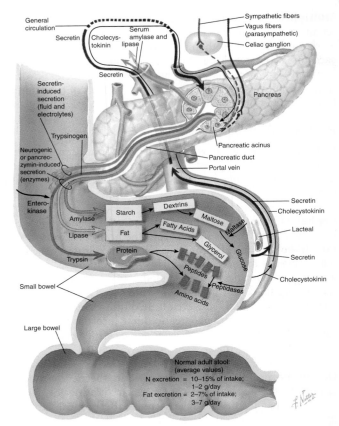

Figure 68-4   Secretion of pancreatic enzymes. *Netter illustration from www.netterimages.com. © Elsevier Inc. All rights reserved.*

BIBLIOGRAPHY

Allen A, Flemström G: Gastroduodenal mucus bicarbonate barrier: protection against acid and pepsin, *Am. J. Physiol. Cell Physiol.* 288:C1, 2005.

Bhattacharyya A, Chattopadhyay R, Mitra S, Crowe SE: Oxidative stress: an essential factor in the pathogenesis of gastrointestinal mucosal diseases, *Physiol. Rev.* 94:329, 2014.

Dockray GJ: Enteroendocrine cell signalling via the vagus nerve, *Curr. Opin. Pharmacol.* 13:954, 2013.

Gareau MG, Barrett KE: Fluid and electrolyte secretion in the inflamed gut: novel targets for treatment of inflammation-induced diarrhea, *Curr. Opin. Pharmacol.* 13:895, 2013.

Heitzmann D, Warth R: Physiology and pathophysiology of potassium channels in gastrointestinal epithelia, *Physiol. Rev.* 88:1119, 2008.

Lee MG, Ohana E, Park HW, et al: Molecular mechanism of pancreatic and salivary gland fluid and HCO$_3^-$ secretion, *Physiol. Rev.* 92:39, 2012.

Lefebvre P, Cariou B, Lien F, et al: Role of bile acids and bile acid receptors in metabolic regulation, *Physiol. Rev.* 89:147, 2009.

Seidler UE: Gastrointestinal HCO$_3^-$ transport and epithelial protection in the gut: new techniques, transport pathways and regulatory pathways, *Curr. Opin. Pharmacol.* 13:900, 2013.

Trauner M, Boyer JL: Bile salt transporters: molecular characterization, function, and regulation, *Physiol. Rev.* 83:633, 2003.

Williams JA, Chen X, Sabbatini ME: Small G proteins as key regulators of pancreatic digestive enzyme secretion, *Am. J. Physiol. Endocrinol. Metab.* 296:E405, 2009.

Functions of the Liver

LEARNING OBJECTIVES

- List the functions of the liver.
- Describe the composition and functions of bile.
- Describe the enterohepatic circulation.
- Describe the types of jaundice.

GLOSSARY OF TERMS

- **Bilirubin:** A pigment that is formed from the heme ring of hemoglobin on destruction of RBCs
- **Gluconeogenesis:** The process of formation of glucose by the liver, from noncarbohydrate sources, such as amino acids and the glycerol portion of fats
- **Jaundice:** Yellowish discoloration of the skin and deeper tissues
- **Kupffer cells:** Liver macrophages that line the sinusoids and are capable of phagocytizing bacteria and other foreign matter
- **Liver lobule:** The basic functional unit of the liver

Although the liver is a discrete organ, it performs many different interrelating functions. This becomes especially evident when abnormalities of the liver occur because many liver functions are disturbed simultaneously. This chapter summarizes the different functions of the liver, including (1) filtration and storage of blood; (2) metabolism of carbohydrates, proteins, fats, hormones, and foreign chemicals; (3) formation of bile; (4) storage of vitamins and iron; and (5) formation of coagulation factors.

Physiological Anatomy of the Liver

The liver is the largest organ in the body, contributing about 2% of the total body weight, or about 1.5 kg (3.3 lb) in the average adult human. The basic functional unit of the liver is the *liver lobule*, which is a cylindrical structure several millimeters in length and 0.8–2 mm in diameter. The human liver contains 50,000–100,000 individual lobules.

The liver lobule, shown in cutaway format in Figure 69-1, is constructed around a *central vein* that empties into the hepatic veins and then into the vena cava. The lobule is composed principally of many liver *cellular plates* (two of which are shown in Figure 69-1) that radiate from the central vein like spokes in a wheel. Each hepatic plate is usually two-cell thick, and between the adjacent cells lie small *bile canaliculi* that empty into *bile ducts* in the fibrous septa separating the adjacent liver lobules.

In the septa are small *portal venules* that receive their blood mainly from the venous outflow of the gastrointestinal tract by way of the portal vein. From these venules blood flows into flat, branching *hepatic sinusoids* that lie between the hepatic plates and then into the central vein. Thus, the hepatic cells are exposed continuously to portal venous blood.

Hepatic arterioles are also present in the interlobular septa. These arterioles supply arterial blood to the septal tissues between the adjacent lobules, and many of the small arterioles also empty directly into the hepatic sinusoids, most frequently emptying into those located about one-third the distance from the interlobular septa, as shown in Figure 69-1.

In addition to the hepatic cells, the venous sinusoids are lined by two other cell types: (1) typical *endothelial cells* and (2) large *Kupffer cells* (also called *reticuloendothelial cells*), which are resident macrophages that line the sinusoids and are capable of phagocytizing bacteria and other foreign matter in the hepatic sinus blood.

The endothelial lining of the sinusoids has extremely large pores, some of which are almost 1 μm in diameter. Beneath this lining, lying between the endothelial cells and the hepatic cells, are narrow tissue spaces called the *spaces of Disse*, also known as the *perisinusoidal spaces*. The millions of spaces of Disse connect with lymphatic vessels in the interlobular septa. Therefore, excess fluid in these spaces is removed through the lymphatics. Because of the large pores in the endothelium, substances in the plasma move freely into the spaces of Disse. Even large portions of the plasma proteins diffuse freely into these spaces.

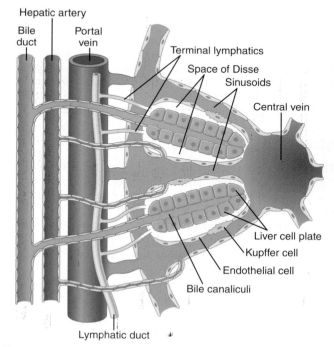

Figure 69-1 Basic structure of a liver lobule, showing the liver cellular plates, the blood vessels, the bile-collecting system, and the lymph flow system composed of the spaces of Disse and the interlobular lymphatics. *Modified from Guyton, A.C., Taylor, A.E., Granger, H.J., 1975. Circulatory Physiology. Vol 2: Dynamics and Control of the Body Fluids. W.B. Saunders, Philadelphia.*

Hepatic Vascular and Lymph Systems

The function of the hepatic vascular system is discussed in Chapter 41 in connection with the portal veins and can be summarized as follows (Box 69-1).

THE LIVER FUNCTIONS AS A BLOOD RESERVOIR

Because the liver is an expandable organ, large quantities of blood can be stored in its blood vessels. Its normal blood volume, including that in both the hepatic veins and the hepatic sinuses, is about 450 mL, or almost 10% of the body's total blood volume. When high pressure in the right atrium causes backpressure in the liver, the liver expands, and 0.5–1 L of extra blood is occasionally stored in the hepatic veins and sinuses. This storage of extra blood occurs especially in cases of cardiac failure with peripheral congestion, which is discussed in Chapter 51.

THE LIVER'S MACROPHAGE SYSTEM SERVES A BLOOD-CLEANSING FUNCTION

Blood flowing through the intestinal capillaries picks up many bacteria from the intestines. Indeed, a sample of blood taken from the portal veins before it enters the liver almost always grows colon bacilli when cultured, whereas growth of colon bacilli from blood in the systemic circulation is extremely rare.

The Kupffer cells, which are large phagocytic macrophages that line the hepatic venous sinuses, efficiently cleanse blood as it passes through the sinuses. Probably less than 1% of the bacteria entering the portal blood from the intestines succeeds in passing through the liver into the systemic circulation.

Metabolic Functions of the Liver

The liver is a large, chemically reactant pool of cells that have a high rate of metabolism. These cells share substrates and energy from one metabolic system to another, process and synthesize multiple substances that are transported to other areas of the body, and perform myriads of other metabolic functions. In this chapter, we summarize the metabolic functions that are especially important in understanding the integrated physiology of the body.

CARBOHYDRATE METABOLISM

In carbohydrate metabolism, the liver performs the following functions:

1. storage of large amounts of glycogen;
2. conversion of galactose and fructose to glucose;
3. gluconeogenesis;
4. formation of many chemical compounds from intermediate products of carbohydrate metabolism.

The liver is especially important for maintaining a normal blood glucose concentration. Storage of glycogen allows the liver to remove excess glucose from the blood, store it, and then return it to the blood when the blood glucose concentration begins to fall too low. This is called the *glucose buffer function* of the liver.

FAT METABOLISM

Although most cells of the body metabolize fat, certain aspects of fat metabolism occur mainly in the liver:

1. oxidation of fatty acids to supply energy for other body functions;
2. synthesis of large quantities of cholesterol, phospholipids, and most lipoproteins;
3. synthesis of fat from proteins and carbohydrates.

To derive energy from neutral fats, the fat is first split into glycerol and fatty acids. The fatty acids are then split by *beta-oxidation* into two-carbon acetyl radicals that form *acetyl coenzyme A* (acetyl-CoA). Acetyl-CoA can enter the citric acid cycle and be oxidized to liberate tremendous amounts of energy. Beta-oxidation can take place in all cells of the body, but it occurs especially rapidly in the hepatic cells.

PROTEIN METABOLISM

The body cannot dispense with the liver's contribution to protein metabolism for more than a few days without death ensuing. The most important functions of the liver in protein metabolism are the following:

1. deamination of amino acids;
2. formation of urea for removal of ammonia from the body fluids;
3. formation of plasma proteins;
4. interconversions of the various amino acids and synthesis of other compounds from amino acids.

OTHER METABOLIC FUNCTIONS OF THE LIVER

The Liver Is a Storage Site for Vitamins. The liver has a particular propensity for storing vitamins and has long been known as an excellent source of certain vitamins in the treatment of patients. The vitamin stored in greatest quantity in the liver is vitamin A, but large quantities of vitamin D and vitamin B_{12} are normally stored there as well.

The Liver Stores Iron as Ferritin. Except for the iron in the hemoglobin of the blood, by far the greatest proportion of iron in the body is stored in the liver in the form of *ferritin*. Thus, the apoferritin–ferritin system of the liver acts as a *blood iron buffer*, as well as an iron storage medium.

The Liver Forms the Blood Substances Used in Coagulation. Substances formed in the liver that are used in the coagulation process include *fibrinogen, prothrombin, accelerator globulin, factor VII,* and several other important factors. Vitamin K is required by the metabolic processes of the liver for the formation of several of these substances, especially prothrombin and factors VII, IX, and X. In the absence of vitamin K, the concentrations of all these substances decrease markedly and almost prevent blood coagulation.

The Liver Removes or Excretes Drugs, Hormones, and Other Substances. The active chemical medium of the liver is well known for its ability to detoxify or excrete many drugs

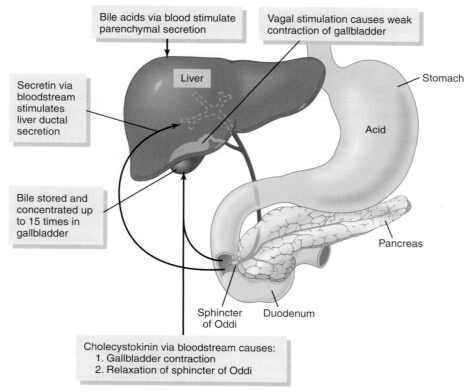

Bile acids via blood stimulate parenchymal secretion

Vagal stimulation causes weak contraction of gallbladder

Secretin via bloodstream stimulates liver ductal secretion

Liver

Stomach

Acid

Bile stored and concentrated up to 15 times in gallbladder

Pancreas

Sphincter of Oddi

Duodenum

Cholecystokinin via bloodstream causes:
1. Gallbladder contraction
2. Relaxation of sphincter of Oddi

Figure 69-2 Liver secretion and gallbladder emptying.

into the bile, including sulfonamides, penicillin, ampicillin, and erythromycin.

Similarly, several of the hormones secreted by the endocrine glands are either chemically altered or excreted by the liver, including thyroxine and essentially all the steroid hormones, such as estrogen, cortisol, and aldosterone. Liver damage can lead to excess accumulation of one or more of these hormones in the body fluids and therefore causes overactivity of the hormonal systems.

Finally, one of the major routes for excreting calcium from the body is secretion by the liver into the bile, which then passes into the gut and is lost in the feces.

Bile Secretion by the Liver

One of the many functions of the liver is to secrete *bile*, normally between 600 and 1000 mL/day. Bile serves two important functions:

1. Bile plays an important role in fat digestion and absorption because *bile acids* in the bile perform two functions:
   a. They help to emulsify the large fat particles of the food into many minute particles, the surface of which can then be attacked by lipase enzymes secreted in pancreatic juice.
   b. They aid in absorption of the digested fat end products through the intestinal mucosal membrane.
2. Bile serves as a means for excretion of several important waste products from the blood. These waste products include in particular *bilirubin*, an end product of hemoglobin destruction, and excesses of *cholesterol*.

PHYSIOLOGICAL ANATOMY OF BILIARY SECRETION

Bile is secreted in two stages by the liver: (1) The initial portion is secreted by the principal functional cells of the liver, the *hepatocytes*; this initial secretion contains large amounts of bile acids, cholesterol, and other organic constituents. It is secreted into minute *bile canaliculi* that originate between the hepatic cells. (2) Next, the bile flows in the canaliculi toward the interlobular septa, where the canaliculi empty into *terminal bile ducts* and then into progressively larger ducts, finally reaching the *hepatic duct* and *common bile duct*. From these the bile either empties directly into the duodenum or is diverted for minutes up to several hours through the *cystic duct* into the *gallbladder*, as shown in Figure 69-2.

In its course through the bile ducts, a second portion of liver secretion is added to the initial bile in response to *secretin*, a local hormone. This additional secretion is a watery solution of sodium and bicarbonate ions secreted by epithelial cells that line the ductules and ducts. This second secretion sometimes increases the total quantity of bile by as much as 100%.

Storing and Concentrating Bile in the Gallbladder. Bile is secreted continually by the liver cells, but most of it is normally stored in the gallbladder until it is needed in the duodenum. The maximum volume that the gallbladder can hold is only 30–60 mL. Nevertheless, as much as 12 hours of bile secretion (usually about 450 mL) can be stored in the gallbladder because water, sodium, chloride, and most other small electrolytes are continually absorbed through the gallbladder mucosa, concentrating the remaining bile constituents that contain the bile salts, cholesterol, lecithin, and bilirubin.

Most of this gallbladder absorption is caused by active transport of sodium through the gallbladder epithelium, and this transport is followed by secondary absorption of chloride ions, water, and most other diffusible constituents. Bile is normally concentrated in this way about 5-fold, but it can be concentrated up to a maximum of 20-fold.

Composition of Bile. Table 69-1 lists the composition of bile when it is first secreted by the liver and then after it has been concentrated in the gallbladder. By far the most abundant substances secreted in the bile are *bile salts*, which account for about one-half of the total solutes also in the bile. Also secreted or excreted in large concentrations are *bilirubin, cholesterol, lecithin*, and the usual *electrolytes* of plasma.

Cholecystokinin Stimulates Gallbladder Emptying. When food begins to be digested in the upper gastrointestinal tract, the gallbladder begins to empty, especially when fatty foods reach the duodenum about 30 minutes after a meal. The mechanism of gallbladder emptying is rhythmic contractions of the gallbladder wall, but effective emptying also requires simultaneous relaxation of the *sphincter of Oddi*, which guards the exit of the common bile duct into the duodenum.

By far the most potent stimulus for causing the gallbladder contractions is the hormone cholecystokinin (*CCK*). This is the same CCK discussed earlier that causes increased secretion of digestive enzymes by the acinar cells of the pancreas. The stimulus for CCK entry into the blood from the duodenal mucosa is mainly the presence of fatty foods in the duodenum.

The gallbladder is also stimulated less strongly by acetylcholine-secreting nerve fibers from both the vagi and the intestinal enteric nervous system. Figure 69-2 summarizes the secretion of bile, its storage in the gallbladder, and its ultimate release from the bladder to the duodenum.

FUNCTION OF BILE SALTS IN FAT DIGESTION AND ABSORPTION

The liver cells synthesize about 6 g of *bile salts* daily. The precursor of the bile salts is *cholesterol*, which is either present in the diet or synthesized in the liver cells during the course of fat metabolism. The cholesterol is first converted to *cholic acid* or *chenodeoxycholic acid* in about equal quantities. These acids in turn combine principally with glycine and to a lesser extent with taurine to form *glyco-* and *tauro-conjugated bile acids*. The salts of these acids, mainly sodium salts, are then secreted in the bile.

The bile salts have two important actions in the intestinal tract.

First, they have a detergent action on the fat particles in the food. This action, which decreases the surface tension of the particles and allows agitation in the intestinal tract to break the fat globules into minute sizes, is called the *emulsifying* or *detergent function* of bile salts.

Second, and even more important than the emulsifying function, bile salts help in the absorption of (1) fatty acids, (2) monoglycerides, (3) cholesterol, and (4) other lipids from the intestinal tract. They help in this absorption by forming small physical complexes with these lipids; the complexes are called *micelles*, and they are semisoluble in the chyme because of the electrical charges of the bile salts. The intestinal lipids are "ferried" in this form to the intestinal mucosa, where they are then absorbed into the blood, as will be described in detail in Chapter 72. Without the presence of bile salts in the intestinal tract, up to 40% of the ingested fats are lost into the feces and a metabolic deficit often develops because of this nutrient loss.

Enterohepatic Circulation of Bile Salts. About 94% of the bile salts are reabsorbed into the blood from the small intestine, about one-half of this by *diffusion* through the mucosa in the early portions of the small intestine and the remainder by an *active transport* process through the intestinal mucosa in the distal ileum. They then enter the portal blood and pass back to the liver. On reaching the liver, and during first passage through the venous sinusoids, these salts are absorbed almost entirely back into the hepatic cells and then resecreted into the bile. This is shown in Figure 69-3.

In this way, about 94% of all the bile salts are recirculated into the bile, so on the average these salts make the entire circuit some 17 times before being carried out in the feces. The small quantities of bile salts lost into the feces are replaced by new amounts formed continually by the liver cells. This recirculation of the bile salts is called the *enterohepatic circulation of bile salts*.

The quantity of bile secreted by the liver each day is highly dependent on the availability of bile salts—the greater the quantity of bile salts in the enterohepatic circulation (usually a total of only about 2.5 g), the greater is the rate of bile secretion. Indeed, ingestion of supplemental bile salts can increase bile secretion by several hundred milliliters per day.

If a bile fistula empties the bile salts to the exterior for several days to several weeks so they cannot be reabsorbed from the ileum, the liver increases its production of bile salts from 6-fold to 10-fold, which increases the rate of bile secretion most of the way back to normal. This demonstrates that the daily rate of liver bile salt secretion is actively controlled by the availability (or lack of availability) of bile salts in the enterohepatic circulation.

Role of Secretin in Controlling Bile Secretion. In addition to the strong stimulating effect of bile acids to cause bile secretion, the hormone *secretin* that also stimulates pancreatic secretion increases bile secretion, sometimes more than doubling its secretion for several hours after a meal. This increase in secretion consists almost entirely of secretion of a sodium bicarbonate–rich watery solution by the epithelial cells of the bile ductules and ducts, and does not represent increased secretion by the liver parenchymal cells themselves. The bicarbonate in turn passes into the small intestine and joins the bicarbonate from the pancreas in neutralizing the hydrochloric acid from the stomach. Thus, the secretin feedback mechanism for neutralizing duodenal acid operates not only through its effects on pancreatic secretion but also to a lesser extent through its effect on secretion by the liver ductules and ducts.

TABLE 69-1	Composition of Bile	
	Liver Bile	**Gallbladder Bile**
Water	97.5 g/dL	92 g/dL
Bile salts	1.1 g/dL	6 g/dL
Bilirubin	0.04 g/dL	0.3 g/dL
Cholesterol	0.1 g/dL	0.3–0.9 g/dL
Fatty acids	0.12 g/dL	0.3–1.2 g/dL
Lecithin	0.04 g/dL	0.3 g/dL
Na^+	145 mEq/L	130 mEq/L
K^+	5 mEq/L	12 mEq/L
Ca^{++}	5 mEq/L	23 mEq/L
Cl^-	100 mEq/L	25 mEq/L
HCO_3^-	28 mEq/L	10 mEq/L

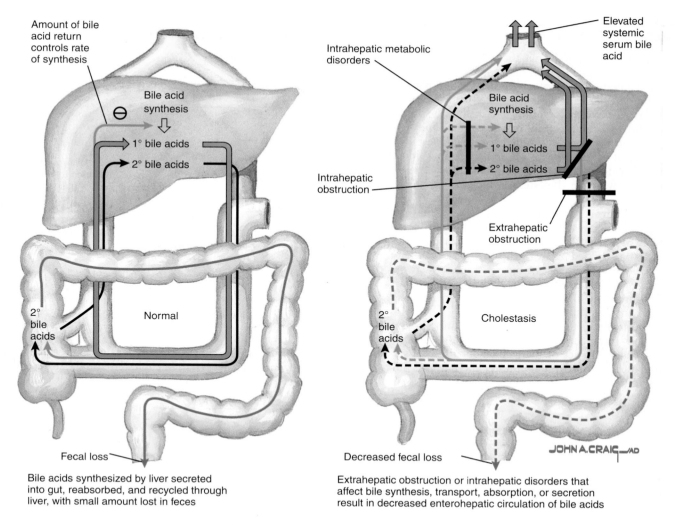

Amount of bile acid return controls rate of synthesis

Bile acid synthesis

⊖

1° bile acids

2° bile acids

2° bile acids

Normal

Fecal loss

Bile acids synthesized by liver secreted into gut, reabsorbed, and recycled through liver, with small amount lost in feces

Intrahepatic metabolic disorders

Elevated systemic serum bile acid

Bile acid synthesis

1° bile acids

2° bile acids

Intrahepatic obstruction

Extrahepatic obstruction

2° bile acids

Cholestasis

JOHN A.CRAIG—AD

Decreased fecal loss

Extrahepatic obstruction or intrahepatic disorders that affect bile synthesis, transport, absorption, or secretion result in decreased enterohepatic circulation of bile acids

Cellular mechanisms of metabolism

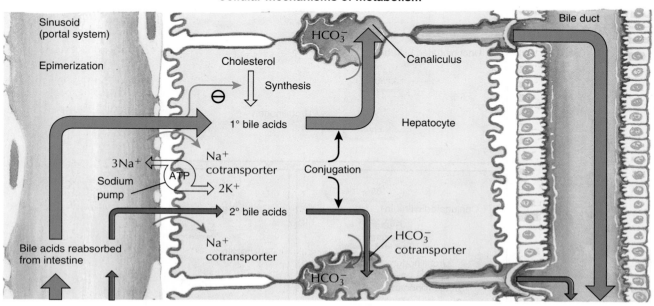

Sinusoid (portal system)

Epimerization

Cholesterol

⊖ Synthesis

1° bile acids

$3Na^+$

Sodium pump   ATP

$2K^+$

Na^+ cotransporter

Conjugation

2° bile acids

Na^+ cotransporter

Bile acids reabsorbed from intestine

HCO_3^-

Canaliculus

Hepatocyte

HCO_3^- cotransporter

HCO_3^-

Bile duct

Primary (1°) acids synthesized, conjugated, and secreted into canaliculi. In gut, portion of bile acid is converted to secondary (2°) bile acids. Bile acids (90%) reabsorbed into portal system and returned to liver; in hepatocytes, primary forms recycled and secondary acids epimerized and excreted.

Figure 69-3   Enterohepatic circulation of bile acids and bile salts. *Netter illustration from www.netterimages.com.*

LIVER SECRETION OF CHOLESTEROL AND GALLSTONE FORMATION

Bile salts are formed in the hepatic cells from cholesterol in the blood plasma. In the process of secreting the bile salts, about 1–2 g of cholesterol is removed from the blood plasma and secreted into the bile each day.

Cholesterol is almost completely insoluble in pure water, but the bile salts and lecithin in bile combine physically with the cholesterol to form ultramicroscopic *micelles* in the form of a colloidal solution. When the bile becomes concentrated in the gallbladder, the bile salts and lecithin become concentrated along with the cholesterol, which keeps the cholesterol in solution.

Under abnormal conditions, the cholesterol may precipitate in the gallbladder, resulting in the formation of *cholesterol gallstones*, as shown in Figure 69-4. The amount of cholesterol in the bile is determined partly by the quantity of fat that the person eats because liver cells synthesize cholesterol as one of the products of fat metabolism in the body. For this reason, people who consume a high-fat diet over a period of years are prone to development of gallstones.

Inflammation of the gallbladder epithelium, often resulting from a low-grade chronic infection, may also change the absorptive characteristics of the gallbladder mucosa, sometimes allowing excessive absorption of water and bile salts but leaving behind the cholesterol in the gallbladder in progressively greater concentrations. The cholesterol then begins to precipitate, first forming many small crystals of cholesterol on the surface of the inflamed mucosa, but then progressing to large gallstones.

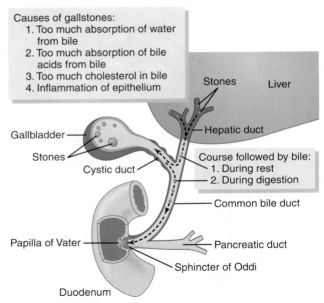

Causes of gallstones:
1. Too much absorption of water from bile
2. Too much absorption of bile acids from bile
3. Too much cholesterol in bile
4. Inflammation of epithelium

Course followed by bile:
1. During rest
2. During digestion

Figure 69-4 Formation of gallstones.

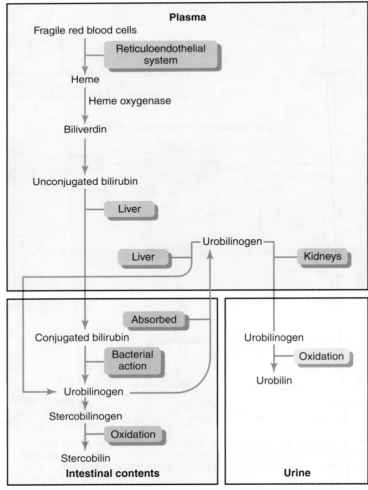

Figure 69-5 Bilirubin formation and secretion.

Measurement of Bilirubin in the Bile as a Clinical Diagnostic Tool

In addition to bile salts, many substances are excreted in the bile and then eliminated in the feces. One of these substances is the greenish yellow pigment *bilirubin*, which is a major end product of hemoglobin degradation, as pointed out in Chapter 19. However, it also provides *an exceedingly valuable tool for diagnosing both hemolytic blood diseases and various types of liver diseases*. Therefore, while referring to Figure 69-5, let us explain this.

Briefly, when the red blood cells have lived out their life span (on average, 120 days) and have become too fragile to exist in the circulatory system, their cell membranes rupture, and the released hemoglobin is phagocytized by tissue macrophages (also called the *reticuloendothelial system*) throughout the body. The hemoglobin is first split into *globin* and *heme*, and the heme ring is opened to give (1) free iron, which is transported in the blood by transferrin, and (2) a straight chain of four pyrrole nuclei, which is the substrate from which bilirubin will eventually be formed. The first substance formed is *biliverdin*, but this substance is rapidly reduced to *free bilirubin*, also called *unconjugated bilirubin*, which is gradually released from the macrophages into the plasma. This form of bilirubin immediately combines strongly with plasma albumin and is transported in this combination throughout the blood and interstitial fluids.

Within hours, the unconjugated bilirubin is absorbed through the hepatic cell membrane. In passing to the inside of the liver cells, it is released from the plasma albumin and soon thereafter conjugated about 80% with glucuronic acid to form *bilirubin glucuronide*, about 10% with sulfate to form *bilirubin sulfate*, and about 10% with a multitude of other substances. In these forms, the bilirubin is excreted from the hepatocytes by an active transport process into the bile canaliculi and then into the intestines.

Formation and Fate of Urobilinogen. Once in the intestine, about half of the "conjugated" bilirubin is converted by bacterial action into the substance *urobilinogen*, which is highly soluble. Some of the urobilinogen is reabsorbed through the intestinal mucosa back into the blood and most is reexcreted by the liver back into the gut, but about 5% is excreted by the kidneys into the urine. After exposure to air in the urine, the urobilinogen becomes oxidized to *urobilin*; alternatively, in the feces, it becomes altered and oxidized to form *stercobilin*. These interrelations of bilirubin and the other bilirubin products are shown in Figure 69-5.

JAUNDICE—EXCESS BILIRUBIN IN THE EXTRACELLULAR FLUID

Jaundice refers to a yellowish tint to the body tissues, including yellowness of the skin and deep tissues. This has been explained in detail in Chapter 23; please refer to this chapter for more details.

BIBLIOGRAPHY

Bernal W, Wendon J: Acute liver failure, *N. Engl. J. Med.* 369:2525, 2013.

Boyer JL: Bile formation and secretion, *Compr. Physiol.* 3:1035, 2013.

DeLeve LD: Liver sinusoidal endothelial cells and liver regeneration, *J. Clin. Invest.* 123:1861, 2013.

Diehl AM, Chute J: Underlying potential: cellular and molecular determinants of adult liver repair, *J. Clin. Invest.* 123:1858, 2013.

Dixon LJ, Barnes M, Tang H, et al: Kupffer cells in the liver, *Compr. Physiol.* 3:785, 2013.

Dockray GJ: Cholecystokinin and gut–brain signalling, *Regul. Pept.* 155:6, 2009.

Erlinger S, Arias IM, Dhumeaux D: Inherited disorders of bilirubin transport and conjugation: new insights into molecular mechanisms and consequences, *Gastroenterology* 146:1625, 2014.

Friedman SL: Hepatic stellate cells: protean, multifunctional, and enigmatic cells of the liver, *Physiol. Rev.* 88:125, 2008.

Gao B, Bataller R: Alcoholic liver disease: pathogenesis and new therapeutic targets, *Gastroenterology* 141:1572, 2011.

Hylemon PB, Zhou H, Pandak WM, Ren S, Gil G, Dent P: Bile acids as regulatory molecules, *J. Lipid Res.* 50:1509, 2009.

Jenne CN, Kubes P: Immune surveillance by the liver, *Nat. Immunol.* 14:996, 2013.

Lefebvre P, Cariou B, Lien F, et al: Role of bile acids and bile acid receptors in metabolic regulation, *Physiol. Rev.* 89:147, 2009.

Malhi H, Guicciardi ME, Gores GJ: Hepatocyte death: a clear and present danger, *Physiol. Rev.* 90:1165, 2010.

Pellicoro A, Ramachandran P, Iredale JP, Fallowfield JA: Liver fibrosis and repair: immune regulation of wound healing in a solid organ, *Nat. Rev. Immunol.* 14:181, 2014.

Perry RJ, Samuel VT, Petersen KF, Shulman GI: The role of hepatic lipids in hepatic insulin resistance and type 2 diabetes, *Nature* 510:84, 2014.

Portincasa P, Moschetta A, Palasciano G: Cholesterol gallstone disease, *Lancet* 368:230, 2006.

Portincasa P, Di Ciaula A, Wang HH, et al: Coordinate regulation of gallbladder motor function in the gut–liver axis, *Hepatology* 47:2112, 2008.

Russell DW: Fifty years of advances in bile acid synthesis and metabolism, *J. Lipid Res.* 50(Suppl.):S120, 2009.

Trauner M, Boyer JL: Bile salt transporters: molecular characterization, function, and regulation, *Physiol. Rev.* 83:633, 2003.

Tripodi A, Mannucci PM: The coagulopathy of chronic liver disease, *N. Engl. J. Med.* 365:147, 2011.

Tsochatzis EA, Bosch J, Burroughs AK: Liver cirrhosis, *Lancet* 383:1749, 2014.

Yin C, Evason KJ, Asahina K, Stainier DY: Hepatic stellate cells in liver development, regeneration, and cancer, *J. Clin. Invest.* 123:1902, 2013.

Digestion and Absorption of Carbohydrates

General Principles of Digestion

The major foods on which the body lives (with the exception of small quantities of substances such as vitamins and minerals) can be classified as *carbohydrates*, *fats*, and *proteins*. They generally cannot be absorbed in their natural forms through the gastrointestinal (GI) mucosa and, for this reason, they are useless as nutrients without preliminary digestion.

Digestion is a process that is characterized by a specific sequence of events following the ingestion of foods. These events allow the foods to interact with the various secretions such as enzymes, emulsifying agents, acid, or alkaline substances thereby facilitating the breakdown of complex molecules into simpler molecules under optimum pH. The various events associated with the process of digestion include the following:

1. Mixing and lubricating the food with secretions of the GI tract ensure uniform homogenization.
2. Enzymatic secretion from various glands and cells lining the GI tract breaks down complex molecules into simpler molecules such as oligomers, dimers, and monomers:
   a. All digestive enzymes act by hydrolysis.
   b. Most GI tract enzymes are secreted as inactive precursors, which are then activated in the GI tract.
3. Secretion of acid or bicarbonate from the GI tract ensures optimal pH for digestion.

4. In the case of fats, secretion of emulsifying agents such as bile acids helps in emulsifying dietary fat thereby promoting fat digestion.
5. Final digestion of most oligomers and dimers occurs at the small intestinal brush border resulting in release of monomers that are finally absorbed.

Therefore, this chapter discusses the processes by which carbohydrates are digested into small enough compounds for absorption and the mechanisms by which the digestive end products, as well as water, electrolytes, and other substances, are absorbed.

Digestion of the Various Foods by Hydrolysis

HYDROLYSIS OF CARBOHYDRATES

Almost all the carbohydrates of the diet are either large *polysaccharides* or *disaccharides*, which are combinations of *monosaccharides* bound to one another by *condensation*. This phenomenon means that a hydrogen ion (H^+) has been removed from one of the monosaccharides, and a hydroxyl ion (OH^-) has been removed from the next one. The two monosaccharides then combine with each other at these sites of removal, and the hydrogen and hydroxyl ions combine to form water (H_2O).

When carbohydrates are digested, this process is reversed and the carbohydrates are converted into monosaccharides. Specific enzymes in the digestive juices of the GI tract return the hydrogen and hydroxyl ions from water to the polysaccharides and thereby separate the monosaccharides from each other. This process, called *hydrolysis*, is the following (in which R''–R' is a disaccharide):

$$R'' - R' + H_2O \xrightarrow[\text{enzyme}]{\text{digestive}} R''OH + R'H$$

DIGESTION OF CARBOHYDRATES

Carbohydrate Foods of the Diet. Only three major sources of carbohydrates exist in the normal human diet. They are as follows:

1. *sucrose*, which is the disaccharide known popularly as cane sugar;
2. *lactose*, which is a disaccharide found in milk;
3. *starches*, which are large polysaccharides present in almost all nonanimal foods, particularly in potatoes and different types of grains;
4. other carbohydrates ingested to a slight extent, which are *amylose*, *glycogen*, *alcohol*, *lactic acid*, *pyruvic acid*, *pectins*, *dextrins*, and minor quantities of *carbohydrate derivatives in meats*.

The diet also contains a large amount of cellulose, which is a carbohydrate. However, no enzymes capable of hydrolyzing cellulose are secreted in the human digestive tract. Consequently, cellulose cannot be considered a food for humans.

Digestion of Carbohydrates Begins in the Mouth and Stomach. When food is chewed, it is mixed with saliva, which contains the digestive enzyme *ptyalin* (an α-amylase) secreted mainly by the parotid glands. This enzyme hydrolyzes starch into the disaccharide *maltose* and other small polymers of glucose that contain three to nine glucose molecules, as shown in Figure 70-1. However, the food remains in the mouth only for a short time, so probably not more than 5% of all the starches will have become hydrolyzed by the time the food is swallowed.

Starch digestion sometimes continues in the body and fundus of the stomach for as long as 1 hour before the food becomes mixed with the stomach secretions. Activity of the salivary amylase is then blocked by acid of the gastric secretions because the amylase is essentially inactive as an enzyme once the pH of the medium falls below about 4.0. Nevertheless, on average, before food and its accompanying saliva become completely mixed with the gastric secretions, as much as 30–40% of the starches will have been hydrolyzed mainly to form *maltose*.

DIGESTION OF CARBOHYDRATES IN THE SMALL INTESTINE

Digestion by Pancreatic Amylase. Pancreatic secretion, like saliva, contains a large quantity of α-amylase that is almost identical in its function to the α-amylase of saliva but is several times as powerful. Therefore, within 15–30 minutes after the chyme empties from the stomach into the duodenum and mixes with pancreatic juice, virtually all the carbohydrates will have become digested.

In general, the carbohydrates are almost totally converted into *maltose* and/or *other small glucose polymers* before passing beyond the duodenum or upper jejunum.

Hydrolysis of Disaccharides and Small Glucose Polymers into Monosaccharides by Intestinal Epithelial Enzymes. The enterocytes lining the villi of the small intestine contain four enzymes (*lactase, sucrase, maltase,* and *α-dextrinase*), which are capable of splitting the disaccharides lactose, sucrose, and maltose, plus other small glucose polymers, into their constituent monosaccharides. These enzymes are located *in the enterocytes covering the intestinal microvilli brush border,* so the disaccharides are digested as they come in contact with these enterocytes.

Lactose splits into a molecule of *galactose* and a molecule of *glucose*. Sucrose splits into a molecule of *fructose* and a molecule of *glucose*. Maltose and all other small glucose polymers split into *multiple molecules of glucose*. Thus, the final products of carbohydrate digestion are all monosaccharides. They are all water soluble and are absorbed immediately into the portal blood (Box 70-1).

The major steps in carbohydrate digestion are summarized in Figure 70-1.

Basic Principles of Gastrointestinal Absorption

It is suggested that the reader review the basic principles of transport of substances through cell membranes discussed in Chapter 4. The following paragraphs present specialized applications of these transport processes during GI absorption.

ANATOMICAL BASIS OF ABSORPTION

The total quantity of fluid that must be absorbed each day by the intestines is equal to the ingested fluid (about 1.5 L) plus that secreted in the various GI secretions (about 7 L), which comes to a total of 8–9 L. All but about 1.5 L of this fluid is absorbed in the small intestine, leaving only 1.5 L to pass through the ileocecal valve into the colon each day.

The stomach is a poor absorptive area of the GI tract because it lacks the typical villus type of absorptive membrane, and also because the junctions between the epithelial cells are tight junctions. Only a few highly lipid-soluble substances, such as alcohol and some drugs (eg, aspirin), can be absorbed in small quantities.

Folds of Kerckring, Villi, and Microvilli Increase the Mucosal Absorptive Area by Nearly 1000-Fold. Figure 70-2 demonstrates the absorptive surface of the small intestinal mucosa, showing many folds called *valvulae conniventes* (or *folds of Kerckring*), which increase the surface area of the absorptive mucosa about threefold.

Also located on the epithelial surface of the small intestine all the way down to the ileocecal valve are millions of small *villi*. These villi project about 1 mm from the surface of the mucosa, as shown on the surfaces of the valvulae conniventes in Figure 70-2 and in individual detail in Figure 70-3. The presence of villi on the mucosal surface enhances the total absorptive area another 10-fold.

Finally, each intestinal epithelial cell on each villus is characterized by a *brush border*, consisting of as many as 1000 *microvilli* that are 1 μm in length and 0.1 μm in diameter and protrude into the intestinal chyme. These microvilli are shown in the electron micrograph in Figure 70-4. This brush border increases the surface area exposed to the intestinal materials at least another 20-fold.

Thus, the combination of the folds of Kerckring, the villi, and the microvilli increases the total absorptive area of the mucosa perhaps 1000-fold, making a tremendous total area of 250 or more square meters for the entire small intestine—about the surface area of a tennis court.

Figure 70-3A shows in longitudinal section the general organization of the villus, emphasizing (1) the advantageous arrangement of the vascular system for absorption of fluid and dissolved material into the portal blood and (2) the arrangement of the "*central lacteal*" lymph vessel for absorption into the lymph. Figure 70-3B shows a cross-section of the villus, and Figure 70-4 shows many small *pinocytic vesicles*, which are pinched-off portions of infolded enterocyte membrane forming vesicles of absorbed fluids that have been entrapped. Small amounts of substances are absorbed by this physical process of *pinocytosis*.

Extending from the epithelial cell body into each microvillus of the brush border are multiple actin filaments that contract rhythmically to cause continual movement of the microvilli, keeping them constantly exposed to new quantities of intestinal fluid.

Absorption in the Small Intestine

Absorption from the small intestine each day consists of several hundred grams of carbohydrates, 100 or more grams of fat, 50–100 g of amino acids, 50–100 g of ions, and 7–8 L of water. The absorptive *capacity* of the normal small intestine is far greater than this; each day as much as several kilograms of

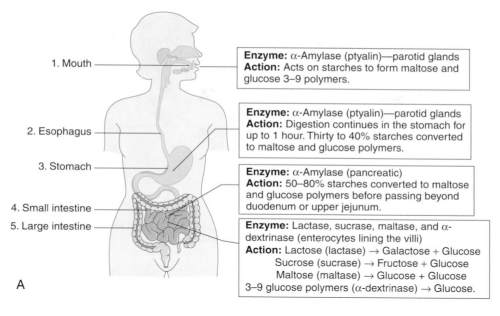

1. Mouth

> **Enzyme:** α-Amylase (ptyalin)—parotid glands
> **Action:** Acts on starches to form maltose and glucose 3–9 polymers.

2. Esophagus

3. Stomach

> **Enzyme:** α-Amylase (ptyalin)—parotid glands
> **Action:** Digestion continues in the stomach for up to 1 hour. Thirty to 40% starches converted to maltose and glucose polymers.

> **Enzyme:** α-Amylase (pancreatic)
> **Action:** 50–80% starches converted to maltose and glucose polymers before passing beyond duodenum or upper jejunum.

4. Small intestine

5. Large intestine

> **Enzyme:** Lactase, sucrase, maltase, and α-dextrinase (enterocytes lining the villi)
> **Action:** Lactose (lactase) → Galactose + Glucose
> Sucrose (sucrase) → Fructose + Glucose
> Maltose (maltase) → Glucose + Glucose
> 3–9 glucose polymers (α-dextrinase) → Glucose.

A

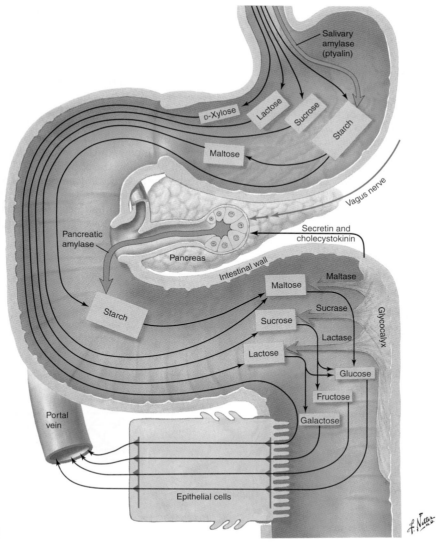

B

Figure 70-1 (A) Digestion of carbohydrates; (B) digestion and absorption of carbohydrates in the GI tract. *GI, gastrointestinal. (B) Netter illustration from www.netterimages.com. © Elsevier Inc. All rights reserved.*

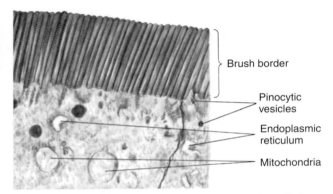

Figure 70-4 Brush border of a gastrointestinal epithelial cell, showing also absorbed pinocytic vesicles, mitochondria, and endoplasmic reticulum lying immediately beneath the brush border. *Courtesy Dr. William Lockwood.*

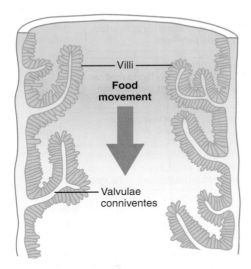

Figure 70-2 Longitudinal section of the small intestine, showing the valvulae conniventes covered by villi.

carbohydrates, 500 g of fat, 500–700 g of proteins, and 20 or more liters of water can be absorbed. The *large* intestine can absorb still more water and ions, although it can absorb very few nutrients.

Isosmotic Absorption of Water. Water is transported through the intestinal membrane entirely by *diffusion*. Furthermore, this diffusion obeys the usual laws of osmosis. Therefore, when the chyme is dilute enough, water is absorbed through the intestinal mucosa into the blood of the villi almost entirely by osmosis.

Conversely, water can also be transported in the opposite direction—from plasma into the chyme. This type of transport occurs especially when hyperosmotic solutions are discharged from the stomach into the duodenum. Within minutes sufficient water usually will be transferred by osmosis to make the chyme isosmotic with the plasma.

ABSORPTION OF IONS

Sodium Is Actively Transported Through the Intestinal Membrane. Twenty to thirty grams of sodium is secreted in the intestinal secretions each day. In addition, the average person eats 5–8 g of sodium each day. Therefore, to prevent net loss of sodium into the feces, the intestines must absorb 25–35 g of sodium each day, which is equal to about one-seventh of all the sodium present in the body.

Whenever significant amounts of intestinal secretions are lost to the exterior, as in extreme diarrhea, the sodium reserves of the body can sometimes be depleted to lethal levels within hours. Normally, however, less than 0.5% of the intestinal

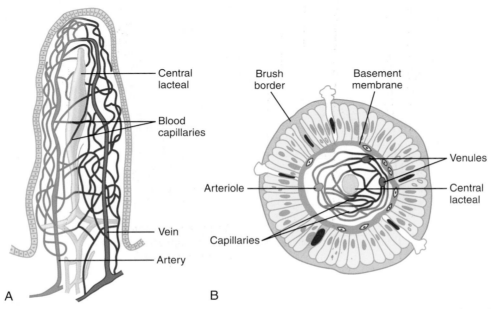

Figure 70-3 Functional organization of the villus. (A) Longitudinal section; (B) Cross-section showing a basement membrane beneath the epithelial cells and a brush border at the other ends of these cells.

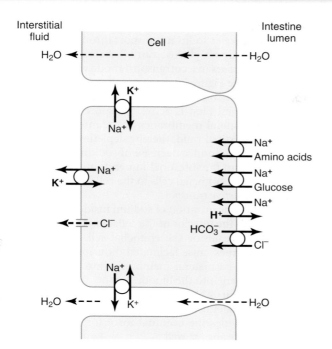

Figure 70-5 Absorption of sodium, chloride, glucose, and amino acids through the intestinal epithelium. Note also osmotic absorption of water (ie, water "follows" sodium through the epithelial membrane).

sodium is lost in the feces each day because it is rapidly absorbed through the intestinal mucosa. Sodium also plays an important role in helping to absorb sugars and amino acids, as subsequent discussions reveal.

The basic mechanism of sodium absorption from the intestine is shown in Figure 70-5.

Sodium absorption is powered by active transport of sodium from inside the epithelial cells through the basal and lateral walls of these cells into paracellular spaces. This active transport obeys the usual laws of active transport: It requires energy, and the energy process is catalyzed by appropriate adenosine triphosphatase (ATPase) enzymes in the cell membrane (see Chapter 4). Part of the sodium is absorbed along with chloride ions; in fact, the negatively charged chloride ions are mainly passively "dragged" by the positive electrical charges of the sodium ions.

Active transport of sodium through the basolateral membranes of the cell reduces the sodium concentration inside the cell to a low value ($\sim$50 mEq/L), as shown in Figure 70-5. Because the sodium concentration in the chyme is normally about 142 mEq/L (ie, about equal to that in plasma), sodium moves down this steep electrochemical gradient from the chyme through the brush border of the epithelial cell into the epithelial cell cytoplasm. Sodium is also cotransported through the brush border membrane by several specific carrier proteins, including (1) the sodium–glucose cotransporter, (2) sodium–amino acid cotransporters, and (3) the sodium–hydrogen exchanger.

Osmosis of the Water. The next step in the transport process is osmosis of water by transcellular and paracellular pathways. This osmosis occurs because a large osmotic gradient has been created by the elevated concentration of ions in the paracellular space. Much of this osmosis occurs through the tight junctions between the apical borders of the epithelial cells (the paracellular pathway), but much also occurs through the cells themselves (the transcellular pathway). Osmotic movement of water creates flow of fluid into and through the paracellular spaces and, finally, into the circulating blood of the villus.

Aldosterone Greatly Enhances Sodium Absorption. When a person becomes dehydrated, large amounts of aldosterone are secreted by the cortices of the adrenal glands. Within 1–3 hours this aldosterone causes increased activation of the enzyme and transport mechanisms for all aspects of sodium absorption by the intestinal epithelium. The increased sodium absorption in turn causes secondary increases in absorption of chloride ions, water, and some other substances.

This effect of aldosterone is especially important in the colon because it allows virtually no loss of sodium chloride in the feces and also little water loss. Thus, the function of aldosterone in the intestinal tract is the same as that achieved by aldosterone in the renal tubules, which also serves to conserve sodium chloride and water in the body when a person becomes depleted of sodium chloride and dehydrated.

Absorption of Chloride Ions in the Small Intestine. In the upper part of the small intestine, chloride ion absorption is rapid and occurs mainly by diffusion (ie, absorption of sodium ions through the epithelium creates electronegativity in the chyme and electropositivity in the paracellular spaces between the epithelial cells). Chloride ions then move along this electrical gradient to "follow" the sodium ions. Chloride is also absorbed across the brush border membrane of parts of the ileum and large intestine by a brush border membrane chloride–bicarbonate exchanger. Chloride exits the cell on the basolateral membrane through chloride channels.

Absorption of Bicarbonate Ions in the Duodenum and Jejunum. Often large quantities of bicarbonate ions must be reabsorbed from the upper small intestine because large amounts of bicarbonate ions have been secreted into the duodenum in both pancreatic secretion and bile. The bicarbonate ion is absorbed in an indirect way as follows: When sodium ions are absorbed, moderate amounts of hydrogen ions are secreted into the lumen of the gut in exchange for some of the sodium. These hydrogen ions in turn combine with the bicarbonate ions to form carbonic acid (H_2CO_3), which then dissociates to form water and carbon dioxide. The water remains as part of the chyme in the intestines, but the carbon dioxide is readily absorbed into the blood and subsequently expired through the lungs. This process is the so-called "active absorption of bicarbonate ions." It is the same mechanism that occurs in the tubules of the kidneys.

Secretion of Bicarbonate and Absorption of Chloride Ions in the Ileum and Large Intestine

The epithelial cells on the surfaces of the villi in the ileum, as well as on all surfaces of the large intestine, have a special capability of secreting bicarbonate ions in exchange for absorption of chloride ions (see Figure 70-5). This capability is important because it provides alkaline bicarbonate ions that neutralize acid products formed by bacteria in the large intestine.

Active Absorption of Calcium, Iron, Potassium, Magnesium, and Phosphate. *Calcium ions* are actively absorbed into the blood, especially from the duodenum, and the amount of calcium ion absorption is exactly controlled to supply the daily need of the body for calcium. One important factor controlling calcium absorption is *parathyroid hormone* secreted by the parathyroid glands and another is *vitamin D*. Parathyroid hormone activates vitamin D, and the activated vitamin D in turn greatly enhances calcium absorption. These effects are discussed in Chapter 90.

Iron ions are also actively absorbed from the small intestine. The principles of iron absorption and regulation of its absorption in proportion to the body's need for iron, especially for the formation of hemoglobin, are discussed in Chapter 21.

Potassium, magnesium, phosphate, and probably *still other ions* can also be actively absorbed through the intestinal mucosa. In general, the monovalent ions are absorbed with ease and in great quantities. Bivalent ions are normally absorbed in only small amounts; for example, maximum absorption of calcium ions is only 1/50 as great as the normal absorption of sodium ions. Fortunately, only small quantities of the bivalent ions are normally required daily by the body.

ABSORPTION OF CARBOHYDRATES

Carbohydrates Are Mainly Absorbed as Monosaccharides

Essentially all the carbohydrates in food are absorbed in the form of monosaccharides; only a small fraction is absorbed as disaccharides and almost none is absorbed as larger carbohydrate compounds. By far the most abundant of the absorbed monosaccharides is *glucose*, which usually accounts for more than 80% of the carbohydrate calories absorbed. The reason for this high percentage is that glucose is the final digestion product of our most abundant carbohydrate food, the starches. The remaining 20% of absorbed monosaccharides is composed almost entirely of *galactose* and *fructose*, the galactose derived from milk and the fructose as one of the monosaccharides digested from cane sugar. The steps in carbohydrate digestion and absorption are summarized in Figure 70-1.

Virtually all the monosaccharides are absorbed by a secondary active transport process. We will first discuss the absorption of glucose.

Glucose Is Transported by a Sodium Cotransport Mechanism. In the absence of sodium transport through the intestinal membrane, virtually no glucose can be absorbed because glucose absorption occurs in a cotransport mode with active transport of sodium (see Figure 70-5).

The transport of sodium through the intestinal membrane occurs in two stages. First is active transport of sodium ions through the basolateral membranes of the intestinal epithelial cells into the interstitial fluid, thereby depleting sodium inside the epithelial cells. Second, a decrease of sodium inside the cells causes sodium from the intestinal lumen to move through the brush border of the epithelial cells to the cell interiors by a process of *secondary active transport.*

Thus, the low concentration of sodium inside the cell literally "drags" sodium to the interior of the cell and glucose is dragged along with it. Once inside the epithelial cell, other transport proteins and enzymes cause facilitated diffusion of the glucose through the cell's basolateral membrane into the paracellular space and from there into the blood.

To summarize, it is the initial active transport of sodium through the basolateral membranes of the intestinal epithelial cells that provides the eventual force for moving glucose through the membranes as well.

Absorption of Other Monosaccharides. Galactose is transported by almost exactly the same mechanism as glucose. Fructose transport does not occur by the sodium cotransport mechanism. Instead, fructose is transported by facilitated diffusion all the way through the intestinal epithelium and is not coupled with sodium transport.

Much of the fructose, on entering the cell, becomes phosphorylated. It is then converted to glucose, and finally transported in the form of glucose the rest of the way into the blood. Because fructose is not cotransported with sodium, its overall rate of transport is only about one-half that of glucose or galactose.

BIBLIOGRAPHY

Bachmann O, Juric M, Seidler U, et al: Basolateral ion transporters involved in colonic epithelial electrolyte absorption, anion secretion and cellular homeostasis, *Acta Physiol. (Oxf.)* 201:33, 2011.

Bronner F: Recent developments in intestinal calcium absorption, *Nutr. Rev.* 67:109, 2009.

Kunzelmann K, Mall M: Electrolyte transport in the mammalian colon: mechanisms and implications for disease, *Physiol. Rev.* 82:245, 2002.

Rothman S, Liebow C, Isenman L: Conservation of digestive enzymes, *Physiol. Rev.* 82:1, 2002.

Seidler UE: Gastrointestinal HCO_3^- transport and epithelial protection in the gut: new techniques, transport pathways and regulatory pathways, *Curr. Opin. Pharmacol.* 13:900, 2013.

Wright EM, Loo DD, Hirayama BA: Biology of human sodium glucose transporters, *Physiol. Rev.* 291:733, 2011.

Digestion and Absorption of Proteins

GLOSSARY OF TERMS

- **Amino acids:** Any group of organic compounds containing one or more amino groups ($-NH_2$), and one or more carboxyl groups ($-COOH$) (they combine together to form proteins)

- **Peptide linkage:** Amino acids bound together by the process of condensation where a peptide linkage is formed when a hydroxyl ion is removed from one amino acid and hydrogen is removed from the succeeding amino acid

- **Peptones:** Derivatives of proteins that are formed by partial hydrolysis of a protein

- **Polypeptides:** Peptides containing many amino acids, typically anything between 10 and 100 amino acids

- **Proteolytic enzymes:** Enzymes that help with hydrolytic breakdown of proteins into simpler, soluble substances, as occurs in digestion

- **Proteoses:** A mixture of split products formed by the hydrolysis of proteins or polypeptides

Hydrolysis of Proteins

Proteins are formed from multiple *amino acids* that are bound together by *peptide linkages*. At each linkage, a hydroxyl ion has been removed from one amino acid and a hydrogen ion has been removed from the succeeding one; thus, the successive amino acids in the protein chain are also bound together by condensation, and digestion occurs by the reverse effect: hydrolysis. That is, the proteolytic enzymes return hydrogen and hydroxyl ions from water molecules to the protein molecules to split them into their constituent amino acids.

Therefore, the chemistry of digestion is simple because in the case of all three major types of food, the same basic process of *hydrolysis* is involved. The only difference lies in the types of enzymes required to promote the hydrolysis reactions for each type of food. All the digestive enzymes are proteins.

DIGESTION OF PROTEINS

Proteins of the Diet. Dietary proteins are chemically long chains of amino acids bound together by *peptide linkages*. A typical linkage is the following:

The characteristics of each protein are determined by the types of amino acids in the protein molecule and by the sequential arrangements of these amino acids.

Digestion of Proteins in the Stomach. *Pepsin*, an important peptic enzyme of the stomach, is most active at a pH of 2.0–3.0 and is inactive at a pH above about 5.0. Consequently, for this enzyme to cause digestion of protein the stomach juices must be acidic. As explained in Chapter 67, the gastric glands secrete a large quantity of hydrochloric acid. This hydrochloric acid is secreted by the parietal (oxyntic) cells in the glands at a pH of about 0.8, but by the time it is mixed with the stomach contents and with secretions from the nonoxyntic glandular cells of the stomach, the pH then averages around 2.0–3.0, a highly favorable range of acidity for pepsin activity.

One of the important features of pepsin digestion is its ability to digest the protein *collagen* that is affected little by other digestive enzymes. Collagen is a major constituent of the intercellular connective tissue of meats; therefore, for the digestive enzymes to penetrate meats and digest the other meat proteins, it is necessary that the collagen fibers be digested. Consequently, in persons who lack pepsin in the stomach juices, the ingested meats are less well penetrated by the other digestive enzymes and, therefore, may be poorly digested.

As shown in Figure 71-1A and B pepsin only initiates the process of protein digestion, usually providing only 10–20% of the total protein digestion to convert the protein to proteoses, peptones, and a few polypeptides. This splitting of proteins occurs as a result of hydrolysis at the peptide linkages between amino acids.

Most Protein Digestion Results from Actions of Pancreatic Proteolytic Enzymes. Most protein digestion occurs in the upper small intestine, in the duodenum and jejunum, under the influence of proteolytic enzymes from pancreatic secretion. Immediately on entering the small intestine from the stomach the partial breakdown products of the protein foods are attacked by the major proteolytic pancreatic enzymes: *trypsin, chymotrypsin, carboxypolypeptidase,* and *elastase,* as shown in Figure 71-1A and B.

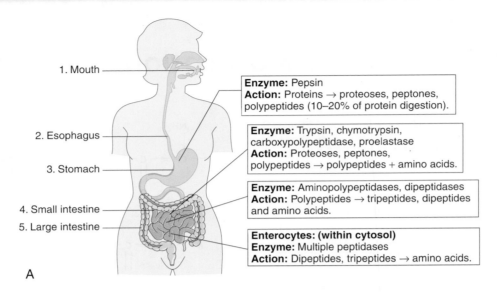

1. Mouth

Enzyme: Pepsin
Action: Proteins → proteoses, peptones, polypeptides (10–20% of protein digestion).

2. Esophagus

3. Stomach

Enzyme: Trypsin, chymotrypsin, carboxypolypeptidase, proelastase
Action: Proteoses, peptones, polypeptides → polypeptides + amino acids.

Enzyme: Aminopolypeptidases, dipeptidases
Action: Polypeptides → tripeptides, dipeptides and amino acids.

4. Small intestine

5. Large intestine

Enterocytes: (within cytosol)
Enzyme: Multiple peptidases
Action: Dipeptides, tripeptides → amino acids.

A

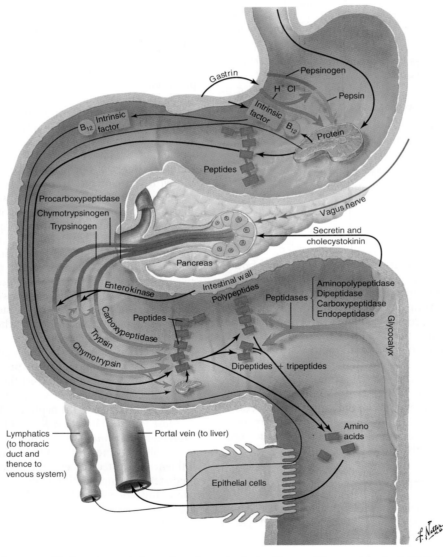

B

Figure 71-1   (A) Digestion of proteins; (B) digestion and absorption of proteins in the GI tract. *GI,* gastrointestinal. *(B) Netter illustration from www. netterimages.com. © Elsevier Inc. All rights reserved.*

Both trypsin and chymotrypsin split protein molecules into small polypeptides; carboxypolypeptidase then cleaves individual amino acids from the carboxyl ends of the polypeptides. *Proelastase*, in turn, is converted into *elastase*, which then digests elastin fibers that partially hold meats together.

Only a small percentage of the proteins are digested all the way to their constituent amino acids by the pancreatic juices. Most remain as dipeptides and tripeptides.

Digestion of Peptides by Peptidases in the Enterocytes that Line the Small Intestinal Villi. The last digestive stage of the proteins in the intestinal lumen is achieved by the enterocytes that line the villi of the small intestine, mainly in the duodenum and jejunum. These cells have a *brush border* that consists of hundreds of *microvilli* projecting from the surface of each cell. In the membrane of each of these microvilli are multiple *peptidases* that protrude through the membranes to the exterior, where they come in contact with the intestinal fluids.

Two types of peptidase enzymes are especially important, *aminopolypeptidase* and several *dipeptidases*. They split the remaining larger polypeptides into tripeptides and dipeptides and a few into amino acids. The amino acids, dipeptides, and tripeptides are easily transported through the microvillar membrane to the interior of the enterocyte.

Finally, inside the cytosol of the enterocyte are multiple other peptidases that are specific for the remaining types of linkages between amino acids. Within minutes, virtually all the last dipeptides and tripeptides are digested to the final stage to form single amino acids, which then pass on through to the other side of the enterocyte and thence into the blood.

More than 99% of the final protein digestive products that are absorbed are individual amino acids, with only rare absorption of peptides and very rare absorption of whole protein molecules. Even these few absorbed molecules of whole protein can sometimes cause serious allergic or immunologic disturbances, as discussed in Chapter 25.

Basic Principles of Gastrointestinal Absorption

The basic principles of gastrointestinal (GI) absorption have been discussed in Chapter 70. Please refer to Chapter 70 for further details.

ABSORPTION OF PROTEINS AS DIPEPTIDES, TRIPEPTIDES, OR AMINO ACIDS

As explained earlier, most proteins after digestion are absorbed through the luminal membranes of the intestinal epithelial cells in the form of dipeptides, tripeptides, and a few free amino acids. The energy for most of this transport is supplied by a sodium cotransport mechanism in the same way that sodium cotransport of glucose occurs. That is, most peptide or amino acid molecules bind in the cell's microvillus membrane with a specific transport protein that requires sodium binding before transport can occur. After binding, the sodium ion then moves down its electrochemical gradient to the interior of the cell and pulls the amino acid or peptide along with it. This process is called *cotransport* (or *secondary active transport*) *of the amino acids and peptides*. A few amino acids do not require this sodium cotransport mechanism but instead are transported by special membrane transport proteins in the same way that fructose is transported, by facilitated diffusion.

At least five types of transport proteins for amino acids and peptides have been found in the luminal membranes of intestinal epithelial cells. This multiplicity of transport proteins is required because of the diverse binding properties of different amino acids and peptides.

BIBLIOGRAPHY

Bachmann O, Juric M, Seidler U, et al: Basolateral ion transporters involved in colonic epithelial electrolyte absorption, anion secretion and cellular homeostasis, *Acta Physiol. (Oxf.)* 201:33, 2011.

Bröer S: Amino acid transport across mammalian intestinal and renal epithelia, *Physiol. Rev.* 88:249, 2008a.

Bröer S: Apical transporters for neutral amino acids: physiology and pathophysiology, *Physiology (Bethesda)* 23:95, 2008b.

Rothman S, Liebow C, Isenman L: Conservation of digestive enzymes, *Physiol. Rev.* 82:1, 2002.

Seidler UE: Gastrointestinal HCO_3^- transport and epithelial protection in the gut: new techniques,

transport pathways and regulatory pathways, *Curr. Opin. Pharmacol.* 13:900, 2013.

Wright EM, Loo DD, Hirayama BA: Biology of human sodium glucose transporters, *Physiol. Rev.* 291:733, 2011.

72

Digestion and Absorption of Fats

LEARNING OBJECTIVE

- Describe the steps involved in the breakdown and absorption of fats.

GLOSSARY OF TERMS

- **Emulsification:** The process of breaking up large fat globules into smaller globules with the help of bile salts and lecithin and agitation

- **Lecithin:** A class of phospholipids containing glycerol, phosphate, choline, and fatty acids (they help in the emulsification of fats during the process of fat digestion)

- **Micelles:** Small spherical, cylindrical globules 3–6 nm in diameter composed of 20–40 molecules of bile salts and help in the digestion and absorption of fats

- **Triglycerides:** The combination of three *fatty acid* molecules condensed with a single *glycerol* molecule

Digestion of the Various Foods by Hydrolysis

HYDROLYSIS OF FATS

Almost the entire fat portion of the diet consists of triglycerides (neutral fats), which are combinations of three *fatty acid* molecules condensed with a single *glycerol* molecule. During condensation, three molecules of water are removed.

Hydrolysis (digestion) of the triglycerides consists of the reverse process: the fat-digesting enzymes return three molecules of water to the triglyceride molecule and thereby split the fatty acid molecules away from the glycerol.

DIGESTION OF FATS

Fats of the Diet. By far the most abundant fats of the diet are the neutral fats, also known as *triglycerides*, each molecule of which is composed of a glycerol nucleus and three fatty acid side chains, as shown in Figure 72-1. Neutral fat is a major constituent in food of animal origin, but much less so in food of plant origin.

Small quantities of phospholipids, cholesterol, and cholesterol esters are also present in the usual diet. The phospholipids and cholesterol esters contain fatty acid and therefore can be considered fats. Cholesterol is a sterol compound that contains no fatty acid, but it does exhibit some of the physical and chemical characteristics of fats; in addition, it is derived from fats and is metabolized similarly to fats. Therefore, cholesterol is considered, from a dietary point of view, to be a fat.

Digestion of Fats Occurs Mainly in the Small Intestine. A small amount of triglycerides is digested *in the stomach* by *lingual lipase* secreted by lingual glands in the mouth and swallowed with the saliva. The stomach also secretes small amounts of gastric lipase from the fundic area. This amount of digestion is less than 10% and is generally unimportant. Instead, essentially all fat digestion occurs in the small intestine as follows.

Steps in Fat Digestion

Emulsification by Bile Acids and Lecithin. The first step in fat digestion is to physically break the fat globules into small sizes so that the water-soluble digestive enzymes can act on the globule surfaces. This process is called *emulsification of the fat*, and it begins by agitation in the stomach to mix the fat with the products of stomach digestion.

Most of the emulsification then occurs in the duodenum under the influence of *bile*, which contains large quantities of *bile salts* as well as the phospholipid *lecithin*. Both of these substances, *but especially the lecithin*, are extremely important for emulsification of the fat. The polar parts (ie, the points where ionization occurs in water) of the bile salts and lecithin molecules are highly soluble in water, whereas most of the remaining portions of their molecules are highly soluble in fat. Therefore, the fat-soluble portions of these liver secretions dissolve in the surface layer of the fat globules, with the polar portions projecting. The polar projections, in turn, are soluble in the surrounding watery fluids, which greatly decreases the interfacial tension of the fat and makes it soluble as well.

When the interfacial tension of a globule of nonmiscible fluid is low, this nonmiscible fluid, on agitation, can be broken up into many tiny particles far more easily than it can when the interfacial tension is great. Consequently, a major function of the bile salts and lecithin (especially the lecithin) in the bile is to make the fat globules readily fragmentable by agitation with the water in the small bowel. This action is the same as that of many detergents that are widely used in household cleaners for removing grease.

Because the average diameter of the fat particles in the intestine after emulsification has occurred is less than 1 μm, this represents an increase of as much as 1000-fold in total surface areas of the fats caused by the emulsification process.

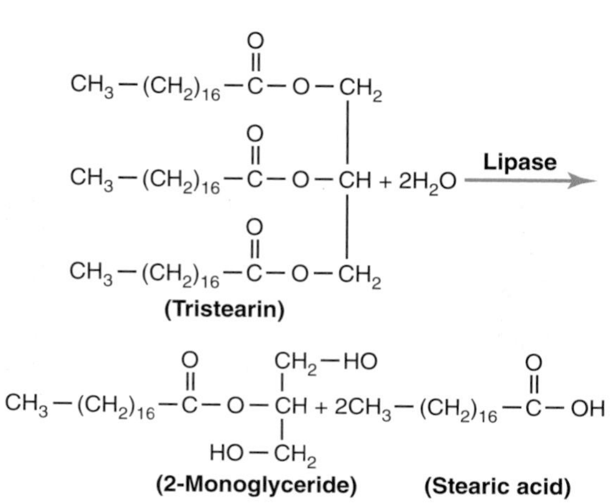

Figure 72-1 Hydrolysis of neutral fat catalyzed by lipase.

457

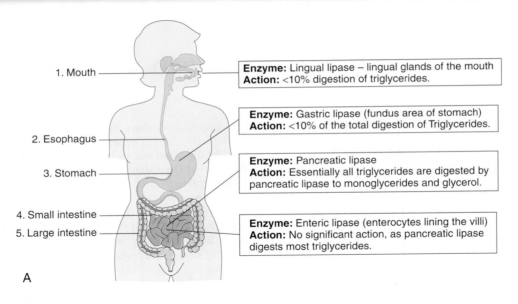

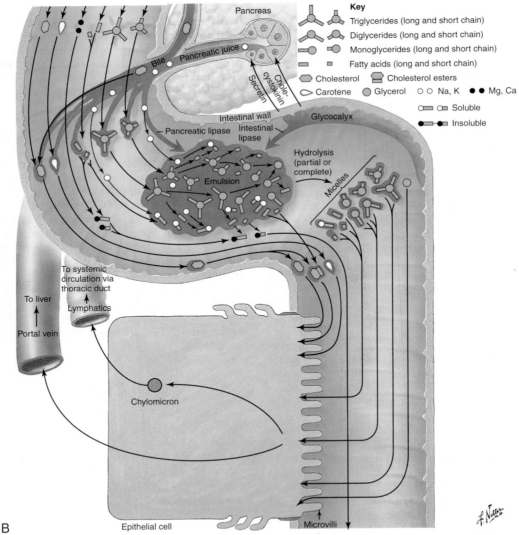

Figure 72-2 (A) Digestion of fats; (B) digestion and absorption of fats. *(B) Netter illustration from www.netterimages.com.*

The lipase enzymes are water-soluble compounds and can attack the fat globules only on their surfaces. Consequently, this detergent function of bile salts and lecithin is very important for digestion of fats.

Triglycerides are Digested by Pancreatic Lipase. By far the most important enzyme for digestion of the triglycerides is *pancreatic lipase*, present in enormous quantities in pancreatic juice, enough to digest within 1 minute all triglycerides that it can reach. The enterocytes of the small intestine contain additional lipase, known as *enteric lipase*, but it is usually not needed.

End Products of Fat Digestion are Free Fatty Acids. Most of the triglycerides of the diet are split by pancreatic lipase into *free fatty acids* and *2-monoglycerides*, as shown in Figure 72-2A and B.

Bile Salts Form Micelles that Accelerate Fat Digestion. The hydrolysis of triglycerides is a highly reversible process; therefore, accumulation of monoglycerides and free fatty acids in the vicinity of digesting fats quickly blocks further digestion. However, the bile salts play the additional important role of removing the monoglycerides and free fatty acids from the vicinity of the digesting fat globules almost as rapidly as these end products of digestion are formed. This process occurs in the following way.

When bile salts are of a high enough concentration in water, they have the propensity to form *micelles*, which are small spherical, cylindrical globules 3–6 nm in diameter composed of 20–40 molecules of bile salt. These micelles develop because each bile salt molecule is composed of a sterol nucleus that is highly fat soluble and a polar group that is highly water soluble. The sterol nucleus encompasses the fat digestate, forming a small fat globule in the middle of a resulting micelle, with polar groups of bile salts projecting outward to cover the surface of the micelle. Because these polar groups are negatively charged, they allow the entire micelle globule to dissolve in the water of the digestive fluids and to remain in stable solution until the fat is absorbed into the blood.

The bile salt micelles also act as a transport medium to carry the monoglycerides and free fatty acids, both of which would otherwise be relatively insoluble to the brush borders of the intestinal epithelial cells where they are absorbed into the blood.

Digestion of Cholesterol Esters and Phospholipids. Most cholesterol in the diet is in the form of cholesterol esters, which are combinations of free cholesterol and one molecule of fatty acid. Phospholipids also contain fatty acid within their molecules. Both the cholesterol esters and the phospholipids are hydrolyzed by two other lipases in the pancreatic secretion that free the fatty acids—the enzyme *cholesterol ester hydrolase* to hydrolyze the cholesterol ester and *phospholipase A₂* to hydrolyze the phospholipid.

The bile salt micelles play the same role in "ferrying" free cholesterol and phospholipid molecule digestates that they play in "ferrying" monoglycerides and free fatty acids. Indeed, essentially no cholesterol is absorbed without this function of the micelles.

Absorption in the Small Intestine
ABSORPTION OF FATS

Earlier in this chapter, it was pointed out that when fats are digested to form monoglycerides and free fatty acids, both of these digestive end products first become dissolved in the central lipid portions of *bile micelles*. Because the molecular dimensions of these micelles are only 3–6 nm in diameter, and because of their highly charged exterior, they are soluble in chyme. In this form, the monoglycerides and free fatty acids are carried to the surfaces of the microvilli of the intestinal cell brush border and then penetrate into the recesses among the moving, agitating microvilli. Here, both the monoglycerides and fatty acids diffuse immediately out of the micelles and into the interior of the epithelial cells, which is possible because the lipids are also soluble in the epithelial cell membrane. This process leaves the bile micelles still in the chyme, where they function again and again to help absorb still more monoglycerides and fatty acids.

Thus, the micelles perform a "ferrying" function that is highly important for fat absorption. In the presence of an abundance of bile micelles about 97% of the fat is absorbed; in the absence of the bile micelles only 40–50% can be absorbed.

After entering the epithelial cell, the fatty acids and monoglycerides are taken up by the cell's smooth endoplasmic reticulum; here they are mainly used to form new triglycerides that are subsequently released in the form of *chylomicrons* through the base of the epithelial cell to flow upward through the thoracic lymph duct and empty into the circulating blood.

Direct Absorption of Fatty Acids into the Portal Blood. Small quantities of short- and medium-chain fatty acids, such as those from butterfat, are absorbed directly into the portal blood rather than being converted into triglycerides and absorbed by way of the lymphatics. The cause of this difference between short- and long-chain fatty acid absorption is that the short-chain fatty acids are more water soluble and mostly are not reconverted into triglycerides by the endoplasmic reticulum. This phenomenon allows direct diffusion of these short-chain fatty acids from the intestinal epithelial cells directly into the capillary blood of the intestinal villi.

BIBLIOGRAPHY

Abumrad NA, Davidson NO: Role of the gut in lipid homeostasis, *Physiol. Rev.* 92:1061, 2012.

Bachmann O, Juric M, Seidler U, et al: Basolateral ion transporters involved in colonic epithelial electrolyte absorption, anion secretion and cellular homeostasis, *Acta Physiol. (Oxf.)* 201:33, 2011.

Black DD: Development and physiological regulation of intestinal lipid absorption. I. Development of intestinal lipid absorption: cellular events in chylomicron assembly and secretion, *Am. J. Physiol. Gastrointest. Liver Physiol.* 293:G519, 2007.

Hamosh M: Lingual and gastric lipases, *Nutrition* 6:421, 1990.

Hui DY, Labonté ED, Howles PN: Development and physiological regulation of intestinal lipid absorption. III. Intestinal transporters and cholesterol absorption, *Am. J. Physiol. Gastrointest. Liver Physiol.* 294:G839, 2008.

Iqbal J, Hussain MM: Intestinal lipid absorption, *Am. J. Physiol. Endocrinol. Metab.* 296:E1183, 2009.

Rothman S, Liebow C, Isenman L: Conservation of digestive enzymes, *Physiol. Rev.* 82:1, 2002.

Seidler UE: Gastrointestinal HCO₃⁻ transport and epithelial protection in the gut: new techniques, transport pathways and regulatory pathways, *Curr. Opin. Pharmacol.* 13:900, 2013.

Williams KJ: Molecular processes that handle—and mishandle—dietary lipids, *J. Clin. Invest.* 118:3247, 2008.

Wright EM, Loo DD, Hirayama BA: Biology of human sodium glucose transporters, *Physiol. Rev.* 291:733, 2011.

73

Functions of the Large Intestine

LEARNING OBJECTIVES

- List the composition of large intestinal secretion.
- List the functions of large intestine in relation to water and electrolyte absorption, and gut fermentation.

GLOSSARY OF TERMS

- **Crypts of Lieberkühn:** Invaginations of the epithelium into the submucosa and contain specialized secretory cells (they are found in the small intestine and the large intestine)
- **Enteritis:** Inflammation of the intestine

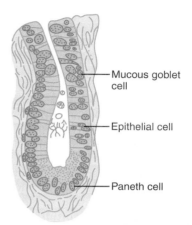

Figure 73-1 A *crypt of Lieberkühn*, found in all parts of the small intestine and large intestine between the villi, which secretes almost pure extracellular fluid.

Secretion of Mucus by the Large Intestine

Mucus Secretion. The mucosa of the large intestine, like that of the small intestine, has many crypts of Lieberkühn; however, unlike the small intestine, it contains no villi (Box 73-1). The epithelial cells secrete almost no digestive enzymes. Instead, they contain mucous cells that secrete only *mucus*. This mucus contains moderate amounts of bicarbonate ions secreted by a few nonmucus-secreting epithelial cells. The rate of secretion of mucus is regulated principally by direct, tactile stimulation of the epithelial cells lining the large intestine and by local nervous reflexes to the mucous cells in the crypts of Lieberkühn (Figure 73-1).

Stimulation of the *pelvic nerves* from the spinal cord, which carry *parasympathetic innervation* to the distal one-half to two-thirds of the large intestine, also can cause marked increase in mucus secretion. This increase occurs along with an increase in peristaltic motility of the colon, which is discussed in Chapter 74.

During extreme parasympathetic stimulation, often caused by emotional disturbances, so much mucus can occasionally be secreted into the large intestine that the person has a bowel movement of ropy mucus as often as every 30 minutes; this mucus often contains little or no fecal material.

BOX 73-1 COMPOSITION OF THE LARGE INTESTINAL SECRETION

The large intestine secretions contain the following:
1. Water
2. Mucus
3. Na^+
4. Cl^-
5. Bicarbonate
6. K^+
7. Ca^{++}

Functions of the Mucus Secretion. Mucus in the large intestine protects the intestinal wall against excoriation.
1. It provides an adherent medium for holding fecal matter together.
2. It protects the intestinal wall from the great amount of bacterial activity that takes place inside the feces.
3. The mucus plus the alkalinity of the secretion (pH of 8.0 caused by large amounts of sodium bicarbonate) provides a barrier to keep acids formed in the feces from attacking the intestinal wall.

Diarrhea Caused by Excess Secretion of Water and Electrolytes in Response to Irritation. Whenever a segment of the large intestine becomes intensely irritated, as occurs when bacterial infection becomes rampant during *enteritis*, the mucosa secretes extra large quantities of water and electrolytes in addition to the normal viscid alkaline mucus. This secretion acts to dilute the irritating factors and to cause rapid movement of the feces toward the anus. The result is *diarrhea*, with loss of large quantities of water and electrolytes. However, the diarrhea also washes away irritant factors, which promotes earlier recovery from the disease than might otherwise occur.

Extreme Secretion of Chloride Ions, Sodium Ions, and Water from the Large Intestinal Epithelium in Some Types of Diarrhea. Immature epithelial cells that continually divide to form new epithelial cells are found deep in the spaces between the intestinal epithelial folds. These new epithelial cells spread outward over the luminal surfaces of the intestines. While still in the deep folds, the epithelial cells secrete sodium chloride and water into the intestinal lumen. This secretion in turn is reabsorbed by the older epithelial cells outside the folds, thus providing flow of water for absorbing intestinal digestates.

The toxins of cholera and of some other types of diarrheal bacteria can stimulate the epithelial fold secretion so greatly

461

that this secretion often becomes much greater than can be re-absorbed, thus sometimes causing a loss of 5–10 L of water and sodium chloride as *diarrhea* each day. Within 1–5 days many severely affected patients die of this loss of fluid alone.

Extreme diarrheal secretion is initiated by entry of a subunit of cholera toxin into the epithelial cells. This subunit stimulates formation of excess cyclic adenosine monophosphate, which opens tremendous numbers of chloride channels, allowing chloride ions to flow rapidly from inside the cell into the intestinal crypts. In turn, this action is believed to activate a sodium pump that pumps sodium ions into the crypts to go along with the chloride ions. Finally, all this extra sodium chloride causes extreme osmosis of water from the blood, thus providing rapid flow of fluid along with the salt. All this excess fluid washes away most of the bacteria and is of value in combating the disease, but too much of a good thing can be lethal because of serious dehydration of the whole body that might ensue. In most instances, the life of a person with cholera can be saved by the administration of tremendous amounts of sodium chloride solution to make up for the loss.

Absorption in the Large Intestine: Formation of Feces

About 1500 mL of chyme normally passes through the ileocecal valve into the large intestine each day. Most of the water and electrolytes in this chyme are absorbed in the colon, usually leaving less than 100 mL of fluid to be excreted in the feces. Also, essentially all the ions are absorbed, leaving only 1–5 mEq each of sodium and chloride ions to be lost in the feces.

Most of the absorption in the large intestine occurs in the proximal one-half of the colon, giving this portion the name *absorbing colon*, whereas the distal colon functions principally for feces storage until a propitious time for feces excretion and is therefore called the *storage colon*.

Absorption and Secretion of Electrolytes and Water. The mucosa of the large intestine, like that of the small intestine, has a high capability for active absorption of sodium, and the electrical potential gradient created by sodium absorption causes chloride absorption as well. The tight junctions between the epithelial cells of the large intestinal epithelium are much tighter than those of the small intestine. This characteristic prevents significant amounts of back diffusion of ions through these junctions, thus allowing the large intestinal mucosa to absorb sodium ions far more completely—that is, against a much higher concentration gradient—than can occur in the small intestine. This is especially true when large quantities of aldosterone are available because aldosterone greatly enhances sodium transport capability.

In addition, as occurs in the distal portion of the small intestine, the mucosa of the large intestine secretes *bicarbonate ions* while it simultaneously absorbs an equal number of chloride ions in an exchange transport process already described. The bicarbonate helps neutralize the acidic end products of bacterial action in the large intestine.

Absorption of sodium and chloride ions creates an osmotic gradient across the large intestinal mucosa, which in turn causes absorption of water.

Maximum Absorption Capacity of the Large Intestine. The large intestine can absorb a maximum of 5–8 L of fluid and

electrolytes each day. When the total quantity entering the large intestine through the ileocecal valve or by way of large intestine secretion exceeds this amount, the excess appears in the feces as diarrhea. As noted earlier, toxins from cholera or certain other bacterial infections often cause the crypts in the terminal ileum and large intestine to secrete 10 or more liters of fluid each day, leading to severe and sometimes lethal diarrhea.

Bacterial Action in the Colon. *Numerous bacteria, especially colon bacilli, are present even normally in the absorbing colon.* They are capable of digesting small amounts of cellulose, in this way providing a few calories of extra nutrition for the body. In herbivorous animals this source of energy is significant, although it is of negligible importance in human beings.

Other substances formed as a result of bacterial activity are vitamin K, vitamin B_{12}, thiamine, riboflavin, and various gases that contribute to *flatus* in the colon, especially carbon dioxide, hydrogen gas, and methane. The bacteria-formed vitamin K is especially important because the amount of this vitamin in the daily ingested foods is normally insufficient to maintain adequate blood coagulation.

Fermentation in the Large Intestine. Fermentation is an important process that occurs in the large intestine. It is a process where bacteria (mainly anaerobic) and yeasts break down dietary substrates and other substrates present in the large intestine to obtain energy for their normal growth and maintenance of cellular functions (Figure 73-2).

Substrates for Fermentation. Many substrates are available for fermentation in the large intestine from dietary and endogenous sources; however the most important ones are starch, dietary fiber (nonstarch polysaccharides), and protein (Table 73-1).

Box 73-2 summarizes the functions of the large intestine.

Composition of the Feces. The feces normally are about three-fourths *water* and one-fourth *solid matter* that is composed of

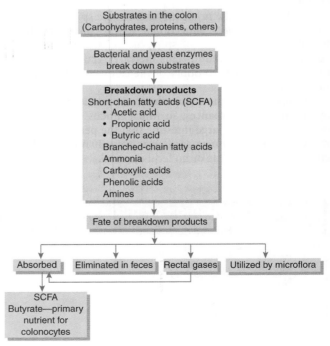

Figure 73-2   Process of gut fermentation.

TABLE 73-1	Probable Substrates for Fermentation	
Carbohydrate	**Protein**	**Others**
Starch	Dietary proteins	Intestinal glycoprotein
Nonstarch polysaccharides (dietary fiber)	Endogenous proteins such as digestive enzymes	Mucopolysaccharides
• Pectin		
• Cellulose		
• Hemicellulose		
Unabsorbed sugars		
Modified cellulose		
Polydextrose		

about 30% *dead bacteria*, 10–20% *fat*, 10–20% *inorganic matter*, 2–3% *protein*, and 30% *undigested roughage* from the food and dried constituents of digestive juices, such as bile pigment and sloughed epithelial cells. The brown color of feces is caused by *stercobilin* and *urobilin*, derivatives of bilirubin. The odor is caused principally by products of bacterial action; these products vary from one person to another, depending on each person's colonic bacterial flora and on the type of food eaten. The actual odoriferous products include *indole, skatole, mercaptans,* and *hydrogen sulfide.*

BIBLIOGRAPHY

Bhattacharyya A, Chattopadhyay R, Mitra S, Crowe SE: Oxidative stress: an essential factor in the pathogenesis of gastrointestinal mucosal diseases, *Physiol. Rev.* 94:329, 2014.

Cummings JH, Englyst HN: Fermentation in the human large intestine and the available substrates, *Am. J. Clin. Nutr.* 45(5 Suppl.):1243, 1987.

Dockray GJ: Enteroendocrine cell signalling via the vagus nerve, *Curr. Opin. Pharmacol.* 13:954, 2013.

FAO, 1997. FAO Food and Nutrition Papers, Physiological effects of dietary fibre. In: Carbohydrates in Human Nutrition, Version 66. <http://www.fao.org/docrep/W8079E/W8079E00.htm> (accessed May 11, 2016).

Gareau MG, Barrett KE: Fluid and electrolyte secretion in the inflamed gut: novel targets for treatment of inflammation-induced diarrhea, *Curr. Opin. Pharmacol.* 13:895, 2013.

Heitzmann D, Warth R: Physiology and pathophysiology of potassium channels in gastrointestinal epithelia, *Physiol. Rev.* 88:1119, 2008.

Kunzelmann K, Mall M: Electrolyte transport in the mammalian colon: mechanisms and implications for disease, *Physiol. Rev.* 82:245, 2002.

Laine L, Takeuchi K, Tarnawski A: Gastric mucosal defense and cytoprotection: bench to bedside, *Gastroenterology* 135:41, 2008.

Lefebvre P, Cariou B, Lien F, et al: Role of bile acids and bile acid receptors in metabolic regulation, *Physiol. Rev.* 89:147, 2009.

Seidler UE: Gastrointestinal HCO_3^- transport and epithelial protection in the gut: new techniques, transport pathways and regulatory pathways, *Curr. Opin. Pharmacol.* 13:900, 2013.

74

Gastrointestinal Motility

The time that food remains in each part of the alimentary tract is critical for optimal processing and absorption of nutrients. In addition, appropriate mixing must be provided. Because the requirements for mixing and propulsion are quite different at each stage of processing, multiple automatic nervous and hormonal mechanisms control the timing of each of these activities so they will occur optimally, not too rapidly and not too slowly.

This chapter discusses these movements, especially the automatic mechanisms of this control.

Functional Types of Movements in the Gastrointestinal Tract

Two types of movements occur in the gastrointestinal (GI) tract:

1. *propulsive movements*, which cause food to move forward along the tract at an appropriate rate to accommodate digestion and absorption;
2. *mixing movements*, which keep the intestinal contents thoroughly mixed at all times.

PROPULSIVE MOVEMENTS—PERISTALSIS

The basic propulsive movement of the GI tract is *peristalsis*, which is illustrated in Figure 74-1. A contractile ring appears around the gut and then moves forward; this mechanism is analogous to putting one's fingers around a thin distended tube, and then constricting the fingers and sliding them forward along the tube. Any material in front of the contractile ring is moved forward.

Peristalsis is an inherent property of many syncytial smooth muscle tubes; it occurs in the bile ducts, glandular ducts, ureters, and many other smooth muscle tubes of the body. The usual stimulus for intestinal peristalsis is *distention of the gut*.

Other stimuli that can initiate peristalsis include chemical or physical irritation of the epithelial lining in the gut. Also, strong parasympathetic nervous signals to the gut will elicit strong peristalsis.

Function of the Myenteric Plexus in Peristalsis. Peristalsis occurs only weakly or not at all in any portion of the GI tract that has congenital absence of the myenteric plexus. Also, it is greatly depressed or completely blocked in the entire gut when a person is treated with atropine to paralyze the cholinergic nerve endings of the myenteric plexus. Therefore, *effectual* peristalsis requires an active myenteric plexus.

Peristaltic Waves Move Toward the Anus with Downstream Receptive Relaxation—"Law of the Gut". Peristalsis, theoretically, can occur in either direction from a stimulated point, but it normally dies out rapidly in the orad (toward the mouth) direction while continuing for a considerable distance toward the anus. The exact cause of this directional transmission of peristalsis has never been ascertained, although it probably results mainly from the fact that the myenteric plexus is "polarized" in the anal direction, which can be explained as follows.

When a segment of the intestinal tract is excited by distention and thereby initiates peristalsis, the contractile ring causing the peristalsis normally begins on the orad side of the distended segment and moves toward the distended segment, pushing the intestinal contents in the anal direction for 5–10 cm before dying out. At the same time, the gut sometimes relaxes several centimeters downstream toward the anus, which is called "receptive relaxation," thus allowing the food to be propelled more easily toward the anus than toward the mouth.

This complex pattern does not occur in the absence of the myenteric plexus. Therefore, the complex is called the *myenteric reflex* or the *peristaltic reflex*. The peristaltic reflex plus the anal direction of movement of the peristalsis is called the "law of the gut."

MIXING MOVEMENTS

Mixing movements differ in different parts of the alimentary tract. In some areas, the peristaltic contractions cause most of the mixing. This is especially true when forward progression of the intestinal contents is blocked by a sphincter so that a peristaltic wave can then only churn the intestinal contents, rather than propelling them forward. At other times, *local intermittent constrictive contractions* occur every few centimeters in the gut wall. These constrictions promote the "chopping" and "shearing" of the contents.

Ingestion of Food

The amount of food that a person ingests is determined principally by an intrinsic desire for food called *hunger*. The type of food that a person preferentially seeks is determined by *appetite*. The current discussion is confined to the mechanics of food ingestion, especially *mastication* and *swallowing*.

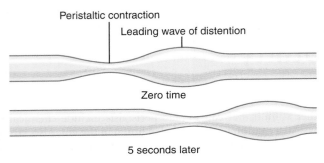

Figure 74-1 Peristalsis.

TABLE 74-1	Stages of Deglutition	
	Stages	**Comment**
1	Voluntary stage	Initiates the swallowing process
2	Pharyngeal stage	Is involuntary and constitutes passage of food through the pharynx into the esophagus
3	Esophageal stage	Another involuntary phase that transports food from the pharynx to the stomach

MASTICATION (CHEWING)

Chewing is important for digestion of all foods, but especially important for most fruits and raw vegetables because these have indigestible cellulose membranes around their nutrient portions that must be broken before the food can be digested. Also, chewing aids the digestion of food for still another simple reason: *Digestive enzymes act only on the surfaces of food particles*; therefore, the rate of digestion is absolutely dependent on the total surface area exposed to the digestive secretions. In addition, grinding the food to a very fine particulate consistency prevents excoriation of the GI tract and increases the ease with which food is emptied from the stomach into the small intestine, and then into all succeeding segments of the gut.

Most of the muscles of chewing are innervated by the motor branch of the fifth cranial nerve, and the chewing process is controlled by nuclei in the brainstem. Stimulation of specific reticular areas in the brainstem taste centers will cause rhythmic chewing movements. Also, stimulation of areas in the hypothalamus, amygdala, and even the cerebral cortex near the sensory areas for taste and smell can often cause chewing.

Chewing Reflex. Much of the chewing process is caused by a *chewing reflex*.

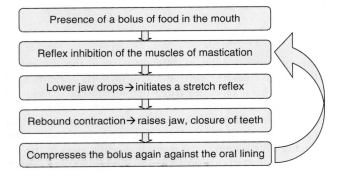

SWALLOWING (DEGLUTITION)

Swallowing is a complicated mechanism, principally because the pharynx subserves respiration and swallowing. The pharynx is converted for only a few seconds at a time into a tract for propulsion of food. It is especially important that respiration not be compromised because of swallowing.

Stages of deglutition have been discussed in Table 74-1.

Voluntary Stage of Swallowing. When the food is ready for swallowing, it is "voluntarily" squeezed or rolled posteriorly into the pharynx by pressure of the tongue upward and backward against the palate, as shown in Figure 74-2. From here on, swallowing becomes entirely—or almost entirely—automatic and ordinarily cannot be stopped.

Involuntary Pharyngeal Stage of Swallowing. As the bolus of food enters the posterior mouth and pharynx, it stimulates *epithelial swallowing receptor areas* all around the opening of the pharynx, especially on the tonsillar pillars, and impulses from these areas pass to the brainstem to initiate a series of automatic pharyngeal muscle contractions as follows:

1. The soft palate is pulled upward to close the posterior nares to prevent reflux of food into the nasal cavities.
2. The palatopharyngeal folds on each side of the pharynx are pulled medially to form a sagittal slit through which the food must pass into the posterior pharynx. Because this stage lasts less than 1 second, any large object is usually impeded too much to pass into the esophagus.
3. The vocal cords of the larynx are strongly approximated, and the larynx is pulled upward and anteriorly by the neck muscles and the epiglottis swings backward over the opening of the larynx. These actions prevent passage of food into the nose and trachea. Most essential is the tight approximation of the vocal cords, but the epiglottis helps to prevent food from ever getting as far as the vocal cords. Destruction of the vocal cords or of the muscles that approximate them can cause strangulation.
4. The upward movement of the larynx also pulls up and enlarges the opening to the esophagus. At the same time, the upper 3–4 cm of the esophageal muscular wall, called the *upper esophageal sphincter* (also called the

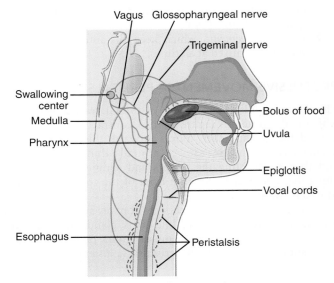

Figure 74-2 Swallowing mechanism.

pharyngoesophageal sphincter), relaxes. Thus, food moves easily and freely from the posterior pharynx into the upper esophagus.

Between swallows this sphincter remains strongly contracted, thereby preventing air from going into the esophagus during respiration. The upward movement of the larynx also lifts the glottis out of the main stream of food flow, so the food mainly passes on each side of the epiglottis rather than over its surface; this action adds still another protection against entry of food into the trachea.

5. Once the larynx is raised and the *upper esophageal sphincter* becomes relaxed, the entire muscular wall of the pharynx contracts, beginning in the superior part of the pharynx, and then spreading downward over the middle and inferior pharyngeal areas, which propels the food by peristalsis into the esophagus.

To summarize the mechanics of the pharyngeal stage of swallowing:

- The trachea is closed.
- The esophagus is opened.
- A fast peristaltic wave initiated by the nervous system of the pharynx forces the bolus of food into the upper esophagus.
- The entire process occurs in less than 2 seconds.

Nervous Initiation of the Pharyngeal Stage of Swallowing. The most sensitive tactile areas of the posterior mouth and pharynx for initiating the pharyngeal stage of swallowing lie in a ring around the pharyngeal opening, with greatest sensitivity on the tonsillar pillars. Impulses are transmitted from these areas through the sensory portions of the trigeminal and glossopharyngeal nerves into the medulla oblongata, either into or closely associated with the *tractus solitarius*, which receives essentially all sensory impulses from the mouth.

The successive stages of the swallowing process are then automatically initiated in orderly sequence by neuronal areas of the reticular substance of the medulla and lower portion of the pons. The areas in the medulla and lower pons that control swallowing are collectively called the *deglutition* or *swallowing center*.

The motor impulses from the swallowing center to the pharynx and upper esophagus that cause swallowing are transmitted successively by the 5th, 9th, 10th, and 12th cranial nerves and even a few of the superior cervical nerves.

In summary, the pharyngeal stage of swallowing is principally a reflex act. It is almost always initiated by voluntary movement of food into the back of the mouth, which in turn excites involuntary pharyngeal sensory receptors to elicit the swallowing reflex.

Effect of the Pharyngeal Stage of Swallowing on Respiration. The entire pharyngeal stage of swallowing usually occurs in less than 6 seconds, thereby interrupting respiration for only a fraction of a usual respiratory cycle. The swallowing center specifically inhibits the respiratory center of the medulla during this time, halting respiration at any point in its cycle to allow swallowing to proceed. Yet even while a person is talking swallowing interrupts respiration for such a short time that it is hardly noticeable.

The Esophageal Stage of Swallowing Involves Two Types of Peristalsis. The esophagus functions primarily to conduct food rapidly from the pharynx to the stomach, and its movements are organized specifically for this function.

The esophagus normally exhibits two types of peristaltic movements: *primary peristalsis* and *secondary peristalsis*.

Primary peristalsis is simply continuation of the peristaltic wave that begins in the pharynx and spreads into the esophagus during the pharyngeal stage of swallowing. This wave passes all the way from the pharynx to the stomach in about 8–10 seconds.

If the primary peristaltic wave fails to move all the food that has entered the esophagus into the stomach, *secondary peristaltic waves* result from distention of the esophagus itself by the retained food; these waves continue until all the food has emptied into the stomach. The secondary peristaltic waves are initiated partly by intrinsic neural circuits in the myenteric nervous system and partly by reflexes that begin in the pharynx and are then transmitted upward through *vagal afferent fibers* to the medulla and back again to the esophagus through *glossopharyngeal* and *vagal efferent nerve fibers*.

The musculature of the pharyngeal wall and upper third of the esophagus is *striated muscle*. Therefore, the peristaltic waves in these regions are controlled by skeletal nerve impulses from the glossopharyngeal and vagus nerves. In the lower two-thirds of the esophagus the musculature is *smooth muscle*, but this portion of the esophagus is also strongly controlled by the vagus nerves that act through connections with the esophageal myenteric nervous system.

Receptive Relaxation of the Stomach. When the esophageal peristaltic wave approaches the stomach, a wave of relaxation, transmitted through myenteric inhibitory neurons, precedes the peristalsis. Furthermore, the entire stomach and, to a lesser extent, even the duodenum become relaxed as this wave reaches the lower end of the esophagus and thus are prepared ahead of time to receive the food propelled into the esophagus during the swallowing act.

Function of the Lower Esophageal Sphincter (Gastroesophageal Sphincter). At the lower end of the esophagus, extending upward about 3 cm above its juncture with the stomach is the broad *lower esophageal sphincter*, also called the *gastroesophageal sphincter*. This sphincter, consisting of circular muscle, normally remains tonically constricted with an intraluminal pressure of about 30 mmHg, in contrast to the midportion of the esophagus, which normally remains relaxed.

When a peristaltic swallowing wave passes down the esophagus, "receptive relaxation" of the lower esophageal sphincter occurs ahead of the peristaltic wave, which allows easy propulsion of the swallowed food into the stomach. Rarely, the sphincter does not relax satisfactorily, resulting in a condition called *achalasia*. This condition is discussed in Chapter 75.

The tonic constriction of the lower esophageal sphincter helps prevent significant reflux of acidic stomach contents into the esophagus except under abnormal conditions.

Additional Prevention of Esophageal Reflux by Valve-Like Closure of the Distal End of the Esophagus. Another factor that helps prevent reflux is a valve-like mechanism of a short portion of the esophagus that extends slightly into the stomach. Increased intraabdominal pressure caves the esophagus inward at this point. Thus, this valve-like closure of the lower esophagus helps to prevent high intraabdominal pressure from forcing stomach contents backward into the esophagus. Otherwise, every time we walked, coughed, or breathed hard, we might expel stomach acid into the esophagus.

Motor Functions of the Stomach

The motor functions of the stomach are threefold:

1. *storage* of large quantities of food until the food can be processed in the stomach, duodenum, and lower intestinal tract;

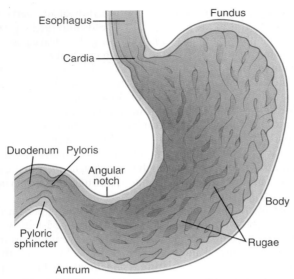

Figure 74-3 Physiological anatomy of the stomach.

2. *mixing* of this food with gastric secretions until it forms a semifluid mixture called *chyme*;

3. *slow emptying* of the chyme from the stomach into the small intestine at a rate suitable for proper digestion and absorption by the small intestine. Figure 74-3 shows the basic anatomy of the stomach. Anatomically, the stomach is usually divided into two major parts: (a) the *body* and (b) the *antrum*. Physiologically, it is more appropriately divided into (a) the "*orad*" portion, comprising about the first two-thirds of the body, and (b) the "*caudad*" portion, comprising the remainder of the body plus the antrum.

STORAGE FUNCTION OF THE STOMACH

As food enters the stomach, it forms concentric circles of the food in the orad portion of the stomach, with the newest food lying closest to the esophageal opening and the oldest food lying nearest the outer wall of the stomach. Normally, when food stretches the stomach, a "vagovagal reflex" from the stomach to the brainstem and then back to the stomach reduces the tone in the muscular wall of the body of the stomach so that the wall bulges progressively outward, accommodating greater and greater quantities of food up to a limit in the completely relaxed stomach of 0.8–1.5 L. The pressure in the stomach remains low until this limit is approached.

MIXING AND PROPULSION OF FOOD IN THE STOMACH—BASIC ELECTRICAL RHYTHM OF THE STOMACH WALL

As long as food is in the stomach, weak peristaltic *constrictor waves*, called *mixing waves*, begin in the mid to upper portions of the stomach wall and move toward the antrum about once every 15–20 seconds. These waves are initiated by the gut wall *basic electrical rhythm*, consisting of electrical "slow waves" that occur spontaneously in the stomach wall. As the constrictor waves progress from the body of the stomach into the antrum they become more intense, some becoming extremely intense and providing powerful *peristaltic action potential*–driven constrictor rings that force the antral contents under higher and higher pressure toward the pylorus.

These constrictor rings also play an important role in mixing the stomach contents by digging deeply into the food contents in the antrum. During gastric motility, most of the antral contents are squeezed upstream through the peristaltic ring toward the body of the stomach, not through the pylorus. Thus, the moving peristaltic constrictive ring, combined with this upstream squeezing action, called "retropulsion," is an exceedingly important mixing mechanism in the stomach.

After food in the stomach has become thoroughly mixed with the stomach secretions, the resulting mixture that passes down the gut is called *chyme*. The appearance of chyme is that of a murky semifluid or paste.

Hunger Contractions. Besides the peristaltic contractions that occur when food is present in the stomach, another type of intense contractions, called *hunger contractions*, often occur *when the stomach has been empty* for several hours or more. These contractions are rhythmic peristaltic contractions in the *body* of the stomach. Hunger contractions are most intense in young, healthy people who have high degrees of GI tonus; they are also greatly increased by the person having lower than normal levels of blood sugar. When hunger contractions occur in the stomach, the person sometimes experiences mild pain in the pit of the stomach, called *hunger pangs*. Hunger pangs usually do not begin until 12–24 hours after the last ingestion of food; in people who are in a state of starvation, they reach their greatest intensity in 3–4 days and gradually weaken in succeeding days.

STOMACH EMPTYING

Stomach emptying is promoted by intense peristaltic contractions in the stomach antrum. At the same time, emptying is opposed by varying degrees of resistance to passage of chyme at the pylorus.

Intense Antral Peristaltic Contractions During Stomach Emptying—"Pyloric Pump". Most of the time, the rhythmic stomach contractions are weak and function mainly to cause mixing of food and gastric secretions. However, for about 20% of the time while food is in the stomach, the contractions become intense, beginning in midstomach and spreading through the caudad stomach; these contractions are strong peristaltic, very tight ring-like constrictions that can cause stomach emptying. These intense peristaltic contractions often create 50–70 cm H_2O pressure, which is about six times as powerful as the usual mixing type of peristaltic waves.

When pyloric tone is normal, each strong peristaltic wave forces up to several milliliters of chyme into the duodenum. Thus, the peristaltic waves, in addition to causing mixing in the stomach, also provide a pumping action called the "pyloric pump."

Role of the Pylorus in Controlling Stomach Emptying. The distal opening of the stomach is the *pylorus* and consists of circular muscle. It remains slightly tonically contracted almost all the time. Therefore, the pyloric circular muscle is called the *pyloric sphincter.*

Despite normal tonic contraction of the pyloric sphincter, the pylorus usually is open enough for water and other fluids to empty from the stomach into the duodenum with ease. The degree of constriction of the pylorus is increased or decreased under the influence of nervous and hormonal signals from both the stomach and the duodenum, as discussed shortly.

TABLE 74-2	Factors that Regulate Gastric Emptying	
Gastric or Duodenal Factors	Description	Action
Gastric factors that promote emptying	Gastric food volume	Increased volume causes stretching of the stomach wall eliciting local myenteric reflexes. This accentuates the pyloric pump and inhibits the pyloric sphincter, which promotes increased emptying
	Gastrin	Gastrin has mild to moderate stimulatory effects on motor functions of the body of the stomach and importantly enhances the activity of the pyloric pump
Powerful duodenal factors that inhibit stomach emptying	Enterogastric nervous reflexes	Strongly inhibits the "pyloric pump" propulsive contractions. Also, increases the tone of the pyloric sphincter
	Hormonal feedback from the duodenum • Cholecystokinin (CCK) • Secretin • Gastric inhibitory peptide (GIP)	Fats entering the duodenum stimulate inhibitory hormones, primarily CCK, which inhibits the pyloric pump and increases the tone of the pyloric sphincter Acidic chyme stimulates the release of secretin, which in turn is a possible inhibitor of gastric motility GIP has a general but weak effect of decreasing gastrointestinal motility

REGULATION OF STOMACH EMPTYING

The rate at which the stomach empties is regulated by signals from both the stomach and the duodenum. However, the duodenum provides by far the more potent of the signals, controlling the emptying of chyme into the duodenum at a rate no greater than the rate at which the chyme can be digested and absorbed in the small intestine. These feedback inhibitory mechanisms work together to slow the rate of emptying when (1) too much chyme is already in the small intestine or (2) the chyme is excessively acidic, contains too much unprocessed protein or fat, is hypotonic or hypertonic, or is irritating.

The factors that regulate gastric emptying are listed in Table 74-2.

Powerful Duodenal Factors that Inhibit Stomach Emptying

Inhibitory Effect of Enterogastric Nervous Reflexes from the Duodenum. When food enters the duodenum, multiple nervous reflexes are initiated from the duodenal wall. These reflexes are mediated by three routes:

1. directly from the duodenum to the stomach through the enteric nervous system in the gut wall;
2. through extrinsic nerves that go to the prevertebral sympathetic ganglia and then back through inhibitory sympathetic nerve fibers to the stomach;
3. probably to a slight extent through the vagus nerves all the way to the brainstem, where they inhibit the normal excitatory signals transmitted to the stomach through the vagi.

All these parallel reflexes have two effects on stomach emptying: First, they strongly inhibit the "pyloric pump" propulsive contractions, and second, they increase the tone of the pyloric sphincter. The types of factors that are continually monitored in the duodenum and that can initiate enterogastric reflexes are summarized in Box 74-1.

Hormonal Feedback from the Duodenum Inhibits Gastric Emptying—Role of Fats and the Hormone Cholecystokinin. Besides the nervous reflexes from the duodenum that inhibit stomach emptying, fats entering the duodenum stimulate inhibitory hormones to be released from the upper intestine. In turn, these hormones are carried by way of the blood to the stomach, where they inhibit the pyloric pump and at the same time increase the strength of contraction of the pyloric sphincter.

The most potent of these hormones appears to be *cholecystokinin* (CCK), which is released from the mucosa of the jejunum in response to fatty substances in the chyme.

Other possible inhibitors of stomach emptying are the hormones *secretin* and *glucose-dependent insulinotropic peptide*, also called *gastric inhibitory peptide* (GIP). Secretin is released mainly from the duodenal mucosa in response to gastric acid passed from the stomach through the pylorus.

GIP is released from the upper small intestine mainly in response to fat in the chyme, but to a lesser extent in response to carbohydrates as well. GIP has a general but weak effect of decreasing GI motility; however, its main effect at physiological concentrations is probably mainly to stimulate secretion of insulin by the pancreas.

Movements of the Small Intestine

The movements of the small intestine, like those elsewhere in the GI tract, can be divided into *mixing contractions* and *propulsive contractions*. To a great extent, this separation is artificial because essentially all movements of the small intestine cause at least some degree of both mixing and propulsion. The usual classification of these processes is described in the following sections.

MIXING CONTRACTIONS (SEGMENTATION CONTRACTIONS)

When a portion of the small intestine becomes distended with chyme, stretching of the intestinal wall elicits localized concentric contractions spaced at intervals along the intestine and

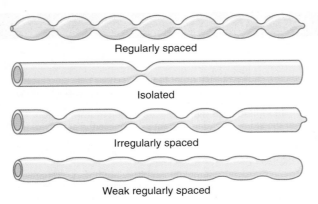

Figure 74-4 Segmentation movements of the small intestine.

lasting a fraction of a minute. The contractions cause "segmentation" of the small intestine, as shown in Figure 74-4, that is, they divide the intestine into spaced segments that have the appearance of a chain of sausages. As one set of segmentation contractions relaxes a new set often begins, but the contractions this time occur mainly at new points between the previous contractions. Therefore, the segmentation contractions "chop" the chyme two to three times per minute, in this way promoting progressive mixing of the food with secretions of the small intestine.

The maximum frequency of the segmentation contractions in the small intestine is determined by the frequency of *electrical slow waves* in the intestinal wall, which is about 12 minute^{-1}, but this maximum frequency occurs only under extreme conditions of stimulation. In the terminal ileum, the maximum frequency is usually eight to nine contractions per minute.

PROPULSIVE MOVEMENTS

Peristalsis in the Small Intestine. Chyme is propelled through the small intestine faster in the proximal intestine and slower in the terminal intestine. Peristaltic waves are normally weak and usually die out after traveling only 3–5 cm. Movement of the chyme is very slow, so slow that *net* movement along the small intestine normally averages only 1 cm/minute. This rate of travel means that 3–5 hours is required for passage of chyme from the pylorus to the ileocecal valve.

Control of Peristalsis by Nervous and Hormonal Signals. Peristaltic activity of the small intestine is greatly increased after a meal. This increased activity is caused partly by the beginning entry of chyme into the duodenum causing stretch of the duodenal wall. In addition, peristaltic activity is increased by the so-called *gastroenteric reflex* that is initiated by distention of the stomach and conducted principally through the myenteric plexus from the stomach down along the wall of the small intestine.

In addition to the nervous signals that may affect small intestinal peristalsis, several hormonal factors also affect peristalsis. These factors include *gastrin, CCK, insulin, motilin,* and *serotonin,* all of which enhance intestinal motility and are secreted during various phases of food processing. Conversely, *secretin* and *glucagon* inhibit small intestinal motility. The physiological importance of each of these hormonal factors for controlling motility is still questionable.

Propulsive Effect of the Segmentation Movements. The segmentation movements, although lasting for only a few seconds at a time, often also travel 1 cm or so in the anal direction and

during that time they help propel the food down the intestine. The difference between the segmentation and the peristaltic movements is not as great as might be implied by their separation into these two classifications.

Peristaltic Rush. Although peristalsis in the small intestine is normally weak, intense irritation of the intestinal mucosa, as occurs in some severe cases of infectious diarrhea, can cause both powerful and rapid peristalsis, called the *peristaltic rush.* This phenomenon is initiated partly by nervous reflexes that involve the autonomic nervous system and brainstem, and partly by intrinsic enhancement of the myenteric plexus reflexes within the gut wall. The powerful peristaltic contractions travel long distances in the small intestine within minutes, sweeping the contents of the intestine into the colon and thereby relieving the small intestine of irritative chyme and excessive distention.

Movements Caused by the Muscularis Mucosae and Muscle Fibers of the Villi. The *muscularis mucosae* can cause short folds to appear in the intestinal mucosa. In addition, individual fibers from this muscle extend into the intestinal villi and cause them to contract intermittently. The mucosal folds increase the surface area exposed to the chyme, thereby increasing absorption. Also, contractions of the villi—shortening, elongating, and shortening again—"milk" the villi so that lymph flows freely from the central lacteals of the villi into the lymphatic system. These mucosal and villous contractions are initiated mainly by local nervous reflexes in the submucosal nerve plexus that occur in response to chyme in the small intestine.

THE ILEOCECAL VALVE PREVENTS BACKFLOW FROM THE COLON TO THE SMALL INTESTINE

A principal function of the ileocecal valve is to prevent backflow of fecal contents from the colon into the small intestine. As shown in Figure 74-5, the ileocecal valve protrudes into the lumen of the cecum and therefore is forcefully closed when excess pressure builds up in the cecum and tries to push cecal contents backward against the valve lips. The valve usually can resist reverse pressure of at least 50–60 cm H_2O.

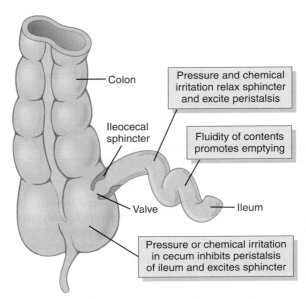

Figure 74-5 Emptying at the ileocecal valve.

TABLE 74-3 | Summary of Intestinal Movements Along the GI Tract

	Segment of GI Tract	Type of Motility	Description
1	Small intestine	Mixing or segmentation contractions	These are localized concentric contractions spaced at intervals along the intestine and lasting a fraction of a minute
		Peristalsis	Propulsive movements of the small intestine that propel the chyme toward the anus
		Movements caused by muscularis mucosae	This muscle can cause short folds to appear in the intestinal mucosa. They can also cause the villi to contract intermittently
		Villi movement	Contractions of the villi by shortening, elongating, and shortening help "milk" the villi to promote lymph flow
2	Large intestine (colon)	Mixing movements—"haustrations"	These are segmentation movements that occur in the colon where the combined contractions of the circular and longitudinal strips of muscle cause the unstimulated portion of the large intestine to bulge outward into bag-like sacs called *haustrations*
		Propulsive movements—"mass movements"	Mass movements are a modified type of peristalsis seen in the colon that helps propel fecal matter

GI, gastrointestinal.

The wall of the ileum for several centimeters immediately upstream from the ileocecal valve has a thickened circular muscle called the *ileocecal sphincter* that normally remains mildly constricted and slows emptying of ileal contents into the cecum.

Normally, only 1500–2000 mL of chyme empties into the cecum each day.

Table 74-3 summarizes the various types of movements along the GI tract. Figure 74-6 summarizes the effect of major GI hormones on GI motility

Feedback Control of the Ileocecal Sphincter. The degree of contraction of the ileocecal sphincter and the intensity of peristalsis in the terminal ileum are controlled significantly by reflexes from the cecum. When the cecum is distended, contraction of the ileocecal sphincter becomes intensified and ileal peristalsis is inhibited, both of which greatly delay emptying of additional chyme into the cecum from the ileum. Also, any irritant in the cecum delays emptying, for example, an inflamed appendix can cause such intense spasm of the ileocecal sphincter and partial

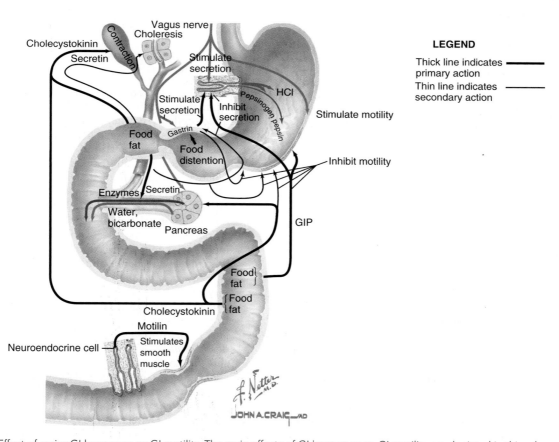

Figure 74-6 Effect of major GI hormones on GI motility. The main effects of GI hormones on GI motility are depicted in this scheme. While many hormones have effects on gastric motility, a few stimulate motility in the small and large intestines, including motilin (small intestine only) and gastrin (both small and large intestines, not shown on figure). GI, gastrointestinal; GIP, gastric inhibitory peptide. *From Netter's Essential Physiology, 2009, Figure 22.11, p. 267.*

paralysis of the ileum that these effects together block emptying of the ileum into the cecum.

The reflexes from the cecum to the ileocecal sphincter and ileum are mediated both by way of the myenteric plexus and by the extrinsic autonomic nerves, especially by way of the prevertebral sympathetic ganglia.

Movements of the Colon

The principal functions of the colon are (1) absorption of water and electrolytes from the chyme to form solid feces (proximal half of the colon) and (2) storage of fecal matter until it can be expelled (distal half of the colon) (Figure 74-7). Although the movements of the colon are normally sluggish, they still have characteristics similar to those of the small intestine and can be divided once again into mixing movements and propulsive movements. Table 74-3 summarizes the various types of movements along the GI tract.

Mixing Movements—"Haustrations". In the same manner that segmentation movements occur in the small intestine, large circular constrictions occur in the large intestine. At each of these constrictions about 2.5 cm of the circular muscle contracts, sometimes constricting the lumen of the colon almost to occlusion. At the same time the longitudinal muscle of the colon, which is aggregated into three longitudinal strips called the *teniae coli*, contracts. These combined contractions of the circular and longitudinal strips of muscle cause the unstimulated portion of the large intestine to bulge outward into bag-like sacs called *haustrations*.

Each haustration usually reaches peak intensity in about 30 seconds and then disappears during the next 60 seconds. Therefore, the fecal material in the large intestine is slowly *dug into and rolled over* in much the same manner that one spades the earth. In this way, all the fecal material is gradually exposed to the mucosal surface of the large intestine, and fluid and dissolved substances are progressively absorbed until only 80–200 mL of feces are expelled each day.

Propulsive Movements—"Mass Movements". Much of the propulsion in the cecum and ascending colon results from the slow but persistent haustral contractions, requiring as many as 8–15 hours to move the chyme from the ileocecal valve through the colon, while the chyme becomes fecal in quality.

From the cecum to the sigmoid, *mass movements* can, for many minutes at a time, take over the propulsive role.

A mass movement is a modified type of peristalsis characterized by the following sequence of events:

1. A *constrictive ring* occurs in response to a distended or irritated point in the colon, usually in the transverse colon.
2. Then, rapidly, the 20 or more centimeters of colon *distal to the constrictive ring* lose their haustrations and instead contract as a unit, propelling the fecal material in this segment *en masse* further down the colon.
3. The contraction develops progressively more force for about 30 seconds, and relaxation occurs during the next 2–3 minutes. Another mass movement then occurs, this time perhaps farther along the colon.

A series of mass movements usually persists for 10–30 minutes. They then cease but return perhaps a half day later. When they have forced a mass of feces into the rectum, the desire for defecation is felt.

Initiation of Mass Movements by Gastrocolic and Duodenocolic Reflexes. The appearance of mass movements after meals is facilitated by *gastrocolic* and *duodenocolic reflexes*. These reflexes result from distention of the stomach and duodenum. They occur either not at all or hardly at all when the extrinsic autonomic nerves to the colon have been removed; therefore, the reflexes almost certainly are transmitted by way of the autonomic nervous system.

Irritation in the colon can also initiate intense mass movements. For instance, a person who has an ulcerated condition of the colon mucosa (*ulcerative colitis*) frequently has mass movements that persist almost all the time.

DEFECATION

Most of the time the rectum is empty of feces partly because a weak functional sphincter exists about 20 cm from the anus at the juncture between the sigmoid colon and the rectum. A sharp angulation is also present here that contributes additional resistance to filling of the rectum.

When a mass movement forces feces into the rectum, the desire for defecation occurs immediately, including reflex contraction of the rectum and relaxation of the anal sphincters.

Continual dribble of fecal matter through the anus is prevented by tonic constriction of:

1. an *internal anal sphincter*, which is a several-centimeters-long thickening of the circular smooth muscle that lies immediately inside the anus;
2. an *external anal sphincter*, composed of striated voluntary muscle that both surrounds the internal sphincter and extends distal to it. The external sphincter is controlled by nerve fibers in the *pudendal nerve*, which is part of the somatic nervous system and therefore is under *voluntary*, *conscious*, or at least *subconscious control*; subconsciously, the external sphincter is usually kept continuously constricted unless conscious signals inhibit the constriction.

Defecation Reflexes. Ordinarily, defecation is initiated by *defecation reflexes*. There are two types of defecation reflexes:

1. One of these reflexes is an *intrinsic reflex* mediated by the local enteric nervous system in the rectal wall. Functioning by itself, this reflex normally is relatively weak.

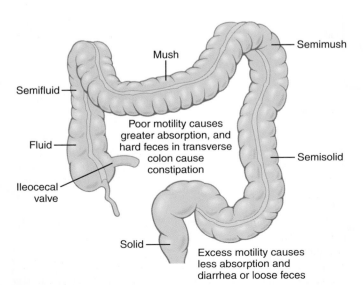

Figure 74-7   Absorptive and storage functions of the large intestine.

This can be described as follows:

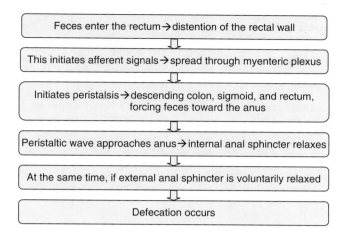

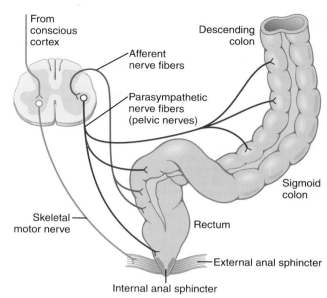

Figure 74-8 Afferent and efferent pathways of the parasympathetic mechanism for enhancing the defecation reflex.

2. The parasympathetic defecation reflex. To be effective in causing defecation, the intrinsic reflex usually must be fortified by a *parasympathetic defecation reflex* that involves the sacral segments of the spinal cord, shown in Figure 74-8. This can be described as follows:

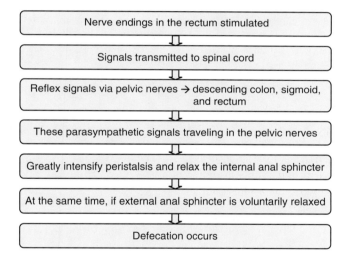

Defecation signals entering the spinal cord initiate other effects, such as taking a deep breath, closure of the glottis, and contraction of the abdominal wall muscles to force the fecal contents of the colon downward, and at the same time they cause the pelvic floor to relax downward and pull outward on the anal ring to evaginate the feces.

In newborn babies and in some people with transected spinal cords, the defecation reflexes cause automatic emptying of the lower bowel at inconvenient times during the day because of lack of conscious control exercised through voluntary contraction or relaxation of the external anal sphincter.

Gastrointestinal Reflexes. The anatomical arrangement of the enteric nervous system and its connections with the sympathetic and parasympathetic systems support three types of GI reflexes that are essential to GI control. They are the following:

1. *Reflexes that are integrated entirely within the gut wall enteric nervous system.* These include reflexes that control

much GI secretion, peristalsis, mixing contractions, local inhibitory effects, and so forth.

2. *Reflexes from the gut to the prevertebral sympathetic ganglia and then back to the GI tract.* These reflexes transmit long-distance signals to other areas of the GI tract, such as signals from the stomach to cause evacuation of the colon (the *gastrocolic reflex*), signals from the colon and small intestine to inhibit stomach motility and stomach secretion (the *enterogastric reflexes*), and reflexes from the colon to inhibit emptying of ileal contents into the colon (the *colonoileal reflex*).

3. *Reflexes from the gut to the spinal cord or brainstem and then back to the GI tract.* These include especially (a) reflexes from the stomach and duodenum to the brainstem and back to the stomach—by way of the vagus nerves—to control gastric motor and secretory activity; (b) pain reflexes that cause general inhibition of the entire GI tract; and (c) defecation reflexes that travel from the colon and rectum to the spinal cord and back again to produce the powerful colonic, rectal, and abdominal contractions required for defecation (the defecation reflexes).

Other Autonomic Reflexes that Affect Bowel Activity

Aside from the duodenocolic, gastrocolic, gastroileal, enterogastric, and defecation reflexes that have been discussed in this chapter, several other important nervous reflexes also can affect the overall degree of bowel activity. They are the peritoneointestinal reflex, renointestinal reflex, and vesicointestinal reflex.

The *peritoneointestinal reflex* results from irritation of the peritoneum; it strongly inhibits the excitatory enteric nerves and thereby can cause intestinal paralysis, especially in patients with peritonitis. The *renointestinal* and *vesicointestinal reflexes* inhibit intestinal activity as a result of kidney or bladder irritation, respectively.

BIBLIOGRAPHY

Boeckxstaens GE, Zaninotto G, Richter JE: Achalasia, *Lancet* 383:83, 2014.

Camilleri M: Pharmacological agents currently in clinical trials for disorders in neurogastroenterology, *J. Clin. Invest.* 123:4111, 2013.

Camilleri M: Physiological underpinnings of irritable bowel syndrome: neurohormonal mechanisms, *J. Physiol.* 592:2967, 2014.

Cooke HJ, Wunderlich J, Christofi FL: "The force be with you": ATP in gut mechanosensory transduction, *News Physiol. Sci.* 18:43, 2003.

Farré R, Tack J: Food and symptom generation in functional gastrointestinal disorders: physiological aspects, *Am. J. Gastroenterol.* 108:698, 2013.

Furness JB: The enteric nervous system and neurogastroenterology, *Nat. Rev. Gastroenterol. Hepatol.* 9:286, 2012.

Huizinga JD, Lammers WJ: Gut peristalsis is governed by a multitude of cooperating mechanisms, *Am. J. Physiol. Gastrointest. Liver Physiol.* 296:G1, 2009.

Miller L, Clavé P, Farré R, et al: Physiology of the upper segment, body, and lower segment of the esophagus, *Ann. N. Y. Acad. Sci.* 1300:261, 2013.

Neunlist M, Schemann M: Nutrient-induced changes in the phenotype and function of the enteric nervous system, *J. Physiol.* 592:2959, 2014.

Ouyang A, Regan J, McMahon BP: Physiology of the upper segment, body, and lower segment of the esophagus, *Ann. N. Y. Acad. Sci.* 1300:261, 2013.

Reimann F, Tolhurst G, Gribble FM: G-protein-coupled receptors in intestinal chemosensation, *Cell Metab.* 15:421, 2012.

Sanders KM, Ward SM, Koh SD: Interstitial cells: regulators of smooth muscle function, *Physiol. Rev.* 94:859, 2014.

Sarna SK: Molecular, functional, and pharmacological targets for the development of gut promotility drugs, *Am. J. Physiol. Gastrointest. Liver Physiol.* 291:G545, 2006.

Sarna SK: Are interstitial cells of Cajal plurifunction cells in the gut? *Am. J. Physiol. Gastrointest. Liver Physiol.* 294:G372, 2008.

Szarka LA, Camilleri M: Methods for measurement of gastric motility, *Am. J. Physiol. Gastrointest. Liver Physiol.* 296:G461, 2009.

Wu T, Rayner CK, Young RL, Horowitz M: Gut motility and enteroendocrine secretion, *Curr. Opin. Pharmacol.* 13:928, 2013.

Physiology of Gastrointestinal Diseases

The purpose of this chapter is to discuss a few representative types of gastrointestinal malfunction that have special physiological bases or consequences.

Disorders of Swallowing and the Esophagus

Paralysis of the Swallowing Mechanism. Damage to the 5th, 9th, or 10th cerebral nerve can cause paralysis of significant portions of the swallowing mechanism. In addition, a few diseases, such as *poliomyelitis* or *encephalitis*, can prevent normal swallowing by damaging the swallowing center in the brainstem. Paralysis of the swallowing muscles, as occurs in persons with *muscle dystrophy* or as a result of failure of neuromuscular transmission in persons with *myasthenia gravis* or *botulism*, can also prevent normal swallowing.

When the swallowing mechanism is partially or totally paralyzed, the abnormalities that can occur include:

- complete abrogation of the swallowing act so that swallowing cannot occur;
- failure of the glottis to close so that food passes into the lungs instead of the esophagus;
- failure of the soft palate and uvula to close the posterior nares so that food refluxes into the nose during swallowing.

One of the most serious instances of paralysis of the swallowing mechanism occurs when patients are in a state of deep anesthesia. While on the operation table, they sometimes vomit large quantities of materials from the stomach into the pharynx; then, instead of swallowing the materials again, they simply suck them into the trachea because the anesthetic has blocked the reflex mechanism of swallowing. As a result, such patients may choke to death on their own vomitus.

Achalasia and Megaesophagus. *Achalasia* is a condition in which the lower esophageal sphincter fails to relax during swallowing. As a result, food swallowed into the esophagus fails to pass from the esophagus into the stomach. Pathological studies have shown damage in the neural network of the myenteric plexus in the lower two-thirds of the esophagus. As a result, the musculature of the lower esophagus remains spastically contracted and the myenteric plexus has lost its ability to transmit a signal to cause "receptive relaxation" of the gastroesophageal sphincter as food approaches this sphincter during swallowing.

When achalasia becomes severe, the esophagus often cannot empty the swallowed food into the stomach for many hours, instead of the few seconds that is the normal time. Over months and years, the esophagus becomes tremendously enlarged until it often can hold as much as 1 L of food, which often becomes putridly infected during the long periods of esophageal stasis. The infection may also cause ulceration of the esophageal mucosa, sometimes leading to severe substernal pain or even rupture and death. Considerable benefit can be achieved by stretching the lower end of the esophagus by means of a balloon inflated on the end of a swallowed esophageal tube. Antispasmodic drugs (ie, drugs that relax smooth muscle) can also be helpful.

Disorders of the Stomach

Gastritis—Inflammation of the Gastric Mucosa. The inflammation of gastritis may be only superficial and therefore not very harmful, or it can penetrate deeply into the gastric mucosa, in many longstanding cases causing almost complete atrophy of the gastric mucosa. In a few cases, gastritis can be acute and severe, with ulcerative excoriation of the stomach mucosa by the stomach's own peptic secretions.

Research suggests that gastritis often is caused by chronic bacterial infection of the gastric mucosa. This condition often can be treated successfully with an intensive regimen of antibacterial therapy.

In addition, certain ingested irritant substances can be especially damaging to the protective gastric mucosal barrier—that is, to the mucous glands and to the tight epithelial junctions between the gastric lining cells—often leading to severe acute or chronic gastritis. Two of the most common of these substances are excesses of *alcohol* or *aspirin*.

Gastric Barrier and its Penetration in Gastritis. Absorption of food from the stomach directly into the blood is normally slight. This low level of absorption is mainly due to two specific features of the gastric mucosa: (1) it is lined with highly resistant mucous cells that secrete viscid and adherent mucus and (2) it has tight junctions between the adjacent epithelial cells. These two features together plus other impediments to gastric absorption are called the "gastric barrier."

The gastric barrier normally is resistant enough to diffusion so that even the highly concentrated hydrogen ions of the gastric juice, averaging about 100,000 times the concentration of hydrogen ions in plasma, seldom diffuse even to the slightest extent through the lining mucus as far as the epithelial membrane itself. In gastritis, the permeability of the barrier is greatly increased. The hydrogen ions do then diffuse into the stomach epithelium, creating additional havoc and leading to a vicious circle of progressive stomach mucosal damage and atrophy. It also makes the mucosa susceptible to digestion by the peptic digestive enzymes, thus frequently resulting in a *gastric ulcer.*

Chronic Gastritis Can Lead to Gastric Atrophy and Loss of Stomach Secretions. In many people who have chronic gastritis, the mucosa gradually becomes more and more atrophic until little or no gastric gland digestive secretion remains. It is also believed that in some people autoimmunity develops against the gastric mucosa, which also leads eventually to gastric atrophy. Loss of the stomach secretions in gastric atrophy leads to *achlorhydria* and, occasionally, to *pernicious anemia.*

Achlorhydria (and Hypochlorhydria). Achlorhydria means simply that the stomach fails to secrete hydrochloric acid; it is diagnosed when the pH of the gastric secretions fails to decrease below 6.5 after maximal stimulation. *Hypochlorhydria* means diminished acid secretion. When acid is not secreted, pepsin also usually is not secreted. Even when it is secreted, the lack of acid prevents it from functioning because pepsin requires an acid medium for activity.

Gastric Atrophy May Cause Pernicious Anemia. Pernicious anemia commonly accompanies gastric atrophy and achlorhydria. Normal gastric secretions contain a glycoprotein called *intrinsic factor,* secreted by the same parietal cells that secrete hydrochloric acid. Intrinsic factor must be present for adequate absorption of vitamin B_{12} from the ileum. That is, intrinsic factor combines with vitamin B_{12} in the stomach and protects it from being digested and destroyed as it passes into the small intestine. Then, when the intrinsic factor–vitamin B_{12} complex reaches the terminal ileum, the intrinsic factor binds with receptors on the ileal epithelial surface, which in turn makes it possible for the vitamin B_{12} to be absorbed.

In the absence of intrinsic factor, only about 1/50 of the vitamin B_{12} is absorbed. In addition without intrinsic factor, an adequate amount of vitamin B_{12} is not made available from the foods to cause young, newly forming red blood cells to mature in the bone marrow. The result is *pernicious anemia.* This is discussed in more detail in Chapter 22.

PEPTIC ULCER

This topic has been discussed in detail in Chapter 67. Please refer to Chapter 67 for further details.

Disorders of the Small Intestine

ABNORMAL DIGESTION OF FOOD IN THE SMALL INTESTINE—PANCREATIC FAILURE

A serious cause of abnormal digestion is failure of the pancreas to secrete pancreatic juice into the small intestine. Lack of pancreatic secretion frequently occurs (1) in persons with *pancreatitis* (discussed later), (2) when the *pancreatic duct is blocked* by a gallstone at the papilla of Vater, or (3) after the *head of the pancreas has been removed* because of malignancy.

Loss of pancreatic juice means loss of trypsin, chymotrypsin, carboxypolypeptidase, pancreatic amylase, pancreatic lipase, and a few other digestive enzymes. Without these enzymes, up to 60% of the fat entering the small intestine may not be absorbed, along with one-third to one-half of the proteins and carbohydrates. As a result, large portions of the ingested food cannot be used for nutrition and copious, fatty feces are excreted.

Pancreatitis—Inflammation of the Pancreas. Pancreatitis can occur in the form of either *acute pancreatitis* or *chronic pancreatitis.*

The most common cause of pancreatitis is *drinking excess alcohol,* and the second most common cause is *blockage of the papilla of Vater* by a gallstone; the two causes together account for more than 90% of all cases. When a gallstone blocks the papilla of Vater, the main secretory duct from the pancreas and the common bile duct are blocked. The pancreatic enzymes are then dammed up in the ducts and acini of the pancreas. Eventually, so much trypsinogen accumulates that it *overcomes the trypsin inhibitor* in the secretions and a small quantity of trypsinogen becomes activated to form trypsin. Once this happens, the trypsin activates still more trypsinogen, as well as chymotrypsinogen and carboxypolypeptidase, resulting in a vicious circle until most of the proteolytic enzymes in the pancreatic ducts and acini become activated. These enzymes rapidly digest large portions of the pancreas, sometimes completely and permanently destroying the ability of the pancreas to secrete digestive enzymes.

MALABSORPTION BY THE SMALL INTESTINAL MUCOSA—SPRUE

Occasionally, nutrients are not adequately absorbed from the small intestine even though the food has been well digested. Several diseases can cause decreased absorption by the mucosa; they are often classified together under the general term "*sprue.*" Malabsorption also can occur when large portions of the small intestine have been removed.

Nontropical Sprue. One type of sprue, called variously *idiopathic sprue, celiac disease* (in children), or *gluten enteropathy,* results from the toxic effects of *gluten* present in certain types of grains, especially wheat and rye. Only some people are susceptible to this effect, but in those who are susceptible, gluten has a direct destructive effect on intestinal enterocytes. In milder forms of the disease, only the microvilli of the absorbing enterocytes on the villi are destroyed, thus decreasing the absorptive surface area as much as twofold. In the more severe forms, the villi become blunted or disappear altogether, thus still further reducing the absorptive area of the gut. Removal of wheat and rye flour from the diet frequently results in cure within weeks, especially in children with this disease.

Tropical Sprue. A different type of sprue called *tropical sprue* frequently occurs in the tropics and can often be treated with antibacterial agents. Even though no specific bacterium has been implicated as the cause, it is believed that this variety of sprue is usually caused by inflammation of the intestinal mucosa resulting from unidentified infectious agents.

Malabsorption in Sprue. In the early stages of sprue, intestinal absorption of fat is more impaired than absorption of other digestive products. The fat that appears in the stools is almost entirely in the form of salts of fatty acids rather than undigested fat, demonstrating that the problem is one of absorption, not of digestion. In fact, the condition is frequently called *steatorrhea,* which means simply excess fats in the stools.

In severe cases of sprue, in addition to malabsorption of fats, impaired absorption of proteins, carbohydrates, calcium, vitamin K, folic acid, and vitamin B_{12} also occurs. As a result, the person experiences (1) severe nutritional deficiency, which often results in wasting of the body; (2) osteomalacia (demineralization of the bones because of lack of calcium); (3) inadequate blood coagulation caused by lack of vitamin K; and (4) macrocytic anemia of the pernicious anemia type, resulting from diminished vitamin B_{12} and folic acid absorption.

Disorders of the Large Intestine

CONSTIPATION

Constipation means *slow movement of feces through the large intestine*. It is often associated with large quantities of dry, hard feces in the descending colon that accumulate because of excess absorption of fluid or insufficient fluid intake. Any pathology of the intestines that obstructs movement of intestinal contents, such as tumors, adhesions that constrict the intestines, or ulcers, can cause constipation. Infants are seldom constipated, but part of their training in the early years of life requires that they learn to control defecation; this control is affected by inhibiting the natural defecation reflexes. Clinical experience shows that if one does not allow defecation to occur when the defecation reflexes are excited or if one overuses laxatives to take the place of natural bowel function, the reflexes become progressively less strong over months or years, and the colon becomes *atonic*. For this reason, if a person establishes regular bowel habits early in life, defecating when the gastrocolic and duodenocolic reflexes cause mass movements in the large intestine, the development of constipation in later life is less likely.

Constipation can also result from spasm of a small segment of the sigmoid colon. Motility normally is weak in the large intestine, so even a slight degree of spasm may cause serious constipation. After the constipation has continued for several days and excess feces have accumulated above a spastic sigmoid colon, excessive colonic secretions often then lead to a day or so of diarrhea. After this, the cycle begins again, with repeated bouts of alternating constipation and diarrhea.

Megacolon (Hirschsprung Disease). Occasionally, constipation is so severe that bowel movements occur only once every several days or sometimes only once a week. This phenomenon allows tremendous quantities of fecal matter to accumulate in the colon, causing the colon sometimes to distend to a diameter of 3–4 in. The condition is called *megacolon*, or *Hirschsprung disease*.

One cause of megacolon is lack of or deficiency *of ganglion cells in the myenteric plexus in a segment of the sigmoid colon.* As a consequence, neither defecation reflexes nor strong peristaltic motility can occur in this area of the large intestine. The sigmoid becomes small and almost spastic while feces accumulate proximal to this area, causing megacolon in the ascending, transverse, and descending colons.

DIARRHEA

Diarrhea results from rapid movement of fecal matter through the large intestine. Several causes of diarrhea with important physiological sequelae are the following.

Enteritis—Inflammation of the Intestinal Tract. Enteritis means inflammation usually caused either by a virus or by bacteria in the intestinal tract. In usual *infectious diarrhea,* the infection is most extensive in the large intestine and the distal end of the ileum. Everywhere the infection is present, the mucosa becomes irritated and its rate of secretion becomes greatly enhanced. In addition, motility of the intestinal wall usually increases markedly. As a result, large quantities of fluid are made available for washing the infectious agent toward the anus, and at the same time strong propulsive movements propel this fluid forward. This mechanism is important for ridding the intestinal tract of a debilitating infection.

Of special interest is diarrhea caused by *cholera* (and less often by other bacteria such as some pathogenic colon bacilli). As explained in Chapter 73, cholera toxin directly stimulates excessive secretion of electrolytes and fluid from the crypts of Lieberkühn in the distal ileum and colon. The amount can be 10–12 L/day, although the colon can usually reabsorb a maximum of only 6–8 L/day. Therefore, loss of fluid and electrolytes can be so debilitating within several days that death can ensue.

The most important physiological basis of therapy in cholera is to replace the fluid and electrolytes as rapidly as they are lost, mainly by giving the patient intravenous solutions. With proper therapy, along with the use of antibiotics, almost no persons with cholera die but without therapy up to 50% of patients die.

Psychogenic Diarrhea. Most people are familiar with the diarrhea that accompanies periods of nervous tension, such as during examination time or when a soldier is about to go into battle. This type of diarrhea, called *psychogenic* emotional diarrhea, is caused by excessive stimulation of the parasympathetic nervous system, which greatly excites both (1) motility and (2) excess secretion of mucus in the distal colon. These two effects added together can cause marked diarrhea.

Ulcerative Colitis. Ulcerative colitis is a disease in which extensive areas of the walls of the large intestine become inflamed and ulcerated. The motility of the ulcerated colon is often so great that *mass movements* occur much of the day rather than for the usual 10–30 minutes. Also, the colon's secretions are greatly enhanced. As a result, the patient has repeated diarrheal bowel movements.

The cause of ulcerative colitis is unknown. Some clinicians believe that it results from an allergic or immune destructive effect, but it also could result from chronic bacterial infection not yet understood. Whatever the cause, there is a strong hereditary tendency for susceptibility to ulcerative colitis. Once the condition has progressed far, the ulcers seldom will heal until an ileostomy is performed to allow the small intestinal contents to drain to the exterior rather than to pass through the colon. Even then the ulcers sometimes fail to heal, and the only solution might be surgical removal of the entire colon.

PARALYSIS OF DEFECATION IN PERSONS WITH SPINAL CORD INJURIES

As discussed in Chapter 74, defecation is normally initiated by accumulating feces in the rectum, which causes a spinal cord–mediated *defecation reflex* passing from the rectum to the *conus medullaris* of the spinal cord and then back to the descending colon, sigmoid, rectum, and anus.

When the spinal cord is injured somewhere between the conus medullaris and the brain, the voluntary portion of the defecation act is blocked while the basic cord reflex for defecation is still intact. Nevertheless, loss of the voluntary aid to defecation—that is, loss of the increased abdominal pressure and relaxation of the voluntary anal sphincter—often makes defecation a difficult process in the person with this type of upper cord injury. However, because the cord defecation reflex can still occur, a small enema to excite action of this cord reflex, usually given in the morning shortly after a meal, can often cause adequate defecation. In this way, people with spinal cord injuries that do not destroy the conus medullaris of the spinal cord can usually control their bowel movements each day.

General Disorders of the Gastrointestinal Tract

VOMITING

Vomiting is the means by which the upper gastrointestinal tract rids itself of its contents when almost any part of the upper tract becomes excessively irritated, overdistended, or even overexcitable. Excessive distention or irritation of the duodenum provides an especially strong stimulus for vomiting.

The sensory signals that initiate vomiting originate mainly from the pharynx, esophagus, stomach, and upper portions of the small intestines. As shown in Figure 75-1, the nerve impulses are transmitted, by both vagal and sympathetic afferent nerve fibers to multiple distributed nuclei in the brainstem, especially the *area postrema* that all together are called the "vomiting center." From here, *motor impulses* that cause the actual vomiting are transmitted from the vomiting center by way of the 5th, 7th, 9th, 10th, and 12th cranial nerves to the upper gastrointestinal

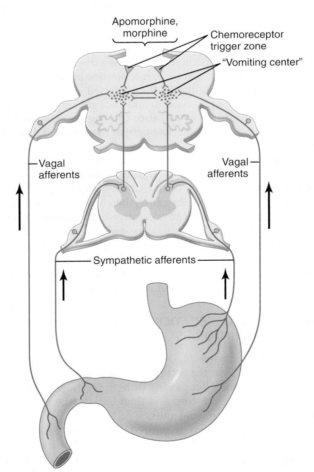

Figure 75-1   Neutral connections of the "vomiting center." This so-called vomiting center includes not only multiple sensory, motor, and control nuclei mainly in the medullary and pontile reticular formation but also extending into the spinal cord.

tract, through vagal and sympathetic nerves to the lower tract, and through spinal nerves to the diaphragm and abdominal muscles.

Antiperistalsis—The Prelude to Vomiting. In the early stages of excessive gastrointestinal irritation or overdistention, *antiperistalsis* begins to occur often many minutes before vomiting appears. Antiperistalsis means peristalsis *up* the digestive tract rather than downward. Antiperistalsis may begin as far down in the intestinal tract as the ileum, and the antiperistaltic wave travels backward up the intestine at a rate of 2–3 cm/second; this process can actually push a large share of the lower small intestine contents all the way back to the duodenum and stomach within 3–5 minutes. Then, as these upper portions of the gastrointestinal tract, especially the duodenum, become overly distended, this distention becomes the exciting factor that initiates the actual vomiting act.

At the onset of vomiting, strong intrinsic contractions occur in both the duodenum and the stomach, along with partial relaxation of the esophageal–stomach sphincter, thus allowing vomitus to begin moving from the stomach into the esophagus. From here, a specific vomiting act involving the abdominal muscles takes over and expels the vomitus to the exterior, as explained in the following.

Vomiting Act. Once the vomiting center has been sufficiently stimulated and the vomiting act has been instituted, the first effects are (1) a deep breath, (2) raising of the hyoid bone and larynx to pull the upper esophageal sphincter open, (3) closing of the glottis to prevent vomitus flow into the lungs, and (4) lifting of the soft palate to close the posterior nares. Next comes a strong downward contraction of the diaphragm along with simultaneous contraction of all the abdominal wall muscles, which squeezes the stomach between the diaphragm and the abdominal muscles, building the intragastric pressure to a high level. Finally, the lower esophageal sphincter relaxes completely, allowing expulsion of the gastric contents upward through the esophagus.

Thus, the vomiting act results from a squeezing action of the muscles of the abdomen associated with simultaneous contraction of the stomach wall and opening of the esophageal sphincters so that the gastric contents can be expelled.

"Chemoreceptor Trigger Zone" in the Brain Medulla for Initiation of Vomiting by Drugs or by Motion Sickness. Aside from the vomiting initiated by irritative stimuli in the gastrointestinal tract, vomiting can also be caused by nervous signals arising in areas of the brain. This mechanism is particularly true for a small area called the *chemoreceptor trigger zone for vomiting* located in the *area postrema* on the lateral walls of the fourth ventricle. Electrical stimulation of this area can initiate vomiting, but, more importantly, administration of certain drugs, including apomorphine, morphine, and some digitalis derivatives, can directly stimulate this chemoreceptor trigger zone and initiate vomiting. Destruction of this area blocks this type of vomiting but does not block vomiting resulting from irritative stimuli in the gastrointestinal tract itself.

Furthermore, it is well known that rapidly changing direction or rhythm of motion of the body can cause certain people to vomit. The mechanism for this phenomenon is the following: The motion stimulates receptors in the vestibular labyrinth of the inner ear, and from here impulses are transmitted mainly by way of the brainstem *vestibular nuclei into the cerebellum*, then to the *chemoreceptor trigger zone*, and finally to the *vomiting center* to cause vomiting.

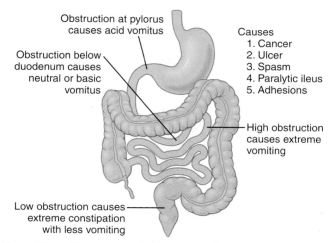

Obstruction at pylorus causes acid vomitus

Obstruction below duodenum causes neutral or basic vomitus

Causes
1. Cancer
2. Ulcer
3. Spasm
4. Paralytic ileus
5. Adhesions

High obstruction causes extreme vomiting

Low obstruction causes extreme constipation with less vomiting

Figure 75-2 Obstruction in different parts of the gastrointestinal tract.

NAUSEA

The sensation of nausea is often a prodrome of vomiting. Nausea is the conscious recognition of subconscious excitation in an area of the medulla closely associated with or part of the vomiting center. It can be caused by (1) irritative impulses coming from the gastrointestinal tract, (2) impulses that originate in the lower brain associated with motion sickness, or (3) impulses from the cerebral cortex to initiate vomiting. Vomiting occasionally occurs without the prodromal sensation of nausea, which indicates that only certain portions of the vomiting center are associated with the sensation of nausea.

GASTROINTESTINAL OBSTRUCTION

The gastrointestinal tract can become obstructed at almost any point along its course, as shown in Figure 75-2. Some common causes of obstruction are (1) *cancer,* (2) *fibrotic constriction resulting from ulceration or from peritoneal adhesions,* (3) *spasm of a segment of the gut,* and (4) *paralysis of a segment of the gut.*

The abnormal consequences of obstruction depend on the point in the gastrointestinal tract that becomes obstructed. If the obstruction occurs at the pylorus, which often results from fibrotic constriction after peptic ulceration, persistent vomiting of stomach contents occurs. This vomiting depresses bodily nutrition; it also causes excessive loss of hydrogen ions from the stomach and can result in various degrees of *whole-body metabolic alkalosis.*

If the obstruction is beyond the stomach, antiperistaltic reflux from the small intestine causes intestinal juices to flow backward into the stomach, and these juices are vomited along with the stomach secretions. In this instance, the person loses large amounts of water and electrolytes. He or she becomes severely dehydrated, but the loss of acid from the stomach and base from the small intestine may be approximately equal, so little change in acid–base balance occurs.

If the obstruction is near the distal end of the large intestine, feces can accumulate in the colon for a week or more. The patient develops an intense feeling of constipation, but at first vomiting is not severe. After the large intestine has become completely filled and it finally becomes impossible for additional chyme to move from the small intestine into the large intestine, severe vomiting then occurs. Prolonged obstruction of the large intestine can finally cause rupture of the intestine or dehydration and circulatory shock resulting from the severe vomiting.

GASES IN THE GASTROINTESTINAL TRACT; "FLATUS"

Gases, called *flatus,* can enter the gastrointestinal tract from three sources: (1) swallowed air, (2) gases formed in the gut as a result of bacterial action, or (3) gases that diffuse from the blood into the gastrointestinal tract. Most gases in the stomach are mixtures of nitrogen and oxygen derived from swallowed air. In the typical person these gases are expelled by belching. Only small amounts of gas normally occur in the small intestine, and much of this gas is air that passes from the stomach into the intestinal tract.

In the large intestine, bacterial action generates most of the gases including especially *carbon dioxide, methane,* and *hydrogen.* When methane and hydrogen become suitably mixed with oxygen, an actual explosive mixture is sometimes formed. Use of the electric cautery during sigmoidoscopy has been known to cause a mild explosion.

Certain foods are known to cause greater expulsion of flatus through the anus than others—beans, cabbage, onion, cauliflower, corn, and certain irritant foods such as vinegar. Some of these foods serve as a suitable medium for gas-forming bacteria, especially unabsorbed fermentable types of carbohydrates. For instance, beans contain an indigestible carbohydrate that passes into the colon and becomes a superior food for colonic bacteria. But in other instances, excess expulsion of gas results from irritation of the large intestine, which promotes rapid peristaltic expulsion of gases through the anus before they can be absorbed.

The amount of gases entering or forming in the large intestine each day averages 7–10 L, whereas the average amount expelled through the anus is usually only about 0.6 L. The remainder is normally absorbed into the blood through the intestinal mucosa and expelled through the lungs.

BIBLIOGRAPHY

Atherton JC, Blaser MJ: Coadaptation of *Helicobacter pylori* and humans: ancient history, modern implications, *J. Clin. Invest.* 119:2475, 2009.

Bassotti G, Blandizzi C: Understanding and treating refractory constipation, *World J. Gastrointest. Pharmacol. Ther.* 5:77, 2014.

Beatty JK, Bhargava A, Buret AG: Post-infectious irritable bowel syndrome: mechanistic insights into chronic disturbances following enteric infection, *World J. Gastroenterol.* 20:3976, 2014.

Bhattacharyya A, Chattopadhyay R, Mitra S, Crowe SE: Oxidative stress: an essential factor in the pathogenesis of gastrointestinal mucosal diseases, *Physiol. Rev.* 94:329, 2014.

Boeckxstaens G, El-Serag HB, Smout AJ, Kahrilas PJ: Symptomatic reflux disease: the present, the past and the future, *Gut* 63:1185, 2014.

Braganza JM, Lee SH, McCloy RF, McMahon MJ: Chronic pancreatitis, *Lancet* 377:1184, 2011.

Camilleri M: Peripheral mechanisms in Crohn's disease, irritable bowel syndrome, *N. Engl. J. Med.* 367:1626, 2012.

Camilleri M: Physiological underpinnings of irritable bowel syndrome: neurohormonal mechanisms, *J. Physiol.* 592:2967, 2014.

Danese, S., Fiocchi, C., 2011. Ulcerative colitis. N. Engl. J. Med. 365, 1713.

Kahrilas PJ, Clinical practice: Gastroesophageal reflux disease, *N. Engl. J. Med.* 359:1700, 2008.

Knights D, Lassen KG, Xavier RJ: Advances in inflammatory bowel disease pathogenesis: linking host genetics and the microbiome, *Gut* 62:1505, 2013.

Kunzelmann K, Mall M: Electrolyte transport in the mammalian colon: mechanisms and implications for disease, *Physiol. Rev.* 82:245, 2002.

Mayer EA, Savidge T, Shulman RJ: Brain–gut microbiome interactions and functional bowel disorders, *Gastroenterology* 146:1500, 2014.

Maynard CL, Elson CO, Hatton RD, Weaver CT: Reciprocal interactions of the intestinal microbiota and immune system, *Nature* 489:231, 2012.

McMahon BP, Jobe BA, Pandolfino JE, Gregersen H: Do we really understand the role of the oesophagogastric junction in disease? *World J. Gastroenterol.* 15:144, 2009.

Morris AM, Regenbogen SE, Hardiman KM, Hendren S: Sigmoid diverticulitis: a systematic review, *JAMA* 311:287, 2014.

Neurath MF: Cytokines in inflammatory bowel disease, *Nat. Rev. Immunol.* 14:329, 2014.

Xavier RJ, Podolsky DK: Unravelling the pathogenesis of inflammatory bowel disease, *Nature* 448:427, 2007.

Renal Physiology

ANURA KURPAD

Functional Anatomy of the Kidney

LEARNING OBJECTIVES

- Describe the functions of the kidney.
- Describe the structure of the nephron.
- Describe the difference between a cortical and a juxtamedullary nephron.

GLOSSARY OF TERMS

- **Angiotensin:** A peptide hormone that is part of the renin–angiotensin system that causes blood vessels to constrict and increases blood pressure

- **Calcitriol:** Hormonally active form of vitamin D

- **Cortical and juxtamedullary nephrons:** Origin of cortical nephrons being in the superficial renal cortex, while that of juxtamedullary nephrons being nearer the renal medulla

- **Erythropoiesis:** The process of red blood cell production

- **Erythropoietin:** Renal hormone that controls erythropoiesis

- **Nephron:** Basic structural and functional unit of the kidney

Multiple Functions of the Kidneys

Most people are familiar with one important function of the kidneys—is to rid the body of waste materials that are either ingested or produced by metabolism. A second function that is especially critical is to control the volume and electrolyte composition of the body fluids. For water and virtually all electrolytes in the body the balance between intake (due to ingestion or metabolic production) and output (due to excretion or metabolic consumption) is maintained largely by the kidneys. This regulatory function of the kidneys maintains the stable internal environment necessary for the cells to perform their various activities.

The kidneys perform their most important functions by filtering the plasma and removing substances from the filtrate at variable rates, depending on the needs of the body. Ultimately, the kidneys "clear" unwanted substances from the filtrate (and therefore from the blood) by excreting them in the urine while returning substances that are needed back to the blood.

Although this chapter and the next few chapters focus mainly on the control of renal excretion of water, electrolytes, and metabolic waste products, the kidneys serve many important homeostatic functions, including the following:

- excretion of metabolic waste products and foreign chemicals
- regulation of water and electrolyte balances
- regulation of body fluid osmolality and electrolyte concentrations

- regulation of arterial pressure
- regulation of acid–base balance
- regulation of erythrocyte production
- secretion, metabolism, and excretion of hormones
- gluconeogenesis

EXCRETION OF METABOLIC WASTE PRODUCTS, FOREIGN CHEMICALS, DRUGS, AND HORMONE METABOLITES

The kidneys are the primary means for eliminating waste products of metabolism that are no longer needed by the body. These products include *urea* (from the metabolism of amino acids), *creatinine* (from muscle creatine), *uric acid* (from nucleic acids), *end products of hemoglobin breakdown* (such as bilirubin), and *metabolites of various hormones*. These waste products must be eliminated from the body as rapidly as they are produced. The kidneys also eliminate most toxins and other foreign substances that are either produced by the body or ingested, such as pesticides, drugs, and food additives.

Regulation of Water and Electrolyte Balances. For maintenance of homeostasis, excretion of water and electrolytes must precisely match intake. If intake exceeds excretion, the amount of that substance in the body will increase. If intake is less than excretion, the amount of that substance in the body will decrease. Although temporary (or cyclic) imbalances of water and electrolytes may occur in various physiological and pathophysiological conditions associated with altered intake or renal excretion, the maintenance of life depends on restoration of water and electrolyte balance.

Intake of water and many electrolytes is governed mainly by a person's eating and drinking habits, requiring the kidneys to adjust their excretion rates to match the intakes of various substances. Figure 76-1 shows the response of the kidneys to a sudden 10-fold increase in sodium intake from a low level of 30 mEq/day to a high level of 300 mEq/day. Within 2–3 days after raising the sodium intake, renal excretion also increases to about 300 mEq/day so that a balance between intake and output is rapidly reestablished. However, during the 2–3 days of renal adaptation to the high sodium intake, there is a modest accumulation of sodium that raises extracellular fluid volume slightly and triggers hormonal changes and other compensatory responses that signal the kidneys to increase their sodium excretion.

The capacity of the kidneys to alter sodium excretion in response to changes in sodium intake is enormous. Experimental studies have shown that in many people sodium intake can be increased to 1500 mEq/day (more than 10 times normal) or decreased to 10 mEq/day (less than one-tenth normal) with relatively small changes in extracellular fluid volume or plasma sodium concentration. This phenomenon is also true for water and for most other electrolytes, such as chloride, potassium, calcium, hydrogen, magnesium, and phosphate ions. In the next few chapters, we discuss the specific mechanisms that permit the kidneys to perform these amazing feats of homeostasis.

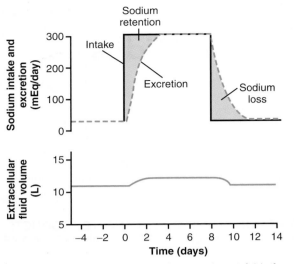

Figure 76-1 Effect of increasing sodium intake 10-fold (from 30 to 300 mEq/day) on urinary sodium excretion and extracellular fluid volume. The shaded areas represent the net sodium retention or the net sodium loss, determined from the difference between sodium intake and sodium excretion.

Regulation of Arterial Pressure. As discussed in Chapter 44, the kidneys play a dominant role in long-term regulation of arterial pressure by excreting variable amounts of sodium and water. The kidneys also contribute to short-term arterial pressure regulation by secreting hormones and vasoactive factors or substances (eg, *renin*) that lead to the formation of vasoactive products (eg, angiotensin II).

Regulation of Acid–Base Balance. The kidneys contribute to acid–base regulation, along with the lungs and body fluid buffers, by excreting acids and by regulating the body fluid buffer stores. The kidneys are the only means of eliminating from the body certain types of acids, such as sulfuric acid and phosphoric acid, generated by the metabolism of proteins.

Regulation of Erythrocyte Production. The kidneys secrete *erythropoietin*, which stimulates the production of red blood cells by *hematopoietic stem cells* in the bone marrow, as discussed in Chapter 20. One important stimulus for erythropoietin se-

cretion by the kidneys is *hypoxia*. The kidneys normally account for almost all the erythropoietin secreted into the circulation. In people with severe kidney disease or who have had their kidneys removed and have been placed on hemodialysis, severe anemia develops as a result of decreased erythropoietin production.

Regulation of 1,25-Dihydroxyvitamin D₃ Production. The kidneys produce the active form of vitamin D, 1,25-dihydroxyvitamin D₃ (*calcitriol*), by hydroxylating this vitamin at the "number 1" position. Calcitriol is essential for normal calcium deposition in bone and calcium reabsorption by the gastrointestinal tract. As discussed in Chapter 90, calcitriol plays an important role in calcium and phosphate regulation.

Glucose Synthesis. The kidneys synthesize glucose from amino acids and other precursors during prolonged fasting, a process referred to as *gluconeogenesis*. The kidneys' capacity to add glucose to the blood during prolonged periods of fasting rivals that of the liver.

With chronic kidney disease or acute failure of the kidneys, these homeostatic functions are disrupted and severe abnormalities of body fluid volumes and composition rapidly occur. With complete renal failure, enough potassium, acids, fluid, and other substances accumulate in the body to cause death within a few days, unless clinical interventions such as hemodialysis are initiated to restore, at least partially, the body fluid and electrolyte balances.

Physiological Anatomy of the Kidneys

GENERAL ORGANIZATION OF THE KIDNEYS AND URINARY TRACT

The two kidneys lie on the posterior wall of the abdomen, outside the peritoneal cavity (Figure 76-2). Each kidney of the adult human weighs about 150 g and is about the size of a clenched fist. The medial side of each kidney contains an indented region called the *hilum* through which pass the renal artery and vein, lymphatics, nerve supply, and ureter, which carries the final urine from the kidney to the bladder, where it is stored until the bladder is emptied. The kidney is surrounded by a tough, fibrous *capsule* that protects its delicate inner structures.

If the kidney is bisected from top to bottom, the two major regions that can be visualized are the outer *cortex* and the inner *medulla* regions. The medulla is divided into 8–10 cone-shaped

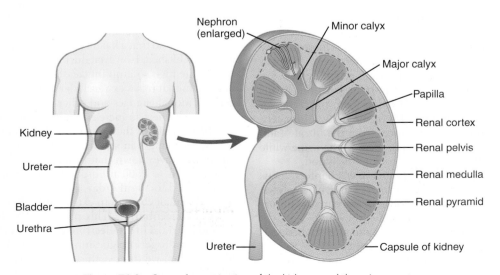

Figure 76-2 General organization of the kidneys and the urinary system.

masses of tissue called *renal pyramids*. The base of each pyramid originates at the border between the cortex and medulla and terminates in the *papilla*, which projects into the space of the *renal pelvis*, a funnel-shaped continuation of the upper end of the ureter. The outer border of the pelvis is divided into open-ended pouches called *major calyces* that extend downward and divide into *minor calyces*, which collect urine from the tubules of each papilla. The walls of the calyces, pelvis, and ureter contain contractile elements that propel the urine toward the *bladder*, where urine is stored until it is emptied by *micturition*, as discussed later in this chapter.

THE NEPHRON IS THE FUNCTIONAL UNIT OF THE KIDNEY

Each kidney in the human contains about 800,000–1,000,000 *nephrons*, each capable of forming urine. The kidney cannot regenerate new nephrons. Therefore, with renal injury, disease, or normal aging, there is a gradual decrease in nephron number. After age 40, the number of functioning nephrons usually decreases about 10% every 10 years; thus, at age 80, many people have 40% fewer functioning nephrons than they did at age 40. This loss is not life threatening because adaptive changes in the remaining nephrons allow them to excrete the proper amounts of water, electrolytes, and waste products, as discussed in Chapter 84.

Each nephron contains (1) a tuft of glomerular capillaries called the *glomerulus*, through which large amounts of fluid are filtered from the blood, and (2) a long *tubule* in which the filtered fluid is converted into urine on its way to the pelvis of the kidney (see Figure 76-3).

The glomerulus contains a network of branching and anastomosing glomerular capillaries that, compared with other capillaries, have high hydrostatic pressure (about 60 mmHg). The glomerular capillaries are covered by epithelial cells, and the total glomerulus is encased in *Bowman capsule*.

Fluid filtered from the glomerular capillaries flows into Bowman capsule and then into the *proximal tubule*, which lies in the cortex of the kidney (Figure 76-4). From the proximal tubule, fluid flows into the *loop of Henle*, which dips into the renal medulla. Each loop consists of a *descending* and an *ascending limb*. The walls of the descending limb and the lower end of the ascending limb are very thin and therefore are called the *thin segment of the loop of Henle*. After the ascending limb of the loop returns partway back to the cortex, its wall becomes much thicker, and it is referred to as the *thick segment of the ascending limb*.

At the end of the thick ascending limb is a short segment that has in its wall a plaque of specialized epithelial cells known as the *macula densa*. As discussed later, the macula densa plays an important role in controlling nephron function. Beyond the macula densa, fluid enters the *distal tubule*, which, like the proximal tubule, lies in the renal cortex. This is followed by the *connecting tubule* and the *cortical collecting tubule*, which lead to the *cortical collecting duct*. The initial parts of 8–10 cortical collecting ducts join to form a single larger collecting duct that runs downward into the medulla and becomes the *medullary collecting duct*. The collecting ducts merge to form progressively larger ducts that eventually empty into the renal pelvis through

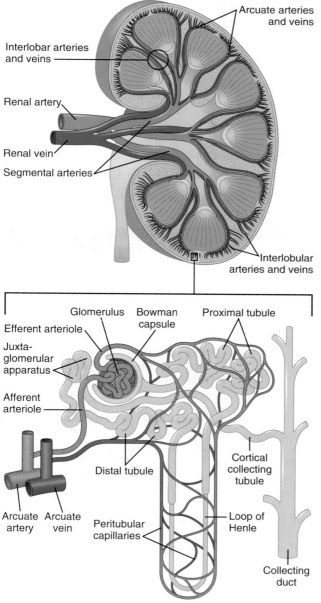

Figure 76-3 Section of the human kidney showing the major vessels that supply the blood flow to the kidney and schematic of the microcirculation of each nephron.

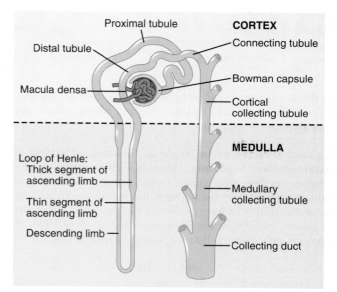

Figure 76-4 Basic tubular segments of the nephron. The relative lengths of the different tubular segments are not drawn to scale.

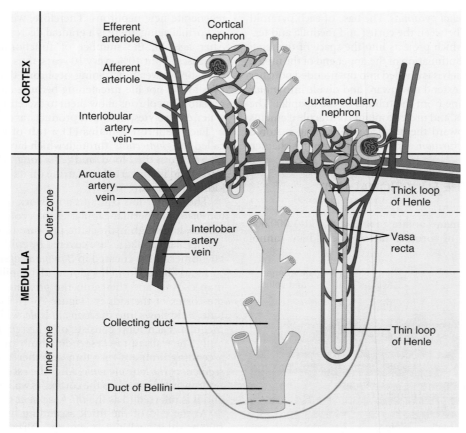

Figure 76-5 Schematic of relations between blood vessels and tubular structures and differences between cortical and juxtamedullary nephrons.

TABLE 76-1	Comparison of Cortical and Juxtamedullary Nephrons	
	Cortical Nephron	**Juxtamedullary Nephron**
Location	Cortex	Medulla–cortex junction
Proportion of total nephrons (%)	85	15
Function	Filtration and reabsorption	Filtration, reabsorption, and creation of medullary osmolar gradient
Length of loop of Henle	Short	Long
Ascending limb of loop	Thin segment only	Thin and thick segments
Vasa recta	Absent	Present, dipping into medulla
Peritubular capillary network	Large	Small

the tips of the *renal papillae*. In each kidney, there are about 250 of the very large collecting ducts, each of which collects urine from about 4000 nephrons.

Regional Differences in Nephron Structure: Cortical and Juxtamedullary Nephrons. Although each nephron has all the components described earlier, there are some differences, depending on how deep the nephron lies within the kidney mass. Those nephrons that have glomeruli located in the outer cortex are called *cortical nephrons*; they have short loops of Henle that penetrate only a short distance into the medulla (Figure 76-5; Table 76-1).

About 20–30% of the nephrons have glomeruli that lie deep in the renal cortex near the medulla and are called *juxtamedullary nephrons*. These nephrons have long loops of Henle that dip

deeply into the medulla, in some cases all the way to the tips of the renal papillae.

The vascular structures supplying the juxtamedullary nephrons also differ from those supplying the cortical nephrons. For the cortical nephrons, the entire tubular system is surrounded by an extensive network of peritubular capillaries. For the juxtamedullary nephrons, long efferent arterioles extend from the glomeruli down into the outer medulla and then divide into specialized peritubular capillaries called *vasa recta* that extend downward into the medulla, lying side by side with the loops of Henle. Like the loops of Henle, the vasa recta return toward the cortex and empty into the cortical veins. This specialized network of capillaries in the medulla plays an essential role in the formation of concentrated urine and is discussed in Chapter 80.

BIBLIOGRAPHY

Beeuwkes R III: The vascular organization of the kidney, *Annu. Rev. Physiol.* 42:531, 1980.

Cupples WA, Braam B: Assessment of renal autoregulation, *Am. J. Physiol. Renal Physiol.* 292:F1105, 2007.

DiBona GF: Physiology in perspective: the wisdom of the body. Neural control of the kidney, *Am. J. Physiol. Regul. Integr. Comp. Physiol.* 289:R633, 2005.

Hall JE, Granger JP, Hall ME: Physiology and pathophysiology of hypertension. In Alpern RJ, Moe OW, Caplan M, editors: *Seldin and Giebisch's The Kidney: Physiology & Pathophysiology*, fifth ed., London, 2013, Elsevier.

Kriz WW, Kaissling B: Structural organization of the mammalian kidney. In Seldin DW, Giebisch G, editors: *The Kidney—Physiology and Pathophysiology*, third ed., Philadelphia, PA, 2000, Lippincott Williams & Wilkins, pp 587–654.

Loutzenhiser R, Griffin K, Williamson G, et al: Renal autoregulation: new perspectives regarding the protective and regulatory roles of the underlying mechanisms, *Am. J. Physiol. Regul. Integr. Comp. Physiol.* 290:R1153, 2006.

Urine Formation by the Kidneys: Renal Blood Flow, Glomerular Filtration, and Their Control

Urine Formation Results From Glomerular Filtration, Tubular Reabsorption, and Tubular Secretion

The rates at which different substances are excreted in the urine represent the sum of three renal processes, shown in Figure 77-1: (1) glomerular filtration, (2) reabsorption of substances from the renal tubules into the blood, and (3) secretion of substances from the blood into the renal tubules. Expressed mathematically,

$$\text{Urinary excretion rate} = \text{Filtration rate} - \text{Reabsorption rate} + \text{Secretion rate}$$

Urine formation begins when a large amount of fluid that is virtually free of protein is filtered from the glomerular capillaries into Bowman's capsule. Most substances in the plasma, except for proteins, are freely filtered, so their concentration in the glomerular filtrate in Bowman's capsule is almost the same as in the plasma. As filtered fluid leaves Bowman's capsule and passes through the tubules, it is modified by reabsorption of water and specific solutes back into the blood or by secretion of other substances from the peritubular capillaries into the tubules.

Figure 77-2 shows the renal handling of four hypothetical substances. The substance shown in panel A is freely filtered by the glomerular capillaries, but is neither reabsorbed nor secreted. Therefore, its excretion rate is equal to the rate at which it was filtered. Certain waste products in the body, such as creatinine, are handled by the kidneys in this manner, allowing excretion of essentially all that is filtered.

In panel B, the substance is freely filtered but is also partly reabsorbed from the tubules back into the blood. Therefore, the rate of urinary excretion is less than the rate of filtration at the glomerular capillaries. In this case, the excretion rate is calculated as the filtration rate minus the reabsorption rate. This pattern is typical for many of the electrolytes of the body such as sodium and chloride ions.

In panel C, the substance is freely filtered at the glomerular capillaries but is not excreted into the urine because all the filtered substance is reabsorbed from the tubules back into the blood. This pattern occurs for some of the nutritional substances in the blood, such as amino acids and glucose, allowing them to be conserved in the body fluids.

The substance in panel D is freely filtered at the glomerular capillaries and is not reabsorbed, but additional quantities of this substance are secreted from the peritubular capillary blood into the renal tubules. This pattern often occurs for organic acids and bases, permitting them to be rapidly cleared from the blood and excreted in large amounts in the urine. The excretion rate in this case is calculated as filtration rate plus tubular secretion rate.

For each substance in the plasma, a particular combination of filtration, reabsorption, and secretion occurs. The rate at which the substance is excreted in the urine depends on the relative rates of these three basic renal processes.

Why Are Large Amounts of Solutes Filtered and Then Reabsorbed by the Kidneys?. One might question the wisdom of filtering such large amounts of water and solutes and then reabsorbing most of these substances. One advantage of a high glomerular filtration rate (GFR) is that it allows the kidneys to rapidly remove waste products from the body that depend mainly on glomerular filtration for their excretion. Most waste products are poorly reabsorbed by the tubules and, therefore, depend on a high GFR for effective removal from the body.

A second advantage of a high GFR is that it allows all the body fluids to be filtered and processed by the kidneys many times each day. Because the entire plasma volume is only about 3 L, whereas the GFR is about 180 L/day, the entire plasma can be filtered and processed about 60 times each day. This high

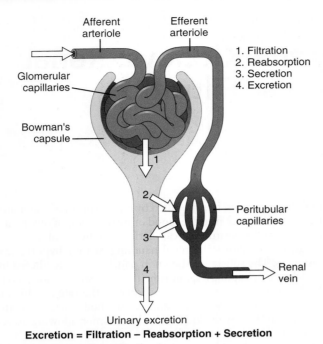

Figure 77-1 Basic kidney processes that determine the composition of the urine. Urinary excretion rate of a substance is equal to the rate at which the substance is filtered minus its reabsorption rate plus the rate at which it is secreted from the peritubular capillary blood into the tubules.

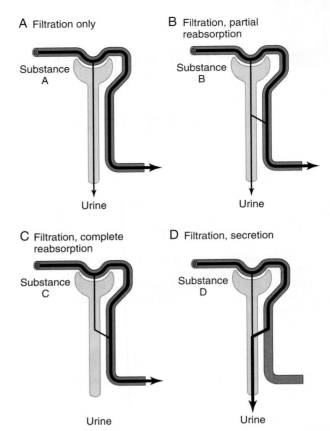

Figure 77-2 Renal handling of four hypothetical substances. (A) The substance is freely filtered but not reabsorbed. (B) The substance is freely filtered, but part of the filtered load is reabsorbed back in the blood. (C) The substance is freely filtered but is not excreted in the urine because all the filtered substance is reabsorbed from the tubules into the blood. (D) The substance is freely filtered and is not reabsorbed but is secreted from the peritubular capillary blood into the renal tubules.

GFR allows the kidneys to precisely and rapidly control the volume and composition of the body fluids.

Renal Blood Flow

RENAL BLOOD SUPPLY

Blood flow to the two kidneys is normally about 22% of the cardiac output or 1100 mL/min. The renal artery enters the kidney through the hilum and then branches progressively to form the *interlobar arteries, arcuate arteries, interlobular arteries* (also called *radial arteries*), and *afferent arterioles*, which lead to the *glomerular capillaries*, where large amounts of fluid and solutes (except the plasma proteins) are filtered to begin urine formation (Figure 76-3). The distal ends of the capillaries of each glomerulus coalesce to form the *efferent arteriole*, which leads to a second capillary network, the *peritubular capillaries*, that surrounds the renal tubules.

The renal circulation is unique in having two capillary beds, the glomerular and peritubular capillaries, which are arranged in series and separated by the efferent arterioles, which help regulate the hydrostatic pressure in both sets of capillaries. High hydrostatic pressure in the glomerular capillaries (about 60 mmHg) causes rapid fluid filtration, whereas a much lower hydrostatic pressure in the peritubular capillaries (about 13 mmHg) permits rapid fluid reabsorption. By adjusting the resistance of the afferent and efferent arterioles, the kidneys can regulate the hydrostatic pressure in both the glomerular and the peritubular capillaries, thereby changing the rate of glomerular filtration, tubular reabsorption, or both in response to body homeostatic demands.

The peritubular capillaries empty into the vessels of the venous system, which run parallel to the arteriolar vessels. The blood vessels of the venous system progressively form the *interlobular vein, arcuate vein, interlobar vein,* and *renal vein,* which leave the kidney beside the renal artery and ureter.

In an average 70-kg man, the combined blood flow through both kidneys is about 1100 mL/min or about 22% of the cardiac output. Considering that the two kidneys constitute only about 0.4% of the total body weight, one can readily see that they receive an extremely high blood flow compared with other organs.

As with other tissues, blood flow supplies the kidneys with nutrients and removes waste products. However, the high flow to the kidneys greatly exceeds this need. The purpose of this additional flow is to supply enough plasma for the high rates of glomerular filtration that are necessary for precise regulation of body fluid volumes and solute concentrations. As might be expected, the mechanisms that regulate renal blood flow are closely linked to the control of GFR and the excretory functions of the kidneys.

RENAL BLOOD FLOW AND OXYGEN CONSUMPTION

On a per-gram-weight basis, the kidneys normally consume oxygen at twice the rate of the brain but have almost seven times the blood flow of the brain. Thus, the oxygen delivered to the kidneys far exceeds their metabolic needs, and the arterial–venous extraction of oxygen is relatively low compared with that of most other tissues.

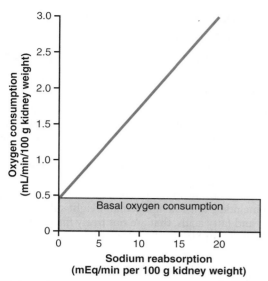

Figure 77-3 Relationship between oxygen consumption and sodium reabsorption in dog kidneys. *(From Kramer, K., Deetjen, P., 1960. Relation of renal oxygen consumption to blood supply and glomerular filtration during variations of blood pressure. Pflugers Arch. Physiol. 271, 782).*

	Pressure in Vessel (mmHg)		
Vessel	**Beginning**	**End**	**Percent of Total Renal Vascular Resistance**
Renal artery	100	100	≈0
Interlobar, arcuate, and interlobular arteries	≈100	85	≈16
Afferent arteriole	85	60	≈26
Glomerular capillaries	60	59	≈1
Efferent arteriole	59	18	≈43
Peritubular capillaries	18	8	≈10
Interlobar, interlobular, and arcuate veins	8	4	≈4
Renal vein	4	≈4	≈0

TABLE 77-1 Approximate Pressures and Vascular Resistances in the Circulation of a Normal Kidney

A large fraction of the oxygen consumed by the kidneys is related to the high rate of active sodium reabsorption by the renal tubules. If renal blood flow and GFR are reduced and less sodium is filtered, less sodium is reabsorbed and less oxygen is consumed. Therefore, renal oxygen consumption varies in proportion to renal tubular sodium reabsorption, which in turn is closely related to GFR and the rate of sodium filtered (Figure 77-3). If glomerular filtration completely ceases, renal sodium reabsorption also ceases and oxygen consumption decreases to about one-fourth normal. This residual oxygen consumption reflects the basic metabolic needs of the renal cells.

DETERMINANTS OF RENAL BLOOD FLOW

Renal blood flow is determined by the pressure gradient across the renal vasculature (the difference between renal artery and renal vein hydrostatic pressures), divided by the total renal vascular resistance:

$$\frac{(\text{Renal artery pressure} - \text{Renal vein pressure})}{\text{Total renal vascular resistance}}$$

Renal artery pressure is about equal to systemic arterial pressure, and renal vein pressure averages about 3–4 mmHg under most conditions. As in other vascular beds, the total vascular resistance through the kidneys is determined by the sum of the resistances in the individual vasculature segments, including the arteries, arterioles, capillaries, and veins (Table 77.1).

Most of the renal vascular resistance resides in three major segments: interlobular arteries, afferent arterioles, and efferent arterioles. Resistance of these vessels is controlled by the sympathetic nervous system, various hormones, and local internal renal control mechanisms, as discussed later. An increase in the resistance of any of the vascular segments of the kidneys tends to reduce the renal blood flow, whereas a decrease in vascular resistance increases renal blood flow if renal artery and renal vein pressures remain constant.

Although changes in arterial pressure have some influence on renal blood flow, the kidneys have effective mechanisms for maintaining renal blood flow and GFR relatively constant over an arterial pressure range between 80 and 170 mmHg, a process called *autoregulation*. This capacity for autoregulation occurs through mechanisms that are completely intrinsic to the kidneys, as discussed later in this chapter.

BLOOD FLOW IN THE VASA RECTA OF THE RENAL MEDULLA IS VERY LOW COMPARED WITH FLOW IN THE RENAL CORTEX

The outer part of the kidney, the renal cortex, receives most of the kidney's blood flow. Blood flow in the renal medulla accounts for only 1–2% of the total renal blood flow. Flow to the renal medulla is supplied by a specialized portion of the peritubular capillary system called the *vasa recta*. These vessels descend into the medulla in parallel with the loops of Henle and then loop back along with the loops of Henle and return to the cortex before emptying into the venous system. As discussed in Chapter 79, the vasa recta play an important role in allowing the kidneys to form concentrated urine.

Autoregulation of GFR and Renal Blood Flow

Feedback mechanisms intrinsic to the kidneys normally keep the renal blood flow and GFR relatively constant, despite marked changes in arterial blood pressure. These mechanisms still function in blood-perfused kidneys that have been removed from the body, independent of systemic influences. This relative constancy of GFR and renal blood flow is referred to as *autoregulation* (Figure 77-4).

The primary function of blood flow autoregulation in most tissues other than the kidneys is to maintain the delivery of oxygen and nutrients at a normal level and to remove the waste products of metabolism, despite changes in the arterial pressure. In the kidneys, the normal blood flow is much higher than that required for these functions. The major function of autoregulation in the kidneys is to maintain a relatively constant GFR and to allow precise control of renal excretion of water and solutes.

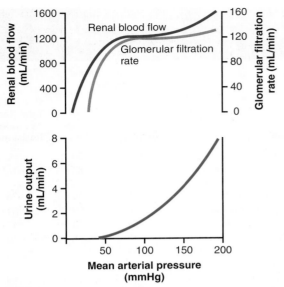

Figure 77-4 Autoregulation of renal blood flow and glomerular filtration rate but lack of autoregulation of urine flow during changes in renal arterial pressure.

The GFR normally remains autoregulated (ie, remains relatively constant), despite considerable arterial pressure fluctuations that occur during a person's usual activities. For instance, a decrease in arterial pressure to as low as 70 to 75 mmHg or an increase to as high as 160 to 180 mmHg usually changes the GFR less than 10%. In general, renal blood flow is autoregulated in parallel with GFR, but GFR is more efficiently autoregulated under certain conditions.

MYOGENIC AUTOREGULATION OF RENAL BLOOD FLOW AND GFR

Another mechanism that contributes to the maintenance of a relatively constant renal blood flow and GFR is the ability of individual blood vessels to resist stretching during increased arterial pressure, a phenomenon referred to as the *myogenic mechanism*. Studies of individual blood vessels (especially small arterioles) throughout the body have shown that they respond to increased wall tension or wall stretch by contraction of the vascular smooth muscle. Stretch of the vascular wall allows increased movement of calcium ions from the extracellular fluid into the vascular smooth muscle cells causing them to contract by combining with intracellular calmodulin and the activation of myosin cross bridges. This contraction prevents excessive stretch of the vessel and at the same time, by raising vascular resistance, helps prevent excessive increases in renal blood flow and GFR when arterial pressure increases.

Although the myogenic mechanism probably operates in most arterioles throughout the body, its importance in renal blood flow and GFR autoregulation has been questioned by some physiologists because this pressure-sensitive mechanism has no means of directly detecting changes in renal blood flow or GFR per se. On the other hand, this mechanism may be more important in protecting the kidney from hypertension-induced injury. In response to sudden increases in blood pressure, the myogenic constrictor response in afferent arterioles occurs within seconds and therefore attenuates transmission of increased arterial pressure to the glomerular capillaries.

Glomerular Filtration—The First Step in Urine Formation

COMPOSITION OF THE GLOMERULAR FILTRATE

Urine formation begins with filtration of large amounts of fluid through the glomerular capillaries into Bowman's capsule. Like most capillaries, the glomerular capillaries are relatively impermeable to proteins, so the filtered fluid (called the *glomerular filtrate*) is essentially protein free and devoid of cellular elements, including red blood cells.

The concentrations of other constituents of the glomerular filtrate, including most salts and organic molecules, are similar to the concentrations in the plasma. Exceptions to this generalization include a few low-molecular-weight substances, such as calcium and fatty acids, that are not freely filtered because they are partially bound to the plasma proteins.

GFR IS ABOUT 20% OF THE RENAL PLASMA FLOW

The GFR is determined by (1) the balance of hydrostatic and colloid osmotic forces acting across the capillary membrane and (2) the capillary filtration coefficient (K_f), the product of the permeability and filtering surface area of the capillaries. The glomerular capillaries have a much higher rate of filtration than most other capillaries because of a high glomerular hydrostatic pressure and a large K_f. In the average adult human, the GFR is about 125 mL/min or 180 L/day. The fraction of the renal plasma flow that is filtered (the filtration fraction) averages about 0.2; this means that about 20% of the plasma flowing through the kidney is filtered through the glomerular capillaries. The filtration fraction is calculated as follows:

$$\text{Filtration fraction} = \text{GFR/Renal plasma flow}$$

GLOMERULAR CAPILLARY MEMBRANE

The glomerular capillary membrane is similar to that of other capillaries, except that it has three (instead of the usual two) major layers: (1) the *endothelium* of the capillary, (2) a *basement membrane*, and (3) a layer of *epithelial cells* (*podocytes*) surrounding the outer surface of the capillary basement membrane (Figure 77-5). Together, these layers make up the filtration barrier, which, despite the three layers, filters several hundred times as much water and solutes as the usual capillary membrane. Even with this high rate of filtration, the glomerular capillary membrane normally prevents filtration of plasma proteins.

The high filtration rate across the glomerular capillary membrane is due partly to its special characteristics. The capillary *endothelium* is perforated by thousands of small holes called *fenestrae*, similar to the fenestrated capillaries found in the liver, although smaller than the fenestrae of the liver. Although the fenestrations are relatively large, endothelial cell proteins are richly endowed with fixed negative charges that hinder the passage of plasma proteins.

Surrounding the endothelium is the *basement membrane*, which consists of a meshwork of collagen and proteoglycan fibrillae that have large spaces through which large amounts of water and small solutes can filter. The basement membrane effectively prevents filtration of plasma proteins, in part because of strong negative electrical charges associated with the proteoglycans.

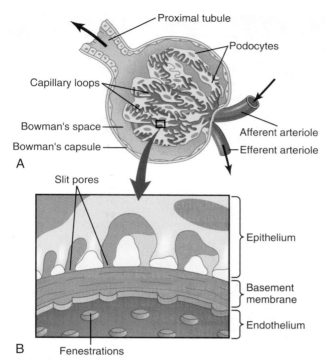

Figure 77-5 (A) Basic ultrastructure of the glomerular capillaries. (B) Cross section of the glomerular capillary membrane and its major components: capillary endothelium, basement membrane, and epithelium (podocytes).

TABLE 77-2	Filterability of Substances by Glomerular Capillaries Based on Molecular Weight		
Substance		Molecular Weight	Filterability
Water		18	1
Sodium		23	1
Glucose		180	1
Inulin		5500	1
Myoglobin		17,000	0.75
Albumin		69,000	0.005

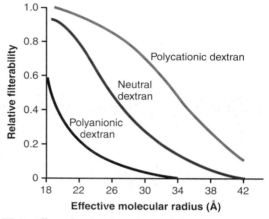

Figure 77-6 Effect of molecular radius and electrical charge of dextran on its filterability by the glomerular capillaries. A value of 1.0 indicates that the substance is filtered as freely as water, whereas a value of 0 indicates that it is not filtered. Dextrans are polysaccharides that can be manufactured as neutral molecules or with negative or positive charges and with varying molecular weights.

The final part of the glomerular membrane is a layer of epithelial cells that line the outer surface of the glomerulus. These cells are not continuous but have long foot-like processes (podocytes) that encircle the outer surface of the capillaries (Figure 77-5). The foot processes are separated by gaps called *slit pores* through which the glomerular filtrate moves. The epithelial cells, which also have negative charges, provide additional restriction to filtration of plasma proteins. Thus, all layers of the glomerular capillary wall provide a barrier to filtration of plasma proteins.

Filterability of Solutes Is Inversely Related to Their Size. The glomerular capillary membrane is thicker than most other capillaries, but it is also much more porous and therefore filters fluid at a high rate. Despite the high filtration rate, the glomerular filtration barrier is selective in determining which molecules will filter, based on their size and electrical charge.

Table 77.2 lists the effect of molecular size on filterability of different molecules. A filterability of 1.0 means that the substance is filtered as freely as water; a filterability of 0.75 means that the substance is filtered only 75% as rapidly as water. Note that electrolytes such as sodium and small organic compounds such as glucose are freely filtered. As the molecular weight of the molecule approaches that of albumin, the filterability rapidly decreases, approaching zero.

Negatively Charged Large Molecules Are Filtered Less Easily Than Positively Charged Molecules of Equal Molecular Size. The molecular diameter of the plasma protein albumin is only about 6 nm, whereas the pores of the glomerular membrane are thought to be about 8 nm (80 Å). Albumin is restricted from filtration, however, because of its negative charge and the electrostatic repulsion exerted by negative charges of the glomerular capillary wall proteoglycans.

Figure 77-6 shows how electrical charge affects the filtration of different molecular weight dextrans by the glomerulus. Dextrans are polysaccharides that can be manufactured as neutral molecules or with negative or positive charges. Note that for any given molecular radius, positively charged molecules are filtered much more readily than are negatively charged molecules. Neutral dextrans are also filtered more readily than are negatively charged dextrans of equal molecular weight. The reason for these differences in filterability is that the negative charges of the basement membrane and the podocytes provide an important means for restricting large negatively charged molecules, including the plasma proteins.

In certain kidney diseases, the negative charges on the basement membrane are lost even before there are noticeable changes in kidney histology, a condition referred to as *minimal change nephropathy*. As a result of this loss of negative charges on the basement membranes some of the lower molecular-weight proteins, especially albumin, are filtered and appear in the urine, a condition known as *proteinuria* or *albuminuria*.

Use of Clearance Methods to Quantify Kidney Function (GFR and RBF)

The rates at which different substances are "cleared" from the plasma provide a useful way of quantitating the effectiveness with which the kidneys excrete various substances (Table A.1).

TABLE A-1	Use of Clearance to Quantify Kidney Function		
Term	**Equation**	**Units**
Clearance rate (C_s)	$C_s = \dfrac{U_s \times \dot{V}}{P_s}$	mL/min
GFR	$GFR = \dfrac{U_{inulin} \times \dot{V}}{P_{inulin}}$	
Clearance ratio	$Clearance\,ratio = \dfrac{C_s}{C_{inulin}}$	None
ERPF	$ERPF = C_{PAH} = \dfrac{U_{PAH} \times \dot{V}}{P_{PAH}}$	mL/min
RPF	$RPF = \dfrac{C_{PAH}}{E_{PAH}} = \dfrac{(U_{PAH} \times \dot{V} / P_{PAH})}{(P_{PAH} - V_{PAH})P_{PAH}} = \dfrac{U_{PAH} \times \dot{V}}{P_{PAH} - V_{PAH}}$	mL/min
RBF	$RBF = \dfrac{RPF}{1 - Hematocrit}$	mL/min
Excretion rate	$Excretion\,rate = U_s \times \dot{V}$	mg/min, mmol/min, or mEq/min
Reabsorption rate	$Reabsorption\,rate = Filtered\,load - Excretion\,rate$ $(GFR \times P_s) - (U_s \times \dot{V})$	mg/min, mmol/min, or mEq/min
Secretion rate	$Secretion\,rate = Excretion\,rate - Filtered\,load$	mg/min, mmol/min, or mEq/min

S, a substance; U, urine concentration; $\dot{V}$, urine flow rate; P, plasma concentration; PAH, para-aminohippuric acid; P_{PAH}, renal arterial PAH concentration; E_{PAH}, PAH extraction ratio; V_{PAH}, renal venous PAH concentration; glomerular filtration rate, GFR; effective renal plasma flow, ERPF; RPF, renal plasma flow; RBF, renal blood flow.

By definition, the *renal clearance of a substance is the volume of plasma that is completely cleared of the substance by the kidneys per unit time.*

This concept is somewhat abstract because there is no single volume of plasma that is *completely* cleared of a substance. However, renal clearance provides a useful way of quantifying the excretory function of the kidneys and, as discussed later, can be used to quantify the rate at which blood flows through the kidneys, as well as the basic functions of the kidneys: glomerular filtration, tubular reabsorption, and tubular secretion.

To illustrate the clearance principle, consider the following example: If the plasma passing through the kidneys contains 1 mg of a substance in each milliliter and if 1 mg of this substance is also excreted into the urine each minute, then 1 mL/min of the plasma is "cleared" of the substance. Thus, clearance refers to the volume of plasma that would be necessary to supply the amount of substance excreted in the urine per unit time. Stated mathematically,

$$C_s \times P_s = U_s \times V,$$

where C_s is the clearance rate of a substance s, P_s is the plasma concentration of the substance, U_s is the urine concentration of that substance, and V is the urine flow rate. Rearranging this equation, clearance can be expressed as

$$C_s = \frac{U_s \times V}{P_s}$$

Thus, renal clearance of a substance is calculated from the urinary excretion rate ($U_s \times V$) of that substance divided by its plasma concentration.

INULIN CLEARANCE CAN BE USED TO ESTIMATE GFR

If a substance is freely filtered (filtered as freely as water) and is not reabsorbed or secreted by the renal tubules, then the rate at which that substance is excreted in the urine ($U_s \times V$) is equal to the filtration rate of the substance by the kidneys (GFR $\times P_s$). Thus,

$$GFR \times P_s = U_s \times V$$

The GFR, therefore, can be calculated as the clearance of the substance as follows:

$$GFR = \frac{U_s \times V}{P_s} = C_s$$

A substance that fits these criteria is *inulin,* a polysaccharide molecule with a molecular weight of about 5200. Inulin, which is not produced in the body, is found in the roots of certain plants and must be administered intravenously to a patient to measure GFR.

Figure A-1 shows the renal handling of inulin. In this example, the plasma concentration is 1 mg/mL, urine concentration is 125 mg/mL, and urine flow rate is 1 mL/min. Therefore, 125 mg/min of inulin passes into the urine. Then, inulin clearance is calculated as the urine excretion rate of inulin divided by the plasma concentration, which yields a value of 125 mL/min. Thus, 125 mL of plasma flowing through the kidneys must be filtered to deliver the inulin that appears in the urine.

Inulin is not the only substance that can be used for determining GFR. Other substances that have been used clinically to estimate GFR include *radioactive iothalamate* and *creatinine.*

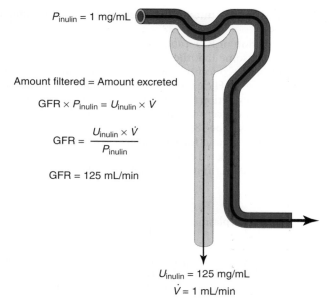

Figure A-1 Measurement of glomerular filtration rate (GFR) from the renal clearance of inulin. Inulin is freely filtered by the glomerular capillaries but is not reabsorbed by the renal tubules. P_{inulin}, plasma inulin concentration; U_{inulin}, urine inulin concentration; $\dot{V}$, urine flow rate.

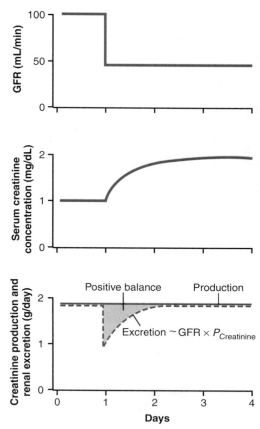

Figure A-2 Effect of reducing glomerular filtration rate (GFR) by 50% on serum creatinine concentration and on creatinine excretion rate when the production rate of creatinine remains constant. $P_{Creatinine}$, plasma creatinine concentration.

CREATININE CLEARANCE AND PLASMA CREATININE CONCENTRATION CAN BE USED TO ESTIMATE GFR

Creatinine is a by-product of muscle metabolism and is cleared from the body fluids almost entirely by glomerular filtration. Therefore, the clearance of creatinine can also be used to assess GFR. Because measurement of creatinine clearance does not require intravenous infusion into the patient, this method is much more widely used than inulin clearance for estimating GFR clinically. However, creatinine clearance is not a perfect marker of GFR because a small amount of it is secreted by the tubules, so the amount of creatinine excreted slightly exceeds the amount filtered. There is normally a slight error in measuring plasma creatinine that leads to an overestimate of the plasma creatinine concentration, and fortuitously, these two errors tend to cancel each other. Therefore, creatinine clearance provides a reasonable estimate of GFR.

In some cases, it may not be practical to collect urine in a patient for measuring creatinine clearance (C_{Cr}). An approximation of changes in GFR, however, can be obtained by simply measuring plasma creatinine concentration (P_{Cr}), which is inversely proportional to GFR:

$$GFR \approx C_{Cr} = \frac{U_{Cr} \times \dot{V}}{P_{Cr}}$$

If GFR suddenly decreases by 50%, the kidneys will transiently filter and excrete only half as much creatinine, causing accumulation of creatinine in the body fluids and raising plasma concentration. Plasma concentration of creatinine will continue to rise until the filtered load of creatinine ($P_{Cr} \times GFR$) and creatinine excretion ($U_{Cr} \times \dot{V}$) return to normal and a balance between creatinine production and creatinine excretion is reestablished. This will occur when plasma creatinine increases to approximately twice normal, as shown in Figure A-2.

If GFR falls to one-fourth normal, plasma creatinine would increase to about four times normal and a decrease of GFR to one-eighth normal would raise plasma creatinine to eight times normal. Thus, under steady-state conditions, the creatinine excretion rate equals the rate of creatinine production, despite reductions in GFR. However, this normal rate of creatinine excretion occurs at the expense of elevated plasma creatinine concentration, as shown in Figure A-3.

PAH CLEARANCE CAN BE USED TO ESTIMATE RENAL PLASMA FLOW

Theoretically, if a substance is completely cleared from the plasma, the clearance rate of that substance is equal to the total renal plasma flow. In other words, the amount of the substance delivered to the kidneys in the blood (renal plasma flow $\times P_s$) would be equal to the amount excreted in the urine ($U_s \times \dot{V}$). Thus, renal plasma flow (RPF) could be calculated as

$$RPF = \frac{U_s \times \dot{V}}{P_s} = C_s$$

Because the GFR is only about 20% of the total plasma flow, a substance that is completely cleared from the plasma must be excreted by tubular secretion, as well as glomerular filtration (Figure A-4). There is no known substance that is completely cleared by the kidneys. One substance, however, PAH, is about 90% cleared from the plasma. Therefore, the clearance of PAH

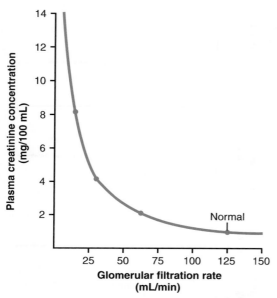

Figure A-3 Approximate relationship between glomerular filtration rate (GFR) and plasma creatinine concentration under steady-state conditions. Decreasing GFR by 50% will increase plasma creatinine to twice normal if creatinine production by the body remains constant.

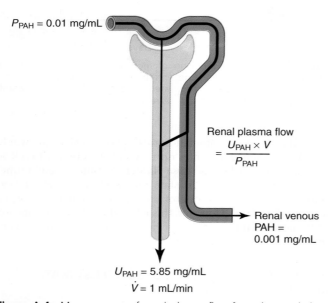

Figure A-4 Measurement of renal plasma flow from the renal clearance of para-aminohippuric acid *(PAH)*. PAH is freely filtered by the glomerular capillaries and is also secreted from the peritubular capillary blood into the tubular lumen. The amount of PAH in the plasma of the renal artery is about equal to the amount of PAH excreted in the urine. Therefore, the renal plasma flow can be calculated from the clearance of PAH (C_{PAH}). To be more accurate, one can correct for the percentage of PAH that is still in the blood when it leaves the kidneys. P_{PAH}, arterial plasma PAH concentration; U_{PAH}, urine PAH concentration; $\dot{V}$, urine flow rate.

can be used as an approximation of renal plasma flow. To be more accurate, one can correct for the percentage of PAH that is still in the blood when it leaves the kidneys. The percentage of PAH removed from the blood is known as the *extraction ratio of PAH* and averages about 90% in normal kidneys. In diseased kidneys, this extraction ratio may be reduced because of

inability of damaged tubules to secrete PAH into the tubular fluid.

The calculation of RPF can be demonstrated by the following example: Assume that the plasma concentration of PAH is 0.01 mg/mL, urine concentration is 5.85 mg/mL, and urine flow rate is 1 mL/min. PAH clearance can be calculated from the rate of urinary PAH excretion (5.85 mg/mL × 1 mL/min) divided by the plasma PAH concentration (0.01 mg/mL). Thus, clearance of PAH calculates to be 585 mL/min.

If the extraction ratio for PAH is 90%, the actual renal plasma flow can be calculated by dividing 585 mL/min by 0.9, yielding a value of 650 mL/min. Thus, total renal plasma flow can be calculated as

$$\text{Total renal plasma flow} = \frac{\text{PAH clearance}}{\text{PAH extraction ratio}}$$

The extraction ratio (E_{PAH}) is calculated as the difference between the renal arterial PAH (P_{PAH}) and renal venous PAH (V_{PAH}) concentrations, divided by the renal arterial PAH concentration:

$$E_{PAH} = \frac{P_{PAH} - V_{PAH}}{P_{PAH}}$$

One can calculate the total blood flow through the kidneys from the total renal plasma flow and hematocrit (the percentage of red blood cells in the blood). If the hematocrit is 0.45 and the total renal plasma flow is 650 mL/min, the total blood flow through both kidneys is 650/(1—0.45), or 1182 mL/min.

FILTRATION FRACTION IS CALCULATED FROM GFR DIVIDED BY RENAL PLASMA FLOW

To calculate the filtration fraction, which is the fraction of plasma that filters through the glomerular membrane, one must first know the renal plasma flow (PAH clearance) and the GFR (inulin clearance). If renal plasma flow is 650 mL/min and GFR is 125 mL/min, the filtration fraction (FF) is calculated as

$$FF = GFR / RPF = 125 / 650 = 0.19$$

Comparisons of Inulin Clearance With Clearances of Different Solutes. The following generalizations can be made by comparing the clearance of a substance with the clearance of inulin, a measure of GFR: (1) if the clearance rate of the substance equals that of inulin, the substance is only filtered and not reabsorbed or secreted; (2) if the clearance rate of a substance is less than inulin clearance, the substance must have been reabsorbed by the nephron tubules; and (3) if the clearance rate of a substance is greater than that of inulin, the substance must be secreted by the nephron tubules. The approximate clearance rates for some of the substances normally handled by the kidneys are listed as follows:

Substance	Clearance Rate (mL/min)
Glucose	0
Sodium	0.9
Chloride	1.3
Potassium	12.0
Phosphate	25.0
Inulin	125.0
Creatinine	140.0

Determinants of the GFR

The GFR is determined by (1) the sum of the hydrostatic and colloid osmotic forces across the glomerular membrane, which gives the *net filtration pressure*, and (2) the glomerular capillary filtration coefficient, K_f. Expressed mathematically, the GFR equals the product of K_f and the net filtration pressure:

$$GFR = K_f \times Net\ filtration\ pressure$$

The net filtration pressure represents the sum of the hydrostatic and colloid osmotic forces that either favor or oppose filtration across the glomerular capillaries (Figure 77-7). These forces include (1) hydrostatic pressure inside the glomerular capillaries (glomerular hydrostatic pressure (P_G), which promotes filtration; (2) the hydrostatic pressure in Bowman's capsule (P_B) outside the capillaries, which opposes filtration; (3) the colloid osmotic pressure of the glomerular capillary plasma proteins (π_G), which opposes filtration; and (4) the colloid osmotic pressure of the proteins in Bowman's capsule (π_B), which promotes filtration. (Under normal conditions, the concentration of protein in the glomerular filtrate is so low that the colloid osmotic pressure of the Bowman's capsule fluid is considered to be zero.)

The GFR can therefore be expressed as

$$GFR = K_f \times (P_G - P_B - \pi_G + \pi_B)$$

Although the normal values for the determinants of GFR have not been measured directly in humans, they have been estimated in animals such as dogs and rats. Based on the results in animals, the approximate normal forces favoring and opposing glomerular filtration in humans are believed to be as follows (Figure 77-7):

Forces Favoring Filtration (mmHg)

Glomerular hydrostatic pressure	60
Bowman's capsule colloid osmotic pressure	0

Forces Opposing Filtration (mmHg)

Bowman's capsule hydrostatic pressure	18
Glomerular capillary colloid osmotic pressure	32

Net filtration = $60 - 18 - 32 = +10$ mmHg

Some of these values can change markedly under different physiologic conditions, whereas others are altered mainly in disease states, as discussed later.

INCREASED GLOMERULAR CAPILLARY FILTRATION COEFFICIENT INCREASES GFR

The K_f is a measure of the product of the hydraulic conductivity and surface area of the glomerular capillaries. The K_f cannot be measured directly, but it is estimated experimentally by dividing the rate of glomerular filtration by net filtration pressure:

$$K_f = GFR/Net\ filtration\ pressure$$

Because the total GFR for both kidneys is about 125 mL/min and the net filtration pressure is 10 mmHg, the normal K_f is calculated to be about 12.5 mL/min/mmHg of filtration pressure. Although increased K_f raises GFR and decreased K_f reduces GFR, changes in K_f probably do not provide a primary mechanism for the normal day-to-day regulation of GFR. Some diseases, however, lower K_f by reducing the number of functional glomerular

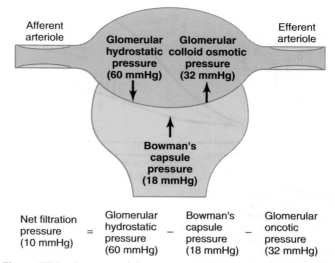

Figure 77-7 Summary of forces causing filtration by the glomerular capillaries. The values shown are estimates for healthy humans.

capillaries (thereby reducing the surface area for filtration) or by increasing the thickness of the glomerular capillary membrane and reducing its hydraulic conductivity. For example, chronic, uncontrolled hypertension and diabetes mellitus gradually reduce K_f by increasing the thickness of the glomerular capillary basement membrane and, eventually, by damaging the capillaries so severely that there is loss of capillary function.

INCREASED BOWMAN'S CAPSULE HYDROSTATIC PRESSURE DECREASES GFR

Direct measurements, using micropipettes, of hydrostatic pressure in Bowman's capsule and at different points in the proximal tubule in experimental animals suggest that a reasonable estimate for Bowman's capsule pressure in humans is about 18 mmHg under normal conditions. Increasing the hydrostatic pressure in Bowman's capsule reduces GFR, whereas decreasing this pressure raises GFR. However, changes in Bowman's capsule pressure normally do not serve as a primary means for regulating GFR.

In certain pathological states associated with obstruction of the urinary tract, Bowman's capsule pressure can increase markedly, causing serious reduction of GFR. For example, precipitation of calcium or of uric acid may lead to "stones" that lodge in the urinary tract, often in the ureter, thereby obstructing outflow of the urinary tract and raising Bowman's capsule pressure. This situation reduces GFR and eventually can cause *hydronephrosis* (distention and dilation of the renal pelvis and calyces) and can damage or even destroy the kidney unless the obstruction is relieved.

INCREASED GLOMERULAR CAPILLARY COLLOID OSMOTIC PRESSURE DECREASES GFR

As blood passes from the afferent arteriole through the glomerular capillaries to the efferent arterioles, the plasma protein concentration increases about 20% (Figure 77-8). The reason for this increase is that about one-fifth of the fluid in the capillaries filters into Bowman's capsule, thereby concentrating the glomerular plasma proteins that are not filtered. Assuming that the normal colloid osmotic pressure of plasma entering the

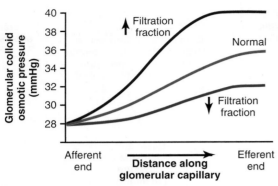

Figure 77-8 Increase in colloid osmotic pressure in plasma flowing through the glomerular capillary. Normally, about one-fifth of the fluid in the glomerular capillaries filters into Bowman's capsule, thereby concentrating the plasma proteins that are not filtered. Increase in the filtration fraction (glomerular filtration rate/renal plasma flow) increases the rate at which the plasma colloid osmotic pressure rises along the glomerular capillary; decrease in the filtration fraction has the opposite effect.

glomerular capillaries is 28 mmHg, this value usually rises to about 36 mmHg by the time the blood reaches the efferent end of the capillaries. Therefore, the average colloid osmotic pressure of the glomerular capillary plasma proteins is midway between 28 and 36 mmHg, or about 32 mmHg.

Thus, two factors that influence the glomerular capillary colloid osmotic pressure are (1) the arterial plasma colloid osmotic pressure and (2) the fraction of plasma filtered by the glomerular capillaries (filtration fraction). Increasing the arterial plasma colloid osmotic pressure raises the glomerular capillary colloid osmotic pressure, which in turn decreases the GFR.

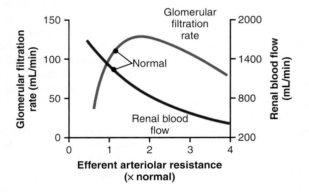

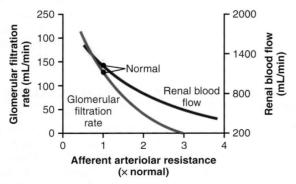

Figure 77-9 Effect of change in afferent arteriolar resistance or efferent arteriolar resistance on glomerular filtration rate and renal blood flow.

TABLE 77-3	Factors That Can Decrease the GFR
Physical Determinants*	**Physiologic/Pathophysiologic Causes**
$\downarrow K_f \rightarrow \downarrow$ GFR	Renal disease, diabetes mellitus, hypertension
$\uparrow P_B \rightarrow \downarrow$ GFR	Urinary tract obstruction (eg, kidney stones)
$\uparrow \pi_G \rightarrow \downarrow$ GFR	$\downarrow$ Renal blood flow, increased plasma proteins
$\downarrow P_G \rightarrow \downarrow$ GFR $\downarrow A_P \rightarrow \downarrow P_G$	$\downarrow$ Arterial pressure (has only small effect due to autoregulation)
$\downarrow R_E \rightarrow \downarrow P_G$	$\downarrow$ Angiotensin II (drugs that block angiotensin II formation)
$\uparrow R_A \rightarrow \downarrow P_G$	$\uparrow$ Sympathetic activity, vasoconstrictor hormones (eg, norepinephrine, endothelin)

K_f, glomerular filtration coefficient; P_B, Bowman's capsule hydrostatic pressure; π_G, glomerular capillary colloid osmotic pressure; P_G, glomerular capillary hydrostatic pressure; A_P, systemic arterial pressure; R_E, efferent arteriolar resistance; R_A, afferent arteriolar resistance; GFR, glomerular filtration rate.
*Opposite changes in the determinants usually increase GFR.

INCREASED GLOMERULAR CAPILLARY HYDROSTATIC PRESSURE INCREASES GFR

The glomerular capillary hydrostatic pressure has been estimated to be about 60 mmHg under normal conditions. Changes in glomerular hydrostatic pressure serve as the primary means for physiological regulation of GFR. Increases in glomerular hydrostatic pressure raise GFR, whereas decreases in glomerular hydrostatic pressure reduce GFR.

Glomerular hydrostatic pressure is determined by three variables, each of which is under physiological control: (1) *arterial pressure*, (2) *afferent arteriolar resistance*, and (3) *efferent arteriolar resistance*.

Increased arterial pressure tends to raise glomerular hydrostatic pressure and, therefore, to increase GFR. (However, as discussed later, this effect is buffered by autoregulatory mechanisms that maintain a relatively constant glomerular pressure as blood pressure fluctuates.)

Increased resistance of afferent arterioles reduces glomerular hydrostatic pressure and decreases GFR. Conversely, dilation of the afferent arterioles increases both glomerular hydrostatic pressure and GFR (Figure 77-9).

Constriction of the efferent arterioles increases the resistance to outflow from the glomerular capillaries. This mechanism raises glomerular hydrostatic pressure, and as long as the increase in efferent resistance does not reduce renal blood flow too much, GFR increases slightly (Figure 77-9). Table 77.3 summarizes the factors that can decrease GFR.

Physiological Control of Glomerular Filtration and Renal Blood Flow

The determinants of GFR that are most variable and subject to physiological control include the glomerular hydrostatic pressure and the glomerular capillary colloid osmotic pressure. These variables, in turn, are influenced by the sympathetic nervous system, hormones and autacoids (vasoactive substances that are released in the kidneys and act locally), and other feedback controls that are intrinsic to the kidneys.

STRONG SYMPATHETIC NERVOUS SYSTEM ACTIVATION DECREASES GFR

Essentially all the blood vessels of the kidneys, including the afferent and the efferent arterioles, are richly innervated by sympathetic nerve fibers. Strong activation of the renal sympathetic nerves can constrict the renal arterioles and decrease renal blood flow and GFR. Moderate or mild sympathetic stimulation has little influence on renal blood flow and GFR. For example, reflex activation of the sympathetic nervous system resulting from moderate decreases in pressure at the carotid sinus baroreceptors or cardiopulmonary receptors has little influence on renal blood flow or GFR.

The renal sympathetic nerves seem to be most important in reducing GFR during severe, acute disturbances lasting for a few minutes to a few hours, such as those elicited by the defense reaction, brain ischemia, or severe hemorrhage. In the healthy resting person, sympathetic tone appears to have little influence on renal blood flow.

HORMONAL AND AUTACOID CONTROL OF RENAL CIRCULATION

Several hormones and autacoids can influence GFR and renal blood flow, as summarized in Table 77-4.

Norepinephrine, Epinephrine, and Endothelin Constrict Renal Blood Vessels and Decrease GFR. Hormones that constrict afferent and efferent arterioles, causing reductions in GFR and renal blood flow, include *norepinephrine* and *epinephrine* released from the adrenal medulla. In general, blood levels of these hormones parallel the activity of the sympathetic nervous system; thus, norepinephrine and epinephrine have little influence on renal hemodynamics except under extreme conditions, such as severe hemorrhage.

Another vasoconstrictor, *endothelin*, is a peptide that can be released by damaged vascular endothelial cells of the kidneys, as well as by other tissues. The physiological role of this autacoid is not completely understood. However, endothelin may contribute to hemostasis (minimizing blood loss) when a blood vessel is severed, which damages the endothelium and releases this powerful vasoconstrictor.

Angiotensin II Preferentially Constricts Efferent Arterioles in Most Physiological Conditions. A powerful renal vasoconstrictor, *angiotensin II*, can be considered a circulating hormone and a locally produced autacoid because it is formed in the kidneys and in the systemic circulation. Receptors for angiotensin II are present in virtually all blood vessels of the kidneys. However, the preglomerular blood vessels, especially the afferent arterioles, appear to be relatively protected from angiotensin II-mediated constriction in most physiological conditions associated with activation of the renin–angiotensin system such as during a low-sodium diet or reduced renal perfusion pressure due to renal artery stenosis. This protection is due to release of vasodilators, especially *nitric oxide* and *prostaglandins*, which counteract the vasoconstrictor effects of angiotensin II in these blood vessels.

The efferent arterioles, however, are highly sensitive to angiotensin II. Because angiotensin II preferentially constricts efferent arterioles in most physiological conditions, increased angiotensin II levels raise glomerular hydrostatic pressure while reducing renal blood flow. It should be kept in mind that increased angiotensin II formation usually occurs in circumstances associated with decreased arterial pressure or volume depletion, which tend to decrease GFR. In these circumstances,

TABLE 77-4	Hormones and Autacoids That Influence GFR	
Hormone or Autacoid	**Effect on GFR**	
Norepinephrine	↓	
Epinephrine	↓	
Endothelin	↓	
Angiotensin II	← (prevents ↓)	
Endothelial-derived nitric oxide	↑	
Prostaglandins	↑	

GFR, glomerular filtration rate.

the increased level of angiotensin II, by constricting efferent arterioles, helps *maintain* glomerular hydrostatic pressure and GFR; at the same time, though, the reduction in renal blood flow caused by efferent arteriolar constriction contributes to decreased flow through the peritubular capillaries, which in turn increases reabsorption of sodium and water, as discussed in Chapter 78.

Endothelial-Derived Nitric Oxide Decreases Renal Vascular Resistance and Increases GFR. An autacoid that decreases renal vascular resistance and is released by the vascular endothelium throughout the body is *endothelial-derived nitric oxide.* A basal level of nitric oxide production appears to be important for maintaining vasodilation of the kidneys because it allows the kidneys to excrete normal amounts of sodium and water. Therefore, administration of drugs that inhibit formation of nitric oxide increases renal vascular resistance and decreases GFR and urinary sodium excretion, eventually causing high blood pressure. In some hypertensive patients or in patients with atherosclerosis, damage of the vascular endothelium and impaired nitric oxide production may contribute to increased renal vasoconstriction and elevated blood pressure.

Prostaglandins and Bradykinin Decrease Renal Vascular Resistance and Tend to Increase GFR. Hormones and autacoids that cause vasodilation and increased renal blood flow and GFR include the prostaglandins (PGE_2 and PGI_2) and bradykinin. These substances are discussed in Chapter 45. Although these vasodilators do not appear to be of major importance in regulating renal blood flow or GFR in normal conditions, they may dampen the renal vasoconstrictor effects of the sympathetic nerves or angiotensin II, especially their effects to constrict the afferent arterioles.

By opposing vasoconstriction of afferent arterioles, the prostaglandins may help prevent excessive reductions in GFR and renal blood flow. Under stressful conditions, such as volume depletion or after surgery, the administration of nonsteroidal antiinflammatory agents, such as aspirin, that inhibit prostaglandin synthesis may cause significant reductions in GFR.

TUBULOGLOMERULAR FEEDBACK AND AUTOREGULATION OF GFR

The kidneys have a special feedback mechanism that links changes in sodium chloride concentration at the macula densa with the control of renal arteriolar resistance and autoregulation of GFR. This feedback helps ensure a relatively constant delivery of sodium chloride to the distal tubule and helps prevent spurious fluctuations in renal excretion that would otherwise occur. In many circumstances, this feedback autoregulates renal blood flow and GFR in parallel. However, because this mechanism is

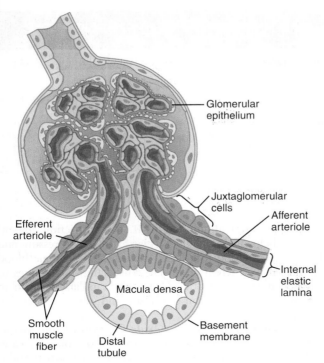

Figure 77-10   Structure of the juxtaglomerular apparatus, demonstrating its possible feedback role in the control of nephron function.

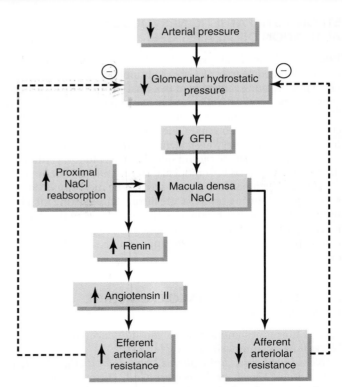

Figure 77-11   Macula densa feedback mechanism for autoregulation of glomerular hydrostatic pressure and glomerular filtration rate (*GFR*) during decreased renal arterial pressure.

specifically directed toward stabilizing sodium chloride delivery to the distal tubule, instances occur when GFR is autoregulated at the expense of changes in renal blood flow, as discussed later. In other instances, this mechanism may actually cause changes in GFR in response to primary changes in renal tubular sodium chloride reabsorption.

The tubuloglomerular feedback mechanism has two components that act together to control GFR: (1) an afferent arteriolar feedback mechanism and (2) an efferent arteriolar feedback mechanism. These feedback mechanisms depend on special anatomical arrangements of the *juxtaglomerular complex* (Figure 77-10).

The juxtaglomerular complex consists of *macula densa cells* in the initial portion of the distal tubule and *juxtaglomerular cells* in the walls of the afferent and efferent arterioles. The macula densa is a specialized group of epithelial cells in the distal tubules that comes in close contact with the afferent and efferent arterioles. The macula densa cells contain Golgi apparatus, which are intracellular secretory organelles directed toward the arterioles, suggesting that these cells may be secreting a substance toward the arterioles.

Decreased Macula Densa Sodium Chloride Causes Dilation of Afferent Arterioles and Increased Renin Release. The macula densa cells sense changes in volume delivery to the distal tubule by way of signals that are not completely understood. Experimental studies suggest that decreased GFR slows the flow rate in the loop of Henle, causing increased reabsorption of the percentage of sodium and chloride ions delivered to the ascending loop of Henle, thereby reducing the concentration of sodium chloride at the macula densa cells. This decrease in sodium chloride concentration initiates a signal from the macula densa that has two effects (Figure 77-11): (1) it decreases resistance to blood flow in the afferent arterioles, which raises glomerular hydrostatic pressure and helps return GFR toward normal and

(2) it increases renin release from the juxtaglomerular cells of the afferent and efferent arterioles, which are the major storage sites for renin. Renin released from these cells then functions as an enzyme to increase the formation of angiotensin I, which is converted to angiotensin II. Finally, the angiotensin II constricts the efferent arterioles, thereby increasing glomerular hydrostatic pressure and helping to return GFR toward normal.

Other Factors That Increase Renal Blood Flow and GFR: High Protein Intake and Increased Blood Glucose. Although renal blood flow and GFR are relatively stable under most conditions, there are circumstances in which these variables change significantly. For example, *a high protein intake is known to increase both renal blood flow and GFR.* With a long-term high-protein diet, such as one that contains large amounts of meat, the increases in GFR and renal blood flow are due partly to growth of the kidneys. However, GFR and renal blood flow also increase 20–30% within 1 or 2 hours after a person eats a high-protein meal.

A similar mechanism may also explain the marked increases in renal blood flow and GFR that occur with large increases in blood glucose levels in persons with uncontrolled diabetes mellitus. Because glucose, like some of the amino acids, is also reabsorbed along with sodium in the proximal tubule, increased glucose delivery to the tubules causes them to reabsorb excess sodium along with glucose. This reabsorption of excess sodium, in turn, decreases the sodium chloride concentration at the macula densa, activating a tubuloglomerular feedback-mediated dilation of the afferent arterioles and subsequent increases in renal blood flow and GFR.

These examples demonstrate that renal blood flow and GFR per se are not the primary variables controlled by the tubuloglomerular feedback mechanism. The main purpose of this feedback is to ensure a constant delivery of sodium chloride to the distal tubule, where final processing of the urine takes place. Thus, disturbances that tend to increase reabsorption of sodium chloride at tubular sites before the macula densa tend to elicit increased renal blood flow and GFR, which helps return distal sodium chloride delivery toward normal so that normal rates of sodium and water excretion can be maintained (Figure 77-11).

BIBLIOGRAPHY

Beeuwkes R III: The vascular organization of the kidney, *Annu. Rev. Physiol.* 42:531, 1980.

Bell PD, Lapointe JY, Peti-Peterdi J: Macula densa cell signaling, *Annu. Rev. Physiol.* 65:481, 2003.

Cowley AW Jr, Mori T, Mattson D, et al: Role of renal NO production in the regulation of medullary blood flow, *Am. J. Physiol. Regul. Integr. Comp. Physiol.* 284:R1355, 2003.

Cupples WA, Braam B: Assessment of renal autoregulation, *Am. J. Physiol. Renal Physiol.* 292:F1105, 2007.

Deen WN: What determines glomerular capillary permeability? *J. Clin. Invest.* 114:1412, 2004.

DiBona GF: Physiology in perspective: the wisdom of the body. Neural control of the kidney, *Am. J. Physiol. Regul. Integr. Comp. Physiol.* 289:R633, 2005.

Drummond HA, Grifoni SC, Jernigan NL: A new trick for an old dogma: ENaC proteins as mechanotransducers in vascular smooth muscle, *Physiology (Bethesda)* 23:23, 2008.

Fowler CJ, Griffiths D, de Groat WC: The neural control of micturition, *Nat. Rev. Neurosci.* 9:453, 2008.

Hall JE: Angiotensin II and long-term arterial pressure regulation: the overriding dominance of the kidney, *J. Am. Soc. Nephrol.* 10(Suppl 12):s258, 1999.

Hall JE, Brands MW, The renin-angiotensin-aldosterone system: renal mechanisms and circulatory homeostasis. In Seldin DW, Giebisch G, editors: third ed. *The Kidney—Physiology and Pathophysiology,* 1992, Raven Press, New York, pp. 1009–1046.

Hall JE, Henegar JR, Dwyer TM, et al: Is obesity a major cause of chronic kidney disease? *Adv. Ren. Replace. Ther.* 11:41, 2004.

Haraldsson B, Sörensson J: Why do we not all have proteinuria? An update of our current understanding of the glomerular barrier, *News Physiol. Sci.* 19:7, 2004.

Kriz W, Kaissling B: Structural organization of the mammalian kidney. In Seldin DW, Giebisch G, editors: third ed. *The Kidney—Physiology and Pathophysiology,* 2000, Raven Press, New York, pp. 587–654.

Loutzenhiser R, Griffin K, Williamson G, et al: Renal autoregulation: new perspectives regarding the protective and regulatory roles of the underlying mechanisms, *Am. J. Physiol. Regul. Integr. Comp. Physiol.* 290:R1153, 2006.

Pallone TL, Zhang Z, Rhinehart K: Physiology of the renal medullary microcirculation, *Am. J. Physiol. Renal Physiol.* 284:F253, 2003.

Roman RJ: P-450 metabolites of arachidonic acid in the control of cardiovascular function, *Physiol. Rev.* 82:131, 2002.

Schnermann J, Levine DZ: Paracrine factors in tubuloglomerular feedback: adenosine, ATP, and nitric oxide, *Annu. Rev. Physiol.* 65:501, 2003.

Tubular Function

Renal Tubular Reabsorption and Secretion

As the glomerular filtrate enters the renal tubules, it flows sequentially through the successive parts of the tubule—the *proximal tubule*, the *loop of Henle*, the *distal tubule*, the *collecting tubule*, and, finally, the *collecting duct*—before it is excreted as urine. Along this course, some substances are selectively reabsorbed from the tubules back into the blood, whereas others are secreted from the blood into the tubular lumen. Eventually, the urine that is formed and all the substances in the urine represent the sum of three basic renal processes—glomerular filtration, tubular reabsorption, and tubular secretion:

$$\text{Urinary excretion} = \text{Glomerular filtration}$$
$$- \text{Tubular reabsorption} + \text{Tubular secretion}$$

For many substances, tubular reabsorption plays a much more important role than secretion in determining the final urinary excretion rate. However, tubular secretion accounts for significant amounts of potassium ions, hydrogen ions, and a few other substances that appear in the urine.

TUBULAR REABSORPTION IS QUANTITATIVELY LARGE AND HIGHLY SELECTIVE

Table 78-1 shows the renal handling of several substances that are all freely filtered in the kidneys and reabsorbed at variable rates. The rate at which each of these substances is filtered is calculated as

$$\text{Filtration} = \text{Glomerular filtration rate} \times \text{Plasma concentration}$$

This calculation assumes that the substance is freely filtered and not bound to plasma proteins. For example, if plasma glucose concentration is 1 g/L, the amount of glucose filtered each day is about 180 L/day × 1 g/L or 180 g/day. Because virtually none of the filtered glucose is normally excreted, the rate of glucose reabsorption is also 180 g/day.

From Table 78-1 two things are immediately apparent. First, the processes of glomerular filtration and tubular reabsorption are quantitatively large relative to urinary excretion for many substances. This situation means that a small change in glomerular filtration or tubular reabsorption can potentially cause a relatively large change in urinary excretion. For example, a 10% decrease in tubular reabsorption, from 178.5 to 160.7 L/day, would increase urine volume from 1.5 to 19.3 L/day (almost a 13-fold increase) if the glomerular filtration rate (GFR) remained constant. In reality, however, changes in tubular reabsorption and glomerular filtration are closely coordinated so that large fluctuations in urinary excretion are avoided.

Second, unlike glomerular filtration, which is relatively nonselective (essentially all solutes in the plasma are filtered except the plasma proteins or substances bound to them), *tubular reabsorption is highly selective*. Some substances, such as glucose and amino acids, are almost completely reabsorbed from the tubules, so the urinary excretion rate is essentially zero. Many of the ions in the plasma, such as sodium, chloride, and bicarbonate, are also highly reabsorbed, but their rates of reabsorption and urinary excretion are variable, depending on the needs of the body. Waste products, such as urea and creatinine, conversely, are poorly reabsorbed from the tubules and are excreted in relatively large amounts.

Therefore, by controlling their reabsorption of different substances, the kidneys regulate the excretion of solutes independently of one another, a capability that is essential for precise control of the body fluid composition. In this chapter, we discuss the mechanisms that allow the kidneys to selectively reabsorb or secrete different substances at variable rates.

Tubular Reabsorption Includes Passive and Active Mechanisms

For a substance to be reabsorbed, it must first be transported (1) across the tubular epithelial membranes into the renal interstitial fluid and then (2) through the peritubular capillary membrane

TABLE 78-1	Filtration, Reabsorption, and Excretion Rates of Different Substances by the Kidneys			
	Amount Filtered	Amount Reabsorbed	Amount Excreted	% of Filtered Load Reabsorbed
Glucose (g/day)	180	180	0	100
Bicarbonate (mEq/day)	4,320	4,318	2	>99.9
Sodium (mEq/day)	25,560	25,410	150	99.4
Chloride (mEq/day)	19,440	19,260	180	99.1
Potassium (mEq/day)	756	664	92	87.8
Urea (g/day)	46.8	23.4	23.4	50
Creatinine (g/day)	1.8	0	1.8	0

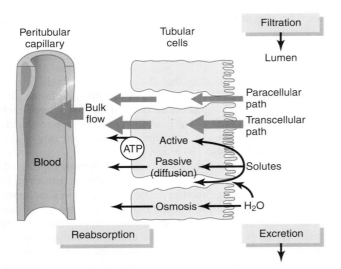

Figure 78-1 Reabsorption of filtered water and solutes from the tubular lumen across the tubular epithelial cells through the renal interstitium and back into the blood. Solutes are transported through the cells (*transcellular path*) by passive diffusion or active transport, or between the cells (*paracellular path*) by diffusion. Water is transported through the cells and between the tubular cells by osmosis. Transport of water and solutes from the interstitial fluid into the peritubular capillaries occurs by ultrafiltration (*bulk flow*).

back into the blood (Figure 78-1). Thus, reabsorption of water and solutes includes a series of transport steps. Reabsorption across the tubular epithelium into the interstitial fluid includes active or passive transport by the same basic mechanisms discussed in Chapter 4 for transport across other cell membranes of the body. For instance, water and solutes can be transported through the cell membranes (*transcellular route*) or through the spaces between the cell junctions (*paracellular route*). Then, after absorption across the tubular epithelial cells into the interstitial fluid, water and solutes are transported through the peritubular capillary walls into the blood by *ultrafiltration* (*bulk flow*) that is mediated by hydrostatic and colloid osmotic forces. The peritubular capillaries behave like the venous ends of most other capillaries because there is a net reabsorptive force that moves the fluid and solutes from the interstitium into the blood.

ACTIVE TRANSPORT

Active transport can move a solute against an electrochemical gradient and requires energy derived from metabolism. Transport that is coupled directly to an energy source, such as the hydrolysis of adenosine triphosphate (ATP), is termed *primary active transport*. An example of this mechanism is the sodium–

potassium adenosine triphosphatase (ATPase) pump that functions throughout most parts of the renal tubule. Transport that is coupled *indirectly* to an energy source, such as that due to an ion gradient, is referred to as *secondary active transport*. Reabsorption of glucose by the renal tubule is an example of secondary active transport. Although solutes can be reabsorbed by active and/or passive mechanisms by the tubule, water is always reabsorbed by a passive (nonactive) physical mechanism called *osmosis*, which means water diffusion from a region of low solute concentration (high water concentration) to one of high solute concentration (low water concentration).

Solutes Can Be Transported Through Epithelial Cells or Between Cells. Renal tubular cells, like other epithelial cells, are held together by *tight junctions*. Lateral intercellular spaces lie behind the tight junctions and separate the epithelial cells of the tubule. Solutes can be reabsorbed or secreted across the cells through the *transcellular pathway* or between the cells by moving across the tight junctions and intercellular spaces by way of the *paracellular pathway*. Sodium is a substance that moves through both routes, although most of the sodium is transported through the transcellular pathway. In some nephron segments, especially the proximal tubule, water is also reabsorbed across the paracellular pathway, and substances dissolved in the water, especially potassium, magnesium, and chloride ions, are carried with the reabsorbed fluid between the cells.

Primary Active Transport Through the Tubular Membrane Is Linked to Hydrolysis of ATP. The special importance of primary active transport is that it can move solutes against an electrochemical gradient. The energy for this active transport comes from the hydrolysis of ATP by way of membrane-bound ATPase, which is also a component of the carrier mechanism that binds and moves solutes across the cell membranes. The primary active transporters in the kidneys that are known include *sodium–potassium ATPase, hydrogen ATPase, hydrogen–potassium ATPase*, and *calcium ATPase*.

A good example of a primary active transport system is the reabsorption of sodium ions across the proximal tubular membrane, as shown in Figure 78-2. On the basolateral sides of the tubular epithelial cell, the cell membrane has an extensive sodium–potassium ATPase system that hydrolyzes ATP and uses the released energy to transport sodium ions out of the cell into the interstitium. At the same time, potassium is transported from the interstitium to the inside of the cell. The operation of this ion pump maintains low intracellular sodium and high intracellular potassium concentrations and creates a net negative charge of about −70 mV within the cell. This active pumping of sodium out of the cell across the *basolateral* membrane of the cell favors passive diffusion of sodium across the *luminal* membrane of the cell, from the tubular lumen into the cell, for two

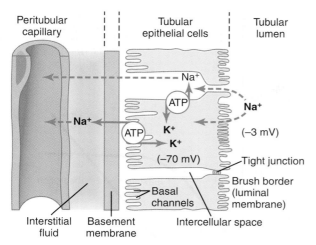

Figure 78-2 Basic mechanism for active transport of sodium through the tubular epithelial cell. The sodium–potassium pump transports sodium from the interior of the cell across the basolateral membrane, creating a low intracellular sodium concentration and a negative intracellular electrical potential. The low intracellular sodium concentration and the negative electrical potential cause sodium ions to diffuse from the tubular lumen into the cell through the brush border.

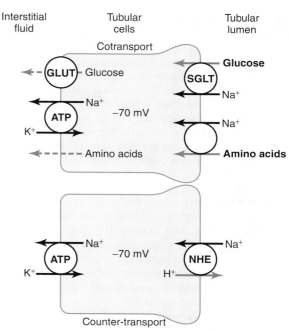

Figure 78-3 Mechanisms of secondary active transport. The upper cell shows the *co-transport* of glucose and amino acids along with sodium ions through the apical side of the tubular epithelial cells, followed by facilitated diffusion through the basolateral membranes. The lower cell shows the *counter-transport* of hydrogen ions from the interior of the cell across the apical membrane and into the tubular lumen; movement of sodium ions into the cell, down an electrochemical gradient established by the sodium–potassium pump on the basolateral membrane, provides the energy for transport of the hydrogen ions from inside the cell into the tubular lumen. *ATP*, adenosine triphosphate; *GLUT*, glucose transporter; *NHE*, sodium–hydrogen exchanger; *SGLT*, sodium–glucose co-transporter.

reasons: (1) there is a concentration gradient favoring sodium diffusion into the cell because intracellular sodium concentration is low (12 mEq/L) and tubular fluid sodium concentration is high (140 mEq/L) and (2) the negative, −70 mV, intracellular potential attracts the positive sodium ions from the tubular lumen into the cell.

Active reabsorption of sodium by sodium–potassium ATPase occurs in most parts of the tubule. In certain parts of the nephron, there are also additional provisions for moving large amounts of sodium into the cell. In the proximal tubule, there is an extensive brush border on the luminal side of the membrane (the side that faces the tubular lumen) that multiplies the surface area to about 20-fold. There are also carrier proteins that bind sodium ions on the luminal surface of the membrane and release them inside the cell, providing *facilitated diffusion* of sodium through the membrane into the cell. These sodium carrier proteins are also important for secondary active transport of other substances, such as glucose and amino acids, as discussed later.

Thus, the net reabsorption of sodium ions from the tubular lumen back into the blood involves at least three steps:

1. Sodium diffuses across the luminal membrane (also called the *apical membrane*) into the cell down an electrochemical gradient established by the sodium–potassium ATPase pump on the basolateral side of the membrane.
2. Sodium is transported across the basolateral membrane against an electrochemical gradient by the sodium–potassium ATPase pump.
3. Sodium, water, and other substances are reabsorbed from the interstitial fluid into the peritubular capillaries by ultrafiltration, a passive process driven by the hydrostatic and colloid osmotic pressure gradients.

Secondary Active Reabsorption Through the Tubular Membrane. In secondary active transport, two or more substances interact with a specific membrane protein (a carrier molecule) and are transported together across the membrane. As one of the substances (for instance, sodium) diffuses down its electrochemical gradient, the energy released is used to drive another substance (for instance, glucose) against its electrochemical gradient. Thus, secondary active transport does not require energy directly from ATP or from other high-energy phosphate sources. Rather, the direct source of the energy is that liberated by the simultaneous facilitated diffusion of another transported substance down its own electrochemical gradient.

Figure 78-3 shows secondary active transport of glucose and amino acids in the proximal tubule. In both instances, specific carrier proteins in the brush border combine with a sodium ion and an amino acid or a glucose molecule at the same time. These transport mechanisms are so efficient that they remove virtually all the glucose and amino acids from the tubular lumen. After entry into the cell, glucose and amino acids exit across the basolateral membranes by diffusion, driven by the high glucose and amino acid concentrations in the cell facilitated by specific transport proteins.

Sodium glucose co-transporters (SGLT2 and SGLT1) are located on the brush border of proximal tubular cells and carry glucose into the cell cytoplasm against a concentration gradient, as described previously. Approximately 90% of the filtered glucose is reabsorbed by SGLT2 in the early part of the proximal tubule (S1 segment) and the residual 10% is transported by SGLT1 in the latter segments of the proximal tubule. On the basolateral side of the membrane, glucose diffuses out of the cell into the interstitial spaces with the help of *glucose transporters—GLUT2* in the S1 segment and *GLUT1* in the latter part (S3 segment) of the proximal tubule.

Although transport of glucose against a chemical gradient does not directly use ATP, the reabsorption of glucose depends on energy expended by the primary active sodium–potassium ATPase pump in the basolateral membrane. Because of the activity of this pump, an electrochemical gradient for facilitated diffusion of sodium across the luminal membrane is maintained, and it is this downhill diffusion of sodium to the interior of the cell that provides the energy for the simultaneous uphill transport of glucose across the luminal membrane. Thus, this reabsorption of glucose is referred to as "secondary active transport" because glucose itself is reabsorbed uphill against a chemical gradient, but it is "secondary" to primary active transport of sodium.

Another important point is that a substance is said to undergo "active" transport when at least one of the steps in the reabsorption involves primary or secondary active transport, even though other steps in the reabsorption process may be passive. For glucose reabsorption, secondary active transport occurs at the luminal membrane, but passive facilitated diffusion occurs at the basolateral membrane, and passive uptake by bulk flow occurs at the peritubular capillaries.

Secondary Active Secretion Into the Tubules. Some substances are secreted into the tubules by secondary active transport which often involves *counter-transport* of the substance with sodium ions. In counter-transport, the energy liberated from the downhill movement of one of the substances (eg, sodium ions) enables uphill movement of a second substance in the opposite direction.

One example of counter-transport, shown in Figure 78-3, is the active secretion of hydrogen ions coupled to sodium reabsorption in the luminal membrane of the proximal tubule. In this case, sodium entry into the cell is coupled with hydrogen extrusion from the cell by sodium–hydrogen counter-transport. This transport is mediated by a specific protein (*sodium–hydrogen exchanger*) in the brush border of the luminal membrane. As sodium is carried to the interior of the cell, hydrogen ions are forced outward in the opposite direction into the tubular lumen. The basic principles of primary and secondary active transport are discussed in additional detail in Chapter 4.

Pinocytosis—An Active Transport Mechanism for Reabsorption of Proteins. Some parts of the tubule, especially the proximal tubule, reabsorb large molecules such as proteins by *pinocytosis*, a type of *endocytosis*. In this process the protein attaches to the brush border of the luminal membrane, and this portion of the membrane then invaginates to the interior of the cell until it is completely pinched off and a vesicle is formed containing the protein. Once inside the cell, the protein is digested into its constituent amino acids, which are reabsorbed through the basolateral membrane into the interstitial fluid. Because pinocytosis requires energy, it is considered a form of active transport.

Transport Maximum for Substances That Are Actively Reabsorbed. For most substances that are actively reabsorbed or secreted, there is a limit to the rate at which the solute can be transported, which is often referred to as the *transport maximum*. This limit is due to saturation of the specific transport systems involved when the amount of solute delivered to the tubule (referred to as *tubular load*) exceeds the capacity of the carrier proteins and specific enzymes involved in the transport process.

The glucose transport system in the proximal tubule is a good example. Normally, measurable glucose does not appear in the urine because essentially all the filtered glucose is reabsorbed in the proximal tubule. However, when the filtered load exceeds the capability of the tubules to reabsorb glucose, urinary excretion of glucose does occur.

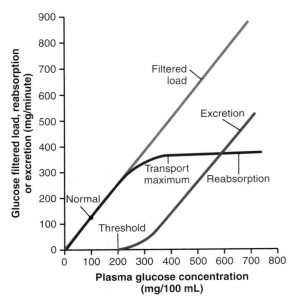

Figure 78-4 Relations among the filtered load of glucose, the rate of glucose reabsorption by the renal tubules, and the rate of glucose excretion in the urine. The *transport maximum* is the maximum rate at which glucose can be reabsorbed from the tubules. The *threshold* for glucose refers to the filtered load of glucose at which glucose first begins to be excreted in the urine.

In the adult human, the transport maximum for glucose averages about 375 mg/min, whereas the filtered load of glucose is only about 125 mg/min (GFR × plasma glucose = 125 mL/min × 1 mg/mL). With large increases in GFR and/or plasma glucose concentration that increase the filtered load of glucose above 375 mg/min, the excess glucose filtered is not reabsorbed and passes into the urine.

Figure 78-4 shows the relation between plasma concentration of glucose, filtered load of glucose, tubular transport maximum for glucose, and rate of glucose loss in the urine. Note that when the plasma glucose concentration is 100 mg/100 mL and the filtered load is at its normal level, 125 mg/min, there is no loss of glucose in the urine. However, when the plasma concentration of glucose rises above about 200 mg/100 mL, increasing the filtered load to about 250 mg/min, a small amount of glucose begins to appear in the urine. This point is termed the *threshold* for glucose. *Note that this appearance of glucose in the urine (at the threshold) occurs before the transport maximum is reached, and represents a "splay" in the otherwise linear relationship between plasma concentration of glucose and the submaximal tubular transport of glucose.* One reason for the difference between threshold and transport maximum is that not all nephrons have the same transport maximum for glucose, and some of the nephrons therefore begin to excrete glucose before others have reached their transport maximum. *The overall transport maximum for the kidneys, which is normally about 375 mg/min, is reached when all nephrons have reached their maximal capacity to reabsorb glucose.*

The plasma glucose of a healthy person almost never becomes high enough to cause glucose excretion in the urine, even after eating a meal. However, in uncontrolled *diabetes mellitus*, plasma glucose may rise to high levels, causing the filtered load of glucose to exceed the transport maximum and resulting in urinary glucose excretion. Some of the important transport maximums for substances *actively reabsorbed* by the tubules are as follows:

Substance	Transport Maximum
Glucose	375 mg/min
Phosphate	0.10 mM/min
Sulfate	0.06 mM/min
Amino acids	1.5 mM/min
Urate	15 mg/min
Lactate	75 mg/min
Plasma protein	30 mg/min

Transport Maximums for Substances That Are Actively Secreted. Substances that are *actively secreted* also exhibit transport maximums as follows:

Substance	Transport Maximum
Creatinine	0.9
Chloride	1.3
Potassium	12.0
Phosphate	25.0
Inulin	125.0
Creatinine	140.0

CALCULATION OF TUBULAR REABSORPTION OR SECRETION FROM RENAL CLEARANCES

If the rates of glomerular filtration and renal excretion of a substance are known, one can calculate whether there is a net reabsorption or a net secretion of that substance by the renal tubules. For example, if the rate of excretion of the substance ($U_s \times \dot{V}$) is less than the filtered load of the substance (GFR $\times P_s$), then some of the substances must have been reabsorbed from the renal tubules.

The following example demonstrates the calculation of tubular reabsorption. Assume the following laboratory values for a patient were obtained:

Urine flow rate = 1 mL/min
Urine concentration of sodium (U_{Na}) = 70 mEq/L = 70 μEq/mL
Plasma sodium concentration = 140 mEq/L = 140 μEq/mL
GFR (inulin clearance) = 100 mL/min

In this example, the filtered sodium load is GFR $\times P_{Na}$, or 100 mL/min $\times$ 140 μEq/mL = 14,000 μEq/min. Urinary sodium excretion ($U_{Na} \times$ urine flow rate) is 70 μEq/min. Therefore, tubular reabsorption of sodium is the difference between the filtered load and urinary excretion, or 14,000 μEq/min − 70 μEq/min = 13,930 μEq/min.

Conversely, if the excretion rate of the substance is greater than its filtered load, then the rate at which it appears in the urine represents the sum of the rate of glomerular filtration plus tubular secretion. Then, the secretion rate is the difference between the urinary excretion and the filtered load.

BIBLIOGRAPHY

Aronson PS: Ion exchangers mediating NaCl transport in the renal proximal tubule, *Cell Biochem. Biophys.* 36:147, 2002.

Benos DJ, Fuller CM, Shlyonsky VG, et al: Amiloride-sensitive Na$^+$ channels: insights and outlooks, *News Physiol. Sci.* 12:55, 1997.

Bröer S: Amino acid transport across mammalian intestinal and renal epithelia, *Physiol. Rev.* 88:249, 2008.

Féraille E, Doucet A: Sodium-potassium-adenosine-triphosphatase–dependent sodium transport in the kidney: hormonal control, *Physiol. Rev.* 81:345, 2001.

Granger JP, Alexander BT, Llinas M: Mechanisms of pressure natriuresis, *Curr. Hypertens. Rep.* 4:152, 2002.

Hall JE, Brands MW: The renin-angiotensin-aldosterone system: renal mechanisms and circulatory homeostasis. In: Seldin, D.W., In Seldin DW, Giebisch G (Eds.): *The Kidney—Physiology and Pathophysiology,* third ed., New York, 2001, Raven Press.

Hall, J.E., Granger, J.P., Regulation of fluid and electrolyte balance in hypertension—role of hormones and peptides. In: Battegay, E.J., Lip, G.Y.H., Bakris, G.L. (Eds.), Hypertension-Principles and Practice. Boca Raton, 2005, Taylor and Francis Group, LLC, pp. 121–142.

Humphreys MH, Valentin J-P: Natriuretic hormonal agents. In Seldin DW, Giebisch G (Eds.): *The Kidney—Physiology and Pathophysiology,* third ed., New York, 1992, Raven Press.

Kellenberger S, Schild L: Epithelial sodium channel/degenerin family of ion channels: a variety of functions for a shared structure, *Physiol. Rev.* 82:735, 2002.

Nielsen S, Frøkiær J, Marples D, et al: Aquaporins in the kidney: from molecules to medicine, *Physiol. Rev.* 82:205, 2002.

Palmer LG, Frindt G: Aldosterone and potassium secretion by the cortical collecting duct, *Kid. Int.* 57:1324, 2000.

Rahn KH, Heidenreich S, Bruckner D: How to assess glomerular function and damage in humans, *J. Hypertens.* 17:309, 1999.

Reeves WB, Andreoli TE: Sodium chloride transport in the loop of Henle, distal convoluted tubule and collecting duct. In Seldin DW, Giebisch G (Eds.) The *Kidney—Physiology and Pathophysiology,* third ed., New York, 1992, Raven Press.

Reilly RF, Ellison DH: Mammalian distal tubule: physiology, pathophysiology, and molecular anatomy, *Physiol. Rev.* 80:277, 2000.

Rossier BC, Praderv S, Schild L, et al: Epithelial sodium channel and the control of sodium balance: interaction between genetic and environmental factors, *Annu. Rev. Physiol.* 64:877, 2002.

Russell JM: Sodium-potassium-chloride cotransport, *Physiol. Rev.* 80:211, 2000.

Schafer JA: Abnormal regulation of ENaC: syndromes of salt retention and salt wasting by the collecting duct, *Am. J. Physiol. Renal. Physiol.* 283:F221, 2002.

Thomson SC, Blantz RC: Glomerulotubular balance, tubuloglomerular feedback, and salt homeostasis, *J. Am. Soc. Nephrol.* 19:2272, 2008.

Verrey F, Ristic Z, Romeo E, et al: Novel renal amino acid transporters, *Annu. Rev. Physiol.* 67:557, 2005.

Weinstein AM: Mathematical models of renal fluid and electrolyte transport: acknowledging our uncertainty, *Am. J. Physiol. Renal Physiol.* 284:F871, 2003.

Wright EM: Renal Na(+)-glucose cotransporters, *Am. J. Physiol. Renal Physiol.* 280:F10, 2001.

Concentration and Dilution of Urine

LEARNING OBJECTIVES

- Describe the functions of antidiuretic hormone.
- Describe the concentration of tubular fluid as it passes through different regions of the nephron.
- Describe the mechanism of creating a hyperosmotic renal medulla—countercurrent multiplier system.
- Describe the countercurrent exchange system—vasa recta.
- Describe disorders of renal concentrating or diluting ability.

GLOSSARY OF TERMS

- **Osmolarity:** Measure of solute concentration, defined as the number of osmoles (Osm) of solute per liter (L) of solution; osmolality is the number of osmoles (Osm) of solute per kg of solution.

- **Clearance:** Measurement of the renal excretion ability and refers to a volume of fluid (usually blood) that is cleaned of the excreted substance per unit time.

- **Free water clearance:** Measurement of the renal ability to clear free water from the blood. It is an indicator of renal function and body water status.

For the cells of the body to function properly, they must be bathed in extracellular fluid with a relatively constant concentration of electrolytes and other solutes. The total concentration of solutes in the extracellular fluid—and therefore the osmolarity—must also be precisely regulated to prevent the cells from shrinking or swelling. The osmolarity is determined by the amount of solute (mainly sodium chloride) divided by the volume of the extracellular fluid. Thus, to a large extent, extracellular fluid osmolarity and sodium chloride concentration are regulated by the amount of extracellular water. The total body water is controlled by (1) fluid intake, which is regulated by factors that determine thirst and (2) renal water excretion, which is controlled by multiple factors that influence glomerular filtration and tubular reabsorption.

In this chapter, we discuss (1) the mechanisms that cause the kidneys to eliminate excess water by excreting a dilute urine; (2) the mechanisms that cause the kidneys to conserve water by excreting a concentrated urine; (3) the renal feedback mechanisms that control the extracellular fluid sodium concentration and osmolarity; and (4) the thirst and salt appetite mechanisms that determine the intakes of water and salt, which also help to control extracellular fluid volume, osmolarity, and sodium concentration.

Antidiuretic Hormone Controls Urine Concentration

The body has a powerful feedback system for regulating plasma osmolarity and sodium concentration that operates by altering renal excretion of water independently of the rate of solute excretion. A primary effector of this feedback is *antidiuretic hormone (ADH)*, also called *vasopressin*.

When osmolarity of the body fluids increases above normal (ie, the solutes in the body fluids become too concentrated), the posterior pituitary gland secretes more ADH, which increases the permeability of the distal tubules and collecting ducts to water, as discussed in Chapter 78. This mechanism increases water reabsorption and decreases urine volume but does not markedly alter the rate of renal excretion of the solutes.

When there is excess water in the body and extracellular fluid osmolarity is reduced, the secretion of ADH by the posterior pituitary decreases, thereby reducing the permeability of the distal tubule and collecting ducts to water, which causes increased amounts of more dilute urine to be excreted. Thus, the rate of ADH secretion determines, to a large extent, whether the kidney excretes dilute or concentrated urine, and this depends on the ability of the kidney to produce a dilute tubular fluid that is delivered to the distal tubules and collecting ducts where ADH acts.

RENAL MECHANISMS FOR EXCRETING DILUTE URINE

When there is a large excess of water in the body, the kidney can excrete as much as 20 L/day of dilute urine, with a concentration as low as 50 mOsm/L. The kidney performs this impressive feat by continuing to reabsorb solutes while failing to reabsorb large amounts of water in the distal parts of the nephron, including the late distal tubule and the collecting ducts.

Figure 79-1 shows the approximate renal responses in a human after ingestion of 1 L of water. Note that urine volume increases to about six times normal within 45 minutes after the water has been drunk. However, the total amount of solute excreted remains relatively constant because the urine formed becomes very dilute and urine osmolarity decreases from 600 to about 100 mOsm/L. Thus, after ingestion of excess water, the kidney rids the body of the excess water but does not excrete excess amounts of solutes.

When the glomerular filtrate is initially formed, its osmolarity is about the same as that of plasma (300 mOsm/L). To excrete excess water, it is necessary to dilute the filtrate as it passes along the tubule. This dilution is achieved by reabsorbing solutes to a greater extent than water, as shown in Figure 79-2, but this occurs only in certain segments of the tubular system as described in the following sections.

Tubular Fluid Remains Isosmotic in the Proximal Tubule. As fluid flows through the proximal tubule, solutes and water are reabsorbed in equal proportions, so little change in osmolarity occurs; thus, the proximal tubule fluid remains isosmotic to the plasma, with an osmolarity of about 300 mOsm/L. As fluid passes down the descending loop of Henle, water is reabsorbed by osmosis and the tubular fluid reaches equilibrium with the surrounding interstitial fluid of the renal medulla, which is very hypertonic—about two to four times the osmolarity of the original glomerular filtrate. Therefore, the tubular fluid becomes more concentrated as it flows into the inner medulla.

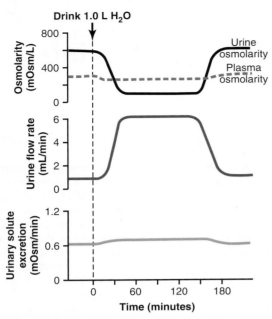

Figure 79-1   Water diuresis in a human after ingestion of 1 L of water. Note that after water ingestion, urine volume increases and urine osmolarity decreases, causing the excretion of a large volume of dilute urine; however, the total amount of solute excreted by the kidneys remains relatively constant. These responses of the kidneys prevent plasma osmolarity from decreasing markedly during excess water ingestion.

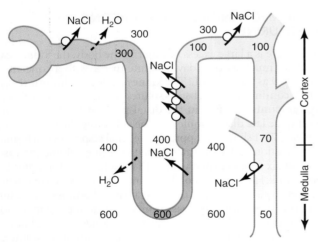

Figure 79-2   Formation of dilute urine when antidiuretic hormone (ADH) levels are very low. Note that in the ascending loop of Henle, the tubular fluid becomes very dilute. In the distal tubules and collecting tubules, the tubular fluid is further diluted by the reabsorption of sodium chloride and the failure to reabsorb water when ADH levels are very low. The failure to reabsorb water and continued reabsorption of solutes lead to a large volume of dilute urine. (Numerical values are in mOsm/L.)

Tubular Fluid Is Diluted in the Ascending Loop of Henle. In the ascending limb of the loop of Henle, especially in the thick segment, sodium, potassium, and chloride are avidly reabsorbed. However, this portion of the tubular segment is impermeable to water, even in the presence of large amounts of ADH. Therefore, the tubular fluid becomes more dilute as it flows up the ascending loop of Henle into the early distal tubule, with the osmolarity decreasing progressively to about 100 mOsm/L by the time the fluid enters the early distal tubular segment. *Thus, regardless of whether ADH is present or absent, fluid leaving the*

early distal tubular segment is hypo-osmotic, with an osmolarity of only about one-third the osmolarity of plasma.

Tubular Fluid in Distal and Collecting Tubules Is Further Diluted in the Absence of ADH. As the dilute fluid in the early distal tubule passes into the late distal convoluted tubule, cortical collecting duct, and collecting duct, there is additional reabsorption of sodium chloride. In the absence of ADH, this portion of the tubule is also impermeable to water, and the additional reabsorption of solutes causes the tubular fluid to become even more dilute, decreasing its osmolarity to as low as 50 mOsm/L. The failure to reabsorb water and the continued reabsorption of solutes leads to a large volume of dilute urine.

To summarize, the mechanism for forming dilute urine is to continue reabsorbing solutes from the distal segments of the tubular system while failing to reabsorb water. In healthy kidneys, fluid leaving the ascending loop of Henle and early distal tubule is always dilute, regardless of the level of ADH. In the absence of ADH, the urine is further diluted in the late distal tubule and collecting ducts and a large volume of dilute urine is excreted.

Kidneys Conserve Water by Excreting Concentrated Urine

The ability of the kidney to form urine more concentrated than plasma is essential for survival of mammals that live on land, including humans. Water is continuously lost from the body through various routes, including the lungs by evaporation into the expired air, the gastrointestinal tract by way of the feces, the skin through evaporation and perspiration, and the kidneys through excretion of urine. Fluid intake is required to match this loss, but the ability of the kidneys to form a small volume of concentrated urine minimizes the intake of fluid required to maintain homeostasis, a function that is especially important when water is in short supply.

When there is a water deficit in the body, the kidneys form concentrated urine by continuing to excrete solutes while increasing water reabsorption and decreasing the volume of urine formed. The human kidney can produce a maximal urine concentration of 1200–1400 mOsm/L, four to five times the osmolarity of plasma.

Some desert animals, such as the Australian hopping mouse, can concentrate urine to as high as 10,000 mOsm/L. This ability allows the mouse to survive in the desert without drinking water; sufficient water can be obtained through the ingested food and water produced in the body by metabolism of the food. Animals adapted to freshwater environments usually have minimal urine concentrating ability. Beavers, for example, can concentrate the urine only to about 500 mOsm/L.

REQUIREMENTS FOR EXCRETING A CONCENTRATED URINE—HIGH ADH LEVELS AND HYPEROSMOTIC RENAL MEDULLA

The basic requirements for forming a concentrated urine are (1) a *high level of ADH*, which increases the permeability of the distal tubules and collecting ducts to water, thereby allowing these tubular segments to avidly reabsorb water and (2) a *high osmolarity of the renal medullary interstitial fluid*, which provides the osmotic gradient necessary for water reabsorption to occur in the presence of high levels of ADH.

The renal medullary interstitium surrounding the collecting ducts is normally hyperosmotic, so when ADH levels are high,

TABLE 79-1	Summary of Tubule Characteristics—Urine Concentration			
	Active NaCl Transport	**Permeability**		
		H₂O	**NaCl**	**Urea**
Proximal tubule	++	++	+	+
Thin descending limb	0	++	+	+
Thin ascending limb	0	0	+	+
Thick ascending limb	++	0	0	0
Distal tubule	+	+ADH	0	0
Cortical collecting tubule	+	+ADH	0	0
Inner medullary collecting duct	+	+ADH	0	++ADH

0, minimal level of active transport or permeability; +, moderate level of active transport or permeability; ++, high level of active transport or permeability; +ADH, permeability to water or urea is increased by ADH.

water moves through the tubular membrane by osmosis into the renal interstitium; from there it is carried away by the vasa recta back into the blood. Thus, the urine concentrating ability is limited by the level of ADH and by the degree of hyperosmolarity of the renal medulla. We discuss the factors that control ADH secretion later, but for now, what is the process by which renal medullary interstitial fluid becomes hyperosmotic? This process involves the operation of the *countercurrent mechanism.*

The countercurrent mechanism depends on the special anatomical arrangement of the loops of Henle and the vasa recta, the specialized peritubular capillaries of the renal medulla. In the human, about 25% of the nephrons are *juxtamedullary nephrons,* with loops of Henle and vasa recta that go deeply into the medulla before returning to the cortex. Some of the loops of Henle dip all the way to the tips of the renal papillae that project from the medulla into the renal pelvis. Paralleling the long loops of Henle are the vasa recta, which also loop down into the medulla before returning to the renal cortex. And finally, the collecting ducts, which carry urine through the hyperosmotic renal medulla before it is excreted, also play a critical role in the countercurrent mechanism.

COUNTERCURRENT MECHANISM PRODUCES A HYPEROSMOTIC RENAL MEDULLARY INTERSTITIUM

The osmolarity of interstitial fluid in almost all parts of the body is about 300 mOsm/L, which is similar to the plasma osmolarity. The osmolarity of the interstitial fluid in the medulla of the kidney is much higher and may increase progressively to about 1200–1400 mOsm/L in the pelvic tip of the medulla. This means that the renal medullary interstitium has accumulated solutes in great excess of water. Once the high solute concentration in the medulla is achieved, it is maintained by a balanced inflow and outflow of solutes and water in the medulla.

The major factors that contribute to the buildup of solute concentration into the renal medulla are as follows:

1. Active transport of sodium ions and co-transport of potassium, chloride, and other ions out of the thick portion of the ascending limb of the loop of Henle into the medullary interstitium.
2. Active transport of ions from the collecting ducts into the medullary interstitium.
3. Facilitated diffusion of urea from the inner medullary collecting ducts into the medullary interstitium.

4. Diffusion of only small amounts of water from the medullary tubules into the medullary interstitium, far less than the reabsorption of solutes into the medullary interstitium.

Special Characteristics of Loop of Henle That Cause Solutes to be Trapped in the Renal Medulla. The transport characteristics of the loops of Henle are summarized in Table 79-1, along with the properties of the proximal tubules, distal tubules, cortical collecting tubules, and inner medullary collecting ducts.

The most important cause of the high medullary osmolarity is active transport of sodium and cotransport of potassium, chloride, and other ions from the thick ascending loop of Henle into the interstitium. Because the thick ascending limb is virtually impermeable to water, the solutes pumped out are not followed by osmotic flow of water into the interstitium. Thus, the active transport of sodium and other ions out of the thick ascending loop adds solutes in excess of water to the renal medullary interstitium. There is some passive reabsorption of sodium chloride from the thin ascending limb of Henle's loop, which is also impermeable to water, adding further to the high solute concentration of the renal medullary interstitium.

The descending limb of Henle's loop, in contrast to the ascending limb, is very permeable to water, and the tubular fluid osmolarity quickly becomes equal to the renal medullary osmolarity. Therefore, water diffuses out of the descending limb of Henle's loop into the interstitium and the tubular fluid osmolarity gradually rises as it flows toward the tip of the loop of Henle.

Steps Involved in Causing Hyperosmotic Renal Medullary Interstitium. Keeping in mind these characteristics of the loop of Henle, let us now discuss how the renal medulla becomes hyperosmotic. First, assume that the loop of Henle is filled with fluid with a concentration of 300 mOsm/L, the same as that leaving the proximal tubule (Figure 79-3, step 1). Next, the active ion pump of the *thick ascending limb* on the loop of Henle reduces the concentration inside the tubule and raises the interstitial concentration; this pump establishes a 200-mOsm/L concentration gradient between the tubular fluid and the interstitial fluid (step 2). Step 3 is that the tubular fluid in the *descending limb of the loop of Henle* and the interstitial fluid quickly reach osmotic equilibrium because of osmosis of water out of the descending limb. The interstitial osmolarity is maintained at 400 mOsm/L because of continued transport of ions out of the thick ascending loop of Henle. Thus, by itself, the active transport of sodium chloride out of the thick ascending limb is capable of establishing

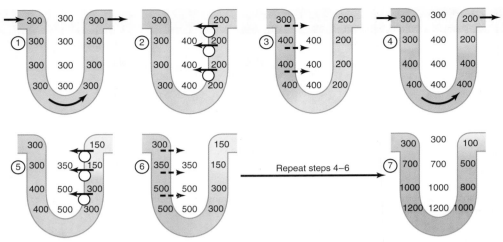

Figure 79-3 Countercurrent multiplier system in the loop of Henle for producing a hyperosmotic renal medulla. (Numerical values are in mOsm/L.)

only a 200-mOsm/L concentration gradient, much less than that achieved by the countercurrent system.

Step 4 is additional flow of fluid into the loop of Henle from the proximal tubule, which causes the hyperosmotic fluid previously formed in the descending limb to flow into the ascending limb. Once this fluid is in the ascending limb, additional ions are pumped into the interstitium, with water remaining in the tubular fluid, until a 200-mOsm/L osmotic gradient is established, with the interstitial fluid osmolarity rising to 500 mOsm/L (step 5). Then, once again, the fluid in the descending limb reaches equilibrium with the hyperosmotic medullary interstitial fluid (step 6), and as the hyperosmotic tubular fluid from the descending limb of the loop of Henle flows into the ascending limb, still more solute is continuously pumped out of the tubules and deposited into the medullary interstitium.

These steps are repeated over and over, with the net effect of adding more and more solute to the medulla in excess of water; with sufficient time, *this process gradually traps solutes in the medulla and multiplies the concentration gradient established by the active pumping of ions out of the thick ascending loop of Henle, eventually raising the interstitial fluid osmolarity to 1200–1400 mOsm/L as shown in step 7.*

Thus, the repetitive reabsorption of sodium chloride by the thick ascending loop of Henle and continued inflow of new sodium chloride from the proximal tubule into the loop of Henle is called the *countercurrent multiplier.* The sodium chloride reabsorbed from the ascending loop of Henle keeps adding to the newly arrived sodium chloride, thus "multiplying" its concentration in the medullary interstitium.

ROLE OF DISTAL TUBULE AND COLLECTING DUCTS IN EXCRETING CONCENTRATED URINE

When the tubular fluid leaves the loop of Henle and flows into the distal convoluted tubule in the renal cortex, the fluid is dilute, with an osmolarity of only about 100 mOsm/L (Figure 79-4). The early distal tubule further dilutes the tubular fluid because this segment, like the ascending loop of Henle, actively transports sodium chloride out of the tubule but is relatively impermeable to water.

As fluid flows into the cortical collecting tubule, the amount of water reabsorbed is critically dependent on the plasma concentration of ADH. In the absence of ADH, this segment is

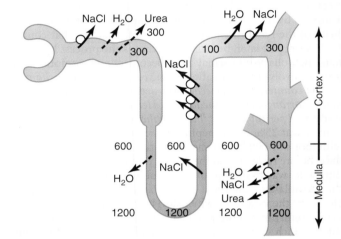

Figure 79-4 Formation of concentrated urine when antidiuretic hormone (ADH) levels are high. Note that the fluid leaving the loop of Henle is dilute but becomes concentrated as water is absorbed from the distal tubules and collecting tubules. With high ADH levels, the osmolarity of the urine is about the same as the osmolarity of the renal medullary interstitial fluid in the papilla, which is about 1200 mOsm/L. (Numerical values are in mOsm/L.)

almost impermeable to water and fails to reabsorb water but continues to reabsorb solutes and further dilutes the urine. When there is a high concentration of ADH, the cortical collecting tubule becomes highly permeable to water, so large amounts of water are now reabsorbed from the tubule into the cortex interstitium, where it is swept away by the rapidly flowing peritubular capillaries. *The fact that these large amounts of water are reabsorbed into the cortex, rather than into the renal medulla, helps to preserve the high medullary interstitial fluid osmolarity.*

As the tubular fluid flows along the medullary collecting ducts, there is further water reabsorption from the tubular fluid into the interstitium, but the total amount of water is relatively small compared with that added to the cortex interstitium. The reabsorbed water is quickly carried away by the vasa recta into the venous blood. When high levels of ADH are present, the collecting ducts become permeable to water, so the fluid at the end of the collecting ducts has essentially the same osmolarity as the interstitial fluid of the renal medulla—about 1200 mOsm/L (Figure 79-3). Thus, by reabsorbing as much water as possible, the kidneys form highly concentrated urine, excreting normal amounts of solutes in the urine while adding water back to the extracellular fluid and compensating for deficits of body water.

UREA CONTRIBUTES TO HYPEROSMOTIC RENAL MEDULLARY INTERSTITIUM AND FORMATION OF CONCENTRATED URINE

Thus far, we have considered only the contribution of sodium chloride to the hyperosmotic renal medullary interstitium. However, urea contributes about 40–50% of the osmolarity (500–600 mOsm/L) of the renal medullary interstitium when the kidney is forming maximally concentrated urine. Unlike sodium chloride, urea is passively reabsorbed from the tubule. When there is water deficit and blood concentration of ADH is high, large amounts of urea are passively reabsorbed from the inner medullary collecting ducts into the interstitium.

The mechanism for reabsorption of urea into the renal medulla is as follows: As water flows up the ascending loop of Henle and into the distal and cortical collecting tubules, little urea is reabsorbed because these segments are impermeable to urea (Table 79-1). In the presence of high concentrations of ADH, water is reabsorbed rapidly from the cortical collecting tubule and the urea concentration increases rapidly because urea is not very permeant in this part of the tubule.

As the tubular fluid flows into the inner medullary collecting ducts, still more water reabsorption takes place, causing an even higher concentration of urea in the fluid. This high concentration of urea in the tubular fluid of the inner medullary collecting duct causes urea to diffuse out of the tubule into the renal interstitial fluid. This diffusion is greatly facilitated by specific *urea transporters, UT-A1, and UT-A3.* One of these urea transporters, UT-A3, is activated by ADH, increasing transport of urea out of the inner medullary collecting duct even more when ADH levels are elevated. The simultaneous movement of water and urea out of the inner medullary collecting ducts maintains a high concentration of urea in the tubular fluid and, eventually, in the urine, even though urea is being reabsorbed.

The fundamental role of urea in contributing to urine concentrating ability is evidenced by the fact that people who ingest a high-protein diet, yielding large amounts of urea as a nitrogenous "waste" product, can concentrate their urine much better than people whose protein intake and urea production are low. Malnutrition is associated with a low urea concentration in the medullary interstitium and considerable impairment of urine concentrating ability.

COUNTERCURRENT EXCHANGE IN THE VASA RECTA PRESERVES HYPEROSMOLARITY OF THE RENAL MEDULLA

Blood flow must be provided to the renal medulla to supply the metabolic needs of the cells in this part of the kidney. Without a special medullary blood flow system, the solutes pumped into the renal medulla by the countercurrent multiplier system would be rapidly dissipated.

There are two special features of the renal medullary blood flow that contribute to the preservation of the high solute concentrations:

1. *The medullary blood flow is low,* accounting for less than 5% of the total renal blood flow. This sluggish blood flow is sufficient to supply the metabolic needs of the tissues but helps to minimize solute loss from the medullary interstitium.

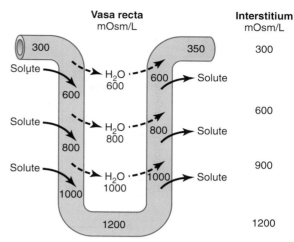

Figure 79-5 Countercurrent exchange in the vasa recta. Plasma flowing down the descending limb of the vasa recta becomes more hyperosmotic because of diffusion of water out of the blood and diffusion of solutes from the renal interstitial fluid into the blood. In the ascending limb of the vasa recta, solutes diffuse back into the interstitial fluid and water diffuses back into the vasa recta. Large amounts of solutes would be lost from the renal medulla without the U shape of the vasa recta capillaries. (Numerical values are in mOsm/L.)

2. *The vasa recta serve as countercurrent exchangers,* minimizing washout of solutes from the medullary interstitium.

The countercurrent exchange mechanism operates as follows (Figure 79-5): Blood enters and leaves the medulla by way of the vasa recta at the boundary of the cortex and renal medulla. The vasa recta, like other capillaries, are highly permeable to solutes in the blood, except for the plasma proteins. As blood descends into the medulla toward the papillae, it becomes progressively more concentrated, partly by solute entry from the interstitium and partly by loss of water into the interstitium. By the time the blood reaches the tips of the vasa recta, it has a concentration of about 1200 mOsm/L, the same as that of the medullary interstitium. As blood ascends back toward the cortex, it becomes progressively less concentrated as solutes diffuse back out into the medullary interstitium and as water moves into the vasa recta.

Although there are large amounts of fluid and solute exchange across the vasa recta, there is little net dilution of the concentration of the interstitial fluid at each level of the renal medulla because of the U shape of the vasa recta capillaries, which act as countercurrent exchangers. Thus, *the vasa recta do not create the medullary hyperosmolarity, but they do prevent it from being dissipated.*

The U-shaped structure of the vessels minimizes loss of solute from the interstitium but does not prevent the bulk flow of fluid and solutes into the blood through the usual colloid osmotic and hydrostatic pressures that favor reabsorption in these capillaries. Under steady-state conditions, the vasa recta carry away only as much solute and water as is absorbed from the medullary tubules and the high concentration of solutes established by the countercurrent mechanism is preserved.

SUMMARY OF URINE CONCENTRATING MECHANISM AND CHANGES IN OSMOLARITY IN DIFFERENT SEGMENTS OF THE TUBULES

The changes in osmolarity and volume of the tubular fluid as it passes through the different parts of the nephron are shown in Figure 79-6.

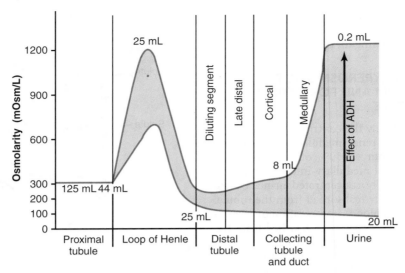

Figure 79-6   Changes in osmolarity of the tubular fluid as it passes through the different tubular segments in the presence of high levels of antidiuretic hormone (*ADH*) and in the absence of ADH. (Numerical values indicate the approximate volumes in mL/min or in osmolarities in mOsm/L of fluid flowing along the different tubular segments.)

Proximal Tubule. About 65% of the filtered electrolytes is reabsorbed in the proximal tubule. However, the proximal tubular membranes are highly permeable to water, so that whenever solutes are reabsorbed water also diffuses through the tubular membrane by osmosis. Therefore, the osmolarity of the fluid remains about the same as the glomerular filtrate, 300 mOsm/L.

Descending Loop of Henle. As fluid flows down the descending loop of Henle, water is absorbed into the medulla. The descending limb is highly permeable to water but much less permeable to sodium chloride and urea. Therefore, the osmolarity of the fluid flowing through the descending loop gradually increases until it is nearly equal to that of the surrounding interstitial fluid, which is about 1200 mOsm/L when the blood concentration of ADH is high.

When dilute urine is being formed, owing to low ADH concentrations, the medullary interstitial osmolarity is less than 1200 mOsm/L; consequently, the descending loop tubular fluid osmolarity also becomes less concentrated. This is due partly to the fact that less urea is absorbed into the medullary interstitium from the collecting ducts when ADH levels are low and the kidney is forming a large volume of dilute urine.

Thin Ascending Loop of Henle. The thin ascending limb is essentially impermeable to water but reabsorbs some sodium chloride. Because of the high concentration of sodium chloride in the tubular fluid, owing to water removal from the descending loop of Henle, there is some passive diffusion of sodium chloride from the thin ascending limb into the medullary interstitium. Thus, the tubular fluid becomes more dilute as the sodium chloride diffuses out of the tubule and water remains in the tubule.

Some of the urea absorbed into the medullary interstitium from the collecting ducts also diffuses into the ascending limb, thereby returning the urea to the tubular system and helping to prevent its washout from the renal medulla. This *urea recycling* is an additional mechanism that contributes to the hyperosmotic renal medulla.

Thick Ascending Loop of Henle. The thick part of the ascending loop of Henle is also virtually impermeable to water, but large amounts of sodium, chloride, potassium, and other ions are actively transported from the tubule into the medullary interstitium. Therefore, fluid in the thick ascending limb of the loop of Henle becomes very dilute, falling to a concentration of about 100 mOsm/L.

Early Distal Tubule. The early distal tubule has properties similar to those of the thick ascending loop of Henle, so further dilution of the tubular fluid to about 50 mOsm/L occurs as solutes are reabsorbed while water remains in the tubule.

Late Distal Tubule and Cortical Collecting Tubules. In the late distal tubule and cortical collecting tubules, the osmolarity of the fluid depends on the level of ADH. With high levels of ADH, these tubules are highly permeable to water and significant amounts of water are reabsorbed. Urea, however, is not very permeant in this part of the nephron, resulting in increased urea concentration as water is reabsorbed. This allows most of the urea delivered to the distal tubule and collecting tubule to pass into the inner medullary collecting ducts, from which it is eventually reabsorbed or excreted in the urine. In the absence of ADH, little water is reabsorbed in the late distal tubule and cortical collecting tubule; therefore, osmolarity decreases even further because of continued active reabsorption of ions from these segments.

Inner Medullary Collecting Ducts. The concentration of fluid in the inner medullary collecting ducts also depends on (1) ADH and (2) the surrounding medullary interstitium osmolarity established by the countercurrent mechanism. In the presence of large amounts of ADH, these ducts are highly permeable to water, and water diffuses from the tubule into the interstitial fluid until osmotic equilibrium is reached, with the tubular fluid having about the same concentration as the renal medullary interstitium (1200–1400 mOsm/L). Thus, a small volume of concentrated urine is produced when ADH levels are high. Because water reabsorption increases urea concentration in the tubular fluid and because the inner medullary collecting ducts have specific urea transporters that greatly facilitate diffusion, much of the highly concentrated urea in the ducts diffuses out of the tubular lumen into the medullary interstitium. This absorption of the urea into the renal medulla contributes to the high osmolarity of the medullary interstitium and the high concentrating ability of the kidney.

Several important points to consider may not be obvious from this discussion. First, although sodium chloride is one of the principal solutes that contribute to the hyperosmolarity of the medullary interstitium, *the kidney can, when needed, excrete highly concentrated urine that contains little sodium chloride.* The hyperosmolarity of the urine in these circumstances is due to high concentrations of other solutes, especially of waste products such as urea. One condition in which this occurs is dehydration accompanied by low sodium intake. As discussed in Chapter 81, low sodium intake stimulates formation of the hormones angiotensin II and aldosterone, which together cause avid sodium reabsorption from the tubules while leaving the urea and other solutes to maintain the highly concentrated urine.

Second, *large quantities of dilute urine can be excreted without increasing the excretion of sodium.* This is accomplished by decreasing ADH secretion, which reduces water reabsorption in the more distal tubular segments without significantly altering sodium reabsorption.

And finally, there is an *obligatory urine volume* that is dictated by the maximum concentrating ability of the kidney and the amount of solute that must be excreted. Therefore, if large amounts of solute must be excreted, they must be accompanied by the minimal amount of water necessary to excrete them.

OBLIGATORY URINE VOLUME

The maximal concentrating ability of the kidney dictates how much urine volume must be excreted each day to rid the body of metabolic waste products and ions that are ingested. A normal 70-kg human must excrete about 600 mOsm of solute each day. If maximal urine concentrating ability is 1200 mOsm/L, the *minimal* volume of urine that must be excreted, called the *obligatory urine volume,* can be calculated as

$$\frac{600 \, \text{mOsm} / \text{day}}{1200 \, \text{mOsm} / \text{L}} = 0.5 \, \text{L/day}$$

This minimal loss of volume in the urine contributes to dehydration, along with water loss from the skin, respiratory tract, and gastrointestinal tract, when water is not available to drink.

The limited ability of the human kidney to concentrate the urine to only about 1200 mOsm/L explains why severe dehydration occurs if one attempts to drink seawater. Sodium chloride concentration in the oceans averages about 3.0–3.5%, with an osmolarity between about 1000 and 1200 mOsm/L. Drinking 1 L of seawater with a concentration of 1200 mOsm/L would provide a total sodium chloride intake of 1200 mOsm. If maximal urine concentrating ability is 1200 mOsm/L, the amount of urine volume needed to excrete 1200 mOsm would be 1200 mOsm divided by 1200 mOsm/L or 1.0 L. Why then does drinking seawater cause dehydration? The answer is that the kidney must also excrete other solutes, especially urea, which contributes about 600 mOsm/L when the urine is maximally concentrated. Therefore, the maximum concentration of sodium chloride that can be excreted by the kidneys is about 600 mOsm/L. Thus, for every liter of seawater drunk, 1.5 L of urine volume would be required to rid the body of 1200 mOsm of sodium chloride ingested in addition to 600 mOsm of other solutes such as urea. This would result in a net fluid loss of 0.5 L for every liter of seawater drunk, explaining the rapid dehydration that occurs in shipwreck victims who drink seawater.

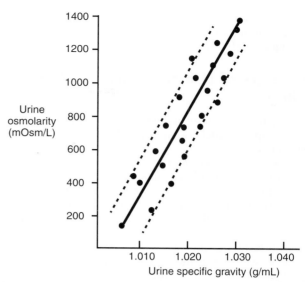

Figure 79-7 Relationship between specific gravity (g/mL) and osmolarity of the urine.

However, a shipwreck victim's pet Australian hopping mouse could drink with impunity all the seawater it wanted.

URINE SPECIFIC GRAVITY

Urine *specific gravity* is often used in clinical settings to provide a rapid estimate of urine solute concentration. The more concentrated the urine, the higher the urine specific gravity. In most cases, urine specific gravity increases linearly with increasing urine osmolarity (Figure 79-7). Urine specific gravity, however, is a measure of the weight of solutes in a given volume of urine and is therefore determined by the number and size of the solute molecules. In contrast, osmolarity is determined only by the number of solute molecules in a given volume.

Urine specific gravity is generally expressed in g/mL and, in humans, normally ranges from 1.002 to 1.028 g/mL, rising by .001 for every 35–40 mOsm/L increase in urine osmolarity.

Quantifying Renal Urine Concentration and Dilution: "Free Water" and Osmolar Clearances

The process of concentrating or diluting the urine requires the kidneys to excrete water and solutes somewhat independently. When the urine is dilute, water is excreted in excess of solutes. Conversely, when the urine is concentrated, solutes are excreted in excess of water.

The total clearance of solutes from the blood can be expressed as the *osmolar clearance* (C_{osm}); this is the volume of plasma cleared of solutes each minute, in the same way that clearance of a single substance is calculated:

$$C_{osm} = \frac{U_{osm} \times \dot{V}}{P_{osm}}$$

where U_{osm} is the urine osmolarity, $\dot{V}$ is the urine flow rate, and P_{osm} is the plasma osmolarity. For example, if plasma osmolarity is 300 mOsm/L, urine osmolarity is 600 mOsm/L, and urine flow rate is 1 mL/min (0.001 L/min), the rate of osmolar excretion is 0.6 mOsm/min (600 mOsm/L × 0.001 L/min) and osmolar clearance is 0.6 mOsm/min divided by 300 mOsm/L, or 0.002 L/min (2.0 mL/min). This means that 2 mL of plasma are being cleared of solute each minute.

Disorders of Urinary Concentrating Ability

Impairment in the ability of the kidneys to concentrate or dilute the urine appropriately can occur with one or more of the following abnormalities:

1. *Inappropriate secretion of ADH.* Either too much or too little ADH secretion results in abnormal water excretion by the kidneys (see Chapter 88).
2. *Impairment of the countercurrent mechanism.* A hyperosmotic medullary interstitium is required for maximal urine concentrating ability. No matter how much ADH is present, maximal urine concentration is limited by the degree of hyperosmolarity of the medullary interstitium.
3. Inability of the distal tubule, collecting tubule, and collecting ducts to respond to ADH.

FAILURE TO PRODUCE ADH: "CENTRAL" DIABETES INSIPIDUS

An inability to produce or release ADH from the posterior pituitary can be caused by head injuries or infections, or it can be congenital (discussed in Chapter 88). Because the distal tubular segments cannot reabsorb water in the absence of ADH, this condition, called *"central" diabetes insipidus*, results in the formation of a large volume of dilute urine with urine volumes that can exceed 15 L/day. The thirst mechanisms, discussed in Chapter 80, are activated when excessive water is lost from the body; therefore, as long as the person drinks enough water, large decreases in body fluid water do not occur. The primary abnormality observed clinically in people with this condition is the large volume of dilute urine. However, if water intake is restricted, as can occur in a hospital setting when fluid intake is restricted or the patient is unconscious (eg, because of a head injury), severe dehydration can rapidly occur.

The treatment for central diabetes insipidus is administration of a synthetic analog of ADH, *desmopressin*, which acts selectively on V_2 receptors to increase water permeability in the late distal and collecting tubules. Desmopressin can be given by injection, as a nasal spray, or orally, and it rapidly restores urine output toward normal.

INABILITY OF THE KIDNEYS TO RESPOND TO ADH: "NEPHROGENIC" DIABETES INSIPIDUS

In some circumstances normal or elevated levels of ADH are present but the renal tubular segments cannot respond appropriately. This condition is referred to as *"nephrogenic" diabetes insipidus* because the abnormality resides in the kidneys. This abnormality can be due to either failure of the countercurrent mechanism to form a hyperosmotic renal medullary interstitium or failure of the distal and collecting tubules and collecting ducts to respond to ADH. In either case, large volumes of dilute urine are formed, which tends to cause dehydration unless fluid intake is increased by the same amount as urine volume is increased.

Many types of renal diseases can impair the concentrating mechanism, especially those that damage the renal medulla (see Chapter 84 for further discussion). Also, impairment of the function of the loop of Henle, as occurs with diuretics that inhibit electrolyte reabsorption by this segment, such as furosemide, can compromise urine concentrating ability. Furthermore, certain drugs, such as lithium (used to treat manic-depressive disorders) and tetracyclines (used as antibiotics), can impair the ability of the distal nephron segments to respond to ADH.

Nephrogenic diabetes insipidus can be distinguished from central diabetes insipidus by administration of desmopressin, the synthetic analog of ADH. Lack of a prompt decrease in urine volume and an increase in urine osmolarity within 2 hours after injection of desmopressin is strongly suggestive of nephrogenic diabetes insipidus. The treatment for nephrogenic diabetes insipidus is to correct, if possible, the underlying renal disorder. The hypernatremia can also be attenuated by a low-sodium diet and administration of a diuretic that enhances renal sodium excretion, such as a thiazide diuretic.

BIBLIOGRAPHY

Antunes-Rodrigues J, de Castro M, Elias LL, et al: Neuroendocrine control of body fluid metabolism, *Physiol. Rev.* 84:169, 2004.

Bourque CW: Central mechanisms of osmosensation and systemic osmoregulation, *Nat. Rev. Neurosci.* 9:519-531, 2008.

Cowley, AW Jr, Mori, T, Mattson, D, et al, 2003. Role of renal NO production in the regulation of medullary blood flow. *Am. J. Physiol. Regul. Integr. Comp. Physiol.* 284, R1355 (Cowen, LE, Hodak, SP, Verbalis, JG, 2013. Age-associated abnormalities of water homeostasis. *Endocrinol. Metab. Clin. North Am.* 42349.

Dwyer TM, Schmidt-Nielsen B: The renal pelvis: machinery that concentrates urine in the papilla, *News Physiol. Sci.* 18:1, 2003.

Fenton RA, Knepper MA: Mouse models and the urinary concentrating mechanism in the new millennium, *Physiol. Rev.* 87:1083, 2007.

Finley JJ 4th, Konstam MA, Udelson JE: Arginine vasopressin antagonists for the treatment of heart failure and hyponatremia, *Circulation* 118:410, 2008.

Geerling JC, Loewy AD: Central regulation of sodium appetite, *Exp. Physiol.* 93:177, 2008.

Klein JD, Blount MA, Sands JM: Molecular mechanisms of urea transport in health and disease, *Pflugers Arch.* 464:561, 2012.

Kortenoeven ML, Fenton RA: Renal aquaporins and water balance disorders, *Biochim. Biophys. Acta.* 1840:1533, 2014.

Kozono D, Yasui M, King LS, et al: Aquaporin water channels: atomic structure molecular dynamics meet clinical medicine, *J. Clin. Invest.* 109:1395, 2002.

Loh JA, Verbalis JG: Disorders of water and salt metabolism associated with pituitary disease, *Endocrinol. Metab. Clin. North Am.* 37:213, 2008.

McKinley MJ, Johnson AK: The physiological regulation of thirst and fluid intake, *News Physiol. Sci.* 19:1, 2004.

Pallone TL, Zhang Z, Rhinehart K: Physiology of the renal medullary microcirculation, *Am. J. Physiol. Renal Physiol.* 284:F253, 2003.

Sands JM, Bichet DG: Nephrogenic diabetes insipidus, *Ann. Intern. Med.* 144:186, 2006.

Schrier RW: Body water homeostasis: clinical disorders of urinary dilution and concentration, *J. Am. Soc. Nephrol.* 17:2006, 1820.

Sharif-Naeini R, Ciura S, Zhang Z, et al: Contribution of TRPV channels to osmosensory transduction, thirst, and vasopressin release, *Kid. Int.* 73:811, 2008.

Control of Extracellular Fluid Osmolarity and Sodium Concentration

Regulation of extracellular fluid osmolarity and sodium concentration are closely linked because sodium is the most abundant ion in the extracellular compartment. Plasma sodium concentration is normally regulated within close limits of 140–145 mEq/L, with an average concentration of about 142 mEq/L. Osmolarity averages about 300 mOsm/L (about 282 mOsm/L when corrected for interionic attraction) and seldom changes more than ±2–3%. As discussed in Chapter 4, these variables must be precisely controlled because they determine the distribution of fluid between the intracellular and extracellular compartments.

Normally, sodium ions and associated anions (primarily bicarbonate and chloride) represent about 94% of the extracellular osmoles, with glucose and urea contributing about 3–5% of the total osmoles. However, because urea easily permeates most cell membranes, it exerts little *effective* osmotic pressure under steady-state conditions. Therefore, the sodium ions in the extracellular fluid and associated anions are the principal determinants of fluid movement across the cell membrane. Consequently, we can discuss the control of osmolarity and control of sodium ion concentration at the same time.

Although multiple mechanisms control the amount of sodium and water excretion by the kidneys, two primary systems are especially involved in regulating the concentration of sodium and osmolarity of extracellular fluid: (1) the osmoreceptor–ADH system and (2) the thirst mechanism.

Osmoreceptor–ADH Feedback System

Figure 80-1 shows the basic components of the osmoreceptor–ADH feedback system for control of extracellular fluid sodium concentration and osmolarity. When osmolarity (plasma sodium concentration) increases above normal because of water deficit, for example, this feedback system operates as follows:

1. An increase in extracellular fluid osmolarity (which in practical terms means an increase in plasma sodium concentration) causes the special nerve cells called *osmoreceptor cells*, located in the *anterior hypothalamus* near the supraoptic nuclei, to shrink.
2. Shrinkage of the osmoreceptor cells causes them to fire, sending nerve signals to additional nerve cells in the supraoptic nuclei, which then relay these signals down the stalk of the pituitary gland to the posterior pituitary.
3. These action potentials conducted to the posterior pituitary stimulate the release of ADH, which is stored in secretory granules (or vesicles) in the nerve endings.
4. ADH enters the blood stream and is transported to the kidneys, where it increases the water permeability of the late distal tubules, cortical collecting tubules, and medullary collecting ducts.
5. The increased water permeability in the distal nephron segments causes increased water reabsorption and excretion of a small volume of concentrated urine.

Thus, water is conserved in the body while sodium and other solutes continue to be excreted in the urine. This causes dilution of the solutes in the extracellular fluid, thereby correcting the initial excessively concentrated extracellular fluid.

The opposite sequence of events occurs when the extracellular fluid becomes too dilute (hypo-osmotic). For example, with excess water ingestion and a decrease in extracellular fluid osmolarity, less ADH is formed, the renal tubules decrease their permeability for water, less water is reabsorbed, and a large volume of dilute urine is formed. This in turn concentrates the body fluids and returns plasma osmolarity toward normal.

ADH SYNTHESIS IN SUPRAOPTIC AND PARAVENTRICULAR NUCLEI OF THE HYPOTHALAMUS AND ADH RELEASE FROM THE POSTERIOR PITUITARY

Figure 80-2 shows the neuroanatomy of the hypothalamus and the pituitary gland, where ADH is synthesized and released. The hypothalamus contains two types of *magnocellular* (*large*) *neurons that synthesize ADH in the supraoptic and paraventricular nuclei of the hypothalamus*, about five-sixths in the supraoptic nuclei and about one-sixth in the paraventricular nuclei. Both of these nuclei have axonal extensions to the posterior pituitary. Once ADH is synthesized, it is transported down the axons of the neurons to their tips, terminating in the posterior pituitary gland. When the supraoptic and paraventricular nuclei are stimulated by increased osmolarity or other factors, nerve impulses pass down these nerve endings, changing their membrane permeability and increasing calcium entry. ADH stored in the secretory granules (also called vesicles) of the nerve endings is released in

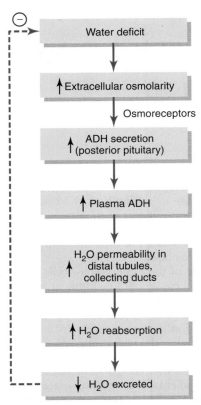

Figure 80-1 Osmoreceptor–ADH feedback mechanism for regulating extracellular fluid osmolarity in response to a water deficit.

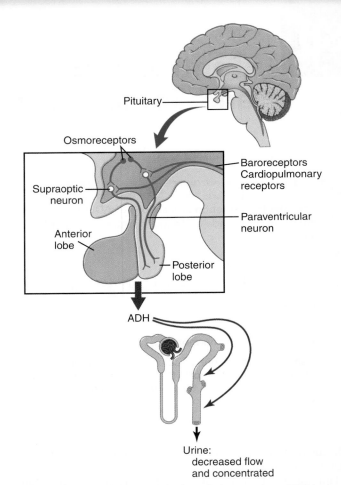

Figure 80-2 Neuroanatomy of the hypothalamus, where ADH is synthesized, and the posterior pituitary gland, where ADH is released.

response to increased calcium entry. The released ADH is then carried away in the capillary blood of the posterior pituitary into the systemic circulation.

Secretion of ADH in response to an osmotic stimulus is rapid, so plasma ADH levels can increase severalfold within minutes, thereby providing a rapid means for altering renal excretion of water.

A second neuronal area important in controlling osmolarity and ADH secretion is located along the *anteroventral region of the third ventricle* called the *AV3V region*. At the upper part of this region is a structure called the *subfornical organ*, and at the inferior part is another structure called the *organum vasculosum* of the *lamina terminalis*. Between these two organs is the *median preoptic nucleus*, which has multiple nerve connections with the two organs, as well as with the supraoptic nuclei and the blood pressure control centers in the medulla of the brain. Lesions of the AV3V region cause multiple deficits in the control of ADH secretion, thirst, sodium appetite, and blood pressure. Electrical stimulation of this region or stimulation by angiotensin II can increase ADH secretion, thirst, and sodium appetite.

In the vicinity of the AV3V region and the supraoptic nuclei are neuronal cells that are excited by small increases in extracellular fluid osmolarity; hence, the term *osmoreceptors* has been used to describe these neurons. These cells send nerve signals to the supraoptic nuclei to control their firing and secretion of ADH. It is also likely that they induce thirst in response to increased extracellular fluid osmolarity.

Both the subfornical organ and the organum vasculosum of the lamina terminalis have vascular supplies that lack the typical blood–brain barrier that impedes the diffusion of most ions from the blood into the brain tissue. This characteristic makes it possible for ions and other solutes to cross between the blood and the local interstitial fluid in this region. As a result, the osmoreceptors rapidly respond to changes in osmolarity of the extracellular fluid, exerting powerful control over the secretion of ADH and over thirst, as discussed later.

STIMULATION OF ADH RELEASE BY DECREASED ARTERIAL PRESSURE AND/OR DECREASED BLOOD VOLUME

ADH release is also controlled by cardiovascular reflexes that respond to decreases in blood pressure and/or blood volume, including (1) the *arterial baroreceptor reflexes* and (2) *the cardiopulmonary reflexes*, both of which are discussed in Chapter 43. These reflex pathways originate in high-pressure regions of the circulation, such as the aortic arch and carotid sinus, and in the low-pressure regions, especially in the cardiac atria. Afferent stimuli are carried by the vagus and glossopharyngeal nerves with synapses in the nuclei of the tractus solitarius. Projections from these nuclei relay signals to the hypothalamic nuclei that control ADH synthesis and secretion.

Thus, in addition to increased osmolarity, two other stimuli increase ADH secretion: (1) decreased arterial pressure and (2) decreased blood volume. Whenever blood pressure and blood volume are reduced, such as occurs during hemorrhage, increased ADH secretion causes increased fluid reabsorption

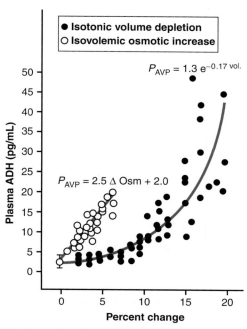

Figure 80-3 The effect of increased plasma osmolarity or decreased blood volume on the level of plasma (*P*) ADH, also called *arginine vasopressin* (*AVP*). (*Modified from Dunn, F.L., Brennan, T.J., Nelson, A.E., et al., 1973. The role of blood osmolality and volume in regulating vasopressin secretion in the rat. J. Clin. Invest. 52 (12), 3212. By copyright permission of the American Society of Clinical Investigation.*)

by the kidneys, helping to restore blood pressure and blood volume toward normal.

QUANTITATIVE IMPORTANCE OF OSMOLARITY AND CARDIOVASCULAR REFLEXES IN STIMULATING ADH SECRETION

As shown in Figure 80-3, either a decrease in effective blood volume or an increase in extracellular fluid osmolarity stimulates ADH secretion. However, ADH is considerably more sensitive to small changes in osmolarity than to similar percentage changes in blood volume. For example, a change in plasma osmolarity of only 1% is sufficient to increase ADH levels. By contrast, after blood loss, plasma ADH levels do not change appreciably until blood volume is reduced by about 10%. With further decreases in blood volume, ADH levels rapidly increase. Thus, with severe decreases in blood volume, the cardiovascular reflexes play a major role in stimulating ADH secretion. The usual day-to-day regulation of ADH secretion during simple dehydration is effected mainly by changes in plasma osmolarity. Decreased blood volume, however, greatly enhances the ADH response to increased osmolarity.

OTHER STIMULI FOR ADH SECRETION

ADH secretion can also be increased or decreased by other stimuli to the central nervous system, as well as by various drugs and hormones, as shown in Table 80-1. For example, *nausea* is a potent stimulus for ADH release, which may increase to as much as 100 times normal after vomiting. Also, drugs such as *nicotine* and *morphine* stimulate ADH release, whereas some

TABLE 80-1	Control of ADH Secretion	
Increase ADH	**Decrease ADH**
↑ Plasma osmolarity	↓ Plasma osmolarity
↓ Blood volume	↑ Blood volume
↓ Blood pressure	↑ Blood pressure
Nausea	
Hypoxia	
Drugs:	Drugs:
Morphine	Alcohol
Nicotine	Clonidine (antihypertensive drug)
Cyclophosphamide	Haloperidol (dopamine blocker)

drugs, such as *alcohol*, inhibit ADH release. The marked diuresis that occurs after ingestion of alcohol is due in part to inhibition of ADH release.

Importance of Thirst in Controlling Extracellular Fluid Osmolarity and Sodium Concentration

The kidneys minimize fluid loss during water deficits through the osmoreceptor–ADH feedback system. Adequate fluid intake, however, is necessary to counterbalance whatever fluid loss does occur through sweating and breathing, and through the gastrointestinal tract. Fluid intake is regulated by the thirst mechanism, which, together with the osmoreceptor–ADH mechanism, maintains precise control of extracellular fluid osmolarity and sodium concentration.

Many of the same factors that stimulate ADH secretion also increase thirst, which is defined as the conscious desire for water.

CENTRAL NERVOUS SYSTEM CENTERS FOR THIRST

Referring again to Figure 80-2, the same area along the anteroventral wall of the third ventricle that promotes ADH release also stimulates thirst. Located anterolaterally in the preoptic nucleus is another small area that, when stimulated electrically, causes immediate drinking that continues as long as the stimulation lasts. All these areas together are called the *thirst center*.

The neurons of the thirst center respond to injections of hypertonic salt solutions by stimulating drinking behavior. These cells almost certainly function as osmoreceptors to activate the thirst mechanism, in the same way that the osmoreceptors stimulate ADH release.

Increased osmolarity of the cerebrospinal fluid in the third ventricle has essentially the same effect to promote drinking. It is likely that the *organum vasculosum of the lamina terminalis*, which lies immediately beneath the ventricular surface at the inferior end of the AV3V region, is intimately involved in mediating this response.

STIMULI FOR THIRST

Table 80-2 summarizes some of the known stimuli for thirst. One of the most important is *increased extracellular fluid osmolarity, which causes intracellular dehydration in the thirst centers*, thereby stimulating the sensation of thirst. *Decreases in extracellular fluid volume and arterial pressure also stimulate*

TABLE 80-2	Control of Thirst	
Increase Thirst	**Decrease Thirst**	
↑ Plasma osmolarity	↓ Plasma osmolarity	
↓ Blood volume	↑ Blood volume	
↓ Blood pressure	↑ Blood pressure	
↑ Angiotensin II	↓ Angiotensin II	
Dry mouth	Gastric distension	

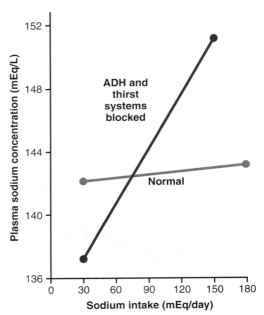

Figure 80-4 Effect of large changes in sodium intake on extracellular fluid sodium concentration in dogs under normal conditions (*red line*) and after the ADH and thirst feedback systems had been blocked (*blue line*). Note that control of extracellular fluid sodium concentration is poor in the absence of these feedback systems. (*Courtesy Dr David B Young.*)

thirst by a pathway that is independent of the one stimulated by increased plasma osmolarity, probably related to neural input from cardiopulmonary and systemic arterial baroreceptors in the circulation.

A third important stimulus for thirst is angiotensin II. Studies in animals have shown that angiotensin II acts on the subfornical organ and on the organum vasculosum of the lamina terminalis. These regions are outside the blood–brain barrier, and peptides such as angiotensin II diffuse into the tissues. Because angiotensin II is also stimulated by factors associated with hypovolemia and low blood pressure, its effect on thirst helps to restore blood volume and blood pressure toward normal, along with the other actions of angiotensin II on the kidneys to decrease fluid excretion.

Dryness of the mouth and mucous membranes of the esophagus can elicit the sensation of thirst. As a result, a thirsty person may receive relief from thirst almost immediately after drinking water, even though the water has not been absorbed from the gastrointestinal tract and has not yet had an effect on extracellular fluid osmolarity.

Gastrointestinal and pharyngeal stimuli influence thirst. In animals that have an esophageal opening to the exterior so that water is never absorbed into the blood, partial relief of thirst occurs after drinking, although the relief is only temporary. Also, gastrointestinal distention may partially alleviate thirst; for instance, simple inflation of a balloon in the stomach can relieve thirst. However, relief of thirst sensations through gastrointestinal or pharyngeal mechanisms is short lived; the desire to drink is completely satisfied only when plasma osmolarity and/or blood volume returns to normal.

The ability of animals and humans to "meter" fluid intake is important because it prevents overhydration. After a person drinks water, 30–60 minutes may be required for the water to be reabsorbed and distributed throughout the body. If the thirst sensation were not temporarily relieved after drinking water, the person would continue to drink more and more, eventually leading to overhydration and excess dilution of the body fluids. Experimental studies have repeatedly shown that animals drink almost exactly the amount necessary to return plasma osmolarity and volume to normal.

INTEGRATED RESPONSES OF OSMORECEPTOR– ADH AND THIRST MECHANISMS IN CONTROLLING EXTRACELLULAR FLUID OSMOLARITY AND SODIUM CONCENTRATION

In a healthy person, the osmoreceptor–ADH and thirst mechanisms work in parallel to precisely regulate extracellular fluid osmolarity and sodium concentration, despite the constant challenges of dehydration. Even with additional challenges,

such as high salt intake, these feedback systems are able to keep plasma osmolarity reasonably constant. Figure 80-4 shows that an increase in sodium intake to as high as six times normal has only a small effect on plasma sodium concentration as long as the ADH and thirst mechanisms are both functioning normally.

When either the ADH or the thirst mechanism fails, the other ordinarily can still control extracellular osmolarity and sodium concentration with reasonable effectiveness, as long as there is enough fluid intake to balance the daily obligatory urine volume and water losses caused by respiration, sweating, or gastrointestinal losses. However, if both the ADH and thirst mechanisms fail simultaneously, plasma sodium concentration and osmolarity are poorly controlled; thus, when sodium intake is increased after blocking the total ADH-thirst system, relatively large changes in plasma sodium concentration occur. In the absence of the ADH–thirst mechanisms, no other feedback mechanism is capable of adequately regulating plasma sodium concentration and osmolarity.

ROLE OF ANGIOTENSIN II AND ALDOSTERONE IN CONTROLLING EXTRACELLULAR FLUID OSMOLARITY AND SODIUM CONCENTRATION

Both angiotensin II and aldosterone play an important role in regulating sodium reabsorption by the renal tubules. When sodium intake is low, increased levels of these hormones stimulate sodium reabsorption by the kidneys and, therefore, prevent large sodium losses, even though sodium intake may be reduced to as low as 10% of normal. Conversely, with high-sodium intake, decreased formation of these hormones permits the kidneys to excrete large amounts of sodium.

Because of the importance of angiotensin II and aldosterone in regulating sodium excretion by the kidneys, one might mistakenly infer that they also play an important role in regulating extracellular fluid sodium concentration. Although these hormones increase the *amount* of sodium in the extracellular fluid, they also increase the extracellular fluid volume by increasing reabsorption of water along with the sodium. Therefore, *angiotensin II and aldosterone have little effect on sodium concentration, except under extreme conditions.*

This relative unimportance of aldosterone in regulating extracellular fluid sodium concentration is shown by the experiment in Figure 80-5. This figure shows the effect on plasma sodium concentration of changing sodium intake more than sixfold under two conditions: (1) under normal conditions and (2) after the aldosterone feedback system was blocked by removing the adrenal glands and infusing the animals with aldosterone at a constant rate so that plasma levels could not increase or decrease. Note that when sodium intake was increased sixfold, plasma concentration changed only about 1–2% in either case. This finding indicates that even without a functional aldosterone feedback system, plasma sodium concentration can be well regulated. The same type of experiment has been conducted after blocking angiotensin II formation, with the same result.

There are two primary reasons why changes in angiotensin II and aldosterone do not have a major effect on plasma sodium concentration. First, as discussed earlier, angiotensin II and aldosterone increase both sodium and water reabsorption by the renal tubules, leading to increases in extracellular fluid volume and sodium *quantity* but little change in sodium *concentration*. Second, as long as the ADH–thirst mechanism is functional, any tendency toward increased plasma sodium concentration is compensated for by increased water intake or increased plasma ADH secretion, which tends to dilute the extracellular fluid back toward normal. The ADH-thirst system far overshadows the angiotensin II and aldosterone systems for regulating sodium concentration under normal conditions. Even in patients with *primary aldosteronism*, who have extremely high levels of aldosterone, the plasma sodium concentration usually increases only about 3–5 mEq/L above normal.

Under extreme conditions, caused by complete loss of aldosterone secretion as a result of adrenalectomy or in patients with Addison's disease (severely impaired secretion or total lack of aldosterone), there is tremendous loss of sodium by the kidneys, which can lead to reductions in plasma sodium concentration. One of the reasons for this is that large losses of sodium eventually cause severe volume depletion and decreased blood pressure, which can activate the thirst mechanism through the cardiovascular reflexes. This activation leads to a further dilution of the plasma sodium concentration, even though the increased water intake helps to minimize the decrease in body fluid volumes under these conditions.

Thus, extreme situations exist in which plasma sodium concentration may change significantly, even with a functional ADH–thirst mechanism. Even so, the ADH–thirst mechanism is by far the most powerful feedback system in the body for controlling extracellular fluid osmolarity and sodium concentration.

Salt-Appetite Mechanism for Controlling Extracellular Fluid Sodium Concentration and Volume

Maintenance of normal extracellular fluid volume and sodium concentration requires a balance between sodium excretion and sodium intake. In modern civilizations, sodium intake is almost always greater than necessary for homeostasis. In fact, the average sodium intake for persons in industrialized cultures who eat processed foods usually ranges between 100 and 200 mEq/day, even though humans can survive and function normally while ingesting only 10–20 mEq/day. Thus, most people eat far more sodium than is necessary for homeostasis, and evidence indicates that our usual high-sodium intake may contribute to cardiovascular disorders such as hypertension.

Salt appetite is due in part to the fact that animals and humans like salt and eat it regardless of whether they are salt deficient. Salt appetite also has a regulatory component in which there is a behavioral drive to obtain salt when a sodium deficiency exists in the body. This behavioral drive is particularly important in herbivores, which naturally eat a low-sodium diet, but salt craving may also be important in humans who have an extreme deficiency of sodium, such as occurs in Addison's disease. In this instance, there is a deficiency of aldosterone secretion, which causes excessive loss of sodium in the urine and leads to decreased extracellular fluid volume and decreased sodium concentration; both of these changes elicit the desire for salt.

In general, the primary stimuli that increase salt appetite are those associated with sodium deficits and decreased blood volume or decreased blood pressure, associated with circulatory insufficiency.

The neuronal mechanism for salt appetite is analogous to that of the thirst mechanism. Some of the same neuronal centers in the AV3V region of the brain seem to be involved because lesions in this region frequently affect both thirst and salt appetite simultaneously in animals. Also, circulatory reflexes elicited by low blood pressure or decreased blood volume affect both thirst and salt appetite at the same time.

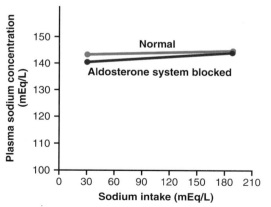

Figure 80-5 Effect of large changes in sodium intake on extracellular fluid sodium concentration in dogs under normal conditions (*red line*) and after the aldosterone feedback system had been blocked (*blue line*). Note that sodium concentration is maintained relatively constant over this wide range of sodium intakes, with or without aldosterone feedback control. (*Courtesy Dr David B Young.*)

BIBLIOGRAPHY

Antunes-Rodrigues J, de Castro M, Elias LL, et al: Neuroendocrine control of body fluid metabolism, *Physiol. Rev.* 84:169, 2004.

Bourque CW: Central mechanisms of osmosensation and systemic osmoregulation, *Nat. Rev. Neurosci.* 9:519-531, 2008.

Finley JJ 4th, Konstam MA, Udelson JE: Arginine vasopressin antagonists for the treatment of heart failure and hyponatremia, *Circulation* 118:410, 2008.

Geerling JC, Loewy AD: Central regulation of sodium appetite, *Exp. Physiol.* 93:177, 2008.

Loh JA, Verbalis JG: Disorders of water and salt metabolism associated with pituitary disease, *Endocrinol. Metab. Clin. North Am.* 37:213, 2008.

McKinley MJ, Johnson AK: The physiological regulation of thirst and fluid intake, *News Physiol. Sci.* 19:1, 2004.

Renal Regulation of Potassium, Calcium, Phosphate, and Magnesium

Regulation of Extracellular Fluid Potassium Concentration and Potassium Excretion

Extracellular fluid potassium concentration normally is regulated at about 4.2 mEq/L, seldom rising or falling more than ±0.3 mEq/L. This precise control is necessary because many cell functions are sensitive to changes in extracellular fluid potassium concentration. For instance, an increase in plasma potassium concentration of only 3–4 mEq/L can cause cardiac arrhythmias, and higher concentrations can lead to cardiac arrest or fibrillation.

A special difficulty in regulating extracellular potassium concentration is the fact that more than 98% of the total body potassium is contained in the cells and only 2% is contained in the extracellular fluid (Figure 81-1). For a 70-kg adult, who has about 28 L of intracellular fluid (40% of body weight) and 14 L of extracellular fluid (20% of body weight), about 3920 mEq of potassium are inside the cells and only about 59 mEq are in the extracellular fluid. Also, the potassium contained in a single meal may be as high as 50 mEq and the daily intake usually ranges between 50 and 200 mEq/day; therefore, failure to rapidly rid the extracellular fluid of the ingested potassium could cause life-threatening *hyperkalemia* (increased plasma potassium concentration). Likewise, a small loss of potassium from the extracellular fluid could cause severe *hypokalemia* (low plasma potassium concentration) in the absence of rapid and appropriate compensatory responses.

Maintenance of balance between intake and output of potassium depends primarily on excretion by the kidneys because the amount excreted in the feces is only about 5–10% of the potassium intake. Thus, the maintenance of normal potassium balance requires the kidneys to adjust their potassium excretion rapidly and precisely in response to wide variations in intake, as is also true for most other electrolytes.

Control of potassium distribution between the extracellular and intracellular compartments also plays an important role in potassium homeostasis. Because more than 98% of the total body potassium is contained in the cells, they can serve as an overflow site for excess extracellular fluid potassium during hyperkalemia or as a source of potassium during hypokalemia. Thus, redistribution of potassium between the intracellular and extracellular fluid compartments provides a first line of defense against changes in extracellular fluid potassium concentration.

REGULATION OF INTERNAL POTASSIUM DISTRIBUTION

After ingestion of a normal meal, extracellular fluid potassium concentration would rise to a lethal level if the ingested potassium did not rapidly move into the cells. For example, absorption of 40 mEq of potassium (the amount contained in a meal rich in vegetables and fruit) into an extracellular fluid volume of 14 L would raise plasma potassium concentration by about 2.9 mEq/L if all the potassium remained in the extracellular compartment. Fortunately, most of the ingested potassium rapidly moves into the cells until the kidneys can eliminate the excess. Table 81-1 summarizes some of the factors that can influence the distribution of potassium between the intracellular and extracellular compartments.

OVERVIEW OF RENAL POTASSIUM EXCRETION

Renal potassium excretion is determined by the sum of three processes: (1) the rate of potassium filtration (glomerular filtration rate [GFR] multiplied by the plasma potassium concentration), (2) the rate of potassium reabsorption by the tubules, and (3) the rate of potassium secretion by the tubules. The normal rate of potassium filtration by the glomerular capillaries is about 756 mEq/day (GFR, 180 L/day multiplied by plasma potassium concentration, 4.2 mEq/L). This rate of filtration is relatively constant in healthy persons because of the autoregulatory mechanisms for GFR discussed previously and the precision with which plasma potassium concentration is regulated. Severe decreases in GFR in certain renal diseases, however, can cause serious potassium accumulation and hyperkalemia.

Figure 81-2 summarizes the tubular handling of potassium under normal conditions. About 65% of the filtered potassium is reabsorbed in the proximal tubule. Another 25–30% of the filtered potassium is reabsorbed in the loop of Henle, especially in the thick ascending part where potassium is actively cotransported along with sodium and chloride. In both the proximal tubule and the loop of Henle, a relatively constant fraction of the filtered potassium load is reabsorbed. Changes in potas-

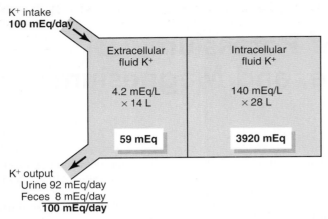

Figure 81-1 Normal potassium intake, distribution of potassium in the body fluids, and potassium output from the body.

TABLE 81-1	**Factors That Can Alter Potassium Distribution Between the Intracellular and Extracellular Fluid**

Factors That Shift K⁺ Into Cells (Decrease Extracellular [K⁺])	Factors That Shift K⁺ Out of Cells (Increase Extracellular [K⁺])
• Insulin	• Insulin deficiency (diabetes mellitus)
• Aldosterone	• Aldosterone deficiency (Addison's disease)
• β-adrenergic stimulation	• β-adrenergic blockade
• Alkalosis	• Acidosis
	• Cell lysis
	• Strenuous exercise
	• Increased extracellular fluid osmolarity

sium reabsorption in these segments can influence potassium excretion, but most of the day-to-day variation of potassium excretion is not due to changes in reabsorption in the proximal tubule or loop of Henle. There is also some potassium reabsorption in the collecting tubules and collecting ducts; the amount reabsorbed in these parts of the nephron varies depending on the potassium intake.

POTASSIUM SECRETION BY PRINCIPAL CELLS OF LATE DISTAL AND CORTICAL COLLECTING TUBULES

The cells in the late distal and cortical collecting tubules that secrete potassium are called *principal cells* and make up the majority of epithelial cells in these regions. Figure 81-3 shows the basic cellular mechanisms of potassium secretion by the principal cells.

Secretion of potassium from the blood into the tubular lumen is a two-step process, beginning with uptake from the interstitium into the cell by the sodium–potassium ATPase pump in the basolateral cell membrane; this pump moves sodium out of the cell into the interstitium and at the same time moves potassium to the interior of the cell.

The second step of the process is passive diffusion of potassium from the interior of the cell into the tubular fluid.

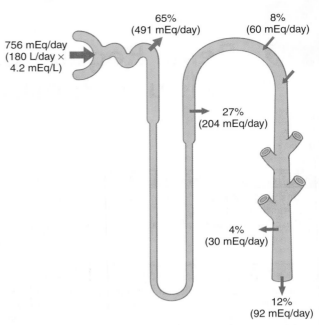

Figure 81-2 Renal tubular sites of potassium reabsorption and secretion . Potassium is reabsorbed in the proximal tubule and in the ascending loop of Henle, so only about 8% of the filtered load is delivered to the distal tubule. Secretion of potassium into the late distal tubules and collecting ducts adds to the amount delivered; therefore, the daily excretion is about 12% of the potassium filtered at the glomerular capillaries. The percentages indicate how much of the filtered load is reabsorbed or secreted into the different tubular segments.

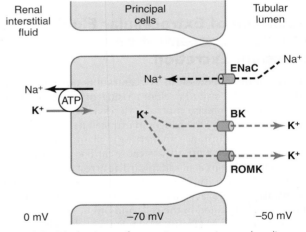

Figure 81-3 Mechanisms of potassium secretion and sodium reabsorption by the principal cells of the late distal and collecting tubules. BK, "big" potassium channel; ENaC, epithelial sodium channel; ROMK, renal outer medullary potassium channel.

The sodium–potassium ATPase pump creates a high intracellular potassium concentration, which provides the driving force for passive diffusion of potassium from the cell into the tubular lumen. The luminal membrane of the principal cells is highly permeable to potassium because there are two types of special channels that allow potassium ions to rapidly diffuse across the membrane: (1) the *renal outer medullary potassium (ROMK) channels*, and (2) high conductance *"big" potassium (BK) channels*. Both types of potassium channels are required for efficient renal potassium excretion, and their abundance in the luminal membrane is increased during high potassium intake.

Control of Potassium Secretion by Principal Cells. The primary factors that control potassium secretion by the principal cells of the late distal and cortical collecting tubules are (1) the activity of the sodium–potassium ATPase pump, (2) the electrochemical gradient for potassium secretion from the blood to the tubular lumen, and (3) the permeability of the luminal membrane for potassium. These three determinants of potassium secretion are in turn regulated by several factors discussed later.

SUMMARY OF MAJOR FACTORS THAT REGULATE POTASSIUM

Because normal regulation of potassium excretion occurs mainly as a result of changes in potassium secretion by the principal cells of the late distal and collecting tubules, in this chapter we discuss the primary factors that influence secretion by these cells. The most important factors that *stimulate* potassium secretion by the principal cells include (1) increased extracellular fluid potassium concentration, (2) increased aldosterone, and (3) increased tubular flow rate.

One factor that *decreases* potassium secretion is increased hydrogen ion concentration (acidosis).

Increased Extracellular Fluid Potassium Concentration Stimulates Potassium Secretion. The rate of potassium secretion in the late distal and cortical collecting tubules is directly stimulated by increased extracellular fluid potassium concentration, leading to increases in potassium excretion, as shown in Figure 81-4. This effect is especially pronounced when extracellular fluid potassium concentration rises above about 4.1 mEq/L, slightly less than the normal concentration. Increased plasma potassium concentration, therefore, serves as one of the most important mechanisms for increasing potassium secretion and regulating extracellular fluid potassium ion concentration.

Increased dietary potassium intake and increased extracellular fluid potassium concentration stimulate potassium secretion by four mechanisms: (1) increased extracellular fluid potassium concentration stimulates the sodium–potassium ATPase pump, thereby increasing potassium uptake across the basolateral membrane. This increased potassium uptake in turn increases intracellular potassium ion concentration, causing potassium to diffuse across the luminal membrane into the tubule. (2) Increased extracellular potassium concentration increases the potassium gradient from the renal interstitial fluid to the interior of the epithelial cell; this reduces back leakage of potassium ions from inside the cells through the basolateral membrane. (3) Increased potassium intake stimulates synthesis of potassium channels and their translocation from the cytosol to the luminal membrane, which, in turn, increases the ease of potassium diffusion through the membrane. (4) Increased potassium concentration stimulates aldosterone secretion by the adrenal cortex, which further stimulates potassium secretion, as discussed next.

Aldosterone Stimulates Potassium Secretion. Aldosterone stimulates active reabsorption of sodium ions by the principal cells of the late distal tubules and collecting ducts (see Chapter 78). This effect is mediated through a sodium–potassium ATPase pump that transports sodium outward through the basolateral membrane of the cell and into the renal interstitial fluid at the same time that it pumps potassium into the cell. Thus, aldosterone also has a powerful effect to control the rate at which the principal cells secrete potassium.

A second effect of aldosterone is to increase the number of potassium channels in the luminal membrane and therefore its permeability for potassium, further adding to the effectiveness of aldosterone in stimulating potassium secretion. Therefore, aldosterone has a powerful effect to increase potassium excretion, as shown in Figure 81-4.

Increased Extracellular Potassium Ion Concentration Stimulates Aldosterone Secretion. In negative feedback control systems, the factor that is controlled usually has a feedback effect on the controller. In the case of the aldosterone–potassium control system, the rate of aldosterone secretion by the adrenal gland is controlled strongly by extracellular fluid potassium ion concentration. Figure 81-5 shows that an increase in plasma potassium concentration of about 3 mEq/L can increase plasma aldosterone concentration from nearly 0 to as high as 60 ng/100 mL, a concentration almost 10 times normal.

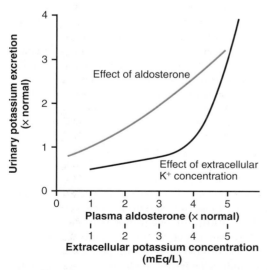

Figure 81-4 Effect of plasma aldosterone concentration (*red line*) and extracellular potassium ion concentration (*black line*) on the rate of urinary potassium excretion. These factors stimulate potassium secretion by the principal cells of the cortical collecting tubules. (*Data from Young, D.B., Paulsen, A.W., 1983. Interrelated effects of aldosterone and plasma potassium on potassium excretion. Am. J. Physiol. 244,F28.*)

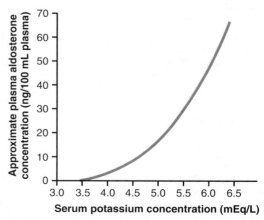

Figure 81-5 Effect of extracellular fluid potassium ion concentration on plasma aldosterone concentration. Note that small changes in potassium concentration cause large changes in aldosterone concentration.

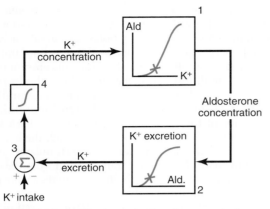

Figure 81-6 Basic feedback mechanism for control of extracellular fluid potassium concentration by aldosterone (*Ald.*).

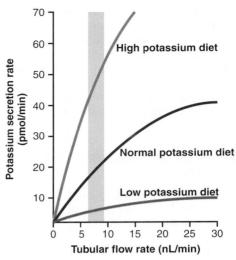

Figure 81-8 Relationship between flow rate in the cortical collecting tubules, and potassium secretion and the effect of changes in potassium intake. Note that a high dietary potassium intake greatly enhances the effect of increased tubular flow rate to increase potassium secretion. The *shaded bar* shows the approximate normal tubular flow rate under most physiological conditions. (*Data from Malnic, G., Berliner, R.W., Giebisch, G., 1989. Flow dependence of K⁺ secretion in cortical distal tubules of the rat. Am. J. Physiol. 256, F932.*)

The effect of potassium ion concentration to stimulate aldosterone secretion is part of a powerful feedback system for regulating potassium excretion, as shown in Figure 81-6. In this feedback system, an increase in plasma potassium concentration stimulates aldosterone secretion and, therefore, increases the blood level of aldosterone (block 1). The increase in blood aldosterone then causes a marked increase in potassium excretion by the kidneys (block 2). The increased potassium excretion then reduces the extracellular fluid potassium concentration back toward normal (circle 3 and block 4). Thus, this feedback mechanism acts synergistically with the direct effect of increased extracellular potassium concentration to elevate potassium excretion when potassium intake is raised (Figure 81-7).

Increased Distal Tubular Flow Rate Stimulates Potassium Secretion. A rise in distal tubular flow rate, as occurs with volume expansion, high sodium intake, or treatment with some diuretics, stimulates potassium secretion (Figure 81-8). Conversely, a decrease in distal tubular flow rate, as caused by sodium depletion, reduces potassium secretion.

The effect of tubular flow rate on potassium secretion in the distal and collecting tubules is strongly influenced by potassium intake. When potassium intake is high, increased tubular flow

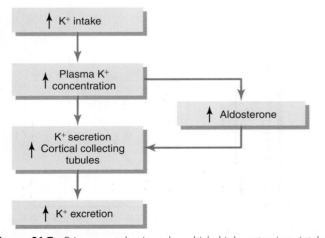

Figure 81-7 Primary mechanisms by which high potassium intake raises potassium excretion. Note that increased plasma potassium concentration directly raises potassium secretion by the cortical collecting tubules and indirectly increases potassium secretion by raising plasma aldosterone concentration.

rate has a much greater effect to stimulate potassium secretion than when potassium intake is low (Figure 81-8).

There are two effects of high-volume flow rate that increase potassium secretion: (1) When potassium is secreted into the tubular fluid the luminal concentration of potassium increases, thereby reducing the driving force for potassium diffusion across the luminal membrane. With increased tubular flow rate, the secreted potassium is continuously flushed down the tubule, so the rise in tubular potassium concentration becomes minimized, and net potassium secretion is increased . (2) A high tubular flow rate also increases the number of high conductance BK channels in the luminal membrane. Although the BK channels are normally quiescent, they become active in response to increases in flow rate, thereby greatly increasing conductance of potassium across the luminal membrane.

The effect of increased tubular flow rate is especially important in helping to preserve normal potassium excretion during changes in sodium intake. For example, with a high sodium intake, there is decreased aldosterone secretion, which by itself would tend to decrease the rate of potassium secretion and, therefore, reduce urinary excretion of potassium. However, the high distal tubular flow rate that occurs with a high sodium intake tends to increase potassium secretion (Figure 81-9), as discussed in the previous paragraph. Therefore, the two effects of high sodium intake, decreased aldosterone secretion and the high tubular flow rate, counterbalance each other, so there is little change in potassium excretion. Likewise, with a low sodium intake, there is little change in potassium excretion because of the counterbalancing effects of increased aldosterone secretion and decreased tubular flow rate on potassium secretion.

Acute Acidosis Decreases Potassium Secretion. Acute increases in hydrogen ion concentration of the extracellular fluid (acidosis) reduce potassium secretion, whereas decreased hydrogen ion concentration (alkalosis) increases potassium secretion. The primary mechanism by which increased hydrogen ion concentration inhibits potassium secretion is by reducing the activity

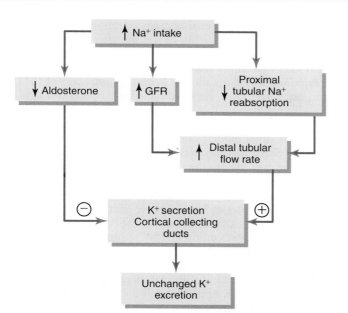

Figure 81-9 Effect of high sodium intake on renal excretion of potassium. Note that a high-sodium diet decreases plasma aldosterone, which tends to decrease potassium secretion by the cortical collecting tubules. However, the high-sodium diet simultaneously increases fluid delivery to the cortical collecting duct, which tends to increase potassium secretion. The opposing effects of a high-sodium diet counterbalance each other, so there is little change in potassium excretion.

of the sodium–potassium ATPase pump. This reduction in turn decreases intracellular potassium concentration and subsequent passive diffusion of potassium across the luminal membrane into the tubule. Acidosis may also reduce the number of potassium channels in the luminal membrane.

With more prolonged acidosis, lasting over a period of several days, there is an increase in urinary potassium excretion. The mechanism for this effect is due in part to an effect of chronic acidosis to inhibit proximal tubular sodium chloride and water reabsorption, which increases distal volume delivery, thereby stimulating potassium secretion. This effect overrides the inhibitory effect of hydrogen ions on the sodium–potassium ATPase pump. *Thus, chronic acidosis leads to a loss of potassium, whereas acute acidosis leads to decreased potassium excretion.*

Beneficial Effects of a Diet High in Potassium and Low in Sodium Content. For most of human history, the typical diet has been one that is low in sodium and high in potassium content, compared with the typical modern diet. In isolated populations that have not experienced industrialization, such as the Yanomamo tribe living in the Amazon of Northern Brazil, sodium intake may be as low as 10–20 mmol/day while potassium intake may be as high as 200 mmol/day. This intake is due to their consumption of a diet containing large amounts of fruits and vegetables and no processed foods. Populations consuming this type of diet typically do not experience age-related increases in blood pressure and cardiovascular diseases.

With industrialization and increased consumption of processed foods, which often have high-sodium and low-potassium content, there have been dramatic increases in sodium intake and decreases in potassium intake. In most industrialized countries potassium consumption averages only 30–70 mmol/day whereas sodium intake averages 140–180 mmol/day.

Experimental and clinical studies have shown that the combination of high sodium and low potassium intake increases the risk for hypertension and associated cardiovascular and kidney diseases. A diet rich in potassium, however, seems to protect against the adverse effects of a high-sodium diet, reducing blood pressure and the risk for stroke, coronary artery disease, and kidney disease. The beneficial effects of increasing potassium intake are especially apparent when combined with a low-sodium diet.

Dietary guidelines published by various international organizations recommend reducing dietary intake sodium chloride to around 65 mmol/day (corresponding to 1.5 g/day of sodium or 3.8 g/day sodium chloride), while increasing potassium intake to 120 mmol/day (4.7 g/day) for healthy adults.

Control of Renal Calcium Excretion and Extracellular Calcium Ion Concentration

The mechanisms for regulating calcium ion concentration are discussed in detail in Chapter 90, along with the endocrinology of the calcium-regulating hormones, parathyroid hormone (PTH), and calcitonin. Therefore, calcium ion regulation is discussed only briefly in this chapter.

Extracellular fluid calcium ion concentration normally remains tightly controlled within a few percentage points of its normal level, 2.4 mEq/L. When calcium ion concentration falls to low levels (*hypocalcemia*), the excitability of nerve and muscle cells increases markedly and can in extreme cases result in *hypocalcemic tetany*. This condition is characterized by spastic skeletal muscle contractions. *Hypercalcemia* (increased calcium concentration) depresses neuromuscular excitability and can lead to cardiac arrhythmias.

About 50% of the total calcium in the plasma (5 mEq/L) exists in the ionized form, which is the form that has biological activity at cell membranes. The remainder is either bound to the plasma proteins (about 40%) or complexed in the nonionized form with anions such as phosphate and citrate (about 10%).

Changes in plasma hydrogen ion concentration can influence the degree of calcium binding to plasma proteins. With acidosis, less calcium is bound to the plasma proteins. Conversely, in alkalosis, a greater amount of calcium is bound to the plasma proteins. Therefore, *patients with alkalosis are more susceptible to hypocalcemic tetany.*

As with other substances in the body, the intake of calcium must be balanced with the net loss of calcium over the long term. Unlike ions such as sodium and chloride, however, a large share of calcium excretion occurs in the feces. The usual rate of dietary calcium intake is about 1000 mg/day, with about 900 mg/day of calcium excreted in the feces. Under certain conditions, fecal calcium excretion can exceed calcium ingestion because calcium can also be secreted into the intestinal lumen. Therefore, the gastrointestinal tract and the regulatory mechanisms that influence intestinal calcium absorption and secretion play a major role in calcium homeostasis, as discussed in Chapter 90.

Almost all the calcium in the body (99%) is stored in the bone, with only about 0.1% in the extracellular fluid and 1.0% in the intracellular fluid and cell organelles. The bone, therefore, acts as a large reservoir for storing calcium and as a source of calcium when extracellular fluid calcium concentration tends to decrease.

One of the most important regulators of bone uptake and release of calcium is PTH. When extracellular fluid calcium concentration falls below normal, the parathyroid glands are

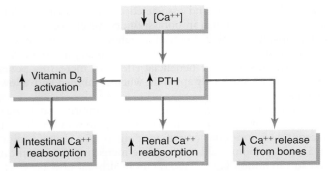

Figure 81-10 Compensatory responses to decreased plasma ionized calcium concentration mediated by parathyroid hormone (PTH) and vitamin D.

directly stimulated by the low calcium levels to promote increased secretion of PTH. This hormone then acts directly on the bones to increase the resorption of bone salts (release of salts from the bones) and to release large amounts of calcium into the extracellular fluid, thereby returning calcium levels back toward normal. When calcium ion concentration is elevated, PTH secretion decreases, so almost no bone resorption occurs; instead, excess calcium is deposited in the bones. Thus, the day-to-day regulation of calcium ion concentration is mediated in large part by the effect of PTH on bone resorption.

The bones, however, do not have an inexhaustible supply of calcium. Therefore, over the long term, the intake of calcium must be balanced with calcium excretion by the gastrointestinal tract and the kidneys. The most important regulator of calcium reabsorption at both of these sites is PTH. *Thus, PTH regulates plasma calcium concentration through three main effects: (1) by stimulating bone resorption; (2) by stimulating activation of vitamin D, which then increases intestinal reabsorption of calcium; and (3) by directly increasing renal tubular calcium reabsorption* (Figure 81-10). The control of gastrointestinal calcium reabsorption and calcium exchange in the bones is discussed elsewhere, and the remainder of this section focuses on the mechanisms that control renal calcium excretion.

CONTROL OF CALCIUM EXCRETION BY THE KIDNEYS

Calcium is both filtered and reabsorbed in the kidneys, but not secreted. Therefore, the rate of renal calcium excretion is calculated as

$$\text{Renal calcium excretion} = \text{Calcium filtered} \\ - \text{Calcium reabsorbed}$$

Only about 60% of the plasma calcium is ionized, with 40% being bound to the plasma proteins and 10 percent complexed with anions such as phosphate. Therefore, only about 60% of the plasma calcium can be filtered at the glomerulus. Normally, about 99% of the filtered calcium is reabsorbed by the tubules, with only about 1% of the filtered calcium being excreted. About 65% of the filtered calcium is reabsorbed in the proximal tubule, 25–30% is reabsorbed in the loop of Henle, and 4–9% is reabsorbed in the distal and collecting tubules. This pattern of reabsorption is similar to that for sodium.

As is true with the other ions, calcium excretion is adjusted to meet the body's needs. With an increase in calcium intake,

there is also increased renal calcium excretion, although much of the increase of calcium intake is eliminated in the feces. With calcium depletion, calcium excretion by the kidneys decreases as a result of enhanced tubular reabsorption.

Proximal Tubular Calcium Reabsorption. Most of the calcium reabsorption in the proximal tubule occurs through the paracellular pathway; it is dissolved in water and carried with the reabsorbed fluid as it flows between the cells. Only about 20% of proximal tubular calcium reabsorption occurs through the transcellular pathway in two steps: (1) calcium diffuses from the tubular lumen into the cell down an electrochemical gradient due to the much higher concentration of calcium in the tubular lumen, compared with the epithelial cell cytoplasm, and because the cell interior has a negative relative to the tubular lumen; (2) calcium exits the cell across the basolateral membrane by a calcium–ATPase pump and by sodium–calcium countertransporter (Figure 81-11).

Loop of Henle and Distal Tubule Calcium Reabsorption. In the loop of Henle, calcium reabsorption is restricted to the thick ascending limb. Approximately 50% of calcium reabsorption in the thick ascending limb occurs through the paracellular route by passive diffusion due to the slight positive charge of the tubular lumen relative to the interstitial fluid. The remaining 50% of calcium reabsorption in the thick ascending limb occurs through the transcellular pathway, a process that is stimulated by PTH.

In the distal tubule, calcium reabsorption occurs almost entirely by active transport through the cell membrane. The mechanism for this active transport is similar to that in the proximal tubule and thick ascending limb, and involves diffusion across the luminal membrane through calcium channels and exits across the basolateral membrane by a calcium–ATPase pump as well as a sodium–calcium counter transport mechanism. In this segment, as well as in the loops of Henle, PTH stimulates calcium reabsorption. Vitamin D (calcitriol) and calcitonin also stimulate calcium reabsorption in the thick ascending limb of Henle's loop and in the distal tubule, although these hormones are not as important quantitatively as PTH in reducing renal calcium excretion.

Factors That Regulate Tubular Calcium Reabsorption. One of the primary controllers of renal tubular calcium reabsorption

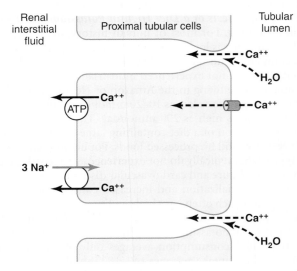

Figure 81-11 Mechanisms of calcium reabsorption by paracellular and transcellular pathways in the proximal tubular cells.

is PTH. Increased levels of PTH stimulate calcium reabsorption in the thick ascending loops of Henle and distal tubules, which reduces urinary excretion of calcium. Conversely, reduction of PTH promotes calcium excretion by decreasing reabsorption in the loops of Henle and distal tubules.

In the proximal tubule, calcium reabsorption usually parallels sodium and water reabsorption, and is independent of PTH. Therefore, in instances of extracellular volume expansion or increased arterial pressure—both of which decrease proximal sodium and water reabsorption—there is also reduction in calcium reabsorption and, consequently, increased urinary excretion of calcium. Conversely, with extracellular volume contraction or decreased blood pressure, calcium excretion decreases primarily because of increased proximal tubular reabsorption.

Another factor that influences calcium reabsorption is the plasma concentration of phosphate. Increased plasma phosphate stimulates PTH, which increases calcium reabsorption by the renal tubules, thereby reducing calcium excretion. The opposite occurs with reduction in plasma phosphate concentration.

Calcium reabsorption is also stimulated by metabolic alkalosis and inhibited by metabolic acidosis. Thus, acidosis tends to increase calcium excretion, whereas alkalosis tends to reduce calcium excretion. Most of the effect of hydrogen ion concentration on calcium excretion results from changes in calcium reabsorption in the distal tubule.

A summary of the factors that are known to influence calcium excretion by the renal tubules is shown in Table 81-2.

REGULATION OF RENAL PHOSPHATE EXCRETION

Phosphate excretion by the kidneys is controlled primarily by an overflow mechanism that can be explained as follows: The renal tubules have a normal transport maximum for reabsorbing phosphate of about 0.1 mM/min. When less than this amount of phosphate is present in the glomerular filtrate, essentially *all* the filtered phosphate is reabsorbed. When more than this amount is present, the *excess* is excreted. Therefore, phosphate normally begins to spill into the urine when its concentration in the extracellular fluid rises above a threshold of about 0.8 mM/L, which gives a tubular load of phosphate of about 0.1 mM/min, assuming a GFR of 125 mL/min. Because most people ingest large quantities of phosphate in milk products and meat, the concentration of phosphate is usually maintained above 1 mM/L, a level at which there is continual excretion of phosphate into the urine.

The proximal tubule normally reabsorbs 75–80% of the filtered phosphate. The distal tubule reabsorbs about 10% of the filtered load, and only very small amounts are reabsorbed in the loop of Henle, collecting tubules, and collecting ducts. Approximately 10% of the filtered phosphate is excreted in the urine.

In the proximal tubule, phosphate reabsorption occurs mainly through the transcellular pathway. Phosphate enters the cell from the lumen by a sodium–phosphate co-transporter and exits the cell across the basolateral membrane by a process that is not well understood but may involve a counter transport mechanism in which phosphate is exchanged for an anion.

Changes in tubular phosphate reabsorptive capacity can also occur in different conditions and influence phosphate excretion. For instance, a diet low in phosphate can, over time, increase the reabsorptive transport maximum for phosphate, thereby reducing the tendency for phosphate to spill over into the urine.

PTH can play a significant role in regulating phosphate concentration through two effects: (1) PTH promotes bone resorption, thereby dumping large amounts of phosphate ions into the extracellular fluid from the bone salts and (2) PTH decreases the transport maximum for phosphate by the renal tubules, so a greater proportion of the tubular phosphate is lost in the urine. *Thus, whenever plasma PTH is increased, tubular phosphate reabsorption is decreased and more phosphate is excreted.* These interrelations among phosphate, PTH, and calcium are discussed in more detail in Chapter 90.

Control of Renal Magnesium Excretion and Extracellular Magnesium Ion Concentration

More than one-half of the body's magnesium is stored in the bones. Most of the rest resides within the cells, with less than 1% located in the extracellular fluid. Although the total plasma magnesium concentration is about 1.8 mEq/L, more than one-half of this is bound to plasma proteins. Therefore, the free ionized concentration of magnesium is only about 0.8 mEq/L.

The normal daily intake of magnesium is about 250–300 mg/day, but only about one-half of this intake is absorbed by the gastrointestinal tract. To maintain magnesium balance, the kidneys must excrete this absorbed magnesium, about one-half the daily intake of magnesium or 125– 150 mg/day. The kidneys normally excrete about 10–15% of the magnesium in the glomerular filtrate.

Renal excretion of magnesium can increase markedly during magnesium excess or decrease to almost nil during magnesium depletion. Because magnesium is involved in many biochemical processes in the body, including activation of many enzymes, its concentration must be closely regulated.

Regulation of magnesium excretion is achieved mainly by changing tubular reabsorption. The proximal tubule usually reabsorbs only about 25% of the filtered magnesium. The primary site of reabsorption is the loop of Henle, where about 65% of the filtered load of magnesium is reabsorbed. Only a small amount (usually <5%) of the filtered magnesium is reabsorbed in the distal and collecting tubules.

The mechanisms that regulate magnesium excretion are not well understood, but the following disturbances lead to increased magnesium excretion: (1) increased extracellular fluid magnesium concentration, (2) extracellular volume expansion, and (3) increased extracellular fluid calcium concentration.

TABLE 81-2	Factors That Alter Renal Calcium Excretion	
↓ Calcium Excretion	↑ Calcium Excretion
↑ PTH	↓ PTH
↓ Extracellular fluid volume	↑ Extracellular fluid volume
↓ Blood pressure	↑ Blood pressure
↑ Plasma phosphate	↓ Plasma phosphate
Metabolic acidosis	Metabolic alkalosis
Vitamin D_3	

Parathyroid hormone, PTH.

BIBLIOGRAPHY

Antunes-Rodrigues J, de Castro M, Elias LL, et al: Neuroendocrine control of body fluid metabolism, *Physiol. Rev.* 84:169, 2004.

Appel LJ, Brands MW, Daniels SR, et al: Dietary approaches to prevent and treat hypertension: a scientific statement from the American Heart Association, *Hypertension* 47:296, 2006.

Cowley AW Jr: Long-term control of arterial pressure, *Physiol. Rev.* 72:231, 1992.

Giebisch G, Hebert SC, Wang WH: New aspects of renal potassium transport, *Pflugers Arch.* 446:289, 2003.

Granger JP, Hall JE: Role of the kidney in hypertension. In: Lip GYH, Hall JE (Eds.), Comprehensive Hypertension. Mosby Elsevier, *Philadelphia*, pp. 241–264.

Guyton AC: Blood pressure control—special role of the kidneys and body fluids, *Science* 252:1813, 1991.

Hall JE: Angiotensin II and long-term arterial pressure regulation: the overriding dominance of the kidney, *J. Am. Soc. Nephrol.* 10(Suppl 12):s258, 1999.

Hall JE, Brands MW: The renin-angiotensin-aldosterone system: renal mechanisms and circulatory homeostasis. In: Seldin DW, Giebisch G, (Eds.), The Kidney—Physiology and Pathophysiology, third ed. *Raven Press, New York*, pp. 1009–1046.

Hall JE, Granger JP, do Carmo JM, et al: Hypertension: physiology and pathophysiology, *Compr. Physiol.* 2:2393, 2012.

Hall JE, Granger JP, Hall ME, et al: Pathophysiology of hypertension. Hurst's The Heart, twelfth ed. McGraw-Hill Medical, New York, pp. 1570–1609.

Hall ME, do Carmo JM, da Silva AA, et al: Obesity, hypertension, and chronic kidney disease, *Int. J. Nephrol. Renovasc. Dis.* 7:75, 2014.

Hebert SC, Desir G, Giebisch G, et al: Molecular diversity and regulation of renal potassium channels, *Physiol. Rev.* 85:319, 2005.

Hoenderop JG, Bindels RJ: Epithelial Ca^{2+} and Mg^{2+} channels in health and disease, *J. Am. Soc. Nephrol.* 16:15, 2005.

Huang CL, Kuo E: Mechanism of hypokalemia in magnesium deficiency, *J. Am. Soc. Nephrol.* 18:2649, 2007.

Murer H, Hernando N, Forster I, et al: Regulation of Na/Pi transporter in the proximal tubule, *Annu. Rev. Physiol.* 65:531, 2003.

Schrier RW: Decreased effective blood volume in edematous disorders: what does this mean? *J. Am. Soc. Nephrol.* 18:2028, 2007.

Suki WN, Lederer ED, Rouse, D: Renal transport of calcium magnesium and phosphate. In: Brenner, BM (Ed.) The Kidney, sixth ed. WB Saunders, *Philadelphia*, pp. 520–574.

Suzuki Y, Landowski CP, Hediger MA: Mechanisms and regulation of epithelial Ca^{2+} absorption in health and disease, *Annu. Rev. Physiol.* 70:257, 2008.

Wall SM: Recent advances in our understanding of intercalated cells, *Curr. Opin. Nephrol. Hypertens.* 14:480, 2005.

Warnock DG: Renal genetic disorders related to K^+ and Mg^{2+}, *Annu. Rev. Physiol.* 64:845, 2002.

Worcester EM, Coe FL: New insights into the pathogenesis of idiopathic hypercalciuria, *Semin. Nephrol.* 28:120, 2008.

Young DB: Analysis of long-term potassium regulation, *Endocr. Rev.* 6:24, 1985.

Young DB: Quantitative analysis of aldosterone's role in potassium regulation, *Am. J. Physiol.* 255:F811, 1988.

82 Acid–Base Regulation

LEARNING OBJECTIVES

- Describe buffer systems in the body.
- Describe renal mechanisms of conserving bicarbonate.
- Describe acidosis and alkalosis.

GLOSSARY OF TERMS

- **Anion gap:** The anion gap is the difference between the sum of the major anions and the major cations in the plasma.
- **Blood pH:** The body maintains the blood at pH 7.4. This is more alkaline than the intracellular pH, which is about 7.0 at body temperature.
- **Neutral pH:** The pH at which there are equal numbers of H^+ ions and OH^- ions. Typically, at room temperature, this has a value of 7.0.
- **PCO₂:** The partial pressure of carbon dioxide. The normal value in arterial blood is 40 mmHg.
- **pH:** The pH is the negative logarithm of the hydrogen ion concentration.

Regulation of hydrogen ion (H^+) balance is similar in some ways to the regulation of other ions in the body. For instance, there must be a balance between the intake or production of H^+ and net removal of H^+ from the body to achieve homeostasis. And, as is true for other ions, the kidneys play a key role in regulating H^+ removal from the body. However, precise control of extracellular fluid H^+ concentration involves much more than simple elimination of H^+ by the kidneys. Multiple acid–base buffering mechanisms involving the blood, cells, and lungs also are essential in maintaining normal H^+ concentrations in both the extracellular and intracellular fluids.

In this chapter, we consider the various mechanisms that contribute to the regulation of H^+ concentration, with special emphasis on control of renal H^+ secretion and renal reabsorption, production, and excretion of bicarbonate ions (HCO_3^-), one of the key components of acid–base control systems in the body fluids.

H^+ Concentration Is Precisely Regulated

Precise H^+ regulation is essential because the activities of almost all enzyme systems in the body are influenced by H^+ concentration. Therefore, changes in H^+ concentration alter virtually all cell and body functions.

Compared with other ions, the H^+ concentration of the body fluids normally is kept at a low level. For example, the concentration of sodium in extracellular fluid (142 mEq/L) is about 3.5 million times as great as the normal concentration of H^+, which averages only 0.00004 mEq/L. Equally important, the normal variation in H^+ concentration in extracellular fluid is only about one millionth as great as the normal variation in sodium ion (Na^+) concentration. Thus, the precision with which H^+ is regulated emphasizes its importance to the various cell functions.

Acids and Bases—Their Definitions and Meanings

A hydrogen ion is a single free proton released from a hydrogen atom. Molecules containing hydrogen atoms that can release hydrogen ions in solutions are referred to as *acids*. An example is hydrochloric acid (HCl), which ionizes in water to form hydrogen ions (H^+) and chloride ions (Cl^-). Likewise, carbonic acid (H_2CO_3) ionizes in water to form H^+ and bicarbonate ions (HCO_3^-).

A *base* is an ion or a molecule that can accept an H^+. For example, HCO_3^- is a base because it can combine with H^+ to form H_2CO_3. Likewise, HPO_4^- is a base because it can accept an H^+ to form H_2PO_4. The proteins in the body also function as bases because some of the amino acids that make up proteins have net negative charges that readily accept H^+. The protein hemoglobin in the red blood cells and proteins in the other cells of the body are among the most important of the body's bases.

The terms *base* and *alkali* are often used synonymously. An *alkali* is a molecule formed by the combination of one or more of the alkaline metals—sodium, potassium, lithium, and so forth—with a highly basic ion such as a hydroxyl ion (OH^-). The base portion of these molecules reacts quickly with H^+ to remove it from solution; they are, therefore, typical bases. For similar reasons, the term *alkalosis* refers to excess removal of H^+ from the body fluids, in contrast to the excess addition of H^+, which is referred to as *acidosis*.

Strong and Weak Acids and Bases. A strong acid is one that rapidly dissociates and releases especially large amounts of H^+ in solution. An example is HCl. Weak acids are less likely to dissociate their ions and, therefore, release H^+ with less vigor. An example is H_2CO_3. A strong base is one that reacts rapidly and strongly with H^+ and, therefore, quickly removes H^+ from a solution. A typical example is OH^-, which reacts with H^+ to form water (H_2O). A typical weak base is HCO_3^- because it binds with H^+ much more weakly than does OH^-. Most acids and bases in the extracellular fluid that are involved in normal acid–base regulation are weak acids and bases. The most important ones that we discuss in detail are carbonic acid (H_2CO_3) and HCO_3^- base.

Normal H^+ Concentration and pH of Body Fluids and Changes That Occur in Acidosis and Alkalosis. Blood H^+ concentration is normally maintained within tight limits around a normal value of about 0.00004 mEq/L (40 nEq/L). Normal variations are only about 3–5 nEq/L, but under extreme conditions

TABLE 82-1	pH and H⁺ Concentration of Body Fluids	
	H⁺ Concentration (mEq/L)	pH
Extracellular fluid		
Arterial blood	4.0×10^{-5}	7.4
Venous blood	4.5×10^{-5}	7.35
Interstitial fluid	4.5×10^{-5}	7.35
Intracellular fluid	1×10^{-3}–4×10^{-5}	6.0–7.4
Urine	3×10^{-2}–1×10^{-5}	4.5–8.0
Gastric HCl	160	0.8

the H⁺ concentration can vary from as low as 10 nEq/L to as high as 160 nEq/L without causing death.

Because H⁺ concentration normally is low, and because these small numbers are cumbersome, it is customary to express H⁺ concentration on a logarithm scale using pH units. pH is related to the actual H⁺ concentration by the following formula (H⁺ concentration [H⁺] is expressed in *equivalents* per liter):

$$pH = \log \frac{1}{[H^+]} = -\log[H^+]$$

For example, normal [H⁺] is 40 nEq/L (0.00000004 Eq/L). Therefore, the normal pH is

$$pH = -\log[0.00000004]$$
$$pH = 7.4$$

From this formula, one can see that pH is inversely related to the H⁺ concentration; therefore, a low pH corresponds to a high H⁺ concentration and a high pH corresponds to a low H⁺ concentration.

The normal pH of arterial blood is 7.4, whereas the pH of venous blood and interstitial fluids is about 7.35 because of the extra amounts of carbon dioxide (CO_2) released from the tissues to form H_2CO_3 in these fluids (Table 82-1). Because the normal pH of arterial blood is 7.4, a person is considered to have *acidosis* when the pH falls below this value and *alkalosis* when the pH rises above 7.4. The lower limit of pH at which a person can live more than a few hours is about 6.8 and the upper limit is about 8.0.

Intracellular pH usually is slightly lower than plasma pH because the metabolism of the cells produces acid, especially H_2CO_3. Depending on the type of cells, the pH of intracellular fluid has been estimated to range between 6.0 and 7.4. Hypoxia of the tissues and poor blood flow to the tissues can cause acid accumulation and decreased intracellular pH.

The pH of urine can range from 4.5 to 8.0, depending on the acid–base status of the extracellular fluid. As discussed later, the kidneys play a major role in correcting abnormalities of extracellular fluid H⁺ concentration by excreting acids or bases at variable rates.

An extreme example of an acidic body fluid is the HCl secreted into the stomach by the oxyntic (parietal) cells of the stomach mucosa, as discussed in Chapter 67. The H⁺ concentration in these cells is about 4 million times greater than the hydrogen concentration in blood, with a pH of 0.8. In the remainder of this chapter, we discuss the regulation of extracellular fluid H⁺ concentration.

Defending Against Changes in H⁺ Concentration: Buffers, Lungs, and Kidneys

Three primary systems regulate the H⁺ concentration in the body fluids to prevent acidosis or alkalosis: (1) the *chemical acid–base buffer systems of the body fluids*, which immediately combine with an acid or a base to prevent excessive changes in H⁺ concentration; (2) the *respiratory center*, which regulates the removal of CO_2 (and, therefore, H_2CO_3) from the extracellular fluid; and (3) the *kidneys*, which can excrete either acid or alkaline urine, thereby readjusting the extracellular fluid H⁺ concentration toward normal during acidosis or alkalosis.

When there is a change in H⁺ concentration, the *buffer systems* of the body fluids react within seconds to minimize these changes. Buffer systems do not eliminate H⁺ from or add H⁺ to the body, but only keep them tied up until balance can be reestablished.

The second line of defense, the *respiratory system*, acts within a few minutes to eliminate CO_2 and, therefore, H_2CO_3 from the body.

These first two lines of defense keep the H⁺ concentration from changing too much until the more slowly responding third line of defense, the *kidneys*, can eliminate the excess acid or base from the body. Although the kidneys are relatively slow to respond compared with the other defenses, over a period of hours to several days, they are by far the most powerful of the acid–base regulatory systems.

Buffering of H⁺ in the Body Fluids

A buffer is any substance that can reversibly bind H⁺. The general form of the buffering reaction is

$$\text{Buffer} + H^+ \rightleftharpoons H\,\text{Buffer}$$

In this example, a free H⁺ combines with the buffer to form a weak acid (H buffer) that can either remain as an unassociated molecule or dissociate back to the buffer and H⁺. When the H⁺ concentration increases, the reaction is forced to the right and more H⁺ binds to the buffer, as long as buffer is available. Conversely, when the H⁺ concentration decreases, the reaction shifts toward the left and H⁺ is released from the buffer. In this way, changes in H⁺ concentration are minimized.

The importance of the body fluid buffers can be quickly realized if one considers the low concentration of H⁺ in the body fluids and the relatively large amounts of acids produced by the body each day. For example, about 80 milliequivalents of H⁺ is either ingested or produced each day by metabolism, whereas the H⁺ concentration of the body fluids normally is only about 0.00004 mEq/L. Without buffering, the daily production and ingestion of acids would cause lethal changes in body fluid H⁺ concentration.

The action of acid–base buffers can perhaps best be explained by considering the buffer system that is quantitatively the most important in the extracellular fluid—the bicarbonate buffer system.

Bicarbonate Buffer System

The bicarbonate buffer system consists of a water solution that contains two ingredients: (1) a weak acid, H_2CO_3, and (2) a bicarbonate salt, such as sodium bicarbonate ($NaHCO_3$).

H_2CO_3 is formed in the body by the reaction of CO_2 with H_2O.

$$CO_2 + H_2O \underset{\text{anhydrase}}{\overset{\text{carbonic}}{\rightleftharpoons}} H_2CO_3$$

This reaction is slow, and exceedingly small amounts of H_2CO_3 are formed unless the enzyme *carbonic anhydrase* is present. This enzyme is especially abundant in the walls of the lung alveoli, where CO_2 is released; carbonic anhydrase is also present in the epithelial cells of the renal tubules, where CO_2 reacts with H_2O to form H_2CO_3.

H_2CO_3 ionizes weakly to form small amounts of H^+ and HCO_3^-.

$$H_2CO_3 \overset{\rightarrow}{\longleftarrow} H^+ + HCO_3^-$$

The second component of the system, bicarbonate salt, occurs predominantly as $NaHCO_3$ in the extracellular fluid. $NaHCO_3$ ionizes almost completely to form HCO_3^- and Na^+, as follows:

$$NaHCO_3 \underset{\leftarrow}{\longrightarrow} Na^+ + HCO_3^-$$

Now, putting the entire system together, we have the following:

$$CO_2 + H_2O \rightleftharpoons H_2CO_3 \overset{\rightarrow}{\longleftarrow} H^+ + \underset{\substack{+ \\ Na^+}}{HCO_3^-}$$

Because of the weak dissociation of H_2CO_3, the H^+ concentration is extremely small.

When a strong acid such as HCl is added to the bicarbonate buffer solution, the increased H^+ released from the acid (HCl $\rightarrow$ H^+ + Cl$^-$) is buffered by HCO_3^-.

$$\uparrow H^+ + HCO_3^- \rightarrow H_2CO_3 \rightarrow CO_2 + H_2O$$

As a result, more H_2CO_3 is formed, causing increased CO_2 and H_2O production. From these reactions, one can see that H^+ from the strong acid HCl reacts with HCO_3^- to form the very weak acid H_2CO_3, which in turn forms CO_2 and H_2O. The excess CO_2 greatly stimulates respiration, which eliminates the CO_2 from the extracellular fluid.

The opposite reactions take place when a strong base, such as sodium hydroxide (NaOH), is added to the bicarbonate buffer solution.

$$NaOH + H_2CO_3 \rightarrow NaHCO_3 + H_2O$$

In this case, the OH$^-$ from the NaOH combines with H_2CO_3 to form additional HCO_3^-. Thus, the weak base $NaHCO_3$ replaces the strong base NaOH. At the same time, the concentration of H_2CO_3 decreases (because it reacts with NaOH), causing more CO_2 to combine with H_2O to replace the H_2CO_3.

$$CO_2 + H_2O \longrightarrow \underset{\substack{+ \\ NaOH}}{H_2CO_3} \longrightarrow \uparrow \underset{\substack{+ \\ Na}}{HCO_3^-} + H^+$$

The net result, therefore, is a tendency for the CO_2 levels in the blood to decrease, but the decreased CO_2 in the blood inhibits respiration and decreases the rate of CO_2 expiration. The rise in blood HCO_3^- that occurs is compensated for by increased renal excretion of HCO_3^-.

QUANTITATIVE DYNAMICS OF THE BICARBONATE BUFFER SYSTEM

All acids, including H_2CO_3, are ionized to some extent. From mass balance considerations, the concentrations of H^+ and HCO_3^- are proportional to the concentration of H_2CO_3.

$$H_2CO_3 \overset{\rightarrow}{\longleftarrow} H^+ + HCO_3^-$$

For any acid, the concentration of the acid relative to its dissociated ions is defined by the *dissociation constant K′.*

$$K' = \frac{H^+ \times HCO_3^-}{H_2CO_3} \tag{82.1}$$

This equation indicates that in an H_2CO_3 solution, the amount of free H^+ is equal to

$$H^+ = \frac{K' \times H_2CO_3}{HCO_3^-} \tag{82.2}$$

The concentration of undissociated H_2CO_3 cannot be measured in solution because it rapidly dissociates into CO_2 and H_2O or to H^+ and HCO_3^-. However, the CO_2 dissolved in the blood is directly proportional to the amount of undissociated H_2CO_3. Therefore, Eq. (82.2) can be rewritten as

$$H^+ = \frac{K \times CO_2}{HCO_3^-} \tag{82.3}$$

The dissociation constant (K) for Eq. (82.3) is only about $\frac{1}{400}$ of the dissociation constant (K') of Eq. (82.2) because the proportionality ratio between H_2CO_3 and CO_2 is 1:400.

Equation (3) is written in terms of the total amount of CO_2 dissolved in solution. However, most clinical laboratories measure the blood CO_2 tension (PCO$_2$) rather than the actual amount of CO_2. Fortunately, the amount of CO_2 in the blood is a linear function of PCO$_2$ multiplied by the solubility coefficient for CO_2; under physiological conditions, the solubility coefficient for CO_2 is 0.03 mmol/mmHg at body temperature. This means that 0.03 mmol of H_2CO_3 is present in the blood for each mmHg PCO$_2$ measured. Therefore, Eq. (82.3) can be rewritten as

$$H^+ = K \times \frac{(0.03 \times PCO_2)}{HCO_3^-} \tag{82.4}$$

Henderson–Hasselbalch Equation. As discussed earlier, it is customary to express H^+ concentration in pH units rather than in actual concentrations. Recall that pH is defined as pH $= -\log H^+$.

The dissociation constant (pK) can be expressed in a similar manner.

$$pK = -\log K$$

Therefore, we can express the H^+ concentration in Eq. (82.4) in pH units by taking the negative logarithm of that equation, which yields

$$-\log H^+ = -\log pK - \log \frac{(0.03 \times PCO_2)}{HCO_3^-} \tag{82.5}$$

Therefore,

$$pH = pK - \log \frac{(0.03 \times PCO_2)}{HCO_3^-} \tag{82.6}$$

Rather than work with a negative logarithm, we can change the sign of the logarithm and invert the numerator and denominator in the last term, using the law of logarithms to yield

$$pH = pK + \log \frac{HCO_3^-}{(0.03 \times PCO_2)} \qquad (82.7)$$

For the bicarbonate buffer system, the pK is 6.1, and Eq. (82.7) can be written as

$$pH = 6.1 + \log \frac{HCO_3^-}{0.03 \times PCO_2} \qquad (82.8)$$

Equation (8) is the Henderson–Hasselbalch equation, and with it, one can calculate the pH of a solution if the molar concentration of HCO_3^- and the PCO_2 are known.

From the Henderson–Hasselbalch equation, it is apparent that an increase in HCO_3^- concentration causes the pH to rise, shifting the acid–base balance toward alkalosis. An increase in PCO_2 causes the pH to decrease, shifting the acid–base balance toward acidosis.

The Henderson–Hasselbalch equation, in addition to defining the determinants of normal pH regulation and acid–base balance in the extracellular fluid, provides insight into the physiological control of acid and base composition of the extracellular fluid. As discussed later, *the HCO_3^- concentration is regulated mainly by the kidneys, whereas the PCO_2 in extracellular fluid is controlled by the rate of respiration.* By increasing the rate of respiration, the lungs remove CO_2 from the plasma, and by decreasing respiration, the lungs elevate PCO_2. Normal physiological acid–base homeostasis results from the coordinated efforts of both of these organs, the lungs and the kidneys, and acid–base disorders occur when one or both of these control mechanisms are impaired, thus altering either the HCO_3^- concentration or the PCO_2 of extracellular fluid.

When disturbances of acid–base balance result from a primary change in extracellular fluid HCO_3^- concentration, they are referred to as *metabolic* acid–base disorders. Therefore, acidosis caused by a primary decrease in HCO_3^- concentration is termed *metabolic acidosis*, whereas alkalosis caused by a primary increase in HCO_3^- concentration is called *metabolic alkalosis*. Acidosis caused by an increase in PCO_2 is called *respiratory acidosis*, whereas alkalosis caused by a decrease in PCO_2 is termed *respiratory alkalosis*.

Bicarbonate Buffer System Titration Curve. Figure 82-1 shows the changes in pH of the extracellular fluid when the ratio of HCO_3^- to CO_2 in extracellular fluid is altered. When the

concentrations of these two components are equal, the right-hand portion of Eq. (82.8) becomes the log of 1, which is equal to 0. Therefore, when the two components of the buffer system are equal, the pH of the solution is the same as the pK (6.1) of the bicarbonate buffer system. When base is added to the system, part of the dissolved CO_2 is converted into HCO_3^- causing an increase in the ratio of HCO_3^- to CO_2 and increasing the pH, as is evident from the Henderson–Hasselbalch equation. When acid is added, it is buffered by HCO_3^-, which is then converted into dissolved CO_2, decreasing the ratio of HCO_3^- to CO_2 and decreasing the pH of the extracellular fluid.

"Buffer Power" Is Determined by the Amount and Relative Concentrations of the Buffer Components. From the titration curve in Figure 82-1, several points are apparent. First, the pH of the system is the same as the pK when each of the components (HCO_3^- and CO_2) constitutes 50% of the total concentration of the buffer system. Second, the buffer system is most effective in the central part of the curve, where the pH is near the pK of the system. This phenomenon means that the change in pH for any given amount of acid or base added to the system is least when the pH is near the pK of the system. The buffer system is still reasonably effective for 1.0 pH unit on either side of the pK, which for the bicarbonate buffer system extends from a pH of about 5.1–7.1 units. Beyond these limits, the buffering power rapidly diminishes. And when all the CO_2 has been converted into HCO_3^- or when all the HCO_3^- has been converted into CO_2, the system has no more buffering power.

The absolute concentration of the buffers is also an important factor in determining the buffer power of a system. With low concentrations of the buffers, only a small amount of acid or base added to the solution changes the pH considerably.

The Bicarbonate Buffer System Is the Most Important Extracellular Buffer. From the titration curve shown in Figure 82-1, one would not expect the bicarbonate buffer system to be powerful, for two reasons: First, the pH of the extracellular fluid is about 7.4, whereas the pK of the bicarbonate buffer system is 6.1 which means that there is about 20 times as much of the bicarbonate buffer system in the form of HCO_3^- as in the form of dissolved CO_2. For this reason, this system operates on the portion of the buffering curve where the slope is low and the buffering power is poor. Second, the concentrations of the two elements of the bicarbonate system, CO_2 and HCO_3^-, are not great.

Despite these characteristics, the bicarbonate buffer system is the most powerful extracellular buffer in the body. This apparent paradox is due mainly to the fact that the two elements of the buffer system, HCO_3^- and CO_2, are regulated, respectively, by the kidneys and the lungs, as discussed later. As a result of this regulation, the pH of the extracellular fluid can be precisely controlled by the relative rate of removal and addition of HCO_3^- by the kidneys and the rate of removal of CO_2 by the lungs.

Phosphate Buffer System

Although the phosphate buffer system is not important as an extracellular fluid buffer, it plays a major role in buffering renal tubular fluid and intracellular fluids.

The main elements of the phosphate buffer system are $H_2PO_4^-$ and HPO_4^-. When a strong acid such as HCl is added to a mixture of these two substances, the hydrogen is accepted by the base HPO_4^- and converted to H_2PO_4.

$$HCl + Na_2HPO_4 \rightarrow NaH_2PO_4 + NaCl$$

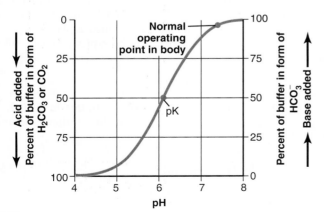

Figure 82-1   Titration curve for bicarbonate buffer system showing the pH of extracellular fluid when the percentages of buffer in the form of HCO_3^- and CO_2 (or H_2CO_3) are altered.

The result of this reaction is that the strong acid, HCl, is replaced by an additional amount of a weak acid, NaH_2PO_4, and the decrease in pH is minimized.

When a strong base, such as NaOH, is added to the buffer system, the OH^- is buffered by the H_2PO_4 to form additional amounts of $HPO_4^- + H_2O$.

$$NaOH + NaH_2PO_4 \rightarrow Na_2HPO_4 + H_2O$$

In this case, a strong base, NaOH, is traded for a weak base, NaH_2PO_4, causing only a slight increase in pH.

The phosphate buffer system has a pK of 6.8, which is not far from the normal pH of 7.4 in the body fluids; this situation allows the system to operate near its maximum buffering power. However, its concentration in the extracellular fluid is low, at only about 8% of the concentration of the bicarbonate buffer. Therefore, the total buffering power of the phosphate system in the extracellular fluid is much less than that of the bicarbonate buffering system.

In contrast to its minor role as an extracellular buffer, *the phosphate buffer is especially important in the tubular fluids of the kidneys,* for two reasons: (1) phosphate usually becomes greatly concentrated in the tubules, thereby increasing the buffering power of the phosphate system, and (2) the tubular fluid usually has a considerably lower pH than the extracellular fluid does, bringing the operating range of the buffer closer to the pK (6.8) of the system.

The phosphate buffer system is also important in buffering intracellular fluid because the concentration of phosphate in this fluid is many times that in the extracellular fluid. Also, the pH of intracellular fluid is lower than that of extracellular fluid and therefore is usually closer to the pK of the phosphate buffer system compared with the extracellular fluid.

Proteins Are Important Intracellular Buffers

Proteins are among the most plentiful buffers in the body because of their high concentrations, especially within the cells.

The pH of the cells, although slightly lower than in the extracellular fluid, nevertheless changes approximately in proportion to extracellular fluid pH changes. There is a slight diffusion of H^+ and HCO_3^- through the cell membrane, although these ions require several hours to come to equilibrium with the extracellular fluid, except for rapid equilibrium that occurs in the red blood cells. CO_2, however, can rapidly diffuse through all the cell membranes. *This diffusion of the elements of the bicarbonate buffer system causes the pH in intracellular fluid to change when there are changes in extracellular pH.* For this reason, the buffer systems within the cells help prevent changes in the pH of extracellular fluid but may take several hours to become maximally effective.

In the red blood cell, hemoglobin (Hb) is an important buffer, as follows:

$$H^+ + Hb \rightleftharpoons HHb$$

Approximately 60–70% of the total chemical buffering of the body fluids is inside the cells, and most of this buffering results from the intracellular proteins. However, except for the red blood cells, the slowness with which H^+ and HCO_3^- move through the cell membranes often delays for several hours the maximum ability of the intracellular proteins to buffer extracellular acid–base abnormalities.

In addition to the high concentration of proteins in the cells, another factor that contributes to their buffering power is the fact that the pKs of many of these protein systems are fairly close to intracellular pH.

Respiratory Regulation of Acid–Base Balance

The second line of defense against acid–base disturbances is control of extracellular fluid CO_2 concentration by the lungs. An increase in ventilation eliminates CO_2 from extracellular fluid, which, by mass action, reduces the H^+ concentration. Conversely, decreased ventilation increases CO_2, thus also increasing H^+ concentration in the extracellular fluid.

PULMONARY EXPIRATION OF CO_2 BALANCES METABOLIC FORMATION OF CO_2

CO_2 is formed continually in the body by intracellular metabolic processes. After it is formed, it diffuses from the cells into the interstitial fluids and blood and the flowing blood transports it to the lungs, where it diffuses into the alveoli and then is transferred to the atmosphere by pulmonary ventilation. About 1.2 mol/L of dissolved CO_2 normally are in the extracellular fluid, corresponding to a PCO_2 of 40 mmHg.

If the rate of metabolic formation of CO_2 increases, the PCO_2 of the extracellular fluid is likewise increased. Conversely, a decreased metabolic rate lowers the PCO_2. If the rate of pulmonary ventilation is increased, CO_2 is blown off from the lungs and the PCO_2 in the extracellular fluid decreases. Therefore, changes in either pulmonary ventilation or the rate of CO_2 formation by the tissues can change the extracellular fluid PCO_2.

INCREASING ALVEOLAR VENTILATION DECREASES EXTRACELLULAR FLUID H^+ CONCENTRATION AND RAISES PH

If the metabolic formation of CO_2 remains constant, the only other factor that affects PCO_2 in extracellular fluid is the rate of alveolar ventilation. The higher the alveolar ventilation the lower the PCO_2. As discussed previously, when CO_2 concentration increases, the H_2CO_3 concentration and H^+ concentration also increase, thereby lowering extracellular fluid pH.

Figure 82-2 shows the approximate changes in blood pH that are caused by increasing or decreasing the rate of alveolar ventilation. Note that increasing alveolar ventilation to about

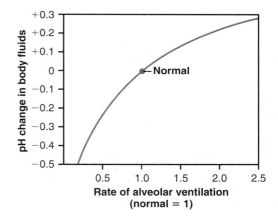

Figure 82-2   Change in extracellular fluid pH caused by increased or decreased rate of alveolar ventilation, expressed as times normal.

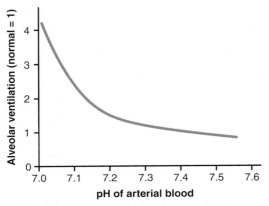

Figure 82-3 Effect of blood pH on the rate of alveolar ventilation.

twice normal raises the pH of the extracellular fluid by about 0.23. If the pH of the body fluids is 7.40 with normal alveolar ventilation, doubling the ventilation rate raises the pH to about 7.63. Conversely, a decrease in alveolar ventilation to one-fourth normal reduces the pH by 0.45. That is, if the pH is 7.4 at a normal alveolar ventilation, reducing the ventilation to one-fourth normal reduces the pH to 6.95. Because the alveolar ventilation rate can change markedly, from as low as 0 to as high as 15 times normal, one can easily understand how much the pH of the body fluids can be changed by the respiratory system.

INCREASED H⁺ CONCENTRATION STIMULATES ALVEOLAR VENTILATION

Not only does the alveolar ventilation rate influence H^+ concentration by changing the PCO_2 of the body fluids, but also the H^+ concentration affects the rate of alveolar ventilation. Thus, Figure 82-3 shows that the alveolar ventilation rate increases four to five times normal as the pH decreases from the normal value of 7.4 to the strongly acidic value of 7.0. Conversely, a rise in plasma pH above 7.4 causes a decrease in the ventilation rate. The change in ventilation rate per unit pH change is much greater at reduced levels of pH (corresponding to elevated H^+ concentration) compared with increased levels of pH. The reason for this phenomenon is that as the alveolar ventilation rate decreases, as a result of to an increase in pH (decreased H^+ concentration), the amount of oxygen added to the blood decreases and the partial pressure of oxygen (PO_2) in the blood also decreases, which stimulates the ventilation rate. Therefore, the respiratory compensation for an increase in pH is not nearly as effective as the response to a marked reduction in pH.

Buffering Power of the Respiratory System. *Respiratory regulation of acid–base balance is a physiological type of buffer system* because it acts rapidly and keeps the H^+ concentration from changing too much until the slowly responding kidneys can eliminate the imbalance. In general, the overall buffering power of the respiratory system is one to two times as great as the buffering power of all other chemical buffers in the extracellular fluid combined. That is, one to two times as much acid or base can normally be buffered by this mechanism as by the chemical buffers.

Impairment of Lung Function Can Cause Respiratory Acidosis. We have discussed thus far the role of the *normal* respiratory mechanism as a means of buffering changes in H^+ concentration. However, *abnormalities of respiration* can also cause changes in

H^+ concentration. For example, an impairment of lung function, such as severe emphysema, decreases the ability of the lungs to eliminate CO_2 which causes a buildup of CO_2 in the extracellular fluid and a tendency toward *respiratory acidosis*. Also, the ability to respond to metabolic acidosis is impaired because the compensatory reductions in PCO_2 that would normally occur by means of increased ventilation are blunted. In these circumstances, the kidneys represent the sole remaining physiologic mechanism for returning pH toward normal after the initial chemical buffering in the extracellular fluid has occurred.

Renal Control of Acid–Base Balance

The kidneys control acid–base balance by excreting either acidic or basic urine. Excreting acidic urine reduces the amount of acid in extracellular fluid, whereas excreting basic urine removes base from the extracellular fluid.

The overall mechanism by which the kidneys excrete acidic or basic urine is as follows: Large numbers of HCO_3^- are filtered continuously into the tubules, and if they are excreted into the urine this removes base from the blood. Large numbers of H^+ are also secreted into the tubular lumen by the tubular epithelial cells, thus removing acid from the blood. If more H^+ is secreted than HCO_3^- is filtered, there will be a net loss of acid from the extracellular fluid. Conversely, if more HCO_3^- is filtered than H^+ is secreted, there will be a net loss of base.

Each day the body produces about 80 mEq of nonvolatile acids, mainly from the metabolism of proteins. These acids are called *nonvolatile* because they are not H_2CO_3 and, therefore, cannot be excreted by the lungs. The primary mechanism for removal of these acids from the body is renal excretion. The kidneys must also prevent the loss of bicarbonate in the urine, a task that is quantitatively more important than the excretion of nonvolatile acids. Each day the kidneys filter about 4320 mEq of HCO_3^- (180 L/day × 24 mEq/L); under normal conditions, almost all this is reabsorbed from the tubules, thereby conserving the primary buffer system of the extracellular fluid.

As discussed later, both the reabsorption of HCO_3^- and the excretion of H^+ are accomplished through the process of H^+ secretion by the tubules. Because the HCO_3^- must react with a secreted H^+ to form H_2CO_3 before it can be reabsorbed, 4320 mEq of H^+ must be secreted each day just to reabsorb the filtered HCO_3^-. Then an additional 80 mEq of H^+ must be secreted to rid the body of the nonvolatile acids produced each day, for a total of 4400 mEq of H^+ secreted into the tubular fluid each day.

When there is a reduction in the extracellular fluid H^+ concentration (alkalosis), the kidneys secrete less H^+ and fail to reabsorb all the filtered HCO_3^-, thereby increasing the excretion of HCO_3^-. Because HCO_3^- normally buffers H^+ in the extracellular fluid, this loss of HCO_3^- is the same as adding an H^+ to the extracellular fluid. Therefore, in alkalosis, the removal of HCO_3^- raises the extracellular fluid H^+ concentration back toward normal.

In acidosis, the kidneys secrete additional H^+ and do not excrete HCO_3^- into the urine but reabsorb all the filtered HCO_3^- and produce new HCO_3^-, which is added back to the extracellular fluid. This action reduces the extracellular fluid H^+ concentration back toward normal.

Thus, the kidneys regulate extracellular fluid H^+ concentration through three fundamental mechanisms: (1) secretion of H^+, (2) reabsorption of filtered HCO_3^-, and (3) production of new HCO_3^-. All these processes are accomplished through the same basic mechanism, as discussed in the next few sections.

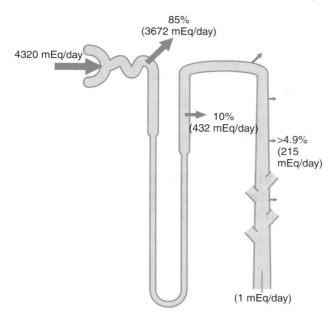

Figure 82-4 Reabsorption of bicarbonate in different segments of the renal tubule. The percentages of the filtered load of HCO_3^- absorbed by the various tubular segments are shown, as well as the number of milliequivalents reabsorbed per day under normal conditions.

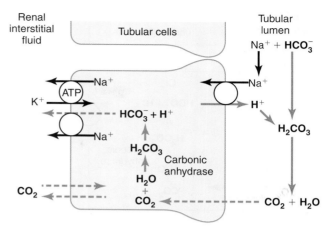

Figure 82-5 Cellular mechanisms for (1) active secretion of H^+ into the renal tubule; (2) tubular reabsorption of HCO_3^- by combination with H^+ to form carbonic acid, which dissociates to form carbon dioxide and water; and (3) sodium ion reabsorption in exchange for H^+ secreted. This pattern of H^+ secretion occurs in the proximal tubule, the thick ascending segment of the loop of Henle, and the early distal tubule.

Secretion of H^+ and Reabsorption of HCO_3^- by the Renal Tubules

Hydrogen ion secretion and HCO_3^- reabsorption occur in virtually all parts of the tubules except the descending and ascending thin limbs of the loop of Henle. Figure 82-4 summarizes HCO_3^- reabsorption along the tubule. Keep in mind that for each HCO_3^- reabsorbed, an H^+ must be secreted.

About 80–90% of the HCO_3^- reabsorption (and H^+ secretion) occurs in the proximal tubule, so only a small amount of HCO_3^- flows into the distal tubules and collecting ducts. In the thick ascending loop of Henle, another 10% of the filtered HCO_3^- is reabsorbed, and the remainder of the reabsorption takes place in the distal tubules and collecting ducts. As discussed previously, the mechanism by which HCO_3^- is reabsorbed also involves tubular secretion of H^+, but different tubular segments accomplish this task differently.

H^+ IS SECRETED BY SECONDARY ACTIVE TRANSPORT IN THE EARLY TUBULAR SEGMENTS

The epithelial cells of the proximal tubule, the thick segment of the ascending loop of Henle, and the early distal tubule all secrete H^+ into the tubular fluid by sodium–hydrogen counter-transport, as shown in Figure 82-5. This secondary active secretion of H^+ is coupled with the transport of Na^+ into the cell at the luminal membrane by the *sodium–hydrogen exchanger* protein, and the energy for H^+ secretion against a concentration gradient is derived from the sodium gradient favoring Na^+ movement into the cell. This gradient is established by the sodium–potassium adenosine triphosphatase (ATPase) pump in the basolateral membrane. About 95% of the bicarbonate is reabsorbed in this manner, requiring about 4000 mEq of H^+ to be secreted each day by the tubules. This mechanism, however, does not establish a very high H^+ concentration in the tubular fluid; the tubular fluid becomes very acidic only in the collecting tubules and collecting ducts.

Figure 82-5 shows how the process of H^+ secretion achieves HCO_3^- reabsorption. The secretory process begins when CO_2 either diffuses into the tubular cells or is formed by metabolism in the tubular epithelial cells. CO_2, under the influence of the enzyme *carbonic anhydrase*, combines with H_2O to form H_2CO_3, which dissociates into HCO_3^- and H^+. The H^+ is secreted from the cell into the tubular lumen by sodium–hydrogen countertransport. That is, when Na^+ moves from the lumen of the tubule to the interior of the cell, it first combines with a carrier protein in the luminal border of the cell membrane; at the same time, a H^+ in the interior of the cells combines with the carrier protein. The Na^+ moves into the cell down a concentration gradient that has been established by the sodium–potassium ATPase pump in the basolateral membrane. The gradient for Na^+ movement into the cell then provides the energy for moving H^+ in the opposite direction from the interior of the cell to the tubular lumen.

The HCO_3^- generated in the cell (when H^+ dissociates from H_2CO_3) then moves downhill across the basolateral membrane into the renal interstitial fluid and the peritubular capillary blood. The net result is that for every H^+ secreted into the tubular lumen, an HCO_3^- enters the blood.

FILTERED HCO_3^- IS REABSORBED BY INTERACTION WITH H^+ IN THE TUBULES

Bicarbonate ions do not readily permeate the luminal membranes of the renal tubular cells; therefore, HCO_3^- that is filtered by the glomerulus cannot be directly reabsorbed. Instead, HCO_3^- is reabsorbed by a special process in which it first combines with H^+ to form H_2CO_3, which eventually becomes CO_2 and H_2O, as shown in Figure 82-5.

This reabsorption of HCO_3^- is initiated by a reaction in the tubules between HCO_3^- filtered at the glomerulus and H^+ secreted by the tubular cells. The H_2CO_3 formed then dissociates into CO_2 and H_2O. The CO_2 can move easily across the tubular membrane; therefore, it instantly diffuses into the tubular cell, where it recombines with H_2O, under the influence of carbonic anhydrase, to generate a new H_2CO_3 molecule. This H_2CO_3 in turn dissociates to form HCO_3^- and H^+; the HCO_3^- then diffuses

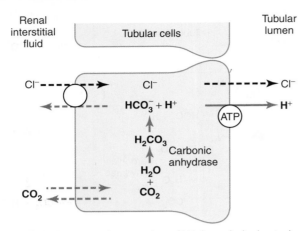

Figure 82-6   Primary active secretion of H⁺ through the luminal membrane of the intercalated epithelial cells of the late distal and collecting tubules. Note that one HCO_3^- is absorbed for each H⁺ secreted, and a chloride ion is passively secreted along with the H⁺.

through the basolateral membrane into the interstitial fluid and is taken up into the peritubular capillary blood. The transport of HCO_3^- across the basolateral membrane is facilitated by two mechanisms: (1) Na^+– HCO_3^- co-transport in the proximal tubules and (2) Cl^- – HCO_3^- exchange in the late segments of the proximal tubule, in the thick ascending loop of Henle, and the collecting tubules and ducts.

Thus, each time a H⁺ is formed in the tubular epithelial cells, a HCO_3^- is also formed and released back into the blood. The net effect of these reactions is "reabsorption" of HCO_3^- from the tubules, although the HCO_3^- that actually enters the extracellular fluid is not the same as that filtered into the tubules. The reabsorption of filtered HCO_3^- does not result in net secretion of H⁺ because the secreted H⁺ combines with the filtered HCO_3^- and is therefore not excreted.

PRIMARY ACTIVE SECRETION OF H⁺ IN THE INTERCALATED CELLS OF LATE DISTAL AND COLLECTING TUBULES

Beginning in the late distal tubules and continuing through the remainder of the tubular system, the tubular epithelium secretes H⁺ by *primary active transport*. The characteristics of this transport are different from those discussed for the proximal tubule, loop of Henle, and early distal tubule.

The mechanism for primary active H⁺ secretion is shown in Figure 82-6. It occurs at the luminal membrane of the tubular cell, where H⁺ is transported directly by a specific protein, a *hydrogen-transporting ATPase* and a *hydrogen-potassium-ATPase transporter*. The energy required for pumping the H⁺ is derived from the breakdown of ATP to adenosine diphosphate.

Primary active secretion of H⁺ occurs in special types of cells called the *type A intercalated cells* of the late distal tubule and in the collecting tubules. Hydrogen ion secretion in these cells is accomplished in two steps: (1) the dissolved CO_2 in this cell combines with H_2O to form H_2CO_3, and (2) the H_2CO_3 then dissociates into HCO_3^-, which is reabsorbed into the blood, plus H⁺, which is secreted into the tubule by means of the hydrogen–ATPase and the hydrogen-potassium-ATPase transporters. For each H⁺ secreted, a HCO_3^- is reabsorbed, similar to the process in the proximal tubules. The main difference is that H⁺ moves across the luminal membrane by an active H⁺ pump instead of by counter-transport, as occurs in the early parts of the nephron.

Although the secretion of H⁺ in the late distal tubule and collecting tubules accounts for only about 5% of the total H⁺ secreted, this mechanism is important in forming maximally acidic urine. In the proximal tubules, H⁺ concentration can be increased only about threefold to fourfold and the tubular fluid pH can be reduced to only about 6.7, although large *amounts* of H⁺ are secreted by this nephron segment. However, H⁺ concentration can be increased as much as 900-fold in the collecting tubules. This mechanism decreases the pH of the tubular fluid to about 4.5, which is the lower limit of pH that can be achieved in normal kidneys.

Combination of Excess H⁺ With Phosphate and Ammonia Buffers in the Tubule Generates "New" HCO_3^-

When H⁺ is secreted in excess of the HCO_3^- filtered into the tubular fluid, only a small part of the excess H⁺ can be excreted in the ionic form (H⁺) in the urine. This is because the minimal urine pH is about 4.5, corresponding to an H⁺ concentration of $10^{-4.5}$ mEq/L or 0.03 mEq/L. Thus, for each liter of urine formed, a maximum of only about 0.03 mEq of free H⁺ can be excreted. To excrete the 80 mEq of nonvolatile acid formed by metabolism each day, about 2667 L of urine would have to be excreted if the H⁺ remained free in solution.

The excretion of large amounts of H⁺ (on occasion as much as 500 mEq/day) in the urine is accomplished primarily by combining the H⁺ with buffers in the tubular fluid. The most important buffers are phosphate buffer and ammonia buffer. Other weak buffer systems, such as urate and citrate, are much less important.

When H⁺ is titrated in the tubular fluid with HCO_3^-, this leads to reabsorption of one HCO_3^- for each H⁺ secreted, as discussed earlier. However when there is excess H⁺ in the tubular fluid, it combines with buffers other than HCO_3^-, and this leads to generation of new HCO_3^- that can also enter the blood. Thus, when there is excess H⁺ in the extracellular fluid, the kidneys not only reabsorb all the filtered HCO_3^- but also generate new HCO_3^-, thereby helping to replenish the HCO_3^- lost from the extracellular fluid in acidosis. In the next two sections, we discuss the mechanisms by which phosphate and ammonia buffers contribute to the generation of new HCO_3^-.

PHOSPHATE BUFFER SYSTEM CARRIES EXCESS H⁺ INTO THE URINE AND GENERATES "NEW" HCO_3^-

The phosphate buffer system is composed of HPO_4^- and $H_2PO_4^-$. Both become concentrated in the tubular fluid because water is normally reabsorbed to a greater extent than phosphate by the renal tubules. Therefore, although phosphate is not an important extracellular fluid buffer, it is much more effective as a buffer in the tubular fluid.

Another factor that makes phosphate important as a tubular buffer is the fact that the pK of this system is about 6.8. Under normal conditions, the urine is slightly acidic, and the urine pH is near the pK of the phosphate buffer system. Therefore, in the tubules, the phosphate buffer system normally functions near its most effective range of pH.

Figure 82-7 shows the sequence of events by which H⁺ is excreted in combination with phosphate buffer and the mechanism by which new HCO_3^- is added to the blood. The process of H⁺ secretion into the tubules is the same as described earlier. As long as there is excess HCO_3^- in the tubular fluid, most of the secreted

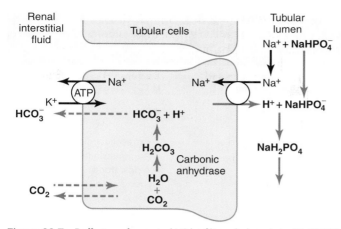

Figure 82-7 Buffering of secreted H^+ by filtered phosphate ($NaHPO_4^-$). Note that a new HCO_3^- is returned to the blood for each $NaHPO_4^-$ that reacts with a secreted H^+.

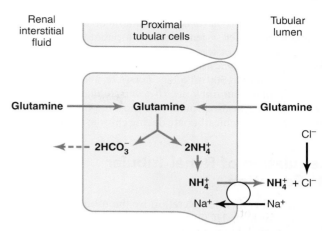

Figure 82-8 Production and secretion of ammonium ion (NH_4^+) by proximal tubular cells. Glutamine is metabolized in the cell, yielding NH_4^+ and bicarbonate. The NH_4^+ is secreted into the lumen by a sodium–NH_4^+ exchanger. For each glutamine molecule metabolized, two NH_4^+ are produced and secreted and two HCO_3^- are returned to the blood.

H^+ combines with HCO_3^-. However, once all the HCO_3^- has been reabsorbed and is no longer available to combine with H^+, any excess H^+ can combine with HPO_4^- and other tubular buffers. After the H^+ combines with HPO_4^- to form $H_2PO_4^-$, it can be excreted as a sodium salt (NaH_2PO_4), carrying with it the excess H^+.

There is one important difference in this sequence of H^+ excretion from that discussed previously. In this case, the HCO_3^- that is generated in the tubular cell and enters the peritubular blood represents a net gain of HCO_3^- by the blood, rather than merely a replacement of filtered HCO_3^-. *Therefore, whenever an H^+ secreted into the tubular lumen combines with a buffer other than HCO_3^-, the net effect is addition of a new HCO_3^- to the blood.* This demonstrates one of the mechanisms by which the kidneys are able to replenish the extracellular fluid stores of HCO_3^-.

Under normal conditions, much of the filtered phosphate is reabsorbed, and only 30–40 mEq/day are available for buffering H^+. Therefore, much of the buffering of excess H^+ in the tubular fluid in acidosis occurs through the ammonia buffer system.

EXCRETION OF EXCESS H^+ AND GENERATION OF NEW HCO_3^- BY THE AMMONIA BUFFER SYSTEM

A second buffer system in the tubular fluid that is even more important quantitatively than the phosphate buffer system is composed of ammonia (NH_3) and the ammonium ion (NH_4^+). Ammonium ion is synthesized from glutamine, which comes mainly from the metabolism of amino acids in the liver. The glutamine delivered to the kidneys is transported into the epithelial cells of the proximal tubules, thick ascending limb of the loop of Henle, and distal tubules (Figure 82-8). Once inside the cell, each molecule of glutamine is metabolized in a series of reactions to ultimately form two NH_4^+ and two HCO_3^- ions. The NH_4^+ is secreted into the tubular lumen by a counter-transport mechanism in exchange for sodium, which is reabsorbed. The HCO_3^- is transported across the basolateral membrane, along with the reabsorbed Na^+, into the interstitial fluid and is taken up by the peritubular capillaries. Thus, for each molecule of glutamine metabolized in the proximal tubules, two NH_4^+ are secreted into the urine and two HCO_3^- are reabsorbed into the blood. *The HCO_3^- generated by this process constitutes new HCO_3^-.*

In the collecting tubules, the addition of NH_4^+ to the tubular fluids occurs through a different mechanism (Figure 82-9). Here, H^+ is secreted by the tubular membrane into the lumen, where it combines with NH_3 to form NH_4^+, which is then excreted. The collecting ducts are permeable to NH_3, which can easily diffuse into the tubular lumen. However, the luminal membrane of this part of the tubules is much less permeable to NH_4^+; therefore, once the H^+ has reacted with NH_3 to form NH_4^+, the NH_4^+ is trapped in the tubular lumen and eliminated in the urine. *For each NH_4^+ excreted, a new HCO_3^- is generated and added to the blood.*

Chronic Acidosis Increases NH_4^+ Excretion. One of the most important features of the renal ammonium–ammonia buffer system is that it is subject to physiological control. An increase in extracellular fluid H^+ concentration stimulates renal glutamine metabolism and, therefore, increases the formation of NH_4^+ and new HCO_3^- to be used in H^+ buffering; a decrease in H^+ concentration has the opposite effect.

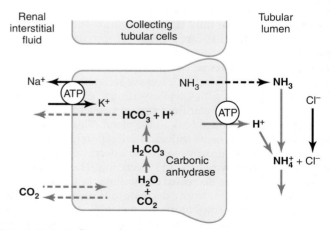

Figure 82-9 Buffering of hydrogen ion secretion by ammonia (NH_3) in the collecting tubules. Ammonia diffuses into the tubular lumen, where it reacts with secreted H^+ to form NH_4^+, which is then excreted. For each NH_4^+ excreted, a new HCO_3^- is formed in the tubular cells and returned to the blood.

Under *normal conditions*, the amount of H$^+$ eliminated by the ammonia buffer system accounts for about 50% of the acid excreted and 50% of the new HCO$_3^-$ generated by the kidneys. However, with *chronic acidosis*, the rate of NH$_4^+$ excretion can increase to as much as 500 mEq/day. *Therefore, with chronic acidosis, the dominant mechanism by which acid is eliminated is excretion of NH$_4^+$.* This process also provides the most important mechanism for generating new bicarbonate during chronic acidosis.

Regulation of Renal Tubular H$^+$ Secretion

As discussed earlier, H$^+$ secretion by the tubular epithelium is necessary for both HCO$_3^-$ reabsorption and generation of new HCO$_3^-$ associated with titratable acid formation. Therefore, the rate of H$^+$ secretion must be carefully regulated if the kidneys are to effectively perform their functions in acid–base homeostasis. Under normal conditions, the kidney tubules must secrete at least enough H$^+$ to reabsorb almost all the HCO$_3^-$ that is filtered, and there must be enough H$^+$ left over to be excreted as titratable acid or NH$_4^+$ to rid the body of the nonvolatile acids produced each day from metabolism.

In alkalosis, tubular secretion of H$^+$ is reduced to a level that is too low to achieve complete HCO$_3^-$ reabsorption, enabling the kidneys to increase HCO$_3^-$ excretion. In this condition, titratable acid and ammonia are not excreted because there is no excess H$^+$ available to combine with nonbicarbonate buffers; therefore, there is no new HCO$_3^-$ added to the blood in alkalosis. During acidosis, the tubular H$^+$ secretion is increased sufficiently to reabsorb all the filtered HCO$_3^-$ with enough H$^+$ left over to excrete large amounts of NH$_4^+$ and titratable acid, thereby contributing large amounts of new HCO$_3^-$ to the total body extracellular fluid. *The most important stimuli for increasing H$^+$ secretion by the tubules in acidosis are (1) an increase in PCO$_2$ of the extracellular fluid in respiratory acidosis and (2) an increase in H$^+$ concentration of the extracellular fluid (decreased pH) respiratory or metabolic acidosis.*

The tubular cells respond directly to an increase in PCO$_2$ of the blood, as occurs in respiratory acidosis, with an increase in the rate of H$^+$ secretion as follows: The increased PCO$_2$ raises the PCO$_2$ of the tubular cells, causing increased formation of H$^+$ in the tubular cells, which in turn stimulates the secretion of H$^+$. The second factor that stimulates H$^+$ secretion is an increase in extracellular fluid H$^+$ concentration (decreased pH).

A special factor that can increase H$^+$ secretion under some pathophysiological conditions is excessive aldosterone secretion. Aldosterone stimulates secretion of H$^+$ by intercalated cells of the collecting duct. Therefore, excessive secretion of aldosterone, as occurs in persons with Conn's syndrome, can increase secretion of H$^+$ into the tubular fluid and, consequently, increase the amount of HCO$_3^-$ added back to the blood. This action usually causes alkalosis in patients with excessive aldosterone secretion.

The tubular cells usually respond to a decrease in H$^+$ concentration (alkalosis) by reducing H$^+$ secretion. The decreased H$^+$ secretion results from decreased extracellular PCO$_2$, as occurs in respiratory alkalosis, or from a decrease in H$^+$ concentration per se, as occurs in both respiratory and metabolic alkalosis.

Table 82-2 summarizes the major factors that influence H$^+$ secretion and HCO$_3^-$ reabsorption. Some of these factors are not directly related to the regulation of acid–base balance. For example, H$^+$ secretion is coupled to Na$^+$ reabsorption by the Na$^+$–H$^+$ exchanger in the proximal tubule and the thick ascending loop of Henle. Therefore, factors that stimulate Na$^+$

TABLE 82-2 Factors That Increase or Decrease H$^+$ Secretion and HCO$_3^-$ Reabsorption by the Renal Tubules

Increase H$^+$ Secretion and HCO$_3^-$ Reabsorption	Decrease H$^+$ Secretion and HCO$_3^-$ Reabsorption
↑ PCO$_2$	↓ PCO$_2$
↑ H$^+$, ↓ HCO$_3^-$	↓ H$^+$, ↑ HCO$_3^-$
↓ Extracellular fluid volume	↑ Extracellular fluid volume
↑ Angiotensin II	↓ Angiotensin II
↑ Aldosterone	↓ Aldosterone
Hypokalemia	Hyperkalemia

reabsorption, such as decreased extracellular fluid volume, may also secondarily increase H$^+$ secretion and HCO$_3^-$ reabsorption.

Extracellular fluid volume depletion stimulates sodium reabsorption by the renal tubules and increases H$^+$ secretion and HCO$_3^-$ reabsorption through multiple mechanisms, including (1) increased angiotensin II levels, which directly stimulate the activity of the Na$^+$–H$^+$ exchanger in the renal tubules, and (2) increased aldosterone levels, which stimulate H$^+$ secretion by the intercalated cells of the cortical collecting tubules. Therefore, extracellular fluid volume depletion tends to cause alkalosis due to excess H$^+$ secretion and HCO$_3^-$ reabsorption.

Changes in plasma potassium concentration can also influence H$^+$ secretion, with hypokalemia stimulating and hyperkalemia inhibiting H$^+$ secretion in the proximal tubule. Decreased plasma potassium concentration tends to increase the H$^+$ concentration in the renal tubular cells. This, in turn, stimulates H$^+$ secretion and HCO$_3^-$ reabsorption and leads to alkalosis. Hyperkalemia decreases H$^+$ secretion and HCO$_3^-$ reabsorption, and tends to cause acidosis.

Renal Correction of Acidosis— Increased Excretion of H$^+$ and Addition of HCO$_3^-$ to the Extracellular Fluid

Now that we have described the mechanisms by which the kidneys secrete H$^+$ and reabsorb HCO$_3^-$, we can explain how the kidneys readjust the pH of the extracellular fluid when it becomes abnormal.

Respiratory and metabolic acidosis both cause a decrease in the ratio of HCO$_3^-$ to H$^+$ in the renal tubular fluid. As a result, there is excess H$^+$ in the renal tubules, causing complete reabsorption of HCO$_3^-$ and still leaving additional H$^+$ available to combine with the urinary buffers NH$_4^+$ and HPO$_4^-$. Thus, in acidosis, the kidneys reabsorb all the filtered HCO$_3^-$ and contribute new HCO$_3^-$ through the formation of NH$_4^+$ and titratable acid.

In metabolic acidosis, an excess of H$^+$ over HCO$_3^-$ occurs in the tubular fluid primarily because of decreased filtration of HCO$_3^-$. This decreased filtration of HCO$_3^-$ is caused mainly by a decrease in the extracellular fluid concentration of HCO$_3^-$.

In respiratory acidosis, the excess H$^+$ in the tubular fluid is due mainly to the rise in extracellular fluid PCO$_2$, which stimulates H$^+$ secretion.

As discussed previously, with chronic acidosis, regardless of whether it is respiratory or metabolic, there is an increase in the production of NH$_4^+$, which further contributes to the excretion of H$^+$ and the addition of new HCO$_3^-$ to the extracellular fluid. With severe chronic acidosis, as much as 500 mEq/day of H$^+$

TABLE 82-3	Characteristics of Primary Acid–Base Disturbances			
	pH	H⁺	PCO₂	HCO₃⁻
Normal	7.4	40 mEq/L	40 mmHg	24 mEq/L
Respiratory acidosis	↓	↑	↑↑	↑
Respiratory alkalosis	↑	↓	↓↓	↓
Metabolic acidosis	↓	↑	↓	↓↓
Metabolic alkalosis	↑	↓	↑	↑↑

The primary event is indicated by the double arrows (↑↑ or ↓↓). Note that respiratory acid–base disorders are initiated by an increase or decrease in PCO_2, whereas metabolic disorders are initiated by an increase or decrease in HCO_3^-.

can be excreted in the urine, mainly in the form of NH_4^+; this, excretion in turn, contributes up to 500 mEq/day of new HCO_3^- that is added to the blood.

Thus, with chronic acidosis, increased secretion of H^+ by the tubules helps eliminate excess H^+ from the body and increases the quantity of HCO_3^- in the extracellular fluid. This process increases the HCO_3^- part of the bicarbonate buffer system, which, in accordance with the Henderson–Hasselbalch equation, helps raise the extracellular pH and corrects the acidosis. If the acidosis is metabolically mediated, additional compensation by the lungs causes a reduction in PCO_2, also helping to correct the acidosis.

Table 82-3 summarizes the characteristics associated with respiratory and metabolic acidosis, as well as respiratory and metabolic alkalosis, which are discussed in the next section. Note that in *respiratory acidosis*, there is a reduction in pH, an increase in extracellular fluid H^+ concentration, and an increase in PCO_2, which is the initial cause of the acidosis. *The compensatory response is an increase in plasma HCO_3^-, caused by the addition of new HCO_3^- to the extracellular fluid by the kidneys.* The rise in HCO_3^- helps offset the increase in PCO_2, thereby returning the plasma pH toward normal.

In *metabolic acidosis*, there is also a decrease in pH and a rise in extracellular fluid H^+ concentration. However, in this case, the primary abnormality is a decrease in plasma HCO_3^-. *The primary compensations include increased ventilation rate, which reduces PCO_2, and renal compensation, which, by adding new HCO_3^- to the extracellular fluid, helps minimize the initial fall in extracellular HCO_3^- concentration.*

Renal Correction of Alkalosis— Decreased Tubular Secretion of H⁺ and Increased Excretion of HCO₃⁻

The compensatory responses to alkalosis are basically opposite to those that occur in acidosis. In alkalosis, the ratio of HCO_3^- to CO_2 in the extracellular fluid increases, causing a rise in pH (a decrease in H^+ concentration), as is evident from the Henderson–Hasselbalch equation.

ALKALOSIS INCREASES THE RATIO OF HCO₃⁻/H⁺ IN RENAL TUBULAR FLUID

Regardless of whether the alkalosis is caused by metabolic or respiratory abnormalities, there is still an increase in the ratio of HCO_3^- to H^+ in the renal tubular fluid. The net effect of this is an excess of HCO_3^- that cannot be reabsorbed from the tubules and is, therefore, excreted in the urine. Thus, in alkalosis, HCO_3^- is removed from the extracellular fluid by renal excretion, which has the same effect as adding an H^+ to the

extracellular fluid. This helps return the H^+ concentration and pH toward normal.

Table 82-3 shows the overall characteristics of respiratory and metabolic alkalosis. In *respiratory alkalosis,* there is an increase in extracellular fluid pH and a decrease in H^+ concentration. *The cause of the alkalosis is decreased plasma PCO_2 caused by hyperventilation.* Reduction in PCO_2 then leads to decreased renal tubular H^+ secretion. Consequently, there is not enough H^+ in the renal tubular fluid to react with all the HCO_3^- that is filtered. Therefore, the HCO_3^- that cannot react with H^+ is not reabsorbed and is excreted in the urine. This results in decreased in plasma HCO_3^- concentration and correction of the alkalosis. *Therefore, the compensatory response to a primary reduction in PCO_2 in respiratory alkalosis is a reduction in plasma HCO_3^- concentration, caused by increased renal excretion of HCO_3^-.*

In *metabolic alkalosis,* there is also decreased in plasma H^+ concentration and increased pH. *The cause of metabolic alkalosis, however, is a rise in the extracellular fluid HCO_3^- concentration.* This rise is partly compensated for by a reduction in the respiration rate, which increases PCO_2 and helps return the extracellular fluid pH toward normal. In addition, increased HCO_3^- concentration in the extracellular fluid increases the filtered load of HCO_3^-, which in turn causes excess HCO_3^- over H^+ secreted in the renal tubular fluid. The excess HCO_3^- in the tubular fluid fails to be reabsorbed because there is no H^+ to react with, and it is excreted in the urine. *In metabolic alkalosis, the primary compensations are decreased ventilation, which raises PCO_2, and increased renal HCO_3^- excretion, which helps compensate for the initial rise in extracellular fluid HCO_3^- concentration.*

Clinical Causes of Acid– Base Disorders

RESPIRATORY ACIDOSIS RESULTS FROM DECREASED VENTILATION AND INCREASED PCO₂

From the previous discussion, it is obvious that any factor that decreases the rate of pulmonary ventilation also increases the PCO_2 of extracellular fluid. This causes an increase in H_2CO_3 and H^+ concentration, thus resulting in acidosis. Because the acidosis is caused by an abnormality in respiration, it is called *respiratory acidosis.*

Respiratory acidosis can occur from pathological conditions that damage the respiratory centers or that decrease the ability of the lungs to eliminate CO_2. For example, damage to the respiratory center in the medulla oblongata can lead to respiratory acidosis. Also, obstruction of the passageways of the respiratory tract, pneumonia, emphysema, or decreased pulmonary membrane surface area, as well as any factor that interferes with the exchange of gases between the blood and the alveolar air, can cause respiratory acidosis.

In respiratory acidosis, the compensatory responses available are (1) the buffers of the body fluids and (2) the kidneys, which require several days to compensate for the disorder.

RESPIRATORY ALKALOSIS RESULTS FROM INCREASED VENTILATION AND DECREASED PCO₂

Respiratory alkalosis is caused by excessive ventilation by the lungs. Rarely does this occur because of physical pathological conditions. However, a psychoneurosis can occasionally increase breathing to the extent that a person becomes alkalotic.

A physiological type of respiratory alkalosis occurs when a person ascends to high altitude. The low oxygen content of the air stimulates respiration, which causes loss of CO_2 and development of mild respiratory alkalosis. Again, the major means for compensation are the chemical buffers of the body fluids and the ability of the kidneys to increase HCO_3^- excretion.

METABOLIC ACIDOSIS RESULTS FROM DECREASED EXTRACELLULAR FLUID HCO_3^- CONCENTRATION

The term *metabolic acidosis* refers to all other types of acidosis besides those caused by excess CO_2 in the body fluids. Metabolic acidosis can result from several general causes: (1) failure of the kidneys to excrete metabolic acids normally formed in the body, (2) formation of excess quantities of metabolic acids in the body, (3) addition of metabolic acids to the body by ingestion or infusion of acids, and (4) loss of base from the body fluids, which has the same effect as adding an acid to the body fluids. Some specific conditions that cause metabolic acidosis are described in the following sections.

Renal Tubular Acidosis. Renal tubular acidosis results from a defect in renal secretion of H^+ or in reabsorption of HCO_3^-, or both. These disorders are generally of two types: (1) impairment of renal tubular HCO_3^- reabsorption, causing loss of HCO_3^- in the urine, or (2) inability of the renal tubular H^+ secretory mechanism to establish normal acidic urine, causing the excretion of alkaline urine. In these cases, inadequate amounts of titratable acid and NH_4^+ are excreted, so there is net accumulation of acid in the body fluids. Some causes of renal tubular acidosis include chronic renal failure, insufficient aldosterone secretion (Addison's disease), and several hereditary and acquired disorders that impair tubular function, such as Fanconi's syndrome (see Chapter 84).

Diarrhea. Severe diarrhea is probably the most frequent cause of metabolic acidosis. *The cause of this acidosis is the loss of large amounts of sodium bicarbonate into the feces.* The gastrointestinal secretions normally contain large amounts of bicarbonate, and diarrhea results in the loss of HCO_3^- from the body, which has the same effect as losing large amounts of bicarbonate in the urine. This form of metabolic acidosis can be particularly serious and can cause death, especially in young children.

Vomiting of Intestinal Contents. Vomiting of gastric contents alone would cause loss of acid and a tendency toward alkalosis because the stomach secretions are highly acidic. However, vomiting large amounts from deeper in the gastrointestinal tract, which sometimes occurs, causes loss of bicarbonate and results in metabolic acidosis in the same way that diarrhea causes acidosis.

Diabetes Mellitus. Diabetes mellitus is caused by lack of insulin secretion by the pancreas (type I diabetes) or by insufficient insulin secretion to compensate for decreased sensitivity to the effects of insulin (type 2 diabetes). In the absence of sufficient insulin, the normal use of glucose for metabolism is prevented. Instead, some of the fats are split into acetoacetic acid, and this acid is metabolized by the tissues for energy in place of glucose. With severe diabetes mellitus, blood acetoacetic acid levels can rise very high, causing severe metabolic acidosis. In an attempt to compensate for this acidosis, large amounts of acid are excreted in the urine, sometimes as much as 500 mmol/day.

Ingestion of Acids. Rarely are large amounts of acids ingested in normal foods. However, severe metabolic acidosis occasionally results from the ingestion of certain acidic poisons. Some of these substances include acetylsalicylics (aspirin) and methyl alcohol (which forms formic acid when it is metabolized).

Chronic Renal Failure. When kidney function declines markedly, there is a buildup of the anions of weak acids in the body fluids that are not being excreted by the kidneys. In addition, the decreased glomerular filtration rate reduces excretion of phosphates and NH_4^+, which reduces the amount of HCO_3^- added back to the body fluids. Thus, chronic renal failure can be associated with severe metabolic acidosis.

METABOLIC ALKALOSIS RESULTS FROM INCREASED EXTRACELLULAR FLUID HCO_3^- CONCENTRATION

Excess retention of HCO_3^- or loss of H^+ from the body causes metabolic alkalosis. Metabolic alkalosis is not nearly as common as metabolic acidosis, but some of the causes of metabolic alkalosis are described in the following sections.

Administration of Diuretics (Except the Carbonic Anhydrase Inhibitors). All diuretics cause increased flow of fluid along the tubules, usually increasing flow in the distal and collecting tubules. This effect leads to increased reabsorption of Na^+ from these parts of the nephrons. Because the sodium reabsorption here is coupled with H^+ secretion, the enhanced sodium reabsorption also leads to an increase in H^+ secretion and an increase in bicarbonate reabsorption. These changes lead to the development of alkalosis, characterized by increased extracellular fluid bicarbonate concentration.

Excess Aldosterone. When large amounts of aldosterone are secreted by the adrenal glands, a mild metabolic alkalosis develops. As discussed previously, aldosterone promotes extensive reabsorption of Na^+ from the distal and collecting tubules, and at the same time stimulates secretion of H^+ by the intercalated cells of the collecting tubules. This increased secretion of H^+ leads to its increased excretion by the kidneys and, therefore, metabolic alkalosis.

Vomiting of Gastric Contents. Vomiting of the gastric contents alone, without vomiting of the lower gastrointestinal contents, causes loss of the HCl secreted by the stomach mucosa. The net result is a loss of acid from the extracellular fluid and development of metabolic alkalosis. This type of alkalosis occurs especially in neonates who have pyloric stenosis caused by hypertrophied pyloric sphincter muscles.

Ingestion of Alkaline Drugs. A common cause of metabolic alkalosis is ingestion of alkaline drugs, such as sodium bicarbonate, for the treatment of gastritis or peptic ulcer.

Treatment of Acidosis or Alkalosis

The best treatment for acidosis or alkalosis is to correct the condition that caused the abnormality. This is often difficult, especially in chronic diseases that cause impaired lung function or kidney failure. In these circumstances, various agents can be used to neutralize the excess acid or base in the extracellular fluid.

To neutralize excess acid, large amounts of *sodium bicarbonate* can be ingested by mouth. The sodium bicarbonate is absorbed from the gastrointestinal tract into the blood and increases the HCO_3^- portion of the bicarbonate buffer system, thereby increasing pH toward normal. Sodium bicarbonate can also be infused intravenously, but because of the potentially dangerous physiological effects of such treatment, other substances are often used instead, such as *sodium lactate* and sodium gluconate. The lactate and gluconate portions of the molecules are metabolized in the body, leaving the sodium in the extracellular fluid in the form of sodium bicarbonate and thereby increasing the pH of the fluid toward normal.

For the treatment of alkalosis, *ammonium chloride* can be administered by mouth. When the ammonium chloride is absorbed into the blood, the ammonia portion is converted by the liver into urea. This reaction liberates HCl, which immediately reacts with the buffers of the body fluids to shift the H^+ concentration in the acidic direction. Ammonium chloride occasionally is infused intravenously, but NH_4^+ is highly toxic and this procedure can be dangerous. The most appropriate treatment is to reverse the underlying cause of the alkalosis. For example, if metabolic alkalosis is associated with extracellular fluid volume depletion, but not heart failure, appropriate repletion of volume by infusion of isotonic saline solution is often beneficial in correcting the alkalosis.

Clinical Measurements and Analysis of Acid–Base Disorders

Appropriate therapy of acid–base disorders requires proper diagnosis. The simple acid–base disorders described previously can be diagnosed by analyzing three measurements from an arterial blood sample: pH, plasma HCO_3^- concentration, and PCO_2.

The diagnosis of simple acid–base disorders involves several steps, as shown in Figure 82-10. By examining the pH, one can determine whether the disorder is acidosis or alkalosis. A pH less than 7.4 indicates acidosis, whereas a pH greater than 7.4 indicates alkalosis.

The second step is to examine the plasma PCO_2 and HCO_3^- concentrations. The normal value for PCO_2 is about 40 mmHg, and for HCO_3^-, it is 24 mEq/L. If the disorder has been characterized as acidosis and the plasma PCO_2 is increased, there must be a respiratory component to the acidosis. After renal compensation, the plasma HCO_3^- concentration in respiratory acidosis would tend to increase above normal. *Therefore, the expected values for a simple respiratory acidosis would be reduced plasma pH, increased PCO_2, and increased plasma HCO_3^- concentration after partial renal compensation.*

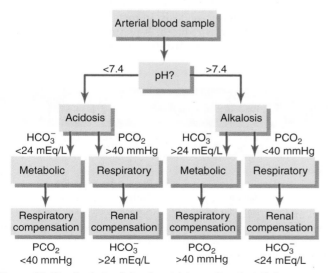

Figure 82-10 Analysis of simple acid–base disorders. If the compensatory responses are markedly different from those shown at the bottom of the figure, one should suspect a mixed acid–base disorder.

For metabolic acidosis, there would also be a decrease in plasma pH. However, with metabolic acidosis, the primary abnormality is a decrease in plasma HCO_3^- concentration. Therefore, if a low pH is associated with a low HCO_3^- concentration, there must be a metabolic component to the acidosis. In simple metabolic acidosis, the PCO_2 is reduced because of partial respiratory compensation, in contrast to respiratory acidosis, in which PCO_2 is increased. *Therefore, in simple metabolic acidosis, one would expect to find a low pH, a low plasma HCO_3^- concentration, and a reduction in PCO_2 after partial respiratory compensation.*

The procedures for categorizing the types of alkalosis involve the same basic steps. First, alkalosis implies that there is an increase in plasma pH. If the increase in pH is associated with decreased PCO_2, there must be a respiratory component to the alkalosis. If the rise in pH is associated with increased HCO_3^-, there must be a metabolic component to the alkalosis. *Therefore, in simple respiratory alkalosis, one would expect to find increased pH, decreased PCO_2, and decreased HCO_3^- concentration in the plasma. In simple metabolic alkalosis, one would expect to find increased pH, increased plasma HCO_3^-, and increased PCO_2.*

COMPLEX ACID–BASE DISORDERS AND USE OF THE ACID–BASE NOMOGRAM FOR DIAGNOSIS

In some instances, acid–base disorders are not accompanied by appropriate compensatory responses. When this situation occurs, the abnormality is referred to as a *mixed acid–base disorder* which means that there are two or more underlying causes for the acid–base disturbance. For example, a patient with low pH would be categorized as acidotic. If the disorder was metabolically mediated, this would also be accompanied by a low plasma HCO_3^- concentration and, after appropriate respiratory compensation, a low PCO_2. However, if the low plasma pH and low HCO_3^- concentration are associated with elevated PCO_2, one would suspect a respiratory component to the acidosis as well as a metabolic component. Therefore, this disorder would be categorized as a mixed acidosis. This disorder could occur, for example, in a patient with acute HCO_3^- loss from the gastrointestinal tract because of diarrhea (metabolic acidosis) and emphysema (respiratory acidosis).

A convenient way to diagnose acid–base disorders is to use an acid–base nomogram, as shown in Figure 82-11. This diagram can be used to determine the type of acidosis or alkalosis, as well as its severity. In this acid–base diagram, pH, HCO_3^- concentration, and PCO_2 values intersect according to the Henderson–Hasselbalch equation. The central open circle shows normal values and the deviations that can still be considered within the normal range. The shaded areas of the diagram show the 95% confidence limits for the normal compensations to simple metabolic and respiratory disorders.

When using this diagram, one must assume that sufficient time has elapsed for a full compensatory response, which is 6–12 hours for the ventilatory compensations in primary metabolic disorders and 3–5 days for the metabolic compensations in primary respiratory disorders. If a value is within the shaded area, this suggests that there is a simple acid–base disturbance. Conversely, if the values for pH, bicarbonate, or PCO_2 lie outside the shaded area, this suggests that the patient may have a mixed acid–base disorder.

It is important to recognize that an acid–base value within the shaded area does not *always* mean that a simple acid–base disorder is present. With this reservation in mind, the acid–base diagrams can be used as a quick means of determining the specific type and severity of an acid–base disorder.

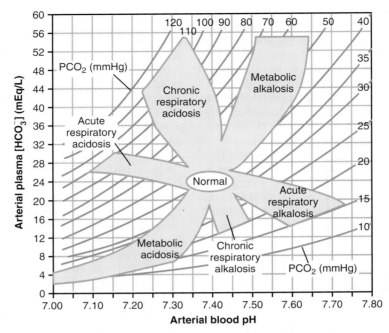

Figure 82-11 Acid–base nomogram showing arterial blood pH, arterial plasma HCO_3^-, and PCO_2 values. The central open circle shows the approximate limits for acid–base status in normal people. The shaded areas in the nomogram show the approximate limits for the normal compensations caused by simple metabolic and respiratory disorders. For values lying outside the shaded areas, one should suspect a mixed acid–base disorder. (*Modified from Cogan, M.G., Rector, Jr, F.C., 1986. Acid–Base Disorders in the Kidney, third ed. WB Saunders, Philadelphia.*)

For example, assume that the arterial plasma from a patient yields the following values: pH 7.30, plasma HCO_3^- concentration 12.0 mEq/L, and plasma PCO_2 25 mmHg. With these values, one can look at the diagram and find that this represents a simple metabolic acidosis, with appropriate respiratory compensation that reduces the PCO_2 from its normal value of 40 mmHg to 25 mmHg.

A second example would be a patient with the following values: pH 7.15, plasma HCO_3^- concentration 7 mEq/L, and plasma PCO_2 50 mmHg. In this example, the patient is acidotic, and there appears to be a metabolic component because the plasma HCO_3^- concentration is lower than the normal value of 24 mEq/L. However, the respiratory compensation that would normally reduce PCO_2 is absent and PCO_2 is slightly increased above the normal value of 40 mmHg. This finding is consistent with a mixed acid–base disturbance consisting of metabolic acidosis, as well as a respiratory component.

The acid–base nomogram serves as a quick way to assess the type and severity of disorders that may be contributing to abnormal pH, PCO_2, and plasma bicarbonate concentrations. In a clinical setting, the patient's history and other physical findings also provide important clues concerning causes and treatment of the acid–base disorders.

USE OF ANION GAP TO DIAGNOSE ACID–BASE DISORDERS

The concentrations of anions and cations in plasma must be equal to maintain electrical neutrality. Therefore, there is no real "anion gap" in the plasma. However, only certain cations and anions are routinely measured in the clinical laboratory. The cation normally measured is Na^+, and the anions are usually Cl^- and HCO_3^-. The "anion gap" (which is only a diagnostic

concept) is the difference between unmeasured anions and unmeasured cations and is estimated as

$$\text{Plasma anion gap} = [Na^+] - [HCO_3^-] - [Cl^-]$$
$$= 144 - 24 - 108 = 12\,\text{mEq/L}$$

The anion gap will increase if unmeasured anions rise or if unmeasured cations fall. The most important unmeasured cations include calcium, magnesium, and potassium, and the major unmeasured anions are albumin, phosphate, sulfate, and other organic anions. Usually the unmeasured anions exceed the unmeasured cations, and the anion gap ranges between 8 and 16 mEq/L.

The plasma anion gap is used mainly in diagnosing different causes of metabolic acidosis. In metabolic acidosis, plasma HCO_3^- concentration is reduced. If plasma sodium concentration is unchanged, the concentration of anions (either Cl^- or an

TABLE 82-4	Metabolic Acidosis Associated with Normal or Increased Plasma Anion Gap
Increased Anion Gap (Normochloremia)	**Normal Anion Gap (Hyperchloremia)**
Diabetes mellitus (ketoacidosis)	Diarrhea
Lactic acidosis	Renal tubular acidosis
Chronic renal failure	Carbonic anhydrase inhibitors
Aspirin (acetylsalicylic acid) poisoning	Addison's disease
Methanol poisoning	
Ethylene glycol poisoning	
Starvation	

unmeasured anion) must increase to maintain electroneutrality. If plasma Cl^- increases in proportion to the fall in plasma HCO_3^-, the anion gap will remain normal. This is often referred to as *hyperchloremic metabolic acidosis.*

If the decrease in plasma HCO_3^- is not accompanied by increased Cl^-, there must be increased levels of unmeasured anions and therefore an increase in the calculated anion gap. Metabolic acidosis caused by excess nonvolatile acids (besides HCl), such as lactic acid or ketoacids, is associated with an increased plasma anion gap because the fall in HCO_3^- is not matched by an equal increase in Cl^-. Some examples of metabolic acidosis associated with a normal or increased anion gap are shown in Table 82-4. By calculating the anion gap, one can narrow some of the potential causes of metabolic acidosis.

BIBLIOGRAPHY

Attmane-Elakeb A, Amlal H, Bichara M: Ammonium carriers in medullary thick ascending limb, *Am. J. Physiol. Renal Physiol.* 280:F1, 2001.

Breton S, Brown D: New insights into the regulation of V-ATPase-dependent proton secretion, *Am. J. Physiol. Renal Physiol.* 292:F1, 2007.

Brown D, Bouley R, Pa unescu TG, et al: New insights into the dynamic regulation of water and acid-base balance by renal epithelial cells, *Am. J. Physiol. Cell Physiol.* 302:C1421, 2012.

Decoursey TE: Voltage-gated proton channels and other proton transfer pathways, *Physiol. Rev.* 83:475, 2003.

Fry AC, Karet FE: Inherited renal acidoses, *Physiology (Bethesda)* 22:202, 2007.

Gennari FJ, Maddox DA, Renal regulation of acid-base homeostasis. In: Seldin DW, Giebisch G. The Kidney—Physiology and Pathophysiology, third ed. Raven Press, New York, pp. 2015–2054.

Good DW: Ammonium transport by the thick ascending limb of Henle's loop, *Ann. Rev. Physiol.* 56:623, 1994.

Igarashi I, Sekine T, Inatomi J, et al: Unraveling the molecular pathogenesis of isolated proximal renal tubular acidosis, *J. Am. Soc. Nephrol.* 13:2171, 2002.

Karet FE: Inherited distal renal tubular acidosis, *J. Am. Soc. Nephrol.* 13:2178, 2002.

Kraut JA, Madias NE: Serum anion gap: its uses and limitations in clinical medicine, *Clin. J. Am. Soc. Nephrol.* 2:162, 2007.

Laffey JG, Kavanagh BP: Hypocapnia, *N. Engl. J. Med.* 347:43, 2002.

Lemann J Jr, Bushinsky DA, Hamm LL: Bone buffering of acid and base in humans, *Am. J. Physiol. Renal Physiol.* 285:F811, 2003.

Madias NE, Adrogue HJ: Cross-talk between two organs: how the kidney responds to disruption of acid-base balance by the lung, *Nephron. Physiol.* 93:61, 2003.

Purkerson JM, Schwartz GJ: The role of carbonic anhydrases in renal physiology, *Kid. Int.* 71:103, 2007.

Wagner CA, Finberg KE, Breton S, et al: Renal vacuolar H^+-ATPase, *Physiol. Rev.* 84:1263, 2004.

Wesson DE, Alpern RJ, Seldin DW. Clinical syndromes of metabolic alkalosis. In: Seldin DW, Giebisch G. The Kidney—Physiology and Pathophysiology, third ed. Raven Press, New York, pp. 2055–2072.

White NH: Management of diabetic ketoacidosis, *Rev. Endocr. Metab. Disord.* 4:343, 2003.

83

Micturition

Micturition is the process by which the urinary bladder empties when it becomes filled. This involves two main steps: First, the bladder fills progressively until the tension in its walls rises above a threshold level; this elicits the second step, which is a nervous reflex called the *micturition reflex* that empties the bladder or, if this fails, at least causes a conscious desire to urinate. Although the micturition reflex is an autonomic spinal cord reflex, it can also be inhibited or facilitated by centers in the cerebral cortex or brain stem.

Physiological Anatomy of the Bladder

The urinary bladder, shown in Figure 83-1, is a smooth muscle chamber composed of two main parts: (1) the *body*, which is the major part of the bladder in which urine collects, and (2) the *neck*, which is a funnel-shaped extension of the body, passing inferiorly and anteriorly into the urogenital triangle and connecting with the urethra. The lower part of the bladder neck is also called the *posterior urethra* because of its relation to the urethra.

The smooth muscle of the bladder is called the *detrusor muscle*. Its muscle fibers extend in all directions and, when contracted, can increase the pressure in the bladder to 40–60 mmHg. Thus, *contraction of the detrusor muscle is a major step in emptying the bladder.* Smooth muscle cells of the detrusor muscle fuse with one another so that low-resistance electrical pathways exist from one muscle cell to the other. Therefore, an action potential can spread throughout the detrusor muscle, from one muscle cell to the next, to cause contraction of the entire bladder at once.

On the posterior wall of the bladder, lying immediately above the bladder neck, is a small triangular area called the *trigone*. At the lowermost apex of the trigone the bladder neck opens into the *posterior urethra* and the two ureters enter the bladder at the uppermost angles of the trigone. The trigone can be identified by the fact that its *mucosa*, the inner lining of the bladder, is smooth, in contrast to the remaining bladder mucosa, which is folded to form *rugae*.

Each ureter, as it enters the bladder, courses obliquely through the detrusor muscle and then passes another 1–2 cm beneath the bladder mucosa before emptying into the bladder.

The bladder neck (posterior urethra) is 2–3 cm long, and its wall is composed of detrusor muscle interlaced with a large amount of elastic tissue. The muscle in this area is called the *internal sphincter*. Its natural tone normally keeps the bladder neck and posterior urethra empty of urine and, therefore, prevents emptying of the bladder until the pressure in the main part of the bladder rises above a critical threshold.

Beyond the posterior urethra, the urethra passes through the *urogenital diaphragm*, which contains a layer of muscle called the *external sphincter* of the bladder. This muscle is a voluntary skeletal muscle, in contrast to the muscle of the bladder body and bladder neck, which is entirely smooth muscle. The external sphincter muscle is under voluntary control of the nervous system and can be used to consciously prevent urination even when involuntary controls are attempting to empty the bladder.

INNERVATION OF THE BLADDER

The principal nerve supply of the bladder is by way of the *pelvic nerves*, which connect with the spinal cord through the *sacral plexus*, mainly connecting with cord segments S2 and S3 (Figure 83-2). Coursing through the pelvic nerves are both *sensory nerve fibers* and *motor nerve fibers*. The sensory fibers detect the degree of stretch in the bladder wall. Stretch signals from the posterior urethra are especially strong and are mainly responsible for initiating the reflexes that cause bladder emptying.

The motor nerves transmitted in the pelvic nerves are *parasympathetic fibers*. These fibers terminate on ganglion cells located in the wall of the bladder. Short postganglionic nerves then innervate the detrusor muscle.

In addition to the pelvic nerves, two other types of innervation are important in bladder function. Most important are the *skeletal motor fibers* transmitted through the *pudendal nerve* to the external bladder sphincter. These fibers are *somatic nerve fibers* that innervate and control the voluntary skeletal muscle of the sphincter. Also, the bladder receives *sympathetic innervation* from the sympathetic chain through the *hypogastric nerves*, connecting mainly with the L2 segment of the spinal cord. These sympathetic fibers stimulate mainly the blood vessels and have little to do with bladder contraction. Some sensory nerve fibers also pass by way of the sympathetic nerves and may be important in the sensation of fullness and, in some instances, pain.

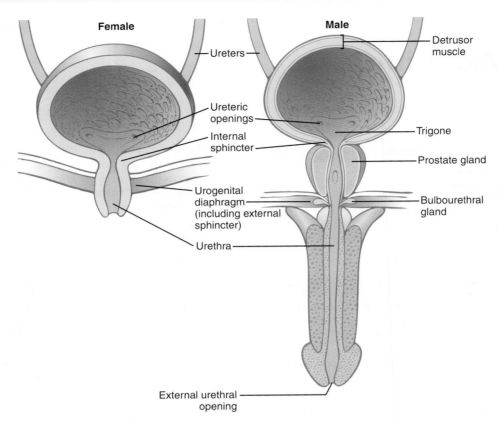

Figure 83-1 Anatomy of the urinary bladder in males and females.

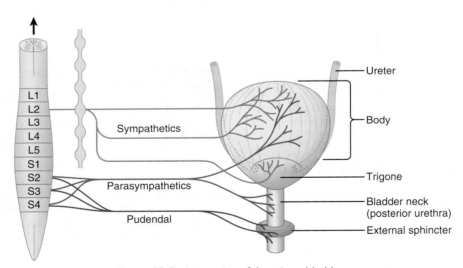

Figure 83-2 Innervation of the urinary bladder.

Transport of Urine From the Kidney Through the Ureters and Into the Bladder

Urine that is expelled from the bladder has essentially the same composition as fluid flowing out of the collecting ducts; there are no significant changes in the composition of urine as it flows through the renal calyces and ureters to the bladder.

Urine flowing from the collecting ducts into the renal calyces stretches the calyces and increases their inherent pacemaker activity, which in turn initiates peristaltic contractions that spread to the renal pelvis and then downward along the length of the ureter, thereby forcing urine from the renal pelvis toward the bladder. In adults, the ureters are normally 25–35 cm (10–inches) long.

The walls of the ureters contain smooth muscle and are innervated by both sympathetic and parasympathetic nerves, as well as by an intramural plexus of neurons and nerve fibers that extends along the entire length of the ureters. As with other visceral smooth muscle, *peristaltic contractions in the ureter are enhanced by parasympathetic stimulation and inhibited by sympathetic stimulation.*

The ureters enter the bladder through the *detrusor muscle* in the trigone region of the bladder, as shown in Figure 83-1. Normally, the ureters course obliquely for several centimeters through the bladder wall. The normal tone of the detrusor muscle in the bladder wall tends to compress the ureter, thereby preventing backflow (reflux) of urine from the bladder when pressure builds up in the bladder during micturition or bladder compression. Each peristaltic wave along the ureter increases the pressure within the ureter so that the region passing through the bladder wall opens and allows urine to flow into the bladder.

In some people, the distance that the ureter courses through the bladder wall is less than normal, and thus contraction of the bladder during micturition does not always lead to complete occlusion of the ureter. As a result, some of the urine in the bladder is propelled backward into the ureter, a condition called *vesicoureteral reflux.* Such reflux can lead to enlargement of the ureters and, if severe, can increase the pressure in the renal calyces and structures of the renal medulla, causing damage to these regions.

Pain Sensation in the Ureters, and the Ureterorenal Reflex. The ureters are well supplied with pain nerve fibers. When a ureter becomes blocked (eg, by a ureteral stone) intense reflex constriction occurs, which is associated with severe pain. Also, the pain impulses cause a sympathetic reflex back to the kidney to constrict the renal arterioles, thereby decreasing urine output from the kidney. This effect is called the *ureterorenal reflex* and is important for preventing excessive flow of fluid into the pelvis of a kidney with a blocked ureter.

Filling of the Bladder and Bladder Wall Tone; the Cystometrogram

Figure 83-3 shows the approximate changes in intravesicular pressure as the bladder fills with urine. When there is no urine in the bladder, the intravesicular pressure is about 0, but by the time 30–50 mL of urine have collected, the pressure rises to 5–10 cm of water. Additional urine—200–300 mL—can collect

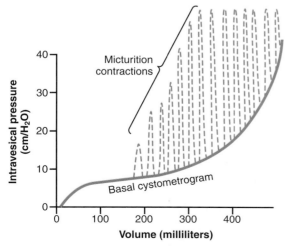

Figure 83-3 A Normal cystometrogram, showing also acute pressure waves (*dashed spikes*) caused by micturition reflexes.

with only a small additional rise in pressure; this constant level of pressure is caused by intrinsic tone of the bladder wall itself. Beyond 300–400 mL, collection of more urine in the bladder causes the pressure to rise rapidly.

Superimposed on the tonic pressure changes during filling of the bladder are periodic acute increases in pressure that last from a few seconds to more than a minute. The pressure peaks may rise only a few centimeters of water or may rise to more than 100 cm of water. These pressure peaks are called *micturition waves* in the cystometrogram and are caused by the micturition reflex.

Micturition Reflex

Referring again to Figure 83-3, one can see that as the bladder fills many superimposed *micturition contractions* begin to appear, as shown by the dashed spikes. They are the result of a stretch reflex initiated by *sensory stretch receptors* in the bladder wall, especially by the receptors in the posterior urethra when this area begins to fill with urine at the higher bladder pressures. Sensory signals from the bladder stretch receptors are conducted to the sacral segments of the cord through the *pelvic nerves* and then reflexively back again to the bladder through the *parasympathetic nerve fibers* by way of these same nerves.

When the bladder is only partially filled, these micturition contractions usually relax spontaneously after a fraction of a minute, the detrusor muscles stop contracting, and pressure falls back to the baseline. As the bladder continues to fill, the micturition reflexes become more frequent and cause greater contractions of the detrusor muscle.

Once a micturition reflex begins, it is "self-regenerative." That is, initial contraction of the bladder activates the stretch receptors to cause a greater increase in sensory impulses from the bladder and posterior urethra, which causes a further increase in reflex contraction of the bladder; thus, the cycle is repeated again and again until the bladder has reached a strong degree of contraction. Then, after a few seconds to more than a minute, the self-regenerative reflex begins to fatigue and the regenerative cycle of the micturition reflex ceases, permitting the bladder to relax.

Thus, the micturition reflex is a single complete cycle of (1) progressive and rapid increase of pressure, (2) a period of sustained pressure, and (3) return of the pressure to the basal tone of the bladder. Once a micturition reflex has occurred but has not succeeded in emptying the bladder, the nervous elements of this reflex usually remain in an inhibited state for a few minutes to 1 hour or more before another micturition reflex occurs. As the bladder becomes more and more filled, micturition reflexes occur more and more often and more and more powerfully.

Once the micturition reflex becomes powerful enough, it causes another reflex, which passes through the *pudendal nerves* to the *external sphincter* to inhibit it. If this inhibition is more potent in the brain than the voluntary constrictor signals to the external sphincter, urination will occur. If not, urination will not occur until the bladder fills still further and the micturition reflex becomes more powerful.

FACILITATION OR INHIBITION OF MICTURITION BY THE BRAIN

The micturition reflex is an autonomic spinal cord reflex, but it can be inhibited or facilitated by centers in the brain. These centers include (1) strong *facilitative* and *inhibitory centers in the brain stem, located mainly in the pons,* and (2) several *centers located in the cerebral cortex* that are mainly inhibitory but can become excitatory.

The micturition reflex is the basic cause of micturition, but the higher centers normally exert final control of micturition as follows:

1. The higher centers keep the micturition reflex partially inhibited, except when micturition is desired.
2. The higher centers can prevent micturition, even if the micturition reflex occurs, by tonic contraction of the external bladder sphincter until a convenient time presents itself.
3. When it is time to urinate, the cortical centers can facilitate the sacral micturition centers to help initiate a micturition reflex and at the same time inhibit the external urinary sphincter so that urination can occur.

Voluntary urination is usually initiated in the following way: First, a person voluntarily contracts his or her abdominal muscles, which increases the pressure in the bladder and allows extra urine to enter the bladder neck and posterior urethra under pressure, thus stretching their walls. This action stimulates the stretch receptors, which excites the micturition reflex and simultaneously inhibits the external urethral sphincter. Ordinarily, all the urine will be emptied, with rarely more than 5–10 mL left in the bladder.

Abnormalities of Micturition

Atonic Bladder and Incontinence Caused by Destruction of Sensory Nerve Fibers. Micturition reflex contraction cannot occur if the sensory nerve fibers from the bladder to the spinal cord are destroyed, thereby preventing transmission of stretch signals from the bladder. When this happens, a person loses bladder control, despite intact efferent fibers from the cord to the bladder and despite intact neurogenic connections within the brain. Instead of emptying periodically, the bladder fills to capacity and overflows a few drops at a time through the urethra. This occurrence is called *overflow incontinence*.

A common cause of atonic bladder is crush injury to the sacral region of the spinal cord. Certain diseases can also cause damage to the dorsal root nerve fibers that enter the spinal cord. For example, syphilis can cause constrictive fibrosis around the dorsal root nerve fibers, destroying them. This condition is called *tabes dorsalis*, and the resulting bladder condition is called *tabetic bladder*.

Automatic Bladder Caused by Spinal Cord Damage Above the Sacral Region. If the spinal cord is damaged above the sacral region but the sacral cord segments are still intact, typical micturition reflexes can still occur. However, they are no longer controlled by the brain. During the first few days to several weeks after the damage to the cord has occurred, the micturition reflexes are suppressed because of the state of "spinal shock" caused by the sudden loss of facilitative impulses from the brain stem and cerebrum. However, if the bladder is emptied periodically by catheterization to prevent bladder injury caused by overstretching of the bladder, the excitability of the micturition reflex gradually increases until typical micturition reflexes return; then, periodic (but unannounced) bladder emptying occurs.

Some patients can still control urination in this condition by stimulating the skin (scratching or tickling) in the genital region, which sometimes elicits a micturition reflex.

Uninhibited Neurogenic Bladder Caused by Lack of Inhibitory Signals From the Brain. Another abnormality of micturition is the so-called uninhibited neurogenic bladder, which results in frequent and relatively uncontrolled micturition. This condition derives from partial damage in the spinal cord or the brain stem that interrupts most of the inhibitory signals. Therefore, facilitative impulses passing continually down the cord keep the sacral centers so excitable that even a small quantity of urine elicits an uncontrollable micturition reflex, thereby promoting frequent urination.

BIBLIOGRAPHY

Beckel JM, Holstege G: Neurophysiology of the lower urinary tract, *Handb. Exp. Pharmacol.* 202:149, 2011.

Fowler CJ, Griffiths D, de Groat WC: The neural control of micturition, *Nat. Rev. Neurosci.* 9:453, 2008.

Holstege G: The emotional motor system and micturition control, *Neurourol. Urodyn.* 29:42, 2010.

Applied Physiology of the Renal System

Diuretics and Their Mechanisms of Action

Diuretics increase the rate of urine volume output, as the name implies. Most diuretics also increase urinary excretion of solutes, especially sodium and chloride. In fact, most diuretics that are used clinically act by decreasing renal tubular sodium reabsorption, which causes natriuresis (increased sodium output), in turn causing diuresis (increased water output). That is, in most cases, increased water excretion occurs secondary to inhibition of tubular sodium reabsorption because sodium remaining in the tubules acts osmotically to decrease water reabsorption. Because renal tubular reabsorption of many solutes, such as potassium, chloride, magnesium, and calcium, is also influenced secondarily by sodium reabsorption, many diuretics raise the renal output of these solutes as well.

The most common clinical use of diuretics is to reduce extracellular fluid volume, especially in diseases associated with edema and hypertension. As discussed in Chapter 80, loss of sodium from the body mainly decreases extracellular fluid volume; therefore, diuretics are most often administered in clinical conditions in which extracellular fluid volume is expanded.

Some diuretics can increase urine output more than 20-fold within a few minutes after they are administered. However, the effect of most diuretics on renal output of salt and water subsides within a few days (Figure 84-1). This is due to activation of compensatory mechanisms initiated by decreased extracellular fluid volume. For example, a decrease in extracellular fluid volume may reduce arterial pressure and the glomerular filtration rate (GFR), and increase renin secretion and angiotensin II formation; all these responses, together, eventually override the chronic effects of the diuretic on urine output. Thus, in the steady state, urine output becomes equal to intake, but only after reductions in arterial pressure and extracellular fluid

volume have occurred, relieving the hypertension or edema that prompted the use of diuretics in the first place.

The many diuretics available for clinical use have different mechanisms of action and, therefore, inhibit tubular reabsorption at different sites along the renal nephron. The general classes of diuretics, their mechanisms, and their tubular sites of action are shown in Table 84-1.

OSMOTIC DIURETICS DECREASE WATER REABSORPTION BY INCREASING THE OSMOTIC PRESSURE OF TUBULAR FLUID

Injection into the blood stream of substances that are not easily reabsorbed by the renal tubules, such as urea, mannitol, and sucrose, causes a marked increase in the concentration of osmotically active molecules in the tubules. The osmotic pressure of these solutes then reduces water reabsorption, flushing large amounts of tubular fluid into the urine.

Large volumes of urine are also formed in certain diseases associated with excess solutes that fail to be reabsorbed from the tubular fluid. For example, when blood glucose concentration rises to high levels in diabetes mellitus, the increased filtered load of glucose into the tubules exceeds their capacity to reabsorb glucose (ie, exceeds their *transport maximum* for glucose). Above a plasma glucose concentration of about 250 mg/dL, little of the extra glucose is reabsorbed by the tubules; instead, the excess glucose remains in the tubules, acts as an osmotic diuretic, and causes rapid loss of fluid into the urine. Therefore, one of the hallmarks of uncontrolled diabetes mellitus is *polyuria* (frequent urination), which is balanced by a high level of fluid intake (*polydipsia*) due to dehydration, increased extracellular fluid osmolarity, and subsequent activation of the thirst mechanism.

"LOOP" DIURETICS DECREASE ACTIVE SODIUM–CHLORIDE–POTASSIUM REABSORPTION IN THE THICK ASCENDING LOOP OF HENLE

Furosemide, ethacrynic acid, and *bumetanide* are powerful diuretics that decrease active reabsorption in the thick ascending limb of the loop of Henle by blocking the 1-sodium, 2-chloride, 1-potassium cotransporter located in the luminal membrane of the epithelial cells. These "loop" diuretics are among the most powerful of the clinically used diuretics.

By blocking sodium–chloride–potassium cotransport in the luminal membrane of the loop of Henle, the loop diuretics increase urine output of sodium, chloride, potassium, and other electrolytes, as well as water, for two reasons: (1) they greatly increase the quantities of solutes delivered to the distal parts of the nephrons, and these solutes act as osmotic agents to prevent water reabsorption as well; and (2) they disrupt the countercurrent multiplier system by decreasing absorption of ions from the loop of Henle into the medullary interstitium, thereby decreasing the osmolarity of the medullary interstitial fluid. Because of this effect, loop diuretics impair the ability of the

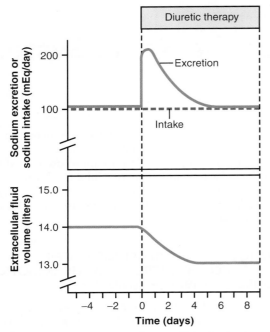

Figure 84-1 Sodium excretion and extracellular fluid volume during diuretic administration. The immediate increase in sodium excretion is accompanied by a decrease in extracellular fluid volume. If sodium intake is held constant, compensatory mechanisms will eventually return sodium excretion to equal sodium intake, thus reestablishing sodium balance.

kidneys to either concentrate or dilute the urine. Urinary dilution is impaired because the inhibition of sodium and chloride reabsorption in the loop of Henle causes more of these ions to be excreted along with increased water excretion. Urinary concentration is impaired because the renal medullary interstitial fluid concentration of these ions, and therefore renal medullary osmolarity, is reduced. Consequently, reabsorption of fluid from the collecting ducts is decreased, so the maximal concentrating ability of the kidneys is also greatly reduced. In addition, decreased renal medullary interstitial fluid osmolarity reduces absorption of water from the descending loop of Henle. Because of these multiple effects, 20–30% of the glomerular filtrate may be delivered into the urine, causing urine output, under acute conditions, to be as great as 25 times normal for at least a few minutes.

THIAZIDE DIURETICS INHIBIT SODIUM–CHLORIDE REABSORPTION IN THE EARLY DISTAL TUBULE

The thiazide derivatives, such as chlorothiazide, act mainly on the early distal tubules to block the sodium–chloride cotransporter in the luminal membrane of the tubular cells. Under favorable conditions, these agents may cause a maximum of 5–10% of the glomerular filtrate to pass into the urine, which is about the same amount of sodium normally reabsorbed by the distal tubules.

CARBONIC ANHYDRASE INHIBITORS BLOCK SODIUM BICARBONATE REABSORPTION IN THE PROXIMAL TUBULES

Acetazolamide inhibits the enzyme *carbonic anhydrase*, which is critical for the reabsorption of bicarbonate (HCO_3^-) in the proximal tubule, as discussed in Chapter 82. Carbonic anhydrase is abundant in the proximal tubule, the primary site of action of carbonic anhydrase inhibitors. Some carbonic anhydrase is also present in other tubular cells, such as in the intercalated cells of the collecting tubule.

Because hydrogen ion (H^+) secretion and HCO_3^- reabsorption in the proximal tubules are coupled to sodium reabsorption through the sodium–hydrogen ion counter-transport mechanism in the luminal membrane, decreasing HCO_3^- reabsorption also reduces sodium reabsorption. The blockage of sodium and HCO_3^- reabsorption from the tubular fluid causes these ions to remain in the tubules and act as an osmotic diuretic. Predictably, a disadvantage of the carbonic anhydrase inhibitors is that they cause some degree of acidosis because of the excessive loss of HCO_3^- in the urine.

MINERALOCORTICOID RECEPTOR ANTAGONISTS DECREASE SODIUM REABSORPTION FROM AND POTASSIUM SECRETION INTO THE COLLECTING TUBULES

Spironolactone and *eplerenone* are mineralocorticoid receptor antagonists that compete with aldosterone for receptor binding sites in the collecting tubule epithelial cells and, therefore, can decrease the reabsorption of sodium and secretion of potassium in this tubular segment. As a consequence, sodium remains in the tubules and acts as an osmotic diuretic, causing increased excretion of water as well as sodium. Because these drugs also

TABLE 84-1	Classes of Diuretics, Their Mechanisms of Action, and Tubular Sites of Action	
Class of Diuretic	**Mechanism of Action**	**Tubular Site of Action**
Osmotic diuretics (mannitol)	Inhibit water and solute reabsorption by increasing osmolarity of tubular fluid	Mainly proximal tubules
Loop diuretics (furosemide, bumetanide)	Inhibit Na^+—K^+—Cl^- cotransport in luminal membrane	Thick ascending loop of Henle
Thiazide diuretics (hydrochlorothiazide, chlorthalidone)	Inhibit Na^+—Cl^- cotransport in luminal membrane	Early distal tubules
Carbonic anhydrase inhibitors (acetazolamide)	Inhibit H^+ secretion and HCO_3^- reabsorption, which reduces Na^+ reabsorption	Proximal tubules
Aldosterone antagonists (spironolactone, eplerenone)	Inhibit action of aldosterone on tubular receptor, decrease Na^+ reabsorption, and decrease K^+ secretion	Collecting tubules
Sodium channel blockers (triamterene, amiloride)	Block entry of Na^+ into Na^+ channels of luminal membrane, decrease Na^+ reabsorption, and decrease K^+ secretion	Collecting tubules

block the effect of aldosterone to promote potassium secretion in the tubules, they decrease the excretion of potassium. Mineralocorticoid receptor antagonists also cause movement of potassium from the cells to the extracellular fluid. In some instances, this movement causes extracellular fluid potassium concentration to increase excessively. For this reason, spironolactone and other mineralocorticoid receptor antagonists are referred to as *potassium-sparing diuretics*. Many of the other diuretics cause loss of potassium in the urine, in contrast to the mineralocorticoid receptor antagonists, which "spare" the loss of potassium.

SODIUM CHANNEL BLOCKERS DECREASE SODIUM REABSORPTION IN THE COLLECTING TUBULES

Amiloride and *triamterene* also inhibit sodium reabsorption and potassium secretion in the collecting tubules, similar to the effects of spironolactone. However, at the cellular level, these drugs act directly to block the entry of sodium into the sodium channels of the luminal membrane of the collecting tubule epithelial cells. Because of this decreased sodium entry into the epithelial cells, there is also decreased sodium transport across the cells' basolateral membranes and, therefore, decreased activity of the sodium–potassium–adenosine triphosphatase pump. This decreased activity reduces the transport of potassium into the cells and ultimately decreases the secretion of potassium into the tubular fluid. For this reason, the sodium channel blockers are also potassium-sparing diuretics and decrease the urinary excretion rate of potassium.

Kidney Diseases

Diseases of the kidneys are among the most important causes of death and disability in many countries throughout the world. For example, in 2014, more than 10% of adults in the United States, or more than 26 million people, were estimated to have chronic kidney disease, and many more millions have acute renal injury or less severe forms of kidney dysfunction.

Severe kidney diseases can be divided into two main categories: (1) *Acute kidney injury (AKI)*, in which there is an abrupt loss of kidney function within a few days; the term *acute renal failure* is usually reserved for severe acute kidney injury where the kidneys may abruptly stop working entirely or almost entirely necessitating renal replacement therapy such as dialysis, as discussed later in the chapter. In some instances, patients with AKI may eventually recover nearly normal kidney function, and (2) *Chronic kidney disease (CKD)*, in which there is progressive loss of function of more and more nephrons that gradually decreases overall kidney function. Within these two general categories, there are many specific kidney diseases that can affect the kidney blood vessels, glomeruli, tubules, renal interstitium, and parts of the urinary tract outside the kidney, including the ureters and bladder. In this chapter, we discuss specific physiologic abnormalities that occur in a few of the more important types of kidney diseases.

Acute Kidney Injury

The causes of AKI can be divided into three main categories:

1. AKI resulting from decreased blood supply to the kidneys. This condition is often referred to as *prerenal AKI* to reflect an abnormality originating outside the kidneys. For example, prerenal AKI can be a consequence of heart failure with reduced cardiac output and low blood pressure or conditions associated with diminished blood volume and low blood pressure, such as severe hemorrhage.
2. *Intrarenal AKI* resulting from abnormalities within the kidney itself, including those that affect the blood vessels, glomeruli, or tubules.
3. *Postrenal AKI* resulting from obstruction of the urinary collecting system anywhere from the calyces to the outflow from the bladder. The most common causes of obstruction of the urinary tract outside the kidney are kidney stones, caused by precipitation of calcium, urate, or cystine.

PHYSIOLOGIC EFFECTS OF ACUTE KIDNEY INJURY

A major physiologic effect of AKI is retention in the blood and extracellular fluid of water, waste products of metabolism, and electrolytes. This can lead to water and salt overload, which, in turn, can lead to edema and hypertension. Excessive retention of potassium, however, is often a more serious threat to patients with AKI because increases in plasma potassium concentration (hyperkalemia) above 8 mEq/L (only twice normal) can be fatal. Because the kidneys are also unable to excrete sufficient hydrogen ions, patients with AKI develop metabolic acidosis, which in itself can be lethal or can aggravate the hyperkalemia.

In the most severe cases of AKI, complete anuria occurs. The patient will die in 8–14 days unless kidney function is restored or unless an artificial kidney is used to rid the body of the excessive retained water, electrolytes, and waste products of metabolism. Other effects of diminished urine output, as well as treatment with an artificial kidney, are discussed in the next section in relation to chronic kidney disease.

Chronic Kidney Disease is Often Associated with Irreversible Loss of Functional Nephrons

CKD is usually defined as the presence of kidney damage or decreased kidney function that persists for at least 3 months. CKD is often associated with progressive and irreversible loss of large numbers of functioning nephrons. Serious clinical symptoms usually do not occur until the number of functional nephrons falls to at least 70–75% below normal. In fact, relatively normal blood concentrations of most electrolytes and normal body fluid volumes can still be maintained until the number of functioning nephrons decreases below 20–25% of normal.

Table 84-2 lists some of the most important causes of CKD. In general, CKD, like AKI, can occur because of disorders of the blood vessels, glomeruli, tubules, renal interstitium, and lower urinary tract. Despite the wide variety of diseases that can lead to CKD, the end result is essentially the same—a decrease in the number of functional nephrons.

VICIOUS CYCLE OF CHRONIC KIDNEY DISEASE LEADING TO END-STAGE RENAL DISEASE

In some cases, an initial insult to the kidney leads to progressive deterioration of kidney function and further loss of nephrons to the point where the person must receive dialysis treatment or undergo transplantation with a functional kidney to survive. This condition is referred to as *end-stage renal disease (ESRD)*.

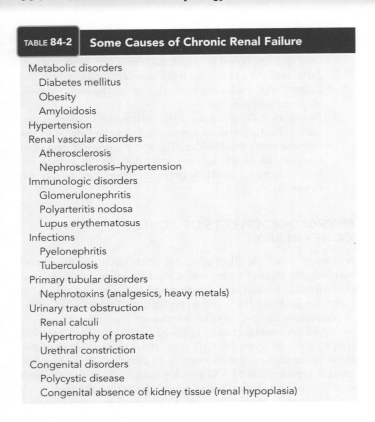

TABLE 84-2	Some Causes of Chronic Renal Failure

Metabolic disorders
    Diabetes mellitus
    Obesity
    Amyloidosis
Hypertension
Renal vascular disorders
    Atherosclerosis
    Nephrosclerosis–hypertension
Immunologic disorders
    Glomerulonephritis
    Polyarteritis nodosa
    Lupus erythematosus
Infections
    Pyelonephritis
    Tuberculosis
Primary tubular disorders
    Nephrotoxins (analgesics, heavy metals)
Urinary tract obstruction
    Renal calculi
    Hypertrophy of prostate
    Urethral constriction
Congenital disorders
    Polycystic disease
    Congenital absence of kidney tissue (renal hypoplasia)

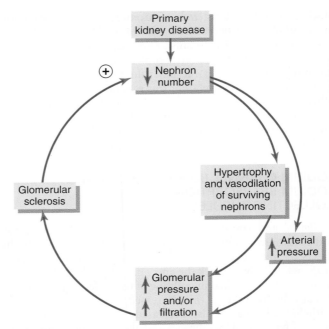

Figure 84-2 The vicious circle that can occur with primary kidney disease. Loss of nephrons because of disease may increase pressure and flow in the surviving glomerular capillaries, which in turn may eventually injure these "normal" capillaries as well, thus causing progressive sclerosis and eventual loss of these glomeruli.

Studies in laboratory animals have shown that surgical removal of large portions of the kidney initially causes adaptive changes in the remaining nephrons that lead to increased blood flow, increased GFR, and increased urine output in the surviving nephrons. The exact mechanisms responsible for these changes are not well understood but involve hypertrophy (growth of the various structures of the surviving nephrons) as well as functional changes that decrease vascular resistance and tubular reabsorption in the surviving nephrons. These adaptive changes permit a person to excrete normal amounts of water and solutes even when kidney mass is reduced to 20–25% of normal. Over a period of several years, however, these renal adaptive changes may lead to further injury of the remaining nephrons, particularly to the glomeruli of these nephrons.

The cause of this additional injury is not fully understood, but some investigators believe it may be related in part to increased pressure or stretch of the remaining glomeruli, which occurs as a result of functional vasodilation or increased blood pressure. The chronic increase in pressure and stretch of the small arterioles and glomeruli are believed to cause injury and sclerosis of these vessels (replacement of normal tissue with connective tissue). These sclerotic lesions can eventually obliterate the glomerulus, leading to further reduction in kidney function, further adaptive changes in the remaining nephrons, and a slowly progressing vicious cycle that eventually terminates in ESRD (Figure 84-2). The most effective method of slowing down this progressive loss of kidney function is to lower arterial pressure and glomerular hydrostatic pressure, especially by using drugs such as angiotensin-converting enzyme inhibitors or angiotensin II receptor antagonists.

Table 84-3 lists the most common causes of ESRD. In the early 1980s, *glomerulonephritis* in all its various forms was believed to be the most common initiating cause of ESRD. In recent years, *diabetes mellitus* and *hypertension* have become recognized as the leading causes of ESRD, together accounting for more than 70% of all ESRD.

Excessive weight gain (obesity) appears to be the most important risk factor for the two main causes of ESRD—diabetes and hypertension. As discussed in Chapter 93, type II diabetes, which is closely linked to obesity, accounts for more than 90% of all cases of diabetes mellitus. Excess weight gain is also a major cause of essential hypertension, accounting for as much as 65–75% of the risk for developing hypertension in adults. In addition to causing renal injury through diabetes and hypertension, obesity may have additive or synergistic effects to worsen renal function in patients with pre-existing kidney disease. In South Asia, infection-related glomerulonephropathies were the main cause of ESRD, but in recent years, owing to the explosion of type II diabetes, diabetic nephropathy has emerged as an important cause of ESRD.

TABLE 84-3	Most Common Causes of ESRD	
Cause		Percentage of Total ESRD Patients
Diabetes mellitus		45
Hypertension		27
Glomerulonephritis		8
Polycystic kidney disease		2
Other/unknown		18

ESRD, end-stage renal disease.

NEPHROTIC SYNDROME—EXCRETION OF PROTEIN IN THE URINE BECAUSE OF INCREASED GLOMERULAR PERMEABILITY

Nephrotic syndrome, which is characterized by loss of large quantities of plasma proteins into the urine develops in many patients with kidney disease. In some instances, this syndrome occurs without evidence of other major abnormalities of kidney function, but more often it is associated with some degree of CKD.

The cause of the protein loss in the urine is increased permeability of the glomerular membrane. Therefore, any disease that increases the permeability of this membrane can cause the nephrotic syndrome. Such diseases include (1) *chronic glomerulonephritis*, which affects primarily the glomeruli and often causes greatly increased permeability of the glomerular membrane; (2) *amyloidosis*, which results from deposition of an abnormal proteinoid substance in the walls of the blood vessels and seriously damages the basement membrane of the glomeruli; and (3) *minimal-change nephrotic syndrome*, which is associated with no major abnormality in the glomerular capillary membrane that can be detected with light microscopy. As discussed in Chapter 77, minimal-change nephropathy has been found to be associated with loss of the negative charges that are normally present in the glomerular capillary basement membrane. Immunological studies have also shown abnormal immune reactions in some cases, suggesting that the loss of the negative charges may have resulted from antibody attack on the membrane. Loss of normal negative charges in the basement membrane of the glomerular capillaries allows proteins, especially albumin, to pass through the glomerular membrane with ease because the negative charges in the basement membrane normally repel the negatively charged plasma proteins.

Minimal-change nephropathy can occur in adults, but more frequently it occurs in children between the ages of 2 and 6 years. Increased permeability of the glomerular capillary membrane occasionally allows as much as 40 g of plasma protein loss into the urine each day, which is an extreme amount for a young child. Therefore, the child's plasma protein concentration often falls below 2 g/dL and the colloid osmotic pressure falls from a normal value of 28 to less than 10 mmHg. As a consequence of this low colloid osmotic pressure in the plasma, large amounts of fluid leak from the capillaries all over the body into most of the tissues, causing severe edema.

EFFECTS OF RENAL FAILURE ON THE BODY FLUIDS—UREMIA

The effect of CKD on the body fluids depends on (1) water and food intake and (2) the degree of impairment of renal function. Assuming that a person with complete renal failure continues to ingest the same amounts of water and food, the concentrations of different substances in the extracellular fluid are approximately those shown in Figure 84-3. Important effects include (1) *generalized edema* resulting from water and salt retention; (2) *acidosis* resulting from failure of the kidneys to rid the body of normal acidic products; (3) *high concentration of the nonprotein nitrogens* (NPN)—especially urea, creatinine, and uric acid—resulting from failure of the body to excrete the metabolic end products of proteins; and (4) *high concentrations of other substances* excreted by the kidney, including *phenols, sulfates, phosphates, potassium,* and *guanidine bases*. This total condition is called *uremia* because of the high concentration of urea in the body fluids.

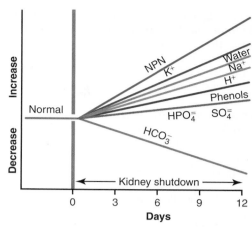

Figure 84-3 Effect of kidney failure on extracellular fluid constituents. NPN, nonprotein nitrogens.

Water Retention and Development of Edema in Chronic Kidney Disease. If water intake is restricted immediately after acute kidney injury begins, the total body fluid content may become only slightly increased. If fluid intake is not limited and the patient drinks in response to the normal thirst mechanisms, the body fluids begin to increase immediately and rapidly.

With CKD, as long as salt and fluid intake are not excessive, accumulation of fluid may not be severe until kidney function falls to 25% of normal or lower. The reason for this, as discussed previously, is that the surviving nephrons excrete larger amounts of salt and water. Even the small fluid retention that does occur, along with increased secretion of renin and angiotensin II that usually occurs in ischemic kidney disease, often causes severe hypertension in persons with CKD. Hypertension develops in almost all patients with kidney function that is so reduced that dialysis is required to preserve life. In many of these patients, severe reduction of salt intake or removal of extracellular fluid by dialysis can control the hypertension. The remaining patients continue to have hypertension even after excess sodium has been removed by dialysis. In this group, removal of the ischemic kidneys usually corrects the hypertension (as long as fluid retention is prevented by dialysis) because it removes the source of excessive renin secretion and subsequent increased angiotensin II formation.

HYPERTENSION AND KIDNEY DISEASE

As discussed earlier in this chapter, hypertension can exacerbate injury to the glomeruli and blood vessels of the kidneys and is a major cause of ESRD. Abnormalities of kidney function can also cause hypertension, as discussed in detail in Chapter 44. Thus, the relation between hypertension and kidney disease can, in some instances, propagate a vicious cycle: primary kidney damage leads to increased blood pressure, which causes further damage to the kidneys, further increases in blood pressure, and so forth, until ESRD develops.

Not all types of kidney disease cause hypertension because damage to certain portions of the kidney causes uremia without hypertension. Nevertheless, some types of renal damage are particularly prone to cause hypertension. A classification of kidney disease relative to hypertensive or nonhypertensive effects is provided in the following sections.

Renal Lesions That Reduce the Ability of the Kidneys to Excrete Sodium and Water Promote Hypertension. Renal lesions that decrease the ability of the kidneys to excrete sodium and water almost invariably cause hypertension. Therefore, lesions that either *decrease GFR* or *increase tubular reabsorption* usually lead to hypertension of varying degrees. Some specific types of renal abnormalities that can cause hypertension are as follows:

1. *Increased renal vascular resistance*, which reduces renal blood flow and GFR. An example is hypertension caused by renal artery stenosis.
2. *Decreased glomerular capillary filtration coefficient, which reduces GFR.* An example is chronic glomerulonephritis, which causes inflammation and thickening of the glomerular capillary membranes, thereby reducing the glomerular capillary filtration coefficient.
3. *Excessive tubular sodium reabsorption.* An example is hypertension caused by excessive aldosterone secretion, which increases sodium reabsorption mainly in the cortical collecting tubules.

Once hypertension has developed, renal excretion of sodium and water returns to normal because the high arterial pressure causes pressure natriuresis and pressure diuresis, so intake and output of sodium and water become balanced once again. Even when there are large increases in renal vascular resistance or decreases in the glomerular capillary coefficient, GFR may still return to nearly normal levels after the arterial blood pressure rises. Likewise, when tubular reabsorption is increased, as occurs with excessive aldosterone secretion, the urinary excretion rate is initially reduced but then returns to normal as arterial pressure rises. Thus, after hypertension develops, there may be no obvious sign of impaired excretion of sodium and water other than the hypertension. As explained in Chapter 44, normal excretion of sodium and water at an elevated arterial pressure means that pressure natriuresis and pressure diuresis have been reset to a higher arterial pressure.

Specific Tubular Disorders

In Chapter 78 we point out that several mechanisms are responsible for transporting different individual substances across the tubular epithelial membranes. In Chapter 3, we also point out that each cellular enzyme and each carrier protein is formed in response to a respective gene in the nucleus. If any required gene happens to be absent or abnormal, the tubules may be deficient in one of the appropriate carrier proteins or one of the enzymes needed for solute transport by the renal tubular epithelial cells. In other instances, too much of the enzyme or carrier protein is produced. Thus, many hereditary tubular disorders occur because of abnormal transport of individual substances or groups of substances through the tubular membrane. In addition, damage to the tubular epithelial membrane by toxins or ischemia can cause important renal tubular disorders.

Renal Glycosuria—Failure of the Kidneys to Reabsorb Glucose. In renal glycosuria, the blood glucose concentration may be normal, but the transport mechanism for tubular reabsorption of glucose is greatly limited or absent. Consequently, despite a normal blood glucose level, large amounts of glucose pass into the urine each day. Because diabetes mellitus is also associated with the presence of glucose in the urine, renal glycosuria, which is a relatively benign condition, must be ruled out before making the diagnosis of diabetes mellitus.

Renal Tubular Acidosis—Failure of the Tubules to Secrete Hydrogen Ions. In renal tubular acidosis, the renal tubules are unable to secrete adequate amounts of hydrogen ions. As a result, large amounts of sodium bicarbonate are continually lost in the urine. This loss causes a continued state of metabolic acidosis, as discussed in Chapter 82. This type of renal abnormality can be caused by hereditary disorders, or it can occur as a result of widespread injury to the renal tubules.

Nephrogenic Diabetes Insipidus—Failure of the Kidneys to Respond to Antidiuretic Hormone. Occasionally, the renal tubules do not respond to antidiuretic hormone, causing large quantities of dilute urine to be excreted. As long as the person is supplied with plenty of water, this condition seldom causes severe difficulty. However, when adequate quantities of water are not available, the person rapidly becomes dehydrated.

Fanconi's Syndrome—A Generalized Reabsorptive Defect of the Renal Tubules. Fanconi's syndrome is usually associated with increased urinary excretion of virtually all amino acids, glucose, and phosphate. In severe cases, other manifestations are also observed, such as (1) failure to reabsorb sodium bicarbonate, which results in metabolic acidosis; (2) increased excretion of potassium and sometimes calcium; and (3) nephrogenic diabetes insipidus.

There are multiple causes of Fanconi's syndrome, which results from a generalized inability of the renal tubular cells to transport various substances. Some of these causes include (1) hereditary defects in cell transport mechanisms, (2) toxins or drugs that injure the renal tubular epithelial cells, and (3) injury to the renal tubular cells as a result of ischemia. The proximal tubular cells are especially affected in Fanconi's syndrome caused by tubular injury because these cells reabsorb and secrete many of the drugs and toxins that can cause damage.

Treatment of Renal Failure by Transplantation or by Dialysis With an Artificial Kidney

Severe loss of kidney function, either acutely or chronically, is a threat to life and requires removal of toxic waste products and restoration of body fluid volume and composition toward normal. This can be accomplished by kidney transplantation or by dialysis with an artificial kidney. Approximately 600,000 patients in the United States are currently receiving some form of ESRD therapy.

Successful transplantation of a single donor kidney to a patient with ESRD can restore kidney function to a level that is sufficient to maintain essentially normal homeostasis of body fluids and electrolytes. Approximately 18,000 kidney transplants are performed each year in the United States. Patients who receive kidney transplants typically live longer and have fewer health problems than do those who are maintained with dialysis. Maintenance of immunosuppressive therapy is required for almost all patients to help prevent acute rejection and loss of the transplanted kidney. The side effects of drugs that suppress the immune system include increased risk for infections and for some cancers, although the amount of immunosuppressive therapy can usually be reduced over time to greatly reduce these risks.

Approximately 400,000 people in the United States who have irreversible renal failure or total kidney removal are being maintained chronically by dialysis with artificial kidneys. Dialysis is also used in certain types of AKI to tide the patient over until the kidneys resume their function. If the loss of kidney function is irreversible, it is necessary to perform dialysis chronically to maintain life. Because dialysis cannot maintain completely normal body fluid composition and cannot replace all the multiple functions performed by the kidneys, the health of patients maintained with use of artificial kidneys usually remains significantly impaired.

Basic Principles of Dialysis. The basic principle of the artificial kidney is to pass blood through minute blood channels bounded by a thin membrane. On the other side of the membrane is a *dialyzing fluid* into which unwanted substances in the blood pass by diffusion.

Figure 84-4 shows the components of one type of artificial kidney in which blood flows continually between two thin membranes of cellophane; outside the membrane is a dialyzing fluid. The cellophane is porous enough to allow the constituents of the plasma, except the plasma proteins, to diffuse in both directions—from plasma into the dialyzing fluid or from the dialyzing fluid back into the plasma. If the concentration of a substance is greater in the plasma than in the dialyzing fluid, there will be a *net* transfer of the substance from the plasma into the dialyzing fluid.

The rate of movement of solute across the dialyzing membrane depends on (1) the concentration gradient of the solute between the two solutions, (2) the permeability of the membrane to the solute, (3) the surface area of the membrane, and (4) the length of time that the blood and fluid remain in contact with the membrane.

Thus, the maximum rate of solute transfer occurs initially when the concentration gradient is greatest (when dialysis is begun) and slows down as the concentration gradient is dissipated. In a flowing system, as is the case with "hemodialysis," in which blood and dialysate fluid flow through the artificial kidney, the dissipation of the concentration gradient can be reduced and diffusion of solute across the membrane can be optimized by increasing the flow rate of the blood, the dialyzing fluid, or both.

In normal operation of the artificial kidney, blood flows continually or intermittently back into the vein. The total amount of blood in the artificial kidney at any one time is usually less than 500 mL, the rate of flow may be several hundred milliliters per minute, and the total diffusion surface area is between 0.6 and 2.5 m^2. To prevent coagulation of the blood in the artificial kidney, a small amount of heparin is infused into the blood as it enters the artificial kidney. In addition to diffusion of solutes, mass transfer of solutes and water can be produced by applying a hydrostatic pressure to force the fluid and solutes across the membranes of the dialyzer; such filtration is called *bulk flow* or *hemofiltration*.

Dialyzing Fluid. Table 84-4 compares the constituents in a typical dialyzing fluid with those in normal plasma and uremic plasma. Note that the concentrations of ions and other substances in dialyzing fluid are not the same as those in normal plasma or in uremic plasma. Instead, they are adjusted to levels that are needed to cause appropriate movement of water and solutes through the membrane during dialysis.

Note that there is no phosphate, urea, urate, sulfate, or creatinine in the dialyzing fluid; however, these substances are present in high concentrations in the uremic blood. Therefore, when a uremic patient undergoes dialysis, these substances are lost in large quantities into the dialyzing fluid.

The effectiveness of the artificial kidney can be expressed in terms of the amount of plasma that is cleared of different substances each minute, which, as discussed in Chapter 77, is the primary means for expressing the functional effectiveness of the kidneys themselves to rid the body of unwanted substances. Most artificial kidneys can clear urea from the plasma

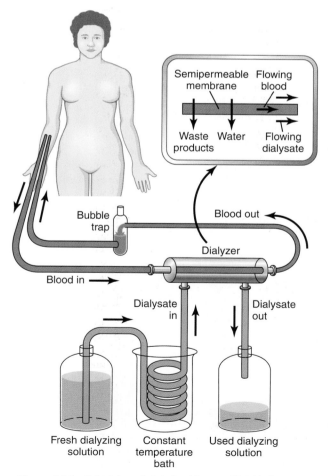

Figure 84-4 Principles of dialysis with an artificial kidney.

TABLE 84-4	Comparison of Dialyzing Fluid With Normal and Uremic Plasma		
Constituent	**Normal Plasma**	**Dialyzing Fluid**	**Uremic Plasma**
Electrolytes (mEq/L)			
Na$^+$	142	133	142
K$^+$	5	1	7
Ca^{++}	3	3	2
Mg^{++}	1.5	1.5	1.5
Cl$^-$	107	105	107
HCO$_3^-$	24	35.7	14
Lactate$^-$	1.2	1.2	1.2
HPO$_4$	3	0	9
Urate$^-$	0.3	0	2
Sulfate$^-$	0.5	0	3
Nonelectrolytes			
Glucose	100	125	100
Urea	26	0	200
Creatinine	1	0	6

at a rate of 100–225 mL/min, which shows that at least for the excretion of urea the artificial kidney can function about twice as rapidly as two normal kidneys together, whose urea clearance is only 70 mL/min. Yet the artificial kidney is used for only 4–6 hours per day, three times a week. Therefore, the overall plasma clearance is still considerably limited when the artificial kidney replaces the normal kidneys. Also, it is important to keep in mind that the artificial kidney cannot replace some of the other functions of the kidneys, such as secretion of erythropoietin, which is necessary for red blood cell production.

BIBLIOGRAPHY

Andreoli TE (Eds.): 2004. Cecil's Essentials of Medicine, sixth ed. Saunders Elsevier, Philadelphia.

Calhoun DA, Jones D, Textor S, et al: 2008. Resistant hypertension: diagnosis, evaluation, and treatment: a scientific statement from the American Heart Association Professional Education Committee of the Council for High Blood Pressure Research. Hypertension 51, 1403.

Devarajan P: Update on mechanisms of ischemic acute kidney injury, *J. Am. Soc. Nephrol.* 17:1503, 2006.

Grantham JJ: Clinical practice, autosomal dominant polycystic kidney disease, *N. Engl. J. Med.* 359:1477, 2008.

Griffin KA, Kramer H, Bidani AK: Adverse renal consequences of obesity, *Am. J. Physiol. Renal Physiol.* 294:F685, 2008.

Hall JE: The kidney, hypertension, and obesity, *Hypertension* 41:625, 2003.

Hall JE, da Silva AA, Brandon E, et al: Pathophysiology of obesity hypertension and target organ injury. In: Lip, GYP, Hall, J.E. (Eds.), Comprehensive Hypertension. Mosby Elsevier, New York, pp. 447–468.

Hall JE, Henegar JR, Dwyer TM, et al: Is obesity a major cause of chronic renal disease? *Adv. Ren. Replace Ther.* 11:41, 2004.

Jha V: Current status of end-stage renal disease care in South Asia, *Ethn. Dis.* 19:S27–32, 2009.

Mitch WE: Acute renal failure. In: Goldman, F., Bennett, J.C. (Eds.): Cecil Textbook of Medicine, twenty-first ed. WB Saunders, Philadelphia, pp. 567–570.

Molitoris BA: Transitioning to therapy in ischemic acute renal failure, *J. Am. Soc. Nephrol.* 14:265, 2003.

Rodriguez-Iturbe B, Musser JM: The current state of poststreptococcal glomerulonephritis, *J. Am. Soc. Nephrol.* 19:1855, 2008.

Rossier BC, Schild L: Epithelial sodium channel: Mendelian versus essential hypertension, *Hypertension* 52:595, 2008.

Sarnak MJ, Levey AS, Schoolwerth AC, et al: Kidney disease as a risk factor for development of cardiovascular disease, *Hypertension* 42:1050, 2003.

Singri N, Ahya SN, Levin ML: Acute renal failure, *JAMA* 289:747, 2003.

United States Renal Data System Available from: http://www.usrds.org/

Wilcox CS: New insights into diuretic use in patients with chronic renal disease, *J. Am. Soc. Nephrol.* 13:798, 2002.

The Endocrine System

TONY RAJ

85 Organization of the Endocrine System

The human body has two major control mechanisms, the *nervous system* and the *endocrine system*. While the *nervous system* can control and communicate rapidly with other systems, the *endocrine system* controls and communicates with the help of chemical messengers and is a much slower system. However, the effects of the endocrine system may be more prolonged and sustained.

Definition of a Hormone

The term "Hormone" is derived from a Greek word meaning "to excite or to arouse." The term was first used by Ernest Henry Starling in 1905 in his first lecture delivered to the Royal Society. Starling along with Bayliss had discovered one of the first hormones called "Secretin" in 1902.

An endocrine hormone is a chemical substance that is produced by endocrine glands or a group of endocrine cells in response to certain stimuli and carried by blood to target tissues, where they exert their physiological actions.

The *endocrine hormones* are carried by the circulatory system to cells throughout the body, including the nervous system in some cases, where they bind with receptors and initiate many cell reactions. Some endocrine hormones affect many different types of cells of the body; for example, *growth hormone* (from the anterior pituitary gland) causes growth in most parts of the body and *thyroxine* (from the thyroid gland) increases the rate of many chemical reactions in almost all the body's cells.

Coordination of Body Functions by Chemical Messengers

The multiple activities of the cells, tissues, and organs of the body are coordinated by the interplay of several types of chemical messenger systems:

1. *Neurotransmitters* are released by axon terminals of neurons into the synaptic junctions and act locally to control nerve cell functions.
2. *Endocrine hormones* are released by glands or specialized cells into the circulating blood and influence the function of target cells at another location in the body.
3. *Neuroendocrine hormones* are secreted by neurons into the circulating blood and influence the function of target cells at another location in the body.
4. *Paracrines* are secreted by cells into the extracellular fluid and affect neighboring target cells of a different type.
5. *Autocrines* are secreted by cells into the extracellular fluid and affect the function of the same cells that produced them.
6. *Cytokines* are peptides secreted by cells into the extracellular fluid and can function as autocrines, paracrines, or endocrine hormones. Examples of cytokines include the *interleukins* and other *lymphokines* that are secreted by helper cells and act on other cells of the immune system (see Chapter 25). Cytokine hormones (eg, *leptin*) produced by adipocytes are sometimes called *adipokines*.

In the next few chapters, we discuss mainly the endocrine and neuroendocrine hormone systems, keeping in mind that many of the body's chemical messenger systems interact with one another to maintain homeostasis. For example, the adrenal medullae and the pituitary gland secrete their hormones primarily in response to neural stimuli.

The multiple hormone systems play a key role in regulating almost all body functions, including metabolism, growth and development, water and electrolyte balance, reproduction, and behavior. For instance, without growth hormone, a person would be a dwarf. Without thyroxine and triiodothyronine from the thyroid gland, almost all the chemical reactions of the body would become sluggish and the person would become sluggish as well. Without insulin from the pancreas, the body's cells could use little of the food carbohydrates for energy. And without the sex hormones, sexual development and sexual functions would be absent.

PARACRINE SECRETIONS

Paracrine secretions (Figure 85-1) are those chemicals when released, exerts its effects on cells and tissues located in the neighborhood of its site of secretion; this by convention includes neurotransmitters. Paracrine hormones are dispersed by simple

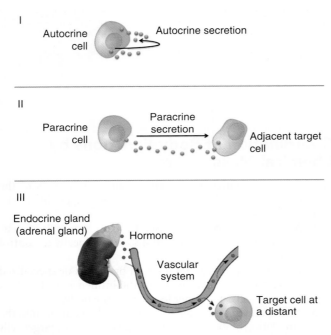

Figure 85-1   Illustration of autocrine (I), paracrine (II), and endocrine (III) secretions.

diffusion in the interstitial fluid and this restricts their action to short distances. Local enzymes in the vicinity usually rapidly inactivate the paracrine secretions thus preventing adequate entry into the blood stream.

Examples of paracrine sections include the following:

1. Histamine released from cells in the stomach mucosa has a direct influence on the parietal cells of the oxyntic glands, causing an increase in acid secretion.
2. Neurotransmitters, such as acetylcholine, act on the parietal cells in the stomach mucosa causing an increase in acid secretion.
3. Prostaglandins—PGE_2 is responsible for cervical dilatation at the time of childbirth (parturition).

AUTOCRINE SECRETIONS

Autocrine secretions are chemicals which are secreted by specific cells into the extracellular fluid surrounding the cell and which acts upon the very cells that secrete it (Figure 85-1).

Examples of autocrine secretions are as follows:

1. Norepinephrine that is released by neurons in the adrenal medulla further inhibits norepinephrine release by those cells.
2. Insulin released from β cells in the pancreas has an inhibitory effect on insulin secreted by these β cells, which is independent of glucose levels in the blood.

LOCATION OF MAJOR ENDOCRINE ORGANS

Figure 85-2 shows the anatomical loci of the major endocrine glands and endocrine tissues of the body, except for the placenta, which is an additional source of the sex hormones. Table 85-1 provides an overview of the different hormone systems and their most important actions.

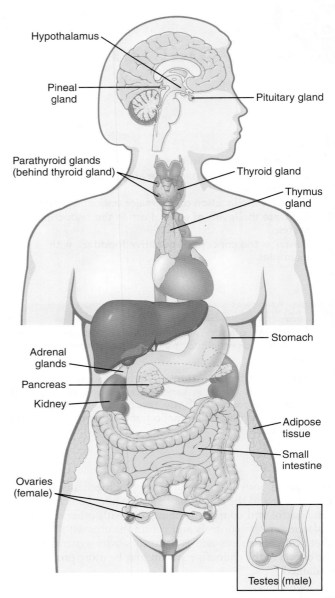

Figure 85-2   Anatomical loci of the principal endocrine glands and tissues of the body.

Feedback Control of Hormone Secretion

LEVELS OF CONTROL WITHIN THE ENDOCRINE SYSTEM

Although the plasma concentrations of many hormones fluctuate in response to various stimuli that occur throughout the day, all hormones studied thus far appear to be closely controlled.

There are several control mechanisms that exist to regulate the levels of hormones very precisely.

An example to review is the hypophysiotrophic hormones with a three-level sequence to understand the different levels of hormonal control.

TABLE 85-1	Endocrine Glands, Hormones, and Their Functions and Structure		
Gland/Tissue	**Hormones**	**Major Functions**	**Chemical Structure**
Hypothalamus (Chapter 87)	Thyrotropin-releasing hormone (TRH)	Stimulates secretion of thyroid-stimulating hormone (TSH) and prolactin	Peptide
	Corticotropin-releasing hormone (CRH)	Causes release of adrenocorticotropic hormone (ACTH)	Peptide
	Growth hormone-releasing hormone (GHRH)	Causes release of growth hormone	Peptide
	Growth hormone-inhibitory hormone (GHIH) (somatostatin)	Inhibits release of growth hormone	Peptide
	Gonadotropin-releasing hormone (GnRH)	Causes release of luteinizing hormone (LH) and follicle-stimulating hormone (FSH)	Peptide
	Dopamine or prolactin-inhibiting factor (PIF)	Inhibits release of prolactin	Amine
Anterior pituitary (Chapter 87)	Growth hormone	Stimulates protein synthesis and overall growth of most cells and tissues	Peptide
	TSH	Stimulates synthesis and secretion of thyroid hormones (thyroxine and triiodothyronine)	Peptide
	ACTH	Stimulates synthesis and secretion of adrenocortical hormones (cortisol, androgens, and aldosterone)	Peptide
	Prolactin	Promotes development of the female breasts and secretion of milk	Peptide
	FSH	Causes growth of follicles in the ovaries and sperm maturation in Sertoli cells of testes	Peptide
	LH	Stimulates testosterone synthesis in Leydig cells of testes; stimulates ovulation, formation of corpus luteum, and estrogen and progesterone synthesis in ovaries	Peptide
Posterior pituitary (Chapter 88)	Antidiuretic hormone (ADH) (also called *vasopressin*)	Increases water reabsorption by the kidneys and causes vasoconstriction and increased blood pressure	Peptide
	Oxytocin	Stimulates milk ejection from breasts and uterine contractions	Peptide
Thyroid (Chapter 89)	Thyroxine (T_4) and triiodothyronine (T_3)	Increases the rates of chemical reactions in most cells, thus increasing body metabolic rate	Amine
	Calcitonin	Promotes deposition of calcium in the bones and decreases extracellular fluid calcium ion concentration	Peptide
Adrenal cortex (Chapter 91)	Cortisol	Has multiple metabolic functions for controlling metabolism of proteins, carbohydrates, and fats; also has antiinflammatory effects	Steroid
	Aldosterone	Increases renal sodium reabsorption, potassium secretion, and hydrogen ion secretion	Steroid
Adrenal medulla (Chapter 92)	Norepinephrine, epinephrine	Same effects as sympathetic stimulation	Amine
Pancreas (Chapter 93)	Insulin (β cells)	Promotes glucose entry in many cells, and in this way controls carbohydrate metabolism	Peptide
	Glucagon (α cells)	Increases synthesis and release of glucose from the liver into the body fluids	Peptide
Parathyroid (Chapter 90)	Parathyroid hormone (PTH)	Controls serum calcium ion concentration by increasing calcium absorption by the gut and kidneys and releasing calcium from bones	Peptide
Testes (Chapter 94)	Testosterone	Promotes development of male reproductive system and male secondary sexual characteristics	Steroid
Ovaries (Chapter 96)	Estrogens	Promotes growth and development of female reproductive system, female breasts, and female secondary sexual characteristics	Steroid
	Progesterone	Stimulates secretion of "uterine milk" by the uterine endometrial glands and promotes development of secretory apparatus of breasts	Steroid

(Continued)

TABLE 85-1	Endocrine Glands, Hormones, and Their Functions and Structure (*cont.*)		
Gland/Tissue	**Hormones**	**Major Functions**	**Chemical Structure**
Placenta (Chapter 98)	Human chorionic gonadotropin (HCG)	Promotes growth of corpus luteum and secretion of estrogens and progesterone by corpus luteum	Peptide
	Human somatomammotropin	Probably helps promote development of some fetal tissues as well as the mother's breasts	Peptide
	Estrogens	See actions of estrogens from ovaries	Steroid
	Progesterone	See actions of progesterone from ovaries	Steroid
Kidney (Chapter 76)	Renin	Catalyzes conversion of angiotensinogen to angiotensin I (acts as an enzyme)	Peptide
	1,25-Dihydroxycholecalciferol	Increases intestinal absorption of calcium and bone mineralization	Steroid
	Erythropoietin	Increases erythrocyte production	Peptide
Heart (Chapter 51)	Atrial natriuretic peptide (ANP)	Increases sodium excretion by kidneys, reduces blood pressure	Peptide
Stomach (Chapter 67)	Gastrin	Stimulates HCl secretion by parietal cells	Peptide
Small intestine (Chapter 68)	Secretin	Stimulates pancreatic acinar cells to release bicarbonate and water	Peptide
	Cholecystokinin (CCK)	Stimulates gallbladder contraction and release of pancreatic enzymes	Peptide
Adipocytes	Leptin	Inhibits appetite, stimulates thermogenesis	Peptide

There are three levels of feedback control as indicated in Figure 85-3; these are as follows:

1. *Long loop feedback control*: In this case, the hormone secreted by the peripheral endocrine gland provides a negative feedback to the hypothalamus or the anterior pituitary gland. For example, excess levels of thyroxine will inhibit both the anterior pituitary gland from secreting thyroid stimulating hormone (TSH) and the hypothalamus from secreting thyrotropin releasing hormone.
2. *Short loop feedback control*: In this mechanism, the anterior pituitary hormone in plasma provides a negative feedback to the hypothalamus, decreasing the secretion of releasing hormones.
3. *Ultrashort loop feedback control:* In this mechanism, the releasing hormones themselves have a negative feedback influence on the hypothalamus thus decreasing the secretion of the hypothalamic hormones.

NEGATIVE FEEDBACK PREVENTS OVERACTIVITY OF HORMONE SYSTEMS

In most instances, hormonal control is exerted through *negative feedback mechanisms* (described in Chapter 1) that ensure a proper level of hormone activity at the target tissue. After a stimulus causes release of the hormone, conditions or products resulting from the action of the hormone tend to suppress its further release. In other words, the hormone (or one of its products) has a negative feedback effect to prevent oversecretion of the hormone or overactivity at the target tissue.

The controlled variable is sometimes not the secretory rate of the hormone but the degree of activity of the target tissue. Therefore, only when the target tissue activity rises to an appropriate level will feedback signals to the endocrine gland become powerful enough to slow further secretion of the hormone. Feedback regulation of hormones can occur at all levels, including gene transcription and translation steps involved in

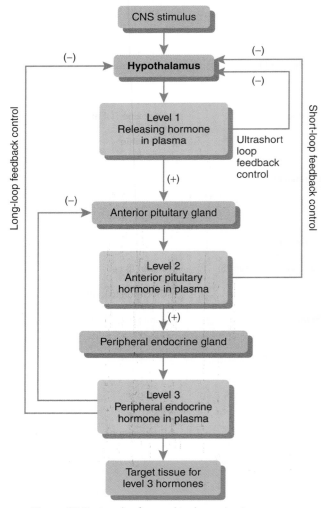

Figure 85-3 Levels of control in the endocrine system.

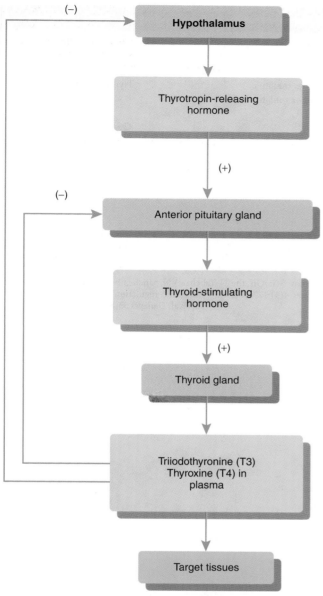

Figure 85-4 Example of negative feedback inhibition.

the synthesis of hormones and steps involved in processing hormones or releasing stored hormones.

Examples of negative feedback mechanisms:

1. Negative feedback by plasma levels of thyroid hormones on the hypothalamus and the anterior pituitary gland (Figure 85-4).
2. Negative feedback by plasma cortisol levels on the hypothalamus and the anterior pituitary gland.

SURGES OF HORMONES CAN OCCUR WITH POSITIVE FEEDBACK

In a few instances, *positive feedback* occurs when the biological action of the hormone causes additional secretion of the hormone. One example of positive feedback is the surge of *luteinizing hormone* (LH) that occurs as a result of the stimulatory effect of estrogen on the anterior pituitary before ovulation. The secreted LH then acts on the ovaries to stimulate additional secretion of estrogen, which in turn causes more secretion of LH. Eventually, LH reaches an appropriate concentration and typical negative feedback control of hormone secretion is then exerted.

CYCLICAL VARIATIONS OCCUR IN HORMONE RELEASE

Superimposed on the negative and positive feedback control of hormone secretion are periodic variations in hormone release that are influenced by seasonal changes, various stages of development and aging, the diurnal (daily) cycle, and sleep. For example, the secretion of growth hormone is markedly increased during the early period of sleep but is reduced during the later stages of sleep. In many cases, these cyclical variations in hormone secretion are due to changes in activity of neural pathways involved in controlling hormone release.

CLINICAL CONDITIONS ASSOCIATED WITH ALTERED HORMONE RELEASE

Various clinical conditions can manifest if the secretion of hormones is altered either due to hyposecretion or hypersecretion. Table 85-2 summarizes the various clinical conditions associated with each endocrine gland.

TABLE 85-2	Clinical Conditions Associated with Hyposecretion and Hypersecretion of Each Endocrine Gland		
S. No.	Endocrine Gland and Hormones	Clinical Conditions Hyposecretion	Clinical Conditions Hypersecretion
1.	Anterior pituitary gland		
	• Growth hormone	Pituitary dwarfism	Gigantism in children
	• All hormones	Panhypopituitarism	Acromegaly in adults
	Posterior pituitary gland		
	• Antidiuretic hormone	Diabetes insipidus	
2.	Thyroid gland	Cretinism in children Myxedema in adults	Graves' disease
3.	Parathyroid gland	Hypoparathyroidism	Hyperparathyroidism

(Continued)

TABLE 85-2	Clinical Conditions Associated with Hyposecretion and Hypersecretion of Each Endocrine Gland (*cont.*)		
S. No.	**Endocrine Gland and Hormones**	**Clinical Conditions Hyposecretion**	**Clinical Conditions Hypersecretion**
4.	Pancreas		
	• Insulin	Type I Diabetes mellitus	Hyperinsulinism
		Type II Diabetes mellitus	
5.	Adrenal gland		
	• Glucocorticoid		Cushing's syndrome
	• Mineralocorticoids and glucocorticoids	Addison's disease	Pheochromocytoma
	• Epinephrine and norepinephrine		

BIBLIOGRAPHY

Aranda A, Pascual A: Nuclear hormone receptors and gene expression, *Physiol. Rev.* 81:1269, 2001.

Evans RM, Mangelsdorf DJ: Nuclear receptors, RXR, and the Big Bang, *Cell* 157:255, 2014.

Henderson J: Ernest Starling and 'hormones': an historical commentary, *J. Endocrinol.* 184:5-10, 2005.

Imai Y, Youn MY, Inoue K, et al: Nuclear receptors in bone physiology and diseases, *Physiol. Rev.* 93:481, 2013.

Rebelakou EP, Tsiamis C, Marketos SG: On the centenary of the term, *Hormones* 4(3):177-179, 2005.

Starling EH: The chemical correlation of the functions of the body, Lecture I, *The Lancet* 2:339-341, 1905.

Tabelros VN, Sanchez-Soto MC, Garcia S, Hiriart M: Autocrine regulation of single pancreatic β-cell survival, *Diabetes* 53(8):2018-2023, 2004.

Hormone–Receptor Interactions

Chemical Structure and Synthesis of Hormones

Hormones can be classified based on their origin or by their chemical structure. Table 85-1 in the previous chapter lists the various hormones based on their site of origin. In the section, the chemical classification of hormones is described (Table 86-1).

Three general classes of hormones exist:

1. *Proteins and polypeptides,* including hormones secreted by the anterior and posterior pituitary gland, the pancreas (insulin and glucagon), the parathyroid gland (parathyroid hormone), and many others (Table 85-1).
2. *Steroids* secreted by the adrenal cortex (cortisol and aldosterone), the ovaries (estrogen and progesterone), the testes (testosterone), and the placenta (estrogen and progesterone).
3. *Derivatives of the amino acid tyrosine,* secreted by the thyroid (thyroxine and triiodothyronine) and the adrenal medullae (epinephrine and norepinephrine).

Polypeptide and Protein Hormones Are Stored in Secretory Vesicles Until Needed. Most of the hormones in the body are polypeptides and proteins. These hormones range in size from small peptides with as few as three amino acids (thyrotropin-releasing hormone) to proteins with almost 200 amino acids (growth hormone and prolactin). In general, polypeptides with 100 or more amino acids are called *proteins,* and those with fewer than 100 amino acids are referred to as *peptides.*

Protein and peptide hormones are synthesized in the same fashion as most other proteins (Figure 86-1).

Steps in the synthesis of protein or peptide hormones are as follows:

1. First synthesized as large biologically inactive proteins *(preprohormones).*
2. Cleaved to form smaller *prohormones* in the endoplasmic reticulum.
3. Then transferred to the Golgi apparatus for packaging into secretory vesicles.
4. Enzymes in the vesicles cleave the prohormones to produce smaller, biologically active hormones and inactive fragments.
5. The vesicles are stored within the cytoplasm, until their secretion is needed.

Secretion of the hormones (as well as the inactive fragments) into the interstitial fluid or directly into the blood stream occurs by *exocytosis.*

In many cases, the stimulus for exocytosis is increased cytosolic calcium concentration caused by depolarization of the plasma membrane. In other instances, stimulation of an endocrine cell surface receptor causes increased cyclic adenosine monophosphate (cAMP) and subsequently activation of protein kinases that initiate secretion of the hormone. The peptide hormones are water soluble, allowing them to enter the circulatory system easily, where they are carried to their target tissues.

Steroid Hormones Are Usually Synthesized From Cholesterol and Are Not Stored. The chemical structure of steroid hormones is similar to that of cholesterol, and in most instances hormones are synthesized from cholesterol. They are lipid soluble and are structurally related to cholesterol (Figure 86-2).

Although there is usually very little hormone storage in steroid-producing endocrine cells, large stores of cholesterol esters in cytoplasm vacuoles can be rapidly mobilized for steroid synthesis after a stimulus. Much of the cholesterol in steroid-producing cells comes from the plasma, but there is also de novo synthesis of cholesterol in steroid-producing cells. Because they are highly lipid soluble, they can simply diffuse across the cell membrane when synthesized and enter the interstitial fluid and then the blood.

Amine Hormones Are Derived From Tyrosine. The two groups of hormones derived from tyrosine are as follows:

1. The thyroid hormones and
2. The adrenal medullary hormones (catecholamines).

TABLE 86-1	Classification of Hormones Based on Chemical Structure	
No.	**Chemical Class**	**Hormones (Examples)**
1.	Proteins and polypeptides	• Anterior pituitary hormones • Posterior pituitary hormones • Insulin • Glucagon • Parathyroid hormones
2.	Steroids	• Cortisol • Aldosterone • Estrogen • Progesterone • Testosterone • Placental estrogen and progesterone
3.	Derivatives of amino acid tyrosine	• Thyroxine • Triiodothyronine • Epinephrine • Norepinephrine

The thyroid hormones are synthesized and stored in the thyroid gland and incorporated into macromolecules of the protein *thyroglobulin* and is stored in large follicles until secretion. After entering the blood, most of the thyroid hormones combine with plasma proteins, especially *thyroxine-binding globulin*, which slowly releases the hormones to the target tissues.

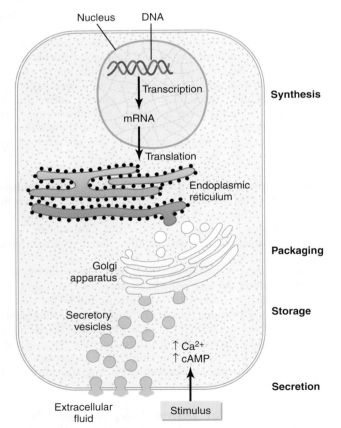

Figure 86-1 Synthesis and secretion of peptide hormones. The stimulus for hormone secretion often involves changes in intracellular calcium or changes in cyclic adenosine monophosphate (cAMP) in the cell.

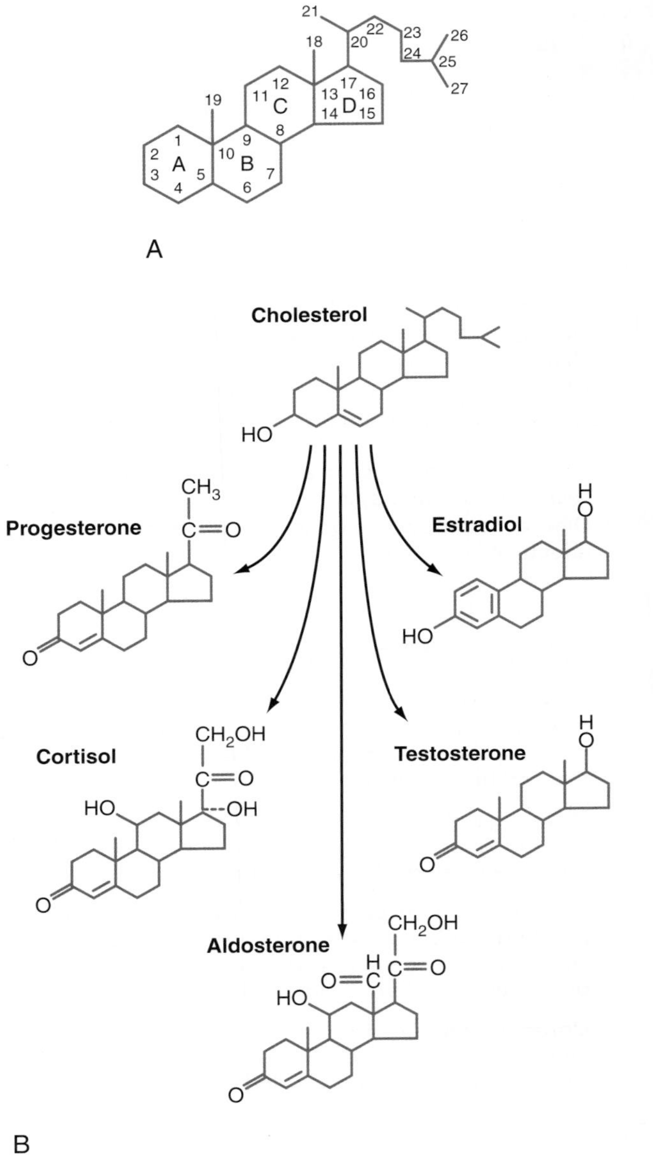

Figure 86-2 (A) Structure of cholesterol, the precursor of steroid hormones (B) Chemical structures of several steroid hormones. (*Source: Figure 37-8 A, B from Chapter 37 Introduction to Endocrinology, Page 659, 6th Ed Berne & Levy Physiology.*)

Epinephrine and norepinephrine are formed in the adrenal medulla. Catecholamines are taken up into preformed vesicles and stored until secreted and released by exocytosis. Once the catecholamines enter the circulation, they can exist in the plasma in free form or in conjugation with other substances.

Hormone Secretion, Transport, and Clearance From the Blood

Hormone Secretion After a Stimulus and Duration of Action of Different Hormones. Some hormones, such as norepinephrine and epinephrine, are secreted within seconds after the gland is stimulated, and may develop full action within another few seconds to minutes; the actions of other hormones, such as thyroxine or growth hormone, may require months for full effect. Thus, each of the different hormones has its own characteristic onset and duration of action—each tailored to perform its specific control function.

Concentrations of Hormones in the Circulating Blood, and Hormonal Secretion Rates. The concentrations of hormones required to control most metabolic and endocrine functions are incredibly small. Their concentrations in the blood range from as little as 1 pg (which is one millionth of one millionth of a gram) in each milliliter of blood up to at most a few micrograms (a few millionths of a gram) per milliliter of blood. Similarly, the rates of secretion of the various hormones are extremely small, usually measured in micrograms or milligrams per day.

TRANSPORT OF HORMONES IN THE BLOOD

Water-Soluble Hormones
- *Peptides* and *Catecholamines* are dissolved in the plasma.
- They are transported from their sites of synthesis to target tissues.
- There they diffuse out of the capillaries into the interstitial fluid and ultimately to target cells.

Steroid and Thyroid Hormones
- These hormones, in contrast, circulate in the blood mainly bound to plasma proteins.
- Usually less than 10% of steroid or thyroid hormones in the plasma exist free in solution (eg, more than 99% of the thyroxine in the blood is bound to plasma proteins).
- However, protein-bound hormones cannot easily diffuse across the capillaries and gain access to their target cells and are therefore biologically inactive until they dissociate from plasma proteins.
- The relatively large amounts of hormones bound to proteins serve as reservoirs, replenishing the concentration of free hormones when they are bound to target receptors or lost from the circulation. Binding of hormones to plasma proteins greatly slows their clearance from the plasma.

"CLEARANCE" OF HORMONES FROM THE BLOOD

Two factors can increase or decrease the concentration of a hormone in the blood.
1. The rate of hormone secretion into the blood.
2. The rate of removal of the hormone from the blood (*metabolic clearance rate*).

Metabolic Clearance Rate. This is usually expressed in terms of the number of milliliters of plasma cleared of the hormone per minute. To calculate this clearance rate, one measures (1) the rate of disappearance of the hormone from the plasma (eg, nanograms per minute) and (2) the plasma concentration of the hormone (eg, nanograms per milliliter of plasma). Then, the metabolic clearance rate is calculated by the following formula:

$$\text{Metabolic clearance rate} = \text{Rate of disappearance of hormone from the plasma}/\text{Concentration of hormone}$$

Hormones are "cleared" from the plasma in several ways, including (1) metabolic destruction by the tissues, (2) binding with the tissues, (3) excretion by the liver into the bile, and (4) excretion by the kidneys into the urine. For certain hormones, a decreased metabolic clearance rate may cause an excessively

high concentration of the hormone in the circulating body fluids. For example, when the liver is diseased, the steroid hormone levels increase because these hormones are conjugated mainly in the liver and then "cleared" into the bile.

Most of the peptide hormones and catecholamines are water soluble and circulate freely in the blood. They are usually degraded by enzymes in the blood and tissues, and rapidly excreted by the kidneys and liver, thus remaining in the blood for only a short time. For example, the half-life of angiotensin II circulating in the blood is less than a minute.

Mechanisms of Action of Hormones

HORMONE RECEPTORS AND THEIR ACTIVATION

The first step of a hormone's action is to bind to specific *receptors* at the target cell. Cells that lack receptors for the hormones do not respond. When the hormone combines with its receptor, this action usually initiates a cascade of reactions in the cell, with each stage becoming more powerfully activated so that even small concentrations of the hormone can have a large effect.

Hormone receptors are large proteins and each cell that is to be stimulated usually has some 2000 to 100,000 receptors. Also, each receptor is usually highly specific for a single hormone, which determines the type of hormone that will act on a particular tissue. The target tissues that are affected by a hormone are those that contain its specific receptors.

Hormone receptors have been classified on the basis of location in Box 86-1.

HORMONE-RECEPTOR INTERACTIONS

The Number and Sensitivity of Hormone Receptors Are Regulated. The number of receptors in a target cell usually does not remain constant from day to day, or even from minute to minute. Receptor proteins are often inactivated or destroyed during the course of their function, and at other times they are reactivated or new ones are manufactured by the cell. For instance, increased hormone concentration and increased binding with its target cell receptors sometimes cause the number of active receptors to decrease.

Downregulation of Receptors. The decrease in the number of receptors in response to a high concentration of circulating hormone is referred to as *downregulation* (Figure 86-3).

Downregulation of the receptors can occur as a result of
1. inactivation of some of the receptor molecules;
2. inactivation of some of the intracellular protein signaling molecules;

BOX 86-1 CLASSIFICATION OF HORMONE RECEPTORS

The locations for the different types of hormone receptors are generally the following:
1. *In or on the surface of the cell membrane.* The membrane receptors are specific mostly for the protein, peptide, and catecholamine hormones.
2. *In the cell cytoplasm.* The primary receptors for the different steroid hormones are found mainly in the cytoplasm.
3. *In the cell nucleus.* The receptors for the thyroid hormones are found in the nucleus and are believed to be located in direct association with one or more of the chromosomes.

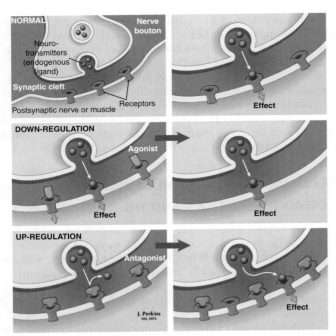

Figure 86-3 Upregulation and downregulation of receptors. (Source: *Netter illustration from www.netterimages.com. © Elsevier Inc. All rights reserved.*)

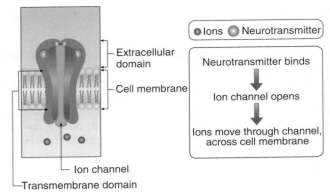

Figure 86-4 Ion channel-linked receptors and their mechanism of action.

3. temporary sequestration of the receptor to the inside of the cell, away from the site of action of hormones that interact with cell membrane receptors;
4. destruction of the receptors by lysosomes after they are internalized; or
5. decreased production of the receptors.

In each case, receptor downregulation decreases the target tissue's responsiveness to the hormone.

Upregulation of Receptors. An increase in the hormone receptor number as a consequence of a sustained low exposure to a particular hormone is called upregulation.

Some hormones cause upregulation of receptors and intracellular signaling proteins; that is, the stimulating hormone induces greater than normal formation of receptor or intracellular signaling molecules by the target cell, or greater availability of the receptor for interaction with the hormone. When upregulation occurs, the target tissue becomes progressively more sensitive to the stimulating effects of the hormone.

INTRACELLULAR SIGNALING AFTER HORMONE RECEPTOR ACTIVATION

Almost without exception, a hormone affects its target tissues by first forming a hormone–receptor complex. Formation of this complex alters the function of the receptor and the activated receptor initiates the hormonal effects. The various mechanisms of hormone–receptor interactions are listed and explained as follows:

1. Ion channel-linked receptors
2. G protein-linked hormone receptors
3. Enzyme-linked hormone receptors
4. Intracellular hormone receptors

Ion Channel-Linked Receptors. Virtually all the neurotransmitter substances, such as acetylcholine and norepinephrine, combine with receptors in the postsynaptic membrane

(Figure 86-4). This combination almost always causes a change in the structure of the receptor, usually opening or closing a channel for one or more ions. Some of these *ion channel-linked receptors* open (or close) channels for sodium ions, others for potassium ions, others for calcium ions, and so forth. The altered movement of these ions through the channels causes the subsequent effects on the postsynaptic cells.

G Protein-Linked Hormone Receptors. Many hormones activate receptors that indirectly regulate the activity of target proteins (eg, enzymes or ion channels) by coupling with groups of cell membrane proteins called *heterotrimeric guanosine triphosphate (GTP)-binding proteins (G proteins)* (Figure 86-5). There are over 1000 known G protein-coupled receptors, all have seven transmembrane segments that loop in and out of the cell membrane. Some parts of the receptor that protrude into the cell cytoplasm (especially the cytoplasmic tail of the receptor) are coupled to G proteins that include three (ie, trimeric) parts—the α, β, and γ subunits.

When the ligand (hormone) binds to the extracellular part of the receptor, a conformational change occurs in the receptor that activates the G proteins and induces intracellular signals that either:

1. open or close cell membrane ion channels or
2. change the activity of an enzyme in the cytoplasm of the cell or
3. activate gene transcription.

The trimeric G proteins are named for their ability to bind *guanosine nucleotides*. In their inactive state, the α, β, and γ subunits of G proteins form a complex that binds *guanosine diphosphate* (GDP) on the α subunit. When the receptor is activated, it undergoes a conformational change that causes the GDP-bound trimeric G protein to associate with the cytoplasmic part of the receptor and to exchange GDP for GTP. Displacement of GDP by GTP causes the α subunit to dissociate from the trimeric complex and to associate with other intracellular signaling proteins; these proteins, in turn, alter the activity of ion channels or intracellular enzymes, such as *adenylyl cyclase* or *phospholipase C*, which alter cell function.

The signaling event is terminated when the hormone is removed and the α subunit inactivates itself by converting its bound GTP to GDP; then the α subunit once again combines with the β and γ subunits to form an inactive, membrane-bound trimeric G protein.

Some hormones are coupled to *inhibitory G proteins* (denoted as G_i proteins), whereas others are coupled to *stimulatory*

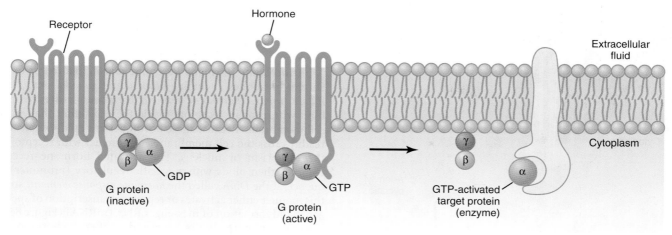

Figure 86-5 Mechanism of activation of a G protein-coupled receptor. When the hormone activates the receptor, the inactive α, β, and γ G protein complex associates with the receptor and is activated, with an exchange of guanosine triphosphate *(GTP)* for guanosine diphosphate *(GDP)*. This causes the α subunit (to which the GTP is bound) to dissociate from the β and γ subunits of the G protein and to interact with membrane-bound target proteins (enzymes) that initiate intracellular signals.

G proteins (denoted G_s proteins). Thus, depending on the coupling of a hormone receptor to an inhibitory or stimulatory G protein, a hormone can either increase or decrease the activity of intracellular enzymes.

Enzyme-Linked Hormone Receptors. Some receptors, when activated, function directly as enzymes or are closely associated with enzymes that they activate. These *enzyme-linked receptors* are proteins that pass through the membrane only once, in contrast to the seven-transmembrane G protein-coupled receptors. Enzyme-linked receptors have their hormone-binding site on the outside of the cell membrane and their catalytic or enzyme-binding site on the inside. When the hormone binds to the extracellular part of the receptor, an enzyme immediately inside the cell membrane is activated (or occasionally inactivated). Although many enzyme-linked receptors have intrinsic enzyme activity, others rely on enzymes that are closely associated with the receptor to produce changes in cell function.

Table 86-2 lists a few of the many peptide growth factors, cytokines, and hormones that use the enzyme-linked receptor tyrosine kinases for cell signaling. One example of an enzyme-linked receptor is the *leptin receptor* (Figure 86-6). Leptin is a hormone secreted by fat cells and has many physiological effects, but it is especially important in regulating appetite and energy balance. The leptin receptor is a member of a large family of *cytokine receptors* that do not themselves contain enzymatic activity but signal through associated enzymes. In the case of the leptin receptor, one of the signaling pathways occurs through a *tyrosine kinase* of the *janus kinase* (JAK) family, *JAK2*. Some of the effects of leptin occur rapidly as a result of activation of

these intracellular enzymes, whereas other actions occur more slowly and require synthesis of new proteins.

Another example, one widely used in hormonal control of cell function, is for the hormone to bind with a special transmembrane receptor, which then becomes the activated enzyme *adenylyl cyclase* at the end that protrudes to the interior of the cell (Figure 86-7). This cyclase catalyzes the formation of cAMP,

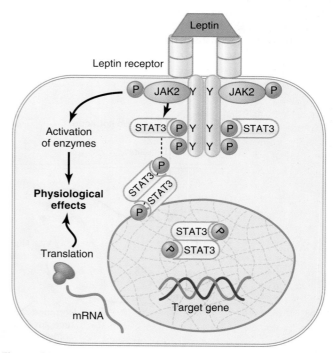

Figure 86-6 An enzyme-linked receptor—the leptin receptor. The receptor exists as a homodimer (two identical parts), and leptin binds to the extracellular part of the receptor, causing phosphorylation and activation of the intracellular associated janus kinase 2 (JAK2). This causes phosphorylation of signal transducer and activator of transcription (STAT) proteins, which then activates the transcription of target genes and the synthesis of proteins. JAK2 phosphorylation also activates several other enzyme systems that mediate some of the more rapid effects of leptin. Y, specific tyrosine phosphorylation sites.

TABLE 86-2	Hormones That Use Receptor Tyrosine Kinase Signaling

1. Fibroblast growth factor
2. Growth hormone
3. Hepatocyte growth factor
4. Insulin
5. Insulin-like growth factor-1
6. Leptin
7. Prolactin
8. Vascular endothelial growth factor

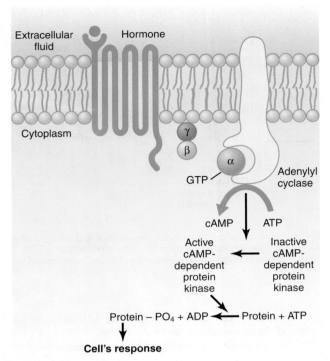

Figure 86-7 Cyclic adenosine monophosphate (cAMP) mechanism by which many hormones exert their control of cell function. Adenosine diphosphate (*ADP*), adenosine triphosphate (*ATP*).

which has a multitude of effects inside the cell to control cell activity, as discussed later. cAMP is called a *second messenger* because it is not the hormone itself that directly institutes the intracellular changes; instead, the cAMP serves as a second messenger to cause these effects.

For a few peptide hormones, such as atrial natriuretic peptide (ANP), *cyclic guanosine monophosphate* (cGMP), which is only slightly different from cAMP, serves in a similar manner as a second messenger.

Intracellular Hormone Receptors and Activation of Genes. Several hormones, including *adrenal* and *gonadal steroid hormones, thyroid hormones, retinoid hormones,* and *vitamin D,* bind with protein receptors inside the cell rather than in the cell membrane. Because these hormones are lipid soluble, they readily cross the cell membrane and interact with receptors in the cytoplasm or nucleus. The activated hormone–receptor complex then binds with a specific regulatory (promoter) sequence of the DNA called the *hormone response element,* and in this manner either activates or represses transcription of specific genes and formation of messenger RNA (mRNA) (Figure 86-8). Therefore, minutes, hours, or even days after the hormone has entered the cell, newly formed proteins appear in the cell and become the controllers of new or altered cellular functions.

Many different tissues have identical intracellular hormone receptors, but the genes that the receptors regulate are different in the various tissues. An intracellular receptor can activate a gene response only if the appropriate combination of gene regulatory proteins is present, and many of these regulatory proteins are tissue specific. Thus, the responses of different tissues to a hormone are determined not only by the specificity of the receptors but also by the expression of genes that the receptor regulates.

GENOMIC AND NONGENOMIC EFFECTS OF HORMONES

The actions of several hormones listed previously which act on receptors within the cell or nucleus causing gene transcription, target gene expression, and ultimately cellular responses are referred to as genomic effects of a hormone.

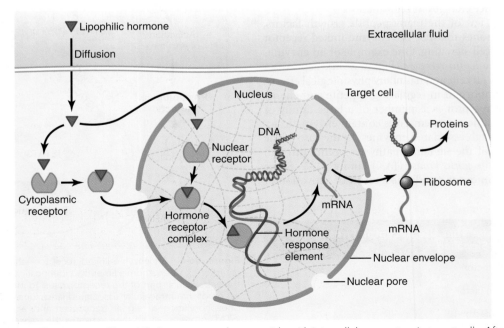

Figure 86-8 Mechanisms of interaction of lipophilic hormones, such as steroids, with intracellular receptors in target cells. After the hormone binds to the receptor in the cytoplasm or in the nucleus, the hormone–receptor complex binds to the hormone response element (promoter) on the DNA. This either activates or inhibits gene transcription, formation of messenger RNA (mRNA), and protein synthesis.

More recently, novel methods of signal transduction through steroid hormone receptors that do not involve gene transcription have been identified for several hormones. These "nongenomic" effects do not depend on gene transcription or protein synthesis. This novel mechanism involves steroid-induced modulation of cytoplasmic or cell membrane-bound regulatory proteins.

The hormones that have both genomic and nongenomic effects include estrogens, progestin, aldosterone, and androgens.

The characteristics of nongenomic effects include the following:

1. The actions are usually too rapid (seconds to minutes) to involve any changes in mRNA and protein synthesis.
2. These actions can be observed even in highly specialized cells that do not accomplish mRNA and protein synthesis (eg, spermatozoa).
3. Nongenomic effects can be elicited even by steroids coupled with high-molecular weight substances that do not pass across the plasma membrane and do not enter into the cell.
4. Nongenomic effects are not blocked by inhibitors of mRNA or protein synthesis.
5. Nongenomic effects are not blocked by antagonists of the classic, genomic steroid receptors.

SECOND MESSENGER MECHANISMS FOR MEDIATING INTRACELLULAR HORMONAL FUNCTIONS

Definition: Second messengers are molecules or substances that help communicate signals from the cell surface to specific target sites within the cell either in the cytoplasm or nucleus. Second messengers help in significantly amplifying the strength of the signals.

There are several types of second messengers and these are listed and explained in Box 86-2.

We noted earlier that one of the means by which hormones exert intracellular actions is to stimulate formation of the second messenger cAMP inside the cell membrane. The cAMP then causes subsequent intracellular effects of the hormone. Thus, the only direct effect that the hormone has on the cell is to activate a single type of membrane receptor. The second messenger does the rest.

cAMP is not the only second messenger used by the different hormones. Two other especially important ones are (1) calcium ions and associated *calmodulin* and (2) products of membrane phospholipid breakdown.

Adenylyl Cyclase–cAMP Second Messenger System

Table 86-3 shows a few of the many hormones that use the adenylyl cyclase–cAMP mechanism to stimulate their target tissues, and Figure 86-7 shows the adenylyl cyclase–cAMP second messenger system. Binding of the hormones with the

| TABLE 86-3 | Hormones That Use the Adenylyl Cyclase–cAMP Second Messenger System |

- ACTH
- Angiotensin II (epithelial cells)
- Calcitonin
- Catecholamines (β receptors)
- CRH
- FSH
- Glucagon
- HCG
- LH
- PTH
- Secretin
- Somatostatin
- TSH
- Vasopressin (V_2 receptor, epithelial cells)

ACTH, adrenocorticotropic hormone; CRH, corticotropin-releasing hormone; FSH, follicle-stimulating hormone; HCG, human chorionic gonadotropin; LH, luteinizing hormone; PTH, parathyroid hormone; TSH, thyroid-stimulating hormone.

receptor allows coupling of the receptor to a *G protein*. If the G protein stimulates the adenylyl cyclase–cAMP system, it is called a G_s *protein*, denoting a stimulatory G protein. Stimulation of adenylyl cyclase, a membrane-bound enzyme, by the G_s protein then catalyzes the conversion of a small amount of cytoplasmic *adenosine triphosphate* into cAMP inside the cell. This then activates *cAMP-dependent protein kinase*, which phosphorylates specific cell proteins, triggering biochemical reactions that ultimately lead to the cell's response to the hormone.

Once cAMP is formed inside the cell, it usually activates a *cascade of enzymes.* In this way, even the slightest amount of hormone acting on the cell surface can initiate a powerful cascading activating force for the entire cell.

If binding of the hormone to its receptors is coupled to an inhibitory G protein (denoted G_i protein), adenylyl cyclase will be inhibited, reducing formation of cAMP and ultimately leading to an inhibitory action in the cell.

Cell Membrane Phospholipid Second Messenger System

Some hormones activate transmembrane receptors that activate the enzyme *phospholipase C* attached to the inside projections of the receptors (Table 86-4). This enzyme catalyzes the breakdown of some phospholipids in the cell membrane, especially *phosphatidylinositol biphosphate* (PIP_2), into two different second messenger products:

1. *Inositol triphosphate* (IP_3) and
2. *Diacylglycerol* (DAG).

| BOX 86-2 | SECOND MESSENGERS MEDIATING HORMONAL FUNCTIONS |

1. cAMP (3′, 5′, adenosine monophosphate)
2. cGMP (Cyclic guanosine monophosphate)
3. Inositol triphosphate (IP_3)
4. Diacylglycerol (DAG)
5. Calcium ions

| TABLE 86-4 | Hormones That Use the Phospholipase C Second Messenger System |

- Angiotensin II (vascular smooth muscle)
- Catecholamines (α receptors)
- GnRH
- GHRH
- Oxytocin
- TRH
- Vasopressin (V_1 receptor, vascular smooth muscle)

GnRH, gonadotropin-releasing hormone; GHRH, growth hormone-releasing hormone; TRH, thyrotropin releasing hormone.

The IP₃ mobilizes calcium ions from mitochondria and the endoplasmic reticulum, and the calcium ions then have their own second messenger effects, such as smooth muscle contraction and changes in cell secretion.

DAG, the other lipid second messenger, activates the enzyme *protein kinase C*, which then phosphorylates a large number of proteins, leading to the cell's response (Figure 86-9). In addition to these effects, the lipid portion of DAG is *arachidonic acid,* which is the precursor for the *prostaglandins* and other local hormones that cause multiple effects in tissues throughout the body.

Calcium–Calmodulin Second Messenger System

Another second messenger system operates in response to the entry of calcium into the cells. Calcium entry may be initiated by (1) changes in membrane potential that open calcium channels or (2) a hormone interacting with membrane receptors that open calcium channels (Figure 86-10).

Upon entering a cell, calcium ions bind with the protein *calmodulin.* The calmodulin changes its shape and initiates multiple effects inside the cell, including activation or inhibition of protein kinases. Activation of calmodulin-dependent protein kinases causes, via phosphorylation, activation or inhibition of proteins involved in the cell's response to the hormone. For example, one specific function of calmodulin is to activate *myosin light chain kinase,* which acts directly on the myosin of smooth muscle to cause smooth muscle contraction.

The normal calcium ion concentration in most cells of the body is 10^{-8} to 10^{-7} mol/L, which is not enough to activate the calmodulin system. But when the calcium ion concentration

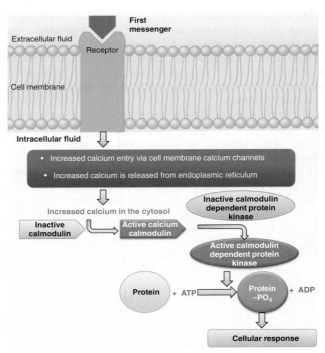

Figure 86-10   Calcium–calmodulin second messenger system. *Modified from Vander's Human Physiology, tenth ed. McGraw Hill, p. 146.*

rises to 10^{-6} to 10^{-5} mol/L, enough binding occurs to cause all the intracellular actions of calmodulin.

HORMONES THAT ACT MAINLY ON THE GENETIC MACHINERY OF THE CELL

Steroid Hormones Increase Protein Synthesis

Another means by which hormones act especially, the steroid hormones, is to cause synthesis of proteins in the target cells. These proteins then function as enzymes, transport proteins, or structural proteins, which in turn provide other functions of the cells.

The sequence of events in steroid function is essentially the following:

1. The steroid hormone diffuses across the cell membrane and enters the cytoplasm of the cell, where it binds with a specific *receptor protein.*
2. The combined receptor protein–hormone then diffuses into or is transported into the nucleus.
3. The combination binds at specific points on the DNA strands in the chromosomes, which activates the transcription process of specific genes to form mRNA.
4. The mRNA diffuses into the cytoplasm, where it promotes the translation process at the ribosomes to form new proteins.

To give an example, *aldosterone,* one of the hormones secreted by the adrenal cortex, enters the cytoplasm of renal tubular cells, which contain a specific receptor protein often called the *mineralocorticoid receptor.* After about 45 minutes, proteins begin to appear in the renal tubular cells and promote sodium reabsorption from the tubules and potassium secretion into the tubules. Thus, the full action of the steroid hormone is characteristically delayed for at least 45 minutes—up to several hours or even days. This action is in marked contrast to the rapid actions of

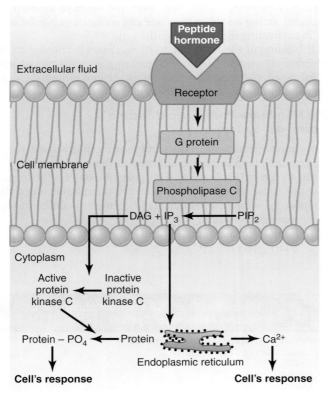

Figure 86-9   The cell membrane phospholipid second messenger system by which some hormones exert their control of cell function. Diacylglycerol *(DAG)*, inositol triphosphate *(IP₃)*, phosphatidylinositol biphosphate *(PIP₂)*.

some of the peptide and amino acid-derived hormones, such as vasopressin and norepinephrine.

Thyroid Hormones Increase Gene Transcription in the Cell Nucleus

The thyroid hormones, *thyroxine* and *triiodothyronine,* cause increased transcription by specific genes in the nucleus. To accomplish this increased transcription, these hormones first bind directly with receptor proteins in the nucleus; these receptors are *activated transcription factors* located within the chromosomal complex, and they control the function of the gene promoters.

The following two features of thyroid hormone function in the nucleus are important:

1. They activate the genetic mechanisms for the formation of many types of intracellular proteins—probably 100 or more. Many of these intracellular proteins are enzymes that promote enhanced intracellular metabolic activity in virtually all cells of the body.
2. Once bound to the intranuclear receptors, the thyroid hormones can continue to express their control functions for days or even weeks.

Measurement of Hormone Concentrations in the Blood

Most hormones are present in the blood in extremely minute quantities; some concentrations are as low as one billionth of a milligram (1 pg) per milliliter. Therefore, it was difficult to measure these concentrations by the usual chemical means. However, an extremely sensitive method, that was developed about 50 years ago revolutionized the measurement of hormones, their precursors, and their metabolic end products. This method is called *radioimmunoassay.* More recently, additional methods, such as *enzyme-linked immunosorbent assays (ELISAs),* have been developed for accurate, high-throughput measurements of hormones.

RADIOIMMUNOASSAY

The method of performing radioimmunoassay is as follows. First, an antibody that is highly specific for the hormone to be measured is produced.

Second, a small quantity of this antibody is (1) mixed with a quantity of fluid from the animal containing the hormone to be measured and (2) mixed simultaneously with an appropriate amount of purified standard hormone that has been tagged with a radioactive isotope. However, one specific condition must be met: there must be too little antibody to bind completely both the radioactively tagged hormone and the hormone in the fluid to be assayed. Therefore, the natural hormone in the assay fluid and the radioactive standard hormone *compete for the binding sites* of the antibody. In the process of competing, the quantity of each of the two hormones, the natural and the radioactive, that binds is proportional to its concentration in the assay fluid.

Third, after binding has reached equilibrium, the antibody–hormone complex is separated from the remainder of the solution, and the quantity of radioactive hormone bound in this complex is measured by radioactive counting techniques. If a large amount of radioactive hormone has bound with the antibody, it is clear that there was only a small amount of natural hormone to compete with the radioactive hormone, and therefore the concentration of the natural hormone in the assayed fluid was small and the converse is also true.

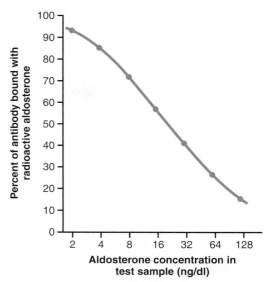

Figure 86-11 "Standard curve" for radioimmunoassay of aldosterone. *(Courtesy Dr Manis Smith.)*

Fourth, to make the assay highly quantitative, the radioimmunoassay procedure is also performed for "standard" solutions of untagged hormone at several concentration levels. Then a "standard curve" is plotted, as shown in Figure 86-11. By comparing the radioactive counts recorded from the "unknown" assay procedures with the standard curve, one can determine within an error of 10–15% the concentration of the hormone in the "unknown" assayed fluid. As little as billionths or even trillionths of a gram of hormone can often be assayed in this way.

ENZYME-LINKED IMMUNOSORBENT ASSAY

ELISAs can be used to measure almost any protein, including hormones. This test combines the specificity of antibodies with the sensitivity of simple enzyme assays. Figure 86-12 shows the

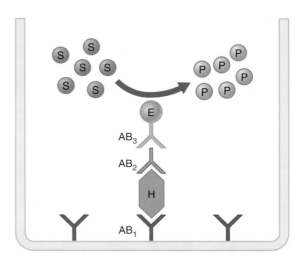

Figure 86-12 Basic principles of the enzyme-linked immunosorbent assay (ELISA) for measuring the concentration of a hormone (H). AB_1 and AB_2 are antibodies that recognize the hormone at different binding sites, and AB_3 is an antibody that recognizes AB_2. E is an enzyme linked to AB_3 that catalyzes the formation of a colored fluorescent product (P) from a substrate (S). The amount of the product is measured using optical methods and is proportional to the amount of hormone in the well if there are excess antibodies in the well.

basic elements of this method, which is often performed on plastic plates that each have 96 small wells. Each well is coated with an antibody (AB_1) that is specific for the hormone being assayed. Samples or standards are added to each of the wells, followed by a second antibody (AB_2) that is also specific for the hormone but binds to a different site of the hormone molecule. A third antibody (AB_3) that is added recognizes AB_2 and is coupled to an enzyme that converts a suitable substrate to a product that can be easily detected by colorimetric or fluorescent optical methods.

Because each molecule of enzyme catalyzes the formation of many thousands of product molecules, even small amounts of hormone molecules can be detected. In contrast to competitive radioimmunoassay methods, ELISA methods use excess antibodies so that all hormone molecules are captured in antibody–hormone complexes. Therefore, the amount of hormone present in the sample or in the standard is proportional to the amount of product formed.

The ELISA method has become widely used in clinical and research laboratories because (1) it does not use radioactive isotopes, (2) much of the assay can be automated using 96-well plates, and (3) it has proved to be a cost-effective and accurate method for assessing hormone levels.

BIBLIOGRAPHY

Aranda A, Pascual A: Nuclear hormone receptors and gene expression, *Physiol. Rev.* 81:1269, 2001.

Brent GA: Mechanisms of thyroid hormone action, *J. Clin. Invest.* 122:3035, 2012.

Chapman K, Holmes M, Seckl J: 11β-hydroxysteroid dehydrogenases: intracellular gate-keepers of tissue glucocorticoid action, *Physiol. Rev.* 93:1139, 2013.

Evans RM, Mangelsdorf DJ: Nuclear receptors, RXR, and the Big Bang, *Cell* 157:255, 2014.

Funder JW: Minireview: aldosterone and the cardiovascular system: genomic and nongenomic effects, *Endocrinology* 147:5564, 2006.

Funder JW: Minireview: aldosterone and mineralocorticoid receptors: past, present, and future, *Endocrinology* 151:5098, 2010.

Heldring N, Pike A, Andersson S, et al: Estrogen receptors: how do they signal and what are their targets? *Physiol. Rev.* 87:905, 2007.

Imai Y, Youn MY, Inoue K, et al: Nuclear receptors in bone physiology and diseases, *Physiol. Rev.* 93:481, 2013.

Morris AJ, Malbon CC: Physiological regulation of G protein-linked signaling, *Physiol. Rev.* 79:1373, 1999.

Mullur R, Liu YY, Brent GA: Thyroid hormone regulation of metabolism, *Physiol. Rev.* 94:355, 2014.

Pascual A, Aranda A: Thyroid hormone receptors, cell growth and differentiation, *Biochim. Biophys. Acta* 1830:3908, 2013.

Revelli A, Massobrio M, Tesarik J: Nongenomic actions of steroid hormones in reproductive tissues, *Endocr. Rev.* 19:3, 1998.

Rieg T, Kohan DE: Regulation of nephron water and electrolyte transport by adenylyl cyclases, *Am. J. Physiol. Renal Physiol.* 306:F701, 2014.

Sarfstein R, Werner H: Minireview: nuclear insulin and insulin-like growth factor-1 receptors: a novel paradigm in signal transduction, *Endocrinology* 154:1672, 2013.

Simoncini T, Mannella P, Fornari L, et al: Genomic and non-genomic effects of estrogens on endothelial cells, *Steroids* 69:537, 2004.

Spat A, Hunyady L: Control of aldosterone secretion: a model for convergence in cellular signaling pathways, *Physiol. Rev.* 84:489, 2004.

Tasken K, Aandahl EM: Localized effects of cAMP mediated by distinct routes of protein kinase A, *Physiol. Rev.* 84:137, 2004.

Vasudevan N, Ogawa S, Pfaff D: Estrogen and thyroid hormone receptor interactions: physiological flexibility by molecular specificity, *Physiol. Rev.* 82:923, 2002.

Wettschureck N, Offermanns S: Mammalian G proteins and their cell type specific functions, *Physiol. Rev.* 85:1159, 2005.

Yen PM: Physiological and molecular basis of thyroid hormone action, *Physiol. Rev.* 81:1097, 2001.

87

Anterior Pituitary Gland and Hypothalamus

LEARNING OBJECTIVES

- Describe the anatomy of the pituitary gland in terms of (a) location, (b) subdivisions, (c) blood supply, and (d) cell types.
- List the hypothalamic hormones involved in the control of pituitary hormone secretion.
- List the hormones secreted by the different parts of the pituitary.
- List the actions of growth hormone.
- List the factors affecting growth hormone (GH) secretion.
- List the clinical features of panhypopituitarism, acromegaly, gigantism, and dwarfism.

GLOSSARY OF TERMS

- **Adenohypophysis:** Refers to the anterior pituitary gland.
- **Neurohypophysis:** Refers to the posterior pituitary gland.
- **Hypophysial:** Derived from the Greek words where *hypo* means "under" and *phyein* means "to grow." The term pertains to the pituitary gland.
- **Acidophils:** Cells that stain strongly with acidic dyes, for example, the somatotrophs.
- **Somatotropin:** Growth hormone is also called somatotropin.

Pituitary Gland and Its Relation to the Hypothalamus

The Anterior and Posterior Lobes of the Pituitary Gland. The *pituitary gland* (Figure 87-1), also called the *hypophysis,* is a small gland—about 1 cm in diameter and 0.5–1 g in weight—that lies in the *sella turcica,* a bony cavity at the base of the brain, and is connected to the hypothalamus by the *pituitary* (or *hypophysial*) stalk. Physiologically, the pituitary gland is divisible into two distinct portions:

1. The *anterior pituitary,* also known as the *adenohypophysis.*
2. The *posterior pituitary,* also known as the *neurohypophysis.*

Between these portions is a small, relatively avascular zone called the *pars intermedia,* which is much less developed in the human being but is larger and much more functional in some animals.

Embryologically, the two portions of the pituitary originate from different sources—the anterior pituitary from *Rathke's pouch,* which is an embryonic invagination of the pharyngeal epithelium, this explains the epithelioid nature of its cells. The posterior pituitary originates from a neural tissue outgrowth from the hypothalamus and this explains the presence of large numbers of glial-type cells in this gland.

Six major peptide hormones plus several other hormones of lesser importance are secreted by the *anterior* pituitary, and two important peptide hormones are secreted by the *posterior* pituitary. The hormones of the anterior pituitary play major roles in the control of metabolic functions throughout the body, as shown in Figure 87-2 and listed in Table 87-1.

The Anterior Pituitary Gland and the Different Cell Types. There is usually one cell type for each major hormone formed in the anterior pituitary gland. With special stains attached to high-affinity antibodies that bind with the distinctive hormones, at least five cell types can be differentiated (Figure 87-3). Table 87-1 provides a summary of these cell types, the hormones they produce, and their physiological actions. These five cell types are as follows:

1. *Somatotropes*—human growth hormone (hGH).
2. *Corticotropes*—adrenocorticotropin (ACTH).
3. *Thyrotropes*—thyroid-stimulating hormone (TSH).
4. *Gonadotropes*—gonadotropic hormones, which include both luteinizing hormone (LH) and follicle-stimulating hormone (FSH).
5. *Lactotropes*—prolactin (PRL).

About 30–40% of the anterior pituitary cells are somatotropes that secrete growth hormone and about 20% are corticotropes that secrete ACTH. Each of the other cell types account for only 3–5% of the total; nevertheless, they secrete powerful hormones for controlling thyroid function, sexual functions, and milk secretion by the breasts.

Somatotropes stain strongly with acid dyes and are therefore called *acidophils.* Thus, pituitary tumors that secrete large quantities of hGH are called *acidophilic tumors.*

Hypothalamus Controls Pituitary Secretion

Almost all secretion by the pituitary is controlled by either hormonal or nervous signals from the hypothalamus. Secretion from the posterior pituitary is controlled by nerve signals that originate in the hypothalamus and terminate in the posterior pituitary.

In contrast, secretion by the anterior pituitary is controlled by hormones called *hypothalamic-releasing* and

577

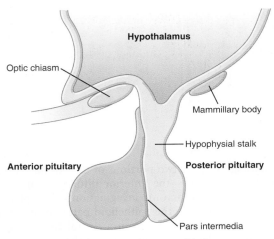

Figure 87-1 Pituitary gland.

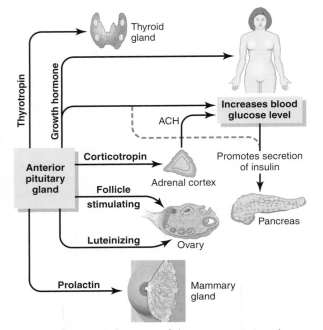

Figure 87-2 Metabolic functions of the anterior pituitary hormones. ACH, adrenal corticosteroid hormones.

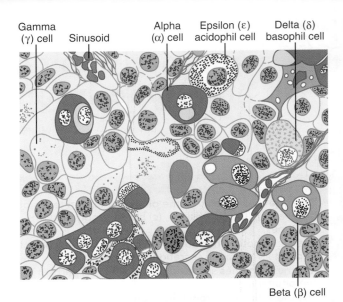

Figure 87-3 Cellular structure of the anterior pituitary gland. (*Modified from Guyton, A.C., 1984. Physiology of the Human Body, sixth ed. Saunders College Publishing, Philadelphia.*)

hypothalamic-inhibitory hormones (or *factors*) secreted within the hypothalamus and then conducted, as shown in Figure 87-4, to the anterior pituitary through minute blood vessels called *hypothalamic–hypophysial portal vessels*. In the anterior pituitary, these releasing and inhibitory hormones act on the glandular cells to control their secretion.

The hypothalamus receives signals from many sources in the nervous system and is a collecting center for information concerning the internal well-being of the body, and much of this information is used to control secretions of the many globally important pituitary hormones.

HYPOTHALAMIC–HYPOPHYSIAL PORTAL BLOOD VESSELS OF THE ANTERIOR PITUITARY GLAND

The anterior pituitary is a highly vascular gland with extensive capillary sinuses among the glandular cells. Almost all the blood that enters these sinuses passes first through another capillary

TABLE 87-1	Cells and Hormones of the Anterior Pituitary Gland and Their Physiological Functions		
Cell	**Hormone**	**Chemistry**	**Physiological Action**
Somatotropes	(GH; somatotropin)	Single chain of 191 amino acids	Stimulates body growth; stimulates secretion of IGF-1; stimulates lipolysis; inhibits actions of insulin on carbohydrate and lipid metabolism
Corticotropes	(ACTH; corticotropin)	Single chain of 39 amino acids	Stimulates production of glucocorticoids and androgens by the adrenal cortex; maintains size of zona fasciculata and zona reticularis of cortex
Thyrotropes	(TSH; thyrotropin)	Glycoprotein of two subunits, α (89 amino acids) and β (112 amino acids)	Stimulates production of thyroid hormones by thyroid follicular cells; maintains size of follicular cells
Gonadotropes	FSH (LH)	Glycoprotein of two subunits, α (89 amino acids) and β (112 amino acids) Glycoprotein of two subunits, α (89 amino acids) and β (115 amino acids)	Stimulates development of ovarian follicles; regulates spermatogenesis in the testis; causes ovulation and formation of the corpus luteum in the ovary; stimulates production of estrogen and progesterone by the ovary; stimulates testosterone production by the testis
Lactotropes Mammotropes	PRL	Single chain of 198 amino acids	Stimulates milk secretion and production

IGF, insulin-like growth factor; GH, growth hormone; ACTH, adrenocorticotropic hormone; TSH, thyroid-stimulating hormone; FSH, follicle-stimulating hormone; LH, luteinizing hormone; PRL, prolactin.

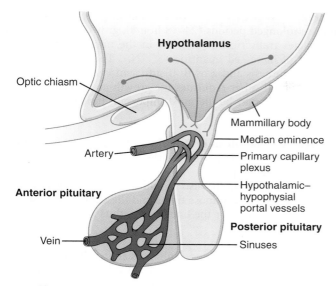

Figure 87-4 Hypothalamic–hypophysial portal system.

TABLE 87-2	Hypothalamic Releasing and Inhibitory Hormones That Control Secretion of the Anterior Pituitary Gland

Hormone	Structure	Primary Action on Anterior Pituitary
TRH	Peptide of 3 amino acids	Stimulates secretion of TSH by thyrotropes
GnRH	Single chain of 10 amino acids	Stimulates secretion of FSH and LH by gonadotropes
CRH	Single chain of 41 amino acids	Stimulates secretion of ACTH by corticotropes
GHRH	Single chain of 44 amino acids	Stimulates secretion of growth hormone by somatotropes
Growth hormone-inhibitory hormone (somatostatin)	Single chain of 14 amino acids	Inhibits secretion of growth hormone by somatotropes
PIH	Dopamine (a catecholamine)	Inhibits synthesis and secretion of PRL by lactotropes

ACTH, adrenocorticotropic hormone; FSH, follicle-stimulating hormone; LH, luteinizing hormone; TSH, thyroid-stimulating hormone; TRH, thyrotropin-releasing hormone; GnRH, gonadotropin-releasing hormone; CRH, corticotropin-releasing hormone; GHRH, growth hormone-releasing hormone, PIH, prolactin-inhibiting hormone.

bed in the lower hypothalamus. The blood then flows through small *hypothalamic–hypophysial portal blood vessels* into the anterior pituitary sinuses. Figure 87-4 shows the lowermost portion of the hypothalamus, called the *median eminence,* which connects inferiorly with the pituitary stalk. Small arteries penetrate into the median eminence and then additional small vessels return to its surface, coalescing to form the hypothalamic–hypophysial portal blood vessels. These vessels pass downward along the pituitary stalk to supply blood to the anterior pituitary sinuses.

Hypothalamic Releasing and Inhibitory Hormones Are Secreted Into the Median Eminence. Special neurons in the hypothalamus synthesize and secrete the *hypothalamic releasing* and *inhibitory hormones* that control secretion of the anterior pituitary hormones. These neurons originate in various parts of the hypothalamus and send their nerve fibers to the median eminence and *tuber cinereum,* an extension of hypothalamic tissue into the pituitary stalk.

The endings of these fibers are different from most endings in the central nervous system, in that their function is not to transmit signals from one neuron to another but rather to secrete the hypothalamic releasing and inhibitory hormones into the tissue fluids. These hormones are immediately absorbed into the hypothalamic–hypophysial portal system and carried directly to the sinuses of the anterior pituitary gland.

Hypothalamic Releasing and Inhibitory Hormones Control Anterior Pituitary Secretion. The function of the releasing and inhibitory hormones is to control secretion of the anterior pituitary hormones. For most of the anterior pituitary hormones, it is the releasing hormones that are important, but for PRL, a hypothalamic inhibitory hormone probably exerts more control. The major hypothalamic releasing and inhibitory hormones, which are summarized in Table 87-2 are the following:

1. *Thyrotropin-releasing hormone* (TRH), which causes release of TSH.
2. *Corticotropin-releasing hormone* (CRH), which causes release of ACTH.
3. *Growth hormone-releasing hormone* (GHRH), which causes release of growth hormone, and *growth hormone-inhibitory hormone* (GHIH), also called *somatostatin,* which inhibits release of growth hormone.

4. *Gonadotropin-releasing hormone* (GnRH), which causes release of the two gonadotropic hormones, LH and FSH.
5. *Prolactin-inhibitory hormone* (PIH), which causes inhibition of PRL secretion.

Additional hypothalamic hormones include one that stimulates PRL secretion and perhaps others that inhibit release of the anterior pituitary hormones. These hormones are also known as *hypophysiotrophic hormones.*

Physiological Functions of Growth Hormone

All the major anterior pituitary hormones, except for growth hormone, exert their principal effects mainly by stimulating target glands, including thyroid gland, adrenal cortex, ovaries, testicles, and mammary glands. Growth hormone, however, does not function through a specific target gland but exerts its effects directly on all or almost all tissues of the body.

Growth Hormone Promotes Growth of Many Body Tissues

Growth hormone, also called *somatotropic hormone* or *somatotropin,* is a small protein molecule that contains 191 amino acids in a single chain and has a molecular weight of 22,005. It causes growth of almost all tissues of the body that are capable of growing. It promotes increased sizes of the cells and increased mitosis, with development of greater numbers of cells and specific differentiation of certain types of cells, such as bone growth cells and early muscle cells. The functions of growth hormone are listed in Table 87-3.

GROWTH HORMONE HAS SEVERAL METABOLIC EFFECTS

Aside from its general effect in causing growth, growth hormone has multiple specific metabolic effects, including the following:

TABLE 87-3	Summary of Growth Hormone Functions	
		Actions
Metabolic functions	Protein metabolism	Enhancement of amino acid transport through cell membranes
		Enhancement of RNA translation to cause protein synthesis by the ribosomes
		Increased nuclear transcription of DNA to form RNA
		Decreased catabolism of protein and amino acids
	Fat metabolism	Growth hormone enhances fat utilization for energy
		"Ketogenic" effect of excessive growth hormone
	Carbohydrate metabolism	Decreased glucose uptake in tissues such as skeletal muscle and fat
		Increased glucose production by the liver
		Increased insulin secretion
Actions on specific tissues	Bone and cartilage	Increased deposition of protein by the chondrocytic and osteogenic cells that cause bone growth
		Increased rate of reproduction of chondrocytic and osteogenic cells
		Specific effect of converting chondrocytes into osteogenic cells
	Muscle	Increases muscle mass
	Organs and soft tissues	Increases the growth of all internal organs and soft tissues

1. increased rate of protein synthesis in most cells of the body;
2. increased mobilization of fatty acids from adipose tissue, increased free fatty acids in the blood, and increased use of fatty acids for energy; and
3. decreased rate of glucose utilization throughout the body.

Thus, in effect, growth hormone *enhances body protein, decreases fat stores,* and *conserves carbohydrates.*

Growth Hormone Promotes Protein Deposition in Tissues

Although the precise mechanisms by which growth hormone increases protein deposition are not fully understood, a series of different effects are known, all of which could lead to enhanced protein deposition.

Enhancement of Amino Acid Transport Through the Cell Membranes. Growth hormone directly enhances transport of most amino acids through the cell membranes to the interior of the cells. This increases the amino acid concentrations in the cells and is presumed to be at least partly responsible for the increased protein synthesis.

Enhancement of RNA Translation to Cause Protein Synthesis by the Ribosomes. Even when the amino acid concentrations are not increased in the cells, growth hormone still increases RNA translation causing protein to be synthesized in greater amounts by the ribosomes in the cytoplasm.

Increased Nuclear Transcription of DNA to Form RNA. Over more prolonged periods (24–48 hours), growth hormone also stimulates transcription of DNA in the nucleus causing formation of increased quantities of RNA. This promotes more protein synthesis and growth if sufficient energy, amino acids, vitamins, and other requisites for growth are available. In the long run, this may be the most important function of growth hormone.

Decreased Catabolism of Protein and Amino Acids. In addition to the increase in protein synthesis, there is a decrease in the breakdown of cell protein. A probable reason for this decrease is that growth hormone also mobilizes large quantities of free fatty acids from the adipose tissue and these are used to supply most of the energy for the body's cells, thus acting as a potent "protein sparer."

Summary. Growth hormone enhances almost all facets of amino acid uptake and protein synthesis by cells, while at the same time reducing the breakdown of proteins.

Growth Hormone Enhances Fat Utilization for Energy

Growth hormone has a specific effect in causing release of fatty acids from adipose tissue and, therefore, increasing the concentration of fatty acids in body fluids. Also, in tissues throughout the body, growth hormone enhances conversion of fatty acids to acetyl coenzyme A (acetyl-CoA) and its subsequent utilization for energy. Therefore, under the influence of growth hormone, fat is used for energy in preference to use of carbohydrates and proteins.

"Ketogenic" Effect of Excessive Growth Hormone. Under the influence of excessive amounts of growth hormone, fat mobilization from adipose tissue sometimes becomes so high that large quantities of acetoacetic acid are formed by the liver and released into the body fluids, thus causing ketosis. This excessive mobilization of fat from the adipose tissue also frequently causes a fatty liver.

Growth Hormone Decreases Carbohydrate Utilization. Growth hormone causes multiple effects that influence carbohydrate metabolism, including (1) decreased glucose uptake in tissues, such as skeletal muscle and fat, (2) increased glucose production by the liver, and (3) increased insulin secretion.

Each of these changes results from growth hormone-induced "insulin resistance," which attenuates insulin's actions to stimulate uptake and utilization of glucose in skeletal muscle and adipose tissue and to inhibit gluconeogenesis (glucose production) by the liver; this leads to increased blood glucose concentration and a compensatory increase in insulin secretion. For these reasons, growth hormone's effects are called *diabetogenic,* and excess secretion of growth hormone can produce metabolic disturbances similar to those found in patients with type II (noninsulin-dependent) diabetes, who are also resistant to the metabolic effects of insulin.

Necessity of Insulin and Carbohydrate for the Growth-Promoting Action of Growth Hormone. Growth hormone fails to cause growth in animals that lack a pancreas; it also fails to cause growth if carbohydrates are excluded from the diet. These phenomena show that adequate insulin activity and adequate availability of carbohydrates are necessary for growth hormone to be effective. Part of this requirement for carbohydrates and insulin is to provide the energy needed for the metabolism of growth, but there seem to be other effects as well. Especially important is the ability of insulin to enhance transport of some amino acids into cells, in the same way that it stimulates glucose transport.

GROWTH HORMONE STIMULATES CARTILAGE AND BONE GROWTH

Although growth hormone stimulates increased deposition of protein and increased growth in almost all tissues of the body, its most obvious effect is to increase growth of the skeletal frame. This results from multiple effects of growth hormone on bone, including the following:

1. increased deposition of protein by the chondrocytic and osteogenic cells that cause bone growth,
2. increased rate of reproduction of these cells, and
3. a specific effect of converting chondrocytes into osteogenic cells, thus causing deposition of new bone.

There are two principal mechanisms of bone growth. First, in response to growth hormone stimulation, the long bones grow in length at the epiphyseal cartilages, where the epiphyses at the ends of the bone are separated from the shaft. This growth first causes deposition of new cartilage, followed by its conversion into new bone, thus elongating the shaft and pushing the epiphyses farther and farther apart. At the same time, the epiphyseal cartilage is progressively used up, so by late adolescence, no additional epiphyseal cartilage remains to provide for further long bone growth. At this time, bony fusion occurs between the shaft and the epiphysis at each end, so no further lengthening of the long bone can occur.

Second, *osteoblasts* in the bone periosteum and in some bone cavities deposit new bone on the surfaces of older bone. Simultaneously, *osteoclasts* in the bone (discussed in detail in Chapter 90) remove old bone. When the rate of deposition is greater than that of resorption, the thickness of the bone increases. *Growth hormone strongly stimulates osteoblasts.* Therefore, the bones can continue to become thicker throughout life under the influence of growth hormone; this is especially true for the membranous bones. For instance, the jaw bones can be stimulated to grow even after adolescence causing forward protrusion of the chin and lower teeth. Likewise, the bones of the skull can grow in thickness and give rise to bony protrusions over the eyes.

GROWTH HORMONE EXERTS MUCH OF ITS EFFECT THROUGH INTERMEDIATE SUBSTANCES CALLED "SOMATOMEDINS"

When growth hormone is supplied directly to cartilage chondrocytes cultured outside the body, proliferation or enlargement of the chondrocytes usually fails to occur. Yet growth hormone injected into the intact animal does cause proliferation and growth of the same cells.

In brief, growth hormone causes the liver (and, to a much less extent, other tissues) to form several small proteins called *somatomedins* that have the potent effect of increasing all aspects of bone growth. Many of the somatomedin effects on growth are similar to the effects of insulin on growth. Therefore, the somatomedins are also called insulin-like growth factors (IGFs).

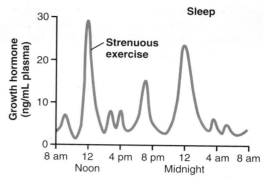

Figure 87-5 Typical variations in growth hormone secretion throughout the day, demonstrating the especially powerful effect of strenuous exercise and also the high rate of growth hormone secretion that occurs during the first few hours of deep sleep.

At least four somatomedins have been isolated, but by far the most important of these is *somatomedin C* (also called insulin-like growth factor-1, or IGF-I). The molecular weight of somatomedin C is about 7500, and its concentration in the plasma closely follows the rate of growth hormone secretion.

The pygmies of Africa have a congenital inability to synthesize significant amounts of somatomedin C. Therefore, even though their plasma concentration of growth hormone is either normal or high, they have diminished amounts of somatomedin C in the plasma, which apparently accounts for the small stature of these people. Some other dwarfs (eg, the Lévi-Lorain dwarf) also have this problem.

It has been postulated that most, if not all, of the growth effects of growth hormone result from somatomedin C and other somatomedins, rather than from direct effects of growth hormone on the bones and other peripheral tissues. Some aspects of the somatomedin hypothesis are still questionable. One possibility is that growth hormone can cause the formation of enough somatomedin C in the local tissue to cause local growth. It is also possible that growth hormone is directly responsible for increased growth in some tissues and that the somatomedin mechanism is an alternative means of increasing growth but not always a necessary one.

Short Duration of Action of Growth Hormone but Prolonged Action of Somatomedin C. Growth hormone attaches only weakly to the plasma proteins in blood. Therefore, it is released from the blood into the tissues rapidly, having a half-time in blood of less than 20 minutes. By contrast, somatomedin C attaches strongly to a carrier protein in the blood that, like somatomedin C, is produced in response to growth hormone. As a result, somatomedin C is released only slowly from the blood to the tissues, with a half-time of about 20 hours. This slow release greatly prolongs the growth-promoting effects of the bursts of growth hormone secretion shown in Figure 87-5.

REGULATION OF GROWTH HORMONE SECRETION

After adolescence, secretion decreases slowly with aging, finally falling to about 25% of the adolescent level in very old age.

Growth hormone is secreted in a pulsatile pattern, increasing and decreasing. The precise mechanisms that control secretion of growth hormone are not fully understood, but several factors related to a person's state of nutrition or stress are known to stimulate secretion such as

TABLE 87-4	Factors That Stimulate or Inhibit Secretion of Growth Hormone

Stimulate Growth Hormone Secretion	Inhibit Growth Hormone Secretion
Decreased blood glucose	Increased blood glucose
Decreased blood free fatty acids	Increased blood free fatty acids
Increased blood amino acids (arginine)	Aging
Starvation or fasting, protein deficiency	Obesity
Trauma, stress, excitement	Growth hormone-inhibitory hormone (somatostatin)
Exercise	Growth hormone (exogenous)
Testosterone, estrogen	Somatomedins (IGFs)
Deep sleep (stages II and IV)	Increased blood glucose
Growth hormone-releasing hormone	Increased blood free fatty acids
Ghrelin	Aging

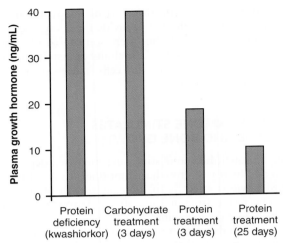

Figure 87-6   Effect of extreme protein deficiency on the plasma concentration of growth hormone in the disease kwashiorkor. Also shown is the failure of carbohydrate treatment but the effectiveness of protein treatment in lowering growth hormone concentration. *(Data from Pimstone, B.L., Barbezat, G., Hansen, J.D. et al., 1968. Studies on growth hormone secretion in protein-calorie malnutrition. Am. J. Clin. Nutr. 21, 482.)*

- *starvation*, especially with severe *protein deficiency*;
- *hypoglycemia* or *low concentration of fatty acids in the blood*;
- *exercise*;
- *excitement*;
- *trauma*; and
- *ghrelin*, a hormone secreted by the stomach before meals.

Growth hormone also characteristically increases during the first 2 hours of *deep sleep*, as shown in Figure 87-5. Table 87-4 summarizes some of the factors that are known to influence growth hormone secretion.

The normal concentration of growth hormone in the plasma of an adult is between 1.6 and 3 ng/mL; in a child or adolescent, it is about 6 ng/mL. These values may increase to as high as 50 ng/mL after depletion of the body stores of proteins or carbohydrates during prolonged starvation.

Under acute conditions, hypoglycemia is a far more potent stimulator of growth hormone secretion than is an acute decrease in protein intake. Conversely, in chronic conditions, growth hormone secretion seems to correlate more with the degree of cellular protein depletion than with the degree of glucose insufficiency. For instance, the extremely high levels of growth hormone that occur during starvation are closely related to the amount of protein depletion.

Figure 87-6 demonstrates the effect of protein deficiency (*kwashiorkor*) on plasma growth hormone and then the effect of adding protein to the diet. These results demonstrate that under severe conditions of protein malnutrition, adequate calories alone are not sufficient to correct the excess production of growth hormone. The protein deficiency must also be corrected before the growth hormone concentration will return to normal.

Role of the Hypothalamus, Growth Hormone-Releasing Hormone, and Somatostatin in Controlling Growth Hormone Secretion

It is known that growth hormone secretion is controlled by two factors secreted in the hypothalamus and then transported to the anterior pituitary gland through the hypothalamic–hypophysial portal vessels. They are *growth hormone-releasing hormone* (GHRH) and *GHIH* (also called *somatostatin*). Both of these are polypeptides; GHRH is composed of 44 amino acids, and somatostatin is composed of 14 amino acids.

The part of the hypothalamus that causes secretion of GHRH is the ventromedial nucleus, which is also sensitive to blood glucose concentration, causing satiety in hyperglycemic states and hunger in hypoglycemic states. The secretion of somatostatin is controlled by other nearby areas of the hypothalamus. Therefore, it is reasonable to expect that some of the same signals that modify a person's behavioral feeding instincts also alter the rate of growth hormone secretion.

In a similar manner, hypothalamic signals depicting emotions, stress, and trauma can all affect hypothalamic control of growth hormone secretion. In fact, experiments have shown that catecholamines, dopamine, and serotonin, each of which is released by a different neuronal system in the hypothalamus, all increase the rate of growth hormone secretion.

When growth hormone is administered directly into the blood of an animal over several hours, the rate of endogenous growth hormone secretion decreases. This decrease demonstrates that growth hormone secretion is subject to typical negative feedback control, as is true for essentially all hormones. The nature of this feedback mechanism and whether it is mediated mainly through inhibition of GHRH or enhancement of somatostatin, which inhibits growth hormone secretion, are uncertain.

Figure 87-7 illustrates the regulation and feedback control of growth hormone secretion.

ABNORMALITIES OF GROWTH HORMONE SECRETION

Panhypopituitarism.   Panhypopituitarism means decreased secretion of all the anterior pituitary hormones. The decrease in secretion may be congenital (present from birth), or it may occur suddenly or slowly at any time during life, most often resulting from a pituitary tumor that destroys the pituitary gland.

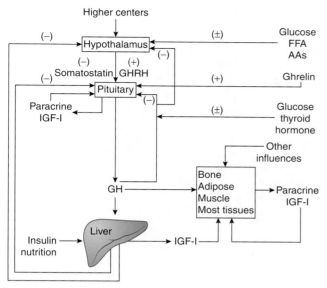

Figure 87-7 Growth hormone regulation.

Panhypopituitarism in the Adult. Panhypopituitarism first occurring in adulthood frequently results from one of three common abnormalities.

1. Craniopharyngiomas—a tumorous condition involving the pituitary gland.
2. Chromophobe tumors may compress the pituitary gland until the functioning anterior pituitary cells are totally or almost totally destroyed.
3. Thrombosis of the pituitary blood vessels. This abnormality occasionally occurs when a new mother develops circulatory shock after the birth of her baby.

The general effects of adult panhypopituitarism are (1) hypothyroidism, (2) depressed production of glucocorticoids by the adrenal glands, and (3) suppressed secretion of the gonadotropic hormones so that sexual functions are lost. Thus, the picture is that of a lethargic person (from lack of thyroid hormones) who is gaining weight (because of lack of fat mobilization by growth, adrenocorticotropic, adrenocortical, and thyroid hormones) and has lost all sexual functions. Except for the abnormal sexual functions, the patient can usually be treated satisfactorily by administering adrenocortical and thyroid hormones.

Dwarfism. Most instances of dwarfism result from generalized deficiency of anterior pituitary secretion (panhypopituitarism) during childhood. In general, all the physical parts of the body develop in appropriate proportion to one another, but the rate of development is greatly decreased.

A person with panhypopituitary dwarfism does not pass through puberty and never secretes sufficient quantities of gonadotropic hormones to develop adult sexual functions. In one-third of such dwarfs, however, only growth hormone is deficient; these persons do mature sexually and occasionally reproduce. In one type of dwarfism (the African pygmy and the Lévi-Lorain dwarf), the rate of growth hormone secretion is normal or high, but there is a hereditary inability to form somatomedin C, which is a key step for the promotion of growth by growth hormone.

Treatment with Human Growth Hormone. Growth hormones from different species of animals are sufficiently different from one another that they will cause growth only in the one species or, at most, closely related species. For this reason, growth hormone prepared from lower animals (except, to some extent, from primates) is not effective in human beings. Therefore, the growth hormone of the human being is called hGH to distinguish it from the others.

hGH is synthesized by *Escherichia coli* bacteria as a result of successful application of recombinant DNA technology and is available in sufficient quantities for treatment purposes. Dwarfs who have pure growth hormone deficiency can be completely cured if treated early in life. hGH may also prove to be beneficial in other metabolic disorders because of its widespread metabolic functions.

Gigantism. Occasionally, the acidophilic, growth hormone-producing cells of the anterior pituitary gland become excessively active, and sometimes even acidophilic tumors occur in the gland. As a result, large quantities of growth hormone are produced. All body tissues grow rapidly, including the bones. If the condition occurs before adolescence, before the epiphyses of the long bones have become fused with the shafts, height increases so that the person becomes a giant—up to 8 feet tall.

The giant ordinarily has *hyperglycemia* and the beta cells of the islets of Langerhans in the pancreas are prone to degenerate because they become overactive owing to the hyperglycemia. Consequently, in about 10% of giants, full-blown *diabetes mellitus* eventually develops.

In most giants, panhypopituitarism eventually develops if they remain untreated because the gigantism is usually caused by a tumor of the pituitary gland that grows until the gland is destroyed. This eventual general deficiency of pituitary hormones usually causes death in early adulthood. However, once gigantism is diagnosed, further effects can often be blocked by microsurgical removal of the tumor or by irradiation of the pituitary gland.

Box 87-1 summarizes clinical features of gigantism.

Acromegaly. If an acidophilic tumor occurs after adolescence—that is, after the epiphyses of the long bones have fused with the shafts—the person cannot grow taller, but the bones can become thicker and the soft tissues can continue to grow. This condition, shown in Figure 87-8, is known as *acromegaly.*

Box 87-2 summarizes clinical features of acromegaly.

BOX 87-1 CLINICAL FEATURES OF GIGANTISM

1. Height increases—up to 8 feet tall
2. Large hands and feet
3. Soft tissues grow rapidly
4. Hyperglycemia usually present leading to full-blown *diabetes mellitus*

5. All features of panhypopituitarism, if the cause is due to a tumor
   a. Weight gain
   b. Loss of sexual functions
   c. Decreased immunity
   d. Features of hypothyroidism
   e. Features of adrenocortical insufficiency

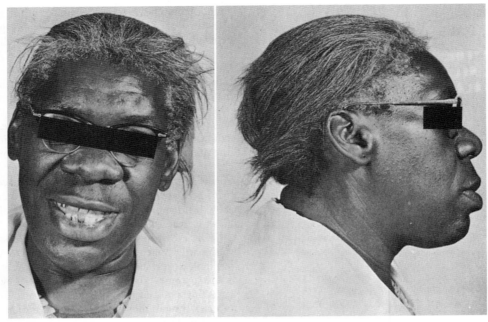

Figure 87-8   Patient with acromegaly.

BOX 87-2   CLINICAL FEATURES OF ACROMEGALY

1. Marked enlargement in the bones of the hands and feet
2. Enlargement of membranous bones:
   a. Cranium
   b. Nose
   c. Bosses on the forehead
   d. Supraorbital ridges become prominent
   e. Protrusion of lower jaw—*Prognathism*
   f. Portions of the vertebrae increase in size

3. Enlargement of soft tissue organs:
   a. Tongue becomes greatly enlarged
   b. Liver becomes greatly enlarged
   c. Kidneys become greatly enlarged

BIBLIOGRAPHY

Allen DB, Cuttler L: Clinical practice. Short stature in childhood—challenges and choices, *N. Engl. J. Med.* 368:1220, 2013.

Bartke A, Sun LY, Longo V: Somatotropic signaling: trade-offs between growth, reproductive development, and longevity, *Physiol. Rev.* 93:571, 2013.

Beltramo M, Dardente H, Cayla X, Caraty A: Cellular mechanisms and integrative timing of neuroendocrine control of GnRH secretion by kisspeptin, *Mol. Cell Endocrinol.* 382:387, 2014.

Chiamolera MI, Wondisford FE: Thyrotropin-releasing hormone and the thyroid hormone feedback mechanism, *Endocrinology* 150:1091, 2009.

Chikani V, Ho KK: Action of GH on skeletal muscle function: molecular and metabolic mechanisms, *J. Mol. Endocrinol.* 52:R107, 2013.

Cohen LE: Idiopathic short stature: a clinical review, *JAMA* 311:1787, 2014.

Freeman ME, Kanyicska B, Lerant A, Nagy G: Prolactin: structure, function, and regulation of secretion, *Physiol. Rev.* 80:1523, 2000.

Gazzaruso C, Gola M, Karamouzis I, et al: Cardiovascular risk in adult patients with growth hormone (GH) deficiency and following substitution with GH—an update, *J. Clin. Endocrinol. Metab.* 99:18, 2014.

Gimpl G, Fahrenholz F: The oxytocin receptor system: structure, function, and regulation, *Physiol. Rev.* 81:629, 2001.

Livingstone C: Insulin-like growth factor-I (IGF-I) and clinical nutrition, *Clin. Sci. (Lond)* 125:265, 2013.

McEwen BS: Physiology and neurobiology of stress and adaptation: central role of the brain, *Physiol. Rev.* 87:873, 2007.

Melmed S: Acromegaly pathogenesis and treatment, *J. Clin. Invest.* 119:3189, 2009.

Møller N, Jørgensen JO: Effects of growth hormone on glucose, lipid, and protein metabolism in human subjects, *Endocr. Rev.* 30:152, 2009.

Nielsen S, Frokiaer J, Marples D, et al: Aquaporins in the kidney: from molecules to medicine, *Physiol. Rev.* 82:205, 2002.

Perez-Castro C, Renner U, Haedo MR, et al: Cellular and molecular specificity of pituitary gland physiology, *Physiol. Rev.* 92:1, 2012.

Zhu X, Gleiberman AS, Rosenfeld MG: Molecular physiology of pituitary development: signaling and transcriptional networks, Physiol. Rev. 87:933, 2007.

88

Posterior Pituitary Gland

LEARNING OBJECTIVES

- List the actions and factors controlling the secretion of oxytocin and vasopressin.
- List the functions of oxytocin.
- List the functions of ADH or vasopressin.
- Describe the disorders of posterior pituitary hormone secretion.

GLOSSARY OF TERMS

- **ADH:** Antidiuretic hormone—it is also called arginine vasopressin (AVP).

- **Diuretic:** Any substance or drug that increases the formation and passage of urine by the kidneys.

- **Euvolemia:** It is a state of balanced body fluid volume, where the fluid intake is balanced by the fluid output.

- **Pituicytes:** These are glial-like cells within the posterior pituitary gland, which mainly act as supportive cells and do not secrete any hormones.

Posterior Pituitary Hormones Are Synthesized by Cell Bodies in the Hypothalamus

The bodies of the cells that secrete the *posterior* pituitary hormones are not located in the pituitary gland but are large neurons, called *magnocellular neurons,* located in
1. The *supraoptic* and
2. *Paraventricular nuclei* of the hypothalamus.

The hormones are then transported in the axoplasm of the neurons' nerve fibers passing from the hypothalamus to the posterior pituitary gland.

Posterior Pituitary Gland and Its Relation to the Hypothalamus

The *posterior pituitary gland,* also called the *neurohypophysis,* is composed mainly of glial-like cells called *pituicytes.* The pituicytes do not secrete hormones; they act simply as a supporting structure for large numbers of *terminal nerve fibers* and *terminal nerve endings* from nerve tracts that originate in the *supraoptic* and *paraventricular nuclei* of the hypothalamus, as shown in Figure 88-1. These tracts pass to the neurohypophysis through the *pituitary stalk* (hypophysial stalk). The nerve endings are bulbous knobs that contain many secretory granules. These endings lie on the surfaces of capillaries, where they secrete two posterior pituitary hormones:
1. *ADH, also called vasopressin,* and
2. *Oxytocin.*

If the pituitary stalk is cut above the pituitary gland but the entire hypothalamus is left intact, the posterior pituitary hormones continue to be secreted normally, after a transient decrease for a few days; they are then secreted by the cut ends of the fibers within the hypothalamus and not by the nerve endings in the posterior pituitary. The reason for this is that the hormones are initially synthesized in the cell bodies of the supraoptic and paraventricular nuclei and are then transported in combination with "carrier" proteins called *neurophysins* down to the nerve endings in the posterior pituitary gland, requiring several days to reach the gland.
1. *ADH is formed primarily in the supraoptic nuclei.*
2. *Oxytocin is formed primarily in the paraventricular nuclei.*

Each of these nuclei can synthesize about one-sixth as much of the second hormone as of its primary hormone.

When nerve impulses are transmitted downward along the fibers from the supraoptic or paraventricular nuclei, the hormone is immediately released from the secretory granules in the nerve endings by the usual secretory mechanism of *exocytosis* and is absorbed into adjacent capillaries. Both the neurophysin and the hormone are secreted together, but because they are only loosely bound to each other, the hormone separates almost immediately. The neurophysin has no known function after leaving the nerve terminals.

ANTIDIURETIC HORMONE

Physiological Functions of Antidiuretic Hormone

The injection of extremely minute quantities of ADH—as small as 2 ng—can cause decreased excretion of water by the kidneys (antidiuresis). Briefly, in the absence of ADH, the collecting tubules and ducts become almost impermeable to water, which prevents significant reabsorption of water and therefore allows extreme loss of water into the urine, also causing extreme dilution of the urine. Conversely, in the presence of ADH, the permeability of the collecting ducts and tubules to water increases greatly and allows most of the water to be reabsorbed as the tubular fluid passes through these ducts, thereby conserving water in the body and producing very concentrated urine.

Without ADH, the luminal membranes of the tubular epithelial cells of the collecting ducts are almost impermeable to water.

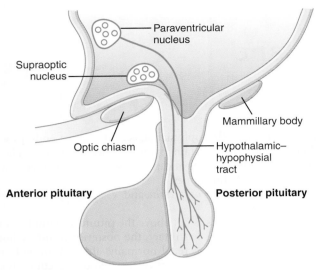

Figure 88-1 Hypothalamic control of the posterior pituitary.

Mechanism of Action of ADH

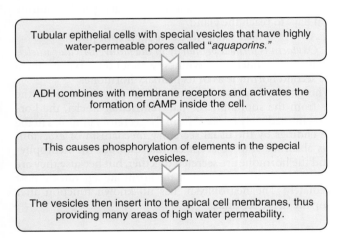

All the events described previously occur within 5–10 minutes. The aforementioned flow charts represent the mechanism of action of ADH. Then, in the absence of ADH, the entire process reverses in another 5–10 minutes. Thus, this process temporarily provides many new pores that allow free diffusion of water from the tubular fluid through the tubular epithelial cells and into the renal interstitial fluid. Water is then absorbed from the collecting tubules and ducts by osmosis, in relation to the urine-concentrating mechanism of the kidneys.

Regulation of Antidiuretic Hormone Production

Increased Extracellular Fluid Osmolarity Stimulates ADH Secretion. When a concentrated electrolyte solution is injected into the artery that supplies the hypothalamus, the ADH neurons in the supraoptic and paraventricular nuclei immediately transmit impulses into the posterior pituitary to release large quantities of ADH into the circulating blood, sometimes increasing the ADH secretion to as high as 20 times normal. Conversely, injection of a dilute solution into this artery causes cessation of the impulses and therefore almost total cessation

of ADH secretion. Thus, the concentration of ADH in the body fluids can change from small amounts to large amounts, or vice versa, in only a few minutes.

Somewhere in or near the hypothalamus are modified neuron receptors called *osmoreceptors* (Figure 88-2). When the extracellular fluid becomes too concentrated, fluid is pulled by osmosis out of the osmoreceptor cell, decreasing its size and initiating appropriate nerve signals in the hypothalamus to cause additional ADH secretion. Conversely, when the extracellular fluid becomes too dilute, water moves by osmosis in the opposite direction into the cell, which decreases the signal for ADH secretion. Although some researchers place these osmoreceptors in the hypothalamus (possibly even in the supraoptic nuclei), others believe that they are located in the *organum vasculosum*, a highly vascular structure in the anteroventral wall of the third ventricle.

Regardless of the mechanism, concentrated body fluids stimulate the supraoptic nuclei, whereas dilute body fluids inhibit them. A feedback control system is available to control the total osmotic pressure of the body fluids.

Further details on the control of ADH secretion and the role of ADH in controlling renal function and body fluid osmolality are presented in Chapter 79.

Low Blood Volume and Low Blood Pressure Stimulate ADH Secretion—Vasoconstrictor Effects of ADH. Although minute concentrations of ADH cause increased water conservation by the kidneys, higher concentrations of ADH have a potent effect of constricting the arterioles throughout the body and therefore increasing the arterial pressure. For this reason, ADH has another name, *vasopressin*.

One of the stimuli for causing intense ADH secretion is decreased blood volume. This occurs strongly when the blood volume decreases 15–25% or more; the secretory rate then sometimes rises to as high as 50 times normal. The cause of this effect is the following.

The atria have stretch receptors that are excited by overfilling. When excited, they send signals to the brain to inhibit ADH secretion. Conversely, when the receptors are unexcited as a result of underfilling, the opposite occurs, with greatly increased ADH secretion. Decreased stretch of the baroreceptors of the carotid, aortic, and pulmonary regions also stimulates ADH secretion. For further details about this blood volume–pressure feedback mechanism, refer to Chapter 79.

OXYTOCIN HORMONE

Oxytocin Causes Contraction of the Pregnant Uterus. The hormone *oxytocin,* in accordance with its name, powerfully stimulates contraction of the pregnant uterus, especially toward the end of gestation. Therefore, many obstetricians believe that this hormone is at least partially responsible for causing birth of the baby. This belief is supported by the following facts: (1) In a hypophysectomized animal, the duration of labor is prolonged, indicating a possible effect of oxytocin during delivery; (2) the amount of oxytocin in the plasma increases during labor, especially during the last stage; and (3) stimulation of the cervix in a pregnant animal elicits nervous signals that pass to the hypothalamus and cause increased secretion of oxytocin. These effects and this possible mechanism for aiding in the birth process are discussed in more detail in Chapters 98 and 99.

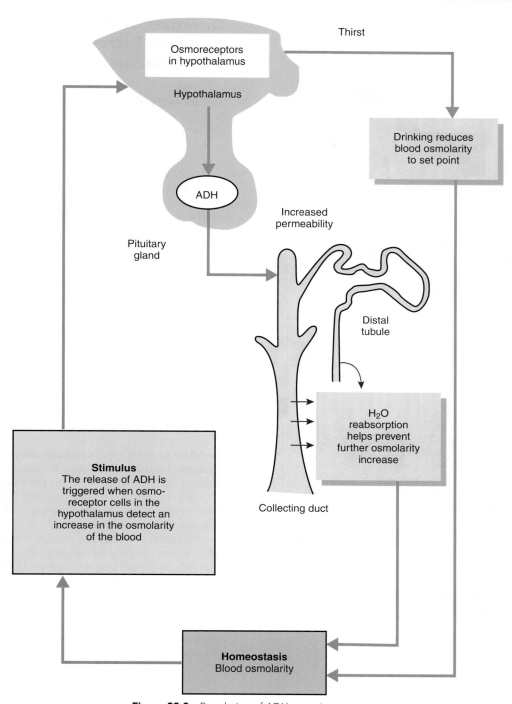

Figure 88-2 Regulation of ADH secretion.

Oxytocin Aids in Milk Ejection by the Breasts. Oxytocin also plays an especially important role in lactation—a role that is far better understood than its role in delivery. In lactation, oxytocin causes milk to be expressed from the alveoli into the ducts of the breast so that the baby can obtain it by suckling.

This mechanism works as follows (Figure 88-3): The suckling stimulus on the nipple of the breast causes signals to be transmitted through sensory nerves to the oxytocin neurons in the paraventricular and supraoptic nuclei in the hypothalamus, which causes release of oxytocin by

the posterior pituitary gland. The oxytocin is then carried by the blood to the breasts, where it causes contraction of *myoepithelial cells* that lie outside and form a latticework surrounding the alveoli of the mammary glands. In less than a minute after the beginning of suckling, milk begins to flow. This mechanism is called *milk letdown* or *milk ejection*. It is discussed further in Chapters 98 and 99 in relation to the physiology of lactation.

Table 88-1 summarizes the functions, regulation, clinical disorders, and clinical tests for the posterior pituitary hormones.

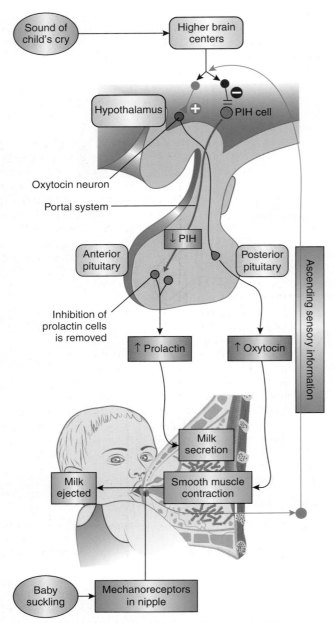

Figure 88-3   Milk ejection reflex.

Disorders of Posterior Pituitary Hormone Secretions

ANTIDIURETIC HORMONE

Failure to Produce ADH: "Central" Diabetes Insipidus. An inability to produce or release ADH from the posterior pituitary can be caused by the following:

1. Head injuries,
2. Infections, or
3. Congenital causes

Because the distal tubular segments cannot reabsorb water in the absence of ADH, this condition, called *"central" diabetes insipidus,* results in the formation of a large volume of dilute urine with urine volumes that can exceed 15 L/day. The thirst mechanisms are activated when excessive water is lost from the body; therefore, as long as the person drinks enough water, large decreases in body fluid water do not occur. The primary abnormality observed clinically in people with this condition is the large volume of dilute urine. However, if water intake is restricted, as can occur in a hospital setting when fluid intake is restricted or the patient is unconscious (eg, because of a head injury), severe dehydration can rapidly occur.

The treatment for central diabetes insipidus is administration of a synthetic analog of ADH, *desmopressin,* which acts selectively on V_2 receptors to increase water permeability in the late distal and collecting tubules. Desmopressin can be given by injection, as a nasal spray, or orally, and it rapidly restores urine output toward normal.

Inability of the Kidneys to Respond to ADH: "Nephrogenic" Diabetes Insipidus. In some circumstances, normal or elevated levels of ADH are present but the renal tubular segments cannot respond appropriately. This condition is referred to as *"nephrogenic" diabetes insipidus* because the abnormality resides in the kidneys. This abnormality can be due to either failure of the countercurrent mechanism to form a hyperosmotic renal medullary interstitium or failure of the distal and collecting tubules and collecting ducts to respond to ADH. In either case, large volumes of dilute urine are formed, which tends to cause dehydration unless fluid intake is increased by the same amount as urine volume is increased.

Many types of renal diseases can impair the concentrating mechanism; especially those that damage the renal medulla. Also, impairment of the function of the loop of Henle, as occurs

TABLE 88-1	Summary of Functions, Regulation, Clinical Disorders, and Clinical Tests for Posterior Pituitary Hormones			
	Functions	**Regulation**	**Clinical Disorders**	**Clinical Tests**
Antidiuretic hormone	• Increase water reabsorption from collecting ducts and distal convoluted tubule • Vasoconstrictor effects that increase arterial pressure	• Increased osmolarity stimulates ADH • Decreased blood volume stimulates ADH in large quantities	Diabetes insipidus SIAD	Water deprivation test Water load test
Oxytocin	• Contraction of the pregnant uterus • Aids in milk ejection by the breasts	• Signals from cervix stimulate hypothalamus. • Suckling stimulus from the nipples initiates the milk ejection reflex		

SIAD, syndrome of inappropriate antidiuresis.

with diuretics that inhibit electrolyte reabsorption by this segment, such as furosemide, can compromise urine concentrating ability. Furthermore, certain drugs, such as lithium (used to treat manic-depressive disorders) and tetracyclines (used as antibiotics), can impair the ability of the distal nephron segments to respond to ADH.

Nephrogenic diabetes insipidus can be distinguished from central diabetes insipidus by administration of desmopressin, the synthetic analog of ADH. Lack of a prompt decrease in urine volume and an increase in urine osmolarity within 2 hours after injection of desmopressin is strongly suggestive of nephrogenic diabetes insipidus. The treatment for nephrogenic diabetes insipidus is to correct, if possible, the underlying renal disorder. The hypernatremia can also be attenuated by a low-sodium diet and administration of a diuretic that enhances renal sodium excretion, such as a thiazide diuretic.

SYNDROME OF INAPPROPRIATE ANTIDIURESIS (SIAD)

In 1957, Schwartz and group described the "syndrome of inappropriate secretion of antidiuretic hormone" (SIADH), which was characterized by inappropriate release of ADH. More recently, it has been observed that not all the affected patients had elevated blood levels of ADH and therefore the term "syndrome of inappropriate antidiuresis" (SIAD) has been proposed.

SIAD is a syndrome of sodium and water imbalance and manifested by *hypotonic hyponatremia* and *impaired urinary dilution*. These features occur in the absence of kidney disorders or any other particular nonosmotic stimulus known to release ADH.

SIAD can be caused by various factors and these are broadly classified as: (1) endogenous causes, (2) exogenous causes, and (3) idiopathic causes. Endogenous causes are further classified as (1) ADH secretion being increased from the hypothalamus, (2) ADH from ectopic production such as carcinomas, and (3) drugs that potentiate ADH effect. Exogenous causes include administration of ADH or analogs such as desmopressin.

SIAD is diagnosed based on certain *essential features*, such as a decrease in effective plasma osmolality (<275 mosm/kg), an increase in urinary osmolality (>100 mosm/kg during hypotonicity), an increase in urinary sodium (>40 mmol/L with normal dietary salt intake), clinical euvolemia, normal thyroid and adrenal function and no history of recent use of diuretic agents.

Other features (*supplemental features*) include a reduced serum uric acid level (<4 mg/dL) and reduced blood urea nitrogen (<10 mg/dL), a fractional sodium excretion >1%, and a fractional urea excretion >55%. There could also be a failure to correct hyponatremia even after infusion of 2 L of 0.9% saline and sometimes hyponatremia can be corrected by fluid restriction. Elevation of ADH levels in plasma even in the presence of hypotonicity and clinical euvolemia is another feature that may be seen.

The management of this condition includes ruling out and addressing all correctable causes, correcting the hyponatremia, restricting fluid intake, encouraging dietary intake of salt and protein, and administering vasopressin receptor antagonists if hyponatremia persists.

BIBLIOGRAPHY

Ellison DH, Berl T: The syndrome of inappropriate antidiuresis, *N. Engl. J. Med.* 356:2064-2072, 2007.

Esposito P, Piotti Stefania G, Malul BY, et al: The syndrome of inappropriate antidiuresis: pathophysiology, clinical management and new therapeutic options, *Nephron. Clin. Pract.* 119:c62-c73, 2011.

Gimpl G, Fahrenholz F: The oxytocin receptor system: structure, function, and regulation, *Physiol. Rev.* 81:629, 2001.

Ho JM, Blevins JE: Coming full circle: contributions of central and peripheral oxytocin actions to energy balance, *Endocrinology* 154:589, 2013.

Juul KV, Bichet DG, Nielsen S, Nørgaard JP: The physiological and pathophysiological functions of renal and extrarenal vasopressin V2 receptors, *Am. J. Physiol. Renal Physiol.* 306:F931, 2014.

Kortenoeven ML, Fenton RA: Renal aquaporins and water balance disorders, *Biochim. Biophys. Acta* 1840:1533, 2014.

Koshimizu TA, Nakamura K, Egashira N, et al: Vasopressin V1a and V1b receptors: from molecules to physiological systems, *Physiol. Rev.* 92:1813, 2012.

McEwen BS: Physiology and neurobiology of stress and adaptation: central role of the brain, *Physiol. Rev.* 87:873, 2007.

McPherson RA, Pincus, MR: Evaluation of endocrine function: arginine vasopressin (AVP)/antidiuretic hormone (ADH), Henry's Clinical Diagnosis and Management by Laboratory Methods, twenty-first ed. Saunders Elsevier, Philadelphia.

Moeller HB, Fenton RA: Cell biology of vasopressin-regulated aquaporin-2 trafficking, *Pflugers Arch.* 464:133, 2012.

Nielsen S, Frokiaer J, Marples D, et al: Aquaporins in the kidney: from molecules to medicine, *Physiol. Rev.* 82:205, 2002.

Perez-Castro C, Renner U, Haedo MR, et al: Cellular and molecular specificity of pituitary gland physiology, *Physiol. Rev.* 92:1, 2012.

Sands JM, Layton HE: The physiology of urinary concentration: an update, *Semin. Nephrol.* 29(3): 178-195, 2009.

Schwartz WB, Bennett W, Curelop S, et al: A syndrome of renal sodium loss and hyponatremia probably resulting from inappropriate secretion of antidiuretic hormone, *Am. J. Med.* 23:529-542, 1957.

Thyroid Gland

The thyroid gland is one of the largest of the endocrine glands, normally weighing 15–20 g in adults. The thyroid secretes two major hormones, *thyroxine* and *triiodothyronine*, commonly called T_4 and T_3, respectively. Both of these hormones profoundly increase the metabolic rate of the body. Thyroid secretion is controlled primarily by *thyroid-stimulating hormone* (TSH) secreted by the anterior pituitary gland.

The thyroid gland also secretes *calcitonin*, a hormone involved in calcium metabolism that is discussed in Chapter 90.

The purpose of this chapter is to discuss the formation and secretion of the thyroid hormones, their metabolic functions, and regulation of their secretion.

Synthesis and Secretion of the Thyroid Metabolic Hormones

About 93% of the metabolically active hormones secreted by the thyroid gland are *thyroxine*, and 7% is *triiodothyronine*. However, almost all the thyroxine is eventually converted to triiodothyronine in the tissues, so both are functionally important. Triiodothyronine is about four times as potent as thyroxine, but it is present in the blood in much smaller quantities and persists for a much shorter time compared with thyroxine.

Physiological Anatomy of the Thyroid Gland. As shown in Figure 89-1, the thyroid gland is composed of large numbers of closed *follicles* (100–300 μm in diameter) that are filled with a secretory substance called *colloid* and lined with *cuboidal epithelial cells* that secrete into the interior of the follicles. The major constituent of colloid is the large glycoprotein *thyroglobulin*, which contains the thyroid hormones. The thyroid gland has a blood flow about five times the weight of the gland each minute, which is a blood supply as great as that of any other area of the body, with the possible exception of the adrenal cortex.

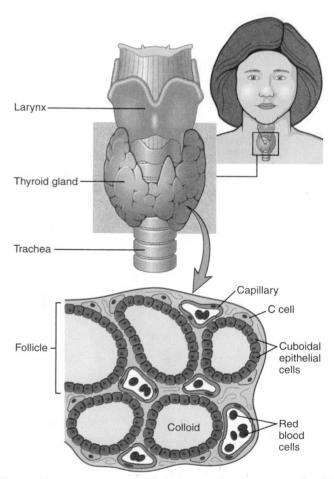

Larynx

Thyroid gland

Trachea

Capillary

C cell

Follicle

Cuboidal epithelial cells

Colloid

Red blood cells

Figure 89-1 Anatomy and microscopic appearance of the thyroid gland, showing secretion of thyroglobulin into the follicles.

The thyroid gland also contains *C cells* that secrete *calcitonin,* a hormone that contributes to regulation of plasma calcium ion concentration, as discussed in Chapter 90.

IODINE IS REQUIRED FOR FORMATION OF THYROXINE

To form normal quantities of thyroxine, about 50 mg of ingested iodine in the form of iodides are required *each year,* or about 1 mg/week. To prevent iodine deficiency, common table salt is iodized with about 1 part sodium iodide to every 100,000 parts sodium chloride.

Fate of Ingested Iodides. Iodides ingested orally are absorbed from the gastrointestinal tract into the blood in about the same manner as chlorides. Normally, most of the iodides are rapidly excreted by the kidneys, but only after about one-fifth are selectively removed from the circulating blood by the cells of the thyroid gland and used for synthesis of the thyroid hormones.

FORMATION AND SECRETION OF THYROGLOBULIN BY THE THYROID CELLS

The thyroid cells are typical protein-secreting glandular cells, as shown in Figure 89-2. *Thyroglobulin,* a large glycoprotein molecule (Mol. Wt. 335,000), is synthesized by the endoplasmic reticulum and Golgi apparatus, and secreted into the follicles.

Each molecule of thyroglobulin contains about 70 tyrosine amino acids, and they are the major substrates that combine with iodine to form the thyroid hormones. Thus, the thyroid hormones form *within* the thyroglobulin molecule.

Various steps in the biosynthesis of thyroid hormone have been summarized in Box 89-1.

Iodide Pump—the Sodium–Iodide Symporter (Iodide Trapping)

The first stage in the formation of thyroid hormones, shown in Figure 89-2, is transport of iodides from the blood into the thyroid glandular cells and follicles. This pumping is achieved

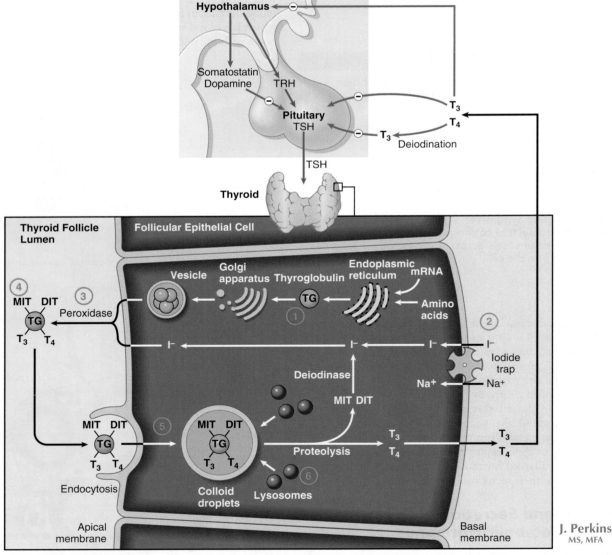

Figure 89-2   Thyroid cellular mechanisms for iodine transport, thyroxine and triiodothyronine formation, and thyroxine and triiodothyronine release into the blood. DIT, diiodotyrosine; I^-, iodide ion; I_2, iodine; MIT, monoiodotyrosine; T_3, triiodothyronine; T_4, thyroxine; T_G, thyroglobulin. *Netter illustration from www.netterimages.com. © Elsevier Inc. All rights reserved.*

BOX 89-1 STEPS IN THE BIOSYNTHESIS OF THYROID HORMONES

1. Iodide trapping
2. Oxidation of the iodide ion
3. "Organification" of thyroglobulin
4. Coupling of iodotyrosine residues
5. Release of T_3 and T_4 into blood

by the action of a *sodium–iodide symporter*, which cotransports one iodide ion along with two sodium ions across the basolateral (plasma) membrane into the cell. The energy for transporting iodide against a concentration gradient comes from the sodium–potassium adenosine triphosphatase (ATPase) pump, which pumps sodium out of the cell, thereby establishing a low intracellular sodium concentration and a gradient for facilitated diffusion of sodium into the cell.

This process of concentrating the iodide in the cell is called *iodide trapping.* The capacity of this pump helps concentrate iodide 30 times that of blood normally and up to 250 times during maximal activity of the gland. The rate of iodide trapping by the thyroid is influenced by the concentration of TSH.

A protein called *pendrin* (chloride–iodide ion counter-transporter) helps transport iodide out of the thyroid cells into the follicle.

Oxidation of the Iodide Ion

The first essential step in the formation of thyroid hormones is conversion of iodide ions to an *oxidized form of iodine,* either nascent iodine (I^0) or I_3-, which is then capable of combining directly with the amino acid tyrosine. This oxidation of iodine is promoted by the enzyme *peroxidase* and its accompanying *hydrogen peroxide,* located in the apical membrane of the cell or attached to it. When the peroxidase system is blocked or when it is hereditarily absent from the cells, the rate of formation of thyroid hormones falls to zero.

Iodination of Tyrosine and Formation of the Thyroid Hormones—"Organification" of Thyroglobulin

The binding of iodine with the thyroglobulin molecule is called *organification* of the thyroglobulin. In thyroid cells, the oxidized iodine with the help of thyroid peroxidase enzyme (Figure 89-2) causes the process to occur within seconds or minutes. Tyrosine is first iodized to *monoiodotyrosine* and then to *diiodotyrosine.*

Figure 89-3 shows the successive stages of iodination of tyrosine and final formation of the two important thyroid hormones, thyroxine and triiodothyronine.

Coupling of Iodotyrosine Residues

Immediately after the formation of *monoiodotyrosine* and *diiodotyrosine,* during the next few minutes, hours, and even days, more and more of the iodotyrosine residues become *coupled* with one another. The major hormonal product of the coupling reaction is the molecule *thyroxine* (T_4), which is formed when two molecules of diiodotyrosine are joined together; the thyroxine then remains part of the thyroglobulin molecule. Or one molecule of monoiodotyrosine couples with one molecule of diiodotyrosine to form *triiodothyronine* (T_3), which represents about one-fifteenth of the final hormones. Small amounts of *reverse* T_3 (RT_3) are formed by coupling of diiodotyrosine with

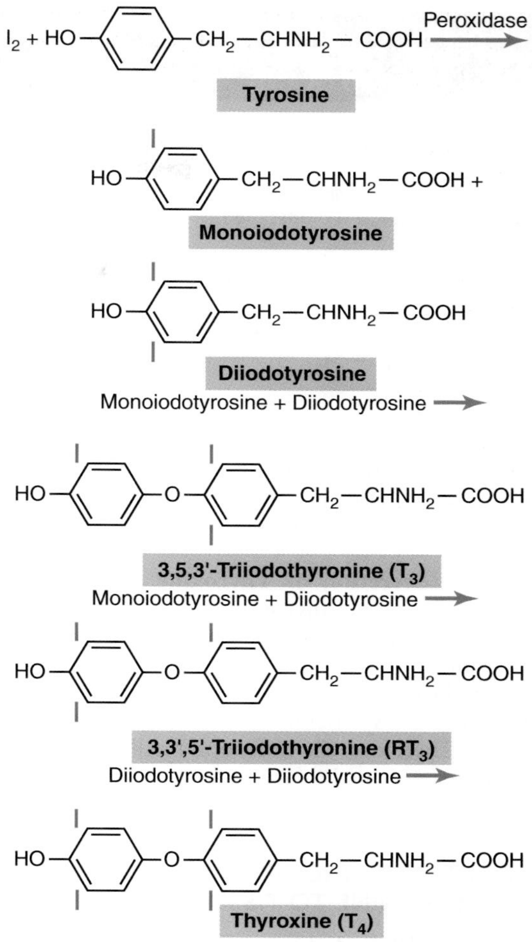

Figure 89-3 Chemistry of thyroxine and triiodothyronine formation.

monoiodotyrosine, but RT_3 does not appear to be of functional significance in humans.

Storage of Thyroglobulin. The thyroid gland is unusual among the endocrine glands in its ability to store large amounts of hormone. After synthesis of the thyroid hormones has run its course, each thyroglobulin molecule contains up to 30 thyroxine molecules and a few triiodothyronine molecules. In this form, the thyroid hormones are stored in the follicles in an amount sufficient to supply the body with its normal requirements of thyroid hormones for 2–3 months. Therefore, when synthesis of thyroid hormone ceases, the physiological effects of deficiency are not observed for several months.

Release of Thyroxine and Triiodothyronine From the Thyroid Gland

Most of the thyroglobulin is not released into the circulating blood; instead, thyroxine and triiodothyronine are cleaved from the thyroglobulin molecule, and then these free hormones are released (Box 89-2).

About three quarters of the iodinated tyrosine in the thyroglobulin never become thyroid hormones but remain monoiodotyrosine and diiodotyrosine. During the digestion of the thyroglobulin molecule, their iodine is cleaved from them

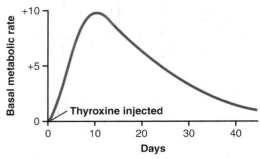

Figure 89-4 Approximate prolonged effect on the basal metabolic rate caused by administering a single large dose of thyroxine.

by a *deiodinase enzyme* that makes virtually all this iodine available again for recycling within the gland. In the congenital absence of this deiodinase enzyme, many persons become iodine deficient because of failure of this recycling process.

Daily Rate of Secretion of Thyroxine and Triiodothyronine. About 93% of the thyroid hormone released is thyroxine and approximately 7% of the thyroid hormone released is triiodothyronine.

However, during the ensuing few days, about one-half of the thyroxine is slowly deiodinated to form additional triiodothyronine. Therefore, the hormone finally delivered to and used by the tissues is mainly triiodothyronine (a total of about 35 µg/day).

TRANSPORT OF THYROXINE AND TRIIODOTHYRONINE TO TISSUES

Thyroxine and Triiodothyronine Are Bound to Plasma Proteins. Upon entering the blood, more than 99% of the thyroxine and triiodothyronine combines immediately with several of the plasma proteins, all of which are synthesized by the liver. They combine mainly with *thyroxine-binding globulin* (TBG) and much less so with *thyroxine-binding prealbumin* (TBPA) and *albumin.*

Thyroxine and Triiodothyronine Are Released Slowly to Tissue Cells. Because of high affinity of the plasma-binding proteins for the thyroid hormones, these substances—in particular, thyroxine—are released to the tissue cells slowly. Half the thyroxine in the blood is released to the tissue cells about every 6 days, whereas half the triiodothyronine—because of its lower affinity—is released to the cells in about 1 day.

Upon entering the tissue cells, both thyroxine and triiodothyronine again bind with intracellular proteins, with the thyroxine binding more strongly than the triiodothyronine. Therefore, they are again stored, but this time in the target cells themselves, and they are used slowly over a period of days or weeks.

Thyroid Hormones Have Slow Onset and Long Duration of Action. After injection of a large quantity of thyroxine into a human being, essentially no effect on the metabolic rate can be discerned for 2–3 days. Once activity does begin, it increases progressively and reaches a maximum in 10–12 days, as shown in Figure 89-4. Thereafter, it decreases with a half-life of about 15 days. Some of the activity persists for as long as 6 weeks to 2 months.

The actions of triiodothyronine occur about four times as rapidly as those of thyroxine, with a latent period as short as 6–12 hours and maximal cellular activity occurring within 2–3 days.

Most of the latency and the prolonged period of action of these hormones are probably caused by their binding with proteins both in the plasma and in the tissue cells, followed by their slow release.

Metabolism and Excretion of the Thyroid Hormones

Most of the Thyroxine Secreted by the Thyroid Is Converted to Triiodothyronine. Before acting on target tissues, one iodide is removed from almost all the thyroxine, thus forming triiodothyronine (T_3). Intracellular thyroid hormone receptors have a high affinity for triiodothyronine. There are three deiodinase enzymes (D1, D2, and D3) of which D1 and D2 are responsible for most of the peripheral conversion of T_4 to T_3. Consequently, more than 90% of the thyroid hormone molecules that bind with the receptors is triiodothyronine.

The third deiodinase enzyme, present in tissues such as the liver, skeletal muscle, and CNS, is responsible for inactivating T_3 and also prevents the activation of T_4 by converting it to reverse T_3.

Following inactivation, these hormones are conjugated with sulfates to form T_4SO_4 or T_3SO_4. Alternatively, they are conjugated with glucuronides to form glucuronidated T4 and T3 and are excreted into the bile. However, in the intestine there may be partial reabsorption after deglucuronidation.

Physiological Functions of the Thyroid Hormones

THYROID HORMONES INCREASE TRANSCRIPTION OF LARGE NUMBERS OF GENES

The general effect of thyroid hormone is to activate nuclear transcription of large numbers of genes (Figure 89-5). Therefore, in virtually all cells of the body, great numbers of protein enzymes, structural proteins, transport proteins, and other substances are synthesized. The net result is generalized increase in functional activity throughout the body.

Thyroid Hormones Activate Nuclear Receptors. The thyroid hormone receptors are either attached to the DNA genetic strands or located in proximity to them. On binding with thyroid hormone, the receptors become activated and initiate the transcription process. Then large numbers of different types of messenger RNA are formed, followed within another few minutes or hours by RNA translation on the cytoplasmic ribosomes

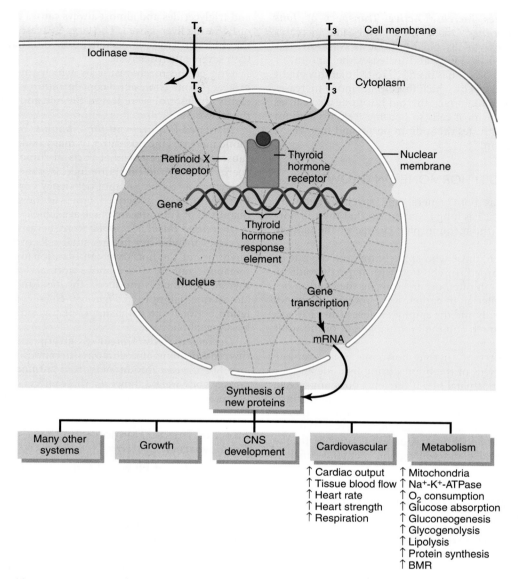

Figure 89-5 Thyroid hormone activation of target cells. Thyroxine (T_4) and triiodothyronine (T_3) enter the cell membrane by a carrier-mediated adenosine triphosphate-dependent transport process. Much of the T_4 is deiodinated to form T_3, which interacts with the thyroid hormone receptor, bound as a heterodimer with a retinoid X receptor, of the thyroid hormone response element of the gene. This action causes either increases or decreases in transcription of genes that lead to the formation of proteins, thus producing the thyroid hormone response of the cell. The actions of thyroid hormone on cells of several different systems are shown. BMR, basal metabolic rate; CNS, central nervous system; mRNA, messenger ribonucleic acid; Na^+-K^+-ATPase, sodium–potassium–adenosine triphosphatase.

to form hundreds of new intracellular proteins, which cause most of the effects of thyroid hormones.

Nongenomic Cellular Effects of Thyroid Hormone. Thyroid hormones also appear to have *nongenomic* cellular effects that are independent of their effects on gene transcription. Nongenomic actions of thyroid hormone include the following:
1. Regulation of ion channels.
2. Regulation of oxidative phosphorylation.
3. Activation of intracellular secondary messengers, such as cyclic AMP or protein kinase signaling cascades.

The site of nongenomic thyroid hormone action appears to be the plasma membrane, cytoplasm, and perhaps some cell organelles such as mitochondria in tissues, such as the heart, pituitary, and adipose tissue.

THYROID HORMONES INCREASE CELLULAR METABOLIC ACTIVITY

The thyroid hormones increase the metabolic activities of almost all the tissues of the body. The basal metabolic rate can increase to 60–100% above normal when large quantities of the hormones are secreted.

Thyroid Hormones Increase the Number and Activity of Mitochondria. One of the principal functions of thyroxine might be simply to increase the number and activity of mitochondria, which in turn increases the rate of formation of adenosine triphosphate (ATP) to energize cellular function. However, the increase in the number and activity of mitochondria could be the *result* of increased activity of the cells as well as the cause of the increase.

Thyroid Hormones Increase Active Transport of Ions Through Cell Membranes. One of the enzymes that increases its activity in response to thyroid hormone is *Na-K-ATPase.* Because this process uses energy and increases the amount of heat produced in the body, it has been suggested that this might be one of the mechanisms by which thyroid hormone increases the body's metabolic rate. In fact, thyroid hormone also causes the cell membranes of most cells to become leaky to sodium ions, which further activates the sodium pump and further increases heat production.

EFFECT OF THYROID HORMONE ON GROWTH

Thyroid hormone has both general and specific effects on growth. For instance, it has long been known that thyroid hormone is essential for the metamorphic change of the tadpole into the frog.

In growing children, those who are hypothyroid, the rate of growth is greatly retarded. In children with hyperthyroidism, excessive skeletal growth often occurs, causing the child to become considerably taller at an earlier age. However, the bones also mature more rapidly and the epiphyses close at an early age, so the duration of growth and the eventual height of the adult actually may be shortened.

An important effect of thyroid hormone is to promote growth and development of the brain during fetal life and for the first few years of postnatal life. If the fetus does not secrete sufficient quantities of thyroid hormone, growth and maturation of the brain both before birth and afterward are greatly retarded and the brain remains smaller than normal. Without specific thyroid therapy within days or weeks after birth, the child without a thyroid gland will remain mentally deficient throughout life.

EFFECTS OF THYROID HORMONE ON SPECIFIC BODY FUNCTIONS

Stimulation of Carbohydrate Metabolism. Thyroid hormone stimulates almost all aspects of carbohydrate metabolism, such as

- rapid glucose uptake by the cells,
- enhanced glycolysis,
- enhanced gluconeogenesis,
- increased rate of absorption from the gastrointestinal tract, and
- even increased insulin secretion with its resultant secondary effects on carbohydrate metabolism.

All these effects probably result from the overall increase in cellular metabolic enzymes caused by thyroid hormone.

Stimulation of Fat Metabolism. Essentially all aspects of fat metabolism are also enhanced under the influence of thyroid hormone. In particular, lipids are mobilized rapidly from the fat tissue, which decreases the fat stores of the body to a greater extent than almost any other tissue element. Mobilization of lipids from fat tissue also increases the free fatty acid concentration in the plasma and greatly accelerates the oxidation of free fatty acids by the cells.

Effect on Plasma and Liver Fats. Increased thyroid hormone decreases the concentrations of cholesterol, phospholipids, and triglycerides in the plasma, even though it increases the free fatty acids. Conversely, decreased thyroid secretion greatly increases the plasma concentrations of cholesterol, phospholipids,

and triglycerides and almost always causes excessive deposition of fat in the liver as well. The large increase in circulating plasma cholesterol in prolonged hypothyroidism is often associated with severe atherosclerosis,

One of the mechanisms by which thyroid hormone decreases plasma cholesterol concentration is to increase significantly cholesterol secretion in the bile and consequent loss in the feces.

Increased Requirement for Vitamins. Because thyroid hormone increases the quantities of many bodily enzymes and because vitamins are essential parts of some of the enzymes or coenzymes, thyroid hormone increases the need for vitamins. Therefore, a relative vitamin deficiency can occur when excess thyroid hormone is secreted, unless at the same time increased quantities of vitamins are made available.

Increased Basal Metabolic Rate. Because thyroid hormone increases metabolism in almost all cells of the body, excessive quantities of the hormone can occasionally increase the basal metabolic rate 60–100% above normal. Conversely, when no thyroid hormone is produced, the basal metabolic rate falls to almost one-half normal. Figure 89-6 shows the approximate relation between the daily supply of thyroid hormones and the basal metabolic rate.

Decreased Body Weight. A greatly increased amount of thyroid hormone almost always decreases body weight, and a greatly decreased amount of thyroid hormone almost always increases body weight; however, these effects do not always occur because thyroid hormone also increases the appetite, which may counterbalance the change in the metabolic rate.

Effect of Thyroid Hormones on the Cardiovascular System

Increased Blood Flow and Cardiac Output. Increased metabolism in the tissues causes release of more metabolic end products from the tissues which in turn causes vasodilation in most body tissues, thus increasing blood flow. This increase in blood flow also meets the need for heat elimination from the body. As a consequence of the increased blood flow, cardiac output also increases above normal (~60%) in hyperthyroid states and decreases to only 50% of normal in severe hypothyroidism.

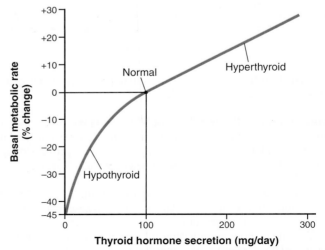

Figure 89-6 Approximate relation of the daily rate of thyroid hormone (T$_4$ and T$_3$) secretion to percent change in basal metabolic rate compared with normal.

Increased Heart Rate. The heart rate increases considerably more under the influence of thyroid hormone than would be expected from the increase in cardiac output, which is an important sensitive physical sign for physicians.

Increased Heart Strength. The increased enzymatic activity caused by increased thyroid hormone production also increases the strength of the heart when only a slight excess of thyroid hormone is secreted. However, when thyroid hormone is increased markedly, the heart muscle strength becomes depressed because of long-term excessive protein catabolism. Indeed, some severely thyrotoxic patients die of cardiac decompensation secondary to myocardial failure and to increased cardiac load imposed by the increase in cardiac output.

Normal Arterial Pressure. The mean arterial pressure usually remains about normal after administration of thyroid hormone. Because of increased blood flow through the tissues between heartbeats, the pulse pressure is often increased, with the systolic pressure elevated 10–15 mmHg in hyperthyroidism and the diastolic pressure reduced a corresponding amount.

Increased Respiration. The increased rate of metabolism increases the utilization of oxygen and the formation of carbon dioxide; these effects activate all the mechanisms that increase the rate and depth of respiration.

Increased Gastrointestinal Motility. In addition to increased appetite and food intake, which has been discussed, thyroid hormone increases both the rate of secretion of the digestive juices and the motility of the gastrointestinal tract. Hyperthyroidism therefore often results in diarrhea, whereas lack of thyroid hormone can cause constipation.

Excitatory Effects on the Central Nervous System. In general, thyroid hormone increases the rapidity of cerebration, although thought processes may be dissociated; conversely, lack of thyroid hormone decreases rapidity of cerebration. A person with hyperthyroidism is likely to be extremely nervous and have many psychoneurotic tendencies, such as anxiety complexes, extreme worry, and paranoia.

Effect on the Function of the Muscles. A slight increase in thyroid hormone usually makes the muscles react with vigor, but when the quantity of hormone becomes excessive, the muscles become weakened because of excess protein catabolism. Conversely, lack of thyroid hormone causes the muscles to become sluggish and they relax slowly after a contraction.

Muscle Tremor. One of the most characteristic signs of hyperthyroidism is a fine muscle tremor. The tremor can be observed easily by placing a sheet of paper on the extended fingers and noting the degree of vibration of the paper. This tremor is believed to be caused by increased reactivity of the neuronal synapses in the areas of the spinal cord that control muscle tone.

Effect on Sleep. Because of the exhausting effect of thyroid hormone on the musculature and on the central nervous system, persons with hyperthyroidism often have a feeling of constant tiredness, but because of the excitable effects of thyroid hormone on the synapses, it is difficult to sleep. Conversely, extreme somnolence is characteristic of hypothyroidism, with sleep sometimes lasting 12–14 hours a day.

Effect on Other Endocrine Glands. Increased thyroid hormone increases the rate of secretion of several other endocrine glands, but it also increases the need of the tissues for the hormones. For instance, increased thyroxine secretion increases the rate of glucose metabolism almost everywhere in the body and therefore causes a corresponding need for increased insulin secretion by the pancreas.

Effect of Thyroid Hormone on Sexual Function. For normal sexual function, thyroid secretion needs to be approximately normal. In men, lack of thyroid hormone is likely to cause loss of libido; a great excess of the hormone, however, sometimes causes impotence.

In women, lack of thyroid hormone often causes *menorrhagia* and *polymenorrhea*—that is, excessive and frequent menstrual bleeding, respectively. However, in some women irregular periods and occasionally even *amenorrhea* (absence of menstrual bleeding) may occur. Greatly decreased libido is also reported in women with hypothyroidism.

In the hyperthyroid woman, *oligomenorrhea*, which means greatly reduced bleeding, is common, and occasionally amenorrhea results. This history may confuse the picture when making a diagnosis. Summary of thyroid hormone actions is given in Table 89-1.

Regulation of Thyroid Hormone Secretion

To maintain normal levels of metabolic activity in the body, precisely the right amount of thyroid hormone must be secreted at all times; to achieve this ideal level of secretion, specific feedback mechanisms operate through the hypothalamus and anterior pituitary gland to control the rate of thyroid secretion. These mechanisms are described in the following sections.

TSH (From the Anterior Pituitary Gland) Increases Thyroid Secretion. TSH, also known as *thyrotropin,* is an anterior pituitary hormone; it is a glycoprotein with a molecular weight of about 28,000. This hormone, also discussed in Chapter 87, increases secretion of thyroxine and triiodothyronine by the thyroid gland. It has the following specific effects on the thyroid gland:

1. *Increased proteolysis of the thyroglobulin* that has already been stored in the follicles, releasing thyroid hormones into the blood.
2. *Increased activity of the iodide pump,* which increases the rate of "iodide trapping" in the glandular cells.
3. *Increased iodination of tyrosine* to form the thyroid hormones.
4. *Increased size and increased secretory activity of the thyroid cells.*
5. *Increased number of thyroid cells* plus a change from cuboidal to columnar cells and much infolding of the thyroid epithelium into the follicles.

In summary, TSH increases all the known secretory activities of the thyroid glandular cells.

The most important early effect after administration of TSH is to initiate proteolysis of thyroglobulin, which causes release of thyroxine and triiodothyronine into the blood within 30 minutes. It is now clear that most of these effects result from activation of the "second messenger" *cyclic adenosine monophosphate* (cAMP) system of the cell. The other effects require hours or even days and weeks to develop fully.

TABLE 89-1	Thyroid Hormone Actions	
		Actions
Metabolic functions	Carbohydrate metabolism	Stimulates all aspects of carbohydrate metabolism Enhanced glucose uptake, glycolysis, gluconeogenesis, increased insulin secretion
	Fat metabolism	Enhanced lipid mobilization from fat tissues Increased free fatty acids Decreases cholesterol, phospholipids, and triglycerides in blood
	Vitamin requirements	Increases vitamin requirements
	Basal metabolic rate	Increases BMR
General features	Body weight	Decreases body weight
Actions on specific systems/ tissues/functions	Cardiovascular system	Increased heart rate Increased cardiac output Increased force of contraction
	Respiratory system	Increased rate of respiration
	Gastrointestinal system	Increased motility of the GI tract
	Central nervous system	Increases rapidity of cerebration
	Musculoskeletal system	Slight increase excites musculoskeletal system Excessive causes muscle weakness
	Endocrine glands	Increases activity in almost all glands

Anterior Pituitary Secretion of TSH Is Regulated by Thyrotropin-Releasing Hormone From the Hypothalamus. Anterior pituitary secretion of TSH is controlled by a hypothalamic hormone, *thyrotropin-releasing hormone* (TRH), which is secreted by nerve endings in the median eminence of the hypothalamus. From the median eminence, TRH is then transported to the anterior pituitary by way of the hypothalamic–hypophysial portal blood.

Effects of Cold and Other Neurogenic Stimuli on TRH and TSH Secretion. One of the best-known stimuli for increasing TRH secretion by the hypothalamus, and therefore TSH secretion by the anterior pituitary gland, is exposure of an animal to cold.

Various emotional reactions can also affect the output of TRH and TSH and therefore indirectly affect the secretion of thyroid hormones. Excitement and anxiety—conditions that greatly stimulate the sympathetic nervous system—cause an acute decrease in secretion of TSH, perhaps because these states increase the metabolic rate and body heat, and therefore exert an inverse effect on the heat control center.

Neither these emotional effects nor the effect of cold is observed after the hypophysial stalk has been cut, demonstrating that both of these effects are mediated by way of the hypothalamus.

FEEDBACK EFFECT OF THYROID HORMONE TO DECREASE ANTERIOR PITUITARY SECRETION OF TSH

Increased thyroid hormone in the body fluids decreases secretion of TSH by the anterior pituitary. As shown in Figure 89-7, it is probable that increased thyroid hormone inhibits anterior pituitary secretion of TSH mainly by a direct effect on the anterior pituitary gland itself.

Figure 85-4 describes the regulation of the secretion of thyroid hormones. Please refer to Chapter 85 for more details.

ANTITHYROID SUBSTANCES SUPPRESS THYROID SECRETION

The best known antithyroid drugs are *thiocyanate, propylthiouracil,* and high concentrations of *inorganic iodides.* The

mechanism by which each of these drugs blocks thyroid secretion is different from the others and can be explained as follows.

Table 89-2 describes the synthesis of thyroid hormones and drugs acting at various steps.

Thiocyanate Ions Decrease Iodide Trapping. The same active pump that transports iodide ions into the thyroid cells can also pump thiocyanate ions, perchlorate ions, and nitrate ions. Therefore, the administration of thiocyanate (or one of the other ions as well) in a high enough concentration can cause competitive inhibition of iodide transport into the cell—that is, inhibition of the iodide-trapping mechanism.

The decreased availability of iodide in the glandular cells does not stop the formation of thyroglobulin; it merely prevents the thyroglobulin that is formed from becoming iodinated and therefore from forming thyroid hormones. This deficiency of thyroid hormones in turn leads to increased secretion of TSH by the anterior pituitary gland, which causes overgrowth of the thyroid gland even though the gland still does not form

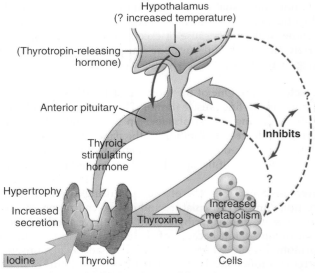

Figure 89-7 Regulation of thyroid secretion.

TABLE 89-2 Synthesis of Thyroid Hormones and Drugs Acting at Various Steps

Steps in the Biosynthesis of Thyroid Hormones	Antithyroid Drug	Actions
1. Iodide trapping	Thiocyanate ions Iodides (High concentration)	Inhibition of the iodide-trapping mechanism Reduces rate of iodide trapping
2. Oxidation of the iodide ion	Propylthiouracil	Block the peroxidase enzyme that is required for iodination of tyrosine
3. "Organification" of thyroglobulin	Methimazole	Partly blocks the coupling reaction
4. Coupling of iodotyrosine residues	Carbimazole	
5. Release of T_3 and T_4 into blood	Iodides (high concentration)	Endocytosis of colloid is paralyzed—thyroid hormone release is shut down

adequate quantities of thyroid hormones. Therefore, the use of thiocyanates and some other ions to block thyroid secretion can lead to the development of a greatly enlarged thyroid gland, which is called a *goiter.*

Propylthiouracil Decreases Thyroid Hormone Formation. Propylthiouracil (along with other, similar compounds, such as methimazole and carbimazole) prevents formation of thyroid hormone from iodides and tyrosine. The mechanism of this action is partly to block the peroxidase enzyme that is required for iodination of tyrosine and partly to block the coupling of two iodinated tyrosines to form thyroxine or triiodothyronine.

Propylthiouracil, like thiocyanate, does not prevent formation of thyroglobulin. The absence of thyroxine and triiodothyronine in the thyroglobulin can lead to tremendous feedback enhancement of TSH secretion by the anterior pituitary gland, thus promoting growth of the glandular tissue and forming a goiter.

Iodides in High Concentrations Decrease Thyroid Activity and Thyroid Gland Size. When iodides are present in the blood in *high concentration* (100 times the normal plasma level), most activities of the thyroid gland are decreased, but often they remain decreased for only a few weeks. The effect is to reduce the rate of iodide trapping so that the rate of iodination of tyrosine to form thyroid hormones is also decreased. Even more important, the normal endocytosis of colloid from the follicles by the thyroid glandular cells is paralyzed by the high iodide concentrations. Because this is the first step in release of thyroid hormones from the storage colloid, there is almost immediate shutdown of thyroid hormone secretion into the blood.

Because iodides in high concentrations decrease all phases of thyroid activity, they slightly decrease the size of the thyroid gland and especially decrease its blood supply, in contradistinction to the opposite effects caused by most of the other antithyroid agents. For this reason, iodides are frequently administered to patients for 2–3 weeks before surgical removal of the thyroid gland to decrease the necessary amount of surgery, and especially to decrease the amount of bleeding.

Diseases of the Thyroid

HYPERTHYROIDISM

Causes of Hyperthyroidism (Toxic Goiter, Thyrotoxicosis, Graves' Disease). In most patients with hyperthyroidism, the thyroid gland is increased to two to three times its normal size, with tremendous hyperplasia and infolding of the follicular cell lining into the follicles.

Graves' disease, the most common form of hyperthyroidism, is an autoimmune disease in which antibodies called *thyroid-stimulating immunoglobulins* (TSIs) form against the TSH receptor in the thyroid gland. These antibodies bind with the same membrane receptors that bind TSH and induce continual activation of the cAMP system of the cells, with resultant development of hyperthyroidism. The TSI antibodies have a prolonged stimulating effect on the thyroid gland, lasting for as long as 12 hours, in contrast to a little over 1 hour for TSH. The high level of thyroid hormone secretion caused by TSI in turn suppresses anterior pituitary formation of TSH. Therefore, TSH concentrations are less than normal (often essentially zero) rather than enhanced in almost all patients with Graves' disease.

The antibodies that cause hyperthyroidism almost certainly occur as the result of autoimmunity that has developed against thyroid tissue. Presumably, at some time in the person's history, an excess of thyroid cell antigens was released from the thyroid cells resulting in the formation of antibodies against the thyroid gland.

Thyroid Adenoma. Hyperthyroidism occasionally results from a localized adenoma (a tumor) that develops in the thyroid tissue and secretes large quantities of thyroid hormone. This presentation is different from the more usual type of hyperthyroidism in that it is usually not associated with evidence of any autoimmune disease. As long as of the adenoma continues to secrete large quantities of thyroid hormone, secretory function in the remainder of the thyroid gland is almost totally inhibited because the thyroid hormone from the adenoma depresses the production of TSH by the pituitary gland.

Symptoms of hyperthyroidism have been summarized in Box 89-3.

Exophthalmos. Most people with hyperthyroidism exhibit some degree of protrusion of the eyeballs, as shown in Figure 89-8. This condition is called *exophthalmos.* As a result, the epithelial surfaces of the eyes become dry and irritated and often infected, resulting in ulceration of the cornea.

The cause of the protruding eyes is edematous swelling of the retro-orbital tissues and degenerative changes in the extraocular muscles. In most patients, immunoglobulins that react

BOX 89-3 SYMPTOMS OF HYPERTHYROIDISM

1. A high state of excitability
2. Intolerance to heat
3. Increased sweating
4. Mild to extreme weight loss (sometimes as much as 100 pounds)
5. Varying degrees of diarrhea
6. Muscle weakness
7. Nervousness or other psychic disorders
8. Extreme fatigue but inability to sleep
9. Tremor of the hands

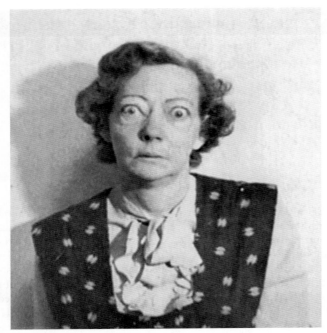

Figure 89-8 A patient with exophthalmic hyperthyroidism. Note protrusion of the eyes and retraction of the superior eyelids. Her basal metabolic rate was +40. *(Courtesy Dr Leonard Posey.)*

with the eye muscles can be found in the blood. Therefore, there is much reason to believe that exophthalmos, like hyperthyroidism itself, is an autoimmune process.

Diagnostic Tests for Hyperthyroidism. For the usual case of hyperthyroidism, the most accurate diagnostic test is direct measurement of the concentration of "free" thyroxine (and sometimes triiodothyronine) in the plasma, using appropriate radioimmunoassay procedures.

The following tests also are sometimes used:
1. The basal metabolic rate is usually increased to +30 to +60 in severe hyperthyroidism.
2. The concentration of TSH in the plasma is measured by radioimmunoassay.
3. The concentration of TSI is measured by radioimmunoassay. This concentration is usually high in thyrotoxicosis but low in thyroid adenoma.

Treatment in Hyperthyroidism. The most direct treatment for hyperthyroidism is surgical removal of most of the thyroid gland. In general, it is desirable to prepare the patient for surgical removal of the gland before the operation by administering propylthiouracil, usually for several weeks, until the basal metabolic rate of the patient has returned to normal. Then, administration of high concentrations of iodides for 1–2 weeks immediately before operation causes the gland to recede in size and its blood supply to diminish. With use of these preoperative procedures, the operative mortality is less than 1 in 1000, whereas before the development of modern procedures, operative mortality was 1 in 25.

Treatment of the Hyperplastic Thyroid Gland With Radioactive Iodine. Eighty to 90% of an injected dose of iodide is absorbed by the hyperplastic, toxic thyroid gland within 1 day after injection. If this injected iodine is radioactive, it can destroy most of the secretory cells of the thyroid gland. Usually 5 mCi of radioactive iodine is given to the patient, whose condition is reassessed several weeks later. If the patient is still in a hyperthyroid state, additional doses are administered until normal thyroid status is reached.

HYPOTHYROIDISM

The effects of hypothyroidism, in general, are opposite to those of hyperthyroidism, a few physiological mechanisms are peculiar to hypothyroidism. Hypothyroidism, like hyperthyroidism, is often initiated by autoimmunity against the thyroid gland (*Hashimoto's disease*), but in this case the autoimmunity destroys the gland rather than stimulates it. The thyroid glands of most of these patients first demonstrate autoimmune "thyroiditis," which means thyroid inflammation. Thyroiditis causes progressive deterioration and finally fibrosis of the gland, with resultant diminished or absent secretion of thyroid hormone. Several other types of hypothyroidism also occur, that are often associated with development of enlarged thyroid glands, called *thyroid goiter,* as described in the following sections.

Endemic Colloid Goiter Caused by Dietary Iodide Deficiency. The term "goiter" means a greatly enlarged thyroid gland. As pointed out in the discussion of iodine metabolism, about 50 mg of iodine are required *each year* for the formation of adequate quantities of thyroid hormone. In certain areas of the world, notably in the Swiss Alps, the Andes, and the Great Lakes region of the United States, insufficient iodine is present in the soil for the foodstuffs to contain even this minute quantity. Therefore, in the days before iodized table salt, many people who lived in these areas developed extremely large thyroid glands, called *endemic goiters.*

The following mechanism results in the development of large endemic goiters: lack of iodine prevents production of both thyroxine and triiodothyronine. As a result, no hormone is available to inhibit production of TSH by the anterior pituitary, which causes the pituitary to secrete excessively large quantities of TSH. The TSH then stimulates the thyroid cells to secrete tremendous amounts of thyroglobulin colloid into the follicles and the gland grows larger and larger. However, because of lack of iodine, thyroxine and triiodothyronine production does not occur in the thyroglobulin molecule and therefore does not cause the normal suppression of TSH production by the anterior pituitary. The follicles become tremendous in size, and the thyroid gland may increase to 10–20 its times normal size.

Finally, some foods contain *goitrogenic substances* that have a propylthiouracil type of antithyroid activity, thus also leading to TSH-stimulated enlargement of the thyroid gland. Such goitrogenic substances are found especially in some varieties of turnips and cabbages.

Physiological Characteristics of Hypothyroidism. Whether hypothyroidism is due to thyroiditis, endemic colloid goiter, idiopathic colloid goiter, destruction of the thyroid gland by irradiation, or surgical removal of the thyroid gland, the physiological effects are the same. Table 89-3 summarizes the comparison between hyperthyroidism and hypothyroidism. Clinical features of hypothyroidism have been summarized in Box 89-4.

Myxedema. *Myxedema* develops in persons who have almost total lack of thyroid hormone function. Figure 89-9 shows such a patient, demonstrating bagginess under the eyes and swelling of the face. In this condition, for reasons that are not explained, greatly increased quantities of hyaluronic acid and chondroitin sulfate bound with protein form excessive tissue gel in the interstitial spaces, which causes the total quantity of interstitial fluid to increase. Because of the gel nature of the excess fluid, it is mainly immobile and the edema is the nonpitting type.

TABLE 89-3 Comparison of Hyperthyroidism and Hypothyroidism

Parameter	Hyperthyroidism	Hypothyroidism
General features	Fatigue High state of excitability Weight loss Increased BMR	Fatigue Extreme sluggishness Weight gain Decreased BMR
Sleep	Decreased sleep	Extreme somnolence
Temperature	Intolerance to heat	Intolerance to cold
Skeletal muscle	Muscle weakness	Extreme muscular sluggishness
Gastrointestinal tract	Mild diarrhea	Constipation
Skin	Increased sweating	Decreased sweating Scaliness of skin
Neurological effects	Fine tremor of the hands Nervousness Other psychic disorders	Mental sluggishness
Cardiac effects	Increased heart rate Increased cardiac output	Decreased heart rate Decreased cardiac output
Menstruation	Oligomenorrhea	Menorrhagia or polymenorrhea
Sexual functions		Men: Loss of libido Women: Decreased libido

---

BOX 89-4 CLINICAL FEATURES OF HYPOTHYROIDISM

1. Fatigue and extreme somnolence with sleeping up to 12–14 hours a day.
2. Extreme muscular sluggishness.
3. Slowed heart rate, decreased cardiac output, decreased blood volume.
4. Sometimes increased body weight.
5. Constipation.
6. Mental sluggishness.
7. Failure of many trophic functions in the body evidenced by depressed growth of hair and scaliness of the skin, development of a frog-like husky voice.
8. In severe cases, development of an edematous appearance throughout the body called myxedema.

Atherosclerosis in Hypothyroidism. As pointed out earlier, lack of thyroid hormone increases the quantity of blood cholesterol because of altered fat and cholesterol metabolism and diminished liver excretion of cholesterol in the bile. The increase in blood cholesterol is usually associated with increased atherosclerosis. Therefore, many hypothyroid patients, particularly those with myxedema, develop atherosclerosis, which in turn results in peripheral vascular disease, deafness, and coronary artery disease with subsequent early death.

Diagnostic Tests for Hypothyroidism. The tests already described for the diagnosis of hyperthyroidism give opposite results in hypothyroidism. The free thyroxine in the blood is low. The basal metabolic rate in myxedema ranges between −30 and −50. In addition, the secretion of TSH by the anterior pituitary when a test dose of TRH is administered is usually greatly increased (except in the rare instances of hypothyroidism caused by depressed response of the pituitary gland to TRH).

Treatment of Hypothyroidism. Figure 89-4 shows the effect of thyroxine on basal metabolic rate, demonstrating that the hormone normally has a duration of action of more than 1 month. Consequently, a steady level of thyroid hormone activity is easily maintained in the body via daily oral ingestion of one or more tablets containing thyroxine. Furthermore, proper treatment of hypothyroidism results in such complete normality that formerly myxedematous patients have lived into their 90s after undergoing treatment for more than 50 years.

CRETINISM

Cretinism is caused by extreme hypothyroidism during fetal life, infancy, or childhood. This condition is characterized especially by failure of body growth and by mental retardation. It results from congenital lack of a thyroid gland (*congenital cretinism*), from failure of the thyroid gland to produce thyroid hormone because of a genetic defect of the gland, or from a lack of iodine in the diet (*endemic cretinism*).

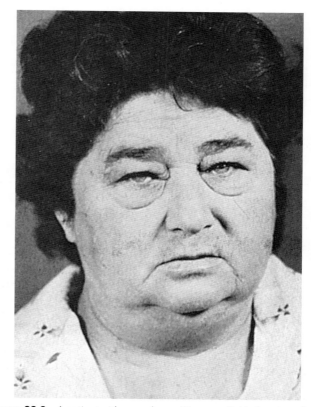

Figure 89-9 A patient with myxedema. (*Courtesy Dr Herbert Langford.*)

A neonate without a thyroid gland may have a normal appearance and function because it was supplied with some (but usually not enough) thyroid hormone by the mother while in utero. A few weeks after birth, however, the neonate's movements become sluggish and both physical and mental growth begin to be greatly retarded. Treatment of the neonate with cretinism at any time with adequate iodine or thyroxine usually causes normal return of physical growth, but unless the cretinism is treated within a few weeks after birth, mental growth remains permanently retarded. This state results from retardation of the growth, branching, and myelination of the neuronal cells of the central nervous system at this critical time in the normal development of the mental powers.

Skeletal growth in a child with cretinism is characteristically more inhibited than is soft tissue growth. As a result of this disproportionate rate of growth, the soft tissues are likely to enlarge excessively, giving the child with cretinism an obese, stocky, and short appearance. Occasionally, the tongue becomes so large in relation to the skeletal growth that it obstructs swallowing and breathing, inducing a characteristic guttural breathing that sometimes chokes the child.

BIBLIOGRAPHY

Bianco AC: Minireview: cracking the metabolic code for thyroid hormone signaling, *Endocrinology* 152:3306, 2011.

Brent GA: Clinical practice. Graves' disease, *N. Engl. J. Med.* 358:2594, 2008.

Brent GA: Mechanisms of thyroid hormone action, *J. Clin. Invest.* 122:3035, 2012.

Cooper DS, Biondi B: Subclinical thyroid disease, *Lancet* 379:1142, 2012.

Danzi S, Klein I: Thyroid hormone and the cardiovascular system, *Med. Clin. North Am.* 96:257, 2012.

De La Vieja A, Dohan O, Levy O, Carrasco N: Molecular analysis of the sodium/iodide symporter: impact on thyroid and extrathyroid pathophysiology, *Physiol. Rev.* 80:1083, 2000.

Franklyn JA, Boelaert K: Thyrotoxicosis, *Lancet* 379:1155, 2012.

Grais IM, Sowers JR: Thyroid and the heart, *Am. J. Med.* 127:691, 2014.

Kharlip J, Cooper DS: Recent developments in hyperthyroidism, *Lancet* 373:1930, 2009.

Klein I, Danzi S: Thyroid disease and the heart, *Circulation* 116:1725, 2007.

Kogai T, Brent GA: The sodium iodide symporter (NIS): regulation and approaches to targeting for cancer therapeutics, *Pharmacol. Ther.* 135:355, 2012.

Mullur R, Liu YY, Brent GA: Thyroid hormone regulation of metabolism, *Physiol. Rev.* 94:355, 2014.

Pearce EN: Update in lipid alterations in subclinical hypothyroidism, *J. Clin. Endocrinol. Metab.* 97:326, 2012.

Ross DS: Radioiodine therapy for hyperthyroidism, *N. Engl. J. Med.* 364:542, 2011.

Sinha RA, Singh BK, Yen PM: Thyroid hormone regulation of hepatic lipid and carbohydrate metabolism, *Trends Endocrinol. Metab.* 25:538, 2014.

Szkudlinski MW, Fremont V, Ronin C, Weintraub BD: Thyroid-stimulating hormone and thyroid-stimulating hormone receptor structure-function relationships, *Physiol. Rev.* 82:473, 2002.

Vasudevan N, Ogawa S, Pfaff D: Estrogen and thyroid hormone receptor interactions: physiological flexibility by molecular specificity, *Physiol. Rev.* 82:923, 2002.

Yen PM: Physiological and molecular basis of thyroid hormone action, *Physiol. Rev.* 81:1097, 2001.

Zimmermann MB: Iodine deficiency, *Endocr. Rev.* 30:376, 2009.

90

Calcium Homeostasis

LEARNING OBJECTIVES

- List the physiological effects of calcium.
- Outline calcium metabolism with regard to:
  - Forms of total serum calcium.
  - Daily calcium requirements.
  - Daily interorgan calcium fluxes.
  - Intestinal absorption of calcium.
  - Role of the kidneys in excretion of calcium.
  - Sites of calcium storage.
- Describe in detail calcium metabolism in bone with regard to:
  - Pools of calcium storage.
  - Cells involved.
  - Functions of each cell type.
- List the mechanism of action of parathormone, calcitonin, and vitamin D_3 in the regulation of calcium homeostasis.
- List the clinical features of (a) hypo- and hypercalcemia, (b) hypo- and hyperparathyroidism, (c) osteoporosis, and (d) osteomalacia.

GLOSSARY OF TERMS

- **Homeostasis:** Homeostasis is a state of internal equilibrium maintained by a cell or organism by adjusting its physiological processes.

- **Steatorrhea:** It is a condition where there is excess discharge of fat in the feces due to a failure to absorb fats.

The physiology of calcium and phosphate metabolism, formation of bone and teeth, and regulation of *vitamin D, parathyroid hormone* (PTH), and *calcitonin* are all closely intertwined. Extracellular calcium ion concentration, for example, is determined by the interplay of calcium absorption from the intestine, renal excretion of calcium, and bone uptake and release of calcium, each of which is regulated by the hormones just noted. Because phosphate homeostasis and calcium homeostasis are closely associated, they are discussed together in this chapter.

Physiological Effects of Calcium

Extracellular fluid calcium concentration is normally regulated precisely, it seldom rises or falls more than a few percent from the normal value of about 9.4 mg/dL, which is equivalent to 2.4 mmol of calcium per liter. This precise control is essential because calcium plays a key role in many physiological processes such as

1. Contraction of skeletal muscles
2. Contraction of cardiac muscles
3. Contraction of smooth muscles

4. Hemostasis and blood clotting
5. Transmission of nerve impulses
6. Acts as a second messenger to initiate various cellular functions

There are several other functions of calcium that are described in Figure 90-1.

Excitable cells, such as neurons, are sensitive to changes in calcium ion concentrations, and increases in calcium ion concentration above normal *(hypercalcemia)* cause progressive depression of the nervous system; conversely, decreases in calcium concentration *(hypocalcemia)* cause the nervous system to become more excited.

An important feature of extracellular calcium regulation is that only about 0.1% of the total body calcium is in the extracellular fluid, about 1% is in the cells and its organelles, and the rest being approximately 99% is stored in bones, which can serve as large reservoirs whenever required.

CALCIUM IN THE PLASMA AND INTERSTITIAL FLUID

The calcium in the plasma is present in three forms, as shown in Figure 90-2:

1. About 41% (1 mmol/L) of the calcium is combined with the plasma proteins and in this form is nondiffusible through the capillary membrane.

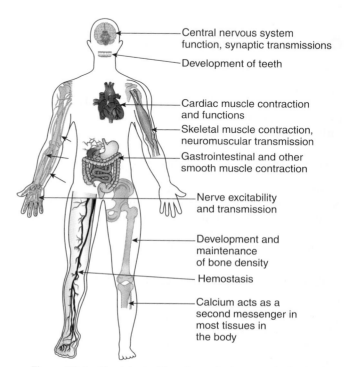

Figure 90-1 Physiological functions of calcium in the body.

Central nervous system function, synaptic transmissions

Development of teeth

Cardiac muscle contraction and functions

Skeletal muscle contraction, neuromuscular transmission

Gastrointestinal and other smooth muscle contraction

Nerve excitability and transmission

Development and maintenance of bone density

Hemostasis

Calcium acts as a second messenger in most tissues in the body

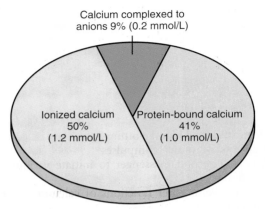

Figure 90-2   Distribution of ionized calcium (Ca++), diffusible but un-ionized calcium complexed to anions, and nondiffusible protein-bound calcium in blood plasma.

2. About 9% of the calcium (0.2 mmol/L) is diffusible; however, it is combined with anionic substances such as citrate and phosphates in such a manner that it is not ionized.
3. The remaining 50% of the calcium in the plasma is both diffusible through the capillary membrane and ionized.

This ionic calcium is the form that is important for most functions of calcium in the body, including the effect of calcium on the heart, the nervous system, and bone formation.

INORGANIC PHOSPHATE IN THE EXTRACELLULAR FLUIDS

Approximately 85% of the body's phosphate is stored in bones, 14–15% is in the cells, and less than 1% is in the extracellular fluid. Although extracellular fluid phosphate concentration is not nearly as well regulated as calcium concentration, phosphate serves several important functions and is controlled by many of the same factors that regulate calcium.

Outline of Calcium Metabolism

DAILY CALCIUM REQUIREMENTS

The usual rates of intake are about 1000 mg/day each for calcium and phosphorus, about the amounts in 1 L of milk (Table 90-1). Normally, divalent cations such as calcium ions are poorly absorbed from the intestines.

DAILY INTERORGAN CALCIUM FLUXES

The daily interorgan calcium fluxes are shown in calcium intake being approximately 1000 mg/day, about 90% (900 mg/day) of the daily intake of calcium is excreted in the feces. The daily interorgan calcium fluxes between extracellular fluid, bone, cells, and the intestines are clearly indicated in Figure 90-3.

INTESTINAL ABSORPTION OF CALCIUM

Vitamin D promotes calcium absorption by the intestines and about 35% (350 mg/day) of the ingested calcium is usually absorbed; the calcium remaining in the intestine is excreted in the feces. An additional 250 mg/day of calcium enters the intestines via secreted gastrointestinal juices and sloughed mucosal cells.

Intestinal absorption of phosphate occurs easily. Except for the portion of phosphate that is excreted in the feces in

Life Stage Group (years)	Recommended Dietary Allowance (mg/day)[a]
1–3 (M or F)	700
4–8 (M or F)	1000
9–13 (M or F)	1300
14–18 (M or F)	1300
19–30 (M or F)	1000
31–50 (M or F)	1000
51–70 (M)	1000
51–70 (F)	1200
71+ (M or F)	1200
Pregnant or Lactating (F)	
14–18	1300
19–50	1000

TABLE 90-1   Recommended Dietary Allowances for Calcium in Different Age Groups

M, Male; F, Female.
[a]Recommended dietary allowance (RDA) intake that meets the needs of 97.5% of the North American population.
Source: Adapted from Ross, A.C., Manson, J.E., Abrams, S.A. et al., 2011. The 2011 dietary reference intakes for calcium and vitamin D: what dietetics practitioners need to know. J. Am. Diet Assoc. 111(4), 524–527.

combination with nonabsorbed calcium, almost all the dietary phosphate is absorbed into the blood from the gut and later excreted in the urine.

RENAL EXCRETION OF CALCIUM

Approximately 10% (100 mg/day) of the ingested calcium is excreted in the urine. About 41% of the plasma calcium is bound to plasma proteins and is therefore not filtered by the glomerular capillaries. The remainder is combined with anions such as phosphate (9%) or ionized (50%) and is filtered through the glomeruli into the renal tubules.

Normally, the renal tubules reabsorb 99% of the filtered calcium and about 100 mg/day are excreted in the urine. Approximately 90% of the calcium in the glomerular filtrate is reabsorbed in the proximal tubules, loops of Henle, and early distal tubules.

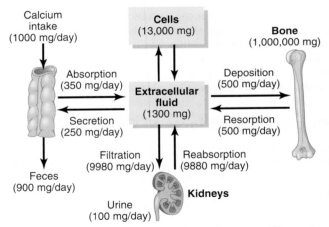

Figure 90-3   Overview of calcium exchange between different tissue compartments in a person ingesting 1000 mg of calcium per day. Note that most of the ingested calcium is normally eliminated in the feces, although the kidneys have the capacity to excrete large amounts by reducing tubular reabsorption of calcium.

In the late distal tubules and early collecting ducts, reabsorption of the remaining 10% is more variable, depending on the calcium ion concentration in the blood.

When calcium concentration is low, this reabsorption is great, and thus almost no calcium is lost in the urine. Conversely, even a minute increase in blood calcium ion concentration above normal increases calcium excretion markedly. The most important factor controlling this reabsorption of calcium in the distal portions of the nephron, and therefore controlling the rate of calcium excretion, is PTH.

SITES OF CALCIUM STORAGE

Bone is composed of a tough *organic matrix* that is greatly strengthened by deposits of *calcium salts*. Average *compact bone* contains by weight about 30% matrix and 70% salts. Approximately 99% of the calcium in the body is stored in bones and teeth. *Newly formed bone* may have a considerably higher percentage of matrix in relation to salts.

Organic Matrix of Bone. The organic matrix of bone is 90–95% *collagen fibers,* and the remainder is a homogeneous gelatinous medium called *ground substance*. The collagen fibers extend primarily along the lines of tensional force and give bone its powerful tensile strength.

The ground substance is composed of extracellular fluid plus *proteoglycans,* especially *chondroitin sulfate* and *hyaluronic acid*. The precise function of each of these proteoglycans is not known, although they do help control the deposition of calcium salts.

Bone Salts. The crystalline salts deposited in the organic matrix of bone are composed principally of *calcium* and *phosphate*. The formula for the major crystalline salt, known as *hydroxyapatite,* is the following:

$$Ca_{10}(PO_4)_6(OH)_2$$

Magnesium, sodium, potassium, and *carbonate* ions are also present among the bone salts, although x-ray diffraction studies fail to show definite crystals formed by them. This ability of many types of ions to conjugate to bone crystals extends to many ions normally foreign to bone, such as *strontium, uranium, plutonium, the other transuranic elements, lead, gold, and other heavy metals*. Deposition of radioactive substances in the bone can cause prolonged irradiation of the bone tissues, and if a sufficient amount is deposited, an osteogenic sarcoma (bone cancer) may eventually develop.

Tensile and Compressional Strength of Bone. The collagen fibers of bone, like those of tendons, have great tensile strength, whereas the calcium salts have great compressional strength. These combined properties plus the degree of bondage between the collagen fibers and the crystals provide a bony structure that has both extreme tensile strength and compressional strength.

Mechanism of Bone Calcification

The initial stage in bone production is the secretion of *collagen molecules* (called collagen monomers) and *ground substance* (mainly proteoglycans) by *osteoblasts*. The collagen monomers polymerize rapidly to form collagen fibers; the resultant tissue becomes *osteoid,* a cartilage-like material differing from cartilage in that calcium salts readily precipitate in it. As the osteoid is formed, some of the osteoblasts become entrapped in the osteoid and become quiescent. At this stage they are called *osteocytes.*

Within a few days after the osteoid is formed, calcium salts begin to precipitate on the surfaces of the collagen fibers. The precipitates first appear at intervals along each collagen fiber, forming minute nidi that rapidly multiply and grow over a period of days and weeks into the finished product, *hydroxyapatite crystals.*

Although the mechanism that causes calcium salts to be deposited in the osteoid is not fully understood, the regulation of this process appears to depend to a great extent on *pyrophosphate,* which inhibits hydroxyapatite crystallization and calcification of the bone. The levels of pyrophosphate, in turn, are regulated by at least three other molecules. One of the most important of these molecules is a substance called *tissue-nonspecific alkaline phosphatase (TNAP),* which breaks down pyrophosphate and keeps its levels in check so that bone calcification can occur as needed. TNAP is secreted by the osteoblasts into the osteoid to neutralize the pyrophosphate, and once the pyrophosphate has been neutralized, the natural affinity of the collagen fibers for calcium salts causes the hydroxyapatite crystallization. The importance of TNAP in bone mineralization is illustrated by the finding that mice with genetic deficiency of TNAP, which causes pyrophosphate levels to rise too high, are born with soft bones that are not adequately calcified.

The osteoblast also secretes at least two other substances that regulate bone calcification: (1) *nucleotide pyrophosphatase phosphodiesterase 1 (NPP1),* which produces pyrophosphate outside the cells, and (2) *ankylosis protein (ANK),* which contributes to the extracellular pool of pyrophosphate by transporting it from the interior to the surface of the cell. Deficiencies of NPP1 or ANK cause decreased extracellular pyrophosphate and excessive calcification of bone, such as bone spurs, or even calcification of other tissues such as tendons and ligaments of the spine, which occurs in people with a form of arthritis called *ankylosing spondylitis.*

CALCIUM EXCHANGE BETWEEN BONE AND EXTRACELLULAR FLUID

If soluble calcium salts are injected intravenously, the calcium ion concentration may increase immediately to high levels. However, within 30–60 minutes, the calcium ion concentration returns to normal. Likewise, if large quantities of calcium ions are removed from the circulating body fluids, the calcium ion concentration again returns to normal within 30 minutes to about 1 hour. These effects result largely from the fact that the bone contains a type of *exchangeable* calcium that is always in equilibrium with calcium ions in the extracellular fluids.

A small portion of this exchangeable calcium is also the calcium found in all tissue cells, especially in highly permeable types of cells such as those of the liver and the gastrointestinal tract. However, most of the exchangeable calcium is in the bone. It normally amounts to about 0.4–1% of the total bone calcium. This calcium is deposited in the bones in a form of readily mobilizable salt, such as $CaHPO_4$ and other amorphous calcium salts.

The importance of exchangeable calcium is that it provides a rapid *buffering* mechanism to keep the calcium ion concentration in the extracellular fluids from rising to excessive levels or falling to low levels under transient conditions of excess or decreased availability of calcium.

DEPOSITION AND RESORPTION OF BONE—REMODELING OF BONE

Deposition of Bone by the Osteoblasts. Bone is continually being deposited by *osteoblasts,* and it is continually being resorbed where *osteoclasts* are active (Figure 90-4). Osteoblasts are found on the outer surfaces of the bones and in the bone cavities. A small amount of osteoblastic activity occurs continually in all living bones (on about 4% of all surfaces at any given time in an adult), so at least some new bone is being formed constantly.

Resorption of Bone—Function of the Osteoclasts. Bone is also being continually resorbed in the presence of osteoclasts, which are large, phagocytic, multinucleated cells (containing as many as 50 nuclei) that are derivatives of monocytes or monocyte-like cells formed in the bone marrow. The osteoclasts are normally active on less than 1% of the bone surfaces of an adult. Later in the chapter, we will see that PTH controls the bone resorptive activity of osteoclasts.

Histologically, bone absorption occurs immediately adjacent to the osteoclasts. The mechanism of this resorption is believed to be the following: the osteoclasts send out villus-like projections toward the bone, forming a ruffled border adjacent to the bone (Figure 90-5). The villi secrete two types of substances: (1) proteolytic enzymes, released from the lysosomes of the osteoclasts, and (2) several acids, including citric acid and lactic acid, released from the mitochondria and secretory vesicles. The enzymes digest or dissolve the organic matrix of the bone, and the acids cause dissolution of the bone salts. The osteoclastic cells also imbibe minute particles of bone matrix and crystals by phagocytosis, eventually also dissoluting these particles and releasing the products into the blood.

PTH stimulates osteoclast activity and bone resorption, but this occurs through an indirect mechanism. The bone-resorbing osteoclast cells do not have PTH receptors. Instead, the osteoblasts signal osteoclast precursors to form mature osteoblasts. Two osteoblast proteins responsible for this signaling are *receptor activator for nuclear factor κ-B ligand (RANKL)* and *macrophage colony-stimulating factor,* which both appear to be necessary for formation of mature osteoclasts.

PTH binds to receptors on the adjacent osteoblasts, stimulating synthesis of RANKL, which is also called *osteoprotegerin*

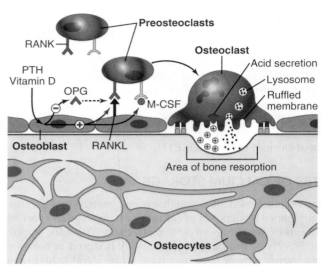

Figure 90-5 Bone resorption by osteoclasts. Parathyroid hormone *(PTH)* binds to receptors on osteoblasts, causing them to form receptor activator for nuclear factor κ-B ligand *(RANKL)* and to release macrophage-colony stimulating factor *(M-CSF)*. RANKL binds to RANK and M-CSF binds to its receptors on preosteoclast cellscausing them to differentiate into mature osteoclasts. PTH also decreases production of osteoprotegerin *(OPG)*, which inhibits differentiation of preosteoclasts into mature osteoclasts by binding to RANKL and preventing it from interacting with its receptor on preosteoclasts. The mature osteoclasts develop a ruffled border and release enzymes from lysosomes, as well as acids that promote bone resorption. Osteocytes are osteoblasts that have become encased in bone matrix during bone tissue production; the osteocytes form a system of interconnected cells that spreads all through the bone.

ligand (OPGL). RANKL binds to its receptors (RANK) on preosteoclast cells, causing them to differentiate into mature multinucleated osteoclasts.Osteoblasts also produce osteoprotegerin (OPG), sometimes called *osteoclastogenesis inhibitory factor* (OCIF), a cytokine that inhibits bone resorption.

Bone Deposition and Resorption Are Normally in Equilibrium. Except in growing bones, the rates of bone deposition and resorption are normally equal, so the total mass of bone remains constant.

Parathyroid Hormone

PTH provides a powerful mechanism for controlling extracellular calcium and phosphate concentrations by regulating intestinal reabsorption, renal excretion, and exchange between the extracellular fluid and bone of these ions. Excess activity of the parathyroid gland causes rapid release of calcium salts from the bones, with resultant *hypercalcemia* in the extracellular fluid; conversely, hypofunction of the parathyroid glands causes *hypocalcemia,* often with resultant tetany.

Physiological Anatomy of the Parathyroid Glands. Normally humans have four parathyroid glands, which are located immediately behind the thyroid gland—one behind each of the upper and each of the lower poles of the thyroid. Each parathyroid gland is about 6 mm long, 3 mm wide, and 2 mm thick and has a macroscopic appearance of dark brown fat. The parathyroid glands are difficult to locate during thyroid operations because they often look like just another lobule of the thyroid gland. For this reason, a total or subtotal thyroidectomy frequently resulted in removal of the parathyroid glands as well leading to hypoparathyroidism.

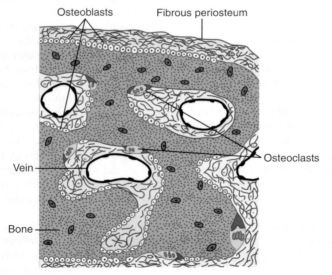

Figure 90-4 Osteoblastic and osteoclastic activity in the same bone.

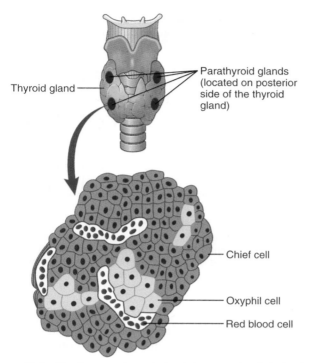

Figure 90-6 The four parathyroid glands lie immediately behind the thyroid gland. Almost all of the PTH is synthesized and secreted by the chief cells. The function of the oxyphil cells is uncertain, but they may be modified or depleted chief cells that no longer secrete PTH.

The parathyroid gland of the adult human being, shown in Figure 90-6, contains mainly *chief cells* and a small to moderate number of *oxyphil cells,* which may be absent in young humans. The chief cells are believed to secrete most, if not all, of the PTH. The function of the oxyphil cells is not certain, but the cells are believed to be modified or depleted chief cells that no longer secrete hormone.

EFFECT OF PARATHYROID HORMONE ON CALCIUM AND PHOSPHATE CONCENTRATIONS IN THE EXTRACELLULAR FLUID

Figure 90-7 shows the approximate effects on the blood calcium and phosphate concentrations caused by suddenly infusing PTH into an animal and continuing this infusion for several hours. Note that at the onset of infusion the calcium ion concentration begins to rise and reaches a plateau in about 4 hours. However, the phosphate concentration, however, falls more rapidly

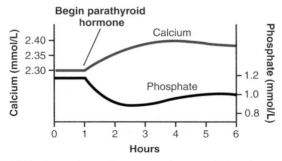

Figure 90-7 Approximate changes in calcium and phosphate concentrations during the first 5 hours of PTH infusion at a moderate rate.

than the calcium rises and reaches a depressed level within 1 or 2 hours. The rise in calcium concentration is caused mainly by two effects:

1. An effect of PTH to increase calcium and phosphate absorption from the bone
2. A rapid effect of PTH to decrease the excretion of calcium by the kidneys.

The decline in phosphate concentration is caused by a strong effect of PTH to increase renal phosphate excretion, an effect that is usually great enough to override increased phosphate absorption from the bone.

Parathyroid Hormone Mobilizes Calcium and Phosphate From the Bone

PTH has two effects to mobilize calcium and phosphate from bone. One is a rapid phase that begins in minutes and increases progressively for several hours. This phase results from activation of the already existing bone cells (mainly the osteocytes) to promote calcium and phosphate release. The second phase is a much slower one, requiring several days or even weeks to become fully developed; it results from proliferation of the osteoclasts, followed by greatly increased osteoclastic reabsorption of the bone itself, not merely release of the calcium phosphate salts from the bone.

Rapid Phase of Calcium and Phosphate Mobilization From Bone—Osteolysis. When large quantities of PTH are injected, the calcium ion concentration in the blood begins to rise within minutes, with studies showing that PTH causes removal of bone salts from two areas in the bone:

- from the bone matrix in the vicinity of the osteocytes lying within the bone itself and
- in the vicinity of the osteoblasts along the bone surface.

In fact, long, filmy processes extend from osteocyte to osteocyte throughout the bone structure, and also connect with the surface osteocytes and osteoblasts. This extensive system is called the *osteocytic membrane system,* and it is believed to provide a membrane that separates the bone itself from the extracellular fluid.

Between the osteocytic membrane and the bone is a small amount of *bone fluid.* Experiments suggest that the osteocytic membrane pumps calcium ions from the bone fluid into the extracellular fluid, creating a calcium ion concentration in the bone fluid only one-third that in the extracellular fluid. When the osteocytic pump becomes excessively activated, the bone fluid calcium concentration falls even lower, and calcium phosphate salts are then released from the bone. This effect is called *osteolysis,* and it occurs without resorption of the bone's fibrous and gel matrix. When the pump is inactivated, the bone fluid calcium concentration rises to a higher level and calcium phosphate salts are redeposited in the matrix.

Where does PTH fit into this picture? First, the cell membranes of both the osteoblasts and the osteocytes have receptor proteins for binding PTH. PTH can activate the calcium pump strongly, thereby causing rapid removal of calcium phosphate salts from the amorphous bone crystals that lie near the cells. PTH is believed to stimulate this pump by increasing the calcium permeability of the bone fluid side of the osteocytic membrane, thus allowing calcium ions to diffuse into the membrane cells from the bone fluid. Then the calcium pump on the other side of the cell membrane transfers the calcium ions the rest of the way into the extracellular fluid.

Slow Phase of Bone Resorption and Calcium Phosphate Release—Activation of the Osteoclasts. A much better known effect of PTH and one for which the evidence is much clearer is its activation of the osteoclasts. Yet the osteoclasts do not themselves have membrane receptor proteins for PTH. Instead, the activated osteoblasts and osteocytes send secondary "signals" to the osteoclasts. As discussed previously, a major secondary signal is *RANKL*, which activates receptors on preosteoclast cells and transforms them into mature osteoclasts that set about their usual task of gobbling up the bone over a period of weeks or months.

Activation of the osteoclastic system occurs in two stages: (1) immediate activation of the osteoclasts that are already formed and (2) formation of new osteoclasts. Several days of excess PTH usually cause the osteoclastic system to become well developed, but it can continue to grow for months under the influence of strong PTH stimulation.

Parathyroid Hormone Decreases Calcium Excretion and Increases Phosphate Excretion by the Kidneys

PTH increases renal tubular reabsorption of calcium at the same time that it diminishes phosphate reabsorption. The increased calcium resorption occurs mainly in the *late distal tubules,* the *collecting tubules,* the early collecting ducts, and possibly the ascending loop of Henle to a lesser extent.

PTH causes rapid loss of phosphate in the urine owing to the effect of the hormone to diminish proximal tubular reabsorption of phosphate ions. Moreover, it increases the rate of reabsorption of magnesium ions and hydrogen ions while it decreases the reabsorption of sodium, potassium, and amino acid ions in much the same way that it affects phosphate.

Parathyroid Hormone Increases Intestinal Absorption of Calcium and Phosphate

At this point, we should be reminded again that PTH greatly enhances both calcium and phosphate absorption from the intestines by increasing the formation in the kidneys of 1,25-dihydroxycholecalciferol from vitamin D, as discussed later in the chapter.

Cyclic Adenosine Monophosphate Mediates the Effects of Parathyroid Hormone. A large share of the effect of PTH on its target organs is mediated by the cyclic adenosine monophosphate (cAMP) second messenger mechanism. Within a few minutes after PTH administration, the concentration of cAMP increases in the osteocytes, osteoclasts, and other target cells. Other direct effects of PTH probably function independently of the second messenger mechanism.

CONTROL OF PARATHYROID SECRETION BY CALCIUM ION CONCENTRATION

Even the slightest decrease in calcium ion concentration in the extracellular fluid causes the parathyroid glands to increase their rate of secretion within minutes. Changes in extracellular fluid calcium ion concentration are detected by a *calcium-sensing receptor* (CaSR) in parathyroid cell membranes.

If the decreased calcium concentration persists, the glands will hypertrophy, for example, they become greatly enlarged in persons *rickets.* They also become greatly enlarged during *pregnancy* and during *lactation.*

Conversely, conditions that increase the calcium ion concentration above normal cause decreased activity and reduced size

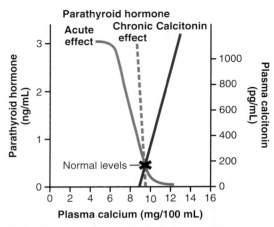

Figure 90-8 The approximate effect of plasma calcium concentration on the plasma concentrations of PTH and calcitonin. Note especially that long-term, changes in calcium concentration of only a few percentage points can cause as much as 100% change in PTH concentration.

of the parathyroid glands. Such conditions include (1) excess quantities of calcium in the diet, (2) increased vitamin D in the diet, and (3) bone resorption caused by factors other than PTH (eg, disuse of the bones).

Figure 90-8 shows the approximate relation between plasma calcium concentration and plasma PTH concentration. The solid red curve shows the acute effect when the calcium concentration is changed over a period of a few hours. The approximate chronic effect is shown by the dashed red line. This is the basis of the body's extremely potent feedback system for long-term control of plasma calcium ion concentration.

Summary of Effects of Parathyroid Hormone. Figure 90-9 summarizes the main effects of increased PTH secretion in response to decreased extracellular fluid calcium ion concentration:

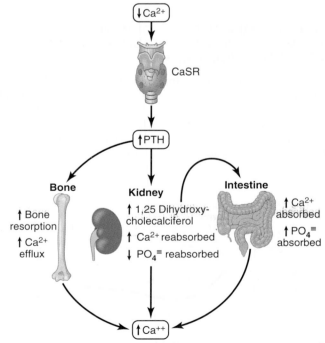

Figure 90-9 Summary of effects of parathyroid hormone (PTH) on bone, the kidneys, and the intestine in response to decreased extracellular fluid calcium ion concentration. CaSR, calcium-sensing receptor.

1. PTH stimulates bone resorption, causing release of calcium into the extracellular fluid.
2. PTH increases reabsorption of calcium and decreases phosphate reabsorption by the renal tubules, leading to decreased excretion of calcium and increased excretion of phosphate.
3. PTH is necessary for conversion of 25-hydroxycholecalciferol to 1,25-dihydroxycholecalciferol, which, in turn, increases calcium absorption by the intestines.

These actions together provide a powerful means of regulating extracellular fluid calcium concentration.

Vitamin D

Vitamin D has a potent effect to increase calcium absorption from the intestinal tract; it also has important effects on bone deposition and bone resorption, as discussed later. However, vitamin D itself is not the active substance that actually causes these effects. Instead, vitamin D must first be converted through a succession of reactions in the liver and the kidneys to the final active product, *1,25-dihydroxycholecalciferol,* also called $1,25(OH)_2D_3$. Figure 90-10 shows the succession of steps that lead to the formation of this substance from vitamin D.

Cholecalciferol (Vitamin D$_3$) Is Formed in the Skin. Vitamin D$_3$ (also called *cholecalciferol*) is the most important of these and is formed in the skin as a result of irradiation of *7-dehydrocholesterol,* a substance normally in the skin, by ultraviolet rays from the sun.

Cholecalciferol Is Converted to 25-Hydroxycholecalciferol in the Liver. The first step in the activation of cholecalciferol is to convert it to 25-hydroxycholecalciferol, which occurs in the

liver. The process is limited because the 25-hydroxycholecalciferol has a feedback inhibitory effect on the conversion reactions. This feedback effect is extremely important for two reasons:

1. Prevents excessive action of vitamin D when intake of vitamin D$_3$ is altered over a wide range.
2. This controlled conversion of vitamin D$_3$ to 25-hydroxycholecalciferol conserves the vitamin D stored in the liver for many months for future use.

Formation of 1,25-Dihydroxycholecalciferol in the Kidneys and Its Control by Parathyroid Hormone. Figure 90-10 also shows the conversion in the proximal tubules of the kidneys of 25-hydroxycholecalciferol to *1,25-dihydroxycholecalciferol.* This latter substance is by far the most active form of vitamin D because the previous products in the scheme of Figure 90-10 have less than 1/1000 of the vitamin D effect. Therefore, in the absence of the kidneys, vitamin D loses almost all its effectiveness.

Note also in Figure 90-10 that the conversion of 25-hydroxycholecalciferol to 1,25-dihydroxycholecalciferol requires PTH. In the absence of PTH, almost none of the 1,25-dihydroxycholecalciferol is formed. Therefore, PTH exerts a potent influence in determining the functional effects of vitamin D in the body.

Calcium Ion Concentration Controls the Formation of 1,25-Dihydroxycholecalciferol. Figure 90-11 demonstrates that the plasma concentration of 1,25-dihydroxycholecalciferol is inversely affected by the concentration of calcium in the plasma. There are two reasons for this:

1. The calcium ion itself has a slight effect in preventing the conversion of 25-hydroxycholecalciferol to 1,25-dihydroxycholecalciferol.
2. The rate of secretion of PTH is greatly suppressed when the plasma calcium ion concentration rises above 9–10 mg/100 mL. Therefore, at calcium concentrations below this level, PTH promotes the conversion of 25-hydroxycholecalciferol to 1,25-dihydroxycholecalciferol in the kidneys.

When the plasma calcium concentration is already too high, the formation of 1,25-dihydroxycholecalciferol is greatly depressed. Lack of 1,25-dihydroxycholecalciferol, in turn, decreases the absorption of calcium from the intestines, bones, and renal tubules, thus causing the calcium ion concentration to fall back toward its normal level.

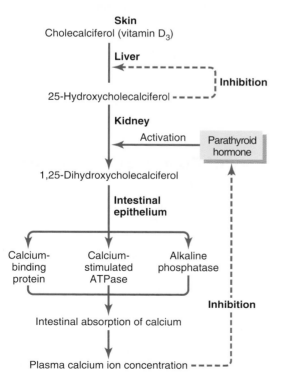

Figure 90-10 Activation of vitamin D$_3$ to form 1,25-dihydroxychole-calciferol and the role of vitamin D in controlling the plasma calcium concentration.

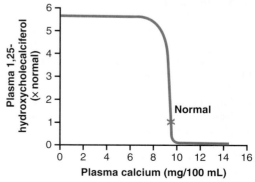

Figure 90-11 Effect of plasma calcium concentration on the plasma concentration of 1,25-dihydroxycholecalciferol. This figure shows that a slight decrease in calcium concentration below normal causes increased formation of activated vitamin D, which in turn leads to greatly increased absorption of calcium from the intestine.

ACTIONS OF VITAMIN D

The active form of vitamin D, 1,25-dihydroxycholecalciferol, has several effects on the intestines, kidneys, and bones that increase absorption of calcium and phosphate into the extracellular fluid and contribute to feedback regulation of these substances.

Vitamin D receptors are present in most cells in the body and are located mainly in the nuclei of target cells. Similar to receptors for steroids and thyroid hormone, the vitamin D receptor has hormone-binding and DNA-binding domains. The affinity of this receptor for 1,25-dihydroxycholecalciferol is roughly 1000 times that for 25-hydroxycholecalciferol, which explains their relative biological potencies.

"Hormonal" Effect of Vitamin D to Promote Intestinal Calcium Absorption. 1,25-Dihydroxycholecalciferol itself functions as a type of "hormone" to promote intestinal absorption of calcium. It promotes this absorption principally by increasing, over a period of about 2 days, formation of *calbindin,* a *calcium-binding protein,* in the intestinal epithelial cells. This protein functions in the brush border of these cells to transport calcium into the cell cytoplasm. The calcium then moves through the basolateral membrane of the cell by facilitated diffusion. The rate of calcium absorption is directly proportional to the quantity of this calcium-binding protein. Furthermore, this protein remains in the cells for several weeks after the 1,25-dihydroxycholecalciferol has been removed from the body, thus causing a prolonged effect on calcium absorption.

Other effects of 1,25-dihydroxycholecalciferol that might play a role in promoting calcium absorption are the formation of (1) a calcium-stimulated adenosine triphosphatase in the brush border of the epithelial cells and (2) an alkaline phosphatase in the epithelial cells. The precise details of all these effects are unclear.

Vitamin D Promotes Phosphate Absorption by the Intestines. Although phosphate is usually absorbed easily, phosphate flux through the gastrointestinal epithelium is enhanced by vitamin D. It is believed that this enhancement results from a direct effect of 1,25-dihydroxycholecalciferol, but it is possible that it results secondarily from this hormone's action on calcium absorption.

Vitamin D Decreases Renal Calcium and Phosphate Excretion. Vitamin D also increases calcium and phosphate reabsorption by the epithelial cells of the renal tubules, thereby tending to decrease excretion of these substances in the urine. However, this effect is weak and probably not of major importance in regulating the extracellular fluid concentration of these substances.

Effect of Vitamin D on Bone and Its Relation to Parathyroid Hormone Activity. Vitamin D plays important roles in bone resorption and bone deposition. The administration of *extreme quantities of vitamin D causes resorption of bone.* In the absence of vitamin D, the effect of PTH in causing bone resorption (discussed in the next section) is greatly reduced or even prevented.

Vitamin D in smaller quantities promotes bone calcification. One of the ways it promotes this calcification is to increase calcium and phosphate absorption from the intestines. However, even in the absence of such an increase, it enhances the mineralization of bone.

Calcitonin

Calcitonin, a peptide hormone secreted by the thyroid gland, tends to *decrease* plasma calcium concentration and, in general, has effects opposite to those of PTH. However, the quantitative role of calcitonin in humans is far less than that of PTH in regulating calcium ion concentration. Synthesis and secretion of calcitonin occur in the *parafollicular cells,* or *C cells,* lying in the interstitial fluid between the follicles of the thyroid gland. Calcitonin is a 32-amino acid peptide with a molecular weight of about 3400.

Increased Plasma Calcium Concentration Stimulates Calcitonin Secretion. The primary stimulus for calcitonin secretion is increased extracellular fluid calcium ion concentration. In contrast, PTH secretion is stimulated by decreased calcium concentration.

In young animals, but much less so in older animals and in humans, an increase in plasma calcium concentration of about 10% causes an immediate twofold or more increase in the rate of secretion of calcitonin, which is shown by the blue line in Figure 90-8. This increase provides a second hormonal feedback mechanism for controlling the plasma calcium ion concentration, but one that is relatively weak and works in a way opposite that of the PTH system.

Calcitonin Decreases Plasma Calcium Concentration. In some young animals, calcitonin decreases blood calcium ion concentration rapidly, beginning within minutes after injection of the calcitonin, in at least two ways:

1. The immediate effect is to decrease the absorptive activities of the osteoclasts and possibly the osteolytic effect of the osteocytic membrane throughout the bone.
2. The second and more prolonged effect of calcitonin is to decrease the formation of new osteoclasts.

Calcitonin also has minor effects on calcium handling in the kidney tubules and the intestines that are opposite those of PTH, but is of little significance.

Calcitonin Has a Weak Effect on Plasma Calcium Concentration in Adult Humans. The reason for the weak effect of calcitonin on plasma calcium is twofold:

1. PTH secretion overrides the calcitonin effect of any reduction of the calcium ion concentration.
2. In the adult human, the daily rates of absorption and deposition of calcium are small, and even after the rate of absorption is slowed by calcitonin, this still has only a small effect on plasma calcium ion concentration.

Summary of Control of Calcium Ion Concentration

For any fluctuations in calcium intake or excretion, there are defense mechanisms to prevent either hypercalcemia or hypocalcemia from occurring even before the parathyroid and calcitonin hormonal feedback systems have a chance to act (Table 90-2).

Buffer Function of the Exchangeable Calcium in Bones—The First Line of Defense. The exchangeable calcium salts in the bones, probably mainly $CaHPO_4$ or some similar compound loosely bound in the bone and in reversible equilibrium with the calcium and phosphate ions in the extracellular fluid act as the first line of defense in buffering ECF calcium ion fluctuations.

In addition to the buffer function of the bones, the *mitochondria* of many of the tissues of the body, especially of the liver and

TABLE 90-2	**Summary of PTH, Calcitonin, and Vitamin D₃ Actions on Calcium Homeostasis**		
Plasma Calcium Levels	**Parathyroid Hormone Actions**	**1,25-Dihydroxycholecalciferol Actions**	**Calcitonin Actions**
Decreased levels of calcium	*Bones* Osteolysis (rapid phase) Increased osteoclastic activity *Kidneys* Increased renal tubular reabsorption of calcium Increased 1,25 (OH)₂ D formation *Intestines* 1,25 (OH)₂ D causes increased intestinal absorption of calcium	*Bones* High quantities: Bone absorption *Kidneys* Increased renal calcium and phosphate reabsorption *Intestines* 1,25 (OH)₂ D causes increased intestinal absorption of calcium	
Increased levels of calcium	Decreased PTH secretion	Decreased 1,25 (OH)₂ D	*Bone* Inhibits osteoclasts and bone resorption

intestine, contain a significant amount of exchangeable calcium (a total of about 10 g in the whole body) that provides an additional buffer system to help maintain constancy of the extracellular fluid calcium ion concentration.

Hormonal Control of Calcium Ion Concentration—The Second Line of Defense. At the same time that the exchangeable calcium mechanism in the bones is "buffering" the calcium in the extracellular fluid, both the parathyroid and the calcitonin hormonal systems are beginning to act (Figure 90-12). Within 3–5 minutes after an acute increase in the calcium ion concentration, the rate of PTH secretion decreases.

At the same time that PTH decreases, calcitonin increases. In young animals and possibly in young children (but probably to a smaller extent in adults), the calcitonin causes rapid deposition of calcium in the bones, and perhaps in some cells of other tissues.

In prolonged calcium excess or prolonged calcium deficiency, only the PTH mechanism seems to be really important in maintaining a normal plasma calcium ion concentration.

NONBONE PHYSIOLOGICAL EFFECTS OF ALTERED CALCIUM CONCENTRATIONS IN THE BODY FLUIDS

Slight increases or decreases of calcium ion in the extracellular fluid can cause extreme immediate physiological effects.

Hypocalcemia Causes Nervous System Excitement and Tetany. When the extracellular fluid concentration of calcium ions falls from its normal level of 9.4 mg/dL to about 6 mg/dL, tetany occurs. This phenomenon is because the nervous system becomes progressively more excitable as the neuronal membrane permeability increases for sodium ions, allowing easy initiation of action potentials.

It also occasionally causes seizures because of its action of increasing excitability in the brain.

Figure 90-13 shows tetany in the hand, which usually occurs before tetany develops in most other parts of the body. This is called "carpopedal spasm." Calcium levels below about 4 mg/dL can be lethal.

Hypercalcemia Depresses Nervous System and Muscle Activity. When the level of calcium in the body fluids rises above about 12 mg/dL, the nervous system becomes depressed and reflex activities of the central nervous system are sluggish.

Also, increased calcium ion concentration decreases the QT interval of the heart and causes lack of appetite and constipation, probably because of depressed contractility of the muscle walls of the gastrointestinal tract.

Pathophysiology of Parathyroid Hormone, Vitamin D, and Bone Disease

HYPOPARATHYROIDISM

When the parathyroid glands do not secrete sufficient PTH, the osteocytic resorption of exchangeable calcium decreases and the osteoclasts become almost totally inactive. As a result, calcium release from the bones is so depressed that the level of calcium in the body fluids decreases. Yet because calcium and phosphates are not being released from the bone, the bone usually remains strong.

When the parathyroid glands are suddenly removed, the calcium level in the blood falls from the normal of 9.4 mg/dL to 6–7 mg/dL within 2–3 days and the blood phosphate concentration may double. When this low calcium level is reached, the usual signs of tetany develop. Among the muscles of the body especially sensitive to tetanic spasm are the laryngeal muscles. Spasm of these muscles obstructs respiration, which is the usual cause of death in persons with tetany unless appropriate treatment is provided.

Treatment of Hypoparathyroidism with PTH and Vitamin D. PTH is occasionally used to treat hypoparathyroidism. However, hyperparathyroidism is usually not treated with PTH because this hormone is expensive, its low duration of action, and the tendency of the body to develop antibodies against it makes it progressively less and less effective. In most patients with hypoparathyroidism, the administration of extremely large quantities of vitamin D, to as high as 100,000 units per day, along with intake of 1–2 g of calcium, keeps the calcium ion concentration in a normal range. At times, it might be necessary to administer 1,25-dihydroxycholecalciferol instead of the nonactivated form of vitamin D because of its much more potent and much more rapid action.

PRIMARY HYPERPARATHYROIDISM

In primary hyperparathyroidism, an abnormality of the parathyroid glands causes inappropriate, excess PTH secretion.

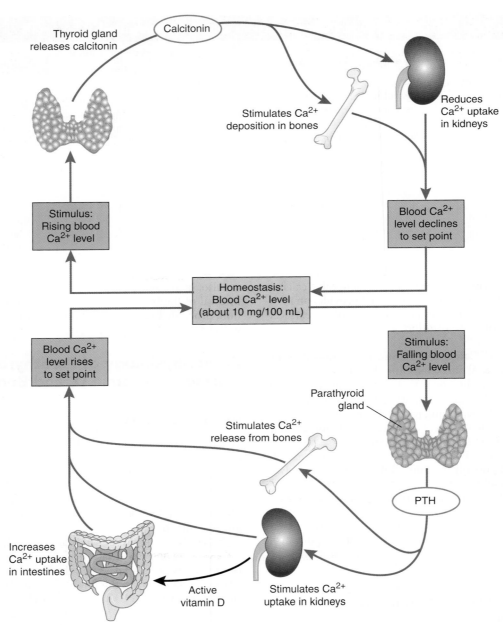

Figure 90-12 Summary of control of calcium homeostasis.

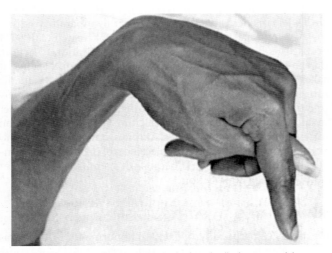

Figure 90-13 Hypocalcemic tetany in the hand called *carpopedal spasm.*

The cause of primary hyperparathyroidism ordinarily is a tumor of one of the parathyroid glands; such tumors occur much more frequently in women, mainly because pregnancy and lactation stimulate the parathyroid glands and therefore predispose to the development of such a tumor.

Hyperparathyroidism causes extreme osteoclastic activity in the bones, which elevates the calcium ion concentration in the extracellular fluid while usually depressing the concentration of phosphate ions because of increased renal excretion of phosphate.

Bone Disease in Hyperparathyroidism. Although new bone can be deposited rapidly enough to compensate for the increased osteoclastic resorption of bone in persons with mild hyperparathyroidism, in severe hyperparathyroidism the osteoclastic absorption soon far outstrips osteoblastic deposition, and the bone may be eaten away almost entirely. This could lead to multiple fractures with mild trauma.

Radiographs of the bone typically show extensive decalcification and, occasionally, large punched-out cystic areas of the bone that are filled with osteoclasts in the form of so-called giant cell osteoclast "tumors." The cystic bone disease of hyperparathyroidism is called *osteitis fibrosa cystica.*

Osteoblastic activity in the bones also increases greatly in a vain attempt to form enough new bone to make up for the old bone absorbed by the osteoclastic activity. When the osteoblasts become active, they secrete large quantities of *alkaline phosphatase.* Therefore, one of the important diagnostic findings in hyperparathyroidism is a high level of plasma alkaline phosphatase.

Effects of Hypercalcemia in Hyperparathyroidism. Hyperparathyroidism can at times cause the plasma calcium level to rise to 12–15 mg/dL and, rarely, leading to effects, such as depression of the central and peripheral nervous systems, muscle weakness, constipation, abdominal pain, peptic ulcer, lack of appetite, and depressed relaxation of the heart during diastole.

Parathyroid Poisoning and Metastatic Calcification. When, on rare occasions, extreme quantities of PTH are secreted, the level of calcium in the body fluids rises rapidly to high values. Even the extracellular fluid phosphate concentration often rises markedly instead of falling, probably because the kidneys cannot excrete all the phosphate being absorbed from the bone rapidly enough. Therefore, the calcium and phosphate in the body fluids become greatly supersaturated, when blood levels rise above 17 mg/dL leading to calcium phosphate ($CaHPO_4$) crystals being deposited in the alveoli of the lungs, the tubules of the kidneys, the thyroid gland, the acid-producing area of the stomach mucosa, and the walls of the arteries throughout the body. This extensive *metastatic* deposition of calcium phosphate can develop within a few days and can be fatal.

Formation of Kidney Stones in Hyperparathyroidism. Most patients with mild hyperparathyroidism tend to have an extreme tendency to form kidney stones due to excess calcium and phosphate eventually being excreted by the kidneys.

As a result, crystals of calcium phosphate tend to precipitate in the kidney, forming calcium phosphate stones. Also, calcium oxalate stones develop because even normal levels of oxalate cause calcium precipitation at high calcium levels.

Because the solubility of most renal stones is slight in alkaline media, the tendency for formation of renal calculi is considerably greater in alkaline urine than in acid urine. For this reason, acidotic diets and acidic drugs are frequently used to treat renal calculi.

SECONDARY HYPERPARATHYROIDISM

In secondary hyperparathyroidism, high levels of PTH occur as a compensation for *hypocalcemia* rather than as a primary abnormality of the parathyroid glands. In contrast, primary hyperparathyroidism is associated with hypercalcemia.

Secondary hyperparathyroidism can be caused by vitamin D deficiency or chronic renal disease, where the damaged kidneys are unable to produce sufficient amounts 1,25-dihydroxycholecalciferol. The vitamin D deficiency leads to *osteomalacia* (inadequate mineralization of the bones) and high levels of PTH cause resorption of the bones.

RICKETS CAUSED BY VITAMIN D DEFICIENCY

Rickets occurs mainly in children. It results from calcium or phosphate deficiency in the extracellular fluid, usually caused by lack of vitamin D. The plasma calcium concentration in rickets is only slightly depressed, but the level of phosphate is greatly depressed. This is because the parathyroid glands prevent the calcium level from falling by promoting bone resorption every time the calcium level begins to fall.

During prolonged cases of rickets, the marked compensatory increase in PTH secretion causes extreme osteoclastic resorption of the bone.This in turn causes the bone to become progressively weaker and imposes marked physical stress on the bone, resulting in rapid osteoblastic activity as well.

When the bones finally become exhausted of calcium, the level of calcium may fall rapidly. As the blood level of calcium falls below 7 mg/dL, the usual signs of tetany develop and the child may die of tetanic respiratory spasm unless calcium is administered intravenously, which relieves the tetany immediately.

Treatment. The treatment of rickets entails supplying adequate calcium and phosphate in the diet and, equally important, administering large amounts of vitamin D. If vitamin D is not administered, little calcium and phosphate are absorbed from the gut.

Osteomalacia—"Adult Rickets". Adults seldom have a serious *dietary* deficiency of vitamin D or calcium because large quantities of calcium are not needed for bone growth as in the case in children. However, serious deficiencies of both vitamin D and calcium occasionally occur as a result of *steatorrhea* (failure to absorb fat). Consequently, in steatorrhea, both vitamin D (being a fat-soluble vitamin) and calcium tend to pass into the feces. Under these conditions, an adult occasionally has such poor calcium and phosphate absorption that rickets can occur. Rickets in adults almost never proceeds to the stage of tetany but often is a cause of severe bone disability.

Osteomalacia and Rickets Caused by Renal Disease. "Renal rickets" is a type of osteomalacia that results from prolonged kidney damage. The cause of this condition is mainly failure of the damaged kidneys to form 1,25-dihydroxycholecalciferol, the active form of vitamin D.

Another type of renal disease that leads to rickets and osteomalacia is *congenital hypophosphatemia*, resulting from congenitally reduced reabsorption of phosphates by the renal tubules. This type of rickets must be treated with phosphate compounds instead of calcium and vitamin D, and it is called *vitamin D-resistant rickets.*

OSTEOPOROSIS—DECREASED BONE MATRIX

Osteoporosis is the most common of all bone diseases in adults, especially in old age. It is different from osteomalacia and rickets because it results from diminished organic bone matrix rather than from poor bone calcification. In persons with osteoporosis, the osteoblastic activity in the bone is usually less than normal, and consequently the rate of bone osteoid deposition is depressed. Occasionally, however, as in hyperparathyroidism, the cause of the diminished bone is excess osteoclastic activity.

The many common causes of osteoporosis are as follows:
1. *Lack of physical stress on the bones* because of inactivity.
2. *Malnutrition* to the extent that sufficient protein matrix cannot be formed.
3. *Lack of vitamin C,* which is necessary for the secretion of intercellular substances by all cells, including formation of osteoid by the osteoblasts.
4. *Postmenopausal lack of estrogen secretion* because estrogens decrease the number and activity of osteoclasts.

5. *Old age,* in which growth hormone and other growth factors diminish greatly, plus the fact that many of the protein anabolic functions also deteriorate with age, so bone matrix cannot be deposited satisfactorily.

6. *Cushing syndrome,* because massive quantities of glucocorticoids secreted in this disease cause decreased deposition of protein throughout the body and increased catabolism of protein and have the specific effect of depressing osteoblastic activity.

7. *Hyperparathyroidism,* where excessive osteoclastic activity can cause increased reabsorption of bone leading to fractures with mild trauma.

BIBLIOGRAPHY

Alfadda TI, Saleh AM, Houillier P, Geibel JP: Calcium-sensing receptor 20 years later, *Am. J. Physiol. Cell Physiol.* 307:C221, 2014.

Bauer DC: Clinical practice. Calcium supplements and fracture prevention, *N. Engl. J. Med.* 369:1537, 2013.

Crane JL, Cao X: Bone marrow mesenchymal stem cells and TGF-β signaling in bone remodeling, *J. Clin. Invest.* 124:466, 2014.

Elder CJ, Bishop NJ: Rickets, *Lancet* 383:1665, 2014.

Hoenderop JG, Nilius B, Bindels RJ: Calcium absorption across epithelia, *Physiol. Rev.* 85:373, 2005.

Holick MF: Vitamin D deficiency, *N. Engl. J. Med.* 357:266, 2007.

Imai Y, Youn MY, Inoue K, et al: Nuclear receptors in bone physiology and diseases, *Physiol. Rev.* 93:481, 2013.

Jones G, Strugnell SA, DeLuca HF: Current understanding of the molecular actions of vitamin D, *Physiol. Rev.* 78:1193, 1998.

Khosla S, Amin S, Orwoll E: Osteoporosis in men, *Endocr. Rev.* 29:441, 2008a.

Khosla S, Oursler MJ, Monroe DG: Estrogen and the skeleton, *Trends Endocrinol. Metab.* 23:576, 2012.

Khosla S, Westendorf JJ, Oursler MJ: Building bone to reverse osteoporosis and repair fractures, *J. Clin. Invest.* 118:421, 2008b.

Kopic S, Geibel JP: Gastric acid, calcium absorption, and their impact on bone health, *Physiol. Rev.* 93:189, 2013.

Marcocci C, Cetani F: Clinical practice. Primary hyperparathyroidism, *N. Engl. J. Med.* 365:2389, 2011.

Martin A, David V, Quarles LD: Regulation and function of the FGF23/klotho endocrine pathways, *Physiol. Rev.* 92:131, 2012.

Marx SJ: Hyperparathyroid and hypoparathyroid disorders, *N. Engl. J. Med.* 343:1863, 2000.

Quarles LD: Endocrine functions of bone in mineral metabolism regulation, *J. Clin. Invest.* 118:3820, 2008.

Ralston SH: Clinical practice. Paget's disease of bone, *N. Engl. J. Med.* 368:644, 2013.

Rosen CJ: Clinical practice. Vitamin D insufficiency, *N. Engl. J. Med.* 364:248, 2011.

Seeman E, Delmas PD: Bone quality—the material and structural basis of bone strength and fragility, *N. Engl. J. Med.* 354:2250, 2006.

Shoback D: Clinical practice. Hypoparathyroidism, *N. Engl. J. Med.* 359:391, 2008.

Silver J, Kilav R, Naveh-Many T: Mechanisms of secondary hyperparathyroidism, *Am. J. Physiol. Renal Physiol.* 283:F367, 2002.

Tordoff MG: Calcium: taste, intake, and appetite, *Physiol. Rev.* 81:1567, 2001.

Zaidi M, Buettner C, Sun L, Iqbal J: Minireview: the link between fat and bone: does mass beget mass? *Endocrinology* 153:2070, 2012.

91

Adrenal Cortex

Anatomy of the Adrenal Glands

Location. The two *adrenal glands*, each of which weighs about 4 g, lie at the superior poles of the two kidneys. As shown in Figure 91-1, each gland is composed of two major parts, the *adrenal medulla* and the *adrenal cortex*. The adrenal medulla is discussed in Chapter 92.

The adrenal cortex secretes an entirely different group of hormones called *corticosteroids*.

Blood Supply. The blood supply to the adrenal gland mainly is from three arteries (Figure 91-2):
1. *Superior adrenal arteries*: Arising from branches of the inferior phrenic artery
2. *Middle adrenal arteries*: Arising directly from the aorta
3. *Inferior adrenal arteries*: Arising from the renal artery on the same side

The venous drainage of the adrenal glands varies on each side. On the left, the *left adrenal vein* joins with the inferior phrenic vein and enters the left renal vein. On the right, the *right adrenal vein* joins directly into the inferior vena cava.

Histology. The adrenal cortex in an adult consists of three distinct zones:
1. the zona glomerulosa—the outermost zone;
2. the zona fasciculata—the middle zone;
3. the zona reticularis—the innermost zone.

The zona glomerulosa consists of cells that are small, with a moderate number of lipid inclusions in the cytoplasm. The nuclei are smaller as compared to the other two zones.

The zona fasciculata consists of cells that are large and have a high cytoplasmic:nuclear ratio with more lipid inclusions. This gives the cytoplasm a foamy appearance. The zona reticularis has comparatively less lipid content in its compact cytoplasm.

Fetal Adrenal Gland. The fetal adrenal gland begins developing at 3–4 weeks of gestation and is seen as the primordium. Around the sixth to eighth weeks of gestation, there is rapid enlargement of the adrenal gland, where cells in the cortex differentiate to form the fetal zone and an outer layer called the definitive zone. About this time, sympathetic neural cells invade the primordium of the adrenal cortex and these cells differentiate into chromaffin cells, which are able to synthesize and store catecholamines. The fetal zone is capable of synthesizing steroids by the 8th to 10th weeks of gestation.

At the time of birth, the fetal adrenal gland consists of the fetal cortex (which is about 80% of the gland) and an outer layer (which is about 20% of the gland) called the "true" cortex. The fetal cortex undergoes a reduction in size to about 50% of its size at birth within the first month. At the same time, the adrenal medulla proportionately increases in size.

Adrenocorticotropic hormone (ACTH) regulates fetal cortisol secretions and the feedback regulation of ACTH by cortisol is established by the 8th to 10th weeks of gestation. The growth and maturation of the fetal adrenal gland is dependent on ACTH secretion. The major precursor substance to synthesize steroids in the fetal adrenal gland is cholesterol bound to low-density lipoproteins (LDLs).

Corticosteroids: Mineralocorticoids, Glucocorticoids, and Androgens

Two major types of adrenocortical hormones, the *mineralocorticoids* and the *glucocorticoids*, are secreted by the adrenal cortex. In addition to these hormones, small amounts of sex hormones are secreted, especially *androgenic hormones*, which exhibit about the same effects in the body as the male sex hormone testosterone. They are normally of only slight importance, although in certain abnormalities of the adrenal cortices, extreme quantities can be secreted (which is discussed later in the chapter) and can result in masculinizing effects.

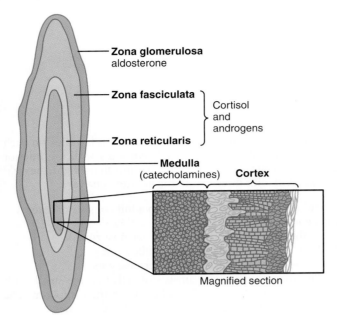

Figure 91-1 Secretion of adrenocortical hormones by the different zones of the adrenal cortex and secretion of catecholamines by the adrenal medulla.

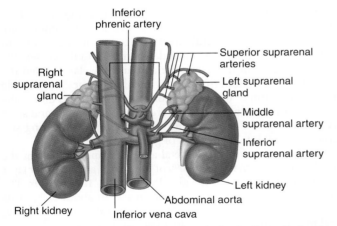

Figure 91-2 Blood supply of the adrenal glands. *From Drake, R.L., Vogl, W., Mitchell, A.W.M., 2005. Gray's Anatomy for Students. Elsevier, Philadelphia.*

The *mineralocorticoids* have gained this name because they especially affect the electrolytes (the "minerals") of the extracellular fluids, especially sodium and potassium. The *glucocorticoids* have gained their name because they exhibit important effects that increase blood glucose concentration. *Aldosterone*, the principal mineralocorticoid, and *cortisol*, the principal glucocorticoid, are the important steroids of over 30 steroids that have been isolated from the adrenal cortex.

Synthesis and Secretion of Adrenocortical Hormones

The Adrenal Cortex Has Three Distinct Layers. Figure 91-1 shows that the adrenal cortex is composed of three relatively distinct layers:

1. The *zona glomerulosa*, a thin layer of cells that lies just underneath the capsule, constitutes about 15% of the

adrenal cortex. These cells are the only ones in the adrenal gland capable of secreting significant amounts of *aldosterone* because they contain the enzyme *aldosterone synthase*, which is necessary for synthesis of aldosterone. The secretion of these cells is controlled mainly by the extracellular fluid concentrations of *angiotensin II* and *potassium*, both of which stimulate aldosterone secretion.

2. The *zona fasciculata*, the middle and widest zone, constitutes about 75% of the adrenal cortex and secretes the glucocorticoids, *cortisol* and *corticosterone*, as well as small amounts of *adrenal androgens* and *estrogens*. The secretion of these cells is controlled in large part by the hypothalamic–pituitary axis via *ACTH*.

3. The *zona reticularis*, the inner zone of the cortex, secretes the adrenal androgens *dehydroepiandrosterone* (DHEA) and *androstenedione*, as well as small amounts of estrogens and some glucocorticoids. ACTH also regulates secretion of these cells, although other factors such as *cortical androgen-stimulating hormone*, released from the pituitary, may also be involved. The mechanisms for controlling adrenal androgen production, however, are not nearly as well understood as those for glucocorticoids and mineralocorticoids.

Aldosterone and cortisol secretion are regulated by independent mechanisms. Factors such as angiotensin II that specifically increase the output of aldosterone and cause hypertrophy of the zona glomerulosa have no effect on the other two zones. Similarly, factors such as ACTH that increase secretion of cortisol and adrenal androgens, and cause hypertrophy of the zona fasciculata and zona reticularis have little effect on the zona glomerulosa.

Adrenocortical Hormones Are Steroids Derived from Cholesterol. All human steroid hormones, including those produced by the adrenal cortex, are synthesized from cholesterol. Although the cells of the adrenal cortex can synthesize de novo small amounts of cholesterol from acetate, approximately 80% of the cholesterol used for steroid synthesis is provided by LDLs in the circulating plasma.

Steps in the Biosynthesis of Adrenal Steroids. Figure 91-3 gives the principal steps in the formation of the important steroid products of the adrenal cortex: aldosterone, cortisol, and the androgens. Essentially all these steps occur in two of the organelles of the cell, the *mitochondria* and the *endoplasmic reticulum*, with some steps occurring in one of these organelles and some in the other. Each step is catalyzed by a specific enzyme system.

In addition to aldosterone and cortisol, other steroids having glucocorticoid or mineralocorticoid activities, or both, are normally secreted in small amounts by the adrenal cortex. Some of the more important of the corticosteroid hormones, including the synthetic ones, are the following, as summarized in Table 91-1.

Mineralocorticoids
- Aldosterone (very potent, accounts for about 90% of all mineralocorticoid activity);
- deoxycorticosterone (1/30 as potent as aldosterone, but very small quantities secreted);
- corticosterone (slight mineralocorticoid activity);
- 9α-fluorocortisol (synthetic, slightly more potent than aldosterone);

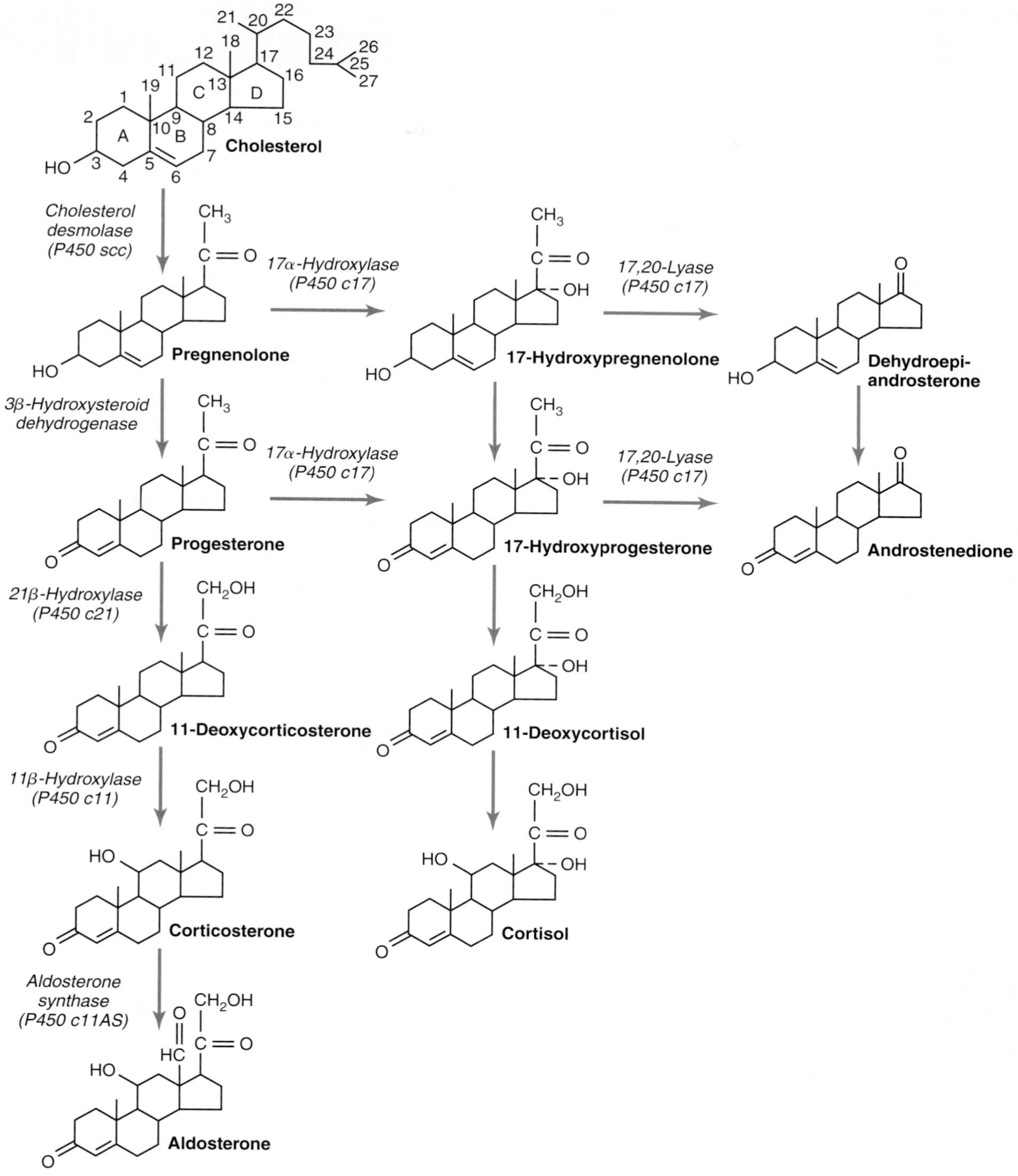

Figure 91-3 Pathways for synthesis of steroid hormones by the adrenal cortex. The enzymes are shown in italics.

- cortisol (very slight mineralocorticoid activity, but large quantity secreted);
- cortisone (slight mineralocorticoid activity).

Glucocorticoids

- Cortisol (very potent, accounts for about 95% of all glucocorticoid activity);
- corticosterone (provides about 4% of total glucocorticoid activity, but much less potent than cortisol);
- cortisone (almost as potent as cortisol);

- prednisone (synthetic, four times as potent as cortisol);
- methylprednisone (synthetic, five times as potent as cortisol);
- dexamethasone (synthetic, 30 times as potent as cortisol).

It is clear from this list that some of these hormones and synthetic steroids have both glucocorticoid and mineralocorticoid activities. It is especially significant that cortisol normally has some mineralocorticoid activity because some syndromes of excess cortisol secretion can cause significant mineralocorticoid effects, along with its much more potent glucocorticoid effects.

TABLE 91-1	Adrenal Steroid Hormones in Adults; Synthetic Steroids and their Relative Glucocorticoid and Mineralocorticoid Activities			
Steroids	Average Plasma Concentration (Free and Bound, mcg/100 mL)	Average Amount Secreted (mg/24 hours)	Glucocorticoid Activity	Mineralocorticoid Activity
Adrenal steroids				
Cortisol	12	15	1	1
Corticosterone	0.4	3	0.3	15
Aldosterone	0.006	0.15	0.3	3000
Deoxycorticosterone	0.006	0.2	0.2	100
Dehydroepiandrosterone	175	20	—	—
Synthetic steroids				
Cortisone	—	—	0.7	0.5
Prednisolone	—	—	4	0.8
Methylprednisone	—	—	5	—
Dexamethasone	—	—	30	—
9α-Fluorocortisol	—	—	10	125

Glucocorticoid and mineralocorticoid activities of the steroids are relative to cortisol, with cortisol being 1.0.

The intense glucocorticoid activity of the synthetic hormone dexamethasone, which has almost zero mineralocorticoid activity, makes it especially important drug for stimulating specific glucocorticoid activity.

Adrenocortical Hormones—Plasma Binding and Excretion

- Approximately 90–95% of the cortisol in the plasma binds to plasma proteins, especially a globulin called *cortisol-binding globulin* or *transcortin*, and, to a lesser extent, to albumin.
- Binding of adrenal steroids to the plasma proteins may serve as a reservoir to lessen rapid fluctuations in free hormone concentrations.
- The adrenal steroids are degraded mainly in the liver and conjugated especially to *glucuronic acid* and, to a lesser extent, sulfates.
- About 25% of these conjugates are excreted in the bile and then in the feces and the remaining excreted in the urine.

Functions of the Mineralocorticoids— Aldosterone

Mineralocorticoid Deficiency Causes Severe Renal Sodium Chloride Wasting and Hyperkalemia. Total loss of adrenocortical secretion may cause death within 3 days to 2 weeks unless the person receives extensive salt therapy or injection of mineralocorticoids.

Without mineralocorticoids, potassium ion concentration of the extracellular fluid rises markedly, sodium and chloride are rapidly lost from the body, and the total extracellular fluid volume and blood volume become greatly reduced. Diminished cardiac output soon develops, which progresses to a shock-like state, followed by death.

This entire sequence can be prevented by the administration of aldosterone or some other mineralocorticoid. Therefore, the mineralocorticoids are said to be the acute "lifesaving" portion of the adrenocortical hormones. The glucocorticoids are equally necessary, however, because they allow the person to resist the destructive effects of life's intermittent physical and mental "stresses," as discussed later in the chapter.

Aldosterone Is the Major Mineralocorticoid Secreted by the Adrenals. In humans, aldosterone exerts nearly 90% of the mineralocorticoid activity of the adrenocortical secretions, while cortisol also provides a significant amount of mineralocorticoid activity (Table 91-2). The mineralocorticoid activity of aldosterone is about 3000 times greater than that of cortisol, but the plasma concentration of cortisol is nearly 2000 times that of aldosterone.

RENAL AND CIRCULATORY EFFECTS OF ALDOSTERONE

Aldosterone Increases Renal Tubular Reabsorption of Sodium and Secretion of Potassium. Aldosterone increases reabsorption of sodium and simultaneously increases secretion of potassium by the renal tubular epithelial cells, especially in the *principal cells of the collecting tubules* and, to a lesser extent, in the distal tubules and collecting ducts. Therefore, aldosterone causes sodium to be conserved in the extracellular fluid while increasing potassium excretion in the urine. The net effect of excess aldosterone in the plasma is to increase the total quantity of sodium in the extracellular fluid while decreasing the potassium.

Conversely, total lack of aldosterone secretion can cause transient loss of 10–20 g of sodium in the urine a day, an amount equal to one-tenth to one-fifth of all the sodium in the body. At the same time, potassium is conserved tenaciously in the extracellular fluid.

Excess Aldosterone Increases Extracellular Fluid Volume and Arterial Pressure but Has Only a Small Effect on Plasma Sodium Concentration. Excess aldosterone causes sodium to be reabsorbed by the tubules, with simultaneous osmotic absorption of almost equivalent amounts of water. Therefore, the extracellular fluid volume increases almost as much as the retained sodium, but without much change in sodium concentration.

An aldosterone-mediated increase in extracellular fluid volume lasting more than 1–2 days also leads to an increase in arterial pressure. The rise in arterial pressure then increases kidney excretion of both sodium and water, called *pressure natriuresis* and *pressure diuresis*, respectively. Thus, after the extracellular fluid volume increases 5–15% above normal, arterial pressure also increases 15–25 mmHg, and this elevated blood pressure

TABLE 91-2	Summary of Actions of Aldosterone
	Aldosterone Actions
Actions on the kidneys	↑ Reabsorption of Na⁺ in renal tubular epithelial cells ↑ Secretion of K⁺ by the renal tubular epithelial cells ↑ Secretion of H⁺ ions in the intercalated cells of the cortical tubules; ↓ H⁺ ions in ECF ↑ ECF volume; ↑ arterial pressure
Sweat glands	↑ Reabsorption of sodium chloride in the ducts ↑ Secretion of K⁺ in the ducts
Salivary glands	↑ Reabsorption of sodium chloride in the ducts ↑ Secretion of K⁺ in the ducts
Intestines; colon	↑ Reabsorption of Na⁺

ECF, extracellular fluid.

returns the renal output of sodium and water to normal despite the excess aldosterone (Figure 91-4).

This return to normal of sodium and water excretion by the kidneys as a result of pressure natriuresis and diuresis is called *aldosterone escape*. Thereafter, the rate of gain of sodium and water by the body is zero, and balance is maintained between sodium and water intake and output by the kidneys despite continued excess aldosterone. In the meantime, however, hypertension has developed hypertension, which lasts as long as the person remains exposed to high levels of aldosterone.

Conversely, when aldosterone secretion becomes zero, large amounts of sodium are lost in the urine, not only diminishing

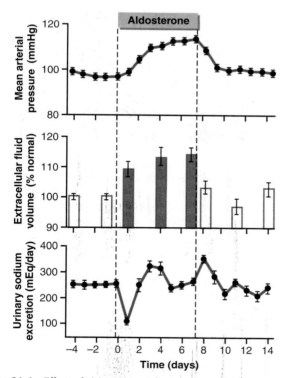

Figure 91-4 Effect of aldosterone infusion on arterial pressure, extracellular fluid volume, and sodium excretion in dogs. Although aldosterone was infused at a rate that raised plasma concentrations to about 20 times normal, note the "escape" from sodium retention on the second day of infusion as arterial pressure increased and urinary sodium excretion returned to normal. *Data from data in Hall, J.E., Granger, J.P., Smith Jr., M.J., et al., 1984. Role of hemodynamics and arterial pressure in aldosterone "escape." Hypertension 6 (Suppl. I), I183–I192.*

the amount of sodium chloride in the extracellular fluid but also decreasing the extracellular fluid volume leading to *circulatory shock*. Without therapy, this usually causes death within a few days after the adrenal glands suddenly stop secreting aldosterone.

Excess Aldosterone Causes Hypokalemia and Muscle Weakness; Aldosterone Deficiency Causes Hyperkalemia and Cardiac Toxicity. Excess aldosterone not only causes loss of potassium ions from the extracellular fluid into the urine but also stimulates transport of potassium from the extracellular fluid into most cells of the body. Therefore, excessive secretion of aldosterone may cause a serious decrease in the plasma potassium concentration, sometimes from the normal value of 4.5 mEq/L to as low as 2 mEq/L. This condition is called *hypokalemia*. When the potassium ion concentration falls below about one-half normal, severe muscle weakness often develops.

Conversely, when aldosterone is deficient, the extracellular fluid potassium ion concentration can rise far above normal. When it rises to 60–100% above normal, serious cardiac toxicity, including weakness of heart contraction and development of arrhythmia, becomes evident, and progressively higher concentrations of potassium lead inevitably to heart failure.

Excess Aldosterone Increases Tubular Hydrogen Ion Secretion and Causes Alkalosis. Aldosterone also causes secretion of hydrogen ions in exchange for sodium in the *intercalated cells* of the cortical collecting tubules. This decreases the hydrogen ion concentration in the extracellular fluid causing a metabolic alkalosis.

ALDOSTERONE STIMULATES SODIUM AND POTASSIUM TRANSPORT IN SWEAT GLANDS, SALIVARY GLANDS, AND INTESTINAL EPITHELIAL CELLS

Sweat and salivary glands form a primary secretion that contains large quantities of sodium chloride, but much of the sodium chloride, on passing through the excretory ducts, is reabsorbed, whereas potassium and bicarbonate ions are secreted. Aldosterone greatly increases the reabsorption of sodium chloride and the secretion of potassium by the ducts.

The effect on the sweat glands is important to conserve body salt in hot environments and the effect on the salivary glands is necessary to conserve salt when excessive quantities of saliva are lost.

Aldosterone also greatly enhances sodium absorption by the intestines, especially in the colon, which prevents loss of sodium in the stools.

CELLULAR MECHANISM OF ALDOSTERONE ACTION

Although for many years we have known the overall effects of mineralocorticoids on the body, the cellular sequence of events that leads to increased sodium reabsorption seems to unfold as follows.

First, because of its lipid solubility in the cellular membranes, aldosterone diffuses readily to the interior of the tubular epithelial cells.

Second, in the cytoplasm of the tubular cells, aldosterone combines with a highly specific cytoplasmic *mineralocorticoid receptor* (MR) protein (Figure 91-5), which has a stereomolecular configuration that allows only aldosterone or similar compounds to combine with it.

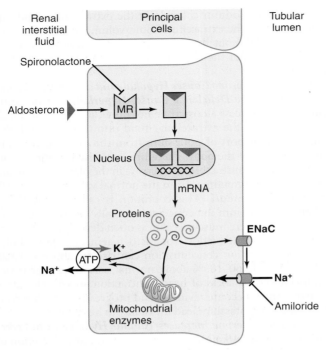

Figure 91-5 Aldosterone-responsive epithelial cell signaling pathways. Activation of the mineralocorticoid receptor (*MR*) by aldosterone can be antagonized with spironolactone. Amiloride is a drug that can be used to block epithelial sodium channel proteins (*ENaC*). *ATP*, adenosine triphosphate; *mRNA*, messenger RNA.

Third, the aldosterone–receptor complex or a product of this complex diffuses into the nucleus, inducing one or more specific portions of the DNA to form one or more types of messenger RNA (mRNA) related to the process of sodium and potassium transport.

Fourth, the mRNA diffuses back into the cytoplasm; it causes protein formation in the ribosomes. The proteins formed are a mixture of (1) one or more enzymes and (2) membrane transport proteins that, all acting together, are required for sodium, potassium, and hydrogen transport through the cell membrane (see Figure 91-5).

Thus, aldosterone does not have a major immediate effect on sodium transport; rather, this effect must await the sequence of events that leads to the formation of the specific intracellular substances required for sodium transport. About 30 minutes is required before new RNA appears in the cells, and about 45 minutes is required before the rate of sodium transport begins to increase; the effect reaches maximum only after several hours.

POSSIBLE NONGENOMIC ACTIONS OF ALDOSTERONE AND OTHER STEROID HORMONES

Some studies suggest that many steroids, including aldosterone, elicit not only slowly developing *genomic* effects that have a latency of 45–60 minutes and require gene transcription and synthesis of new proteins but also more rapid *nongenomic* effects that take place in a few seconds or minutes.

These nongenomic actions are believed to be mediated by binding of steroids to cell membrane receptors that are coupled to second messenger systems. Examples include:

1. Aldosterone increases formation of cyclic adenosine monophosphate (cAMP) in vascular smooth muscle cells and in epithelial cells of the renal collecting tubules in less than 2 minutes.

2. In other cell types, aldosterone has been shown to rapidly stimulate the phosphatidylinositol, second messenger system.

However, the precise structure of receptors responsible for the rapid effects of aldosterone has not been determined, nor is the physiological significance of these nongenomic actions of steroids well understood.

REGULATION OF ALDOSTERONE SECRETION

Regulation of aldosterone secretion is so deeply intertwined with regulation of extracellular fluid electrolyte concentrations, extracellular fluid volume, blood volume, arterial pressure, and many special aspects of renal function that it is difficult to discuss control of aldosterone secretion independently of all these other factors. This subject is presented in more detail in Chapters 79 and 81, to which the reader is referred. However, it is important to list here some of the more important points of aldosterone secretion control.

Regulation of aldosterone secretion by the zona glomerulosa cells is almost entirely independent of regulation of cortisol and androgens by the zona fasciculata and zona reticularis.

The following four factors are known to play essential roles in regulation of aldosterone:

1. Increased potassium ion concentration in the extracellular fluid greatly *increases* aldosterone secretion.
2. Increased angiotensin II concentration in the extracellular fluid also greatly *increases* aldosterone secretion.
3. Increased sodium ion concentration in the extracellular fluid *very slightly decreases* aldosterone secretion.
4. ACTH from the anterior pituitary gland is necessary for aldosterone secretion but has little effect in controlling the rate of secretion in most physiological conditions.

Of these factors, *potassium ion concentration* and the *renin–angiotensin system* are by far the most potent in regulating aldosterone secretion. Figure 91-6 shows the effects on plasma aldosterone concentration caused by blocking the formation of angiotensin II with an angiotensin-converting enzyme inhibitor after several weeks of a low-sodium diet that increases plasma aldosterone concentration. Note that blockade of angiotensin II formation markedly decreases plasma aldosterone concentration without significantly changing cortisol concentration, which indicates the important role of angiotensin II in stimulating aldosterone secretion when sodium intake and extracellular fluid volume are reduced.

By contrast, the effects of sodium ion concentration per se and of ACTH in controlling aldosterone secretion are usually minor.

Functions of Glucocorticoids

At least 95% of the glucocorticoid activity of the adrenocortical secretions results from the secretion of *cortisol*, known also as *hydrocortisone*. In addition, a small but significant amount of glucocorticoid activity is provided by *corticosterone*.

Glucocorticoids have functions just as important as those of the mineralocorticoids. These are explained in the following sections (Table 91-3; Figure 91-7).

EFFECTS OF CORTISOL ON CARBOHYDRATE METABOLISM

Stimulation of Gluconeogenesis. The best-known metabolic effect of cortisol and other glucocorticoids on metabolism is the ability to stimulate gluconeogenesis (ie, the formation

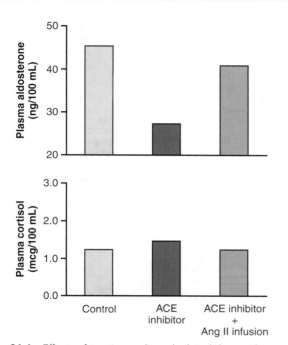

Figure 91-6 Effects of treating sodium-depleted dogs with an angiotensin-converting enzyme (ACE) inhibitor for 7 days to block formation of angiotensin II (Ang II) and of infusing exogenous Ang II to restore plasma Ang II levels after ACE inhibition. Note that blocking Ang II formation reduced plasma aldosterone concentration with little effect on cortisol, demonstrating the important role of Ang II in stimulating aldosterone secretion during sodium depletion. *Data from Hall, J.E., Guyton, A.C., Smith Jr., M.J., et al., 1979. Chronic blockade of angiotensin II formation during sodium deprivation. Am. J. Physiol. 237, F424.*

of carbohydrate from proteins and some other substances) as much as 6- to 10-fold by the liver. This increased rate of gluconeogenesis results mainly from direct effects of cortisol on the liver, as well as by antagonizing the effects of insulin.

1. *Cortisol increases the enzymes required to convert amino acids into glucose in the liver cells.*
2. *Cortisol causes mobilization of amino acids from the extrahepatic tissues mainly from muscle.*
3. *Cortisol antagonizes insulin's effects to inhibit gluconeogenesis in the liver.*

As discussed in Chapter 93 insulin stimulates glycogen synthesis in the liver and inhibits enzymes involved in glucose production by the liver. The net effect of cortisol is to increase glucose production by the liver.

The marked increase in glycogen storage in liver cells that accompanies increased gluconeogenesis potentiates the effects of other glycolytic hormones, such as epinephrine and glucagon, to mobilize glucose in times of need, such as between meals.

Decreased Glucose Utilization by Cells. Cortisol also causes a moderate decrease in glucose utilization by most cells in the body. Although the precise cause of this decrease is unclear, one important effect of cortisol is to decrease translocation of the glucose transporters *GLUT 4* to the cell membrane, especially in skeletal muscle cells, leading to *insulin resistance.* Glucocorticoids may also depress the expression and phosphorylation of other signaling cascades that influence glucose utilization directly or indirectly by affecting protein and lipid metabolism.

Elevated Blood Glucose Concentration and "Adrenal Diabetes". Both the increased rate of gluconeogenesis and the moderate reduction in the rate of glucose utilization by the cells cause the blood glucose concentrations to rise. The rise in blood glucose in turn stimulates secretion of insulin. The increased plasma levels of insulin, however, are not as effective in maintaining plasma glucose as they are under normal conditions.

For reasons that were discussed previously, high levels of glucocorticoid reduce the sensitivity of many tissues, especially skeletal muscle and adipose tissue, to the stimulatory effects of insulin on glucose uptake and utilization.

The increase in blood glucose concentration is occasionally great enough (50% or more above normal) that the condition is called *adrenal diabetes.* Administration of insulin lowers the blood glucose concentration only a moderate amount in adrenal diabetes—not nearly as much as it does in pancreatic diabetes—because the tissues are resistant to the effects of insulin.

EFFECTS OF CORTISOL ON PROTEIN METABOLISM

Reduction in Cellular Protein. One of the principal effects of cortisol on the metabolic systems of the body is reduction of the protein stores in essentially all cells of the body except those of the liver. This reduction is caused by both decreased protein synthesis and increased catabolism of protein already in the cells.

In the presence of great excesses of cortisol, the muscles can become so weak that the person cannot rise from the squatting

TABLE 91-3	Summary of Actions of Cortisol and Integration of Features of Cushing Syndrome	
	Cortisol Actions	**Features of Cushing Syndrome**
Carbohydrate metabolism	Stimulates gluconeogenesis ↑ Glycogen storage in liver cells ↓ Glucose utilization in cells ↑ Blood glucose levels	↑ Blood glucose levels
Protein metabolism	↓ Protein stores in all cells except liver cells ↑ Catabolism of protein in cells ↑ Protein in liver ↑ Amino acids in plasma	↓ Protein from muscles causes severe muscle weakness ↓ Protein in lymphoid tissue causes suppressed immune system ↓ Protein in collagen fibers leads to purplish striae ↓ Protein in bones leads to weak bones and osteoporosis
Fat metabolism	↑ Mobilization of fatty acids ↑ Oxidation of fatty acid in cells	Moon face and buffalo torso occur due to an abnormal mobilization of fat from the lower part of the body and deposition in the thoracic and upper abdominal regions
Anti-inflammatory effects	Stabilizes lysosomal enzymes ↓ Migration of WBCs ↓ Phagocytosis Suppresses the immune system	Suppression of the immune system

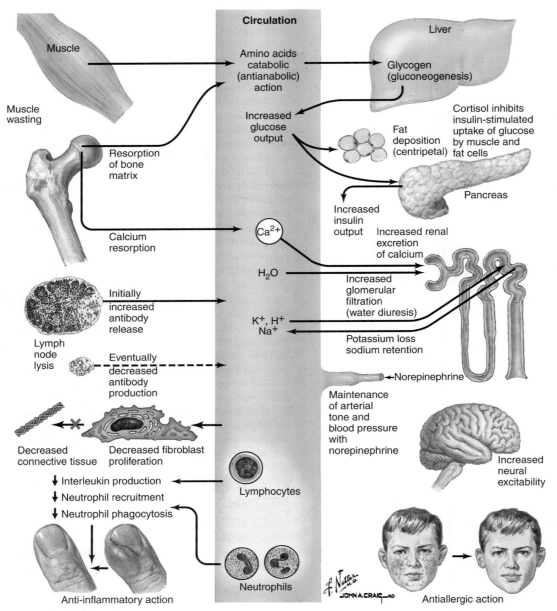

Figure 91-7 Actions of cortisol. Cortisol has a wide array of actions, including muscle wasting, gluconeogenesis, hyperglycemia, anti-inflammatory and anti-immune effects, and insulin resistance. It also has mineralocorticoid-like effects on the kidney at high concentrations. *From Netter's Essential Physiology, 2009, p. 333, Figure 28-4.*

position. In addition, the immunity functions of the lymphoid tissue can be decreased to a small fraction of normal.

Cortisol Increases Liver and Plasma Proteins. Coincidentally with the effect of glucocorticoids to reduce proteins elsewhere in the body, the liver proteins are increased. Furthermore, the plasma proteins (which are produced by the liver and then released into the blood) are also increased. These increases are exceptions to the protein depletion that occurs elsewhere in the body. It is believed that this difference results from a possible effect of cortisol to enhance amino acid transport into liver cells (but not into most other cells) and to enhance the liver enzymes required for protein synthesis.

Increased Blood Amino Acids, Diminished Transport of Amino Acids into Extrahepatic Cells, and Enhanced Transport into Hepatic Cells. Studies in isolated tissues have demonstrated that cortisol depresses amino acid transport into muscle cells and perhaps into other extrahepatic cells.

Cortisol mobilizes amino acids from the nonhepatic tissues and in doing so diminishes the tissue stores of protein.

The increased plasma concentration of amino acids and enhanced transport of amino acids into the hepatic cells by cortisol could also account for enhanced utilization of amino acids by the liver to cause such effects as (1) increased rate of deamination of amino acids by the liver, (2) increased protein synthesis in the liver, (3) increased formation of plasma proteins by the liver, and (4) increased conversion of amino acids to glucose—that is, enhanced gluconeogenesis.

EFFECTS OF CORTISOL ON FAT METABOLISM

Mobilization of Fatty Acids. In much the same manner that cortisol promotes amino acid mobilization from muscle, it also promotes mobilization of fatty acids from adipose tissue. This mobilization increases the concentration of free fatty acids in the plasma, which also increases their utilization for energy. Cortisol also seems to have a direct effect to enhance the oxidation of fatty acids in the cells.

The increased mobilization of fats by cortisol, combined with increased oxidation of fatty acids in the cells, helps shift the metabolic systems of the cells from utilization of glucose for energy to utilization of fatty acids in times of starvation or other stresses. Nevertheless, the increased use of fatty acids for metabolic energy is an important factor for long-term conservation of body glucose and glycogen.

Excess Cortisol Causes Obesity. Despite the fact that cortisol can cause a moderate degree of fatty acid mobilization from adipose tissue, a peculiar type of obesity develops in many people with excess cortisol secretion, with excess deposition of fat in the chest and head regions of the body, giving a buffalo-like torso and a rounded "moon face." Although the cause is unclear, it has been suggested that this peculiar type of obesity may occur because fat is generated in some tissues of the body more rapidly than it is mobilized and oxidized.

CORTISOL IS IMPORTANT IN RESISTING STRESS AND INFLAMMATION

Almost any type of stress, whether physical or neurogenic, causes an immediate and marked increase in ACTH secretion by the anterior pituitary gland, followed within minutes by greatly increased adrenocortical secretion of cortisol. This effect is demonstrated dramatically by the experiment shown in Figure 91-8, in which corticosteroid formation and secretion increased sixfold in a rat within 4–20 minutes after fracture of two leg bones.

The following list details some of the different types of stress that increase cortisol release:

1. trauma of almost any type
2. infection
3. intense heat or cold
4. injection of norepinephrine and other sympathomimetic drugs
5. surgery
6. injection of necrotizing substances beneath the skin
7. restraining an animal so it cannot move
8. debilitating diseases

Even though cortisol secretion often increases greatly in stressful situations, we are not sure why this is of significant benefit to the animal. One possibility is that the glucocorticoids cause rapid mobilization of amino acids and fats from their cellular stores, making them immediately available both for energy and for synthesis of other compounds, including glucose, needed by the different tissues of the body.

Cortisol usually does not mobilize the basic functional proteins of the cells, such as the muscle contractile proteins and the proteins of neurons, until almost all other proteins have been released. This preferential effect of cortisol in mobilizing labile proteins could make amino acids available to needy cells to synthesize substances essential to life.

ANTI-INFLAMMATORY EFFECTS OF HIGH LEVELS OF CORTISOL

When tissues are damaged by trauma, by infection with bacteria, or in other ways, they almost always become "inflamed." Administration of large amounts of cortisol can usually block this inflammation or even reverse many of its effects once it has begun. Before attempting to explain the way in which cortisol functions to block inflammation, let us review the basic steps in the inflammation process, which are discussed in more detail in Chapters 24 and 25.

Five main stages of inflammation occur:

1. release from the damaged tissue cells of chemicals such as histamine, bradykinin, proteolytic enzymes, prostaglandins, and leukotrienes that activate the inflammation process;
2. an increase in blood flow in the inflamed area caused by some of the released products from the tissues, an effect called *erythema*;
3. leakage of large quantities of almost pure plasma out of the capillaries into the damaged areas because of increased capillary permeability, followed by clotting of the tissue fluid, thus causing a *nonpitting type of edema*;
4. infiltration of the area by leukocytes;
5. after days or weeks, ingrowth of fibrous tissue that often helps in the healing process.

When large amounts of cortisol are secreted or injected into a person, the glucocorticoid has two basic *anti-inflammatory effects*: (1) it can block the early stages of the inflammation process before noticeable inflammation even begins or (2) if inflammation has already begun, it causes rapid resolution of the inflammation and increased rapidity of healing. These effects are explained further in the following sections.

Cortisol Prevents the Development of Inflammation by Stabilizing Lysosomes and by Other Effects. Cortisol has the following effects in preventing inflammation:

1. *Cortisol stabilizes lysosomal membranes.* This stabilization is one of its most important anti-inflammatory effects where the lysosomes are released in greatly decreased quantities.
2. *Cortisol decreases permeability of the capillaries*, probably as a secondary effect of the reduced release of proteolytic enzymes. This decrease in permeability prevents loss of plasma into the tissues.

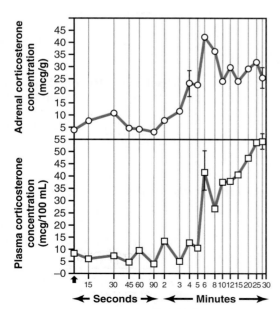

Figure 91-8 Rapid reaction of the adrenal cortex of a rat to stress caused by fracture of the tibia and fibula at time zero. (In the rat, corticosterone is secreted in place of cortisol.)

3. *Cortisol decreases both migration of white blood cells into the inflamed area and phagocytosis of the damaged cells.* Cortisol diminishes the formation of prostaglandins and leukotrienes that otherwise would increase vasodilation, capillary permeability, and mobility of white blood cells.

4. *Cortisol suppresses the immune system causing lymphocyte reproduction to decrease markedly.* The T lymphocytes are especially suppressed that lessen tissue reactions that would otherwise promote inflammation.

5. *Cortisol attenuates fever mainly because it reduces release of interleukin-1 from white blood cells,* which is one of the principal excitants to the hypothalamic temperature control system. The decreased temperature in turn reduces the degree of vasodilation.

Thus, cortisol has an almost global effect in reducing all aspects of the inflammatory process.

Cortisol Causes Resolution of Inflammation. Regardless of the precise mechanisms by which the anti-inflammatory effect occurs, this effect of cortisol plays a major role in combating certain types of diseases, such as rheumatoid arthritis, rheumatic fever, and acute glomerulonephritis.

When cortisol or other glucocorticoids are administered to patients with these diseases, almost invariably the inflammation begins to subside within 24 hours. Even though cortisol does not correct the basic disease condition, preventing the damaging effects of the inflammatory response can often be a lifesaving measure.

OTHER EFFECTS OF CORTISOL

Cortisol Blocks the Inflammatory Response to Allergic Reactions. The basic allergic reaction between antigen and antibody is not affected by cortisol, and even some of the secondary effects of the allergic reaction still occur. However, because the inflammatory response is responsible for many of the serious and sometimes lethal effects of allergic reactions, administration of cortisol, followed by its effect in reducing inflammation and the release of inflammatory products, can be lifesaving. For instance, cortisol effectively prevents shock or death as a result of anaphylaxis, a condition that otherwise kills many people, as explained in Chapters 24 and 25.

Effect on Blood Cells and on Immunity in Infectious Diseases. Cortisol decreases the number of eosinophils and lymphocytes in the blood; administration of large doses of cortisol causes significant atrophy of all the lymphoid tissue throughout the body. Indeed, a finding of lymphocytopenia or eosinopenia is an important diagnostic criterion for overproduction of cortisol by the adrenal gland.

As a result, the level of immunity for almost all foreign invaders of the body is decreased.

However, this ability of cortisol and other glucocorticoids to suppress immunity makes them useful drugs in preventing immunological rejection of transplanted hearts, kidneys, and other tissues.

Cortisol increases the production of red blood cells by mechanisms that are unclear. When excess cortisol is secreted by the adrenal glands, polycythemia often results, and conversely, when the adrenal glands secrete no cortisol, anemia often results.

CELLULAR MECHANISM OF CORTISOL ACTION

Cortisol, like other steroid hormones, exerts its effects by first interacting with intracellular receptors in target cells and the mechanism is similar to aldosterone. Once inside the cell, the hormone–receptor complex then interacts with specific regulatory DNA sequences, called *glucocorticoid response elements*, to induce or repress gene transcription. Certain proteins in the cell, called *transcription factors*, are also necessary for this interaction.

Glucocorticoids increase or decrease transcription of many genes to alter synthesis of mRNA for the proteins that mediate their multiple physiological effects. The metabolic effects of cortisol are not immediate but require 45–60 minutes for proteins to be synthesized, and up to several hours or days to fully develop. Recent evidence suggests that glucocorticoids, especially at high concentrations, may also have some rapid *nongenomic effects* on cell membrane ion transport that may contribute to their therapeutic benefits.

REGULATION OF CORTISOL SECRETION BY ADRENOCORTICOTROPIC HORMONE FROM THE PITUITARY GLAND

ACTH Stimulates Cortisol Secretion. Unlike aldosterone secretion by the zona glomerulosa, which is controlled mainly by potassium and angiotensin II acting directly on the adrenocortical cells, secretion of cortisol is controlled almost entirely by ACTH that is secreted by the anterior pituitary gland. This hormone, also called *corticotropin* or *adrenocorticotropin*, also enhances the production of adrenal androgens.

ACTH secretion is further controlled by *corticotropin-releasing factor* (CRF) from the hypothalamus.

ACTH Activates Adrenocortical Cells to Produce Steroids by Increasing Cyclic Adenosine Monophosphate. The principal effect of ACTH on the adrenocortical cells is to activate *adenylyl cyclase* in the cell membrane. This then induces the formation of cAMP in the cell cytoplasm, reaching its maximal effect in about 3 minutes. The cAMP in turn activates the intracellular enzymes that cause formation of the adrenocortical hormones. This is another example of cAMP as a *second messenger* signal system.

Long-term stimulation of the adrenal cortex by ACTH not only increases secretory activity but also causes hypertrophy and proliferation of the adrenocortical cells, especially in the zona fasciculata and zona reticularis, where cortisol and the androgens are secreted.

Inhibitory Effect of Cortisol on the Hypothalamus and on the Anterior Pituitary to Decrease ACTH Secretion. Cortisol has direct negative feedback effects on (1) the hypothalamus to decrease the formation of CRF and (2) the anterior pituitary gland to decrease the formation of ACTH. Both of these feedbacks help regulate the plasma concentration of cortisol.

Summary of the Cortisol Control System

Figure 91-9 shows the overall system for control of cortisol secretion. The key to this control is the excitation of the hypothalamus by different types of stress. Stress stimuli activate the entire system to cause rapid release of cortisol, and the cortisol in turn initiates a series of metabolic effects directed toward relieving the damaging nature of the stressful state.

Direct feedback of the cortisol to both the hypothalamus and the anterior pituitary gland also occurs to decrease the concentration of cortisol in the plasma at times when the body is not experiencing stress. However, the stress stimuli are the most potent ones; they can always break through this

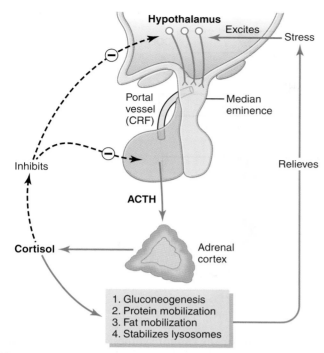

Figure 91-9 Mechanism for regulation of glucocorticoid secretion. *ACTH*, adrenocorticotropic hormone; *CRF*, corticotropin-releasing factor.

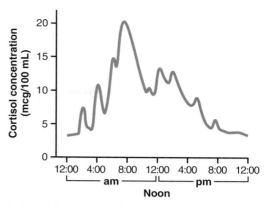

Figure 91-10 Typical pattern of cortisol concentration during the day. Note the oscillations in secretion as well as a daily secretory surge an hour or so after waking in the morning.

direct inhibitory feedback of cortisol, causing either periodic exacerbations of cortisol secretion at multiple times during the day (Figure 91-10) or prolonged cortisol secretion in times of chronic stress.

Circadian Rhythm of Glucocorticoid Secretion. The secretory rates of CRF, ACTH, and cortisol are high in the early morning but low in the late evening, as shown in Figure 91-10. This effect results from a 24-hour cyclic alteration in the signals from the hypothalamus that cause cortisol secretion. When a person changes daily sleeping habits, the cycle changes correspondingly. Therefore, measurements of blood cortisol levels are meaningful only when expressed in terms of the time in the cycle at which the measurements are made.

Synthesis and Secretion of ACTH in Association with Melanocyte-Stimulating Hormone, Lipotropin, and Endorphin

When ACTH is secreted by the anterior pituitary gland, several other hormones that have similar chemical structures are secreted simultaneously. The reason for this secretion is that the gene that is transcribed to form the RNA molecule that causes ACTH synthesis initially causes the formation of a considerably larger protein, a preprohormone called *proopiomelanocortin* (POMC), which is the precursor of ACTH and several other peptides, including *melanocyte-stimulating hormone* (MSH), β-*lipotropin*, β-*endorphin*, and a few others (Figure 91-11). Under normal conditions, most of these hormones are not secreted in enough quantity by the pituitary to have a major effect on the human body, but when the rate of secretion of ACTH is high, as may occur in persons with Addison disease, formation of some of the other POMC-derived hormones may also be increased.

In *melanocytes*, located in abundance between the dermis and epidermis of the skin, MSH stimulates formation of the black pigment *melanin* and disperses it to the epidermis.

ACTH, because it contains an MSH sequence, has about 1/30 as much melanocyte-stimulating effect as MSH. Furthermore, because the quantities of pure MSH secreted in humans are extremely small, whereas those of ACTH are large, it is likely that ACTH is normally more important than MSH in determining the amount of melanin in the skin.

Adrenal Androgens

Several moderately active male sex hormones called *adrenal androgens* (the most important of which is *DHEA*) are continually secreted by the adrenal cortex, especially during fetal life, as discussed in Chapter 98. Also, progesterone and estrogens, which are female sex hormones, are secreted in minute quantities.

Normally, the adrenal androgens have only weak effects in humans. It is possible that part of the early development of the male sex organs results from childhood secretion of adrenal androgens. The adrenal androgens also exert mild effects in the female, not only before puberty but also throughout life. Much of the growth of the pubic and axillary hair in the female results from the action of these hormones.

In extraadrenal tissues, some of the adrenal androgens are converted to testosterone, the primary male sex hormone, which probably accounts for much of their androgenic activity. The physiological effects of androgens are discussed in Chapter 94 in relation to male sexual function.

Abnormalities of Adrenocortical Secretion

HYPOADRENALISM (ADRENAL INSUFFICIENCY)—ADDISON DISEASE

Addison disease results from an inability of the adrenal cortices to produce sufficient adrenocortical hormones. Features of Addison disease have been provided in Box 91-1.

Causes
1. Addison disease is most frequently caused by *primary atrophy or injury* of the adrenal cortices. In about 80% of the cases, the atrophy is caused by autoimmunity against the cortices.
2. It can also be caused by tuberculous destruction of the adrenal glands.
3. Invasion of the adrenal cortices by cancer is another cause of Addison disease.

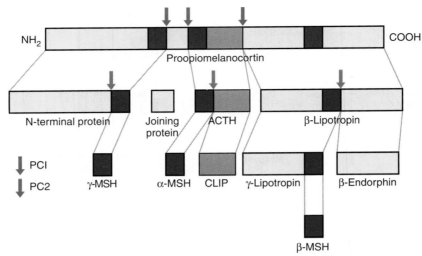

Figure 91-11   Proopiomelanocortin processing by prohormone convertase 1 (PC1, *red arrows*) and PC2 (*blue arrows*). Tissue-specific expression of these two enzymes results in different peptides produced in various tissues. *ACTH*, adrenocorticotropic hormone; *CLIP*, corticotropin-like intermediate peptide; *MSH*, melanocyte-stimulating hormone.

BOX 91-1   FEATURES OF ADDISON DISEASE

- Fatigue and weakness
- Loss of appetite (anorexia)
- Symptoms related to the gastrointestinal (GI) tract:
  - Vomiting
  - Nausea
  - Diarrhea
  - Constipation
  - Abdominal pain
- Dizziness due to decreased blood pressure
- Hyperpigmentation
- Loss of weight
- Vitiligo

In some cases, adrenal insufficiency is secondary to impaired function of the pituitary gland, which fails to produce sufficient ACTH. When ACTH output is too low, cortisol and aldosterone production decreases and, eventually, the adrenal glands may atrophy because of a lack of ACTH stimulation. Secondary adrenal insufficiency is much more common than Addison disease, which is sometimes called *primary adrenal insufficiency*. Disturbances in severe adrenal insufficiency are described in the following sections.

Mineralocorticoid Deficiency. Lack of aldosterone secretion greatly decreases renal tubular sodium reabsorption and consequently allows sodium ions, chloride ions, and water to be lost into urine in great profusion. The net result is a greatly decreased extracellular fluid volume. Furthermore, hyponatremia, hyperkalemia, and mild acidosis develop because of failure of potassium and hydrogen ions to be secreted in exchange for sodium reabsorption.

As the extracellular fluid becomes depleted, plasma volume falls, red blood cell concentration rises markedly, cardiac output and blood pressure decrease, and the patient dies in shock, with death usually occurring in the untreated patient 4 days to 2 weeks after complete cessation of mineralocorticoid secretion.

Glucocorticoid Deficiency. Loss of cortisol secretion makes it impossible for a person with Addison disease to maintain normal blood glucose concentration between meals because he or she cannot synthesize significant quantities of glucose by gluconeogenesis. Furthermore, lack of cortisol reduces the mobilization of both proteins and fats from the tissues, thereby depressing many other metabolic functions of the body. Even when excess quantities of glucose and other nutrients are available, the person's muscles are weak, indicating that glucocorticoids are necessary to maintain other metabolic functions of the tissues in addition to energy metabolism.

Lack of adequate glucocorticoid secretion also makes a person with Addison disease highly susceptible to the deteriorating effects of different types of stress, and even a mild respiratory infection can cause death.

Melanin Pigmentation. Another characteristic of most people with Addison disease is melanin pigmentation of the mucous membranes and skin. This melanin is not always deposited evenly but occasionally is deposited in blotches, and it is deposited especially in the thin skin areas, such as the mucous membranes of the lips and the thin skin of the nipples.

The melanin deposition is believed to have the following cause: When cortisol secretion is depressed, this causes tremendous rates of ACTH secretion, as well as simultaneous secretion of increased amounts of MSH. Probably the tremendous amounts of ACTH cause most of the pigmenting effect because they can stimulate formation of melanin by the melanocytes in the same way that MSH does.

Treatment of People with Addison Disease. An untreated person with total adrenal destruction dies within a few days to a few weeks because of weakness and usually circulatory shock. Yet such a person can live for years if small quantities of mineralocorticoids and glucocorticoids are administered daily.

Addisonian Crisis. In a person with Addison disease, the output of glucocorticoids does not increase during stress. Yet during different types of trauma, disease, or other stresses, such as surgical operations, a person is likely to have an acute need for excessive amounts of glucocorticoids and often must be given 10 or more times the normal quantities of glucocorticoids to prevent death.

This critical need for extra glucocorticoids and the associated severe debility in times of stress is called an *Addisonian crisis*.

CLINICAL FINDINGS OF CUSHING'S SYNDROME

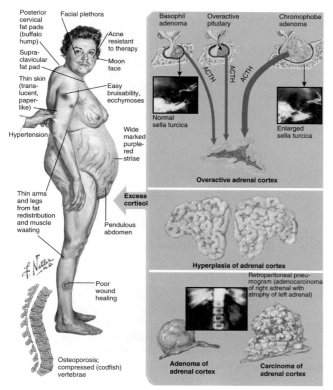

Figure 91-12 Patient with features of Cushing syndrome. *ACTH*, adrenocorticotropic hormone. *Netter illustration from www.netterimages.com. © Elsevier Inc. All rights reserved.*

HYPERADRENALISM—CUSHING SYNDROME

Hypersecretion by the adrenal cortex causes a complex cascade of hormone effects called *Cushing syndrome* (Figure 91-12). Many of the abnormalities of Cushing syndrome can be ascribed to abnormal amounts of cortisol, but excess secretion of androgens may also cause important effects. Hypercortisolism

can occur from multiple causes, including (1) adenomas of the anterior pituitary that secrete large amounts of ACTH; (2) abnormal function of the hypothalamus that causes high levels of corticotropin-releasing hormone (CRH) causing excess ACTH release; (3) "ectopic secretion" of ACTH by a tumor elsewhere in the body, such as an abdominal carcinoma; and (4) adenomas of the adrenal cortex. When Cushing syndrome is secondary to excess secretion of ACTH by the anterior pituitary, this condition is referred to as *Cushing disease.*

Excess ACTH secretion is the most common cause of Cushing syndrome and is characterized by high plasma levels of ACTH and cortisol. Primary overproduction of cortisol by the adrenal glands accounts for about 20–25% of clinical cases of Cushing syndrome and is usually associated with reduced ACTH levels due to cortisol feedback inhibition of ACTH secretion by the anterior pituitary gland.

Administration of large doses of dexamethasone, a synthetic glucocorticoid, can be used to distinguish between *ACTH-dependent* and *ACTH-independent* Cushing syndrome. This test is called the *dexamethasone test* and is usually considered to be a first step in the differential diagnosis of Cushing syndrome.

Cushing syndrome can also occur when large amounts of glucocorticoids are administered over prolonged periods for therapeutic purposes. For example, patients with chronic inflammation associated with diseases such as rheumatoid arthritis are often treated with glucocorticoids and may develop some of the clinical symptoms of Cushing syndrome.

A special characteristic of Cushing syndrome is mobilization of fat from the lower part of the body, with concomitant extra deposition of fat in the thoracic and upper abdominal regions, giving rise to a buffalo torso. The excess secretion of steroids also leads to an edematous appearance of the face, and the androgenic potency of some of the hormones sometimes causes acne and hirsutism (excess growth of facial hair). The appearance of the face is frequently described as a "moon face," as demonstrated in the untreated patient with Cushing syndrome to the left in Figure 91-13. About 80% of patients have hypertension, presumably because of the mineralocorticoid effects of cortisol.

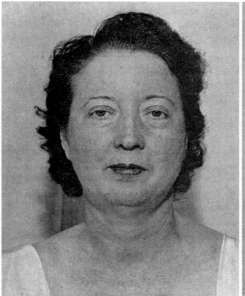
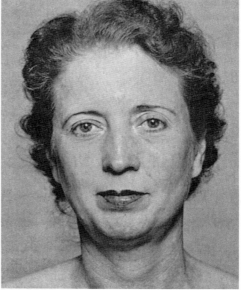

Figure 91-13 A person with Cushing syndrome before (*left*) and after (*right*) subtotal adrenalectomy. *Courtesy Dr. Leonard Posey.*

Effects on Carbohydrate and Protein Metabolism. The abundance of cortisol secreted in Cushing syndrome can increase blood glucose concentration, sometimes to values as high as 200 mg/dL after meals due to the enhanced gluconeogenesis and decreased glucose utilization by the tissues.

The effects of glucocorticoids on protein catabolism are often profound in Cushing syndrome, causing greatly decreased tissue proteins almost everywhere in the body with the exception of the liver; the plasma proteins also remain unaffected. The loss of protein from the muscles in particular causes severe weakness. The loss of protein synthesis in the lymphoid tissues leads to a suppressed immune system, and thus many of these patients die of infections. Even the protein collagen fibers in the subcutaneous tissue are diminished so that the subcutaneous tissues tear easily, resulting in development of large *purplish striae* where they have torn apart. In addition, severely diminished protein deposition in the bones often causes severe *osteoporosis* with consequent weakness of the bones.

Treatment of Cushing Syndrome. Treatment of Cushing syndrome consists of removing an adrenal tumor if this is the cause or decreasing the secretion of ACTH, if possible. Hypertrophied pituitary glands or even small tumors in the pituitary that oversecrete ACTH can sometimes be surgically removed or destroyed by radiation. Drugs that block steroidogenesis, such as *metyrapone*, *ketoconazole*, and *aminoglutethimide*, or that inhibit ACTH secretion, such as *serotonin antagonists* and *gamma-aminobutyric acid (GABA)-transaminase inhibitors*, can also be used when surgery is not feasible. If ACTH secretion cannot easily be decreased, the only satisfactory treatment is usually bilateral partial (or even total) adrenalectomy, followed by administration of adrenal steroids to make up for any insufficiency that develops.

PRIMARY ALDOSTERONISM (CONN SYNDROME)

Occasionally, a small tumor of the zona glomerulosa cells occurs and secretes large amounts of aldosterone; the resulting condition is called "primary aldosteronism" or "Conn syndrome." Also, in a few instances, hyperplastic adrenal cortices secrete aldosterone rather than cortisol. The effects of the excess aldosterone are discussed in detail earlier in the chapter. The most important effects are hypokalemia, mild metabolic alkalosis, a slight increase in extracellular fluid volume and blood volume, a modest increase in plasma sodium concentration (usually <4 to 6 mEq/L increase), and, almost always, hypertension. Especially interesting in persons with primary aldosteronism are occasional periods of muscle paralysis caused by the hypokalemia. The paralysis is caused by a depressant effect of low extracellular potassium concentration on action potential transmission by the nerve fibers, as explained in Chapter 9.

One of the diagnostic criteria of primary aldosteronism is a decreased plasma renin concentration. This decrease results from feedback suppression of renin secretion caused by the excess aldosterone or by the excess extracellular fluid volume and arterial pressure resulting from the aldosteronism. Treatment of primary aldosteronism may include surgical

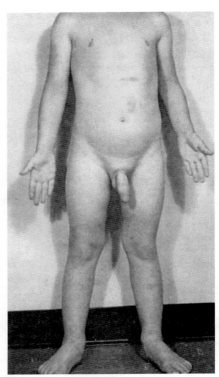

Figure 91-14   Adrenogenital syndrome in a 4-year-old boy. *Courtesy Dr. Leonard Posey.*

removal of the tumor or of most of the adrenal tissue when hyperplasia is the cause. Another option for treatment is pharmacological antagonism of the MR with spironolactone or eplerenone.

ADRENOGENITAL SYNDROME

Occasionally an adrenocortical tumor secretes excessive quantities of androgens that cause intense masculinizing effects throughout the body. If this phenomenon occurs in a female, virile characteristics develop, including growth of a beard, a much deeper voice, occasionally baldness if she also has the genetic trait for baldness, masculine distribution of hair on the body and the pubis, growth of the clitoris to resemble a penis, and deposition of proteins in the skin and especially in the muscles to give typical masculine characteristics.

In the prepubertal male, a virilizing adrenal tumor causes the same characteristics as in the female plus rapid development of the male sexual organs, as shown in Figure 91-14, which depicts a 4-year-old boy with adrenogenital syndrome. In the adult male, the virilizing characteristics of adrenogenital syndrome are usually obscured by the normal virilizing characteristics of the testosterone secreted by the testes. It is often difficult to make a diagnosis of adrenogenital syndrome in the adult male. In adrenogenital syndrome, the excretion of 17-ketosteroids (which are derived from androgens) in the urine may be 10–15 times normal. This finding can be used in diagnosing the disease.

BIBLIOGRAPHY

Baker ME, Funder JW, Kattoula SR: Evolution of hormone selectivity in glucocorticoid and mineralocorticoid receptors, *J. Steroid Biochem. Mol. Biol.* 137:57, 2013.

Biller BM, Grossman AB, Stewart PM, et al: Treatment of adrenocorticotropin-dependent Cushing's syndrome: a consensus statement, *J. Clin. Endocrinol. Metab.* 93:2454, 2008.

Bornstein SR: Predisposing factors for adrenal insufficiency, *N. Engl. J. Med.* 360:2328, 2009.

Boscaro M, Arnaldi G: Approach to the patient with possible Cushing's syndrome, *J. Clin. Endocrinol. Metab.* 94:3121, 2009.

Chapman K, Holmes M, Seckl J: 11β-Hydroxysteroid dehydrogenases: intracellular gate-keepers of tissue glucocorticoid action, *Physiol. Rev.* 93:1139, 2013.

Charmandari E, Nicolaides NC, Chrousos GP: Adrenal insufficiency, *Lancet* 383:2152, 2014.

Feelders RA, Hofland LJ: Medical treatment of Cushing disease, *J. Clin. Endocrinol. Metab.* 98:425, 2013.

Fuller PJ: Adrenal diagnostics: an endocrinologist's perspective focused on hyperaldosteronism, *Clin. Biochem. Rev.* 34:111, 2013.

Fuller PJ, Young MJ: Mechanisms of mineralocorticoid action, *Hypertension* 46:1227, 2005.

Funder JW: Aldosterone and the cardiovascular system: genomic and nongenomic effects, *Endocrinology* 147:5564, 2006.

Funder JW: The genetic basis of primary aldosteronism, *Curr. Hypertens. Rep.* 14:120, 2012.

Gomez-Sanchez CE, Oki K: Minireview: potassium channels and aldosterone dysregulation: is primary aldosteronism a potassium channelopathy? *Endocrinology* 155:47, 2014.

Hall JE, Granger JP, Smith MJ Jr, Premen AJ: Role of renal hemodynamics and arterial pressure in aldosterone "escape", *Hypertension* 6:I183, 1984.

Hammes SR, Levin ER: Minireview: recent advances in extranuclear steroid receptor actions, *Endocrinology* 152:4489, 2011.

Mazziotti G, Giustina A: Glucocorticoids and the regulation of growth hormone secretion, *Nat. Rev. Endocrinol.* 9:265, 2013.

Pimenta E, Wolley M, Stowasser M: Adverse cardiovascular outcomes of corticosteroid excess, *Endocrinology* 153:5137, 2012.

Prague JK, May S, Whitelaw BC: Cushing's syndrome, *BMJ* 346:f945, 2013.

Spat A, Hunyady L: Control of aldosterone secretion: a model for convergence in cellular signaling pathways, *Physiol. Rev.* 84:489, 2004.

Speiser PW, White PC: Congenital adrenal hyperplasia, *N. Engl. J. Med.* 349:776, 2003.

Tritos NA, Biller BM: Advances in medical therapies for Cushing's syndrome, *Discov. Med.* 13:171, 2012.

Vinson GP: The adrenal cortex and life, *Mol. Cell. Endocrinol.* 300:2, 2009.

Wendler A, Albrecht C, Wehling M: Nongenomic actions of aldosterone and progesterone revisited, *Steroids* 77:1002, 2012.

Adrenal Medulla

The adrenal medulla occupies the central 20% of the adrenal gland and is functionally related to the sympathetic nervous system; it secretes the hormones *epinephrine* and *norepinephrine* in response to sympathetic stimulation. In turn, these hormones cause almost the same effects as direct stimulation of the sympathetic nerves in all parts of the body.

Special Nature of the Sympathetic Nerve Endings in the Adrenal Medullae

Preganglionic sympathetic nerve fibers pass, *without synapsing*, all the way from the intermediolateral horn cells of the spinal cord, through the sympathetic chains, then through the splanchnic nerves, and finally into the two adrenal medullae. There they end directly on modified neuronal cells that secrete *epinephrine* and *norepinephrine* into the bloodstream. These secretory cells embryologically are derived from nervous tissue and are actually postganglionic neurons; indeed, they even have rudimentary nerve fibers and it is the endings of these fibers that secrete the adrenal hormones *epinephrine* and *norepinephrine*.

Biosynthesis of Epinephrine and Norepinephrine, its Removal, and its Duration of Action

Synthesis of norepinephrine begins in the axoplasm of the terminal nerve endings of adrenergic nerve fibers but is completed inside the secretory vesicles. The basic steps are illustrated in Figure 92-1.

After secretion of norepinephrine by the terminal nerve endings, it is removed from the secretory site in three ways: (1) reuptake into the adrenergic nerve endings by an active transport process—accounting for removal of 50–80% of the secreted norepinephrine; (2) diffusion away from the nerve endings into the surrounding body fluids and then into the blood—accounting for removal of most of the remaining norepinephrine; and (3) destruction of small amounts by tissue enzymes (one of these enzymes is *monoamine oxidase*, which is found in the nerve endings, and another is *catechol-O-methyl transferase*, which is present diffusely in tissues).

Ordinarily, the norepinephrine secreted directly into a tissue remains active for only a few seconds, demonstrating that its reuptake and diffusion away from the tissue are rapid. However, the norepinephrine and epinephrine secreted into the blood by the adrenal medullae remain active until they diffuse into some tissue, where they can be destroyed by catechol-O-methyl transferase; this action occurs mainly in the liver. Therefore, when secreted into the blood, both norepinephrine and epinephrine remain active for 10–30 seconds, but their activity declines to extinction over 1 to several minutes.

Factors that Control the Secretion of Catecholamines from the Adrenal Medulla

Several stressful stimuli can activate the catecholamine secretion from the adrenal medulla. Some of the important stimuli are listed as follows:

1. position of the individual (standing increases norepinephrine secretion)
2. exercise (varying degrees of exercise can cause catecholamine secretions)
3. hypoglycemia (strongly stimulates epinephrine secretions)
4. cigarette smoking
5. surgery (causes both epinephrine and norepinephrine secretions)
6. ketoacidosis
7. myocardial infarction
8. anesthesia

The chromaffin cells in the adrenal medulla are stimulated by acetylcholine released from the preganglionic sympathetic fibers. These chromaffin cells have nicotinic cholinergic receptors and depolarize on contact with acetylcholine leading to activation of voltage-gated calcium channels.

The result of this activation causes the release of the vesicle contents by a process of exocytosis into the extracellular space. The release of norepinephrine is controlled by the activation of α_2 receptors that are located on the presynaptic membrane. The stimulation of these receptors inhibits the release of norepinephrine. This mechanism is used by certain drugs such as clonidine to treat hypertension.

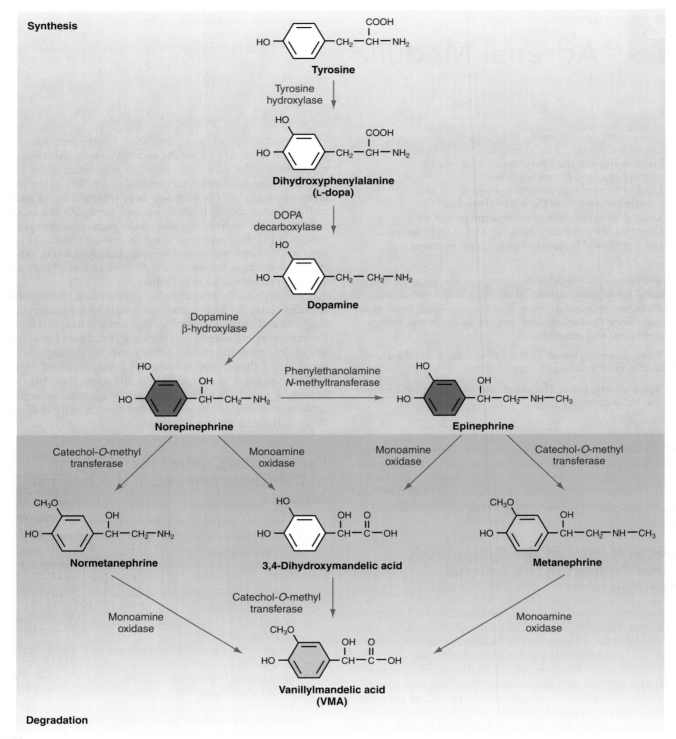

Figure 92-1 Catecholamine biosynthesis and metabolism. Synthetic steps are shaded orange; degradative steps are shaded turquoise. Major catecholamines are indicated in green, major metabolites in yellow. *Netter illustration from www.netterimages.com. © Elsevier Inc. All rights reserved.*

Adrenergic Receptors—Alpha and Beta Receptors

Two major classes of adrenergic receptors also exist; they are called *alpha receptors* and *beta receptors*. There are two major types of alpha receptors, alpha$_1$ and alpha$_2$, which are linked to different G proteins. The beta receptors are divided into *beta$_1$*, *beta$_2$*, and *beta$_3$* receptors because certain chemicals affect only

certain beta receptors. The beta receptors also use G proteins for signaling.

Norepinephrine and epinephrine, both of which are secreted into the blood by the adrenal medulla, have slightly different effects in exciting the alpha and beta receptors. Norepinephrine excites mainly alpha receptors but excites the beta receptors to a lesser extent as well. Epinephrine excites both types of receptors approximately equally. Therefore, the relative effects

TABLE 92-1	Adrenergic Receptors and Function
Alpha Receptor	**Beta Receptor**
Vasoconstriction	Vasodilation (β_2)
Iris dilation	Cardioacceleration (β_1)
Intestinal relaxation	Increased myocardial strength (β_1)
Intestinal sphincter contraction	Intestinal relaxation (β_2)
	Uterus relaxation (β_2)
Pilomotor contraction	Bronchodilation (β_2)
Bladder sphincter contraction	Calorigenesis (β_2)
Inhibits neurotransmitter release (α_2)	Glycogenolysis (β_2)
	Lipolysis (β_1)
	Bladder wall relaxation (β_2)
	Thermogenesis (β_3)

TABLE 92-2	Autonomic Effects on Various Organs of the Body	
Organ	**Effect of Sympathetic Stimulation**	
Eye		
Pupil	Dilated	
Ciliary muscle	Slight relaxation (far vision)	
Glands	Vasoconstriction and slight secretion	
Nasal		
Lacrimal		
Parotid		
Submandibular		
Gastric		
Pancreatic		
Sweat glands	Copious sweating (cholinergic)	
Apocrine glands	Thick, odoriferous secretion	
Blood vessels	Most often constricted	
Heart		
Muscle	Increased rate	
Increased force of contraction	Decreased force of contraction (especially of atria)	
Coronaries	Dilated (β_2); constricted (α)	
Lungs		
Bronchi	Dilated	
Blood vessels	Mildly constricted	
Gut		
Lumen	Decreased peristalsis and tone	
Sphincter	Increased tone (most times)	
Liver	Glucose released	
Gallbladder and bile ducts	Relaxed	
Kidney	Decreased urine output and increased renin secretion	
Bladder		
Detrusor	Relaxed (slight)	
Trigone	Contracted	
Penis	Ejaculation	
Systemic arterioles		
Abdominal viscera	Constricted	
Muscle	Constricted (adrenergic α) Dilated (adrenergic β_2) Dilated (cholinergic)	
Skin	Constricted	
Blood		
Coagulation	Increased	
Glucose	Increased	
Lipids	Increased	
Basal metabolism	Increased up to 100%	
Adrenal medullary secretion	Increased	
Mental activity	Increased	
Piloerector muscles	Contracted	
Skeletal muscle	Increased glycogenolysis Increased strength	
Fat cells	Lipolysis	

of norepinephrine and epinephrine on different effector organs are determined by the types of receptors in the organs. If they are all beta receptors, epinephrine will be the more effective excitant.

Table 92-1 lists the distribution of alpha and beta receptors in some of the organs and systems controlled by the sympathetic nerves. Note that certain alpha functions are excitatory, whereas others are inhibitory. Likewise, certain beta functions are excitatory and others are inhibitory. Therefore, alpha and beta receptors are not necessarily associated with excitation or inhibition but simply with the affinity of the hormone for the receptors in the given effector organ.

A synthetic hormone chemically similar to epinephrine and norepinephrine, *isopropyl norepinephrine*, has an extremely strong action on beta receptors but essentially no action on alpha receptors.

Physiological Effects of Catecholamines

EXCITATORY AND INHIBITORY ACTIONS OF SYMPATHETIC STIMULATION

Table 92-2 lists the effects on different visceral functions of the body caused by stimulating the sympathetic nerves. Note again that *sympathetic stimulation causes excitatory effects in some organs but inhibitory effects in others.*

FUNCTION OF THE ADRENAL MEDULLAE

Stimulation of the sympathetic nerves to the adrenal medullae causes large quantities of epinephrine and norepinephrine to be released into the circulating blood, and these two hormones in turn are carried in the blood to all tissues of the body. On average, about 80% of the secretion is epinephrine and 20% is norepinephrine, although the relative proportions can change considerably under different physiological conditions.

The circulating epinephrine and norepinephrine have almost the same effects on the different organs as the effects caused by direct sympathetic stimulation, except that *the effects last 5–10 times as long* because both of these hormones are removed from the blood slowly over a period of 2–4 minutes.

The circulating norepinephrine causes constriction of most of the blood vessels of the body; it also causes increased activity of the heart, inhibition of the gastrointestinal tract, dilation of the pupils of the eyes, and so forth.

Epinephrine causes almost the same effects as those caused by norepinephrine, but the effects differ in the following respects (Table 92-3): First, epinephrine, because of its greater effect in stimulating the beta receptors, has a greater effect on cardiac stimulation than does norepinephrine. Second, epinephrine causes only weak constriction of the blood vessels in the muscles, in comparison with much stronger constriction caused by norepinephrine. Because the muscle vessels represent a major segment of the vessels of the body, this difference is

TABLE 92-3	Difference in Actions Between Epinephrine and Norepinephrine		
No.	Function	Epinephrine	Norepinephrine
1	Predilection for type of receptor	Excites both types of receptors equally with a preference for beta receptors	Alpha receptors mainly Beta receptors to a lesser extent
2	Cardiac stimulation	Greater effect due to action on beta receptors	Lesser effect as compared to epinephrine
3	Blood vessels in muscles	Weak constriction	Much stronger constriction increasing peripheral resistance
4	Tissue metabolism	Increases metabolic rate to as much as 100% above normal	Increases metabolic rate to a lesser extent

of special importance because norepinephrine greatly increases the total peripheral resistance and elevates arterial pressure, whereas epinephrine raises the arterial pressure to a lesser extent but increases the cardiac output more.

A third difference between the actions of epinephrine and norepinephrine relates to their effects on tissue metabolism. Epinephrine has 5–10 times as great a metabolic effect as norepinephrine. Indeed, the epinephrine secreted by the adrenal medullae can increase the metabolic rate of the whole body often to as much as 100% above normal, in this way increasing the activity and excitability of the body. It also increases the rates of other metabolic activities, such as glycogenolysis in the liver and muscle, and glucose release into the blood.

In summary, stimulation of the adrenal medullae causes release of the hormones epinephrine and norepinephrine, which together have almost the same effects throughout the body as direct sympathetic stimulation, except that the effects are greatly prolonged, lasting 2–4 minutes after the stimulation is over.

Value of the Adrenal Medullae to the Function of the Sympathetic Nervous System. Epinephrine and norepinephrine are almost always released by the adrenal medullae at the same time that the different organs are stimulated directly by generalized sympathetic activation. Therefore, the organs are actually stimulated in two ways: directly by the sympathetic nerves and indirectly by the adrenal medullary hormones. The two means of stimulation support each other, and either can, in most instances, substitute for the other. For instance, the loss of the two adrenal medullae usually has little effect on the operation of the sympathetic nervous system because the direct pathways can still perform almost all the necessary duties. Thus, the dual mechanism of sympathetic stimulation provides a safety factor, with one mechanism substituting for the other if it is missing.

Another important value of the adrenal medullae is the capability of epinephrine and norepinephrine to stimulate structures of the body that are not innervated by direct sympathetic fibers. For instance, the metabolic rate of almost every cell of the body is increased by these hormones, especially by epinephrine, even though only a small proportion of all the cells in the body are innervated directly by sympathetic fibers.

SYMPATHETIC "TONE"

Normally, the sympathetic and parasympathetic systems are continually active, and the basal rates of activity are known, respectively, as *sympathetic tone* and *parasympathetic tone*.

The value of tone is that *it allows a single nervous system to both increase and decrease the activity of a stimulated organ.*

Tone Caused by Basal Secretion of Epinephrine and Norepinephrine by the Adrenal Medullae. The normal resting rate

of secretion by the adrenal medullae is about 0.2 mcg/kg per minute of epinephrine and about 0.05 mcg/kg per minute of norepinephrine. These quantities are considerable—indeed, enough to maintain the blood pressure almost normal even if all direct sympathetic pathways to the cardiovascular system are removed. Therefore, it is obvious that much of the overall tone of the sympathetic nervous system results from basal secretion of epinephrine and norepinephrine in addition to the tone resulting from direct sympathetic stimulation.

"ALARM" OR "STRESS" RESPONSE OF THE SYMPATHETIC NERVOUS SYSTEM

When large portions of the sympathetic nervous system discharge at the same time—that is, a *mass discharge*—this action increases the ability of the body to perform vigorous muscle activity in many ways, as summarized in the following list:

1. increased arterial pressure;
2. increased blood flow to active muscles concurrent with decreased blood flow to organs such as the gastrointestinal tract and the kidneys that are not needed for rapid motor activity;
3. increased rates of cellular metabolism throughout the body;
4. increased blood glucose concentration;
5. increased glycolysis in the liver and muscles;
6. increased muscle strength;
7. increased mental activity;
8. increased rate of blood coagulation.

The sum of these effects permits a person to perform far more strenuous physical activity than would otherwise be possible. Because either *mental* or *physical stress* can excite the sympathetic system, it is frequently said that the purpose of the sympathetic system is to provide extra activation of the body in states of stress, which is called the sympathetic *stress response*.

PHEOCHROMOCYTOMA

Pheochromocytomas are tumors that arise from the chromaffin cells that secrete catecholamines. About 90% of these tumors occur in the adrenal medulla; however, occasionally they arise in the abdominal sympathetic ganglia close to the aorta and inferior mesenteric artery. When they occur in the sympathetic ganglia, they are referred to as *catecholamine-secreting paragangliomas.*

Clinical Features. Pheochromocytomas are rare; however, the occurrence is equal in males and females. If they occur in children, they may be associated with hereditary syndromes with multifocal manifestations. The most common feature of

BOX 92-1   CLINICAL FEATURES OF PHEOCHROMOCYTOMA

1. Hypertension
2. Headache
3. Palpitations—sense of one's own forceful heartbeat
4. Chest pain
5. Difficulty in breathing (dyspnea)
6. Dizziness
7. Excessive sweating (diaphoresis)
8. Sensation of nausea or vomiting
9. Sensation of anxiety and fear
10. Tremors

If this condition is chronic, then additional features listed as follows may manifest:
1. Constipation
2. Orthostatic hypotension
3. Fatigue
4. Fever
5. Retinopathy
6. Congestive cardiac failure
7. Weight loss

this condition is hypertension due to excess levels of catecholamines in the blood and this associated hypertension may be sustained or may occur as spells or paroxysms along with other features listed in Box 92-1.

Pheochromocytomas, if diagnosed early and accurately, can be managed with both medical and surgical interventions and can be cured. If the disease is malignant or not managed or detected early, it could be fatal.

BIBLIOGRAPHY

Cannon WB: Organization for physiological homeostasis, *Physiol. Rev.* 9:399, 1929.

Dajas-Bailador F, Wonnacott S: Nicotinic acetylcholine receptors and the regulation of neuronal signalling, *Trends Pharmacol. Sci.* 25:317, 2004.

DiBona GF: Sympathetic nervous system and hypertension, *Hypertension* 61:556, 2013.

Eisenhofer G, Kopin IJ, Goldstein DS: Catecholamine metabolism: a contemporary view with implications for physiology and medicine, *Pharmacol. Rev.* 56:331, 2004.

Goldstein DS, Sharabi Y: Neurogenic orthostatic hypotension: a pathophysiological approach, *Circulation* 119:139, 2009.

Guyenet PG: The sympathetic control of blood pressure, *Nat. Rev. Neurosci.* 7:335, 2006.

Guyenet PG, Stornetta RL, Bochorishvili G, et al: C1 neurons: the body's EMTs, *Am. J. Physiol. Regul. Integr. Comp. Physiol.* 305:R187, 2013.

Hall JE, da Silva AA, do Carmo JM, et al: Obesity-induced hypertension: role of sympathetic nervous system, leptin, and melanocortins, *J. Biol. Chem.* 285(23):17271, 2010.

Kvetnansky R, Sabban EL, Palkovits M: Catecholaminergic systems in stress: structural and molecular genetic approaches, *Physiol. Rev.* 89:535, 2009.

Lohmeier TE, Iliescu R: Lowering of blood pressure by chronic suppression of central sympathetic outflow: insight from prolonged baroreflex activation, *J. Appl. Physiol.* 113:1652, 2012.

Lymperopoulos A, Rengo G, Koch WJ: Adrenergic nervous system in heart failure: pathophysiology and therapy, *Circ. Res.* 113:739, 2013.

Malpas SC: Sympathetic nervous system overactivity and its role in the development of cardiovascular disease, *Physiol. Rev.* 90:513, 2010.

Mancia G, Grassi G: The autonomic nervous system and hypertension, *Circ. Res.* 114:1804, 2014.

Melmed S: Endocrine hypertension, thirteenth ed., Williams Textbook of Endocrinology. Philadelphia, 2015, Saunders Elsevier.

Taylor EW, Jordan D, Coote JH: Central control of the cardiovascular and respiratory systems and their interactions in vertebrates, *Physiol. Rev.* 79:855, 1999.

Ulrich-Lai YM, Herman JP: Neural regulation of endocrine and autonomic stress responses, *Nat. Rev. Neurosci.* 10:397, 2009.

Young WF Jr: Pheochromocytoma, 1926–1993, *Trends Endocrinol. Metab.* 4:122-127, 1993.

Young WF Jr, Maddox DE: Spells: in search of a cause, *Mayo Clin. Proc.* 70:757-765, 1995.

93

Endocrine Pancreas and Glucose Homeostasis

LEARNING OBJECTIVES

- List the cells of the pancreatic islets and the hormones secreted.
- Describe the steps involved in the biosynthesis of insulin.
- Describe the biological actions of insulin with regard to the three important target organs: muscle, liver, and adipose tissue.
- List the factors affecting insulin secretion.
- Describe the biological actions of glucagon.
- List the factors affecting glucagon secretion.
- Describe the role of other hormones in maintaining glucose homeostasis.
- Describe the salient clinical features of diabetes mellitus.
- Describe the effects of insulin excess.

GLOSSARY OF TERMS

- **Catabolism:** The breakdown of complex molecules into simpler forms during metabolism (this is usually associated with release of energy)
- **Gluconeogenesis:** The process of formation of glucose from sources other than carbohydrates such as amino acids or glycerol from triglycerides
- **Glycogenolysis:** The process of breaking down glycogen to glucose
- **Hyperglycemia:** A condition where the level of glucose in blood is abnormally above the normal range
- **Hypoglycemia:** A state where the level of glucose in blood is abnormally lower than the normal range
- **Ketosis:** A condition where there is an abnormal increase of ketone bodies in the blood
- **Polyphagia:** Excessive sense of hunger perceived by diabetic patients
- **Polyuria:** Excessive excretion of urine
- **Triglycerides:** Esters consisting of three fatty acids joined to glycerol molecule

The pancreas, in addition to its digestive functions, secretes two important hormones, *insulin* and *glucagon*, that are crucial for normal regulation of glucose, lipid, and protein metabolism. Although the pancreas secretes other hormones, such as *amylin*, *somatostatin*, and *pancreatic polypeptide*, their functions are not as well established. The main purpose of this chapter is to discuss the physiological roles of insulin and glucagon, and the pathophysiology of diseases, especially *diabetes mellitus*, caused by abnormal secretion or activity of these hormones.

Physiological Anatomy of the Pancreas. The pancreas is composed of two major types of tissues, as shown in Figure 93-1: (1) the *acini*, which secrete digestive juices into the duodenum, and (2) the *islets of Langerhans*, which secrete insulin and glucagon directly into the blood. The digestive secretions of the pancreas are discussed in Chapter 68.

The human pancreas has 1–2 million islets of Langerhans. Each islet is only about 0.3 mm in diameter and is organized around small capillaries into which its cells secrete their hormones. The islets contain three major types of cells, *alpha*, *beta*, and *delta* cells that are distinguished from one another by their morphological and staining characteristics (Box 93-1).

The close interrelations among these cell types in the islets of Langerhans allow cell-to-cell communication and direct control of secretion of some of the hormones by the other hormones. For instance, insulin inhibits glucagon secretion, amylin inhibits insulin secretion, and somatostatin inhibits the secretion of both insulin and glucagon.

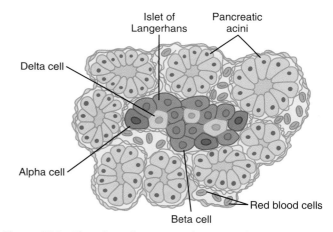

Figure 93-1 Physiological anatomy of an islet of Langerhans in the pancreas.

BOX 93-1 TYPE OF CELLS AND THEIR SECRETIONS

Type of Cell	Proportion (%)	Secretions
Beta cells	60	Insulin
		Amylin
Alpha cells	25	Glucagon
Delta cells	10	Somatostatin
PP cells	5	Pancreatic polypeptide

Insulin and its Metabolic Effects

Insulin was first isolated from the pancreas in 1922 by Banting and Best, and almost overnight the outlook for patients with severe cases of diabetes changed from one of rapid decline and death to that of nearly normal persons. Although, historically, insulin has been associated with "blood sugar," and has profound effects on carbohydrate metabolism, its deficiency also causes abnormalities of fat metabolism and protein metabolism leading to wasting of the tissues and many cellular functional disorders. Therefore, it is clear that insulin affects fat and protein metabolism almost as much as it affects carbohydrate metabolism.

INSULIN CHEMISTRY AND SYNTHESIS

Insulin is a small protein. Human insulin, which has a molecular weight of 5808, is composed of two amino acid chains, shown in Figure 93-2, that are connected to each other by disulfide linkages. When the two amino acid chains are split apart, the functional activity of the insulin molecule is lost.

Insulin is synthesized in beta cells by the usual cell machinery for protein synthesis in the following steps:

1. Initially *preproinsulin* is formed in the ribosomes (molecular weight of about 11,500).
2. Preproinsulin is then cleaved in the endoplasmic reticulum to form a *proinsulin* with a molecular weight of about 9000 and consisting of three chains of peptides, A, B, and C.

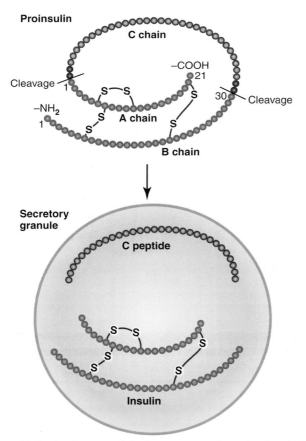

Figure 93-2   A schematic of the human proinsulin molecule, which is cleaved in the Golgi apparatus of the pancreatic beta cells to form connecting peptide (C peptide), and insulin, which is composed of the A and B chains connected by disulfide bonds. The C peptide and insulin are packaged in granules and secreted in equimolar amounts, along with a small amount of proinsulin.

3. Most of the proinsulin is further cleaved in the Golgi apparatus to form insulin, which is composed of the A and B chains connected by disulfide linkages, and the C chain peptide, called *connecting peptide* (*C peptide*).
4. The insulin and C peptide are packaged in the secretory granules and secreted in equimolar amounts. About 5–10% of the final secreted product is still in the form of proinsulin.

The proinsulin and C peptide have virtually no insulin activity. However, C peptide binds to a membrane structure, activating at least two enzyme systems:

- sodium–potassium adenosine triphosphatase (ATPase);
- endothelial nitric oxide synthase.

Although both of these enzymes have multiple physiological functions, the importance of C peptide in regulating these enzymes is still uncertain.

C peptide levels can be measured by radioimmunoassay in insulin-treated diabetic patients to determine how much of their own natural insulin they are still producing. Patients with type 1 diabetes who are unable to produce insulin will usually have greatly decreased levels of C peptide.

INSULIN IN THE CIRCULATION AND ITS METABOLISM

When insulin is secreted into the blood, it circulates almost entirely in an unbound form. Because it has a plasma half-life of approximately 6 minutes, it is cleared from the circulation within 10–15 minutes. Insulin that is not bound with receptors in the target cells is degraded by the enzyme *insulinase* mainly in the liver, to a lesser extent in the kidneys and muscles, and slightly in most other tissues.

ACTIVATION OF TARGET CELL RECEPTORS BY INSULIN AND THE RESULTING CELLULAR EFFECTS

To initiate its effects on target cells, insulin first binds with and activates a membrane receptor protein that has a molecular weight of about 300,000 (Figure 93-3). It is the activated receptor that causes the subsequent effects.

The insulin receptor is a combination of four subunits held together by disulfide linkages: *two alpha subunits* that lie entirely outside the cell membrane and *two beta subunits* that penetrate through the membrane protruding into the cell cytoplasm. The insulin binds with the alpha subunits on the outside of the cell, but because of the linkages with the beta subunits, the portions of the beta subunits protruding into the cell become autophosphorylated, which activates a local *tyrosine kinase*. Thus, the insulin receptor is an example of an *enzyme-linked receptor*. Tyrosine kinase in turn causes phosphorylation of multiple other intracellular enzymes including a group called *insulin receptor substrates* (*IRS*). In this way, insulin directs the intracellular metabolic machinery to produce the desired effects on carbohydrate, fat, and protein metabolism. The following are the main end effects of insulin stimulation:

1. Within seconds after insulin binds with its membrane receptors, there is a marked increase in uptake of glucose in most cells, especially *muscle cells* and *adipose cells*. The increased glucose uptake is caused due to mobilization and translocation of multiple glucose transporters to the cell membrane that facilitates glucose uptake into the cells.
2. The cell membrane becomes more permeable to many of the amino acids, potassium ions, and phosphate ions, causing increased transport of these substances into the cell.

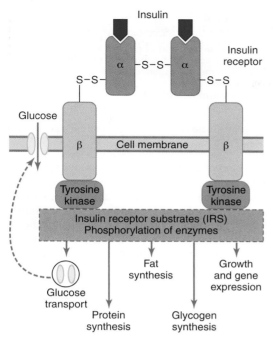

Figure 93-3 A schematic of the insulin receptor. Insulin binds to the α-subunit of its receptor, which causes autophosphorylation of the β-subunit receptor, which in turn induces tyrosine kinase activity. The receptor tyrosine kinase activity begins a cascade of cell phosphorylation that increases or decreases the activity of enzymes, including insulin receptor substrates, that mediate the effects on glucose, fat, and protein metabolism. For example, glucose transporters are moved to the cell membrane to assist glucose entry into the cell.

3. Slower effects occur during the next 10–15 minutes to change the activity levels of many more intracellular metabolic enzymes. These effects result mainly from the changed states of phosphorylation of the enzymes.
4. Much slower effects continue to occur for hours and even several days. New proteins are formed, which helps insulin remold much of the cellular enzymatic machinery to achieve its metabolic goals.

EFFECTS OF INSULIN ON THE MUSCLE

Immediately after a high-carbohydrate meal, the high blood glucose causes rapid secretion of insulin (Box 93-2). The insulin in turn causes rapid uptake, storage, and use of glucose by almost all tissues of the body, but especially by the muscles, adipose tissue, and liver.

Insulin Promotes Muscle Glucose Uptake and Metabolism

During much of the day, muscle tissue depends not on glucose but on fatty acids for its energy. The *resting muscle* membrane is only slightly permeable to glucose without the influence of insulin.

> **BOX 93-2 EFFECTS OF INSULIN ON MUSCLE**
>
> 1. Promotes glucose uptake by muscle cells
> 2. Promotes muscle glycogen synthesis
> 3. Promotes protein synthesis and storage in muscles:
>   a. Increases amino acid transport into cells
>   b. Stimulates transcription and translation
>   c. Inhibits catabolism of muscle proteins
> 4. Increased transport of potassium into cells

However, under two conditions the muscles do use large amounts of glucose:
1. During moderate or heavy exercise, the exercising muscle fibers become more permeable to glucose. This usage of glucose does not require large amounts of insulin because muscle contraction increases translocation of *glucose transporter 4 (GLUT 4)* from intracellular storage depots to the cell membrane, which, in turn, facilitates diffusion of glucose into the cell.
2. During the few hours after a meal, the blood glucose concentration is high and the pancreas is secreting large quantities of insulin causing rapid transport of glucose into the muscle cells, which causes the muscle cell to use glucose preferentially over fatty acids during this period, as will be discussed later.

Storage of Glycogen in Muscle. If the muscles are not exercised after a meal and yet glucose is transported into the muscle cells in abundance, instead of being used for energy, most of the glucose is stored in the form of muscle glycogen, up to a limit of 2–3% concentration. The glycogen can be used by the muscle later for energy.

Insulin Promotes Protein Synthesis and Storage

1. *Insulin stimulates transport of many of the amino acids into the cells.* Among the amino acids most strongly transported are *valine, leucine, isoleucine, tyrosine,* and *phenylalanine.*
2. *Insulin increases translation of messenger RNA,* thus forming new proteins.
3. Over a longer period, *insulin also increases the rate of transcription of selected DNA genetic sequences* in the cell nuclei, thus promoting protein synthesis.
4. *Insulin inhibits catabolism of proteins,* thus decreasing the rate of amino acid release from the cells, especially from muscle cells.

Insulin Promotes Increased Transport of Potassium into Cells

Insulin increases the transport of potassium into muscle cells by stimulating the activity of Na^+–K^+ ATPase present on the cell membranes. This could result in lower potassium concentrations in the blood.

EFFECTS OF INSULIN ON THE LIVER

Insulin Promotes Liver Uptake, Storage, and Use of Glucose

One of the most important of all the effects of insulin is to cause most of the glucose absorbed after a meal to be stored almost immediately in the liver in the form of glycogen (Box 93-3).
1. Insulin *inactivates liver phosphorylase,* the principal enzyme that causes liver glycogen to split into glucose. This inactivation prevents breakdown of the glycogen that has been stored in liver cells.
2. Insulin causes *enhanced uptake of glucose* from the blood by the liver cells by *increasing the activity of the enzyme glucokinase.*
3. Insulin stimulates *glycogen synthase,* which promotes glycogen synthesis.
4. *In the liver, insulin depresses the rate of gluconeogenesis* by decreasing the activity of the enzymes that promote gluconeogenesis. This suppression of gluconeogenesis

conserves the amino acids in the protein stores of the body as they form the major substrate for gluconeogenesis.

The net effect of all these actions is to increase the amount of glycogen in the liver, which can store up to 100 g in the entire liver (Box 93-4).

Thus, the liver removes glucose from the blood when it is present in excess after a meal and returns it to the blood when the blood glucose concentration falls between meals. Ordinarily, about 60% of the glucose in the meal is stored in this way in the liver and then returned later.

Insulin Promotes Conversion of Excess Glucose into Fatty Acids. When the quantity of glucose entering the liver cells is more than can be stored as glycogen or can be used for local hepatocyte metabolism, *insulin promotes the conversion of all this excess glucose into fatty acids*. These fatty acids are subsequently packaged as triglycerides in very low-density lipoproteins, transported in this form by way of the blood to the adipose tissue, and deposited as fat.

Insulin Promotes Protein Synthesis in the Liver

Insulin promotes protein synthesis in the liver by similar actions as seen in the muscle cells.

EFFECT OF INSULIN ON THE ADIPOSE TISSUE

Insulin has several effects that lead to fat storage in adipose tissue (Box 93-5). First, insulin increases the utilization of glucose by most of the body's tissues, which automatically decreases the utilization of fat, thus functioning as a fat sparer.

Role of Insulin in Storage of Fat in the Adipose Cells

Insulin has other essential effects that are required for fat storage in adipose cells:

1. *Insulin inhibits the action of hormone-sensitive lipase* that causes hydrolysis of triglycerides stored in fat cells. This inhibits the release of fatty acids from the adipose tissue into the circulating blood.

2. *Insulin promotes glucose transport through the cell membrane into fat cells* similar to muscle cells. Some of this glucose is then used to synthesize minute amounts of fatty acids.
3. *Insulin promotes the formation of large quantities of α-glycerol phosphate from glucose.* This substance supplies the *glycerol* that combines with fatty acids to form the triglycerides that are the storage form of fat in adipose cells.
4. *Insulin promotes triglyceride formation* in the liver that is transported to the adipose tissue and deposited there.
5. *Insulin increases the transport of K^+ ions into the adipose tissue cells.*

EFFECTS OF INSULIN DEFICIENCY ON FAT AND PROTEIN METABOLISM

All aspects of fat breakdown and use for providing energy are greatly enhanced in the absence of insulin. This occurs even normally between meals when secretion of insulin is minimal, but it becomes extreme in diabetes mellitus when secretion of insulin is almost zero. The resulting effects are as follows:

1. *Insulin deficiency causes lipolysis of storage fat and release of free fatty acids.* This is because the enzyme *hormone-sensitive lipase* in the fat cells becomes strongly activated. This causes hydrolysis of the stored triglycerides, releasing large quantities of fatty acids and glycerol into the circulating blood.

Figure 93-4 shows the effect of insulin lack on the plasma concentrations of free fatty acids, glucose, and acetoacetic acid. Note that almost immediately after removal of the pancreas, the free fatty acid concentration in the plasma begins to rise, more rapidly even than the concentration of glucose.

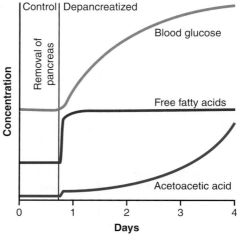

Figure 93-4 The effect of removing the pancreas on the approximate concentrations of blood glucose, plasma free fatty acids, and acetoacetic acid.

2. *Insulin deficiency increases plasma cholesterol and phospholipid concentrations.* These two substances are then discharged into the blood along with the excess triglycerides formed. This high lipid concentration—especially the high concentration of cholesterol—promotes the development of atherosclerosis in people with serious diabetes.

3. *Excess usage of fats during insulin lack causes ketosis and acidosis.* Insulin lack also causes excessive amounts of acetoacetic acid to be formed in the liver cells from acetyl coenzyme A (CoA) (Figure 93-4). Some of the acetoacetic acid is also converted into β-hydroxybutyric acid and acetone. These two substances, along with the acetoacetic acid, are called ketone bodies, and their presence in large quantities in the body fluids is called ketosis, which can cause severe acidosis and coma, which may lead to death.

4. *Insulin deficiency causes protein depletion and increased plasma amino acids.* Virtually all protein storage comes to a halt when insulin is not available. The catabolism of proteins increases, protein synthesis stops, and large quantities of amino acids are dumped into the plasma. The resulting protein wasting is one of the most serious of all the effects of severe diabetes mellitus. It can lead to extreme weakness and many deranged functions of the organs.

EFFECT OF INSULIN ON PROTEIN METABOLISM AND GROWTH

Insulin and Growth Hormone Interact Synergistically to Promote Growth

Because insulin is required for the synthesis of proteins, it is as essential as growth hormone for growth of an animal. As demonstrated in Figure 93-5, a depancreatized, hypophysectomized rat that does not undergo therapy hardly grows at all. Furthermore, administration of either growth hormone or insulin one at a time causes almost no growth. However, a combination of these hormones causes dramatic growth. Thus, it appears that the two hormones function synergistically to promote growth, with each performing a specific function separate from that of the other.

MECHANISMS OF INSULIN SECRETION

Figure 93-6 shows the basic cellular mechanisms for insulin secretion by the pancreatic beta cells in response to increased blood glucose concentration.

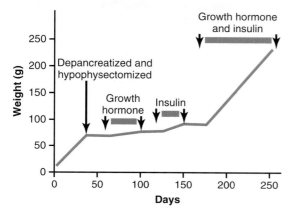

Figure 93-5 The effect of growth hormone, insulin, and growth hormone plus insulin on growth in a depancreatized and hypophysectomized rat.

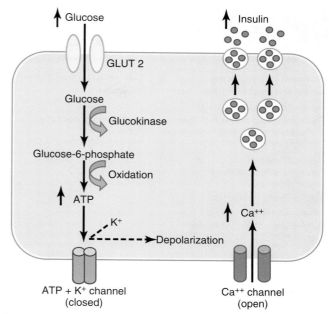

Figure 93-6 The basic mechanisms of glucose stimulation of insulin secretion by beta cells of the pancreas. *ATP*, adenosine triphosphate; *GLUT*, glucose transporter.

1. The beta cells have a large number of *glucose transporters* that permit a rate of glucose influx that is proportional to the blood concentration in the physiological range.

2. Glucose inside the cells is phosphorylated to glucose-6-phosphate by *glucokinase*. This appears to be the rate-limiting step for glucose metabolism in the beta cell.

3. The glucose-6-phosphate is subsequently oxidized to form adenosine triphosphate (ATP).

4. ATP inhibits the *ATP-sensitive potassium channels* of the cell. Closure of the potassium channels depolarizes the cell membrane, thereby opening *voltage-gated calcium channels*.

5. The influx of calcium stimulates fusion of the docked insulin-containing vesicles with the cell membrane and secretion of insulin into the extracellular fluid by *exocytosis*.

Sulfonylurea drugs stimulate insulin secretion by binding to the ATP-sensitive potassium channels and blocking their activity. This mechanism results in a depolarizing effect that triggers insulin secretion, making these drugs useful in stimulating insulin secretion in patients with type 2 diabetes. Table 93-1 summarizes some of the factors that can increase or decrease secretion of insulin.

CONTROL OF INSULIN SECRETION

At one time, it was believed that insulin secretion was controlled almost entirely by the concentration of glucose in the blood. However, as more has been learned about the metabolic functions of insulin for protein and fat metabolism, it has become apparent that blood amino acids and other factors also play important roles in controlling the secretion of insulin as listed in Table 93-1.

Increased Blood Glucose Stimulates Insulin Secretion. At the normal *fasting* level of blood glucose of 80–90 mg/100 mL, the rate of insulin secretion is minimal—on the order of 25 ng/minute per kilogram of body weight, a level that has only slight physiological activity. If the blood glucose concentration is suddenly increased to a level two to three times normal and is kept at this high level thereafter, insulin secretion increases markedly in two stages, as shown by the changes in plasma insulin concentration in Figure 93-7.

TABLE 93-1	Factors and Conditions that Increase or Decrease Insulin Secretion
Increase Insulin Secretion	**Decrease Insulin Secretion**
Increased blood glucose	Decreased blood glucose
Increased blood free fatty acids	Fasting
Increased blood amino acids	Somatostatin
Gastrointestinal hormones (gastrin, cholecystokinin, secretin, gastric inhibitory peptide)	α-Adrenergic activity
	Leptin
Glucagon, growth hormone, cortisol	
Parasympathetic stimulation; acetylcholine	
β-Adrenergic stimulation	
Insulin resistance; obesity	
Sulfonylurea drugs (glyburide, tolbutamide)	

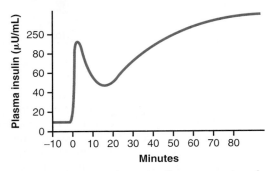

Figure 93-7 An increase in plasma insulin concentration after a sudden increase in blood glucose to two to three times the normal range. Note an initial rapid surge in insulin concentration and then a delayed but higher and continuing increase in concentration beginning 15–20 minutes later.

OTHER FACTORS THAT STIMULATE INSULIN SECRETION

Amino Acids

Some of the amino acids have a similar effect as glucose in stimulating the beta cells. The most potent of these are *arginine* and *lysine*.

Gastrointestinal Hormones

A mixture of several important gastrointestinal hormones—*gastrin, secretin, cholecystokinin, glucagon-like peptide-1 (GLP-1)*, and *glucose-dependent insulinotropic peptide (GIP)*—can cause moderate increases in insulin secretion. Two of these hormones, GLP-1 and GIP, appear to be the most potent and are often called *incretins* because they enhance the rate of insulin release from the pancreatic beta cells in response to an increase in plasma glucose. They also inhibit glucagon secretion from the alpha cells of the islets of Langerhans.

These hormones are released after a person eats a meal and causes an "anticipatory" increase in blood insulin in preparation for the glucose and amino acids to be absorbed from the meal.

Other Hormones and the Autonomic Nervous System

Other hormones that either directly increase insulin secretion or potentiate the glucose stimulus for insulin secretion include *glucagon, growth hormone, cortisol*, and, to a lesser extent, *progesterone* and *estrogen*.

1. *Growth hormone* from the anterior pituitary gland
2. *Cortisol* from the adrenal cortex
3. *Epinephrine* from the adrenal medulla
4. *Glucagon* from the alpha cells of the islets of Langerhans

THE ROLE OF INSULIN (AND OTHER HORMONES) IN "SWITCHING" BETWEEN CARBOHYDRATE AND LIPID METABOLISM

When glucose concentration is low, insulin secretion is suppressed and fat is used almost exclusively for energy everywhere except in the brain. When the glucose concentration is high, insulin secretion is stimulated and carbohydrate is used instead of fat. The excess blood glucose is stored in the form of liver glycogen, liver fat, and muscle glycogen. Therefore, one of the most important functional roles of insulin in the body is to control which of these two foods will be used by the cells for energy from moment to moment.

At least four other known hormones also play important roles in this switching mechanism (Box 93-6).

Both growth hormone and cortisol are secreted in response to hypoglycemia, and both inhibit cellular utilization of glucose while promoting fat utilization.

Epinephrine is especially important in increasing plasma glucose concentration during periods of stress when the sympathetic nervous system is excited. However, epinephrine acts differently from the other hormones in that it increases plasma fatty acid concentration at the same time. Therefore, epinephrine especially enhances the utilization of fat in such stressful states as exercise, circulatory shock, and anxiety.

Glucagon and its Functions

Glucagon, a hormone secreted by the *alpha cells* of the islets of Langerhans when the blood glucose concentration falls, has several functions that are diametrically opposed to those of insulin (Table 93-2).

Like insulin, glucagon is a large polypeptide. It has a molecular weight of 3485 and is composed of a chain of 29 amino acids. Glucagon is also called the *hyperglycemic hormone*.

TABLE 93-2	Comparison of the Metabolic Actions of Insulin and Glucagon	
	Insulin Actions	**Glucagon Actions**
Muscle tissue		
• Glycogen synthesis	↑ Glycogen synthesis	No response
• Amino acid uptake	↑ Amino acid uptake	No response
• Glucose uptake	↑ Glucose uptake	No response
• K+ transport into cells	↑ K+ into cells	↓ K+ into cells
Liver		
• Glycogenolysis	Prevents glycogenolysis	↑ Glycogenolysis
• Gluconeogenesis	↓ Gluconeogenesis	↑ Gluconeogenesis
• Protein synthesis	↓ Gluconeogenesis ↑ Protein synthesis	↓ Protein synthesis
Adipose tissue		
• Fatty acid synthesis	↑ Fatty acid synthesis	↓ Fatty acid synthesis
• Lipolysis	↓ Lipolysis	↑ Lipolysis
• Triglycerides	↑ Storage of triglycerides	↓ Storage of triglycerides

EFFECTS ON GLUCOSE METABOLISM

The major effects of glucagon on glucose metabolism are (1) breakdown of liver glycogen (*glycogenolysis*) and (2) increased *gluconeogenesis* in the liver. Both of these effects greatly enhance the availability of glucose to the other organs of the body.

Glucagon Causes Glycogenolysis and Increased Blood Glucose Concentration. The most dramatic effect of glucagon is its ability to cause glycogenolysis in the liver, which in turn increases the blood glucose concentration within minutes.

Only a few micrograms of glucagon can cause the blood glucose level to double or increase even more within a few minutes.

Glucagon Increases Gluconeogenesis

Even after all the glycogen in the liver has been exhausted under the influence of glucagon, continued infusion of this hormone still causes continued hyperglycemia. This hyperglycemia results from the effect of glucagon to increase the rate of amino acid uptake by the liver cells and then the conversion of many of the amino acids to glucose by gluconeogenesis.

This effect is achieved by activating multiple enzymes that are required for amino acid transport and gluconeogenesis, especially activation of the enzyme system for converting pyruvate to phosphoenolpyruvate, a rate-limiting step in gluconeogenesis.

Other Effects of Glucagon

Most other effects of glucagon occur only when its concentration rises well above the maximum normally found in the blood. Perhaps the most important effect is that *glucagon activates adipose cell lipase*, making increased quantities of fatty acids available to the energy systems of the body. Glucagon also inhibits the storage of triglycerides in the liver, which prevents the liver from removing fatty acids from the blood; this also helps make additional amounts of fatty acids available for the other tissues of the body.

Glucagon in high concentrations also:
* enhances the strength of the heart;
* increases blood flow in some tissues, especially the kidneys;
* enhances bile secretion;
* inhibits gastric acid secretion.

These effects of glucagon are probably of much less importance in the normal function of the body compared with its effects on glucose.

REGULATION OF GLUCAGON SECRETION

Increased Blood Glucose Inhibits Glucagon Secretion. The blood glucose concentration is by far the most potent factor that controls glucagon secretion. Note specifically, however, that *the effect of blood glucose concentration on glucagon secretion is in exactly the opposite direction from the effect of glucose on insulin secretion.*

This is demonstrated in Figure 93-8, which shows that a *decrease* in the blood glucose concentration from its normal fasting level of about 90 mg/100 mL of blood down to hypoglycemic levels can increase the plasma concentration of glucagon severalfold.

Thus, in hypoglycemia, glucagon is secreted in large amounts; it then greatly increases the output of glucose from the liver and thereby serves the important function of correcting the hypoglycemia.

Increased Blood Amino Acids Stimulate Secretion of Glucagon. High concentrations of amino acids, such as those that occur in the blood after a meal containing protein (especially the amino acids *alanine* and *arginine*), *stimulate* the

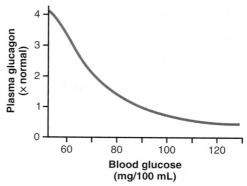

Figure 93-8 The approximate plasma glucagon concentration at different blood glucose levels.

secretion of glucagon. This is the same effect that amino acids have in stimulating insulin secretion. Thus, in this instance, the glucagon and insulin responses are not opposites. The importance of amino acid stimulation of glucagon secretion is that the glucagon then promotes rapid conversion of the amino acids to glucose, thus making even more glucose available to the tissues.

EXERCISE STIMULATES SECRETION OF GLUCAGON

During exhaustive exercise, the blood concentration of glucagon often increases fourfold to fivefold. The cause of this increase is not well understood because the blood glucose concentration does not necessarily fall. A beneficial effect of the glucagon is that it prevents a decrease in blood glucose.

One of the factors that might increase glucagon secretion during exercise is increased circulating amino acids. Other factors, such as β-adrenergic stimulation of the islets of Langerhans, may also play a role.

Somatostatin Inhibits Glucagon and Insulin Secretion

The *delta cells* of the islets of Langerhans secrete the hormone *somatostatin*, a 14–amino acid polypeptide that has an extremely short half-life of only 3 minutes in the circulating blood. Almost all factors related to the ingestion of food stimulate somatostatin secretion. These factors include (1) increased blood glucose, (2) increased amino acids, (3) increased fatty acids, and (4) increased concentrations of several of the gastrointestinal hormones released from the upper gastrointestinal tract in response to food intake.

In turn, somatostatin has multiple inhibitory effects as follows:

1. Somatostatin acts locally within the islets of Langerhans themselves to depress secretion of both insulin and glucagon.
2. Somatostatin decreases motility of the stomach, duodenum, and gallbladder.
3. Somatostatin decreases both secretion and absorption in the gastrointestinal tract.

In putting all this information together, it has been suggested that the principal role of somatostatin is to extend the period over which the food nutrients are assimilated into the blood. At the same time, the effect of somatostatin in depressing insulin and glucagon secretion decreases utilization of the absorbed nutrients by the tissues, thus preventing rapid exhaustion of the food and therefore making it available over a longer period.

It should also be recalled that somatostatin is the same chemical substance as *growth hormone inhibitory hormone*, which is secreted in the hypothalamus and suppresses secretion of growth hormone by the anterior pituitary gland.

Summary of Blood Glucose Regulation

In a normal person, the blood glucose concentration is narrowly controlled, usually between 80 and 90 mg/100 mL of blood in the fasting person each morning before breakfast. This concentration increases to 120–140 mg/100 mL during the first hour or so after a meal, but the feedback systems for control of blood glucose rapidly return glucose concentration back to the control level, usually within 2 hours after the last absorption of carbohydrates. Conversely, in a state of starvation, the gluconeogenesis function of the liver provides the glucose that is required to maintain the fasting blood glucose level.

IMPORTANCE OF BLOOD GLUCOSE REGULATION

One might ask: Why is it so important to maintain a constant blood glucose concentration, particularly because most tissues can shift to utilization of fats and proteins for energy in the absence of glucose? The answer is that glucose is the only nutrient that normally can be used by the *brain, retina,* and *germinal epithelium of the gonads* in sufficient quantities to supply them optimally with their required energy. Therefore, it is important to maintain the blood glucose concentration at a level sufficient to provide this necessary nutrition.

Most of the glucose formed by gluconeogenesis during the interdigestive period is used for metabolism in the brain. Indeed, it is important that the pancreas not secrete insulin during this time; otherwise, the scant supplies of glucose that are available would all go into the muscles and other peripheral tissues, leaving the brain without a nutritive source.

Diabetes Mellitus

Diabetes mellitus is a syndrome of impaired carbohydrate, fat, and protein metabolism caused by either lack of insulin secretion or decreased sensitivity of the tissues to insulin. There are two general types of diabetes mellitus:

1. *Type 1 diabetes*, also called *insulin-dependent diabetes mellitus* (IDDM), is caused by lack of insulin secretion.
2. *Type 2 diabetes*, also called *noninsulin-dependent diabetes mellitus* (NIDDM), is initially caused by decreased sensitivity of target tissues to the metabolic effect of insulin. This reduced sensitivity to insulin is often called *insulin resistance*.

In both types of diabetes mellitus, metabolism of all the main foodstuffs is altered. The basic effect of insulin deficiency or insulin resistance on glucose metabolism is to prevent the efficient uptake and utilization of glucose by most cells of the body, except those of the brain. As a result, blood glucose concentration increases, cell utilization of glucose falls increasingly lower, and utilization of fats and proteins increases.

TYPE 1 DIABETES—DEFICIENCY OF INSULIN PRODUCTION BY BETA CELLS OF THE PANCREAS

Injury to the beta cells of the pancreas or diseases that impair insulin production can lead to type 1 diabetes. The causes of destruction of beta cells in type 1 diabetes could be:

1. *viral infections*;
2. *autoimmune disorders*;
3. *heredity* determining the susceptibility of the beta cells to destruction by these insults.

Clinical Features. The usual onset of type 1 diabetes occurs at about 14 years of age in the United States, and for this reason it is often called *juvenile diabetes mellitus*. However, type 1 diabetes can occur at any age, including adulthood, following disorders that lead to the destruction of pancreatic beta cells. Type 1 diabetes may develop abruptly, over a period of a few days or weeks, with three principal sequelae:

- increased blood glucose levels, raising plasma glucose to 300–1200 mg/100 mL;
- increased utilization of fats for energy and for formation of cholesterol by the liver;
- depletion of the body's proteins.

Approximately 5–10% of people with diabetes mellitus have the type 1 form of the disease.

Increased Blood Glucose Causes Loss of Glucose in the Urine. High levels of blood glucose cause more glucose to filter into the renal tubules than can be reabsorbed and the excess glucose spills into the urine. This spillage normally occurs when the blood glucose concentration rises above 180 mg/100 mL, a level that is called the blood "threshold" for the appearance of glucose in the urine. When the blood glucose level rises to 300–500 mg/100 mL—common values in people with severe untreated diabetes—100 or more grams of glucose can be lost into the urine each day.

Increased Blood Glucose Causes Dehydration. The very high levels of blood glucose (sometimes as high as 8–10 times normal in severe untreated diabetes) can cause severe cell dehydration throughout the body.

In addition to the direct cellular dehydrating effect of excessive glucose, the loss of glucose in the urine causes *osmotic diuresis*, that is, the osmotic effect of glucose in the renal tubules greatly decreases tubular reabsorption of fluid. The overall effect is massive loss of fluid in the urine, causing dehydration of the extracellular fluid, which in turn causes compensatory dehydration of the intracellular fluid. Thus, *polyuria* (excessive urine excretion), *intracellular and extracellular dehydration*, and *increased thirst* are classic symptoms of diabetes.

Chronic High Glucose Concentration Causes Tissue Injury. Poor blood glucose control over long periods in diabetes mellitus affects blood vessels in multiple tissues throughout the body leading to structural changes and inadequate blood supply to the tissues. This situation in turn leads to increased risk for heart attack, stroke, end-stage kidney disease, retinopathy and blindness, and ischemia and gangrene of the limbs.

Chronic high glucose concentration also causes damage to many other tissues, such as *peripheral neuropathy* and *autonomic nervous system dysfunction*. These abnormalities can result in impaired cardiovascular reflexes, impaired bladder control, decreased sensation in the extremities, and other symptoms of peripheral nerve damage.

In addition, *hypertension*, secondary to renal injury, and *atherosclerosis*, secondary to abnormal lipid metabolism, often develop in patients with diabetes and amplify the tissue damage caused by elevated glucose levels.

Diabetes Mellitus Causes Increased Utilization of Fats and Metabolic Acidosis. The shift from carbohydrate to fat metabolism in diabetes increases the release of keto acids, such as acetoacetic acid and β-hydroxybutyric acid, into the plasma resulting in severe *metabolic acidosis*. This scenario leads rapidly to *dia-*

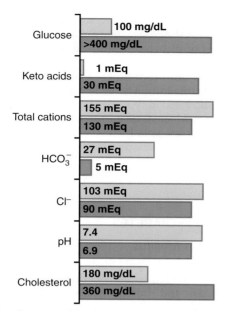

Figure 93-9 Changes in blood constituents in diabetic coma, showing normal values (*purple bars*) and diabetic coma values (*red bars*).

betic coma and death unless the patient is treated immediately with large amounts of insulin.

The overall changes in the electrolytes of the blood as a result of severe diabetic acidosis are shown in Figure 93-9.

Excess fat utilization in the liver that occurs over a long time causes large amounts of cholesterol in the circulating blood and increased deposition of cholesterol in the arterial walls. This situation leads to severe *arteriosclerosis* and other vascular lesions, as discussed earlier.

Diabetes Causes Depletion of the Body's Proteins. Failure to use glucose for energy leads to increased utilization and decreased storage of proteins and fat. Therefore, a person with severe untreated diabetes mellitus experiences rapid weight loss and *asthenia* (lack of energy) despite eating large amounts of food (*polyphagia*). Without treatment, these metabolic abnormalities can cause severe wasting of the body tissues and death within a few weeks.

TYPE 2 DIABETES—RESISTANCE TO THE METABOLIC EFFECTS OF INSULIN

Type 2 diabetes is far more common than type 1, accounting for about 90–95% of all cases of diabetes mellitus. The age of onset of type 2 diabetes is usually after 30 years, often between the ages of 50 and 60 years. Therefore, this syndrome is often referred to as *adult-onset diabetes*. More recently, this disease is seen in some younger than 20 years old perhaps due to the increasing prevalence of *obesity, the most important risk factor for type 2 diabetes* in children and adults.

Obesity, Insulin Resistance, and "Metabolic Syndrome" Usually Precede the Development of Type 2 Diabetes. In contrast to type 1 diabetes, type 2 diabetes is associated with *increased* plasma insulin concentration (*hyperinsulinemia*). Hyperinsulinemia occurs as a compensatory response by the pancreatic beta cells for *insulin resistance*, a diminished sensitivity of target tissues to insulin. The development of insulin resistance and impaired glucose metabolism is usually a gradual process, beginning with excess weight gain and obesity.

Insulin resistance is part of a cascade of disorders that is often called the "*metabolic syndrome*" (Box 93-7).

Several of the metabolic abnormalities associated with the syndrome increase the risk for cardiovascular disease, and insulin resistance predisposes to the development of type 2 diabetes mellitus, which is also a major cause of cardiovascular disease.

Other Factors that Can Cause Insulin Resistance and Type 2 Diabetes. Although most patients with type 2 diabetes are overweight or have substantial accumulation of visceral fat, severe insulin resistance and type 2 diabetes can also occur as a result of other acquired or genetic conditions that impair insulin signaling in peripheral tissues as detailed in Table 93-3.

Development of Type 2 Diabetes During Prolonged Insulin Resistance. With prolonged and severe insulin resistance, even the increased levels of insulin are not sufficient to maintain normal glucose regulation. As a result, moderate hyperglycemia occurs after ingestion of carbohydrates in the early stages of the disease.

In the later stages of type 2 diabetes, the pancreatic beta cells become "exhausted" or damaged and are unable to produce enough insulin to prevent more severe hyperglycemia, especially after the person ingests a carbohydrate-rich meal.

PHYSIOLOGY OF DIAGNOSIS OF DIABETES MELLITUS

Table 93-4 compares some of the clinical features of type 1 and type 2 diabetes mellitus. The usual methods for diagnosing diabetes are based on various chemical tests of the urine and the blood.

Urinary Glucose. Simple office tests or more complicated quantitative laboratory tests may be used to determine urinary glucose. A normal person loses undetectable amounts of glucose, whereas a diabetic individual loses glucose in small to large amounts, in proportion to the severity of the disease and the intake of carbohydrates.

TABLE 93-3 Some Causes of Insulin Resistance

- Obesity/overweight (especially excess visceral adiposity)
- Excess glucocorticoids (Cushing syndrome or steroid therapy)
- Excess growth hormone (acromegaly)
- Pregnancy, gestational diabetes
- Polycystic ovary disease
- Lipodystrophy (acquired or genetic; associated with lipid accumulation in liver)
- Autoantibodies to the insulin receptor
- Mutations of insulin receptor
- Mutations of the peroxisome proliferator-activated receptor γ (PPARγ)
- Mutations that cause genetic obesity (eg, melanocortin receptor mutations)
- Hemochromatosis (a hereditary disease that causes tissue iron accumulation)

TABLE 93-4	Clinical Characteristics of Patients with Type 1 and Type 2 Diabetes Mellitus	
Feature	Type 1	Type 2
Age at onset	Usually <20 years	Usually >30 years
Body mass	Low (wasted) to normal	Obese
Plasma insulin	Low or absent	Normal to high initially
Plasma glucagon	High, can be suppressed	High, resistant to suppression
Plasma glucose	Increased	Increased
Insulin sensitivity	Normal	Reduced
Therapy	Insulin	Weight loss, thiazolidinediones, metformin, sulfonylureas, insulin

Fasting Blood Glucose and Insulin Levels. The fasting blood glucose level in the early morning is normally 80–90 mg/100 mL, and 110 mg/100 mL is considered to be the upper limit of normal. A fasting blood glucose level above this value often indicates diabetes mellitus or at least marked insulin resistance.

In persons with type 1 diabetes, plasma insulin levels are very low or undetectable during fasting and even after a meal. In persons with type 2 diabetes, plasma insulin concentration may be severalfold higher than normal and usually increases to a greater extent after ingestion of a standard glucose load during a glucose tolerance test (see the next section).

Glucose Tolerance Test. As demonstrated by the bottom curve in Figure 93-10, called a "glucose tolerance curve," when a normal, fasting person ingests 1 g of glucose per kilogram of body weight, the blood glucose level rises from about 90 mg/100 mL to 120–140 mg/100 mL and falls back to below normal in about 2 hours.

In a person with diabetes, the fasting blood glucose concentration is almost always above 110 mg/100 mL and often is above 140 mg/100 mL. In addition, results of the glucose tolerance test are almost always abnormal. After ingestion of glucose, these people exhibit a much greater than normal rise in blood glucose level, as demonstrated by the upper curve in Figure 93-10, and the glucose level falls back to the control value only after 4–6 hours; furthermore, it fails to fall *below* the control level.

The slow fall of this curve and its failure to fall below the control level demonstrate that either (1) the normal increase in insulin secretion after glucose ingestion does not occur or (2) the person has decreased sensitivity to insulin.

A diagnosis of diabetes mellitus can usually be established on the basis of such a curve, and type 1 and type 2 diabetes can be distinguished from each other by measurements of plasma insulin, with plasma insulin being low or undetectable in type I diabetes and increased in type 2 diabetes.

Acetone Breath. Small quantities of acetoacetic acid in the blood, which increase greatly in severe diabetes, are converted to acetone, which is volatile and vaporized into the expired air. Consequently, one can frequently make a diagnosis of type 1 diabetes mellitus simply by smelling acetone on the breath of a patient.

TREATMENT OF DIABETES

Type 1 Diabetes Mellitus

Effective treatment of type 1 diabetes mellitus requires administration of enough insulin so that the patient will have carbohydrate, fat, and protein metabolism that is as normal as possible. Insulin is available in several forms, such as "regular" and "longer-acting" (precipitated with zinc or with various protein derivatives). "Regular" insulin's actions last from 3 to 8 hours, whereas longer-acting insulin actions last as long as 10–48 hours. Each patient is provided with an individualized pattern of treatment with a combination of longer-acting and regular insulin. In the past, the insulin used for treatment was derived from animal pancreata. However, human insulin produced by the recombinant DNA process has become more widely used because immunity and sensitization against animal insulin develops in some patients, thus limiting its effectiveness.

Type 2 Diabetes Mellitus

In many instances, type 2 diabetes can be effectively treated, at least in the early stages, with exercise, caloric restriction, and weight reduction, and no exogenous administration of insulin is required. Drugs that increase insulin sensitivity (eg, *thiazolidinediones*), drugs that suppress liver glucose production (eg, *metformin*), or drugs that cause additional release of insulin by the pancreas (eg, *sulfonylureas*) may also be used. However, in the later stages of type 2 diabetes, insulin administration is usually required to control plasma glucose levels.

Drugs that mimic the actions of the incretin GLP-1 have been developed for the treatment of type 2 diabetes. These drugs enhance the secretion of insulin and are intended to be used in conjunction with other antidiabetic drugs. Another therapeutic approach is to inhibit the enzyme *dipeptidyl peptidase 4 (DPP-4)*, which inactivates GLP-1 and GIP. By blocking the actions of DPP-4, the incretin effects of GLP-1 and GIP can be prolonged, leading to increased insulin secretion and improved control of blood glucose levels.

Relation of Treatment to Arteriosclerosis. Mainly because of the hypertension and high levels of circulating cholesterol and other lipids in diabetic patients, atherosclerosis, arteriosclerosis, severe coronary heart disease, and multiple microcirculatory lesions develop far more easily than in normal people.

Because complications of diabetes, such as atherosclerosis, increased susceptibility to infection, diabetic retinopathy, cataracts, hypertension, and chronic renal disease, are closely associated with the levels of lipids and glucose in the blood, most physicians also prescribe lipid-lowering drugs to help prevent these disturbances. The common complications of diabetes are depicted in Figure 93-11.

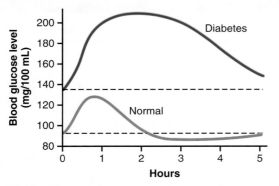

Figure 93-10 Glucose tolerance curve in a normal person and in a person with diabetes.

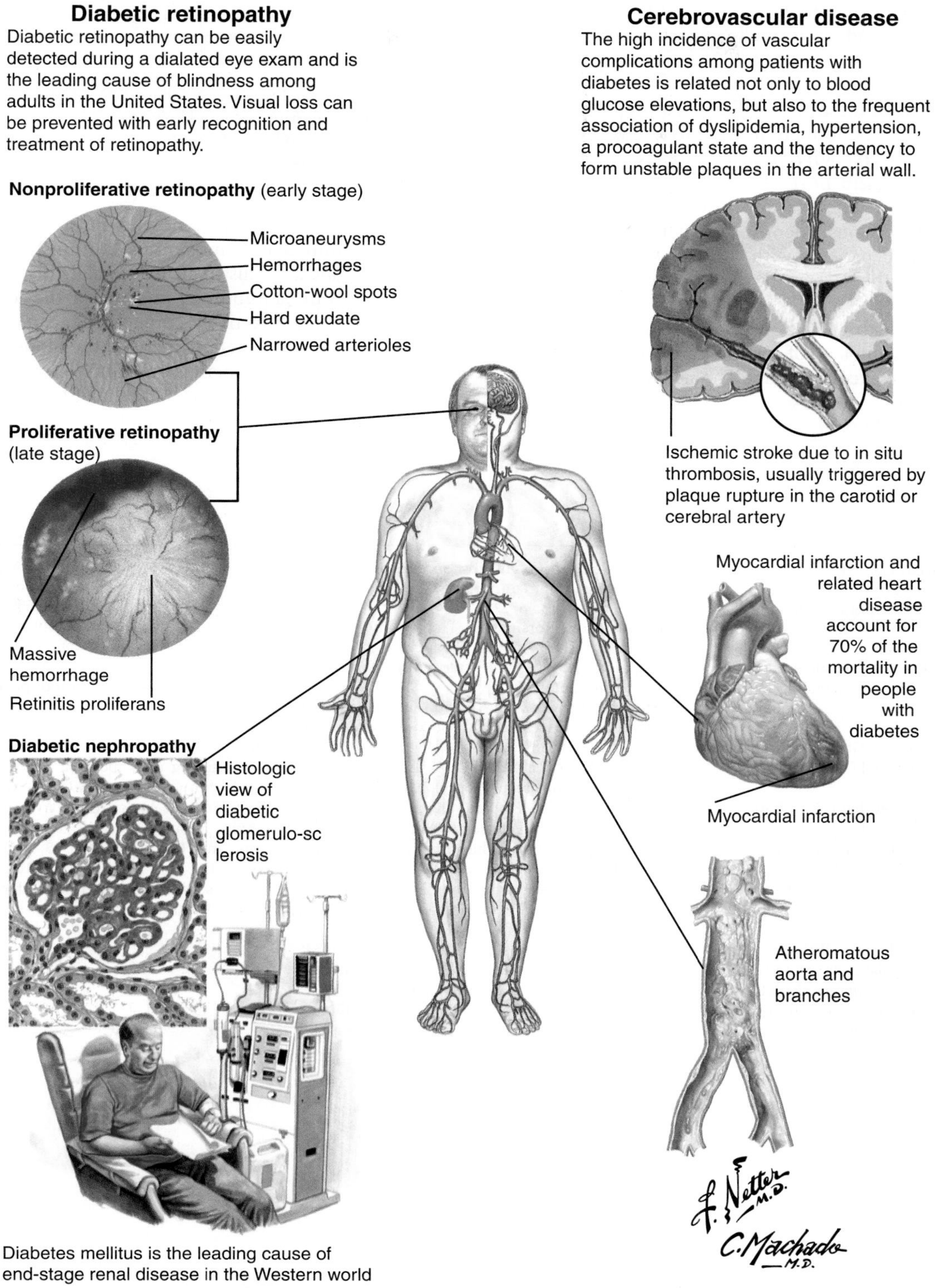

Diabetic retinopathy

Diabetic retinopathy can be easily detected during a dialated eye exam and is the leading cause of blindness among adults in the United States. Visual loss can be prevented with early recognition and treatment of retinopathy.

Nonproliferative retinopathy (early stage)

— Microaneurysms
— Hemorrhages
— Cotton-wool spots
— Hard exudate
— Narrowed arterioles

Proliferative retinopathy (late stage)

Massive hemorrhage

Retinitis proliferans

Diabetic nephropathy

Histologic view of diabetic glomerulo-sclerosis

Diabetes mellitus is the leading cause of end-stage renal disease in the Western world

Cerebrovascular disease

The high incidence of vascular complications among patients with diabetes is related not only to blood glucose elevations, but also to the frequent association of dyslipidemia, hypertension, a procoagulant state and the tendency to form unstable plaques in the arterial wall.

Ischemic stroke due to in situ thrombosis, usually triggered by plaque rupture in the carotid or cerebral artery

Myocardial infarction and related heart disease account for 70% of the mortality in people with diabetes

Myocardial infarction

Atheromatous aorta and branches

Figure 93-11 Microvascular and macrovascular complications of diabetes. Vascular complications can occur with either type 1 or type 2 diabetes and include retinopathy (which can lead to blindness), cardiovascular disease, cerebrovascular disease, and diabetic nephropathy. These complications are responsible for the high morbidity in diabetes. *Netter's Essential Physiology, 2009, p. 346.*

INSULINOMA—HYPERINSULINISM

Although excessive insulin production occurs much more rarely than does diabetes, it occasionally can be a consequence of an adenoma of an islet of Langerhans. About 10–15% of these adenomas are malignant, and occasionally metastases from the islets of Langerhans spread throughout the body, causing tremendous production of insulin by both the primary and metastatic cancers. Indeed, some of these patients have required more than 1000 g of glucose every 24 hours to prevent hypoglycemia.

Insulin Shock and Hypoglycemia. As already emphasized, the central nervous system normally derives essentially all its energy from glucose metabolism and insulin is not necessary for this use of glucose. Consequently, in patients with insulin-secreting tumors or in patients with diabetes who administer too much insulin to themselves, the syndrome called *insulin shock* may occur (Box 93-8).

It is important to distinguish between diabetic coma as a result of acidosis caused by lack of insulin and coma due to hypoglycemia caused by excess insulin. The acetone breath and the rapid, deep breathing of persons in a diabetic coma are not present in persons in a hypoglycemic coma.

BOX 93-8   EFFECTS OF EXCESS INSULIN

1. Blood glucose level falls into the range of 50–70 mg/100 mL
2. The hypoglycemia sensitizes neuronal activity causing the central nervous system to become excitable
3. Hallucinations or extreme nervousness may result
4. Increase in tremors may be seen
5. Increased sweating also occurs
6. If glucose level falls to 20–50 mg/100 mL, clonic seizures and loss of consciousness are likely to occur
7. If glucose levels fall further, the seizures cease and only a state of coma remains

---

Proper treatment for a patient who has hypoglycemic shock or coma is immediate intravenous administration of large quantities of glucose. This treatment usually brings the patient out of shock within a minute or more. Also, the administration of glucagon (or, less effectively, epinephrine) can cause glycogenolysis in the liver and thereby increase the blood glucose level extremely rapidly. If treatment is not administered immediately, permanent damage to the neuronal cells of the central nervous system often occurs.

BIBLIOGRAPHY

Atkinson MA, Eisenbarth GS, Michels AW: Type 1 diabetes, *Lancet* 383:69, 2014.

Bansal P, Wang Q: Insulin as a physiological modulator of glucagon secretion, *Am. J. Physiol. Endocrinol. Metab.* 295:E751, 2008.

Bashan N, Kovsan J, Kachko I, et al: Positive and negative regulation of insulin signaling by reactive oxygen and nitrogen species, *Physiol. Rev.* 89:27, 2009.

Bryant NJ, Govers R, James DE: Regulated transport of the glucose transporter GLUT4, *Nat. Rev. Mol. Cell Biol.* 3:267, 2002.

Forbes JM, Cooper ME: Mechanisms of diabetic complications, *Physiol. Rev.* 93:137, 2013.

Hall JE, Summers RL, Brands MW, et al: Resistance to the metabolic actions of insulin and its role in hypertension, *Am. J. Hypertens.* 7:772, 1994.

Holst JJ: The physiology of glucagon-like peptide 1, *Physiol. Rev.* 87:1409, 2007.

Kahn SE, Cooper ME, Del Prato S: Pathophysiology and treatment of type 2 diabetes: perspectives on the past, present, and future, *Lancet* 383:1068, 2014.

Konrad D, Wueest S: The gut–adipose–liver axis in the metabolic syndrome, *Physiology (Bethesda)* 29:304, 2014.

Leto D, Saltiel AR: Regulation of glucose transport by insulin: traffic control of GLUT4, *Nat. Rev. Mol. Cell Biol.* 13:383, 2012.

MacDonald PE, Rorsman P: The ins and outs of secretion from pancreatic beta-cells: control of single-vesicle exo- and endocytosis, *Physiology (Bethesda)* 22:113, 2007.

Morton GJ, Schwartz MW: Leptin and the central nervous system control of glucose metabolism, *Physiol. Rev.* 91:389, 2011.

Mussa BM, Verberne AJ: The dorsal motor nucleus of the vagus and regulation of pancreatic secretory function, *Exp. Physiol.* 98:25, 2013.

Perry RJ, Samuel VT, Petersen KF, Shulman GI: The role of hepatic lipids in hepatic insulin resistance and type 2 diabetes, *Nature* 510:84, 2014.

Richter EA, Hargreaves M: Exercise, GLUT4, and skeletal muscle glucose uptake, *Physiol. Rev.* 93:993, 2013.

Ruderman NB, Carling D, Prentki M, Cacicedo JM: AMPK, insulin resistance, and the metabolic syndrome, *J. Clin. Invest.* 123:2764, 2013.

Samuel VT, Shulman GI: Mechanisms for insulin resistance: common threads and missing links, *Cell* 148:852, 2012.

Schwartz MW, Seeley RJ, Tschöp MH, et al: Cooperation between brain and islet in glucose homeostasis and diabetes, *Nature* 503:59, 2013.

Tchernof A, Després JP: Pathophysiology of human visceral obesity: an update, *Physiol. Rev.* 93:359, 2013.

Thorens B: Neural regulation of pancreatic islet cell mass and function, *Diabetes Obes. Metab.* 16(Suppl. 1):87, 2014.

Unger RH, Cherrington AD: Glucagonocentric restructuring of diabetes: a pathophysiologic and therapeutic makeover, *J. Clin. Invest.* 122:4, 2012.

Westermark P, Andersson A, Westermark GT: Islet amyloid poly peptide, islet amyloid, and diabetes mellitus, *Physiol. Rev.* 91:795, 2011.

Wright EM, Loo DD, Hirayama BA: Biology of human sodium glucose transporters, *Physiol. Rev.* 91:733, 2011.

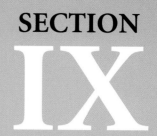

SECTION IX

Reproductive Physiology

MARIO VAZ

94

Physiological Anatomy of the Male Sexual Organs and Spermatogenesis

LEARNING OBJECTIVES

- Describe the physiological anatomy of the male sexual organs.
- Describe the steps of spermatogenesis.
- List the hormones that stimulate spermatogenesis.
- Describe the structure of the mature sperm.
- Describe the role of the prostate gland and seminal vesicle.
- Describe the composition of semen.
- Define the following terms: cryptorchidism, oligospermia, and azoospermia.

GLOSSARY OF TERMS

- **Azoospermia:** Absence of sperm in the ejaculate
- **Cryptorchidism:** Failure of testis to descend from the abdomen into the scrotum at or near the time of birth
- **Oligospermia:** Low sperm count in the ejaculate
- **Spermatogenesis:** The proliferation and differentiation of spermatogonia through definite stages of development to form sperm
- **Spermatogonia:** Immature germ cells in the testes
- **Spermiogenesis:** The process by which spermatids mature into spermatozoa

Figure 94-1A shows the various portions of the male reproductive system and Figure 94-1B gives a more detailed structure of the testis and epididymis. The testis is composed of up to 900 coiled *seminiferous tubules*, each averaging more than 0.5 m long, in which the sperms are formed. The sperms then empty into the *epididymis*, which is another coiled tube about 6 m long. The epididymis leads into the *vas deferens*, which enlarges into the *ampulla of the vas deferens* immediately before the vas enters the body of the *prostate gland*.

Two *seminal vesicles*, one located on each side of the prostate, empty into the prostatic end of the ampulla and the contents from both the ampulla and the seminal vesicles pass into an *ejaculatory duct* leading through the body of the prostate gland and then emptying into the *internal urethra*. *Prostatic ducts* also empty from the prostate gland into the ejaculatory duct and from there into the prostatic urethra.

Finally, the *urethra* is the last connecting link from the testis to the exterior. The urethra is supplied with mucus derived from a large number of minute *urethral glands* located along its entire extent and even more so from bilateral *bulbourethral glands* (Cowper glands) located near the origin of the urethra.

Spermatogenesis

During formation of the embryo, the *primordial germ cells* migrate into the testes and become immature germ cells called *spermatogonia*, which lie in two or three layers of the inner surfaces of the *seminiferous tubules* (a cross-section of a tubule is shown in Figure 94-2A). At puberty, the spermatogonia begin to undergo mitotic division, and continually proliferate and differentiate through definite stages of development to form sperms, as shown in Figure 94-2B.

STEPS OF SPERMATOGENESIS

Spermatogenesis occurs in the seminiferous tubules during active sexual life as the result of stimulation by anterior pituitary gonadotropic hormones. Spermatogenesis begins at an average

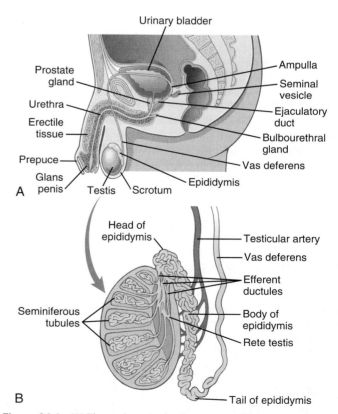

Figure 94-1 (A) The male reproduction system; (B) the internal structure of the testis and the relation of the testis to the epididymis. (*A, Modified from Bloom V, Fawcett DW: Textbook of Histology, 10th ed. Philadelphia: WB Saunders, 1975. B, Modified from Guyton AC: Anatomy and Physiology. Philadelphia: Saunders College Publishing, 1985*)

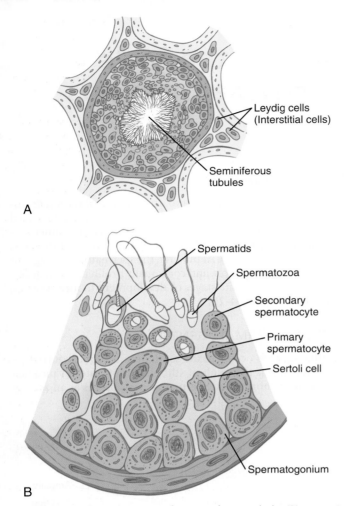

A

B

Figure 94-2 (A) Cross-section of a seminiferous tubule; (B) stages in the development of sperm from spermatogonia.

age of 13 years and continues throughout most of the remainder of life but decreases markedly in old age.

In the first stage of spermatogenesis, the spermatogonia migrate among *Sertoli cells* toward the central lumen of the seminiferous tubule. The Sertoli cells are large with overflowing cytoplasmic envelopes that surround the developing spermatogonia all the way to the central lumen of the tubule.

Meiosis. Spermatogonia that cross the barrier into the Sertoli cell layer become progressively modified and enlarged to form large *primary spermatocytes* (Figure 94-3). Each of these primary spermatocytes, in turn, undergoes meiotic division to form two *secondary spermatocytes*. After another few days, these secondary spermatocytes also divide to form *spermatids* that are eventually modified to become *spermatozoa* (sperms).

During the change from the spermatocyte stage to the spermatid stage, the 46 chromosomes (23 pairs of chromosomes) of the spermatocyte are divided, and, thus, 23 chromosomes go to one spermatid and the other 23 go to the second spermatid. The chromosomal genes are also divided so that only one-half of the genetic characteristics of the eventual fetus are provided by the father, with the other half being derived from the oocyte of the mother.

The entire period of spermatogenesis, from spermatogonia to spermatozoa, takes about 74 days.

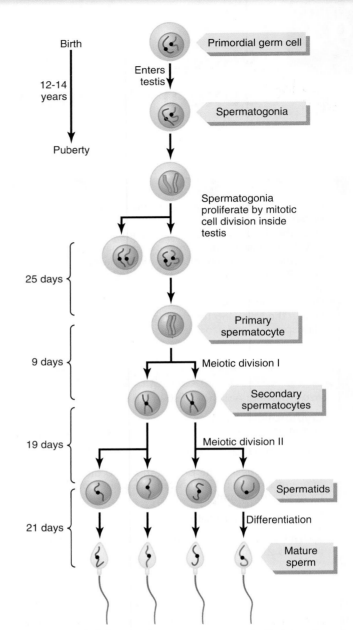

Figure 94-3 Cell divisions during spermatogenesis. During embryonic development the primordial germ cells migrate to the testis, where they become spermatogonia. At puberty (usually 12–14 years after birth), the spermatogonia proliferate rapidly by mitosis. Some begin meiosis to become primary spermatocytes and continue through meiotic division I to become secondary spermatocytes. After completion of meiotic division II, the secondary spermatocytes produce spermatids, which differentiate to form spermatozoa.

Sex Chromosomes. In each spermatogonium, 1 of the 23 pairs of chromosomes carries the genetic information that determines the sex of each eventual offspring. This pair is composed of one X chromosome, which is called the *female chromosome*, and one Y chromosome, the *male chromosome*. During meiotic division, the male Y chromosome goes to one spermatid that then becomes a *male sperm*, and the female X chromosome goes to another spermatid that becomes a *female sperm*. The sex of the eventual offspring is determined by which of these two types of sperm fertilizes the ovum. Fertilization is discussed further in Chapter 98.

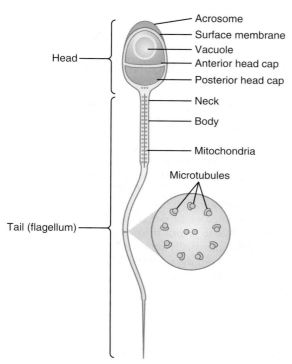

Head
— Acrosome
— Surface membrane
— Vacuole
— Anterior head cap
— Posterior head cap

— Neck
— Body
— Mitochondria

Microtubules

Tail (flagellum)

Figure 94-4   Structure of the human spermatozoon.

Formation of Sperm. When the spermatids are first formed, they still have the usual characteristics of epithelioid cells, but soon they begin to differentiate and elongate into spermatozoa (*spermiogenesis*). As shown in Figure 94-4, each spermatozoon is composed of a *head* and a *tail*. The head comprises the condensed nucleus of the cell with only a thin cytoplasmic and cell membrane layer around its surface. On the outside of the anterior two-thirds of the head is a thick cap called the *acrosome* that is formed mainly from the Golgi apparatus. The acrosome contains several enzymes similar to those found in lysosomes of the typical cell, including *hyaluronidase* (which can digest proteoglycan filaments of tissues) and powerful *proteolytic enzymes* (which can digest proteins). These enzymes play important roles in allowing the sperm to enter the ovum and fertilize it.

The tail of the sperm, called the *flagellum*, has three major components: (1) a central skeleton constructed of 11 microtubules, collectively called the *axoneme* (the structure of the axoneme is similar to that of cilia found on the surfaces of other types of cells); (2) a thin cell membrane covering the axoneme; and (3) a collection of mitochondria surrounding the axoneme in the proximal portion of the tail (called the *body of the tail*).

Back-and-forth movement of the tail (flagellar movement) provides motility for the sperm. This movement results from a rhythmic longitudinal sliding motion between the anterior and posterior tubules that make up the axoneme. The energy for this process is supplied in the form of adenosine triphosphate, which is synthesized by the mitochondria in the body of the tail.

Normal sperms move in a fluid medium at a velocity of 1–4 mm/minute, which allows them to move through the female genital tract in quest of the ovum.

Hormonal Factors that Stimulate Spermatogenesis

The role of hormones in reproduction is discussed in later chapters in detail; for now let us note that several hormones play essential roles in spermatogenesis. Some of these roles are as follows:

1. *Testosterone*, secreted by the *Leydig cells* located in the interstitium of the testis (see Figure 94-2), is essential for growth and division of the testicular germinal cells, which is the first stage in forming sperm.
2. *Luteinizing hormone*, secreted by the anterior pituitary gland, stimulates the Leydig cells to secrete testosterone.
3. *Follicle-stimulating hormone*, also secreted by the anterior pituitary gland, stimulates the *Sertoli cells*; without this stimulation, the conversion of the spermatids to sperm (the process of spermiogenesis) will not occur.
4. *Estrogens*, formed from testosterone by the Sertoli cells when they are stimulated by follicle-stimulating hormone, are probably also essential for spermiogenesis.
5. *Growth hormone* (as well as most of the other body hormones) is necessary for controlling background metabolic functions of the testes. Growth hormone specifically promotes early division of the spermatogonia themselves; in its absence, as in pituitary dwarfs, spermatogenesis is severely deficient or absent, thus causing infertility.

Maturation of Sperm in the Epididymis

After formation in the seminiferous tubules, the sperms require several days to pass through the 6-m-long tubule of the *epididymis*. Sperms removed from the seminiferous tubules and from the early portions of the epididymis are nonmotile, and cannot fertilize an ovum. However, after the sperm have been in the epididymis for 18–24 hours, they develop the *capability of motility*, even though several inhibitory proteins in the epididymal fluid still prevent final motility until after ejaculation.

Storage of Sperms in the Testes. The two testes of the human adult form up to 120 million sperms each day. Most of these sperm can be stored in the epididymis, although a small quantity is stored in the vas deferens. They can remain stored, while maintaining their fertility, for at least a month. During this time, they are kept in a deeply suppressed, inactive state by multiple inhibitory substances in the secretions of the ducts. Conversely, with a high level of sexual activity and ejaculations, they may be stored no longer than a few days.

After ejaculation, the sperms become motile and capable of fertilizing the ovum, a process called *maturation*. The Sertoli cells and the epithelium of the epididymis secrete a special nutrient fluid that is ejaculated along with the sperm. This fluid contains hormones (including both testosterone and estrogens), enzymes, and special nutrients that are essential for sperm maturation.

Physiology of the Mature Sperm. The normal motile, fertile sperms are capable of flagellated movement through the fluid medium at velocities of 1–4 mm/minute. The activity of sperms is greatly enhanced in a neutral and slightly alkaline medium, as exists in the ejaculated semen, but it is greatly depressed in a mildly acidic medium. A strong acidic medium can cause the rapid death of sperm.

The activity of sperms increases markedly with increasing temperature, but so does the rate of metabolism, causing the life of the sperms to be considerably shortened. Although sperms can live for many weeks in the suppressed state in the genital ducts of the testes, the life expectancy of ejaculated sperm in the female genital tract is only 1–2 days.

FUNCTION OF THE SEMINAL VESICLES

Each seminal vesicle is a tortuous, loculated tube lined with a secretory epithelium that secretes a mucoid material containing an abundance of *fructose*, *citric acid*, and other nutrient substances, as well as large quantities of *prostaglandins* and *fibrinogen*. During the process of emission and ejaculation, each seminal vesicle empties its contents into the ejaculatory duct shortly after the vas deferens empties the sperms. This action adds greatly to the bulk of the ejaculated semen, and the fructose and other substances in the seminal fluid are of considerable nutrient value for the ejaculated sperms until one of the sperm fertilizes the ovum.

Prostaglandins are believed to aid fertilization in two ways: (1) by reacting with the female cervical mucus to make it more receptive to sperm movement and (2) by possibly causing backward, reverse peristaltic contractions in the uterus and fallopian tubes to move the ejaculated sperms toward the ovaries (a few sperms reach the upper ends of the fallopian tubes within 5 minutes).

FUNCTION OF THE PROSTATE GLAND

The prostate gland secretes a thin, milky fluid that contains calcium, citrate ion, phosphate ion, a clotting enzyme, and a profibrinolysin. During emission, the capsule of the prostate gland contracts simultaneously with the contractions of the vas deferens so that the thin, milky fluid of the prostate gland adds further to the bulk of the semen. A slightly alkaline characteristic of the prostatic fluid may be quite important for the successful fertilization of the ovum because the fluid of the vas deferens is relatively acidic owing to the presence of citric acid and metabolic end products of the sperm and, consequently, helps inhibit sperm fertility. Also, the vaginal secretions of the female are acidic (with a pH of 3.5–4.0). Sperms do not become optimally motile until the pH of the surrounding fluids rises to about 6.0–6.5. Consequently, it is probable that the slightly alkaline prostatic fluid helps neutralize the acidity of the other seminal fluids during ejaculation and thus enhances the motility and fertility of the sperms.

SEMEN

Semen, which is ejaculated during the male sexual act, is composed of the fluid and sperm from the vas deferens (about 10% of the total), fluid from the seminal vesicles (almost 60%), fluid from the prostate gland (about 30%), and small amounts from the mucous glands, especially the bulbourethral glands. Thus, the bulk of the semen is seminal vesicle fluid, which is the last to be ejaculated and serves to wash the sperm through the ejaculatory duct and urethra.

The average pH of the combined semen is about 7.5, with the alkaline prostatic fluid having more than neutralized the mild acidity of the other portions of the semen. The prostatic fluid gives the semen a milky appearance, and fluid from the seminal vesicles and mucous glands gives the semen a mucoid consistency. Also, a clotting enzyme from the prostatic fluid causes the fibrinogen of the seminal vesicle fluid to form a weak fibrin coagulum that holds the semen in the deeper regions of the vagina where the uterine cervix lies. The coagulum then dissolves during the next 15–30 minutes because of lysis by fibrinolysin formed from the prostatic profibrinolysin. In the early minutes after ejaculation, the sperms remain relatively immobile, possibly because of the viscosity of the coagulum. As the coagulum dissolves, the sperms simultaneously become highly motile.

ABNORMAL SPERMATOGENESIS AND MALE FERTILITY

The seminiferous tubular epithelium can be destroyed by a number of diseases. For instance, bilateral *orchitis* (inflammation) of the testes resulting from *mumps* causes sterility in some affected males.

Effect of Temperature on Spermatogenesis. Increasing the temperature of the testes can prevent spermatogenesis by causing degeneration of most cells of the seminiferous tubules besides the spermatogonia. It has often been stated that the reason the testes are located in the dangling scrotum is to maintain the temperature of these glands below the internal temperature of the body, although usually only about 2°C below the internal temperature. On cold days, scrotal reflexes cause the musculature of the scrotum to contract, pulling the testes close to the body to maintain this 2°C differential. Thus, the scrotum acts as a cooling mechanism for the testes (but a *controlled* cooling), without which spermatogenesis might be deficient during hot weather.

Cryptorchidism

Cryptorchidism means failure of a testis to descend from the abdomen into the scrotum at or near the time of birth of a fetus. During development of the male fetus, the testes are derived from the genital ridges in the abdomen. However, at about 3 weeks to 1 month before birth of the baby, the testes normally descend through the inguinal canals into the scrotum. Occasionally, this descent does not occur or occurs incompletely, and as a result one or both testes remain in the abdomen, in the inguinal canal, or elsewhere along the route of descent.

A testis that remains in the abdominal cavity throughout life is incapable of forming sperms. The tubular epithelium becomes degenerate, leaving only the interstitial structures of the testis. It has been claimed that even the few "degrees" higher temperature in the abdomen than in the scrotum is sufficient to cause this degeneration of the tubular epithelium and, consequently, to cause sterility, although this effect is not certain. Nevertheless, for this reason, operations to relocate the cryptorchid testes from the abdominal cavity into the scrotum before the beginning of adult sexual life can be performed on boys who have undescended testes.

Testosterone secretion by the fetal testes is the normal stimulus that causes the testes to descend into the scrotum from the abdomen. Therefore, many, if not most, instances of cryptorchidism are caused by abnormally formed testes that are unable to secrete enough testosterone. The surgical operation for cryptorchidism in these patients is unlikely to be successful.

Effect of Sperm Count on Fertility. The usual quantity of semen ejaculated during each coitus averages about 3.5 mL, and each milliliter of semen on average contains about 120 million sperms, although even in "normal" males this quantity can vary from 35 to 200 million. This means an average total of 400 million sperms are usually present in the several milliliters of each ejaculate. When the number of sperms in each milliliter falls below about 20 million, the person is likely to be infertile. A reduction in the sperm count below 20 million is referred to as oligospermia while the absence of sperm in the ejaculate is called azoospermia. Thus, even though only a single sperm is necessary to fertilize the ovum, for reasons that are not understood,

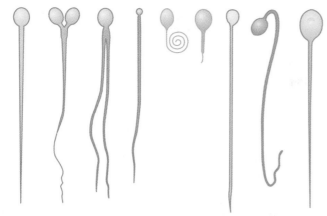

Figure 94-5 Abnormal infertile sperm compared with a normal sperm on the right.

TABLE 94-1	Composition of Semen
Appearance	Translucent, thick, with a whitish tint
Volume	~3.5 mL (1–6.5 mL)
pH	~7.5
Number of sperms	~35–200 million/mL (>15 million is normal)
Percent of motile sperms	>50, measured within 60 minutes of collection of the sample
Contribution by	
Vas deferens	~10%
Seminal vesicle	~60%
Prostate	~30%
Bulbourethral glands	Minimal, ~1%

the ejaculate usually must contain a tremendous number of sperm for only one sperm to fertilize the ovum. There are many causes of low counts and these include hormonal imbalances, infections or tumors involving the testes, exposure to environmental toxins, and lifestyle issues (chronic alcoholism, smoking, and substance abuse) among others.

Effect of Sperm Morphology and Motility on Fertility. Occasionally, a man has a normal number of sperms but is still infertile. When this situation occurs, sometimes as many as one-half of the sperms are found to be abnormal physically, having two heads, abnormally shaped heads, or abnormal tails, as shown in Figure 94-5. At other times, the sperms appear to be structurally normal, but for reasons not understood, they are either entirely nonmotile or relatively nonmotile. Whenever most of the sperms are morphologically abnormal or are nonmotile, the person is likely to be infertile, even though the remainder of the sperms appear to be normal.

Table 94-1 summarizes the composition of the semen that has been discussed in the earlier sections.

BIBLIOGRAPHY

Basaria S: Reproductive aging in men, *Endocrinol. Metab. Clin. North Am.* 42:255, 2013.

Basaria S: Male hypogonadism, *Lancet* 383:1250, 2014.

Darszon A, Nishigaki T, Beltran C, Treviño CL: Calcium channels in the development, maturation, and function of spermatozoa, *Physiol. Rev.* 91:1305, 2011.

Feng CW, Bowles J, Koopman P: Control of mammalian germ cell entry into meiosis, *Mol. Cell. Endocrinol.* 382:488, 2014.

Groth KA, Skakkebæk A, Høst C, et al: Clinical review: Klinefelter syndrome—a clinical update, *J. Clin. Endocrinol. Metab.* 98:20, 2013.

Guerrero-Bosagna C, Skinner MK: Environmentally induced epigenetic transgenerational inheritance of male infertility, *Curr. Opin. Genet. Dev.* 26C:79, 2014.

Matzuk M, Lamb D: The biology of infertility: research advances and clinical challenges, *Nat. Med.* 14:1197, 2008.

Michels G, Hoppe UC: Rapid actions of androgens, *Front. Neuroendocrinol.* 29:182, 2008.

Plant TM, Marshall GR: The functional significance of FSH in spermatogenesis and the control of its secretion in male primates, *Endocr. Rev.* 22:764, 2001.

Shamloul R, Ghanem H: Erectile dysfunction, *Lancet.* 381:153, 2013.

Svingen T, Koopman P: Building the mammalian testis: origins, differentiation, and assembly of the component cell populations, *Genes Dev.* 27:2409, 2013.

Wilhelm D, Palmer S, Koopman P: Sex determination and gonadal development in mammals, *Physiol. Rev.* 87:1, 2007.

95

Testosterone and Other Male Sex Hormones

The testes secrete several male sex hormones, which are collectively called *androgens*, including *testosterone, dihydrotestosterone,* and *androstenedione.* Testosterone is so much more abundant than the others that one can consider it to be the primary testicular hormone, although much of the testosterone is eventually converted into the more active hormone dihydrotestosterone in the target tissues.

Testosterone is formed by the *interstitial cells of Leydig,* which lie in the interstices between the seminiferous tubules and constitute about 20% of the mass of the adult testes, as shown in Figure 95-1. Leydig cells are almost nonexistent in the testes during childhood when the testes secrete almost no testosterone, but they are numerous in the newborn male infant for the first few months of life and in the adult male after puberty; at both these times the testes secrete large quantities of testosterone. Furthermore, when tumors develop from the interstitial cells of Leydig, great quantities of testosterone are secreted. Finally, when the germinal epithelium of the testes is destroyed by X-ray treatment or excessive heat, the Leydig cells, which are less easily destroyed, often continue to produce testosterone.

Secretion of Androgens Elsewhere in the Body. The term "androgen" means any steroid hormone that has masculinizing effects, including testosterone; it also includes male sex hormones produced elsewhere in the body besides the testes. For instance, the adrenal glands secrete at least five androgens, although the total masculinizing activity of all these androgens is normally so slight (<5% of the total in the adult male) that even in women they do not cause significant masculine characteristics, except for causing growth of pubic and axillary hair. However, when a tumor of the adrenal androgen-producing cells occurs,

the quantity of androgenic hormones may then become great enough to cause all the usual male secondary sexual characteristics to occur even in the female, the *adrenogenital syndrome.*

Chemistry of the Androgens. All androgens are steroid compounds. Both in the testes and in the adrenals, the androgens can be synthesized either from cholesterol or directly from acetyl coenzyme A.

Metabolism of Testosterone. After secretion by the testes, about 97% of the testosterone becomes either loosely bound with plasma albumin or more tightly bound with a beta globulin called *sex hormone–binding globulin* and circulates in the blood in these states for 30 minutes to several hours. By that time, the testosterone is either transferred to the tissues or degraded into inactive products that are subsequently excreted.

Much of the testosterone that becomes fixed to the tissues is converted within the tissue cells to *dihydrotestosterone,* especially in certain target organs such as the prostate gland in the adult and the external genitalia of the male fetus. Some, but not all, actions of testosterone depend on this conversion. The intracellular functions are discussed later in this chapter.

Degradation and Excretion of Testosterone. The testosterone that does not become fixed to the tissues is rapidly converted, mainly by the liver, into *androsterone* and *dehydroepiandrosterone* and simultaneously conjugated as either glucuronides or sulfates (glucuronides, particularly). These substances are excreted either into the gut by way of the liver bile or into the urine through the kidneys.

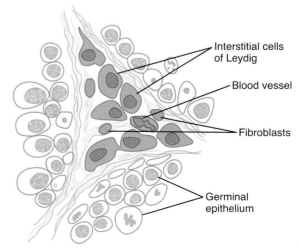

Figure 95-1 Interstitial cells of Leydig, the cells that secrete testosterone, located in the interstices between the seminiferous tubules.

Production of Estrogen in the Male. In addition to testosterone, small amounts of estrogens are formed in the male (about one-fifth the amount in the nonpregnant female) and a reasonable quantity of estrogens can be recovered from a man's urine. The exact source of estrogens in the male is unclear, but the following information is known: (1) The concentration of estrogens in the fluid of the seminiferous tubules is quite high and probably plays an important role in spermiogenesis. This estrogen is believed to be formed by the Sertoli cells by converting testosterone to estradiol. (2) Much larger amounts of estrogens are formed from testosterone and androstanediol in other tissues of the body, especially the liver, probably accounting for as much as 80% of the total male estrogen production.

Functions of Testosterone

In general, testosterone is responsible for the distinguishing characteristics of the masculine body. Even during fetal life, the testes are stimulated by chorionic gonadotropin from the placenta to produce moderate quantities of testosterone throughout the entire period of fetal development and for 10 or more weeks after birth; thereafter, essentially no testosterone is produced during childhood until about the ages of 10–13 years. Testosterone production then increases rapidly under the stimulus of anterior pituitary gonadotropic hormones at the onset of puberty and lasts throughout most of the remainder of life, as shown in Figure 95-2, dwindling rapidly beyond age 50 to become 20–50% of the peak value by age 80.

FUNCTIONS OF TESTOSTERONE DURING FETAL DEVELOPMENT

Testosterone begins to be elaborated by the male fetal testes at about the seventh week of embryonic life. Indeed, one of the major functional differences between the female and the male sex chromosome is that the male chromosome has the *sex-determining region Y (SRY) gene* that encodes a protein called the *testis-determining factor* (also called the *SRY protein*). The SRY protein initiates a cascade of gene activations that cause the genital ridge cells to differentiate into cells that secrete testosterone and eventually become the testes, whereas the female chromosome causes this ridge to differentiate into cells that secrete estrogens.

Injection of large quantities of male sex hormone into pregnant animals causes development of male sexual organs even though the fetus is female. Also, early removal of the testes in the male fetus causes development of female sexual organs.

Thus, testosterone secreted first by the genital ridges and later by the fetal testes is responsible for the development of the male body characteristics, including the formation of a penis and a scrotum rather than formation of a clitoris and a vagina. It also causes formation of the prostate gland, seminal vesicles, and male genital ducts, while at the same time suppressing the formation of female genital organs.

Effect of Testosterone to Cause Descent of the Testes

The testes usually descend into the scrotum during the last 2–3 months of gestation when the testes begin secreting reasonable quantities of testosterone. If a male child is born with undescended but otherwise normal testes, administration of testosterone usually causes the testes to descend in the usual manner if the inguinal canals are large enough to allow the testes to pass.

Administration of gonadotropic hormones, which stimulate the Leydig cells of the newborn child's testes to produce testosterone, can also cause the testes to descend. Thus, the stimulus for descent of the testes is testosterone, indicating again that testosterone is an important hormone for male sexual development during fetal life.

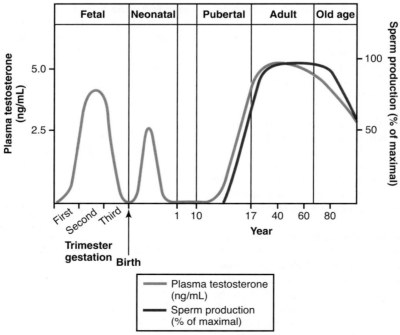

Figure 95-2 The different stages of male sexual function as reflected by average plasma testosterone concentrations (*red line*) and sperm production (*blue line*) at different ages. *Modified from Griffin, J.F., Wilson, J.D., 1980. The testis. In: Bondy, P.K., Rosenberg, L.E. (Eds.), Metabolic Control and Disease, eighth ed. W.B. Saunders, Philadelphia.*

EFFECT OF TESTOSTERONE ON DEVELOPMENT OF ADULT PRIMARY AND SECONDARY SEXUAL CHARACTERISTICS

After puberty, increasing amounts of testosterone secretion cause the penis, scrotum, and testes to enlarge about eightfold before the age of 20 years. In addition, testosterone causes the secondary sexual characteristics of the male to develop, beginning at puberty and ending at maturity. These secondary sexual characteristics, in addition to the sexual organs themselves, distinguish the male from the female as follows.

Effect on the Distribution of Body Hair

Testosterone causes growth of hair (1) over the pubis, (2) upward along the linea alba of the abdomen sometimes to the umbilicus and above, (3) on the face, (4) usually on the chest, and (5) less often on other regions of the body, such as the back. It also causes the hair on most other portions of the body to become more prolific.

Male Pattern Baldness

Testosterone decreases the growth of hair on the top of the head; a man who does not have functional testes does not become bald. However, many virile men never become bald because baldness is a result of two factors: first, a genetic background for the development of baldness and, second, superimposed on this genetic background, large quantities of androgenic hormones.

Effect on the Voice

Testosterone secreted by the testes or injected into the body causes hypertrophy of the laryngeal mucosa and enlargement of the larynx. The effects at first cause a relatively discordant, "cracking" voice that gradually changes into the typical adult masculine voice.

Testosterone Increases Thickness of the Skin and Can Contribute to Development of Acne

Testosterone increases the thickness of the skin over the entire body and the ruggedness of the subcutaneous tissues. Testosterone also increases the rate of secretion by some or perhaps all of the body's sebaceous glands. Especially important is excessive secretion by the sebaceous glands of the face, which can result in *acne*. Therefore, acne is one of the most common features of male adolescence. After several years of testosterone secretion, the skin normally adapts to the testosterone in a way that allows it to overcome the acne.

Testosterone Increases Protein Formation and Muscle Development

One of the most important male characteristics is development of increasing musculature after puberty, averaging about a 50% increase in muscle mass over that in the female. Because of the great effect that testosterone and other androgens have on the body musculature, synthetic androgens are widely used by athletes to improve their muscular performance. This practice is to be severely deprecated because of prolonged harmful effects of excess androgens.

Testosterone Increases Bone Matrix and Causes Calcium Retention

After the great increase in circulating testosterone that occurs at puberty (or after prolonged injection of testosterone), the bones grow considerably thicker and deposit considerable additional calcium salts. Thus, testosterone increases the total quantity of bone matrix and causes calcium retention. The increase in bone matrix is believed to result from the general protein anabolic function of testosterone plus deposition of calcium salts in response to the increased protein.

Testosterone has a specific effect on the pelvis to (1) narrow the pelvic outlet, (2) lengthen it, (3) cause a funnel-like shape instead of the broad ovoid shape of the female pelvis, and (4) greatly increase the strength of the entire pelvis for load-bearing. In the absence of testosterone, the male pelvis develops into a pelvis that is similar to that of the female.

When great quantities of testosterone (or any other androgen) are secreted abnormally in the still-growing child, the rate of bone growth increases markedly, causing a spurt in total body height. However, the testosterone also causes the epiphyses of the long bones to unite with the shafts of the bones at an early age. Therefore, despite the rapidity of growth, this early uniting of the epiphyses prevents the person from growing as tall as he would have grown had testosterone not been secreted at all.

Testosterone Increases the Basal Metabolic Rate

Injection of large quantities of testosterone can increase the basal metabolic rate by as much as 15%. Also, even the usual quantity of testosterone secreted by the testes during adolescence and early adult life increases the rate of metabolism some 5–10% above the value that it would be were the testes not active. This increased rate of metabolism is possibly an indirect result of the effect of testosterone on protein anabolism, with the increased quantity of proteins—the enzymes especially—increasing the activities of all cells.

Testosterone Increases Red Blood Cells

When normal quantities of testosterone are injected into a castrated adult, the number of red blood cells per cubic millimeter of blood increases 15–20%. Also, the average man has about 700,000 more red blood cells per cubic millimeter than the average woman. Despite the strong association of testosterone and increased hematocrit, testosterone does not appear to directly increase erythropoietin levels or have a direct effect on red blood cell production. The effect of testosterone to increase red blood cell production may be at least partly indirect because of the increased metabolic rate that occurs after testosterone administration.

Effect on Electrolyte and Water Balance

Many steroid hormones can increase the reabsorption of sodium in the distal tubules of the kidneys. Testosterone also has such an effect, but only to a minor degree in comparison with the adrenal mineralocorticoids.

Basic Intracellular Mechanism of Action of Testosterone

Most of the effects of testosterone result basically from increased rate of protein formation in the target cells. This phenomenon has been studied extensively in the prostate gland, which is one of the organs that is most affected by testosterone. In this gland, testosterone enters the prostatic cells within a few minutes after secretion. Then it is most often converted, under the influence of the intracellular enzyme 5α-reductase, to *dihydrotestosterone*, which in turn binds with a cytoplasmic "receptor protein." This combination migrates to the cell nucleus, where it binds with a nuclear protein and induces DNA–RNA transcription. Within 30 minutes, RNA polymerase has become activated and the concentration of RNA begins to increase in the prostatic cells, which is followed by a progressive increase in cellular protein. After several days, the quantity of DNA in the prostate gland has also increased and there has been a simultaneous increase in the number of prostatic cells.

Testosterone stimulates production of proteins virtually everywhere in the body, although more specifically affecting the proteins in "target" organs or tissues responsible for the development of both primary and secondary male sexual characteristics.

Recent studies suggest that testosterone, like other steroidal hormones, may also exert some rapid, *nongenomic effects* that do not require synthesis of new proteins. The physiological role of these nongenomic actions of testosterone, however, has yet to be determined.

Control of Male Sexual Functions by Hormones from the Hypothalamus and Anterior Pituitary Gland

A major share of the control of sexual functions in both the male and the female begins with secretion of *gonadotropin-releasing hormone* (GnRH) by the hypothalamus (Figure 95-3). This hormone in turn stimulates the anterior pituitary gland to secrete two other hormones called *gonadotropic hormones*: (1) *luteinizing hormone* (LH) and (2) *follicle-stimulating hormone* (FSH). In turn, LH is the primary stimulus for the secretion of testosterone by the testes and FSH mainly stimulates spermatogenesis.

GnRH AND ITS EFFECT IN INCREASING THE SECRETION OF LUTEINIZING HORMONE AND FOLLICLE-STIMULATING HORMONE

GnRH is a 10–amino acid peptide secreted by neurons whose cell bodies are located in the *arcuate nuclei of the hypothalamus*. The endings of these neurons terminate mainly in the median eminence of the hypothalamus, where they release GnRH into the hypothalamic–hypophysial portal vascular system. The GnRH is then transported to the anterior pituitary gland in the hypophysial portal blood and stimulates the release of the two gonadotropins, LH and FSH.

GnRH is secreted intermittently a few minutes at a time once every 1–3 hours. The intensity of this hormone's stimulus is determined in two ways: (1) by the frequency of these cycles of secretion and (2) by the quantity of GnRH released with each cycle.

The secretion of LH by the anterior pituitary gland is also cyclic, with LH following fairly faithfully the pulsatile release of GnRH. Conversely, FSH secretion increases and decreases only slightly with each fluctuation of GnRH secretion; instead, it changes more slowly over a period of many hours in response to longer-term changes in GnRH. Because of the much closer relation between GnRH secretion and LH secretion, GnRH is also widely known as *LH-releasing hormone*.

GONADOTROPIC HORMONES: LUTEINIZING HORMONE AND FOLLICLE-STIMULATING HORMONE

Both of the gonadotropic hormones, LH and FSH, are secreted by the same cells, called *gonadotropes*, in the anterior pituitary gland.

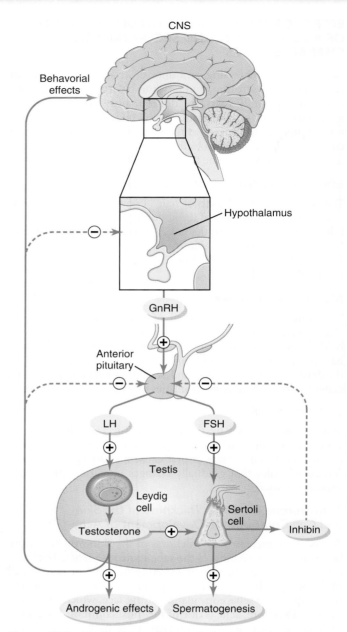

Figure 95-3 Feedback regulation of the hypothalamic–pituitary–testicular axis in males. Stimulatory effects are shown by plus signs and negative feedback inhibitory effects are shown by minus signs. *CNS,* central nervous system; *FSH,* follicle-stimulating hormone; *GnRH,* gonadotropin-releasing hormone; *LH,* luteinizing hormone.

In the absence of GnRH secretion from the hypothalamus, the gonadotropes in the pituitary gland secrete almost no LH or FSH.

LH and FSH are *glycoproteins*. They exert their effects on their target tissues in the testes mainly by *activating the cyclic adenosine monophosphate second messenger system*, which in turn activates specific enzyme systems in the respective target cells.

Regulation of Testosterone Production by Luteinizing Hormone

Testosterone is secreted by the *interstitial cells of Leydig* in the testes, but only when they are stimulated by LH from the anterior pituitary gland. Furthermore, the quantity of testosterone that is secreted increases approximately in direct proportion to the amount of LH that is available.

Mature Leydig cells are normally found in a child's testes for a few weeks after birth but then disappear until after the age of about 10 years. However, injection of purified LH into a child at any age or secretion of LH at puberty causes testicular interstitial cells that look like fibroblasts to evolve into functioning Leydig cells.

Inhibition of Anterior Pituitary Secretion of LH and FSH by Testosterone-Negative Feedback Control of Testosterone Secretion

The testosterone secreted by the testes in response to LH has the reciprocal effect of inhibiting anterior pituitary secretion of LH (see Figure 95-3). Most of this inhibition probably results from a direct effect of testosterone on the hypothalamus to decrease the secretion of GnRH. This effect in turn causes a corresponding decrease in secretion of both LH and FSH by the anterior pituitary, and the decrease in LH reduces the secretion of testosterone by the testes. Thus, whenever secretion of testosterone becomes too great, this automatic negative feedback effect, operating through the hypothalamus and anterior pituitary gland, reduces the testosterone secretion back toward the desired operating level. Conversely, too little testosterone allows the hypothalamus to secrete large amounts of GnRH, with a corresponding increase in anterior pituitary LH and FSH secretion and consequent increase in testicular testosterone secretion.

REGULATION OF SPERMATOGENESIS BY FOLLICLE-STIMULATING HORMONE AND TESTOSTERONE

FSH binds with specific FSH receptors attached to the Sertoli cells in the seminiferous tubules, which causes the Sertoli cells to grow and secrete various spermatogenic substances. Simultaneously, testosterone (and dihydrotestosterone) diffusing into the seminiferous tubules from the Leydig cells in the interstitial spaces also has a strong tropic effect on spermatogenesis. Thus, both FSH and testosterone are necessary to initiate spermatogenesis.

Role of Inhibin in Negative Feedback Control of Seminiferous Tubule Activity

When the seminiferous tubules fail to produce sperm, secretion of FSH by the anterior pituitary gland increases markedly. Conversely, when spermatogenesis proceeds too rapidly, pituitary secretion of FSH diminishes. The cause of this negative feedback effect on the anterior pituitary is believed to be the secretion by the Sertoli cells of still another hormone called *inhibin* (see Figure 95-3). This hormone has a strong direct effect on the anterior pituitary gland to inhibit the secretion of FSH.

Inhibin is a glycoprotein, like both LH and FSH, with a molecular weight between 10,000 and 30,000. It has been isolated from cultured Sertoli cells. Its potent inhibitory feedback effect on the anterior pituitary gland provides an important negative feedback mechanism for control of spermatogenesis, operating simultaneously with and in parallel to the negative feedback mechanism for control of testosterone secretion.

HUMAN CHORIONIC GONADOTROPIN SECRETED BY THE PLACENTA DURING PREGNANCY STIMULATES TESTOSTERONE SECRETION BY THE FETAL TESTES

During pregnancy, the hormone *human chorionic gonadotropin* (hCG) is secreted by the placenta, and it circulates both in the mother and in the fetus. This hormone has almost the same effects on the sexual organs as LH.

During pregnancy, if the fetus is a male, hCG from the placenta causes the testes of the fetus to secrete testosterone. This testosterone is critical for promoting formation of the male sexual organs, as pointed out earlier. We discuss hCG and its functions during pregnancy in greater detail in Chapter 98.

PUBERTY AND REGULATION OF ITS ONSET

Initiation of the onset of puberty has long been a mystery, but it has now been determined that *during childhood the hypothalamus simply does not secrete significant amounts of GnRH*. One of the reasons for this is that, during childhood, the slightest secretion of any sex steroid hormones exerts a strong inhibitory effect on hypothalamic secretion of GnRH. Yet for reasons still not understood, at the time of puberty, the secretion of hypothalamic GnRH breaks through the childhood inhibition and adult sexual life begins.

Male Adult Sexual Life and Male Climacteric

After puberty, gonadotropic hormones are produced by the male pituitary gland for the remainder of life, and at least some spermatogenesis usually continues until death. Most men, however, begin to exhibit slowly decreasing sexual functions in their late 50s or 60s. There is considerable variation in this decline, with some men continuing to be virile until their 80s and 90s. This decline in sexual function is related, in part, to a decrease in testosterone secretion, as shown in Figure 95-2. The decrease in male sexual function is called the *male climacteric*.

Abnormalities of Male Sexual Function

THE PROSTATE GLAND AND ITS ABNORMALITIES

The prostate gland remains relatively small throughout childhood and begins to grow at puberty under the stimulus of testosterone. This gland reaches an almost stationary size by the age of 20 years and remains at this size up to the age of about 50 years. At that time, in some men it begins to involute, along with decreased production of testosterone by the testes.

A benign prostatic fibroadenoma frequently develops in the prostate in many older men and can cause urinary obstruction. This hypertrophy is caused not by testosterone but instead by abnormal overgrowth of prostate tissue.

Cancer of the prostate gland is a different problem that accounts for about 2–3% of all male deaths. Once cancer of the prostate gland occurs, the cancerous cells are usually stimulated to more rapid growth by testosterone and are inhibited by removal of both testes so that testosterone cannot be formed. Prostatic cancer usually can be inhibited by administration of estrogens.

HYPOGONADISM IN THE MALE

When the testes of a male fetus are nonfunctional during fetal life, none of the male sexual characteristics develop in the fetus. Instead, female organs are formed. The reason for this is that the basic genetic characteristic of the fetus, whether male or female, is to form female sexual organs if there are no sex hormones. However, in the presence of testosterone, formation of female sexual organs is suppressed and male organs are induced instead.

When a boy loses his testes before puberty, a state of eunuchism ensues in which he continues to have infantile sex organs and other infantile sexual characteristics throughout life. The height of an adult eunuch is slightly greater than that of a normal man because the bone epiphyses are slow to unite, although the bones are quite thin and the muscles are considerably weaker than those of a normal man. The voice is child-like, there is no loss of hair on the head, and the normal adult masculine hair distribution on the face and elsewhere does not occur.

When a man is castrated after puberty, some of his male secondary sexual characteristics revert to those of a child and others remain of adult masculine character. The sexual organs regress slightly in size but not to a child-like state, and the voice regresses from the bass quality only slightly. However, there is loss of masculine hair production, loss of the thick masculine bones, and loss of the musculature of the virile male.

Also in a castrated adult male, sexual desires are decreased but not lost, provided sexual activities have been practiced previously. Erection can still occur as before, although with less ease, but it is rare that ejaculation can take place, primarily because the semen-forming organs degenerate and there has been a loss of the testosterone-driven psychic desire.

Some instances of hypogonadism are caused by a genetic inability of the hypothalamus to secrete normal amounts of GnRH. This condition is often associated with a simultaneous abnormality of the feeding center of the hypothalamus, causing the person to greatly overeat. Consequently, obesity occurs along with eunuchism. A patient with this condition is shown in Figure 95-4; the condition is called *adiposogenital syndrome*, *Fröhlich syndrome*, or *hypothalamic eunuchism*.

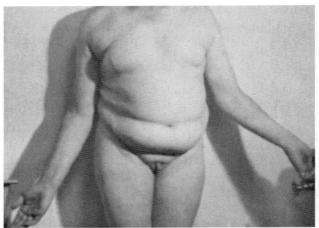

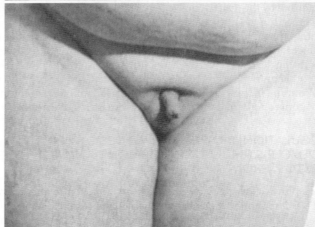

Figure 95-4 Adiposogenital syndrome in an adolescent male. Note the obesity and child-like sexual organs. *Courtesy Dr. Leonard Posey.*

BIBLIOGRAPHY

Barakat B, Itman C, Mendis SH, Loveland KL: Activins and inhibins in mammalian testis development: new models, new insights, *Mol. Cell. Endocrinol.* 359:66, 2012.

Basaria S: Reproductive aging in men, *Endocrinol. Metab. Clin. North Am.* 42:255, 2013.

Basaria S: Male hypogonadism, *Lancet* 383:1250, 2014.

Guerrero-Bosagna C, Skinner MK: Environmentally induced epigenetic transgenerational inheritance of male infertility, *Curr. Opin. Genet. Dev.* 26C:79, 2014.

Kovac JR, Pan MM, Lipshultz LI, Lamb DJ: Current state of practice regarding testosterone supplementation therapy in men with prostate cancer, *Steroids* 89C:27, 2014.

Michels G, Hoppe UC: Rapid actions of androgens, *Front. Neuroendocrinol.* 29:182, 2008.

Nelson WG, De Marzo AM, Isaacs WB: Prostate cancer, *N. Engl. J. Med.* 349:366, 2003.

Oatley JM, Brinster RL: The germline stem cell niche unit in mammalian testes, *Physiol. Rev.* 92:577, 2012.

Female Physiology Before Pregnancy and Female Hormones

GLOSSARY OF TERMS

- **Amenorrhea:** Absence of menstruation (typically when three or more periods have been missed)

- **Anovulatory menstrual cycle:** A menstrual cycle in which ovulation does not occur

- **Follicular phase:** The first half of the menstrual cycle that extends from the stoppage of menstruation (bleeding) to the luteinizing hormone (LH) surge that precedes ovulation

- **Luteal phase:** The second half of the menstrual cycle from ovulation to the start of menstruation (progesterone is secreted from the corpus luteum during this phase)

- **Menarche:** The time of the first menstrual cycle

- **Menopause:** The permanent cessation of menstrual cycles, typically in middle age (usually identified when menstruation has ceased for 12 months)

Female reproductive functions can be divided into two major phases: (1) preparation of the female body for conception and pregnancy and (2) the period of pregnancy itself. This chapter is concerned with preparation of the female body for pregnancy, which is described in detail in Chapter 98.

Physiological Anatomy of the Female Sexual Organs

Figures 96-1 and 96-2 show the principal organs of the human female reproductive tract, including the *ovaries, fallopian tubes* (also called *uterine tubes*), *uterus*, and *vagina*. Reproduction

begins with the development of ova in the ovaries. In the middle of each monthly sexual cycle, a single ovum is expelled from an ovarian follicle into the abdominal cavity near the open fimbriated ends of the two fallopian tubes. This ovum then passes through one of the fallopian tubes into the uterus; if it has been fertilized by a sperm, it implants in the uterus, where it develops into a fetus, a placenta, and fetal membranes—and eventually into a baby.

Oogenesis and Follicular Development in the Ovaries

A developing egg (*oocyte*) differentiates into a mature egg (*ovum*) through a series of steps called *oogenesis* (Figure 96-3). During early embryonic development, *primordial germ cells* from the dorsal endoderm of the yolk sac migrate along the mesentery of the hindgut to the outer surface of the ovary, which is covered by a germinal epithelium, derived embryologically from the epithelium of the germinal ridges. During this migration, the germ cells divide repeatedly. Once these primordial germ cells reach the germinal epithelium, they migrate into the substance of the ovarian cortex and become *oogonia* or *primordial ova*.

Each primordial ovum then collects around it a layer of spindle cells from the ovarian *stroma* (the supporting tissue of the ovary) and causes them to take on epithelioid characteristics; these epithelioid-like cells are then called *granulosa cells*. The ovum surrounded by a single layer of granulosa cells is called a *primordial follicle*. At this stage the ovum is still immature and is called a *primary oocyte*, requiring two more cell divisions before it can be fertilized by a sperm.

The oogonia in the embryonic ovary complete mitotic replication and the first stage of meiosis by the fifth month of fetal development. The germ cell mitosis then ceases and no additional oocytes are formed. At birth the ovary contains about 1–2 million primary oocytes.

The first meiotic division of the oocyte occurs after puberty. Each oocyte divides into two cells, a large ovum (*secondary oocyte*) and a small first *polar body*. Each of these cells contains 23 duplicated chromosomes. The first polar body may or may not undergo a second meiotic division and then disintegrates. The ovum undergoes a second meiotic division, and after the sister chromatids separate, there is a pause in meiosis. If the ovum is fertilized, the final step in meiosis occurs and the sister chromatids in the ovum go to separate cells.

When the ovary releases the ovum (*ovulation*) and if the ovum is fertilized, the final meiosis occurs. Half of the sister chromatids remain in the fertilized ovum and the other half are released in a second polar body, which then disintegrates.

At puberty, only about 300,000 oocytes remain in the ovaries, and only a small percentage of these oocytes become mature. The many thousands of oocytes that do not mature degenerate.

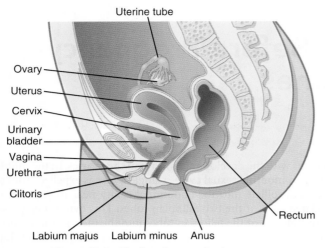

Figure 96-1   The female reproductive organs.

During all the reproductive years of adult life, between about 13 and 46 years of age, only 400–500 of the primordial follicles develop enough to expel their ova—1 each month; the remainder degenerate (ie, become *atretic*). At the end of reproductive capability (at *menopause*), only a few primordial follicles remain in the ovaries, and even these follicles degenerate soon thereafter.

Female Hormonal System

The female hormonal system, like that of the male hormonal system, consists of three hierarchies of hormones, as follows:

1. a hypothalamic-releasing hormone called *gonadotropin-releasing hormone* (GnRH);
2. the anterior pituitary sex hormones, *follicle-stimulating hormone* (FSH) and *luteinizing hormone* (LH), both of which are secreted in response to the release of GnRH from the hypothalamus;
3. the ovarian hormones, *estrogen* and *progesterone*, which are secreted by the ovaries in response to the two female sex hormones from the anterior pituitary gland.

These various hormones are secreted at drastically differing rates during different parts of the female monthly sexual cycle. Figure 96-4 shows the approximate changing concentrations of the anterior pituitary gonadotropic hormones FSH and LH (bottom two curves) and of the ovarian hormones estradiol (estrogen) and progesterone (top two curves).

The amount of GnRH released from the hypothalamus increases and decreases much less drastically during the monthly sexual cycle. It is secreted in short pulses averaging once every 90 minutes, as occurs in the male.

Female Monthly Sexual Cycle (Menstrual Cycle)

THE OVARIAN CYCLE

The normal reproductive years of the female are characterized by monthly rhythmic changes in the rates of secretion of the female hormones and corresponding physical changes in the ovaries and other sexual organs. This rhythmic pattern is called the *female monthly sexual cycle* (or, less accurately, the *menstrual cycle*). The duration of the cycle averages 28 days. It may be as short as 20 days or as long as 45 days in some women, although abnormal cycle length is frequently associated with decreased fertility.

The female sexual cycle has two significant results. First, only a *single* ovum is normally released from the ovaries each month, so normally only a single fetus will begin to grow at a time. Second, the uterine endometrium is prepared in advance for implantation of the fertilized ovum at the required time of the month.

GONADOTROPIC HORMONES AND THEIR EFFECTS ON THE OVARIES

The ovarian changes that occur during the sexual cycle depend completely on the gonadotropic hormones *FSH* and *LH*, which are secreted by the anterior pituitary gland. Both FSH and LH are small glycoproteins that have molecular weights of about 30,000. In the absence of these hormones, the ovaries remain inactive, which is the case throughout childhood, when almost no pituitary gonadotropic hormones are secreted. At age 9–12 years, the pituitary begins to secrete progressively more FSH and LH, which leads to onset of normal monthly sexual cycles beginning between the ages of 11 and 15 years. This period of change is called *puberty*, and the time of the first menstrual cycle is called *menarche*.

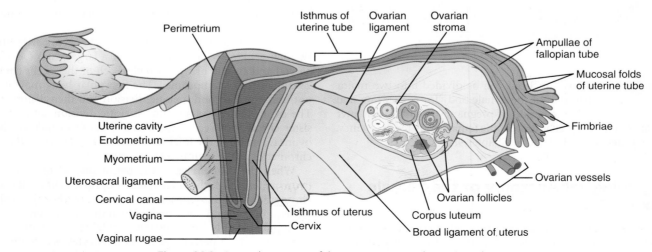

Figure 96-2   Internal structures of the uterus, ovary, and a uterine tube.

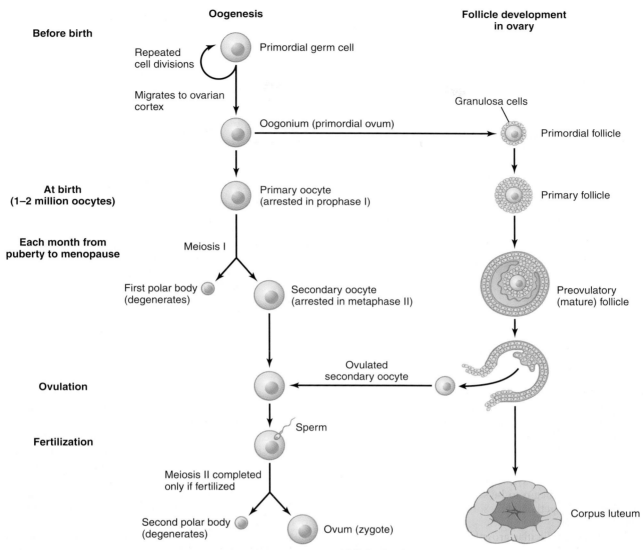

Figure 96-3 Oogenesis and follicle development.

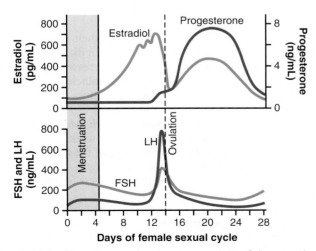

Figure 96-4 Approximate plasma concentrations of the gonadotropins and ovarian hormones during the normal female sexual cycle. *FSH,* follicle-stimulating hormone; *LH,* luteinizing hormone.

During each month of the female sexual cycle, there is a cyclic increase and decrease of FSH and LH, as shown in the bottom of Figure 96-4. These cyclic variations cause cyclic ovarian changes, which are explained in the following sections.

Both FSH and LH stimulate their ovarian target cells by combining with highly specific FSH and LH receptors in the ovarian target cell membranes. In turn, the activated receptors increase the cells' rates of secretion and usually the growth and proliferation of the cells as well. Almost all these stimulatory effects result from *activation of the cyclic adenosine monophosphate second messenger system* in the cell cytoplasm, which causes the formation of *protein kinase* and multiple *phosphorylations of key enzymes* that stimulate sex hormone synthesis.

OVARIAN FOLLICLE GROWTH—THE "FOLLICULAR" PHASE OF THE OVARIAN CYCLE

Figure 96-5 shows the progressive stages of follicular growth in the ovaries. When a female child is born, each ovum is surrounded by a single layer of granulosa cells; the ovum, with this

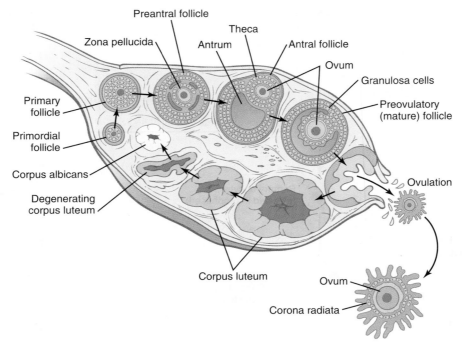

Figure 96-5 Stages of follicular growth in the ovary, also showing formation of the corpus luteum.

granulosa cell sheath, is called a *primordial follicle*, as shown in the figure. Throughout childhood, the granulosa cells are believed to provide nourishment for the ovum and to secrete an *oocyte maturation-inhibiting factor* that keeps the ovum suspended in its primordial state in the prophase stage of meiotic division. Then, after puberty, when FSH and LH from the anterior pituitary gland begin to be secreted in significant quantities, the ovaries (together with some of the follicles within them) begin to grow.

The first stage of follicular growth is moderate enlargement of the ovum, which increases in diameter twofold to threefold. That stage is followed by growth of additional layers of granulosa cells in some of the follicles. These follicles are known as *primary follicles*.

Development of Antral and Vesicular Follicles. During the first few days of each monthly female sexual cycle, the concentrations of both FSH and LH secreted by the anterior pituitary gland increase slightly to moderately, with the increase in FSH slightly greater than that of LH and preceding it by a few days. These hormones, especially FSH, cause accelerated growth of 6–12 primary follicles each month. The initial effect is rapid proliferation of the granulosa cells, giving rise to many more layers of these cells. In addition, spindle cells derived from the ovary interstitium collect in several layers outside the granulosa cells, giving rise to a second mass of cells called the *theca*. The theca is divided into two layers. In the *theca interna*, the cells take on epithelioid characteristics similar to those of the granulosa cells and develop the ability to secrete additional steroid sex hormones (estrogen and progesterone). The outer layer, the *theca externa*, develops into a highly vascular connective tissue capsule that becomes the capsule of the developing follicle.

After the early proliferative phase of growth, which lasts for a few days, the mass of granulosa cells secretes a *follicular fluid* that contains a high concentration of estrogen, one of the important female sex hormones (discussed later). Accumulation of this fluid causes an *antrum* to appear within the mass of granulosa cells, as shown in Figure 96-5.

The early growth of the primary follicle up to the antral stage is stimulated mainly by FSH alone. Greatly accelerated growth then occurs, leading to still larger follicles called *vesicular follicles*. This accelerated growth is caused by the following mechanisms: (1) estrogen is secreted into the follicle and causes the granulosa cells to form increasing numbers of FSH receptors, which causes a positive feedback effect because it makes the granulosa cells even more sensitive to FSH; (2) the pituitary FSH and the estrogens combine to promote LH receptors on the original granulosa cells, thus allowing LH stimulation to occur in addition to FSH stimulation and creating an even more rapid increase in follicular secretion; (3) the increasing estrogens from the follicle plus the increasing LH from the anterior pituitary gland act together to cause proliferation of the follicular thecal cells and increase their secretion as well.

Once the antral follicles begin to grow, their growth occurs almost explosively. The ovum also enlarges in diameter another 3- to 4-fold, giving a total ovum diameter increase up to 10-fold, or a mass increase of 1000-fold. As the follicle enlarges, the ovum remains embedded in a mass of granulosa cells located at one pole of the follicle.

Only One Follicle Fully Matures Each Month and the Remainder Undergoes Atresia. After a week or more of growth—but before ovulation occurs—1 of the follicles begins to outgrow all the others and the remaining 5–11 developing follicles involute (a process called *atresia*); these follicles are said to become *atretic*.

The cause of the atresia is unclear, but it has been postulated to be the following: the large amounts of estrogen from the most rapidly growing follicle act on the hypothalamus to depress further enhancement of FSH secretion by the anterior pituitary gland, in this way blocking further growth of the less well-developed follicles. Therefore, the largest follicle continues to grow because of its intrinsic positive feedback effects, while all the other follicles stop growing and actually involute.

This process of atresia is important because it normally allows only one of the follicles to grow large enough each month to ovulate, which usually prevents more than one child from developing with each pregnancy. The single follicle reaches a diameter of 1–1.5 cm at the time of ovulation and is called the *mature follicle.*

Ovulation

Ovulation in a woman who has a normal 28-day female sexual cycle occurs 14 days after the onset of menstruation. Shortly before ovulation the protruding outer wall of the follicle swells rapidly, and a small area in the center of the follicular capsule, called the *stigma*, protrudes like a nipple. In another 30 minutes or so, fluid begins to ooze from the follicle through the stigma, and about 2 minutes later, the stigma ruptures widely, allowing a more viscous fluid, which has occupied the central portion of the follicle, to evaginate outward. This viscous fluid carries with it the ovum surrounded by a mass of several thousand small granulosa cells, called the *corona radiata.*

A Surge of Luteinizing Hormone Is Necessary for Ovulation. LH is necessary for final follicular growth and ovulation. Without this hormone, even when large quantities of FSH are available, the follicle will not progress to the stage of ovulation.

About 2 days before ovulation (for reasons that are not completely understood but are discussed later in this chapter), the rate of secretion of LH by the anterior pituitary gland increases markedly, rising 6- to 10-fold and peaking about 16 hours before ovulation. FSH also increases about twofold to threefold at the same time, and the FSH and LH act synergistically to cause rapid swelling of the follicle during the last few days before ovulation. The LH also has a specific effect on the granulosa and theca cells, converting them mainly to progesterone-secreting cells. Therefore, the rate of secretion of estrogen begins to fall about 1 day before ovulation, while increasing amounts of progesterone begin to be secreted.

It is in this environment of (1) rapid growth of the follicle, (2) diminishing estrogen secretion after a prolonged phase of excessive estrogen secretion, and (3) initiation of secretion of progesterone that ovulation occurs. Without the initial preovulatory surge of LH, ovulation will not take place.

Initiation of Ovulation. Figure 96-6 provides a schema for the initiation of ovulation, showing the role of the large quantity of LH secreted by the anterior pituitary gland. This LH causes rapid secretion of follicular steroid hormones that contain progesterone. Within a few hours, two events occur, both of which are necessary for ovulation: (1) the *theca externa* (ie, the capsule of the follicle) begins to release proteolytic enzymes from lysosomes and these enzymes cause dissolution of the follicular capsular wall and consequent weakening of the wall, resulting in further swelling of the entire follicle and degeneration of the stigma; (2) simultaneously, there is rapid growth of new blood vessels into the follicle wall, and at the same time, prostaglandins (local hormones that cause vasodilation) are secreted into the follicular tissues. These two effects cause plasma transudation into the follicle, which contributes to follicle swelling. Finally, the combination of follicle swelling and simultaneous degeneration of the stigma causes follicle rupture with discharge of the ovum.

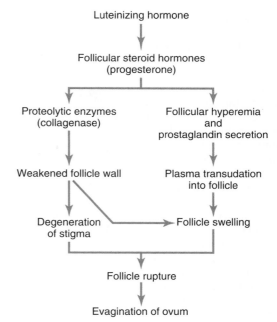

Figure 96-6   The postulated mechanism of ovulation.

CORPUS LUTEUM—THE "LUTEAL" PHASE OF THE OVARIAN CYCLE

During the first few hours after expulsion of the ovum from the follicle, the remaining granulosa and theca interna cells change rapidly into *lutein cells.* They enlarge in diameter two or more times and become filled with lipid inclusions that give them a yellowish appearance. This process is called *luteinization*, and the total mass of cells together is called the *corpus luteum*, which is shown in Figure 96-5. A well-developed vascular supply also grows into the corpus luteum.

The *granulosa cells* in the corpus luteum develop extensive intracellular smooth endoplasmic reticula that form large amounts of the female sex hormones *progesterone* and *estrogen* (with more progesterone than estrogen during the luteal phase). The *theca cells* form mainly the androgens *androstenedione* and *testosterone* rather than female sex hormones. However, most of these hormones are also converted by the enzyme *aromatase* in the granulosa cells into estrogens, the female hormones.

The corpus luteum normally grows to about 1.5 cm in diameter, reaching this stage of development 7–8 days after ovulation. Then the corpus luteum begins to involute and eventually loses its secretory function and its yellowish, lipid characteristic about 12 days after ovulation, becoming the *corpus albicans*; during the ensuing few weeks, the corpus luteum is replaced by connective tissue and over months is absorbed.

Luteinizing Function of Luteinizing Hormone. The change of granulosa and theca interna cells into lutein cells is dependent mainly on LH secreted by the anterior pituitary gland. In fact, this function gives LH its name—"luteinizing," for "yellowing." Luteinization also depends on extrusion of the ovum from the follicle. A yet uncharacterized local hormone in the follicular fluid, called *luteinization-inhibiting factor*, seems to hold the luteinization process in check until after ovulation.

Secretion by the Corpus Luteum: An Additional Function of Luteinizing Hormone. The corpus luteum is a highly secretory organ, secreting large amounts of both *progesterone* and *estrogen.* Once LH (mainly that secreted during the ovulatory surge) has acted on the granulosa and theca cells to cause luteinization, the newly formed lutein cells seem to be programmed to go through a preordained sequence of (1) proliferation, (2) enlargement, and (3) secretion, followed by (4) degeneration. All this occurs in about 12 days. We shall see in the discussion of pregnancy in Chapter 98 that another hormone with almost exactly the same properties as LH, *chorionic gonadotropin*, which is secreted by the placenta, can act on the corpus luteum to prolong its life—usually maintaining it for at least the first 2–4 months of pregnancy.

Involution of the Corpus Luteum and Onset of the Next Ovarian Cycle. Estrogen in particular and progesterone to a lesser extent, secreted by the corpus luteum during the luteal phase of the ovarian cycle, have strong feedback effects on the anterior pituitary gland to maintain low secretory rates of both FSH and LH.

In addition, the lutein cells secrete small amounts of the hormone *inhibin*, the same as the inhibin secreted by the Sertoli cells of the male testes. This hormone inhibits FSH secretion by the anterior pituitary gland. Low blood concentrations of both FSH and LH result, and loss of these hormones finally causes the corpus luteum to degenerate completely, a process called *involution* of the corpus luteum.

Final involution normally occurs at the end of almost exactly 12 days of corpus luteum life, which is around the 26th day of the normal female sexual cycle, 2 days before menstruation begins. At this time, the sudden cessation of secretion of estrogen, progesterone, and inhibin by the corpus luteum removes the feedback inhibition of the anterior pituitary gland, allowing it to begin secreting increasing amounts of FSH and LH again. FSH and LH initiate the growth of new follicles, beginning a new ovarian cycle. The paucity of secretion of progesterone and estrogen at this time also leads to menstruation by the uterus, which will be explained later.

SUMMARY

About every 28 days, gonadotropic hormones from the anterior pituitary gland cause 8–12 new follicles to begin to grow in the ovaries. One of these follicles finally becomes "mature" and ovulates on the 14th day of the cycle. During growth of the follicles, estrogen is mainly secreted.

After ovulation, the secretory cells of the ovulating follicle develop into a corpus luteum that secretes large quantities of the major female hormones, progesterone and estrogen. After another 2 weeks, the corpus luteum degenerates, whereupon the ovarian hormones estrogen and progesterone decrease greatly and menstruation begins. A new ovarian cycle then follows.

MONTHLY ENDOMETRIAL CYCLE AND MENSTRUATION

Associated with the monthly cyclic production of estrogens and progesterone by the ovaries is an endometrial cycle in the lining of the uterus that operates through the following stages: (1) proliferation of the uterine endometrium; (2) development of secretory changes in the endometrium; and (3) desquamation of the endometrium, which is known as *menstruation*. The various phases of this endometrial cycle are shown in Figure 96-7.

Proliferative Phase (Estrogen Phase) of the Endometrial Cycle, Occurring Before Ovulation. At the beginning of each monthly cycle, most of the endometrium has been desquamated by menstruation. After menstruation, only a thin layer

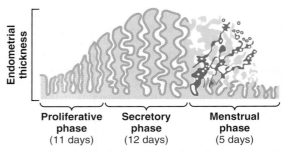

Figure 96-7 Phases of endometrial growth and menstruation during each monthly female sexual cycle.

of endometrial stroma remains and the only epithelial cells that are left are those located in the remaining deeper portions of the glands and crypts of the endometrium. *Under the influence of estrogens*, secreted in increasing quantities by the ovary during the first part of the monthly ovarian cycle, the stromal cells and the epithelial cells proliferate rapidly. The endometrial surface is reepithelialized within 4–7 days after the beginning of menstruation.

Then, during the next week and a half, before ovulation occurs, the endometrium increases greatly in thickness, owing to increasing numbers of stromal cells and to progressive growth of the endometrial glands and new blood vessels into the endometrium. At the time of ovulation, the endometrium is 3–5 mm thick.

The endometrial glands, especially those of the cervical region, secrete a thin, stringy mucus. The mucus strings actually align themselves along the length of the cervical canal, forming channels that help guide sperm in the proper direction from the vagina into the uterus.

Secretory Phase (Progestational Phase) of the Endometrial Cycle, Occurring After Ovulation. During most of the latter half of the monthly cycle, after ovulation has occurred, progesterone and estrogen together are secreted in large quantities by the corpus luteum. The estrogens cause slight additional cellular proliferation in the endometrium during this phase of the cycle, whereas progesterone causes marked swelling and secretory development of the endometrium. The glands increase in tortuosity and an excess of secretory substances accumulates in the glandular epithelial cells. In addition, the cytoplasm of the stromal cells increases; lipid and glycogen deposits increase greatly in the stromal cells; and the blood supply to the endometrium further increases in proportion to the developing secretory activity, with the blood vessels becoming highly tortuous. At the peak of the secretory phase, about 1 week after ovulation, the endometrium has a thickness of 5–6 mm.

The whole purpose of all these endometrial changes is to produce a highly secretory endometrium that contains large amounts of stored nutrients to provide appropriate conditions for implantation of a *fertilized* ovum during the latter half of the monthly cycle. From the time a fertilized ovum enters the uterine cavity from the fallopian tube (which occurs 3–4 days after ovulation) until the time the ovum implants (7–9 days after ovulation), the uterine secretions, called "uterine milk," provide nutrition for the early dividing ovum. Then, once the ovum implants in the endometrium, the trophoblastic cells on the surface of the implanting ovum (in the blastocyst stage) begin to digest the endometrium and absorb the endometrial stored substances, thus making great quantities of nutrients available to the early implanting embryo.

Menstruation. If the ovum is not fertilized, about 2 days before the end of the monthly cycle, the corpus luteum in the ovary involutes and the ovarian hormones (estrogens and progesterone) decrease to low levels of secretion, as shown in Figure 96-4. Menstruation follows.

Menstruation is caused by the reduction of estrogens and progesterone, especially progesterone, at the end of the monthly ovarian cycle. The first effect is decreased stimulation of the endometrial cells by these two hormones, followed rapidly by involution of the endometrium to about 65% of its previous thickness. Then, during the 24 hours preceding the onset of menstruation, the tortuous blood vessels leading to the mucosal layers of the endometrium become vasospastic, presumably because of some effect of involution, such as release of a vasoconstrictor material—possibly one of the vasoconstrictor types of prostaglandins that are present in abundance at this time.

The vasospasm, the decrease in nutrients to the endometrium, and the loss of hormonal stimulation initiate necrosis in the endometrium, especially of the blood vessels. As a result, blood at first seeps into the vascular layer of the endometrium and the hemorrhagic areas grow rapidly over a period of 24–36 hours. Gradually, the necrotic outer layers of the endometrium separate from the uterus at the sites of the hemorrhages until, about 48 hours after the onset of menstruation, all the superficial layers of the endometrium have desquamated. The mass of desquamated tissue and blood in the uterine cavity, plus contractile effects of prostaglandins or other substances in the decaying desquamate, all acting together, initiate uterine contractions that expel the uterine contents.

During normal menstruation, approximately 40 mL of blood and an additional 35 mL of serous fluid are lost. The menstrual fluid is normally nonclotting because a *fibrinolysin* is released along with the necrotic endometrial material. If excessive bleeding occurs from the uterine surface, the quantity of fibrinolysin may not be sufficient to prevent clotting. The presence of clots during menstruation is often clinical evidence of uterine disease.

Within 4–7 days after menstruation starts, the loss of blood ceases because, by this time, the endometrium has become reepithelialized.

Leukorrhea During Menstruation. During menstruation, large numbers of leukocytes are released along with the necrotic material and blood. A substance liberated by the endometrial necrosis likely causes this outflow of leukocytes. As a result of these leukocytes and possibly other factors, the uterus is highly resistant to infection during menstruation, even though the endometrial surfaces are denuded. This resistance to infection is of extreme protective value.

Regulation of the Female Monthly Rhythm—Interplay Between the Ovarian and Hypothalamic–Pituitary Hormones

Now that we have presented the major cyclic changes that occur during the monthly female sexual cycle, we can attempt to explain the basic rhythmic mechanism that causes the cyclic variations.

THE HYPOTHALAMUS SECRETES GnRH, WHICH CAUSES THE ANTERIOR PITUITARY GLAND TO SECRETE LH AND FSH

As pointed out in Chapter 86, secretion of most of the anterior pituitary hormones is controlled by "releasing hormones" formed in the hypothalamus and then transported to the anterior pituitary gland by way of the hypothalamic–hypophysial portal system. In the case of the gonadotropins, one releasing hormone, *GnRH*, is important. This hormone has been purified and has been found to be a decapeptide with the following formula:

$$Glu - His - Trp - Ser - Tyr - Gly - Leu - Arg - Pro - Gly - NH_2$$

Intermittent, Pulsatile Secretion of GnRH by the Hypothalamus Stimulates Pulsatile Release of LH from the Anterior Pituitary Gland. The hypothalamus does not secrete GnRH continuously but instead secretes it in pulses lasting 5 to 25 minutes that occur every 1–2 hours. The lower curve in Figure 96-8 shows the electrical pulsatile signals in the hypothalamus that cause the hypothalamic pulsatile output of GnRH.

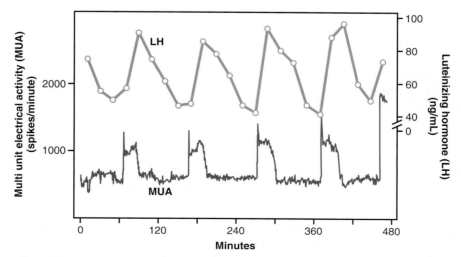

Figure 96-8 *(Red line)* Pulsatile change in luteinizing hormone (LH) in the peripheral circulation of a pentobarbital-anesthetized ovariectomized rhesus monkey. *(Blue line)* Minute-by-minute recording of multiunit electrical activity (MUA) in the mediobasal hypothalamus. *Data from Wilson, R.C., Kesner, J.S., Kaufman, J.M., et al., 1984. Central electrophysiologic correlates of pulsatile luteinizing hormone secretion. Neuroendocrinology 39, 256.*

It is intriguing that when GnRH is infused continuously so that it is available all the time rather than in pulses, its ability to cause the release of LH and FSH by the anterior pituitary gland is lost. Therefore, for reasons that are unknown, the pulsatile nature of GnRH release is essential to its function.

The pulsatile release of GnRH also causes intermittent output of LH secretion about every 90 minutes, which is shown by the upper curve in Figure 96-8.

Hypothalamic Centers for Release of Gonadotropin-Releasing Hormone. The neuronal activity that causes pulsatile release of GnRH occurs primarily in the mediobasal hypothalamus, especially in the arcuate nuclei of this area. Therefore, it is believed that these arcuate nuclei control most female sexual activity, although neurons located in the preoptic area of the anterior hypothalamus also secrete GnRH in moderate amounts. Multiple neuronal centers in the higher brain's "limbic" system (the system for psychic control) transmit signals into the arcuate nuclei to modify both the intensity of GnRH release and the frequency of the pulses, thus providing a partial explanation of why psychic factors often modify female sexual function.

NEGATIVE FEEDBACK EFFECTS OF ESTROGEN AND PROGESTERONE TO DECREASE LH AND FSH SECRETION

Estrogen in small amounts has a strong inhibitory effect on the production of both LH and FSH. Also, when progesterone is available, the inhibitory effect of estrogen is multiplied, even though progesterone by itself has little effect (Figure 96-9).

These feedback effects seem to operate mainly on the anterior pituitary gland directly, but they also operate to a lesser extent on the hypothalamus to decrease secretion of GnRH, especially by altering the frequency of the GnRH pulses.

Inhibin from the Corpus Luteum Inhibits Follicle-Stimulating Hormone and Luteinizing Hormone Secretion. In addition to the feedback effects of estrogen and progesterone, other hormones seem to be involved, especially *inhibin*, which is secreted along with the steroid sex hormones by the granulosa cells of the ovarian corpus luteum in the same way that Sertoli cells secrete inhibin in the male testes (see Figure 96-9). This hormone has the same effect in the female as in the male, that is, inhibiting the secretion of FSH and, to a lesser extent, LH by the anterior pituitary gland. Therefore, it is believed that inhibin might be especially important in causing the decrease in secretion of FSH and LH at the end of the monthly female sexual cycle.

POSITIVE FEEDBACK EFFECT OF ESTROGEN BEFORE OVULATION—THE PREOVULATORY LUTEINIZING HORMONE SURGE

For reasons that are not completely understood, the anterior pituitary gland secretes greatly increased amounts of LH for 1–2 days beginning 24–48 hours before ovulation. This effect is demonstrated in Figure 96-4. The figure shows a much smaller preovulatory surge of FSH as well.

Experiments have shown that infusion of estrogen into a female above a critical rate for 2–3 days during the latter part of the first half of the ovarian cycle will cause rapidly accelerating growth of the ovarian follicles, as well as rapidly accelerating secretion of ovarian estrogens. During this period, secretions of both FSH and LH by the anterior pituitary gland are at first slightly suppressed. Secretion of LH then increases abruptly

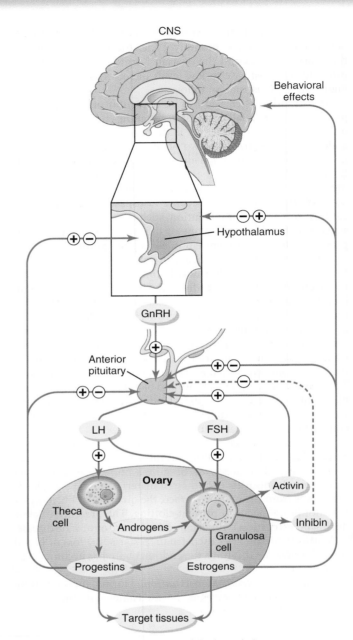

Figure 96-9 Feedback regulation of the hypothalamic–pituitary–ovarian axis in females. Stimulatory effects are shown by plus signs, and negative feedback inhibitory effects are shown by minus signs. Estrogens and progestins exert both negative and positive feedback effects on the anterior pituitary and hypothalamus depending on the stage of the ovarian cycle. Inhibin has a negative feedback effect on the anterior pituitary, whereas activin has the opposite effect, stimulating FSH secretion by the anterior pituitary. *CNS*, central nervous system; *FSH*, follicle-stimulating hormone; *GnRH*, gonadotropin-releasing hormone; *LH*, luteinizing hormone.

sixfold to eightfold, and secretion of FSH increases about twofold. The greatly increased secretion of LH causes ovulation to occur.

The cause of this abrupt surge in LH secretion is not known. However, the following explanations are possible: (1) it has been suggested that at this point in the cycle estrogen has a peculiar *positive feedback* effect of stimulating pituitary secretion of LH and, to a lesser extent, FSH (see Figure 96-9), which is in sharp contrast to the normal negative feedback of estrogen that occurs during the remainder of the female monthly cycle; (2) the granulosa cells of the follicles begin to secrete small but increasing quantities of progesterone a day or so before the preovulatory LH surge, and it has been suggested that this secretion might be the factor that stimulates the excess LH secretion.

Without this normal preovulatory surge of LH, ovulation will not occur.

FEEDBACK OSCILLATION OF THE HYPOTHALAMIC–PITUITARY–OVARIAN SYSTEM

The feedback oscillation that controls the rhythm of the female sexual cycle seems to operate in approximately the following sequence of three events:

1. *Postovulatory secretion of the ovarian hormones, and depression of the pituitary gonadotropins.* Between ovulation and the beginning of menstruation the corpus luteum secretes large quantities of progesterone and estrogen, as well as the hormone inhibin. All these hormones together have a combined negative feedback effect on the anterior pituitary gland and hypothalamus, causing the suppression of both FSH and LH secretion. These effects are shown in Figure 96-4.
2. *Follicular growth phase.* Two to 3 days before menstruation, the corpus luteum has regressed to almost total involution and the secretion of estrogen, progesterone, and inhibin from the corpus luteum decreases to a low ebb, which releases the hypothalamus and anterior pituitary from the negative feedback effect of these hormones. Therefore, a day or so later, at about the time that menstruation begins, pituitary secretion of FSH begins to increase again, as much as twofold; then, several days after menstruation begins, LH secretion increases slightly as well. These hormones initiate new ovarian follicle growth and a progressive increase in the secretion of estrogen, reaching a peak estrogen secretion at about 12.5–13 days after the onset of the new female monthly sexual cycle. During the first 11–12 days of this follicle growth, the rates of pituitary secretion of the gonadotropins, FSH and LH, decrease slightly because of the negative feedback effect, mainly of estrogen, on the anterior pituitary gland. Then there is a sudden, marked increase in the secretion of LH and, to a lesser extent, FSH. This increased secretion is the preovulatory surge of LH and FSH, which is followed by ovulation.
3. *Preovulatory surge of LH and FSH causes ovulation.* About 11.5–12 days after the onset of the monthly cycle, the decline in secretion of FSH and LH comes to an abrupt halt. The high level of estrogens at this time (or the beginning of progesterone secretion by the follicles) is believed to cause a positive feedback stimulatory effect on the anterior pituitary, as explained earlier, which leads to a large surge in the secretion of LH and, to a lesser extent, FSH. Whatever the cause of this preovulatory LH and FSH surge, the great excess of LH leads to both ovulation and subsequent development of and secretion by the corpus luteum. Thus, the hormonal system begins its new round of secretions until the next instance of ovulation.

Anovulatory Cycles—Sexual Cycles at Puberty

If the preovulatory surge of LH is not of sufficient magnitude, ovulation will not occur and the cycle is said to be "anovulatory." The phases of the sexual cycle continue, but they are altered in the following ways: First, lack of ovulation causes failure of development of the corpus luteum, so there is almost no secretion of progesterone during the latter portion of the cycle. Second, the cycle is shortened by several days but the rhythm continues. Therefore, it is likely that progesterone is not required for maintenance of the cycle itself, although it can alter the cycle's rhythm.

The first few cycles after the onset of puberty are usually anovulatory, as are the cycles occurring several months to years before menopause, presumably because the LH surge is not potent enough at these times to cause ovulation.

Tests of Ovulation. There are several tests that indicate if ovulation has taken place. These include:

1. Maintenance of a basal body temperature chart. Here temperature is recorded every morning before getting out of bed. Following ovulation there is a small increment in the temperature of 0.5°F due to the thermogenic effect of progesterone (Figure 96-10).
2. Physical testing of the cervical mucus. This becomes profuse and tenacious at the time of ovulation so that the mucus can be stretched between the fingers—a property called "spinnbarkeit."
3. Microscopic evaluation of the cervical mucus reveals a "ferning" pattern around the time of ovulation.
4. Hormonal tests include the measurement of LH around the expected time of ovulation to capture the LH surge and the measurement of progesterone levels (in blood or urine; pregnanediol) during the luteal phase.

Functions of the Ovarian Hormones— Estradiol and Progesterone

The two types of ovarian sex hormones are the *estrogens* and the *progestins*. By far the most important of the estrogens is the hormone *estradiol*, and by far the most important progestin is *progesterone*. The estrogens mainly promote proliferation and growth of specific cells in the body that are responsible for the development of most secondary sexual characteristics of the female. The progestins function mainly to prepare the uterus for pregnancy and the breasts for lactation.

CHEMISTRY OF THE SEX HORMONES

Estrogens. In the normal *nonpregnant* female, estrogens are secreted in significant quantities only by the ovaries, although

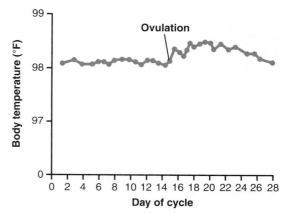

Figure 96-10 Elevation in body temperature shortly after ovulation.

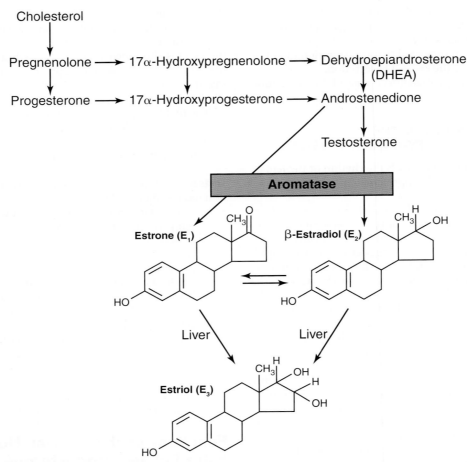

Figure 96-11 Synthesis of the principal female hormones. The chemical structures of the precursor hormones, including progesterone, are shown in Figure 91-3.

minute amounts are also secreted by the adrenal cortices. During *pregnancy*, large quantities of estrogens are also secreted by the placenta, as discussed in Chapter 98.

Only three estrogens are present in significant quantities in the plasma of the human female: β-*estradiol*, *estrone*, and *estriol*, the formulas for which are shown in Figure 96-11. The principal estrogen secreted by the ovaries is β-estradiol. The estrogenic potency of β-estradiol is 12 times that of estrone and 80 times that of estriol. Considering these relative potencies, one can see that the total estrogenic effect of β-estradiol is usually many times that of the other two together. For this reason, β-estradiol is considered the major estrogen, although the estrogenic effects of estrone are not negligible.

Progestins. By far the most important of the progestins is progesterone. However, small amounts of another progestin, 17-α-hydroxyprogesterone, are secreted along with progesterone and have essentially the same effects. Yet for practical purposes, it is usually reasonable to consider progesterone to be the only important progestin.

In the nonpregnant female, progesterone is usually secreted in significant amounts only during the latter half of each ovarian cycle, when it is secreted by the corpus luteum.

As we shall see in Chapter 98, large amounts of progesterone are also secreted by the placenta during pregnancy, especially after the fourth month of gestation.

Synthesis of the Estrogens and Progestins. Estrogens and progesterone are all steroids. They are synthesized in the ovaries mainly from cholesterol derived from the blood but also to a slight extent from acetyl coenzyme A, multiple molecules of which can combine to form the appropriate steroid nucleus.

During synthesis, mainly progesterone and androgens (testosterone and androstenedione) are synthesized first; then, during the follicular phase of the ovarian cycle, before these two initial hormones can leave the ovaries, almost all the androgens and much of the progesterone are converted into estrogens by the enzyme aromatase in the granulosa cells. Because the theca cells lack aromatase, they cannot convert androgens to estrogens. However, androgens diffuse out of the theca cells into the adjacent granulosa cells, where they are converted to estrogens by aromatase, the activity of which is stimulated by FSH (Figure 96-12).

During the luteal phase of the cycle, far too much progesterone is formed for all of it to be converted, which accounts for the large secretion of progesterone into the circulating blood at this time. Also, about one-fifteenth as much testosterone is secreted into the plasma of the female by the ovaries as is secreted into the plasma of the male by the testes.

Estrogens and Progesterone Are Transported in the Blood Bound to Plasma Proteins. Both estrogens and progesterone are transported in the blood bound mainly with plasma albumin and with specific estrogen- and progesterone-binding globulins. The binding between these hormones and the plasma proteins is loose enough that they are rapidly released to the tissues over a period of 30 minutes or so.

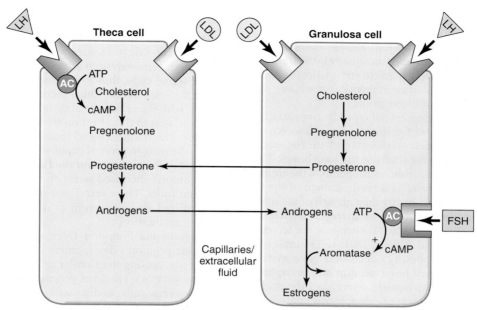

Figure 96-12 Interaction of follicular theca and granulosa cells for production of estrogens. The theca cells, under the control of luteinizing hormone (LH), produce androgens that diffuse into the granulosa cells. In mature follicles, follicle-stimulating hormone (FSH) acts on granulosa cells to stimulate aromatase activity, which converts the androgens to estrogens. *AC,* adenylate cyclase; *ATP,* adenosine triphosphate; *cAMP,* cyclic adenosine monophosphate; *LDL,* low-density lipoproteins.

Functions of the Liver in Estrogen Degradation. The liver conjugates the estrogens to form glucuronides and sulfates, and about one-fifth of these conjugated products is excreted in the bile; most of the remainder is excreted in the urine. Also, the liver converts the potent estrogens, estradiol and estrone, into the almost totally impotent estrogen estriol. Therefore, diminished liver function actually *increases* the activity of estrogens in the body, sometimes causing *hyperestrinism.*

Fate of Progesterone. Within a few minutes after secretion, almost all the progesterone is degraded to other steroids that have no progestational effect. As with the estrogens, the liver is especially important for this metabolic degradation.

The major end product of progesterone degradation is *pregnanediol.* About 10% of the original progesterone is excreted in the urine in this form. Therefore, one can estimate the rate of progesterone formation in the body from the rate of this excretion.

FUNCTIONS OF THE ESTROGENS—THEIR EFFECTS ON THE PRIMARY AND SECONDARY FEMALE SEX CHARACTERISTICS

A primary function of the estrogens is to cause cellular proliferation and growth of the tissues of the sex organs and other tissues related to reproduction.

Effect of Estrogens on the Uterus and External Female Sex Organs. During childhood, estrogens are secreted only in minute quantities, but at puberty, the quantity secreted in the female under the influence of the pituitary gonadotropic hormones increases 20-fold or more. At this time, the female sex organs change from those of a child to those of an adult. The ovaries, fallopian tubes, uterus, and vagina all increase several times in size. Also, the external genitalia enlarge, with deposition of fat in the mons pubis and labia majora and enlargement of the labia minora.

In addition, estrogens change the vaginal epithelium from a cuboidal into a stratified type, which is considerably more resistant to trauma and infection than is the prepubertal cuboidal cell epithelium. Vaginal infections in children can often be cured by the administration of estrogens simply because of the resulting increased resistance of the vaginal epithelium.

During the first few years after puberty, the size of the uterus increases twofold to threefold, but more important than the increase in uterus size are the changes that take place in the uterine endometrium under the influence of estrogens. Estrogens cause marked proliferation of the endometrial stroma and greatly increased development of the endometrial glands, which will later aid in providing nutrition to the implanted ovum. These effects are discussed later in the chapter in connection with the endometrial cycle.

Effect of Estrogens on the Fallopian Tubes. The estrogens' effect on the mucosal lining of the fallopian tubes is similar to their effects on the uterine endometrium. They cause the glandular tissues of this lining to proliferate and, especially important, they cause the number of ciliated epithelial cells that line the fallopian tubes to increase. Also, activity of the cilia is considerably enhanced. These cilia always beat toward the uterus, which helps propel the fertilized ovum in that direction.

Effect of Estrogens on the Breasts. The primordial breasts of females and males are exactly alike. In fact, under the influence of appropriate hormones, the masculine breast during the first two decades of life can develop sufficiently to produce milk in the same manner as the female breast.

Estrogens cause (1) development of the stromal tissues of the breasts, (2) growth of an extensive ductile system, and (3) deposition of fat in the breasts. The lobules and alveoli of the breast develop to a slight extent under the influence of estrogens alone, but it is progesterone and prolactin that cause the ultimate determinative growth and function of these structures.

In summary, the estrogens initiate growth of the breasts and of the milk-producing apparatus. They are also responsible for the characteristic growth and external appearance of the mature female breast. However, they do not complete the job of converting the breasts into milk-producing organs.

Effect of Estrogens on the Skeleton. Estrogens inhibit osteoclastic activity in the bones and therefore stimulate bone growth. At least part of this effect is due to stimulation of *osteoprotegerin*, which is also called *osteoclastogenesis-inhibitory factor*, a cytokine that inhibits bone resorption.

At puberty, when the female enters her reproductive years, her growth in height becomes rapid for several years. However, estrogens have another potent effect on skeletal growth. They cause uniting of the epiphyses with the shafts of the long bones. This effect of estrogen in the female is much stronger than the similar effect of testosterone in the male. As a result, growth of the female usually ceases several years earlier than growth of the male.

Osteoporosis of the Bones Caused by Estrogen Deficiency in Old Age. After menopause, almost no estrogens are secreted by the ovaries. This estrogen deficiency leads to (1) increased osteoclastic activity in the bones, (2) decreased bone matrix, and (3) decreased deposition of bone calcium and phosphate. In some women this effect is extremely severe, and the resulting condition is *osteoporosis*. Because osteoporosis can greatly weaken the bones and lead to bone fracture, especially fracture of the vertebrae, many postmenopausal women are treated prophylactically with estrogen replacement to prevent the osteoporotic effects.

Estrogens Slightly Increase Protein Deposition. Estrogens cause a slight increase in total body protein, which is evidenced by a slight positive nitrogen balance when estrogens are administered. The enhanced protein deposition caused by testosterone is much more general and much more powerful than that caused by estrogens.

Estrogens Increase Body Metabolism and Fat Deposition. Estrogens increase the whole-body metabolic rate slightly, but only about one-third as much as the increase caused by the male sex hormone testosterone. Estrogens also cause deposition of increased quantities of fat in the subcutaneous tissues. As a result, the percentage of body fat in the female body is considerably greater than that in the male body, which contains more protein. In addition to deposition of fat in the breasts and subcutaneous tissues, estrogens cause the deposition of fat in the buttocks and thighs, which is characteristic of the feminine figure.

Estrogens Have Little Effect on Hair Distribution. Estrogens do not greatly affect hair distribution. However, hair does develop in the pubic region and in the axillae after puberty. Androgens formed in increased quantities by the female adrenal glands after puberty are mainly responsible for this development of hair.

Effect of Estrogens on the Skin. Estrogens cause the skin to develop a texture that is soft and usually smooth, but even so, the skin of a woman is thicker than that of a child or a castrated female. Estrogens also cause the skin to become more vascular, which is often associated with increased warmth of the skin and also promotes greater bleeding of cut surfaces than is observed in men.

Effect of Estrogens on Electrolyte Balance. The chemical similarity of estrogenic hormones to adrenocortical hormones has been pointed out. Estrogens, like aldosterone and some other adrenocortical hormones, cause sodium and water retention by the kidney tubules. This effect of estrogens is normally slight and rarely of significance, but during pregnancy, the tremendous formation of estrogens by the placenta may contribute to body fluid retention in pregnancy (see Chapter 98).

FUNCTIONS OF PROGESTERONE

Progesterone Promotes Secretory Changes in the Uterus. A major function of progesterone is *to promote secretory changes in the uterine endometrium* during the latter half of the monthly female sexual cycle, thus preparing the uterus for implantation of the fertilized ovum. This function is discussed later in connection with the endometrial cycle of the uterus.

In addition to this effect on the endometrium, progesterone decreases the frequency and intensity of uterine contractions, thereby helping to prevent expulsion of the implanted ovum.

Effect of Progesterone on the Fallopian Tubes. Progesterone also promotes increased secretion by the mucosal lining of the fallopian tubes. These secretions are necessary for nutrition of the fertilized, dividing ovum as it traverses the fallopian tube before implantation.

Progesterone Promotes Development of the Breasts. Progesterone promotes development of the lobules and alveoli of the breasts, causing the alveolar cells to proliferate, enlarge, and become secretory. However, progesterone does not cause the alveoli to secrete milk; as discussed in Chapter 99 milk is secreted only after the prepared breast is further stimulated by *prolactin* from the anterior pituitary gland.

Progesterone also causes the breasts to swell. Part of this swelling is due to the secretory development in the lobules and alveoli, but part also results from increased fluid in the tissue.

Puberty and Menarche

Puberty means the onset of adult sexual life, and *menarche* means the beginning of the cycle of menstruation. The period of puberty is caused by a gradual increase in gonadotropic hormone secretion by the pituitary, beginning in about the eighth year of life, as shown in Figure 96-13, and usually culminating in the onset of puberty and menstruation between ages 11 and 16 years in girls (average, 13 years).

In the female, as in the male, the infantile pituitary gland and ovaries are capable of full function if they are appropriately stimulated. However, as is also true in the male, and for reasons that are not understood, the hypothalamus does not secrete significant quantities of GnRH during childhood. Experiments have shown that the hypothalamus is capable of secreting this hormone, but the appropriate signal from some other area of

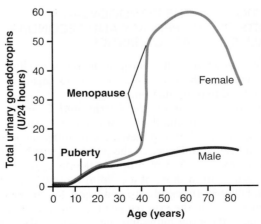

Figure 96-13 Total rates of secretion of gonadotropic hormones throughout the sexual lives of female and male human beings, showing an especially abrupt increase in gonadotropic hormones at menopause in the female.

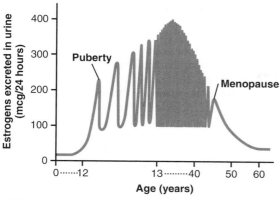

Figure 96-14 Estrogen secretion throughout the sexual life of the female human being.

the brain to cause the secretion is lacking. Therefore, it is now believed that the onset of puberty is initiated by some maturation process that occurs elsewhere in the brain, perhaps somewhere in the limbic system.

Figure 96-14 shows (1) the increasing levels of estrogen secretion at puberty, (2) the cyclic variation during the monthly sexual cycle, (3) the further increase in estrogen secretion during the first few years of reproductive life, (4) the progressive decrease in estrogen secretion toward the end of reproductive life, and, finally, (5) almost no estrogen or progesterone secretion beyond menopause.

Menopause

At age 40–50 years, the sexual cycle usually becomes irregular and ovulation often fails to occur. After a few months to a few years, the cycle ceases altogether, as shown in Figure 96-14. The period during which the cycle ceases and the female sex hormones diminish to almost none is called *menopause*.

The cause of menopause is "burning out" of the ovaries. Throughout a woman's reproductive life, about 400 of the primordial follicles grow into mature follicles and ovulate, and hundreds of thousands of ova degenerate. At about age 45 years, only a few primordial follicles remain to be stimulated by FSH and LH, and, as shown in Figure 96-14, the production of estrogens by the ovaries decreases as the number of primordial follicles approaches zero. When estrogen production falls below a critical value, the estrogens can no longer inhibit the production of the gonadotropins FSH and LH. Instead, as shown in Figure 96-13, the gonadotropins FSH and LH (mainly FSH) are produced after menopause in large and continuous quantities, but as the remaining primordial follicles become atretic, the production of estrogens by the ovaries falls virtually to zero.

At the time of menopause, a woman must readjust her life from one that has been physiologically stimulated by estrogen and progesterone production to one devoid of these hormones. The loss of estrogens often causes marked physiological changes in the function of the body, including (1) "hot flushes" characterized by extreme flushing of the skin, (2) psychic sensations of dyspnea, (3) irritability, (4) fatigue, (5) anxiety, and (6) decreased strength and calcification of bones throughout the body. These symptoms are of sufficient magnitude in about 15% of women to warrant treatment. Daily estrogen in small quantities usually reverses the symptoms, and by gradually decreasing the dose, postmenopausal women can likely avoid severe symptoms.

Large clinical trials have provided evidence that administration of estrogen after menopause, although ameliorating many of the symptoms of menopause, may increase the risk for cardiovascular disease. As a result, hormone replacement therapy with estrogen is no longer routinely prescribed for postmenopausal women. Some studies, however, suggest that estrogen therapy may actually reduce the risk for cardiovascular disease if it is begun early in the postmenopausal years. Therefore, it is currently recommended that postmenopausal women who are considering hormone replacement therapy should discuss with their physicians whether the benefits outweigh the risks.

Rhythm Method of Contraception

FERTILE PERIOD OF EACH SEXUAL CYCLE

The ovum remains viable and capable of being fertilized probably no longer than 24 hours after it is expelled from the ovary. Therefore, sperm must be available soon after ovulation if fertilization is to take place. A few sperm can remain fertile in the female reproductive tract for up to 5 days. Therefore, for fertilization to take place, intercourse must occur sometime between 4 and 5 days before ovulation up to a few hours after ovulation. Thus, the period of female fertility during each month is short—about 4–5 days.

ABSTINENCE FROM SEXUAL INTERCOURSE DURING THE FERTILE PERIOD IS THE BASIS OF THE RHYTHM METHOD OF FAMILY PLANNING

One commonly practiced method of contraception is to avoid intercourse near the time of ovulation. The difficulty with this method of contraception is predicting the exact time of ovulation. Yet the interval from ovulation until the next succeeding onset of menstruation is almost always between 13 and 15 days. Therefore, if the menstrual cycle is regular, with an exact periodicity of 28 days, ovulation usually occurs within 1 day of the 14th day of the cycle. If, in contrast, the periodicity of the cycle is 40 days, ovulation usually occurs within 1 day of the 26th day of the cycle. Finally, if the periodicity of the cycle is 21 days, ovulation usually occurs within 1 day of the 7th day of the cycle. Therefore, it is usually stated that avoidance of intercourse for 4 days before the calculated day of ovulation and 3 days afterward prevents conception. However, such a method of contraception can be used only when the periodicity of the menstrual cycle is regular. The failure rate of this method of contraception, resulting in an unintentional pregnancy, may be as high as 20–25% per year.

Hormonal Suppression of Fertility— "The Pill"

It has long been known that administration of either estrogen or progesterone, if given in appropriate quantities during the first half of the monthly cycle, can inhibit ovulation. The reason for this is that appropriate administration of either of these hormones can prevent the preovulatory surge of LH secretion by the pituitary gland, which is essential in causing ovulation.

It is not clearly understood why administration of estrogen or progesterone prevents the preovulatory surge of LH secretion. However, experimental work has suggested that immediately before the surge occurs, a sudden depression of estrogen secretion by the ovarian follicles probably occurs, which might be the necessary signal that causes the subsequent feedback effect on the anterior pituitary that leads to the LH surge. The administration of sex hormones (estrogens or progesterone) could prevent the initial ovarian hormonal depression that might be the initiating signal for ovulation.

The challenge in devising methods for the hormonal suppression of ovulation has been in developing appropriate combinations of estrogens and progestins that suppress ovulation but do not cause other, unwanted effects. For instance, too much of either hormone can cause abnormal menstrual bleeding patterns. However, use of certain synthetic progestins in place of progesterone, especially the 19-norsteroids, along with small amounts of estrogens usually prevents ovulation yet allows an almost normal pattern of menstruation. Therefore, almost all "pills" used for the control of fertility consist of some combination of synthetic estrogens and synthetic progestins. The main reason for using synthetic estrogens and progestins

is that the *natural* hormones are almost entirely destroyed by the liver within a short time after they are absorbed from the gastrointestinal tract into the portal circulation. However, many of the *synthetic* hormones can resist this destructive propensity of the liver, thus allowing oral administration.

Two of the most commonly used synthetic estrogens are *ethinyl estradiol* and *mestranol*. Among the most commonly used progestins are *norethindrone*, *norethynodrel*, *ethynodiol*, and *norgestrel*. The drug is usually begun in the early stages of the monthly cycle and continued beyond the time that ovulation would normally occur. Then the drug is stopped, allowing menstruation to occur and a new cycle to begin.

The failure rate, resulting in an unintentional pregnancy, for hormonal suppression of fertility using various forms of the "pill" is about 8–9% per year.

Table 96-1 provides a brief summary of various methods of contraception in the female and male.

TABLE 96-1	Summary of Methods of Contraception in the Male and Female			
Method	**Process**	**Mechanism**	**Advantages**	**Disadvantages**
IN THE FEMALE				
Natural family planning	Sexual abstinence during the "fertile" phase of the menstrual cycle	The limited viability of the ovum and the limited duration of the survival of sperm is the basis of this method	Empowers the woman to make decisions Cost-effective No externally administered hormones	Higher failure rate Difficult for women with irregular menstrual cycles
Diaphragm, cervical cap, female condom	Positioned prior to sexual intercourse	Barrier to the meeting of ovum and sperm	Woman in charge of placement No hormones	Can be improperly used with increase in failure of contraception Availability at time of intercourse
Intrauterine device	A T or other shaped device is placed in the uterus	May contain copper or a progestin Thickens the cervical mucus/reduces chances of fertilization or implantation	Long acting—can be kept in place for several years Suitable for women who cannot take estrogen	Insertion may be uncomfortable or painful Small risk of infection May "fall" out of the uterus
Contraceptive pill	May contain progestin only (minipill) or both estrogen and progestin (combined pill) Taken daily	Prevents release of ovum Thickens cervical mucus Prevents implantation	Depends on the type of pill used Minipill can be used in women who cannot take estrogen Combined pill can reduce menstrual cramps and regulate the menstrual cycle	Depends on the type of pill used Minipill associated with headaches, breast tenderness, acne Combined pill increases the risk of blood clots
Contraceptive injection	Injection of progesterone given once in 12–13 weeks	Prevents an ovum being released Thickens cervical mucus Changes the uterine surface to prevent implantation	Daily contraceptive methods not required (four injections a year) Suitable for women who cannot take estrogen	Once stopped, release of ovum takes several months Menstrual cycles may be irregular Gain in weight
Tubectomy	Surgical section/closure/block of the fallopian tube	Does not allow ovum and sperm to meet—prevents fertilization	Permanent No hormones No significant long-term side effects	Later regret Difficult to reverse Possible short-term complications of surgery
IN THE MALE				
Male condom	Placed over the erect penis during intercourse	Barrier to the movement of sperm into the female genital tract	Inexpensive Allows male to assume responsibility for birth control Protects against sexually transmitted diseases	Availability at intercourse May slip or break during intercourse Some are allergic to latex
Withdrawal (coitus interruptus)	Man withdraws penis prior to ejaculation	Sperm does not enter the female genital tract	Cost-effective Can be used in the absence of other methods	Risky, requires self-control, higher failure rate
Vasectomy	Surgical procedure to close or block the vas deferens	Sperm is not released into the female genital tract	Permanent Less invasive than tubectomy No significant long-term effects	Later regret Difficult to reverse Possible short-term complications of surgery

Abnormal Conditions that Cause Female Sterility

About 5–10% of women are infertile. Occasionally, no abnormality can be discovered in the female genital organs, in which case it must be assumed that the infertility is due to either abnormal physiological function of the genital system or abnormal genetic development of the ova themselves.

The most common cause of female sterility is failure to ovulate. This failure can result from hyposecretion of gonadotropic hormones, in which case the intensity of the hormonal stimuli is simply insufficient to cause ovulation, or it can result from abnormal ovaries that do not allow ovulation. For instance, thick ovarian capsules occasionally exist on the outsides of the ovaries, making ovulation difficult. Because of the high incidence of anovulation in sterile women, special methods are often used to determine whether ovulation occurs; these have been described earlier.

Lack of ovulation caused by hyposecretion of the pituitary gonadotropic hormones can sometimes be treated by appropriately timed administration of *human chorionic gonadotropin*, a hormone (discussed in Chapter 98) that is extracted from the human placenta. This hormone, although secreted by the placenta, has almost the same effects as LH and is therefore a powerful stimulator of ovulation.

One of the most common causes of female sterility is *endometriosis*, a common condition in which endometrial tissue almost identical to that of the normal uterine endometrium grows and even menstruates in the pelvic cavity surrounding the uterus, fallopian tubes, and ovaries. Endometriosis causes fibrosis throughout the pelvis, and this fibrosis sometimes so enshrouds the ovaries that an ovum cannot be released into the abdominal cavity. Another common cause of female infertility is *salpingitis*, that is, *inflammation of the fallopian tubes*, which causes fibrosis in the tubes, thereby occluding them. Still another cause of infertility is secretion of abnormal mucus by the uterine cervix. Abnormalities of the cervix itself, such as low-grade infection or inflammation, or abnormal hormonal stimulation of the cervix, can lead to a viscous mucous plug that prevents fertilization.

BIBLIOGRAPHY

Barros RP, Gustafsson JÅ: Estrogen receptors and the metabolic network, *Cell Metab.* 14:289, 2011.

Blaustein JD: Progesterone and progestin receptors in the brain: the neglected ones, *Endocrinology* 149:2737, 2008.

Campbell RE, Herbison AE: Gonadal steroid neuromodulation of developing and mature hypothalamic neuronal networks, *Curr. Opin. Neurobiol.* 29C:96, 2014.

Crandall CJ, Barrett-Connor E: Endogenous sex steroid levels and cardiovascular disease in relation to the menopause: a systematic review, *Endocrinol. Metab. Clin. North Am.* 42:227, 2013.

de la Iglesia HO, Schwartz WJ: Minireview: timely ovulation: circadian regulation of the female hypothalamo-pituitary–gonadal axis, *Endocrinology* 147:1148, 2006.

Federman DD: The biology of human sex differences, *N. Engl. J. Med.* 354:1507, 2006.

Gordon CM: Clinical practice. Functional hypothalamic amenorrhea, *N. Engl. J. Med.* 363:365, 2010.

Heldring N, Pike A, Andersson S, et al: Estrogen receptors: how do they signal and what are their targets, *Physiol. Rev.* 87:905, 2007.

Hodis HN, Mack WJ: Hormone replacement therapy and the association with coronary heart disease and overall mortality: clinical application of the timing hypothesis, *J. Steroid Biochem. Mol. Biol.* 142:68, 2014.

Kelly MJ, Zhang C, Qiu J, Rønnekleiv OK: Pacemaking kisspeptin neurons, *Exp. Physiol.* 98:1535, 2013.

Maranon R, Reckelhoff JF: Sex and gender differences in control of blood pressure, *Clin. Sci. (Lond.)* 125:311, 2013.

Nilsson S, Makela S, Treuter E, et al: Mechanisms of estrogen action, *Physiol. Rev.* 81:1535, 2001.

Niswender GD, Juengel JL, Silva PJ, et al: Mechanisms controlling the function and life span of the corpus luteum, *Physiol. Rev.* 80:1, 2000.

Palmert MR, Dunkel L: Clinical practice. Delayed puberty, *N. Engl. J. Med.* 366:443, 2012.

Pavone ME, Bulun SE: Clinical review: the use of aromatase inhibitors for ovulation induction and superovulation, *J. Clin. Endocrinol. Metab.* 98:1838, 2013.

Pfaff D, Waters E, Khan Q, et al: Minireview: estrogen receptor-initiated mechanisms causal to mammalian reproductive behaviors, *Endocrinology* 152:1209, 2011.

Pinilla L, Aguilar E, Dieguez C, et al: Kisspeptins and reproduction: physiological roles and regulatory mechanisms, *Physiol. Rev.* 92:1235, 2012.

Riggs BL: The mechanisms of estrogen regulation of bone resorption, *J. Clin. Invest.* 106:1203, 2000.

Santen RJ, Kagan R, Altomare CJ, et al: Current and evolving approaches to individualizing estrogen receptor-based therapy for menopausal women, *J. Clin. Endocrinol. Metab.* 99:733, 2014.

Vasudevan N, Ogawa S, Pfaff D: Estrogen and thyroid hormone receptor interactions: physiological flexibility by molecular specificity, *Physiol. Rev.* 82:923, 2002.

Xing D, Nozell S, Chen YF, et al: Estrogen and mechanisms of vascular protection, *Arterioscler. Thromb. Vasc. Biol.* 29:289, 2009.

The Sexual Act and Fertilization

LEARNING OBJECTIVES

- Describe the stages in the male sexual act.
- Describe the changes that the female undergoes during the sexual act.
- Describe the processes involved in fertilization of the ovum.

GLOSSARY OF TERMS

- **Acrosome reaction:** The release of the enzymes of the acrosome of the sperm that allow the sperm to penetrate the zona pellucida of the ovum

- **Capacitation:** The collective changes that activate the sperm on coming in contact with the fluids of the female genital tract

- **Fertilization:** Fusion of the sperm and the ovum to form a diploid zygote

The most important source of sensory nerve signals for initiating the male sexual act is the *glans penis*. The glans contains an especially sensitive sensory end-organ system that transmits into the central nervous system and that special modality of sensation is called *sexual sensation*. The slippery massaging action of intercourse on the glans stimulates the sensory end organs, and the sexual signals in turn pass through the pudendal nerve, then through the sacral plexus into the sacral portion of the spinal cord, and finally up the cord to undefined areas of the brain.

Impulses may also enter the spinal cord from areas adjacent to the penis to aid in stimulating the sexual act. For instance, stimulation of the anal epithelium, the scrotum, and perineal structures in general can send signals into the cord that add to the sexual sensation. Sexual sensations can even originate in internal structures, such as in areas of the urethra, bladder, prostate, seminal vesicles, testes, and vas deferens. Indeed, one of the causes of "sexual drive" is filling of the sexual organs with secretions. Mild infection and inflammation of these sexual organs may sometimes stimulate sexual desire.

Psychic Element of Male Sexual Stimulation

Appropriate psychic stimuli can greatly enhance the ability of a person to perform the sexual act. Simply thinking sexual thoughts or even dreaming that the act of intercourse is being performed can initiate the male act, culminating in ejaculation. Indeed, *nocturnal emissions, sometimes called "wet dreams,"* occur in many males during some stages of sexual life, especially during the teens.

Integration of the Male Sexual Act in the Spinal Cord

Although psychic factors usually play an important part in the male sexual act and can initiate or inhibit it, brain function is probably not necessary for its performance because appropriate genital stimulation can cause ejaculation in some animals and occasionally in humans after their spinal cords have been cut above the lumbar region. The male sexual act results from inherent reflex mechanisms integrated in the sacral and lumbar spinal cord, and these mechanisms can be initiated by either psychic stimulation from the brain or actual sexual stimulation from the sex organs, but usually it is a combination of both.

Stages of the Male Sexual Act

PENILE ERECTION—ROLE OF THE PARASYMPATHETIC NERVES

Penile erection is the first effect of male sexual stimulation and the degree of erection is proportional to the degree of stimulation, whether psychic or physical. Erection is caused by parasympathetic impulses that pass from the sacral portion of the spinal cord through the pelvic nerves to the penis. These parasympathetic nerve fibers, in contrast to most other parasympathetic fibers, are believed to release *nitric oxide* and/or *vasoactive intestinal peptide* in addition to acetylcholine. Nitric oxide activates the enzyme *guanylyl cyclase* causing increased formation of *cyclic guanosine monophosphate* (GMP). The cyclic GMP especially relaxes the arteries of the penis and the trabecular meshwork of smooth muscle fibers in the *erectile tissue* of the *corpora cavernosa* and *corpus spongiosum* in the shaft of the penis, shown in Figure 97-1. As the vascular smooth muscles relax, blood flow into the penis increases, causing release of nitric oxide from the vascular endothelial cells and further vasodilation.

The erectile tissue of the penis consists of large cavernous sinusoids that are normally relatively empty of blood but become dilated tremendously when arterial blood flows rapidly into them under pressure while the venous outflow is partially occluded. Also, the erectile bodies, especially the two corpora cavernosa, are surrounded by strong fibrous coats; therefore, high pressure within the sinusoids causes ballooning of the erectile tissue to such an extent that the penis becomes hard and elongated, which is the phenomenon of *erection*.

LUBRICATION IS A PARASYMPATHETIC FUNCTION

During sexual stimulation, the parasympathetic impulses, in addition to promoting erection, cause the urethral glands and the bulbourethral glands to secrete mucus. This mucus flows through the urethra during intercourse to aid in the lubrication during coitus. However, most of the lubrication of coitus is provided by the female sexual organs rather than by the male organs.

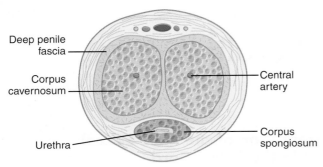

Figure 97-1 Erectile tissue of the penis.

Without satisfactory lubrication, the male sexual act is seldom successful because unlubricated intercourse causes grating, painful sensations that inhibit rather than excite sexual sensations.

EMISSION AND EJACULATION ARE FUNCTIONS OF THE SYMPATHETIC NERVES

Emission and ejaculation are the culmination of the male sexual act. When the sexual stimulus becomes extremely intense, the reflex centers of the spinal cord begin to emit *sympathetic impulses* that leave the cord at T-12 to L-2 and pass to the genital organs through the hypogastric and pelvic sympathetic nerve plexuses to initiate *emission,* the forerunner of ejaculation.

Emission begins with contraction of the vas deferens and the ampulla to cause expulsion of sperms into the internal urethra. Then, contractions of the muscular coat of the prostate gland followed by contraction of the seminal vesicles expel prostatic and seminal fluid also into the urethra, forcing the sperms forward. All these fluids mix in the internal urethra with mucus already secreted by the bulbourethral glands to form the semen. The process to this point is *emission.*

The filling of the internal urethra with semen elicits sensory signals that are transmitted through the pudendal nerves to the sacral regions of the cord, giving the feeling of sudden fullness in the internal genital organs. Also, these sensory signals further excite rhythmic contraction of the internal genital organs and cause contraction of the ischiocavernosus and bulbocavernosus muscles that compress the bases of the penile erectile tissue. These effects together cause rhythmic, wave-like increases in pressure in both the erectile tissue of the penis and the genital ducts and urethra, which "ejaculate" the semen from the urethra to the exterior. This final process is called *ejaculation.* At the same time, rhythmic contractions of the pelvic muscles and even of some of the muscles of the body trunk cause thrusting movements of the pelvis and penis, which also help propel the semen into the deepest recesses of the vagina and perhaps even slightly into the cervix of the uterus.

This entire period of emission and ejaculation is called the *male orgasm.* At its termination, the male sexual excitement disappears almost entirely within 1–2 minutes and erection ceases, a process called *resolution.*

Erectile Dysfunction in the Male

Erectile dysfunction, also called "impotence," is characterized by an inability of the man to develop or maintain an *erection* of sufficient rigidity for satisfactory sexual intercourse. Neurological problems, such as trauma to the parasympathetic nerves from prostate surgery, deficient levels of testosterone, and some drugs (eg, *nicotine, alcohol, and antidepressants),* can also contribute to erectile dysfunction.

In men older than 40 years, erectile dysfunction is most often caused by underlying vascular disease. As discussed previously, adequate blood flow and nitric oxide formation are essential for penile erection. Vascular disease, which can occur as a result of uncontrolled *hypertension, diabetes,* and *atherosclerosis,* reduces the ability of the body's blood vessels, including those in the penis, to dilate. Part of this impaired vasodilation is due to decreased release of nitric oxide.

Erectile dysfunction caused by vascular disease can often be successfully treated with *phosphodiesterase-5 (PDE-5) inhibitors,* such as sildenafil (Viagra), vardenafil (Levitra), or tadalafil (Cialis). These drugs increase cyclic GMP levels in the erectile tissue by inhibiting the enzyme *PDE-5,* which rapidly degrades cyclic GMP. Thus, by inhibiting the degradation of cyclic GMP, the PDE-5 inhibitors enhance and prolong the effect of cyclic GMP to cause erection.

Female Sexual Act

STIMULATION OF THE FEMALE SEXUAL ACT

As is true in the male sexual act, successful performance of the female sexual act depends on both psychic stimulation and local sexual stimulation.

Thinking sexual thoughts can lead to female sexual desire, and this aids greatly in the performance of the female sexual act. Such desire is based on psychological and physiological drive, although sexual desire does increase in proportion to the level of sex hormones secreted. Desire also changes during the monthly sexual cycle, reaching a peak near the time of ovulation, probably because of the high levels of estrogen secretion during the preovulatory period.

Local sexual stimulation in women occurs in more or less the same manner as in men because massage and other types of stimulation of the vulva, vagina, and other perineal regions can create sexual sensations. The glans of the *clitoris* is especially sensitive for initiating sexual sensations.

As in the male, the sexual sensory signals are transmitted to the sacral segments of the spinal cord through the pudendal nerve and sacral plexus. Once these signals have entered the spinal cord, they are transmitted to the cerebrum. Also, local reflexes integrated in the sacral and lumbar spinal cord are at least partly responsible for some of the reactions in the female sexual organs.

FEMALE ERECTION AND LUBRICATION

Located around the introitus and extending into the clitoris is erectile tissue almost identical to the erectile tissue of the penis. This erectile tissue, like that of the penis, is controlled by the parasympathetic nerves that pass through the nervi erigentes from the sacral plexus to the external genitalia. In the early phases of sexual stimulation, parasympathetic signals dilate the arteries of the erectile tissue, probably resulting from release of acetylcholine, nitric oxide, and vasoactive intestinal polypeptide at the nerve endings. This allows rapid accumulation of blood in the erectile tissue so that the introitus tightens around the penis, which aids the male in his attainment of sufficient sexual stimulation for ejaculation to occur.

Parasympathetic signals also pass to the bilateral Bartholin glands located beneath the labia minora and cause them to secrete mucus immediately inside the introitus. This mucus is responsible for much of the lubrication during sexual intercourse, although much lubrication is also provided by mucus secreted by the vaginal epithelium and a small amount is provided from the male urethral glands. This lubrication is necessary during intercourse to establish a satisfactory massaging sensation rather than an irritative sensation, which may be provoked by a dry vagina. A massaging sensation constitutes the optimal stimulus for evoking the appropriate reflexes that culminate in both the male and female climaxes.

FEMALE ORGASM

When local sexual stimulation reaches maximum intensity, and especially when the local sensations are supported by appropriate psychic conditioning signals from the cerebrum, reflexes are initiated that cause the female orgasm, also called the *female climax*. The female orgasm is analogous to emission and ejaculation in the male, and it may help promote fertilization of the ovum. Indeed, the human female is known to be somewhat more fertile when inseminated by normal sexual intercourse rather than by artificial methods, thus indicating an important function of the female orgasm. Possible reasons for this phenomenon are as follows.

First, during the orgasm, the perineal muscles of the female contract rhythmically, which results from spinal cord reflexes similar to those that cause ejaculation in the male. It is possible that these reflexes increase uterine and fallopian tube motility during the orgasm, thus helping to transport the sperms upward through the uterus toward the ovum; however, information on this subject is scanty. Also, the orgasm seems to cause dilation of the cervical canal for up to 30 minutes, thus allowing easy transport of the sperms.

Second, in many animals, copulation causes the posterior pituitary gland to secrete oxytocin; this effect is probably mediated through the brain amygdaloid nuclei and then through the hypothalamus to the pituitary. The oxytocin causes increased rhythmic contractions of the uterus, which have been postulated to cause increased transport of the sperms. A few sperms have been shown to traverse the entire length of the fallopian tube in the cow in about 5 minutes, a rate at least 10 times as fast as the swimming motions of the sperms could possibly achieve. Whether this effect occurs in the human female is unknown.

In addition to the possible effects of the orgasm on fertilization, the intense sexual sensations that develop during the orgasm also pass to the cerebrum and cause intense muscle tension throughout the body. After culmination of the sexual act, this tension gives way during the succeeding minutes to a sense of satisfaction characterized by relaxed peacefulness, an effect called *resolution*.

Fertilization

FERTILE PERIOD OF EACH SEXUAL CYCLE

The ovum remains viable and capable of being fertilized probably no longer than 24 hours after it is expelled from the ovary. Therefore, sperms must be available soon after ovulation if fertilization is to take place. A few sperms can remain fertile in the female reproductive tract for up to 5 days. Therefore, for fertilization to take place, intercourse must occur sometime between 4 and 5 days before ovulation up to a few hours after ovulation.

Thus, the period of female fertility during each month is short, about 4–5 days.

"CAPACITATION" OF SPERMATOZOA IS REQUIRED FOR FERTILIZATION OF THE OVUM

Although spermatozoa are said to be "mature" when they leave the epididymis, their activity is held in check by multiple inhibitory factors secreted by the genital duct epithelia. Therefore, when they are first expelled in the semen, they are unable to fertilize the ovum. However, on coming in contact with the fluids of the female genital tract, multiple changes occur that activate the sperms for the final processes of fertilization. These collective changes are called *capacitation of the spermatozoa*, which normally requires from 1 to 10 hours. The following changes are believed to occur:

1. The uterine and fallopian tube fluids wash away the various inhibitory factors that suppress sperm activity in the male genital ducts.
2. While the spermatozoa remain in the fluid of the male genital ducts, they are continually exposed to many floating vesicles from the seminiferous tubules containing large amounts of cholesterol. This cholesterol is continually added to the cellular membrane covering the sperm acrosome, toughening this membrane and preventing release of its enzymes. After ejaculation, the sperms deposited in the vagina swim away from the cholesterol vesicles upward into the uterine cavity and they gradually lose much of their other excess cholesterol during the next few hours. In doing so, the membrane at the head of the sperm (the acrosome) becomes much weaker.
3. The membrane of the sperm also becomes much more permeable to calcium ions, so calcium now enters the sperm in abundance and changes the activity of the flagellum, giving it a powerful whiplash motion in contrast to its previously weak undulating motion. In addition, the calcium ions cause changes in the cellular membrane that cover the leading edge of the acrosome, making it possible for the acrosome to release its enzymes rapidly and easily as the sperm penetrates the granulosa cell mass surrounding the ovum, and even more so as it attempts to penetrate the zona pellucida of the ovum.

Thus, multiple changes occur during the process of capacitation. Without these changes the sperm cannot make its way to the interior of the ovum to cause fertilization.

ACROSOME ENZYMES, THE "ACROSOME REACTION," AND PENETRATION OF THE OVUM

Stored in the acrosome of the sperm are large quantities of *hyaluronidase* and *proteolytic enzymes*. Hyaluronidase depolymerizes the hyaluronic acid polymers in the intercellular cement that holds the ovarian granulosa cells together. The proteolytic enzymes digest proteins in the structural elements of tissue cells that still adhere to the ovum.

When the ovum is expelled from the ovarian follicle into the fallopian tube, it still carries with it multiple layers of granulosa cells. Before a sperm can fertilize the ovum, it must dissolute these granulosa cell layers and then it must penetrate through the thick covering of the ovum itself, the *zona pellucida* (Figure 97-2A–C). To achieve this penetration, the stored enzymes in the acrosome begin to be released. It is believed that the hyaluronidase among these enzymes is especially important

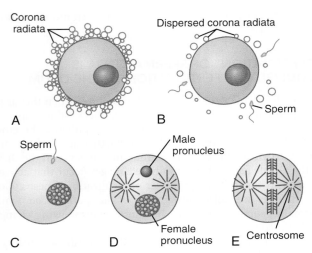

Figure 97-2 Fertilization of the ovum. (A) The mature ovum surrounded by the corona radiata; (B) dispersal of the corona radiata; (C) entry of the sperm; (D) formation of the male and female pronuclei; (E) reorganization of a full complement of chromosomes and beginning division of the ovum. *Modified from Arey, L.B., 1974. Developmental Anatomy: A Textbook and Laboratory Manual of Embryology, seventh ed. W.B. Saunders, Philadelphia.*

in opening pathways between the granulosa cells so that the sperm can reach the ovum.

When the sperm reaches the zona pellucida of the ovum, the anterior membrane of the sperm binds specifically with receptor proteins in the zona pellucida. Next, the entire acrosome rapidly dissolves and all the acrosomal enzymes are released. Within minutes, these enzymes open a penetrating pathway for passage of the sperm head through the zona pellucida to the inside of the ovum. Within another 30 minutes, the cell membranes of the sperm head and of the oocyte fuse with each other to form a single cell. At the same time, the genetic material of the sperm and the oocyte combine to form a completely new cell genome containing equal numbers of chromosomes and genes from mother and father. This is the process of *fertilization*.

Once a sperm has entered the ovum (which is still in the secondary oocyte stage of development), the oocyte divides again to form the *mature ovum* plus a *second polar body* that is expelled. The mature ovum still carries in its nucleus (now called the *female pronucleus*) 23 chromosomes. One of these chromosomes is the female chromosome known as the *X chromosome*.

In the meantime, the fertilizing sperm has also changed. On entering the ovum, its head swells to form a *male pronucleus*, shown in Figure 97-2D. Later, the 23 unpaired chromosomes of the male pronucleus and the 23 unpaired chromosomes of the female pronucleus align themselves to reform a complete complement of 46 chromosomes (23 pairs) in the *fertilized ovum* (Figure 97-2E).

Why Does Only One Sperm Enter the Oocyte? With as many sperms as there are, why does only one enter the oocyte? The reason is not entirely known, but within a few minutes after the first sperm penetrates the zona pellucida of the ovum, calcium ions diffuse inward through the oocyte membrane and cause multiple cortical granules to be released by exocytosis from the oocyte into the perivitelline space. These granules contain substances that permeate all portions of the zona pellucida and prevent binding of additional sperms and they even cause any sperm that have already begun to bind to fall off. Thus, almost never does more than one sperm enter the oocyte during fertilization.

What Determines the Sex of the Fetus that Is Created?

After formation of the mature sperm, half of these carry in their genome an X chromosome (the female chromosome) and half carry a Y chromosome (the male chromosome). Therefore, if an X chromosome from a sperm combines with an X chromosome from an ovum, giving an XX combination, a female child will be born. But if a Y chromosome from a sperm is paired with an X chromosome from an ovum, giving an XY combination, a male child will be born.

BIBLIOGRAPHY

Also refer to Bibliography of Chapters 95 and 96.
Ikawa M, Inoue N, Benham AM, et al: Fertilization: a sperm's journey to and interaction with the oocyte, *J. Clin. Invest.* 120:984, 2010.

Matzuk M, Lamb D: The biology of infertility: research advances and clinical challenges, *Nat. Med.* 14:1197, 2008.

Physiology of Pregnancy

If the ovum becomes fertilized, a new sequence of events called *gestation*, or *pregnancy*, takes place, and the fertilized ovum eventually develops into a full-term fetus. The purpose of this chapter is to discuss the early stages of ovum development after fertilization and then to discuss the physiology of pregnancy.

Entry of the Ovum into the Fallopian Tube (Uterine Tube)

When ovulation occurs, the ovum, along with a hundred or more attached granulosa cells that constitute the *corona radiata*, is expelled directly into the peritoneal cavity and must then enter one of the fallopian tubes (also called uterine tubes) to reach the cavity of the uterus. The fimbriated ends of each fallopian tube fall naturally around the ovaries. The inner surfaces of the fimbriated tentacles are lined with ciliated epithelium, and the *cilia* are activated by estrogen from the ovaries, which causes the cilia to beat toward the opening, or *ostium*, of the involved fallopian tube. One can actually see a slow fluid current flowing toward the ostium. By this means, the ovum enters one of the fallopian tubes.

Although one might suspect that many ova fail to enter the fallopian tubes, conception studies suggest that up to 98% of ova succeed in this task. Indeed, in some recorded cases, women with one ovary removed and the opposite fallopian tube removed have had several children with relative ease of conception, thus demonstrating that ova can even enter the opposite fallopian tube.

Fertilization of the Ovum

After the male ejaculates semen into the vagina during intercourse, a few sperm are transported within 5–10 minutes upward from the vagina and through the uterus and fallopian tubes to the *ampullae* of the fallopian tubes near the ovarian ends of the tubes. This transport of the sperm is aided by contractions of the uterus and fallopian tubes stimulated by prostaglandins in the male seminal fluid and also by oxytocin released from the posterior pituitary gland of the female during her orgasm. Of the almost half a billion sperm deposited in the vagina, a few thousand succeed in reaching each ampulla.

Fertilization of the ovum normally takes place in the ampulla of one of the fallopian tubes soon after both the sperm and the ovum enter the ampulla. Before a sperm can enter the ovum, however, it must first penetrate the multiple layers of granulosa cells attached to the outside of the ovum (the *corona radiata*) and then bind to and penetrate the *zona pellucida* surrounding the ovum. The mechanisms used by the sperm for these purposes are presented in Chapter 97.

Transport of the Fertilized Ovum in the Fallopian Tube

After fertilization has occurred, an additional 3–5 days is normally required for transport of the fertilized ovum through the remainder of the fallopian tube into the cavity of the uterus (Figure 98-1). This transport is affected:
- mainly by a feeble fluid current in the tube resulting from epithelial secretion;
- by action of the ciliated epithelium that lines the tube (the cilia always beat toward the uterus);
- by weak contractions of the fallopian tube.

The fallopian tubes are lined with a rugged, cryptoid surface that impedes passage of the ovum despite the fluid current. Also, the *isthmus* of the fallopian tube (the last 2 cm before the tube enters the uterus) remains spastically contracted for about the first 3 days after ovulation. After this time, the rapidly increasing progesterone secreted by the ovarian corpus luteum first promotes increasing progesterone receptors on the fallopian tube smooth muscle cells; then the progesterone activates the receptors, exerting a tubular relaxing effect that allows entry of the ovum into the uterus.

This delayed transport of the fertilized ovum through the fallopian tube allows several stages of cell division to occur before the dividing ovum—now called a *blastocyst*, with about 100

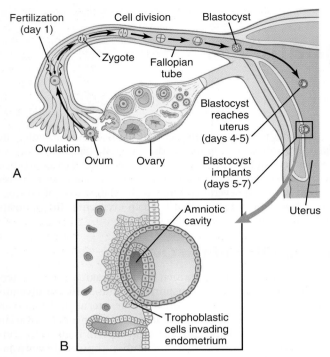

Figure 98-1   (A) Ovulation, fertilization of the ovum in the fallopian tube, and implantation of the blastocyst in the uterus; (B) the action of trophoblast cells in implantation of the blastocyst in the uterine endometrium.

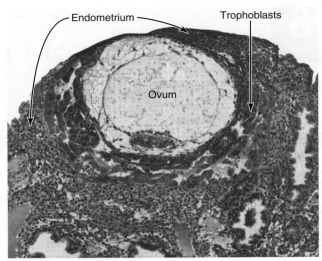

Figure 98-2   Implantation of the early human embryo, showing trophoblastic digestion and invasion of the endometrium. *Courtesy Dr. Arthur Hertig.*

cells—enters the uterus. During this time, the fallopian tube secretory cells produce large quantities of secretions used for the nutrition of the developing blastocyst.

Implantation of the Blastocyst in the Uterus

After reaching the uterus, the developing blastocyst usually remains in the uterine cavity an additional 1–3 days before it implants in the endometrium; thus, implantation ordinarily occurs on about the fifth to seventh days after ovulation. Before implantation, the blastocyst obtains its nutrition from the uterine endometrial secretions called "uterine milk."

Implantation results from the action of *trophoblast cells* that develop over the surface of the blastocyst. These cells secrete proteolytic enzymes that digest and liquefy the adjacent cells of the uterine endometrium. Some of the fluid and nutrients released are actively transported by the same trophoblast cells into the blastocyst, adding more sustenance for growth. Figure 98-2 shows an early implanted human blastocyst, with a small embryo. Once implantation has taken place, the trophoblast cells and other adjacent cells (from the blastocyst and the uterine endometrium) proliferate rapidly, forming the placenta and the various membranes of pregnancy.

Early Nutrition of the Embryo

In Chapter 96, we pointed out that the progesterone secreted by the ovarian corpus luteum during the latter half of each monthly sexual cycle has an effect on the uterine endometrium, converting the endometrial stromal cells into large swollen cells containing extra quantities of glycogen, proteins, lipids, and

even some minerals necessary for development of the *conceptus* (the embryo and its adjacent parts or associated membranes). Then, when the conceptus implants in the endometrium, the continued secretion of progesterone causes the endometrial cells to swell further and to store even more nutrients. These cells are now called *decidual cells*, and the total mass of cells is called the *decidua*.

As the trophoblast cells invade the decidua, digesting and imbibing it, the stored nutrients in the decidua are used by the embryo for growth and development. During the first week after implantation, this is the only means by which the embryo can obtain nutrients; the embryo continues to obtain at least some of its nutrition in this way for up to 8 weeks, although the placenta also begins to provide nutrition after about the 16th day beyond fertilization (a little more than 1 week after implantation). Figure 98-3 shows this trophoblastic period of nutrition, which gradually gives way to placental nutrition.

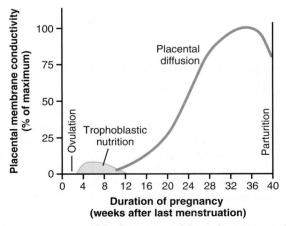

Figure 98-3   Nutrition of the fetus. Most of the early nutrition is due to trophoblastic digestion and absorption of nutrients from the endometrial decidua, and essentially all the later nutrition results from diffusion through the placental membrane.

Anatomy and Function of the Placenta

While the trophoblastic cords from the blastocyst are attaching to the uterus, blood capillaries grow into the cords from the vascular system of the newly forming embryo. About 21 days after fertilization, blood also begins to be pumped by the heart of the human embryo. Simultaneously, *blood sinuses* supplied with blood from the mother develop around the outsides of the trophoblastic cords. The trophoblast cells send out more and more projections, which become *placental villi* into which fetal capillaries grow. Thus, the villi, carrying fetal blood, are surrounded by sinuses that contain maternal blood.

The final structure of the placenta is shown in Figure 98-4. The lower part of Figure 98-4 shows the relationship between the fetal blood of each fetal placental villus and the blood of the mother surrounding the outsides of the villus in the fully developed placenta.

The total surface area of all the villi of the mature placenta is only a few square meters—many times less than the area of the pulmonary membrane in the lungs. Nevertheless, nutrients and other substances pass through this placental membrane mainly by diffusion in much the same manner that diffusion occurs through the alveolar membranes of the lungs and the capillary membranes elsewhere in the body.

Diffusion of Oxygen Through the Placental Membrane. Almost the same principles for diffusion of oxygen through the pulmonary membrane (discussed in detail in Chapter 58) are applicable for diffusion of oxygen through the placental membrane. The dissolved oxygen in the blood of the large maternal sinuses passes into the fetal blood by *simple diffusion*, driven by an oxygen pressure gradient from the mother's blood to the fetus's blood. Near the end of pregnancy, the mean partial pressure of oxygen (PO_2) of the mother's blood in the placental sinuses is about 50 mmHg and the mean PO_2 in the fetal blood after it becomes oxygenated in the placenta is about 30 mmHg. Therefore, the mean pressure gradient for diffusion of oxygen through the placental membrane is about 20 mmHg.

One might wonder how it is possible for a fetus to obtain sufficient oxygen when the fetal blood leaving the placenta has a PO_2 of only 30 mmHg. There are three reasons why even this low PO_2 is capable of allowing the fetal blood to transport almost as much oxygen to the fetal tissues as is transported by the mother's blood to her tissues:

1. The hemoglobin of the fetus is mainly *fetal hemoglobin*. Figure 98-5 shows the comparative oxygen dissociation curves for maternal hemoglobin and fetal hemoglobin, demonstrating that the curve for fetal hemoglobin is shifted to the left of that for maternal hemoglobin. This means that at the low PO_2 levels in fetal blood, the fetal hemoglobin can carry 20–50% more oxygen than can maternal hemoglobin.
2. The *hemoglobin concentration of fetal blood is about 50% greater than that of the mother*, which is an even more important factor in enhancing the amount of oxygen transported to the fetal tissues.
3. The *Bohr effect*, which is explained in relation to the exchange of carbon dioxide and oxygen in the lung in Chapter 59. Hemoglobin can carry more oxygen at a low PCO_2 than it can at a high PCO_2. The fetal blood entering the placenta carries large amounts of carbon dioxide, but much of this carbon dioxide diffuses from the fetal blood into the maternal blood. Loss of the carbon dioxide makes the fetal blood more alkaline, whereas the increased carbon dioxide in the maternal blood makes it more acidic.

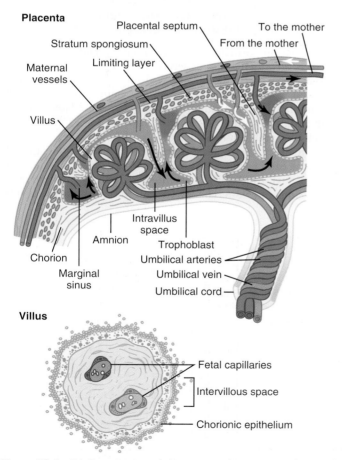

Placenta

Placental septum
Stratum spongiosum
Limiting layer
To the mother
From the mother
Maternal vessels
Villus
Intravillus space
Amnion
Trophoblast
Chorion
Umbilical arteries
Marginal sinus
Umbilical vein
Umbilical cord

Villus

Fetal capillaries
Intervillous space
Chorionic epithelium

Figure 98-4 (A) Organization of the mature placenta; (B) relation of the fetal blood in the villus capillaries to the mother's blood in the intervillous spaces.

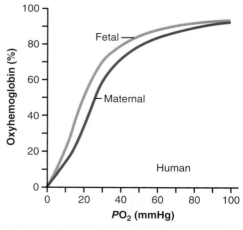

Figure 98-5 Oxygen–hemoglobin dissociation curves for maternal and fetal blood, showing that fetal blood can carry a greater quantity of oxygen than can maternal blood for a given blood PO_2. *Data from Metcalfe, J., Moll, W., Bartels, H., 1964. Gas exchange across the placenta. Fed. Proc. 23, 775.*

These changes cause the capacity of fetal blood to combine with oxygen to increase and that of maternal blood to decrease, which forces still more oxygen from the maternal blood, while enhancing oxygen uptake by the fetal blood. Thus, the Bohr shift operates in one direction in the maternal blood and in the other direction in the fetal blood. These two effects make the Bohr shift twice as important here as it is for oxygen exchange in the lungs; therefore, it is called the *double Bohr effect.*

By these three means, the fetus is capable of receiving more than adequate oxygen through the placental membrane, despite the fact that the fetal blood leaving the placenta has a PO_2 of only 30 mmHg.

Diffusion of Carbon Dioxide Through the Placental Membrane. Carbon dioxide is continually formed in the tissues of the fetus in the same way that it is formed in maternal tissues, and the only means for excreting the carbon dioxide from the fetus is through the placenta into the mother's blood. The partial pressure of carbon dioxide (PCO_2) of the fetal blood is 2–3 mmHg higher than that of the maternal blood. This small pressure gradient for carbon dioxide across the membrane is more than sufficient to allow adequate diffusion of carbon dioxide because the extreme solubility of carbon dioxide in the placental membrane allows carbon dioxide to diffuse about 20 times as rapidly as oxygen.

Diffusion of Foodstuffs Through the Placental Membrane. Other metabolic substrates needed by the fetus diffuse into the fetal blood in the same manner as oxygen does. For instance, in the late stages of pregnancy, the fetus often uses as much glucose as is used by the entire body of the mother. To provide this much glucose, the trophoblast cells lining the placental villi provide for *facilitated diffusion* of glucose through the placental membrane, that is, the glucose is transported by carrier molecules in the trophoblast cells of the membrane. Even so, the glucose level in the fetal blood is 20–30% lower than that in the maternal blood.

Because of the high solubility of fatty acids in cell membranes, these fatty acids also diffuse from the maternal blood into the fetal blood, but more slowly than glucose, so glucose is used more easily by the fetus for nutrition. Also, such substances as ketone bodies and potassium, sodium, and chloride ions diffuse with relative ease from the maternal blood into the fetal blood.

Excretion of Waste Products Through the Placental Membrane. In the same manner that carbon dioxide diffuses from the fetal blood into the maternal blood, other excretory products formed in the fetus also diffuse through the placental membrane into the maternal blood and are then excreted along with the excretory products of the mother. These products include especially the *nonprotein nitrogens,* such as *urea, uric acid,* and *creatinine.* The level of urea in fetal blood is only slightly greater than that in maternal blood because urea diffuses through the placental membrane with great ease. However, creatinine, which does not diffuse as easily, has a fetal blood concentration considerably higher than that in the mother's blood. Therefore, excretion from the fetus depends mainly, if not entirely, on the diffusion gradients across the placental membrane and its permeability. Because there are higher concentrations of the excretory products in the fetal blood than in the maternal blood, there is continual diffusion of these substances from the fetal blood to the maternal blood.

Hormonal Factors in Pregnancy

In pregnancy, the placenta forms especially large quantities of *human chorionic gonadotropin* (hCG), *estrogens, progesterone,* and *human chorionic somatomammotropin,* the first three of which, and probably the fourth as well, are all essential to a normal pregnancy.

HUMAN CHORIONIC GONADOTROPIN CAUSES PERSISTENCE OF THE CORPUS LUTEUM AND PREVENTS MENSTRUATION

Menstruation normally occurs in a nonpregnant woman about 14 days after ovulation, at which time most of the endometrium of the uterus sloughs away from the uterine wall and is expelled to the exterior. If this should happen after an ovum has implanted, the pregnancy would terminate. However, this sloughing is prevented by the secretion of hCG by the newly developing embryonic tissues.

Coincidental with the development of the trophoblast cells from the early fertilized ovum, the hormone *hCG* is secreted by the syncytial trophoblast cells into the fluids of the mother, as shown in Figure 98-6. The secretion of this hormone can first be

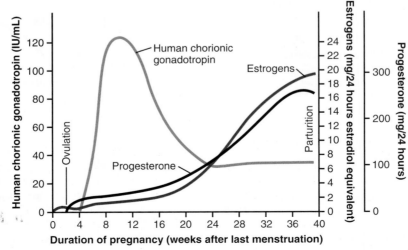

Figure 98-6   Rates of secretion of estrogens and progesterone, and concentration of human chorionic gonadotropin at different stages of pregnancy.

measured in the blood 8–9 days after ovulation, shortly after the blastocyst implants in the endometrium, and the appearance of this hormone in urine is used as the basis of a test for pregnancy. Then the rate of secretion rises rapidly to reach a maximum at about 10–12 weeks of pregnancy and decreases back to a lower value by 16–20 weeks. It continues at this level for the remainder of the pregnancy.

Function of Human Chorionic Gonadotropin. hCG is a glycoprotein having a molecular weight of about 39,000 and much the same molecular structure and function as luteinizing hormone secreted by the pituitary gland. By far, the most important function of hCG is to prevent involution of the corpus luteum at the end of the monthly female sexual cycle. Instead, it causes the corpus luteum to secrete even larger quantities of its sex hormones—progesterone and estrogens—for the next few months. These sex hormones prevent menstruation and cause the endometrium to continue to grow and store large amounts of nutrients rather than being shed in the menstruum. As a result, the *decidua-like cells* that develop in the endometrium during the normal female sexual cycle become actual *decidual cells*—greatly swollen and nutritious—at about the time that the blastocyst implants.

Under the influence of hCG, the corpus luteum in the mother's ovary grows to about twice its initial size by a month or so after pregnancy begins. Its continued secretion of estrogens and progesterone maintains the decidual nature of the uterine endometrium, which is necessary for the early development of the fetus.

If the corpus luteum is removed before approximately the 7th week of pregnancy, spontaneous abortion almost always occurs, sometimes even up to the 12th week. After that time, the placenta secretes sufficient quantities of progesterone and estrogens to maintain pregnancy for the remainder of the gestation period. The corpus luteum involutes slowly after the 13th to 17th weeks of gestation.

Human Chorionic Gonadotropin Stimulates the Fetal Testes to Produce Testosterone. hCG also exerts an *interstitial cell-*stimulating effect on the testes of the male fetus, resulting in the production of testosterone in male fetuses until the time of birth. This small secretion of testosterone during gestation is what causes the fetus to grow male sex organs instead of female organs. Near the end of pregnancy, the testosterone secreted by the fetal testes also causes the testes to descend into the scrotum.

SECRETION OF ESTROGENS BY THE PLACENTA

The placenta, like the corpus luteum, secretes both estrogens and progesterone. Histochemical and physiological studies show that these two hormones, like most other placental hormones, are secreted by the *syncytial trophoblast* cells of the placenta.

Figure 98-6 shows that toward the end of pregnancy, the daily production of placental estrogens increases to about 30 times the mother's normal level of production. However, the secretion of estrogens by the placenta is quite different from secretion by the ovaries. Most important, the estrogens secreted by the placenta are not synthesized de novo from basic substrates in the placenta. Instead, they are formed almost entirely from androgenic steroid compounds, *dehydroepiandrosterone* and *16-hydroxydehydroepiandrosterone,* which are formed both in the mother's adrenal glands and in the adrenal glands of the fetus.

Function of Estrogen in Pregnancy. In Chapter 96, we pointed out that estrogens exert mainly a proliferative function on most reproductive and associated organs of the mother. During pregnancy, the extreme quantities of estrogens cause (1) enlargement of the mother's uterus, (2) enlargement of the mother's breasts and growth of the breast ductal structure, and (3) enlargement of the mother's female external genitalia.

The estrogens also relax the pelvic ligaments of the mother, so the sacroiliac joints become relatively limber and the symphysis pubis becomes elastic. These changes allow easier passage of the fetus through the birth canal. There is much reason to believe that estrogens also affect many general aspects of fetal development during pregnancy, for example, by affecting the rate of cell reproduction in the early embryo.

SECRETION OF PROGESTERONE BY THE PLACENTA

Progesterone is also essential for a successful pregnancy—in fact, it is just as important as estrogen. In addition to being secreted in moderate quantities by the corpus luteum at the beginning of pregnancy, progesterone is secreted later in tremendous quantities by the placenta as shown in Figure 98-6.

The special effects of progesterone that are essential for the normal progression of pregnancy are as follows:

1. Progesterone causes decidual cells to develop in the uterine endometrium. These cells play an important role in the nutrition of the early embryo.
2. Progesterone decreases the contractility of the pregnant uterus, thus preventing uterine contractions from causing spontaneous abortion.
3. Progesterone contributes to the development of the conceptus even before implantation because it specifically increases the secretions of the mother's fallopian tubes and uterus to provide appropriate nutritive matter for the developing *morula* (the spherical mass of 16–32 blastomeres formed before the blastula) and *blastocyst.* There is also reason to believe that progesterone affects cell cleavage in the early developing embryo.
4. The progesterone secreted during pregnancy helps estrogen prepare the mother's breasts for lactation, which is discussed later in this chapter.

HUMAN CHORIONIC SOMATOMAMMOTROPIN

Human chorionic somatomammotropin, a protein hormone with a molecular weight of about 22,000, begins to be secreted by the placenta at about the fifth week of pregnancy. Secretion of this hormone increases progressively throughout the remainder of pregnancy in direct proportion to the weight of the placenta. Although the functions of chorionic somatomammotropin are uncertain, it is secreted in quantities several times greater than that of all the other pregnancy hormones combined. It has several possible important effects:

1. The first function of the hormone discovered was the development of breasts and sometimes lactation in animals; it was thus first named *human placental lactogen.* However, attempts to use it to promote lactation in humans have not been successful.
2. Weak actions similar to those of growth hormone, causing the formation of protein tissues in the same way that growth hormone does. While it has a chemical structure similar to that of growth hormone, 100 times as much

human chorionic somatomammotropin as growth hormone is required to promote growth.

3. Decreased insulin sensitivity and decreased utilization of glucose in the mother, thereby making larger quantities of glucose available to the fetus. Further, the hormone promotes the release of free fatty acids from the fat stores of the mother, thus providing this alternative source of energy for the mother's metabolism during pregnancy.

OTHER HORMONAL FACTORS IN PREGNANCY

Almost all the nonsexual endocrine glands of the mother also react markedly to pregnancy. This reaction results mainly from the increased metabolic load on the mother but also, to some extent, from the effects of placental hormones on the pituitary and other glands. The following effects are some of the most notable.

Pituitary Secretion. The anterior pituitary gland of the mother enlarges at least 50% during pregnancy and increases its production of *corticotropin*, *thyrotropin*, and *prolactin*. Conversely, pituitary secretion of follicle-stimulating hormone and luteinizing hormone is almost totally suppressed as a result of the inhibitory effects of estrogens and progesterone from the placenta.

Increased Corticosteroid Secretion. The rate of adrenocortical secretion of the *glucocorticoids* is moderately increased throughout pregnancy. It is possible that these glucocorticoids help mobilize amino acids from the mother's tissues so these amino acids can be used for the synthesis of tissues in the fetus.

Pregnant women usually have about a twofold increase in *aldosterone*, secretion reaching a peak at the end of gestation. This increase, along with the actions of estrogens, causes a tendency for even a normal pregnant woman to reabsorb excess sodium from her renal tubules and, therefore, to retain fluid, which occasionally leads to *pregnancy-induced hypertension*.

Increased Thyroid Gland Secretion. The mother's thyroid gland ordinarily enlarges up to 50% during pregnancy and increases its production of thyroxine a corresponding amount. The increased thyroxine production is caused at least partly by a thyrotropic effect of *hCG* secreted by the placenta and by small quantities of a specific thyroid-stimulating hormone, *human chorionic thyrotropin*, also secreted by the placenta.

Increased Parathyroid Gland Secretion. The mother's parathyroid glands usually enlarge during pregnancy; this enlargement especially occurs if the mother's diet is deficient in calcium. Enlargement of these glands causes calcium absorption from the mother's bones, thereby maintaining normal calcium ion concentration in the mother's extracellular fluid even while the fetus removes calcium to ossify its own bones. This secretion of parathyroid hormone is even more intensified during lactation after the baby's birth because the growing baby requires many times more calcium than does the fetus.

Secretion of "Relaxin" by the Ovaries and Placenta. Another substance besides the estrogens and progesterone, a hormone called *relaxin*, is secreted by the corpus luteum of the ovary and by placental tissues. Its secretion is increased by a stimulating effect of hCG at the same time that the corpus luteum and the placenta secrete large quantities of estrogens and progesterone.

Relaxin is a 48–amino acid polypeptide with a molecular weight of about 9000. This hormone, when injected, causes relaxation of the ligaments of the symphysis pubis in the estrous rat and guinea pig. This effect is weak or possibly even absent in pregnant women. Instead, this role is probably played mainly by the estrogens, which also cause relaxation of the pelvic ligaments. It has also been claimed that relaxin softens the cervix of the pregnant woman at the time of delivery. Relaxin is also thought to serve as a vasodilator, contributing to increased blood flow in various tissues, including the kidneys, and increasing venous return and cardiac output in pregnancy.

Response of the Mother's Body to Pregnancy

Most apparent among the many reactions of the mother to the fetus and to the excessive hormones of pregnancy is the increased size of the various sexual organs. For instance, the uterus increases from about 50 to 1100 g, and the breasts approximately double in size. At the same time, the vagina enlarges and the introitus opens more widely. Also, the various hormones can cause marked changes in a pregnant woman's appearance, sometimes resulting in the development of edema, acne, and masculine or acromegalic features.

WEIGHT GAIN IN THE PREGNANT WOMAN

The average weight gain during pregnancy is about 25–35 lb (2.2 lb = 1 kg), with most of this gain occurring during the last two trimesters. Of this added weight, about 8 lb is fetus and 4 lb is amniotic fluid, placenta, and fetal membranes. The uterus increases about 3 lb and the breasts another 2 lb, still leaving an average weight increase of 8–18 lb. About 5 lb of this added weight is extra fluid in the blood and extracellular fluid, and the remaining 3–13 lb is generally fat accumulation. The extra fluid is excreted in the urine during the first few days after birth, that is, after loss of the fluid-retaining hormones from the placenta.

During pregnancy, a woman often has a greatly increased desire for food, partly as a result of removal of food substrates from the mother's blood by the fetus and partly because of hormonal factors.

METABOLISM DURING PREGNANCY

As a consequence of the increased secretion of many hormones during pregnancy, including thyroxine, adrenocortical hormones, and the sex hormones, the basal metabolic rate of the pregnant woman increases about 15% during the latter half of pregnancy.

NUTRITION DURING PREGNANCY

By far the greatest growth of the fetus occurs during the last trimester of pregnancy; its weight almost doubles during the last 2 months of pregnancy. Ordinarily, the mother does not absorb sufficient protein, calcium, phosphates, and iron from her diet during the last months of pregnancy to supply these extra needs of the fetus. However, in anticipation of these extra needs, the mother's body has already been storing these substances—some in the placenta, but most in the normal storage depots of the mother.

If appropriate nutritional elements are not present in a pregnant woman's diet, several maternal deficiencies can occur, especially in calcium, phosphates, iron, and the vitamins. For example, the fetus needs about 375 mg of iron to form its blood, and the mother needs an additional 600 mg to form her own extra blood. The normal store of nonhemoglobin iron in the mother at the outset of pregnancy is often only 100 mg and almost never more than 700 mg. Therefore, without sufficient iron in her food, a pregnant woman usually develops *hypochromic anemia*. Also, it is especially important that she receive vitamin D, because although the total quantity of calcium used by the fetus is small, calcium is normally poorly absorbed by the mother's gastrointestinal tract without vitamin D. Finally, shortly before birth of the baby, vitamin K is often added to the mother's diet so the baby will have sufficient prothrombin to prevent hemorrhage, particularly brain hemorrhage, caused by the birth process.

CHANGES IN THE MATERNAL CIRCULATORY SYSTEM DURING PREGNANCY

The maternal circulatory system undergoes profound changes during pregnancy in order to deal with the increasing demands of a growing fetus.

Blood Flow Through the Placenta and Maternal Cardiac Output Increases During Pregnancy. About 625 mL of blood flows through the maternal circulation of the placenta each minute during the last month of pregnancy. This flow, plus the general increase in the mother's metabolism, increases the mother's cardiac output to 30–40% above normal by the 27th week of pregnancy; then, for unexplained reasons, the cardiac output falls to only a little above normal during the last 8 weeks of pregnancy, despite the high uterine blood flow, indicating that blood flow in some other tissue(s) may be reduced.

Maternal Blood Volume Increases During Pregnancy. The maternal blood volume shortly before term is about 30% above normal. This increase occurs mainly during the latter half of pregnancy, as shown by the curve of Figure 98-7. The cause of the increased volume is likely due, at least in part, to aldosterone and estrogens, which are greatly increased in pregnancy, and to increased fluid retention by the kidneys. In addition, the bone marrow becomes increasingly active and produces extra red blood cells to go with the excess fluid volume. Therefore, at the time of the birth of the baby, the mother has about 1–2 L of extra blood in her circulatory system. Only about one-fourth of this amount is normally lost through bleeding during delivery of the baby, thereby allowing a considerable safety factor for the mother.

Maternal Respiration Increases During Pregnancy

Because of the increased basal metabolic rate of a pregnant woman and because of her greater size, the total amount of oxygen used by the mother shortly before birth of the baby is about 20% above normal and a commensurate amount of carbon dioxide is formed. These effects cause the mother's minute ventilation to increase. It is also believed that the high levels of

progesterone during pregnancy increase the minute ventilation even more because progesterone increases the sensitivity of the respiratory center to carbon dioxide. The net result is an increase in minute ventilation of about 50% and a decrease in arterial PCO_2 to several millimeters of mercury below that in a nonpregnant woman. Simultaneously, the growing uterus presses upward against the abdominal contents, which press upward against the diaphragm, so the total excursion of the diaphragm is decreased. Consequently, the respiratory rate is increased to maintain the extra ventilation.

Maternal Kidney Function During Pregnancy

The rate of urine formation by a pregnant woman is usually slightly increased because of increased fluid intake and increased load of excretory products. In addition, several special alterations of kidney function occur.

First, the renal tubules' reabsorptive capacity for sodium, chloride, and water is increased as much as 50% as a consequence of increased production of salt- and water-retaining hormones, especially steroid hormones by the placenta and adrenal cortex.

Second, the renal blood flow and glomerular filtration rate increase up to 50% during normal pregnancy as a result of renal vasodilation. Although the mechanisms that cause renal vasodilation in pregnancy are still unclear, some studies suggest that increased levels of nitric oxide or the ovarian hormone relaxin may contribute to these changes. The increased glomerular filtration rate likely occurs, at least in part, as a compensation for increased tubular reabsorption of salt and water. Thus, the *normal* pregnant woman ordinarily accumulates only about 5 lb of extra water and salt.

An overall summary of the maternal changes in pregnancy is given in Table 98-1.

Amniotic Fluid and its Formation

Normally, the volume of *amniotic fluid* (the fluid inside the uterus in which the fetus floats) is between 500 mL and 1 L, but it can be only a few milliliters or as much as several liters. Isotope studies of the rate of formation of amniotic fluid show that, on average, the water in amniotic fluid is replaced once every 3 hours and the electrolytes sodium and potassium are replaced an average of once every 15 hours. A large portion of the fluid is derived from renal excretion by the fetus. Likewise, a certain amount of absorption occurs by way of the gastrointestinal tract and lungs of the fetus. However, even after in utero death of a fetus, some turnover of the amniotic fluid still occurs, which indicates that some of the fluid is formed and absorbed directly through the amniotic membranes.

Preeclampsia and Eclampsia

About 5% of all pregnant women experience *pregnancy-induced hypertension*, that is, a rapid rise in arterial blood pressure to hypertensive levels during the last few months of pregnancy that is also associated with leakage of large amounts of protein into the urine. This condition is called *preeclampsia* or *toxemia of pregnancy*. It is often characterized by excess salt and water retention by the mother's kidneys and by weight gain and the development of edema and hypertension in the mother. Various attempts have been made to prove that preeclampsia is caused by excessive secretion of placental or adrenal hormones, but proof of a hormonal basis is still lacking. Another theory is that preeclampsia results from some type of autoimmunity or allergy in the mother caused by the presence of the fetus. In support of

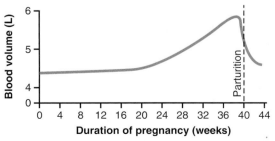

Figure 98-7 The effect of pregnancy in increasing the mother's blood volume.

TABLE 98-1	Summary of Maternal Changes During Pregnancy
Weight gain	11–15 kg: depending on the height and prepregnant weight of the woman
Body fluid	Increase in total body water; water retention increases and exceeds sodium retention resulting in a small drop in plasma osmolality
Cardiovascular system	Cardiac output increases by about 30–40% by 27th week of pregnancy and then begins to fall to a little over normal by term Blood volume increases by about 30% by term BP decreases up to about 24 weeks, and then rises toward normal at term. Some women experience postural hypotension during pregnancy
Respiratory system	Tidal volume and minute ventilation increase Total lung capacity and residual volume decrease, in part because the diaphragm is moved up due to the developing fetus
Renal changes	Renal blood flow and GFR increase Ureteral and renal pelvis dilatation (partly because of the mechanical compression of the uterus)
Hematological changes	Red cell mass increases but due to greater plasma volume expansion there is hemodilution resulting in physiological anemia of pregnancy
Endocrine changes	Glucocorticoids, thyroxine, aldosterone, and parathormone all increased
Gastrointestinal changes	Changes in appetite—*pica* Nausea and vomiting in early pregnancy ("morning sickness") Reduced GI motility sometimes leading to constipation Gastroesophageal reflux due to increased intraabdominal pressure
Skeletal–muscular	Relaxin in later pregnancy results in relaxation of pubic symphysis and sacroiliac joints Lordosis (increased curving of the lumbar spine)—to compensate for the shift in center of gravity brought on by the enlarging uterus

GFR, glomerular filtration rate; GI, gastrointestinal.

this theory, the acute symptoms usually disappear within a few days after birth of the baby.

Evidence also indicates that preeclampsia is initiated by *insufficient blood supply to the placenta*, resulting in the placenta's release of substances that cause widespread dysfunction of the maternal vascular endothelium.

Eclampsia is an extreme degree of preeclampsia, characterized by vascular spasm throughout the body; clonic seizures in the mother, sometimes followed by coma; greatly decreased kidney output; malfunction of the liver; often extreme hypertension; and a generalized toxic condition of the body. It usually occurs shortly before the birth of the baby. Without treatment, a high percentage of mothers with eclampsia die. However, with optimal and immediate use of rapidly acting vasodilating drugs to reduce the arterial pressure to normal, followed by immediate termination of pregnancy—by cesarean section if necessary—the mortality even in mothers with eclampsia has been reduced to 1% or less.

BIBLIOGRAPHY

Anand-Ivell R, Ivell R: Regulation of the reproductive cycle and early pregnancy by relaxin family peptides, *Mol. Cell. Endocrinol.* 382:472, 2014.

Arck PC, Hecher K: Fetomaternal immune crosstalk and its consequences for maternal and offspring's health, *Nat. Med.* 19:548, 2013.

August P: Preeclampsia: a "nephrocentric" view, *Adv. Chronic Kidney Dis.* 20:280, 2013.

Augustine RA, Ladyman SR, Grattan DR: From feeding one to feeding many: hormone-induced changes in bodyweight homeostasis during pregnancy, *J. Physiol.* 586:387, 2008.

Bertram R, Helena CV, Gonzalez-Iglesias AE, et al: A tale of two rhythms: the emerging roles of oxytocin in rhythmic prolactin release, *J. Neuroendocrinol.* 22:778, 2010.

Carter AM: Evolution of placental function in mammals: the molecular basis of gas and nutrient transfer, hormone secretion, and immune responses, *Physiol. Rev.* 92:1543, 2010.

Conrad KP, Davison JM: The renal circulation in normal pregnancy and preeclampsia: is there a place for relaxin? *Am. J. Physiol. Renal Physiol.* 306:F1121, 2014.

Freeman ME, Kanyicska B, Lerant A, Nagy G: Prolactin: structure, function, and regulation of secretion, *Physiol. Rev.* 80:1523, 2000.

Gimpl G, Fahrenholz F: The oxytocin receptor system: structure, function, and regulation, *Physiol. Rev.* 81:629, 2001.

Iams JD: Clinical practice. Prevention of preterm parturition, *N. Engl. J. Med.* 370:254, 2014.

LaMarca B, Cornelius D, Wallace K: Elucidating immune mechanisms causing hypertension during pregnancy, *Physiology (Bethesda)* 28:225, 2013.

Maltepe E, Bakardjiev AI, Fisher SJ: The placenta, transcriptional, epigenetic, and physiological integration during development, *J. Clin. Invest.* 120:1016, 2010.

Osol G, Mandala M: Maternal uterine vascular remodeling during pregnancy, *Physiology (Bethesda)* 24:58, 2009.

Palei AC, Spradley FT, Warrington JP, et al: Pathophysiology of hypertension in pre-eclampsia: a lesson in integrative physiology, *Acta Physiol. (Oxf.)* 208:224, 2013.

Rana S, Karumanchi SA, Lindheimer MD: Angiogenic factors in diagnosis, management, and research in preeclampsia, *Hypertension* 63:198, 2014.

Roberts JM, Gammill HS: Preeclampsia: recent insights, *Hypertension* 46:1243, 2005.

Smith R: Parturition, *N. Engl. J. Med.* 356:271, 2007.

Wang A, Rana S, Karumanchi SA: Preeclampsia: the role of angiogenic factors in its pathogenesis, *Physiology (Bethesda)* 24:147, 2009.

Parturition and Lactation

Parturition

Parturition means birth of the baby. Toward the end of pregnancy, the uterus becomes progressively more excitable, until finally it develops such strong rhythmic contractions that the baby is expelled. The exact cause of the increased activity of the uterus is not known, but at least two major categories of effects lead up to the intense contractions responsible for parturition: (1) progressive hormonal changes that cause increased excitability of the uterine musculature and (2) progressive mechanical changes.

Hormonal Factors that Increase Uterine Contractility

Increased Ratio of Estrogens to Progesterone. Progesterone inhibits uterine contractility during pregnancy, thereby helping to prevent expulsion of the fetus. Conversely, estrogens have a definite tendency to increase the degree of uterine contractility, partly because estrogens increase the number of gap junctions between the adjacent uterine smooth muscle cells, but also because of other poorly understood effects. Both progesterone and estrogen are secreted in progressively greater quantities

throughout most of pregnancy, but from the seventh month onward, estrogen secretion continues to increase while progesterone secretion remains constant or perhaps even decreases slightly. Therefore, it has been postulated that the *estrogen-to-progesterone ratio* increases sufficiently toward the end of pregnancy to be at least partly responsible for the increased contractility of the uterus.

Oxytocin Causes Contraction of the Uterus. Oxytocin, a hormone secreted by the neurohypophysis, specifically causes uterine contraction (see Chapter 88). There are four reasons to believe that oxytocin might be important in increasing the contractility of the uterus near term:

1. The uterine muscle increases its oxytocin receptors and, therefore, increases its responsiveness to a given dose of oxytocin during the latter few months of pregnancy.
2. The rate of oxytocin secretion by the neurohypophysis is considerably increased at the time of labor.
3. Although hypophysectomized animals can still deliver their young at term, labor is prolonged.
4. Experiments in animals indicate that irritation or stretching of the uterine cervix, as occurs during labor, can cause a neurogenic reflex through the paraventricular and supraoptic nuclei of the hypothalamus that causes the posterior pituitary gland (the neurohypophysis) to increase its secretion of oxytocin.

Effect of Fetal Hormones on the Uterus. The fetus's pituitary gland secretes increasing quantities of oxytocin, which might play a role in exciting the uterus. Also, the fetus's adrenal glands secrete large quantities of cortisol, another possible uterine stimulant. In addition, the fetal membranes release prostaglandins in high concentration at the time of labor. These prostaglandins, too, can increase the intensity of uterine contractions.

Mechanical Factors that Increase Uterine Contractility

Stretch of the Uterine Musculature. Simply stretching smooth muscle organs usually increases their contractility. Further, intermittent stretch, which occurs repeatedly in the uterus because of fetal movements, can also elicit smooth muscle contraction. Note especially that twins are born, on average, *19 days* earlier than a single child, which emphasizes the importance of mechanical stretch in eliciting uterine contractions.

Stretch or Irritation of the Cervix. There is reason to believe that stretching or irritating the uterine cervix is particularly important in eliciting uterine contractions. For instance, obstetricians frequently induce labor by rupturing the membranes so that the head of the baby stretches the cervix more forcefully than usual or irritates it in other ways.

The mechanism by which cervical irritation excites the body of the uterus is not known. It has been suggested that stretching or irritation of nerves in the cervix initiates reflexes to the body of the uterus, but the effect could also result simply from myogenic transmission of signals from the cervix to the body of the uterus.

ONSET OF LABOR—A POSITIVE FEEDBACK MECHANISM FOR ITS INITIATION

During most of the months of pregnancy, the uterus undergoes periodic episodes of weak and slow rhythmic contractions called *Braxton–Hicks contractions*. These contractions become progressively stronger toward the end of pregnancy; then they change suddenly, within hours, to become exceptionally strong contractions that start stretching the cervix and later force the baby through the birth canal, thereby causing parturition. This process is called *labor*, and the strong contractions that result in final parturition are called *labor contractions*.

We do not know what suddenly changes the slow, weak rhythmicity of the uterus into strong labor contractions. However, on the basis of experience with other types of physiological control systems, a theory has been proposed to explain the onset of labor. The *positive feedback* theory suggests that stretching of the cervix by the fetus's head finally becomes great enough to elicit a strong reflex increase in contractility of the uterine body. This pushes the baby forward, which stretches the cervix more and initiates more positive feedback to the uterine body. Thus, the process repeats until the baby is expelled. This theory is shown in Figure 99-1 and the following observations support this theory.

First, labor contractions obey all the principles of positive feedback. That is, once the strength of uterine contraction becomes greater than a critical value, each contraction leads to subsequent contractions that become stronger and stronger until maximum effect is achieved. By referring to the discussion in Chapter 1 of positive feedback in control systems, one can see that this is the precise nature of all positive feedback

1. Baby's head stretches cervix
2. Cervical stretch excites fundic contraction
3. Fundic contraction pushes baby down and stretches cervix some more
4. Cycle repeats over and over again

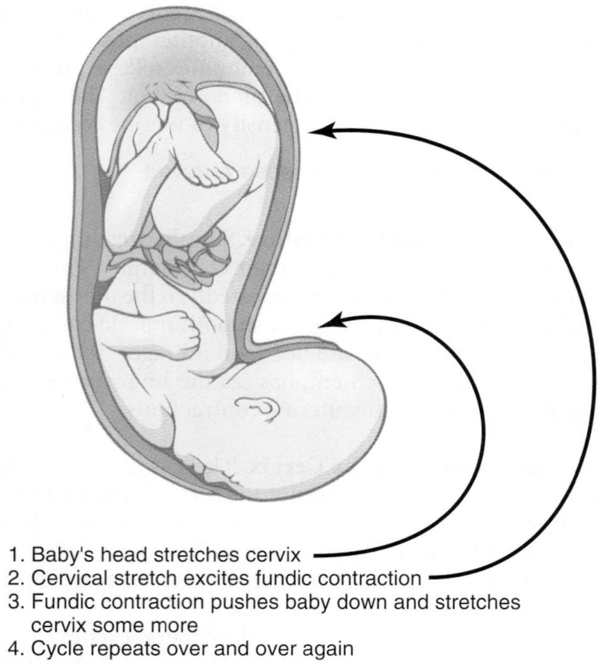

Figure 99-1 Theory for the onset of intensely strong contractions during labor.

mechanisms when the feedback gain becomes greater than a critical value.

Second, two known types of positive feedback increase uterine contractions during labor: (1) stretching of the cervix causes the entire body of the uterus to contract, and this contraction stretches the cervix even more because of the downward thrust of the baby's head, and (2) cervical stretching also causes the pituitary gland to secrete oxytocin, which is another means for increasing uterine contractility.

To summarize, we can assume that multiple factors increase the contractility of the uterus toward the end of pregnancy. Eventually, a uterine contraction becomes strong enough to irritate the uterus, especially at the cervix, and this irritation increases uterine contractility still more because of positive feedback, resulting in a second uterine contraction stronger than the first, a third stronger than the second, and so forth. Once these contractions become strong enough to cause this type of feedback, with each succeeding contraction greater than the preceding one, the process proceeds to completion.

One might ask about the many instances of false labor, in which the contractions become stronger and stronger and then fade away. Remember that for a positive feedback to continue, *each* new cycle of the positive feedback must be stronger than the previous one. If at any time after labor starts some contractions fail to reexcite the uterus sufficiently, the positive feedback could go into a retrograde decline and the labor contractions would fade away.

ABDOMINAL MUSCLE CONTRACTIONS DURING LABOR

Once uterine contractions become strong during labor, pain signals originate both from the uterus and from the birth canal. These signals, in addition to causing suffering, elicit neurogenic reflexes in the spinal cord to the abdominal muscles, causing intense contractions of these muscles. The abdominal contractions add greatly to the force that causes expulsion of the baby.

MECHANICS OF PARTURITION

The uterine contractions during labor begin mainly at the top of the uterine fundus and spread downward over the body of the uterus. Also, the intensity of contraction is great in the top and body of the uterus but weak in the lower segment of the uterus adjacent to the cervix. Therefore, each uterine contraction tends to force the baby downward toward the cervix.

In the early part of labor, the contractions might occur only once every 30 minutes. As labor progresses, the contractions finally appear as often as once every 1–3 minutes and the intensity of contraction increases greatly, with only a short period of relaxation between contractions. The combined contractions of the uterine and abdominal musculature during delivery of the baby cause a downward force on the fetus of about 25 lb during each strong contraction.

It is fortunate that the contractions of labor occur intermittently because strong contractions impede or sometimes even stop blood flow through the placenta and would cause death of the fetus if the contractions were continuous. Indeed, overuse of various uterine stimulants, such as oxytocin, can cause uterine spasm rather than rhythmic contractions and can lead to death of the fetus.

In more than 95% of births, the head is the first part of the baby to be expelled, and in most of the remaining instances, the buttocks are presented first. Entering the birth canal with the buttocks or feet first is called a *breech* presentation.

The head acts as a wedge to open the structures of the birth canal as the fetus is forced downward. The first major obstruction to expulsion of the fetus is the uterine cervix. Toward the end of pregnancy, the cervix becomes soft, which allows it to stretch when labor contractions begin in the uterus. The so-called *first stage of labor* is a period of progressive cervical dilation, lasting until the cervical opening is as large as the head of the fetus. This stage usually lasts for 8–24 hours in the first pregnancy but often only a few minutes after many pregnancies.

Once the cervix has dilated fully, the fetal membranes usually rupture and the amniotic fluid is lost suddenly through the vagina. Then the head of the fetus moves rapidly into the birth canal and with additional force from above, it continues to wedge its way through the canal until delivery occurs. This is called the *second stage of labor*, and it may last from as little as 1 minute after many pregnancies to 30 minutes or more in the first pregnancy.

SEPARATION AND DELIVERY OF THE PLACENTA

For 10–45 minutes after birth of the baby, the uterus continues to contract to a smaller and smaller size, which causes a *shearing* effect between the walls of the uterus and the placenta, thus separating the placenta from its implantation site. Separation of the placenta opens the placental sinuses and causes bleeding. The amount of bleeding is limited to an average of 350 mL by the following mechanism: the smooth muscle fibers of the uterine musculature are arranged in figures of eight around the blood vessels as the vessels pass through the uterine wall. Therefore, contraction of the uterus after delivery of the baby constricts the vessels that had previously supplied blood to the placenta. In addition, it is believed that vasoconstrictor prostaglandins formed at the placental separation site cause additional blood vessel spasm.

LABOR PAINS

With each uterine contraction, the mother experiences considerable pain. The cramping pain in early labor is probably caused mainly by hypoxia of the uterine muscle resulting from compression of the blood vessels in the uterus. This pain is not felt when the visceral sensory *hypogastric nerves*, which carry the visceral sensory fibers leading from the uterus, have been sectioned.

During the second stage of labor, when the fetus is being expelled through the birth canal, much more severe pain is caused by cervical stretching, perineal stretching, and stretching or tearing of structures in the vaginal canal itself. This pain is conducted to the mother's spinal cord and brain by somatic nerves instead of by the visceral sensory nerves.

INVOLUTION OF THE UTERUS AFTER PARTURITION

During the first 4–5 weeks after parturition, the uterus involutes. Its weight becomes less than half its immediate postpartum weight within 1 week, and in 4 weeks, if the mother lactates, the uterus may become as small as it was before pregnancy. This effect of lactation results from the suppression of pituitary gonadotropin and ovarian hormone secretion during the first few months of lactation, as discussed later. During early involution

of the uterus, the placental site on the endometrial surface autolyzes, causing a vaginal discharge known as "lochia," which is first bloody and then serous in nature, and continues for a total of about 10 days. After this time, the endometrial surface becomes reepithelialized and ready for normal, nongravid sex life again.

Lactation

DEVELOPMENT OF THE BREASTS

The breasts, shown in Figure 99-2, begin to develop at puberty. This development is stimulated by the estrogens of the monthly female sexual cycle; estrogens stimulate growth of the *mammary glands* plus the deposition of fat to give the breasts mass. In addition, far greater growth occurs during the high-estrogen state of pregnancy, and only then does the glandular tissue become completely developed for the production of milk.

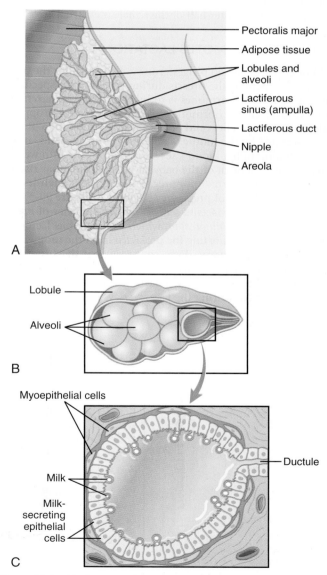

Figure 99-2   The breast and its secretory lobules, alveoli, and lactiferous ducts (milk ducts) that constitute its mammary gland (A). The enlargements show a lobule (B) and milk-secreting cells of an alveolus (C).

Estrogens Stimulate Growth of the Ductal System of the Breasts. All through pregnancy, the large quantities of estrogens secreted by the placenta cause the ductal system of the breasts to grow and branch. Simultaneously, the stroma of the breasts increases in quantity, and large quantities of fat are laid down in the stroma.

Also important for growth of the ductal system are at least four other hormones: *growth hormone, prolactin,* the *adrenal glucocorticoids,* and *insulin.* Each of these hormones is known to play at least some role in protein metabolism, which presumably explains their function in the development of the breasts.

Progesterone Is Required for Full Development of the Lobule–Alveolar System. Final development of the breasts into milk-secreting organs also requires *progesterone.* Once the ductal system has developed, progesterone—acting synergistically with estrogen, as well as with the other hormones just mentioned—causes additional growth of the breast lobules, with budding of alveoli and development of secretory characteristics in the cells of the alveoli. These changes are analogous to the secretory effects of progesterone on the endometrium of the uterus during the latter half of the female menstrual cycle.

PROLACTIN PROMOTES LACTATION

Although estrogen and progesterone are essential for the physical development of the breasts during pregnancy, a specific effect of both these hormones is to inhibit *the actual secretion of milk.* Conversely, the hormone *prolactin* has exactly the opposite effect on milk secretion and promotes milk production. Prolactin is secreted by the mother's anterior pituitary gland, and its concentration in her blood rises steadily from the fifth week of pregnancy until birth of the baby, at which time it has risen to 10–20 times the normal nonpregnant level. This high level of prolactin at the end of pregnancy is shown in Figure 99-3.

In addition, the placenta secretes large quantities of *human chorionic somatomammotropin,* which probably has lactogenic properties, thus supporting the prolactin from the mother's pituitary during pregnancy. Even so, because of the suppressive effects of estrogen and progesterone, no more than a few milliliters of fluid are secreted each day until after the baby is born. The fluid secreted during the last few days before and the first few days after parturition is called *colostrum*; it contains essentially the same concentrations of proteins and lactose as milk, but it has almost no fat and its maximum rate of production is about 1/100 the subsequent rate of milk production.

Immediately after the baby is born, the sudden loss of both estrogen and progesterone secretion from the placenta allows the lactogenic effect of prolactin from the mother's pituitary gland to assume its natural milk-promoting role, and during the next 1–7 days, the breasts begin to secrete copious quantities of milk instead of colostrum. This secretion of milk requires an adequate background secretion of most of the mother's other hormones as well, but most important are *growth hormone, cortisol, parathyroid hormone,* and *insulin.* These hormones are necessary to provide the amino acids, fatty acids, glucose, and calcium required for the formation of milk.

After the birth of the baby, the *basal level* of prolactin secretion returns to the nonpregnant level during the next few weeks, as shown in Figure 99-3. However, each time the mother nurses her baby, nervous signals from the nipples to the hypothalamus cause a 10- to 20-fold surge in prolactin secretion that lasts for about 1 hour, which is also shown in Figure 99-3. This prolactin acts on the mother's breasts to keep the mammary glands secreting milk into the alveoli for the subsequent nursing periods. If this prolactin surge is absent or blocked as a result of hypothalamic or pituitary damage or if nursing does not continue, the breasts lose their ability to produce milk within 1 week or so. However, milk production can continue for several years if the child continues to suckle, although the rate of milk formation normally decreases considerably after 7–9 months.

The Hypothalamus Secretes Prolactin-Inhibitory Hormone. The hypothalamus plays an essential role in controlling prolactin secretion, as it does for almost all the other anterior pituitary hormones. However, this control is different in one aspect: The hypothalamus mainly *stimulates* production of all the other hormones, but it mainly *inhibits* prolactin production. Consequently, damage to the hypothalamus or blockage of the hypothalamic–hypophysial portal system often increases prolactin secretion while it depresses secretion of the other anterior pituitary hormones.

Therefore, it is believed that anterior pituitary secretion of prolactin is controlled either entirely or almost entirely by

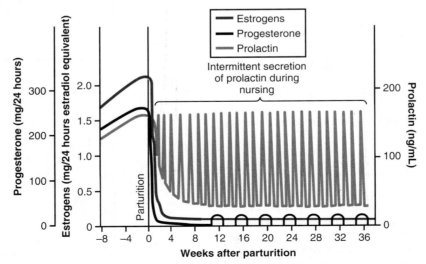

Figure 99-3   Changes in rates of secretion of estrogens, progesterone, and prolactin for 8 weeks before parturition and 36 weeks thereafter. Note especially the decrease of prolactin secretion back to basal levels within a few weeks after parturition, but also the intermittent periods of marked prolactin secretion (for about 1 hour at a time) during and after periods of nursing.

an inhibitory factor formed in the hypothalamus and transported through the hypothalamic–hypophysial portal system to the anterior pituitary gland. This factor is sometimes called *prolactin-inhibitory hormone* but it is almost certainly the same as the catecholamine *dopamine*, which is known to be secreted by the arcuate nuclei of the hypothalamus and can decrease prolactin secretion as much as 10-fold.

Suppression of the Female Ovarian Cycles in Nursing Mothers for Many Months After Delivery. In most nursing mothers, the ovarian cycle (and ovulation) does not resume until a few weeks after cessation of nursing. The reason seems to be that the same nervous signals from the breasts to the hypothalamus that cause prolactin secretion during suckling—either because of the nervous signals or because of a subsequent effect of increased prolactin—inhibit secretion of gonadotropin-releasing hormone by the hypothalamus. This inhibition, in turn, suppresses formation of the pituitary gonadotropic hormones—luteinizing hormone and follicle-stimulating hormone. However, after several months of lactation, in some mothers (especially in those who nurse their babies only some of the time) the pituitary begins to secrete sufficient gonadotropic hormones to reinstate the monthly sexual cycle, even though nursing continues.

EJECTION (OR "LET-DOWN") PROCESS IN MILK SECRETION—FUNCTION OF OXYTOCIN

Milk is secreted continuously into the alveoli of the breasts, but it does not flow easily from the alveoli into the ductal system and, therefore, does not continually leak from the nipples. Instead, the milk must be *ejected* from the alveoli into the ducts before the baby can obtain it. This ejection is caused by a combined neurogenic and hormonal reflex that involves the posterior pituitary hormone *oxytocin*.

When the baby suckles, it receives virtually no milk for the first half minute or so. Sensory impulses must first be transmitted through somatic nerves from the nipples to the mother's spinal cord and then to her hypothalamus, where they cause nerve signals that promote *oxytocin* secretion at the same time that they cause prolactin secretion. The oxytocin is carried in the blood to the breasts, where it causes *myoepithelial cells* (which surround the outer walls of the alveoli) to contract, thereby expressing the milk from the alveoli into the ducts at a pressure of +10 to 20 mmHg. Then the baby's suckling becomes effective in removing the milk. Thus, within 30 seconds to 1 minute after a baby begins to suckle, milk begins to flow. This process is called *milk ejection* or *milk letdown*. The milk ejection reflex is illustrated in Figure 99-4.

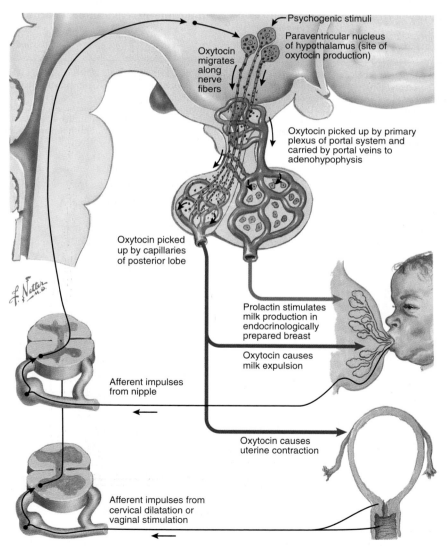

Figure 99-4 Secretion and action of oxytocin. *Netter illustration from www.netterimages.com.* © Elsevier Inc. All rights reserved.

Suckling on one breast causes milk flow not only in that breast but also in the opposite breast. It is especially interesting that fondling of the baby by the mother or hearing the baby crying often gives enough of an emotional signal to the hypothalamus to cause milk ejection. Additional information about oxytocin is given in Chapter 88.

Inhibition of Milk Ejection. A particular problem in nursing a baby comes from the fact that many psychogenic factors or even generalized sympathetic nervous system stimulation throughout the mother's body can inhibit oxytocin secretion and consequently depress milk ejection. For this reason, many mothers must have an undisturbed period of adjustment after childbirth if they are to be successful in nursing their babies.

MILK COMPOSITION

Table 99-1 lists the contents of human milk and cow's milk. The concentration of lactose in human milk is about 50% greater than in cow's milk, but the concentration of protein in cow's milk is ordinarily two or more times greater than in human milk. Finally, only one-third as much ash, which contains calcium and other minerals, is found in human milk compared with cow's milk.

Antibodies and Other Anti-Infectious Agents in Milk. Not only does milk provide the newborn baby with needed nutrients,

TABLE 99-1	Composition of Milk	
Constituent	Human Milk (%)	Cow's Milk (%)
Water	88.5	87
Fat	3.3	3.5
Lactose	6.8	4.8
Casein	0.9	2.7
Lactalbumin and other proteins	0.4	0.7
Ash	0.2	0.7

but it also provides important protection against infection. For instance, multiple types of *antibodies* and other anti-infectious agents are secreted in milk along with the nutrients. Also, several different types of white blood cells are secreted, including both *neutrophils* and *macrophages*, some of which are especially lethal to bacteria that could cause deadly infections in newborn babies. Particularly important are antibodies and macrophages that destroy *Escherichia coli* bacteria, which often cause lethal diarrhea in newborns.

When cow's milk is used to supply nutrition for the baby in place of mother's milk, the protective agents in it are usually of little value because they are normally destroyed within minutes in the internal environment of the human being.

BIBLIOGRAPHY

Ben-Jonathan N, Hnasko R: Dopamine as a prolactin (PRL) inhibitor, *Endocr. Rev.* 22:724, 2001.

Freeman ME, Kanyicska B, Lerant A, et al: Prolactin: structure, function, and regulation of secretion, *Physiol. Rev.* 80:1523, 2000.

Gimpl G, Fahrenholz F: The oxytocin receptor system: structure, function, and regulation, *Physiol. Rev.* 81:629, 2001.

Labbok MH, Clark D, Goldman AS: Breastfeeding: maintaining an irreplaceable immunological resource, *Nat. Rev. Immunol.* 4:565, 2004.

LaMarca HL, Rosen JM: Hormones and mammary cell fate—what will I become when I grow up? *Endocrinology* 149:4317, 2008.

Shennan DB, Peaker M: Transport of milk constituents by the mammary gland, *Physiol. Rev.* 80:925, 2000.

Sherwood OD: Relaxin's physiological roles and other diverse actions, *Endocr. Rev.* 25:205, 2004.

Smith R: Parturition, *N. Engl. J. Med.* 356:271, 2007.

Central Nervous System

SECTION OUTLINE

100

Organization of the Central Nervous System

The nervous system is unique in the vast complexity of thought processes and control actions it can perform. Each minute it receives literally millions of bits of information from the different sensory nerves and sensory organs, and then integrates all these to determine responses to be made by the body.

Before beginning this discussion of the nervous system, the reader should review Chapters 9 and 12, which present the principles of membrane potentials and transmission of signals in nerves and through neuromuscular junctions.

General Design of the Nervous System

CENTRAL NERVOUS SYSTEM NEURON: THE BASIC FUNCTIONAL UNIT

The central nervous system contains more than 100 billion neurons. Figure 100-1 shows a typical neuron of a type found in the brain motor cortex. Incoming signals enter this neuron through synapses located not only mostly on the neuronal dendrites but also on the cell body. For different types of neurons, there may be only a few hundred or as many as 200,000 such synaptic connections from input fibers. Conversely, the output signal travels by way of a single axon leaving the neuron. Then, this axon may have many separate branches to other parts of the nervous system or peripheral body.

A special feature of most synapses is that the signal normally passes only in the forward direction, from the axon of a preceding neuron to dendrites on cell membranes of subsequent neurons. This feature forces the signal to travel in required directions to perform specific nervous functions.

SENSORY PART OF THE NERVOUS SYSTEM— SENSORY RECEPTORS

Most activities of the nervous system are initiated by sensory experiences that excite *sensory receptors*, whether visual receptors in the eyes, auditory receptors in the ears, tactile receptors on the surface of the body, or other kinds of receptors. Either of these sensory experiences can cause immediate reactions from the brain or memories of the experiences can be stored in the brain for minutes, weeks, or years and bodily reactions determined at some future date.

Figure 100-2 shows the *somatic* portion of the sensory system, which transmits sensory information from the receptors of the entire body surface and some deep structures. This information enters the central nervous system through peripheral nerves and is conducted immediately to multiple sensory areas in (1) the spinal cord at all levels; (2) the reticular substance of the medulla, pons, and mesencephalon of the brain; (3) the cerebellum; (4) the thalamus; and (5) areas of the cerebral cortex.

MOTOR PART OF THE NERVOUS SYSTEM—EFFECTORS

The most important eventual role of the nervous system is to control the various bodily activities. This is achieved by controlling (1) contraction of appropriate skeletal muscles throughout the body, (2) contraction of smooth muscle in the internal organs, and (3) secretion of active chemical substances by both exocrine and endocrine glands in many parts of the body. These activities are collectively called *motor functions* of the nervous system, and the muscles and glands are called *effectors* because they are the actual anatomical structures that perform the functions dictated by the nerve signals.

Figure 100-3 shows the *"skeletal" motor nerve axis* of the nervous system for controlling skeletal muscle contraction. Operating parallel to this axis is another system, called the *autonomic nervous system*, for controlling smooth muscles, glands, and other internal bodily systems; this system is discussed in Chapter 119.

Note in Figure 100-3 that the skeletal muscles can be controlled from many levels of the central nervous system, including (1) the spinal cord; (2) the reticular substance of the medulla, pons, and mesencephalon; (3) the basal ganglia; (4) the cerebellum; and (5) the motor cortex. Each of these areas plays its own specific role.,The lower regions are concerned primarily with automatic, instantaneous muscle responses to sensory stimuli, and the higher regions are concerned with deliberate complex muscle movements controlled by the thought processes of the brain.

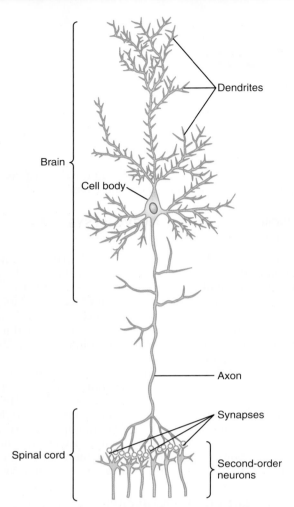

Figure 100-1 Structure of a large neuron in the brain, showing its important functional parts. *Modified from Guyton, A.C., 1987. Basic Neuroscience: Anatomy and Physiology. W.B. Saunders, Philadelphia.*

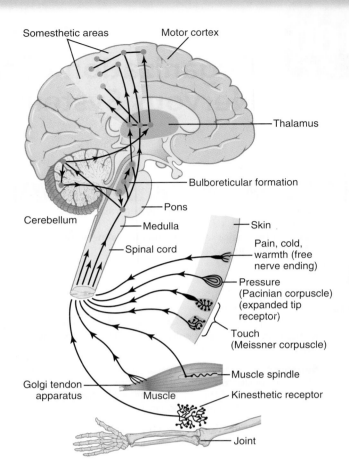

Figure 100-2 Somatosensory axis of the nervous system.

PROCESSING OF INFORMATION—"INTEGRATIVE" FUNCTION OF THE NERVOUS SYSTEM

One of the most important functions of the nervous system is to process incoming information in such a way that *appropriate* mental and motor responses will occur. More than 99% of all sensory information is discarded by the brain as irrelevant and unimportant. For instance, one is ordinarily unaware of the parts of the body that are in contact with clothing, as well as of the seat pressure when sitting. Likewise, attention is drawn only to an occasional object in one's field of vision, and even the perpetual noise of our surroundings is usually relegated to the subconscious.

However, when important sensory information excites the mind, it is immediately channeled into proper integrative and motor regions of the brain to cause desired responses. This channeling and processing of information is called the *integrative function* of the nervous system. Thus, if a person places a hand on a hot stove, the desired instantaneous response is to lift the hand. Other associated responses follow, such as moving the entire body away from the stove and perhaps even shouting with pain.

Role of Synapses in Processing Information. The synapse is the junction point from one neuron to the next. Later in this

chapter, we discuss the details of synaptic function. However, it is important to point out here that synapses determine the directions that the nervous signals will spread through the nervous system. Some synapses transmit signals from one neuron to the next with ease, whereas others transmit signals only with difficulty. Also, *facilitatory* and *inhibitory* signals from other areas in the nervous system can control synaptic transmission, sometimes opening the synapses for transmission and at other times closing them. In addition, some postsynaptic neurons respond with large numbers of output impulses, and others respond with only a few. Thus, the synapses perform a selective action, often blocking weak signals while allowing strong signals to pass, but at other times selecting and amplifying certain weak signals, and often channeling these signals in many directions rather than in only one direction.

STORAGE OF INFORMATION—MEMORY

Only a small fraction of even the most important sensory information usually causes immediate motor response. But much of the information is stored for future control of motor activities and for use in the thinking processes. Most storage occurs in the *cerebral cortex*, but even the basal regions of the brain and the spinal cord can store small amounts of information.

The storage of information is the process we call *memory*, and this, too, is a function of the synapses. Each time certain

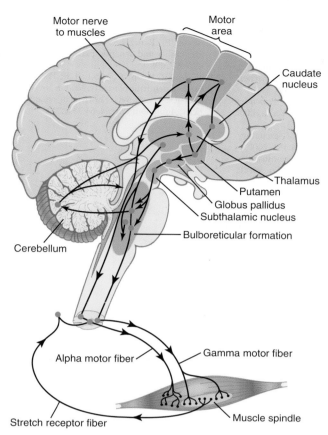

Figure 100-3 Skeletal motor nerve axis of the nervous system.

types of sensory signals pass through sequences of synapses, these synapses become more capable of transmitting the same type of signal the next time, a process called *facilitation*. After the sensory signals have passed through the synapses a large number of times, the synapses become so facilitated that signals generated within the brain itself can also cause transmission of impulses through the same sequences of synapses, even when the sensory input is not excited. This process gives the person a perception of experiencing the original sensations, although the perceptions are only memories of the sensations.

The precise mechanisms by which long-term facilitation of synapses occurs in the memory process are still uncertain, but what is known about this and other details of the sensory memory process is discussed in Chapter 125.

Once memories have been stored in the nervous system, they become part of the brain processing mechanism for future "thinking." That is, the thinking processes of the brain compare new sensory experiences with stored memories; the memories then help to select the important new sensory information and to channel this into appropriate memory storage areas for future use or into motor areas to cause immediate bodily responses.

Major Levels of Central Nervous System Function

The human nervous system has inherited special functional capabilities from each stage of human evolutionary development. From this heritage, three major levels of the central nervous

system have specific functional characteristics: (1) the *spinal cord level*, (2) the *lower brain* or *subcortical level*, and (3) the *higher brain* or *cortical level*.

SPINAL CORD LEVEL

We often think of the spinal cord as being only a conduit for signals from the periphery of the body to the brain, or in the opposite direction from the brain back to the body. This is far from the truth. Even after the spinal cord has been cut in the high neck region, many highly organized spinal cord functions still occur. For instance, neuronal circuits in the cord can cause (1) walking movements, (2) reflexes that withdraw portions of the body from painful objects, (3) reflexes that stiffen the legs to support the body against gravity, and (4) reflexes that control local blood vessels, gastrointestinal movements, or urinary excretion. In fact, the upper levels of the nervous system often operate not by sending signals directly to the periphery of the body but by sending signals to the control centers of the cord, simply "commanding" the cord centers to perform their functions.

LOWER BRAIN OR SUBCORTICAL LEVEL

Many, if not most, of what we call subconscious activities of the body are controlled in the lower areas of the brain—that is, in the medulla, pons, mesencephalon, hypothalamus, thalamus, cerebellum, and basal ganglia. For instance, subconscious control of arterial pressure and respiration is achieved mainly in the medulla and pons. Control of equilibrium is a combined function of the older portions of the cerebellum and the reticular substance of the medulla, pons, and mesencephalon. Feeding reflexes, such as salivation and licking of the lips in response to the taste of food, are controlled by areas in the medulla, pons, mesencephalon, amygdala, and hypothalamus. In addition, many emotional patterns, such as anger, excitement, sexual response, reaction to pain, and reaction to pleasure, can still occur after destruction of much of the cerebral cortex.

HIGHER BRAIN OR CORTICAL LEVEL

After the preceding account of the many nervous system functions that occur at the cord and lower brain levels, one may ask, what is left for the cerebral cortex to do? The answer to this question is complex, but it begins with the fact that the cerebral cortex is an extremely large memory storehouse. The cortex never functions alone but always in association with lower centers of the nervous system.

Without the cerebral cortex, the functions of the lower brain centers are often imprecise. The vast storehouse of cortical information usually converts these functions to determinative and precise operations.

Finally, the cerebral cortex is essential for most of our thought processes, but it cannot function by itself. In fact, it is the lower brain centers, not the cortex, that initiate *wakefulness* in the cerebral cortex, thus opening its bank of memories to the thinking machinery of the brain. Thus, each portion of the nervous system performs specific functions. But it is the cortex that opens a world of stored information for use by the mind.

BIBLIOGRAPHY

Bloodgood BL, Sabatini BL: Regulation of synaptic signalling by postsynaptic, non-glutamate receptor ion channels, *J. Physiol.* 586:1475, 2008.

Clarke LE, Barres BA: Emerging roles of astrocytes in neural circuit development, *Nat. Rev. Neurosci.* 14:311, 2013.

Conde C, Cáceres A: Microtubule assembly, organization and dynamics in axons and dendrites, *Nat. Rev. Neurosci.* 10:319, 2009.

Jacob TC, Moss SJ, Jurd R: GABA(A) receptor trafficking and its role in the dynamic modulation of neuronal inhibition, *Nat. Rev. Neurosci.* 9(5):331-343, 2008.

Kandel ER: The molecular biology of memory storage: a dialogue between genes and synapses, *Science* 294:1030, 2001.

Kandel ER, Schwartz JH, Jessell TM: *Principles of Neural Science*, fourth ed., New York, 2000, McGraw-Hill.

Magee JC: Dendritic integration of excitatory synaptic input, *Nat. Rev. Neurosci.* 1:181, 2000.

Ruff RL: Neurophysiology of the neuromuscular junction: overview, *Ann. N. Y. Acad. Sci.* 998:1, 2003.

Sjöström PJ, Rancz EA, Roth A, et al: Dendritic excitability and synaptic plasticity, *Physiol. Rev.* 88:769, 2008.

Williams SR, Wozny C, Mitchell SJ: The back and forth of dendritic plasticity, *Neuron* 56:947, 2007.

Zucker RS, Regehr WG: Short-term synaptic plasticity, *Annu. Rev. Physiol.* 64:355, 2002.

Sensory System

ANURA KURPAD

101 Synapses

Information is transmitted in the central nervous system mainly in the form of nerve action potentials, called "nerve impulses," through a succession of neurons, one after another. However, in addition, each impulse (1) may be blocked in its transmission from one neuron to the next, (2) may be changed from a single impulse into repetitive impulses, or (3) may be integrated with impulses from other neurons to cause highly intricate patterns of impulses in successive neurons. All these functions can be classified as *synaptic functions of neurons*.

Types of Synapses—Chemical and Electrical

There are two major types of synapses: (1) *chemical* and (2) *electrical*.

Most of the synapses used for signal transmission in the central nervous system of the human being are *chemical synapses*. In these synapses, the first neuron secretes at its nerve ending synapse a chemical substance called a *neurotransmitter* (often called a *transmitter substance*), and this transmitter in turn acts on receptor proteins in the membrane of the next neuron to excite the neuron, inhibit it, or modify its sensitivity in some other way. More than 40 important neurotransmitters have been discovered thus far. Some of the best known are acetylcholine, norepinephrine, epinephrine, histamine, gamma-aminobutyric acid (GABA), glycine, serotonin, and glutamate.

In electrical synapses, the cytoplasms of adjacent cells are directly connected by clusters of ion channels called *gap junctions* that allow free movement of ions from the interior of one cell to the interior of the next cell. Such junctions were discussed in Chapter 4and it is by way of gap junctions and other similar junctions that action potentials are transmitted from one smooth muscle fiber to the next in visceral smooth muscle (see Chapter 30) and from one cardiac muscle cell to the next in cardiac muscle (see Chapter 65).

Although most synapses in the brain are chemical, electrical and chemical synapses may coexist and interact in the central nervous system. The bidirectional transmission of electrical synapses permits them to help coordinate the activities of large groups of interconnected neurons. For example, electrical synapses are useful in detecting the coincidence of simultaneous subthreshold depolarizations within a group of interconnected neurons; this enables increased neuronal sensitivity and promotes synchronous firing of a group of interconnected neurons.

"One-Way" Conduction at Chemical Synapses. Chemical synapses have one exceedingly important characteristic that makes them highly desirable for transmitting nervous system signals. This characteristic is that they always transmit the signals in one direction: that is, from the neuron that secretes theneurotransmitter, called the *presynaptic neuron*, to the neuron on which the transmitter acts, called the *postsynaptic neuron*. This phenomenon is the *principle of one-way conduction* at chemical synapses, and it is quite different from conduction through electrical synapses, which often transmit signals in either direction.

A one-way conduction mechanism allows signals to be directed toward specific goals. Indeed, it is this specific transmission of signals to discrete and highly focused areas, both within the nervous system and at the terminals of the peripheral nerves, that allows the nervous system to perform its myriad functions of sensation, motor control, memory, and many other functions.

Physiological Anatomy of the Synapse

Figure 101-1 shows a typical *anterior motor neuron* in the anterior horn of the spinal cord. It is composed of three major parts: the *soma*, which is the main body of the neuron; a single *axon*, which extends from the soma into a peripheral nerve that leaves the spinal cord; and the *dendrites*, which are great numbers of

branching projections of the soma that extend as much as 1 mm into the surrounding areas of the cord.

As many as 10,000–200,000 minute synaptic knobs called *presynaptic terminals* lie on the surfaces of the dendrites and soma of the motor neuron, about 80–95% of them on the dendrites and only 5–20% on the soma. These presynaptic terminals are the ends of nerve fibrils that originate from many other neurons. Many of these presynaptic terminals are *excitatory*—that is, they secrete a neurotransmitter that excites the postsynaptic neuron. However other presynaptic terminals are *inhibitory*—that is they secrete a neurotransmitter that inhibits the postsynaptic neuron.

Neurons in other parts of the cord and brain differ from the anterior motor neuron in (1) the size of the cell body; (2) the length, size, and number of dendrites, ranging in length from almost zero to many centimeters; (3) the length and size of the axon; and (4) the number of presynaptic terminals, which may range from only a few to as many as 200,000. These differences make neurons in different parts of the nervous system react differently to incoming synaptic signals and, therefore, perform many different functions.

Presynaptic Terminals

Electron microscopic studies of the presynaptic terminals show that they have varied anatomical forms, but most of them resemble small round or oval knobs and, therefore, are sometimes called *terminal knobs, boutons, end-feet,* or *synaptic knobs.*

Figure 101-2 illustrates the basic structure of a chemical synapse, showing a single presynaptic terminal on the membrane surface of a postsynaptic neuron. The presynaptic terminal is separated from the postsynaptic neuronal soma by a *synaptic cleft* having a width usually of 200–300 Å. The terminal has two internal structures important to the excitatory or inhibitory function of the synapse: the *transmitter vesicles* and the *mitochondria.* The transmitter vesicles contain the *neurotransmitter* that, when released into the synaptic cleft, either *excites* or *inhibits* the postsynaptic neuron.—It excites the postsynaptic neuron if the neuronal membrane contains *excitatory receptors*, and it inhibits the neuron if the membrane contains *inhibitory receptors.* The mitochondria provide adenosine triphosphate (ATP),

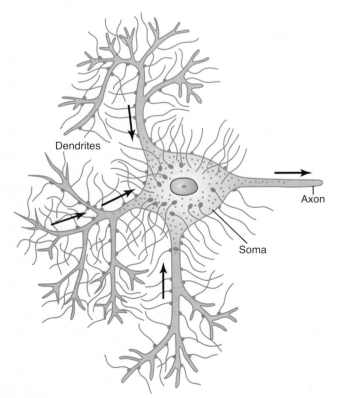

Figure 101-1   A typical anterior motor neuron, showing presynaptic terminals on the neuronal soma and dendrites. Note also the single axon.

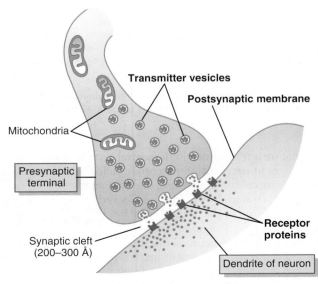

Figure 101-2   Physiological anatomy of the synapse.

which in turn supplies the energy for synthesizing new transmitter substance.

When an action potential spreads over a presynaptic terminal, depolarization of its membrane causes a small number of vesicles to empty into the cleft. The released transmitter in turn causes an immediate change in permeability characteristics of the postsynaptic neuronal membrane, which leads to excitation or inhibition of the postsynaptic neuron, depending on the neuronal receptor characteristics.

MECHANISM BY WHICH AN ACTION POTENTIAL CAUSES TRANSMITTER RELEASE FROM THE PRESYNAPTIC TERMINALS—ROLE OF CALCIUM IONS

The membrane of the presynaptic terminal is called the *presynaptic membrane*. It contains large numbers of *voltage-gated calcium channels*. When an action potential depolarizes the presynaptic membrane, these calcium channels open and allow large numbers of calcium ions to flow into the terminal. The quantity of neurotransmitter that is then released from the terminal into the synaptic cleft is directly related to the number of calcium ions that enter. The precise mechanism by which the calcium ions cause this release is not known, but it is believed to be the following.

When the calcium ions enter the presynaptic terminal, they bind with special protein molecules on the inside surface of the presynaptic membrane called *release sites*. This binding in turn causes the release sites to open through the membrane, allowing a few transmitter vesicles to release their transmitter into the cleft after each single action potential. For the vesicles that store the neurotransmitter acetylcholine, between 2000 and 10,000 molecules of acetylcholine are present in each vesicle, and there are enough vesicles in the presynaptic terminal to transmit from a few hundred to more than 10,000 action potentials.

ACTION OF THE TRANSMITTER SUBSTANCE ON THE POSTSYNAPTIC NEURON—FUNCTION OF "RECEPTOR PROTEINS"

The membrane of the postsynaptic neuron contains large numbers of *receptor proteins*, also shown in Figure 101-2. The molecules of these receptors have two important components: (1) a *binding component* that protrudes outward from the membrane into the synaptic cleft—here it binds the neurotransmitter coming from the presynaptic terminal—and (2) an *intracellular component* that passes all the way through the postsynaptic membrane to the interior of the postsynaptic neuron. Receptor activation controls the opening of ion channels in the postsynaptic cell in one of two ways: (1) by *gating ion channels directly* and allowing passage of specified types of ions through the membrane or (2) by activating a *"second messenger"* that is not an ion channel but instead is a molecule that protrudes into the cell cytoplasm and activates one or more substances inside the postsynaptic neuron. These second messengers increase or decrease specific cellular functions.

Neurotransmitter receptors that directly gate ion channels are often called *ionotropic receptors,* whereas those that act through second messenger systems are called *metabotropic receptors.*

Ion Channels

The ion channels in the postsynaptic neuronal membrane are usually of two types: (1) *cation channels* that most often allow sodium ions to pass when opened, but sometimes also allow potassium and/or calcium ions to pass, and (2) *anion channels* that mainly allow chloride ions to pass but allow minute quantities of other anions to pass as well.

The *cation channels* that conduct sodium ions are lined with negative charges. These charges attract the positively charged sodium ions into the channel when the channel diameter increases to a size larger than that of the hydrated sodium ion. However those same negative charges *repel chloride ions and other anions* and prevent their passage.

For the *anion channels*, when the channel diameters become large enough, chloride ions pass into the channels and on through to the opposite side, whereas sodium, potassium, and calcium cations are blocked, mainly because their hydrated ions are too large to pass.

We will learn later that when cation channels open and allow positively charged sodium ions to enter, the positive electrical charges of the sodium ions will in turn excite this neuron. Therefore, a neurotransmitter that opens cation channels is called an *excitatory transmitter.* Conversely, opening anion channels allows negative electrical charges to enter, which inhibits the neuron. Therefore, neurotransmitter that open these channels are called *inhibitory transmitters.*

When a neurotransmitter activates an ion channel, the channel usually opens within a fraction of a millisecond; when the transmitter substance is no longer present, the channel closes equally rapidly. The opening and closing of ion channels provide a means for very rapid control of postsynaptic neurons.

"Second Messenger" System in the Postsynaptic Neuron

Many functions of the nervous system—for instance, the process of memory—require prolonged changes in neurons for seconds to months after the initial transmitter substance is gone. The ion channels are not suitable for causing prolonged postsynaptic neuronal changes because these channels close within milliseconds after the transmitter substance is no longer present. However, in many instances, prolonged postsynaptic neuronal excitation or inhibition is achieved by activating a "second messenger" chemical system inside the postsynaptic neuronal cell itself, and then it is the second messenger that causes the prolonged effect.

There are several types of second messenger systems. One of the most common types uses a group of proteins called *G-proteins.* Figure 101-3 shows a membrane receptor G protein. The inactive G-protein complex is free in the cytosol and consists of guanosine diphosphate (GDP) plus three components: an alpha component that is the *activator* portion of the G-protein, and beta and gamma components that are attached to the alpha component As long as the G-protein complex is bound to GDP, it remains inactive.

When the receptor is activated by a neurotransmitter, following a nerve impulse, the receptor undergoes a conformational change, exposing a binding site for the G protein complex, which then binds to the portion of the receptor that protrudes into the interior of the cell. This process permits the α subunit to release GDP and simultaneously bind guanosine triphosphate (GTP) while separating from the β and γ portions of the complex. The separated GTP complex is then free to move within the cytoplasm of the cell and perform one or more of multiple functions, depending on the specific characteristic of each type of neuron. The following four changes that can occur are shown in Figure 101-3:

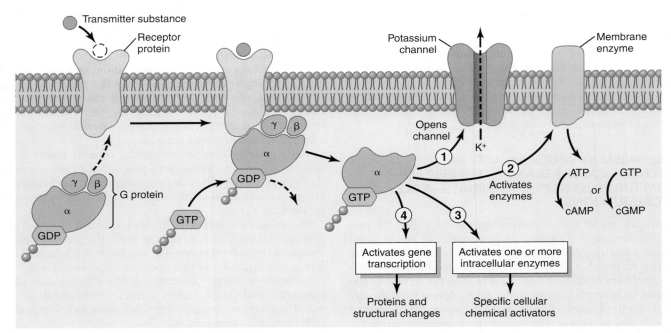

Figure 101-3 The "Second messenger" system by which a transmitter substance from an initial neuron can activate a second neuron by first releasing a "G-protein" into the second neuron's cytoplasm. Four subsequent possible effects of the G-protein are shown, including (1) opening an ion channel in the membrane of the second neuron; (2) activating an enzyme system in the neuron's membrane; (3) activating an intracellular enzyme system; and/or (4) causing gene transcription in the second neuron. Return of the G protein to the inactive state occurs when guanosine triphosphate (*GTP*) bound to the α subunit is hydrolyzed to guanosine diphosphate (*GDP*) and the β and γ subunits are reattached to the α subunit.

1. *Opening specific ion channels through the postsynaptic cell membrane.* Shown in the upper right of the figure is a potassium channel that is opened in response to the G-protein; this channel often stays open for a prolonged time in contrast to rapid closure of directly activated ion channels that do not use the second messenger system.

2. *Activation of cyclic adenosine monophosphate (cAMP) or cyclic guanosine monophosphate (cGMP) in the neuronal cell.* Recall that either cAMP or cGMP can activate highly specific metabolic machinery in the neuron and, therefore, can initiate any one of many chemical results, including long-term changes in cell structure itself, which in turn alters long-term excitability of the neuron.

3. *Activation of one or more intracellular enzymes.* The G-protein can directly activate one or more intracellular enzymes. In turn the enzymes can cause any one of many specific chemical functions in the cell.

4. *Activation of gene transcription.* Activation of gene transcription is one of the most important effects of activation of the second messenger systems because gene transcription can cause formation of new proteins within the neuron, thereby changing its metabolic machinery or its structure. Indeed, it is well known that structural changes of appropriately activated neurons do occur, especially in long-term memory processes.

Inactivation of the G protein occurs when the GTP bound to the α subunit is hydrolyzed to GDP. This action causes the α subunit to release from its target protein, thereby inactivating the second messenger systems, and then to combine again with the β and γ subunits, returning the G protein complex to its inactive state.

It is clear that activation of second messenger systems within the neuron, whether they be of the G-protein type or of other types, is extremely important for changing the long-term response characteristics of different neuronal pathways. We will

return to this subject in more detail in Chapter 125 when we discuss memory functions of the nervous system.

EXCITATORY OR INHIBITORY RECEPTORS IN THE POSTSYNAPTIC MEMBRANE

Upon activation, some postsynaptic receptors cause excitation of the postsynaptic neuron, and others cause inhibition. The importance of having inhibitory, as well as excitatory, types of receptors is that this feature gives an additional dimension to nervous function, allowing restraint of nervous action and excitation.

The different molecular and membrane mechanisms used by the different receptors to cause excitation or inhibition include the following.

EXCITATION

1. Opening of sodium channels to allow large numbers of positive electrical charges to flow to the interior of the postsynaptic cell. This action raises the intracellular membrane potential in the positive direction up toward the threshold level for excitation. It is by far the most widely used means for causing excitation.

2. Depressed conduction through chloride or potassium channels, or both. This action decreases the diffusion of negatively charged chloride ions to the inside of the postsynaptic neuron or decreases the diffusion of positively charged potassium ions to the outside. In either instance, the effect is to make the internal membrane potential more positive than normal, which is excitatory.

3. Various changes in the internal metabolism of the postsynaptic neuron to excite cell activity or, in some instances, to increase the number of excitatory membrane receptors or decrease the number of inhibitory membrane receptors.

INHIBITION

1. *Opening of chloride ion channels through the postsynaptic neuronal membrane.* This action allows rapid diffusion of negatively charged chloride ions from outside the post-synaptic neuron to the inside, thereby carrying negative charges inward and increasing the negativity inside, which is inhibitory.
2. *Increase in conductance of potassium ions out of the neuron.* This action allows positive ions to diffuse to the exterior, which causes increased negativity inside the neuron; this is inhibitory.
3. *Activation of receptor enzymes* that inhibit cellular metabolic functions that increase the number of inhibitory synaptic receptors or decrease the number of excitatory receptors.

Chemical Substances that Function as Synaptic Transmitters

More than 50 chemical substances have been proved or postulated to function as synaptic transmitters. Many of them are listed in Tables 101-1 and 101-2, which provide two groups of synaptic transmitters. One group comprises *small-molecule, rapidly acting transmitters.* The other is made up of a large number of *neuropeptides* of much larger molecular size that usually act much more slowly.

The small-molecule, rapidly acting transmitters cause most acute responses of the nervous system, such as transmission of sensory signals to the brain and of motor signals back to the muscles. The neuropeptides, in contrast, usually cause more prolonged actions, such as long-term changes in numbers of neuronal receptors, long-term opening or closure of certain ion channels, and possibly even long-term changes in numbers of synapses or sizes of synapses.

SMALL-MOLECULE, RAPIDLY ACTING TRANSMITTERS

In most cases, the small-molecule types of transmitters are synthesized in the cytosol of the presynaptic terminal and are absorbed by means of active transport into the many transmitter

TABLE 101-1	Small-Molecule, Rapidly Acting Transmitters

Class I
Acetylcholine
Class II: the amines
Norepinephrine
Epinephrine
Dopamine
Serotonin
Histamine
Class III: amino acids
Gamma-aminobutyric acid (GABA)
Glycine
Glutamate
Aspartate
Class IV
Nitric oxide (NO)

TABLE 101-2	Neuropeptide, Slowly Acting Transmitters or Growth Factors

Hypothalamic-releasing hormones
Thyrotropin-releasing hormone
Luteinizing hormone–releasing hormone
Somatostatin (growth hormone inhibitory factor)
Pituitary peptides
Adrenocorticotropic hormone (ACTH)
β-Endorphin
α-Melanocyte-stimulating hormone
Prolactin
Luteinizing hormone
Thyrotropin
Growth hormone
Vasopressin
Oxytocin
Peptides that act on gut and brain
Leucine enkephalin
Methionine enkephalin
Substance P
Gastrin
Cholecystokinin
Vasoactive intestinal polypeptide (VIP)
Nerve growth factor
Brain-derived neurotropic factor
Neurotensin
Insulin
Glucagon
From other tissues
Angiotensin II
Bradykinin
Carnosine
Sleep peptides
Calcitonin

vesicles in the terminal. Then, each time an action potential reaches the presynaptic terminal, a few vesicles at a time release their transmitter into the synaptic cleft. This action usually occurs within a millisecond or less by the mechanism described earlier. The subsequent action of the small-molecule transmitter on the membrane receptors of the postsynaptic neuron usually also occurs within another millisecond or less. Most often the effect is to increase or decrease conductance through ion channels; an example is to increase sodium conductance, which causes excitation, or to increase potassium or chloride conductance, which causes inhibition.

Characteristics of Some Important Small-Molecule Transmitters

Acetylcholine is secreted by neurons in many areas of the nervous system but specifically by (1) the terminals of the large pyramidal cells from the motor cortex, (2) several different types of neurons in the basal ganglia, (3) the motor neurons that innervate the skeletal muscles, (4) the preganglionic neurons of the autonomic nervous system, (5) the postganglionic neurons of the parasympathetic nervous system, and (6) some of the postganglionic neurons of the sympathetic nervous system. In most instances, acetylcholine has an excitatory effect; however, it is known to have inhibitory effects at some peripheral parasympathetic nerve endings, such as inhibition of the heart by the vagus nerves.

Norepinephrine is secreted by the terminals of many neurons whose cell bodies are located in the brainstem and hypothalamus. Specifically, norepinephrine-secreting neurons located in the *locus ceruleus* in the pons send nerve fibers to widespread areas of the brain to help control overall activity and mood of the mind, such as increasing the level of wakefulness. In most of these areas, norepinephrine probably activates excitatory receptors, but in a few areas, it activates inhibitory receptors instead. Norepinephrine is also secreted by most postganglionic neurons of the sympathetic nervous system, where it excites some organs but inhibits others.

Dopamine is secreted by neurons that originate in the substantia nigra. The termination of these neurons is mainly in the striatal region of the basal ganglia. The effect of dopamine is usually inhibition.

Glycine is secreted mainly at synapses in the spinal cord. It is believed to always act as an inhibitory transmitter.

GABA is secreted by nerve terminals in the spinal cord, cerebellum, basal ganglia, and many areas of the cortex. It is believed always to cause inhibition.

Glutamate is secreted by the presynaptic terminals in many of the sensory pathways entering the central nervous system, as well as in many areas of the cerebral cortex. It probably always causes excitation.

Serotonin is secreted by nuclei that originate in the median raphe of the brainstem and project to many brain and spinal cord areas, especially to the dorsal horns of the spinal cord and to the hypothalamus. Serotonin acts as an inhibitor of pain pathways in the cord, and an inhibitor action in the higher regions of the nervous system is believed to help control the mood of the person, perhaps even to cause sleep.

Nitric oxide is especially secreted by nerve terminals in areas of the brain responsible for long-term behavior and memory. Therefore, this transmitter system might in the future explain some behavior and memory functions that thus far have defied understanding. Nitric oxide is different from other small-molecule transmitters in its mechanism of formation in the presynaptic terminal and in its actions on the postsynaptic neuron. It is not preformed and stored in vesicles in the presynaptic terminal as are other transmitters. Instead, it is synthesized almost instantly as needed, and it then diffuses out of the presynaptic terminals over a period of seconds rather than being released in vesicular packets. Next, it diffuses into postsynaptic neurons nearby. In the postsynaptic neuron, it usually does not greatly alter the membrane potential but instead changes intracellular metabolic functions that modify neuronal excitability for seconds, minutes, or perhaps even longer.

NEUROPEPTIDES

Neuropeptides are synthesized differently and have actions that are usually slow and in other ways quite different from those of the small-molecule transmitters. The neuropeptides are not synthesized in the cytosol of the presynaptic terminals. Instead, they are synthesized as integral parts of large-protein molecules by ribosomes in the neuronal cell body.

The protein molecules then enter the spaces inside the endoplasmic reticulum of the cell body and subsequently inside the Golgi apparatus, where two changes occur: First, the neuropeptide-forming protein is enzymatically split into smaller fragments, some of which are either the neuropeptide itself or a precursor of it. Second, the Golgi apparatus packages the neuropeptide into minute transmitter vesicles that are released into

the cytoplasm. Then the transmitter vesicles are transported all the way to the tips of the nerve fibers by *axonal streaming* of the axon cytoplasm, traveling at the slow rate of only a few centimeters per day. Finally, these vesicles release their transmitter at the neuronal terminals in response to action potentials in the same manner as for small-molecule transmitters. However, the vesicle is autolyzed and is not reused.

Because of this laborious method of forming the neuropeptides, much smaller quantities of neuropeptides than of the small-molecule transmitters are usually released. This difference is partly compensated for by the fact that the neuropeptides are generally a thousand or more times as potent as the small-molecule transmitters. Another important characteristic of the neuropeptides is that they often cause much more prolonged actions. Some of these actions include prolonged closure of calcium channels, prolonged changes in the metabolic machinery of cells, prolonged changes in activation or deactivation of specific genes in the cell nucleus, and/or prolonged alterations in numbers of excitatory or inhibitory receptors. Some of these effects last for days, but others last perhaps for months or years. Our knowledge of the functions of the neuropeptides is only beginning to develop.

EFFECT OF SYNAPTIC EXCITATION ON THE POSTSYNAPTIC MEMBRANE—EXCITATORY POSTSYNAPTIC POTENTIAL

Figure 101-4A shows the resting neuron with an unexcited presynaptic terminal resting on its surface. The resting membrane potential everywhere in the soma is −65 mV.

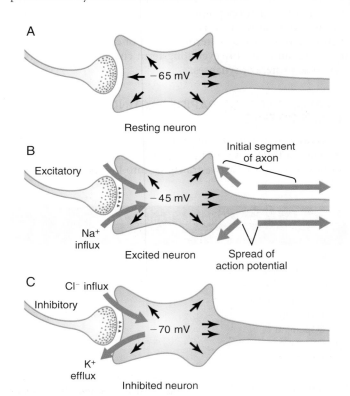

Figure 101-4 Three states of a neuron: (A) *resting neuron*, with a normal intraneuronal potential of −65 mV; (B) neuron in an *excited state*, with a less negative intraneuronal potential (−45 mV) caused by sodium influx; (C) neuron in an *inhibited state*, with a more negative intraneuronal membrane potential (−70 mv) caused by potassium ion efflux, chloride ion influx, or both.

Figure 101-4B shows a presynaptic terminal that has secreted an excitatory transmitter into the cleft between the terminal and the neuronal somal membrane. This transmitter acts on the membrane excitatory receptor *to increase the membrane's permeability to Na⁺*. Because of the large sodium concentration gradient and large electrical negativity inside the neuron, sodium ions diffuse rapidly to the inside of the membrane.

The rapid influx of positively charged sodium ions to the interior neutralizes part of the negativity of the resting membrane potential. Thus, in Figure 101-4B, the resting membrane potential has increased in the positive direction from −65 to −45 mV. This positive increase in voltage above the normal resting neuronal potential—that is, to a less negative value—is called the *excitatory postsynaptic potential* (or EPSP) because if this potential rises high enough in the positive direction, it will elicit an action potential in the postsynaptic neuron, thus exciting it. (In this case, the EPSP is +20 mV—that is, 20 mV more positive than the resting value.)

Discharge of a single presynaptic terminal can never increase the neuronal potential from −65 mV all the way up to −45 mV. An increase of this magnitude requires simultaneous discharge of many terminals—about 40–80 for the usual anterior motor neuron—at the same time or in rapid succession. This simultaneous discharge occurs by a process called *summation*, which is discussed in detail in the next sections.

GENERATION OF ACTION POTENTIALS IN THE INITIAL SEGMENT OF THE AXON LEAVING THE NEURON—THRESHOLD FOR EXCITATION

When the EPSP rises high enough in the positive direction, there comes a point at which this initiates an action potential in the neuron. However, the action potential does not begin adjacent to the excitatory synapses. Instead, *it begins in the initial segment of the axon* where the axon leaves the neuronal soma. The main reason for this point of origin of the action potential is that the soma has relatively few voltage-gated sodium channels in its membrane, which makes it difficult for the EPSP to open the required number of sodium channels to elicit an action potential. Conversely, *the membrane of the initial segment* has seven times as great a concentration of voltage-gated sodium channels as does the soma and, therefore, can generate an action potential with much greater ease than can the soma. The EPSP that will elicit an action potential in the axon initial segment is between +10 and +20 mV in contrast to the +30 or +40 mV or more required on the soma.

Once the action potential begins, it travels peripherally along the axon and usually also backward over the soma. In some instances it travels backward into the dendrites but not into all of them because they, like the neuronal soma, have very few voltage-gated sodium channels and therefore frequently cannot generate action potentials at all. Thus, in Figure 101-4B, the *threshold* for excitation of the neuron is shown to be about −45 mV, which represents an EPSP of +20 mV—that is, 20 mV more positive than the normal resting neuronal potential of −65 mV.

Electrical Events During Neuronal Inhibition

Effect of Inhibitory Synapses on the Postsynaptic Membrane—Inhibitory Postsynaptic Potential. The inhibitory synapses *open mainly chloride channels*, allowing easy passage of chloride ions. To understand how the inhibitory synapses inhibit the postsynaptic neuron, we must recall what we learned about the Nernst potential for chloride ions. We calculated the Nernst potential for chloride ions to be about −70 mV. This potential is more negative than the −65 mV normally present inside the resting neuronal membrane. Therefore, opening the chloride channels will allow negatively charged chloride ions to move from the extracellular fluid to the interior, which will make the interior membrane potential more negative than normal, approaching the −70 mV level.

Opening potassium channels will allow positively charged potassium ions to move to the exterior, and this will also make the interior membrane potential more negative than usual. Thus, both chloride influx and potassium efflux increase the degree of intracellular negativity, which is called *hyperpolarization*. This inhibits the neuron because the membrane potential is even more negative than the normal intracellular potential. Therefore, an increase in negativity beyond the normal resting membrane potential level is called an *inhibitory postsynaptic potential* (IPSP).

Figure 101-4C shows the effect on the membrane potential caused by activation of inhibitory synapses, allowing chloride influx into the cell and/or potassium efflux out of the cell, with the membrane potential decreasing from its normal value of −65 mV to the more negative value of −70 mV. This membrane potential is 5 mV more negative than normal and is therefore an IPSP of −5 mV, which inhibits transmission of the nerve signal through the synapse.

PRESYNAPTIC INHIBITION

In addition to inhibition caused by inhibitory synapses operating at the neuronal membrane, which is called *postsynaptic inhibition*, another type of inhibition often occurs at the presynaptic terminals before the signal ever reaches the synapse. This type of inhibition is called *presynaptic inhibition*.

Presynaptic inhibition is caused by release of an inhibitory substance onto the outsides of the presynaptic nerve fibrils before their own endings terminate on the postsynaptic neuron. *In most instances, the inhibitory transmitter substance is GABA.* This release has a specific effect of opening anion channels, allowing large numbers of chloride ions to diffuse into the terminal fibril. The negative charges of these ions inhibit synaptic transmission because they cancel much of the excitatory effect of the positively charged sodium ions that also enter the terminal fibrils when an action potential arrives.

Presynaptic inhibition occurs in many of the sensory pathways in the nervous system. In fact, adjacent sensory nerve fibers often mutually inhibit one another, which minimizes sideways spread and mixing of signals in sensory tracts. We discuss the importance of this phenomenon more fully in subsequent chapters.

TIME COURSE OF POSTSYNAPTIC POTENTIALS

When an excitatory synapse excites the anterior motor neuron, the neuronal membrane becomes highly permeable to sodium ions for 1–2 milliseconds. During this very short time, enough sodium ions diffuse rapidly to the interior of the postsynaptic motor neuron to increase its intraneuronal potential by a few millivolts, thus creating the EPSP shown by the blue and green curves of Figure 101-5. This potential then slowly declines over the next 15 milliseconds because this is the time required for the

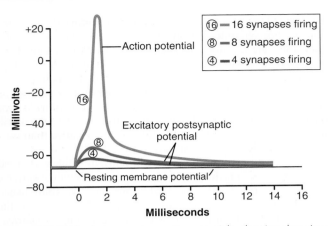

Figure 101-5 Excitatory postsynaptic potentials, showing that simultaneous firing of only a few synapses will not cause sufficient summated potential to elicit an action potential, but that simultaneous firing of many synapses will raise the summated potential to threshold for excitation and cause a superimposed action potential.

excess positive charges to leak out of the excited neuron and to reestablish the normal resting membrane potential.

Precisely the opposite effect occurs for an IPSP; that is, the inhibitory synapse increases the permeability of the membrane to potassium or chloride ions, or both, for 1–2 milliseconds, and this action decreases the intraneuronal potential to a more negative value than normal, thereby creating the IPSP. This potential also dies away in about 15 milliseconds.

Other types of transmitter substances can excite or inhibit the postsynaptic neuron for much longer periods—for hundreds of milliseconds or even for seconds, minutes, or hours. This is especially true for some of the neuropeptide transmitters.

Some Special Characteristics of Synaptic Transmission (Box 101-1)

Fatigue of Synaptic Transmission. When excitatory synapses are repetitively stimulated at a rapid rate, the number of discharges by the postsynaptic neuron is at first very great, but the firing rate becomes progressively less in succeeding milliseconds or seconds. This phenomenon is called *fatigue* of synaptic transmission.

Fatigue is an exceedingly important characteristic of synaptic function because when areas of the nervous system become overexcited, fatigue causes them to lose this excess excitability after a while. For example, fatigue is probably the most important means by which the excess excitability of the brain during an epileptic seizure is finally subdued so that the seizure ceases. Thus, the development of fatigue is a protective mechanism against excess neuronal activity.

BOX 101-1 SUMMARY OF PROPERTIES OF SYNAPSE

- Unidirectional propagation of the nervous impulse
- Delay
- Subliminal fringe
- Temporal summation
- Occlusion
- Inhibitory (IPSP) or excitatory (EPSP) postsynaptic events
- Ionotropic—fast transmission
- Metabotropic—slower transmission—neuromodulatory role
- Fatigue

The mechanism of fatigue is mainly exhaustion or partial exhaustion of the stores of transmitter substance in the presynaptic terminals. The excitatory terminals on many neurons can store enough excitatory transmitter to cause only about 10,000 action potentials, and the transmitter can be exhausted in only a few seconds to a few minutes of rapid stimulation. Part of the fatigue process probably results from two other factors as well: (1) progressive inactivation of many of the postsynaptic membrane receptors and (2) slow development of abnormal concentrations of ions inside the *postsynaptic* neuronal cell.

Effect of Acidosis or Alkalosis on Synaptic Transmission. Most neurons are highly responsive to changes in pH of the surrounding interstitial fluids. *Normally, alkalosis greatly increases neuronal excitability.* For instance, a rise in arterial blood pH from the normal 7.4 to 7.8–8.0 often causes cerebral epileptic seizures because of increased excitability of some or all of the cerebral neurons. In a person who is predisposed to epileptic seizures even a short period of hyperventilation, which blows off carbon dioxide and elevates the pH may precipitate an epileptic attack.

Conversely, *acidosis greatly depresses neuronal activity*; a fall in pH from 7.4 to below 7.0 usually causes a comatose state. For instance, in very severe diabetic or uremic acidosis coma virtually alomost always develops.

Effect of Hypoxia on Synaptic Transmission. Neuronal excitability is also highly dependent on an adequate supply of oxygen. Cessation of oxygen for only a few seconds can cause complete inexcitability of some neurons. This effect is observed when the brain's blood flow is temporarily interrupted because within 3–7 seconds the person becomes unconscious.

Effect of Drugs on Synaptic Transmission. Many drugs are known to increase the excitability of neurons, and others are known to decrease excitability. For instance, *caffeine, theophylline*, and *theobromine*, which are found in coffee, tea, and cocoa, respectively, all *increase* neuronal excitability, presumably by reducing the threshold for excitation of neurons.

Strychnine is one of the best known of all agents that increase excitability of neurons. However, it does not do this by reducing the threshold for excitation of the neurons; instead, it *inhibits the action of some normally inhibitory transmitter substances*, especially the inhibitory effect of glycine in the spinal cord. Therefore, the effects of the excitatory transmitters become overwhelming, and the neurons become so excited that they go into rapidly repetitive discharge, resulting in severe tonic muscle spasms.

Most anesthetics increase the neuronal membrane threshold for excitation and thereby decrease synaptic transmission at many points in the nervous system. Because many of the anesthetics are especially lipid soluble, it has been reasoned that some of them might change the physical characteristics of the neuronal membranes, making them less responsive to excitatory agents.

Synaptic Delay. During transmission of a neuronal signal from a presynaptic neuron to a postsynaptic neuron, a certain amount of time is consumed in the process of (1) discharge of the transmitter substance by the presynaptic terminal, (2) diffusion of the transmitter to the postsynaptic neuronal membrane, (3) action of the transmitter on the membrane receptor, (4) action of the receptor to increase the membrane permeability, and (5) inward diffusion of sodium to raise the EPSP to a high enough level to elicit an action potential. The *minimal* period of time required for all these events to take place, even when large numbers of excitatory synapses are stimulated simultaneously, is about 0.5 millisecond which is called the *synaptic delay*. Neurophysiologists can measure the *minimal* delay time between an input volley of impulses into a pool of neurons and the consequent output volley. From the measure of delay time one can then estimate the number of series neurons in the circuit.

Convergence and Divergence. Convergence occurs when multiple presynaptic neurons terminate on a single synapse. The presynaptic neurons can be inhibitory or excitatory but offer a method of integrating several responses. Spatial summation (later), for example, requires convergence. Divergence occurs when one synapse has connections with two or more postsynaptic neurons, thereby offering a method to amplify the incoming signal to many downstream neurons.

Spatial and Temporal Summation. Spatial summation occurs when two or more separate presynaptic stimuli arrive at the synapse simultaneously. In this case, the individual postsynaptic potentials summate to give a threshold response. Temporal summation occurs when the presynaptic neuronal stimuli arrive at the synapse rapidly one after the other, in quick succession. The postsynaptic potential summates if the presynaptic stimuli are frequent enough.

Occlusion and Subliminal Fringe. The subliminal fringe occurs when a neuron receiving an excitatory input can affect synapses in its fringe (adjacent) area. While this level of stimulation may not be enough on its own, to generate a threshold response from the subliminal fringe neuron, a summated threshold response can be observed if the subliminal fringe neuron also received excitatory inputs from other neighboring neurons simultaneously. In effect, this is a form of spatial summation leading to facilitation. If two neighboring neurons are excited separately, they have summed effects that are less than if they were excited at the same time; this is because these neighboring neurons can facilitate additional threshold responses from their overlapping fringe neurons. Neurons are said to be in the subliminal fringe if they are affected by excitatory input of an adjacent neuron, but not brought to their firing threshold.

In a similar fashion, occlusion occurs when two adjacent neurons are given stronger excitatory inputs. This causes an overlap of excitation in the subliminal fringes of each neuron, such that the result of stimulating both adjacent neurons simultaneously would lead to a lesser than expected response (in contrast to the facilitation earlier).

Clearly, the difference between the facilitation and occlusion is related to the strength of the incoming excitatory signal on two neurons that have an overlapping subliminal fringe area: when the incoming excitation is weak, summation can occur in the fringe neurons, such that the response of simultaneous excitation of the two adjacent neurons is greater than their summed individual excitation. However, when the incoming excitation signal is stronger, overlap of excitation areas can occur, such that a smaller than expected response is obtained when both adjacent neurons are stimulated simultaneously.

BIBLIOGRAPHY

Alberini CM: Transcription factors in long-term memory and synaptic plasticity, *Physiol. Rev.* 89:121, 2009.

Ariel P, Ryan TA: New insights into molecular players involved in neurotransmitter release, *Physiology (Bethesda)* 27:15, 2012.

Ben-Ari Y, Gaiarsa JL, Tyzio R, et al: GABA: a pioneer transmitter that excites immature neurons and generates primitive oscillations, *Physiol. Rev.* 87:1215, 2007.

Bloodgood BL, Sabatini BL: Regulation of synaptic signalling by postsynaptic, non-glutamate receptor ion channels, *J. Physiol.* 586:1475, 2008.

Boehning D, Snyder SH: Novel neural modulators, *Annu. Rev. Neurosci.* 26:105, 2003.

Gassmann M, Bettler B: Regulation of neuronal GABA(B) receptor functions by subunit composition, *Nat. Rev. Neurosci.* 13:380, 2012.

Haines DE, Lancon JA: *Review of Neuroscience*, New York, 2003, Churchill Livingstone.

Kandel ER: The molecular biology of memory storage: a dialogue between genes and synapses, *Science* 294:1030, 2001.

Kandel ER, Schwartz JH, Jessell TM: *Principles of Neural Science*, fourth ed., New York, 2000, McGraw-Hill.

Kerchner GA, Nicoll RA: Silent synapses and the emergence of a postsynaptic mechanism for LTP, *Nat. Rev. Neurosci.* 9:813, 2008.

O'Rourke NA, Weiler NC, Micheva KD, Smith SJ: Deep molecular diversity of mammalian synapses: why it matters and how to measure it, *Nat. Rev. Neurosci.* 13:365, 2012.

Pereda AE: Electrical synapses and their functional interactions with chemical synapses, *Nat. Rev. Neurosci.* 15:250, 2014.

Sjöström PJ, Rancz EA, Roth A, et al: Dendritic excitability and synaptic plasticity, *Physiol. Rev.* 88:769, 2008.

van den Pol AN: Neuropeptide transmission in brain circuits, *Neuron* 76:98, 2012.

Sensory Receptors

Our perceptions of signals within our bodies and of the world around us are mediated by a complex system of sensory receptors that detect such stimuli as touch, sound, light, pain, cold, and warmth. The purpose of this chapter is to discuss the basic mechanisms by which these receptors change sensory stimuli into nerve signals that are then conveyed to and processed in the central nervous system.

Types of Sensory Receptors and the Stimuli they Detect

Table 102-1 lists and classifies five basic types of sensory receptors: (1) *mechanoreceptors*, which detect mechanical compression or stretching of the receptor or of tissues adjacent to the receptor; (2) *thermoreceptors*, which detect changes in temperature, with some receptors detecting cold and others warmth; (3) *nociceptors* (pain receptors), which detect physical or chemical damage occurring in the tissues; (4) *electromagnetic receptors*, which detect light on the retina of the eye; and (5) *chemoreceptors*, which detect taste in the mouth, smell in the nose, oxygen level in the arterial blood, osmolality of the body fluids, carbon dioxide concentration, and other factors that make up the chemistry of the body.

In this chapter, we discuss the function of a few specific types of receptors, primarily peripheral mechanoreceptors, to illustrate some of the principles by which receptors operate. Other receptors are discussed in other chapters in relation to the sensory systems that they subserve. Figure 102-1 shows some of the types of mechanoreceptors found in the skin or in deep tissues of the body.

DIFFERENTIAL SENSITIVITY OF RECEPTORS

How do two types of sensory receptors detect different types of sensory stimuli? The answer is, by "*differential sensitivities.*"

That is, each type of receptor is highly sensitive to one type of stimulus for which it is designed and yet is almost nonresponsive to other types of sensory stimuli. Thus, the rods and cones of the eyes are highly responsive to light but are almost completely nonresponsive to normal ranges of heat, cold, pressure on the eyeballs, or chemical changes in the blood. The osmoreceptors of the supraoptic nuclei in the hypothalamus detect minute changes in the osmolality of the body fluids but have never been known to respond to sound. Finally, pain receptors in the skin are almost never stimulated by usual touch or pressure stimuli but do become highly active the moment tactile stimuli become severe enough to damage the tissues.

Modality of Sensation—The "Labeled Line" Principle

Each of the principal types of sensation that we can experience—pain, touch, sight, sound, and so forth—is called a *modality* of sensation. Yet despite the fact that we experience these different modalities of sensation, nerve fibers transmit only impulses. Therefore, how do different nerve fibers transmit different modalities of sensation?

The answer is that each nerve tract terminates at a specific point in the central nervous system, and the type of sensation felt when a nerve fiber is stimulated is determined by the point in the nervous system to which the fiber leads. For instance, if a pain fiber is stimulated, the person perceives pain regardless of what type of stimulus excites the fiber. The stimulus can be electricity, overheating of the fiber, crushing of the fiber, or stimulation of the pain nerve ending by damage to the tissue cells. In all these instances, the person perceives pain. Likewise, if a touch fiber is stimulated by electrical excitation of a touch receptor or in any other way, the person perceives touch because touch fibers lead to specific touch areas in the brain. Similarly, fibers from the retina of the eye terminate in the vision areas of the brain, fibers from the ear terminate in the auditory areas of the brain, and temperature fibers terminate in the temperature areas.

This specificity of nerve fibers for transmitting only one modality of sensation is called the *labeled line principle*, and the impression of the specific stimulus arising when the specific nerve fiber is stimulated anywhere along its path to the brain is called the *law of projection*.

Transduction of Sensory Stimuli into Nerve Impulses

LOCAL ELECTRICAL CURRENTS AT NERVE ENDINGS—RECEPTOR POTENTIALS

All sensory receptors have one feature in common. Whatever the type of stimulus that excites the receptor, its immediate effect is to change the membrane electrical potential of the receptor. This change in potential is called a *receptor potential*.

TABLE 102-1	Classification of Sensory Receptors

I. *Mechanoreceptor*
   Skin tactile sensibilities (epidermis and dermis)
      Free nerve endings
      Expanded tip endings
         Merkel discs
         Plus several other variants
      Spray endings
         Ruffini endings
      Encapsulated endings
         Meissner corpuscles
         Krause corpuscles
      Hair end organs
   Deep tissue sensibilities
      Free nerve endings
      Expanded tip endings
      Spray endings
         Ruffini endings
      Encapsulated endings
         Pacinian corpuscles
         Plus a few other variants
      Muscle endings
         Muscle spindles
         Golgi tendon receptors
   Hearing
      Sound receptors of cochlea
   Equilibrium
      Vestibular receptors
   Arterial pressure
      Baroreceptors of carotid sinuses and aorta

II. *Thermoreceptors*
   Cold
      Cold receptors
   Warmth
      Warm receptors

III. *Nociceptors*
   Pain
      Free nerve endings

IV. *Electromagnetic receptors*
   Vision
      Rods
      Cones

V. *Chemoreceptors*
   Taste
      Receptors of taste buds
   Smell
      Receptors of olfactory epithelium
   Arterial oxygen
      Receptors of aortic and carotid bodies
   Osmolality
      Neurons in or near supraoptic nuclei
   Blood CO_2
      Receptors in or on surface of medulla and in aortic and
         carotid bodies
   Blood glucose, amino acids, fatty acids
      Receptors in hypothalamus

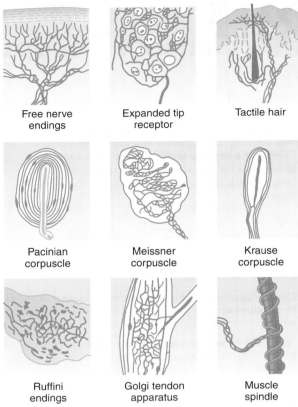

Free nerve endings   Expanded tip receptor   Tactile hair

Pacinian corpuscle   Meissner corpuscle   Krause corpuscle

Ruffini endings   Golgi tendon apparatus   Muscle spindle

Figure 102-1   Several types of somatic sensory nerve endings.

Mechanisms of Receptor Potentials. Different receptors can be excited in one of several ways to cause receptor potentials: (1) by mechanical deformation of the receptor, which stretches the receptor membrane and opens ion channels; (2) by application of a chemical to the membrane, which also opens ion channels; (3) by change of the temperature of the membrane, which alters the permeability of the membrane; or (4) by the effects of electromagnetic radiation, such as light on a retinal visual receptor, which either directly or indirectly changes the receptor membrane characteristics and allows ions to flow through membrane channels.

These four means of exciting receptors correspond in general to the different types of known sensory receptors. In all instances, the basic cause of the change in membrane potential is a change in membrane permeability of the receptor, which allows ions to diffuse more or less readily through the membrane and thereby to change the *transmembrane potential*.

Maximum Receptor Potential Amplitude. The maximum amplitude of most sensory receptor potentials is about 100 mV, but this level occurs only at an extremely high intensity of sensory stimulus. This is about the same maximum voltage recorded in action potentials and is also the change in voltage when the membrane becomes maximally permeable to sodium ions.

Relation of the Receptor Potential to Action Potentials. When the receptor potential rises above the *threshold* for eliciting action potentials in the nerve fiber attached to the receptor, action potentials occur, as illustrated in Figure 102-2. Note also that the more the receptor potential rises above the threshold level, the greater becomes the *action potential frequency*.

Receptor Potential of the Pacinian Corpuscle—An Example of Receptor Function

Note in Figure 102-1 that the Pacinian corpuscle has a central nerve fiber extending through its core. Surrounding this central nerve fiber are multiple concentric capsule layers, and thus compression anywhere on the outside of the corpuscle will elongate, indent, or otherwise deform the central fiber.

Figure 102-3 shows only the central fiber of the Pacinian corpuscle after all capsule layers but one have been removed. The tip of the central fiber inside the capsule is unmyelinated, but the fiber does become myelinated (the blue sheath shown in the figure) shortly before leaving the corpuscle to enter a peripheral sensory nerve.

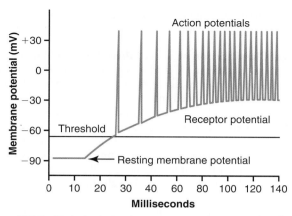

Figure 102-2 Typical relation between receptor potential and action potentials when the receptor potential rises above threshold level.

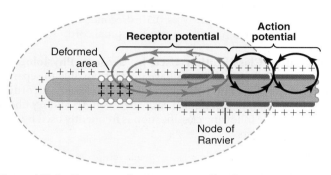

Figure 102-3 Excitation of a sensory nerve fiber by a receptor potential produced in a Pacinian corpuscle. *Modified from Loëwenstein, W.R., 1961. Excitation and inactivation in a receptor membrane. Ann. N. Y. Acad. Sci. 94, 510.*

Figure 102-3 also shows the mechanism by which a receptor potential is produced in the Pacinian corpuscle. Observe the small area of the terminal fiber that has been deformed by compression of the corpuscle, and note that ion channels have opened in the membrane, allowing positively charged sodium ions to diffuse to the interior of the fiber. This action creates increased positivity inside the fiber, which is the "receptor potential." The receptor potential in turn induces a *local circuit* of current flow, shown by the arrows, that spreads along the nerve fiber. At the first node of Ranvier, which lies inside the capsule of the Pacinian corpuscle, the local current flow depolarizes the fiber membrane at this node, which then sets off typical action potentials that are transmitted along the nerve fiber toward the central nervous system.

Relation Between Stimulus Intensity and the Receptor Potential. Figure 102-4 shows the changing amplitude of the receptor potential caused by progressively stronger mechanical compression (increasing "stimulus strength") applied experimentally to the central core of a Pacinian corpuscle. Note that the amplitude increases rapidly at first but then progressively less rapidly at high stimulus strength.

In turn, the *frequency of repetitive action potentials* transmitted from sensory receptors increases approximately in proportion to the increase in receptor potential. Putting this principle together with the data in Figure 102-4, one can see that very intense stimulation of the receptor causes progressively less and less additional increase in numbers of action potentials. This

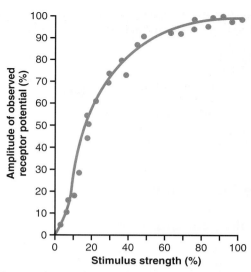

Figure 102-4 Relation of amplitude of receptor potential to strength of a mechanical stimulus applied to a Pacinian corpuscle. *Data from Loëwenstein, W.R., 1961. Excitation and inactivation in a receptor membrane. Ann. N. Y. Acad. Sci. 94, 510.*

exceedingly important principle is applicable to almost all sensory receptors. It allows the receptor to be sensitive to very weak sensory experience and yet not reach a maximum firing rate until the sensory experience is extreme. This feature allows the receptor to have an extreme range of response, from very weak to very intense.

ADAPTATION OF RECEPTORS

Another characteristic of all sensory receptors is that they *adapt* either partially or completely to any constant stimulus after a period of time. That is, when a continuous sensory stimulus is applied, the receptor responds at a high impulse rate at first and then at a progressively slower rate until finally the rate of action potentials decreases to very few or often to none at all.

Figure 102-5 shows typical adaptation of certain types of receptors. Note that the Pacinian corpuscle adapts very rapidly, hair receptors adapt within a second or so, and some joint capsule and muscle spindle receptors adapt slowly.

Furthermore, some sensory receptors adapt to a far greater extent than do others. For example, the Pacinian corpuscles adapt to "extinction" within a few hundredths of a second, and

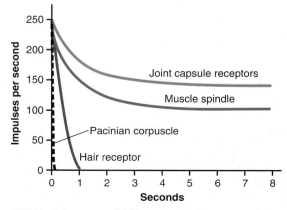

Figure 102-5 Adaptation of different types of receptors, showing rapid adaptation of some receptors and slow adaptation of others.

the receptors at the bases of the hairs adapt to extinction within a second or more. It is probable that all other *mechanoreceptors* eventually adapt almost completely, but some require hours or days to do so, for which reason they are called "nonadapting" receptors. The longest measured time for almost complete adaptation of a mechanoreceptor is about 2 days, which is the adaptation time for many carotid and aortic baroreceptors; however, some physiologists believe that these specialized baroreceptors never fully adapt. Some of the nonmechanoreceptors—the chemoreceptors and pain receptors, for instance—probably never adapt completely.

Nerve Fibers that Transmit Different Types of Signals and their Physiological Classification

Some signals need to be transmitted to or from the central nervous system extremely rapidly; otherwise, the information would be useless. An example of this is the sensory signals that apprise the brain of the momentary positions of the legs at each fraction of a second during running. At the other extreme, some types of sensory information, such as that depicting prolonged, aching pain, do not need to be transmitted rapidly, and thus slowly conducting fibers will suffice. As shown in Figure 102-6, nerve fibers come in all sizes between 0.5 and 20 μm in diameter—the larger the diameter, the greater is the conducting velocity. The range of conducting velocities is between 0.5 and 120 m/second.

General Classification of Nerve Fibers. Shown in Figure 102-6 is a "general classification" and a "sensory nerve classification" of the different types of nerve fibers. In the general classification, the fibers are divided into types A and C, and the type A fibers are further subdivided into α, β, γ, and δ fibers.

Type A fibers are the typical large- and medium-sized *myelinated* fibers of spinal nerves. Type C fibers are the small *unmyelinated* nerve fibers that conduct impulses at low velocities. The C fibers constitute more than one-half of the sensory fibers in most peripheral nerves, as well as all the postganglionic autonomic fibers.

The sizes, velocities of conduction, and functions of the different nerve fiber types are also given in Figure 102-6. Note that a few large myelinated fibers can transmit impulses at velocities as great as 120 m/second, covering a distance that is longer than a football field in 1 second. Conversely, the smallest fibers transmit impulses as slowly as 0.5 m/second, requiring about 2 seconds to go from the big toe to the spinal cord.

Alternative Classification Used by Sensory Physiologists. Certain recording techniques have made it possible to separate the type Aα fibers into two subgroups; yet these same recording techniques cannot distinguish easily between Aβ and Aγ fibers. Therefore, the following classification is frequently used by sensory physiologists.

Group Ia

Fibers from the annulospiral endings of muscle spindles (about 17 μm in diameter on average; these fibers are α-type A fibers in the general classification).

Group Ib

Fibers from the Golgi tendon organs (about 16 μm in diameter on average; these fibers also are α-type A fibers).

Group II

Fibers from most discrete cutaneous tactile receptors and from the flower-spray endings of the muscle spindles (about 8 μm in diameter on average; these fibers are β- and γ-type A fibers in the general classification).

Group III

Fibers carrying temperature, crude touch, and pricking pain sensations (about 3 μm in diameter on average; they are δ-type A fibers in the general classification).

Group IV

Unmyelinated fibers carrying pain, itch, temperature, and crude touch sensations (0.5–2 μm in diameter; they are type C fibers in the general classification).

Transmission of Signals of Different Intensity in Nerve Tracts—Spatial and Temporal Summation

One of the characteristics of each signal that always must be conveyed is signal intensity—for instance, the intensity of pain. The different gradations of intensity can be transmitted either by using increasing numbers of parallel fibers or by sending

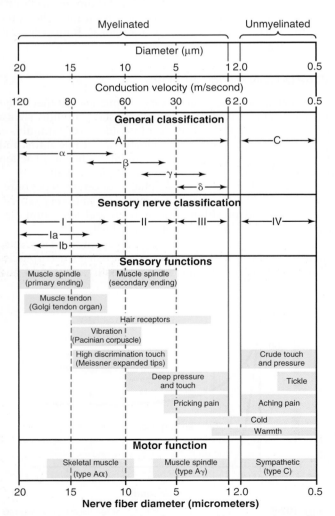

Figure 102-6 Physiological classifications and functions of nerve fibers.

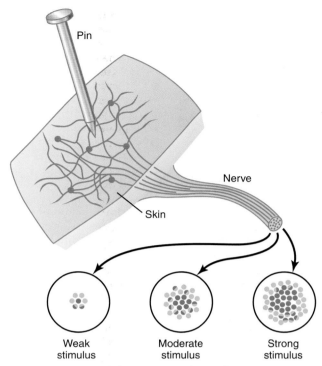

Figure 102-7 Pattern of stimulation of pain fibers in a nerve leading from an area of skin pricked by a pin. This is an example of *spatial summation*.

more action potentials along a single fiber. These two mechanisms are called, respectively, *spatial summation* and *temporal summation*.

Spatial Summation. Figure 102-7 shows the phenomenon of *spatial summation*, whereby increasing signal strength is transmitted by using progressively greater numbers of fibers. This figure shows a section of skin innervated by a large number of parallel pain fibers. Each of these fibers arborizes into hundreds of minute *free nerve endings* that serve as pain receptors. The entire cluster of fibers from one pain fiber frequently covers an area of skin as large as 5 cm in diameter. This area is called the *receptor field* of that fiber. The number of endings is large in the center of the field but diminishes toward the periphery. One can also see from the figure that the arborizing fibrils overlap those from other pain fibers. Therefore, a pinprick of the skin usually stimulates endings from many different pain fibers simultaneously. When the pinprick is in the center of the receptive field of a particular pain fiber, the degree of stimulation of that fiber is far greater than when it is in the periphery of the field because

the number of free nerve endings in the middle of the field is much greater than at the periphery.

Thus, the lower part of Figure 102-7 shows three views of the cross-section of the nerve bundle leading from the skin area. To the left is the effect of a weak stimulus, with only a single nerve fiber in the middle of the bundle stimulated strongly (represented by the red-colored fiber), whereas several adjacent fibers are stimulated weakly (half-red fibers). The other two views of the nerve cross-section show the effect of a moderate stimulus and a strong stimulus, with progressively more fibers being stimulated. Thus, the stronger signals spread to more and more fibers. This process is the phenomenon of *spatial summation*.

Temporal Summation. A second means for transmitting signals of increasing strength is by increasing the *frequency* of nerve impulses in each fiber, which is called *temporal summation*. Figure 102-8 demonstrates this phenomenon, showing in the upper part a changing strength of signal and in the lower part the actual impulses transmitted by the nerve fiber.

A summary of the properties of receptors is provided in Box 102-1.

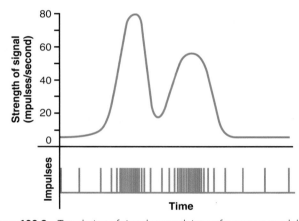

Figure 102-8 Translation of signal strength into a frequency-modulated series of nerve impulses, showing the strength of signal (*above*) and the separate nerve impulses (*below*). This is an example of *temporal summation*.

BOX 102-1   **SUMMARY OF PROPERTIES OF RECEPTORS**
• Differential sensitivities • Ordered projection to the cortex-labeled line • Graded responses • Adaptable

BIBLIOGRAPHY

Bautista DM, Wilson SR, Hoon MA: Why we scratch an itch: the molecules, cells and circuits of itch, *Nat. Neurosci.* 17:175, 2014.

Bensmaia SJ: Tactile intensity and population codes, *Behav. Brain Res.* 190:165, 2008.

Gebhart GF: Descending modulation of pain, *Neurosci. Biobehav. Rev.* 27:729, 2004.

Hamill OP, Martinac B: Molecular basis of mechanotransduction in living cells, *Physiol. Rev.* 81:685, 2001.

Kandel ER, Schwartz JH, Jessell TM: *Principles of Neural Science*, fourth ed., New York, 2000, McGraw-Hill.

Katz DB, Matsunami H, Rinberg D, et al: Receptors, circuits, and behaviors: new directions in chemical senses, *J. Neurosci.* 28:11802, 2008.

Lumpkin EA, Caterina MJ: Mechanisms of sensory transduction in the skin, *Nature* 445:858, 2007.

Schepers RJ, Ringkamp M: Thermoreceptors and thermosensitive afferents, *Neurosci. Biobehav. Rev.* 33:205, 2009.

Stein BE, Stanford TR: Multisensory integration: current issues from the perspective of the single neuron, *Nat. Rev. Neurosci.* 9:255, 2008.

103

Somatic Sensory Pathways

LEARNING OBJECTIVES

- Describe tactile receptors.
- Describe the Weber–Fechner law and power law.
- Enumerate the characteristics of sensory transmission.
- Trace the ascending pathways and describe the sensations carried by them.

GLOSSARY OF TERMS

- **Anterolateral system:** A tract carrying sensory signals upward, which immediately cross to the opposite side of the cord and ascend through the anterior and lateral white columns of the cord
- **Dorsal column–medial lemniscal system:** A tract carrying sensory signals upward mainly in the dorsal columns of the cord (the tract crosses to the opposite side in the medulla, and continues upward through the brainstem to the thalamus by way of the medial lemniscus)
- **Proprioception:** Relating the sense of position
- **Somatic:** Relating to "the body"
- **Tactile:** Relating to the sense of touch

The *somatic senses* are the nervous mechanisms that collect sensory information from all over the body. These senses are in contradistinction to the *special senses*, which mean specifically vision, hearing, smell, taste, and equilibrium. The attributes of sensations are their quality (or types, as described later), intensity, duration, and localization.

Classification of Somatic Senses

The somatic senses can be classified into three physiological types: (1) the *mechanoreceptive somatic senses*, which include both *tactile* and *position* sensations that are stimulated by mechanical displacement of some tissue of the body; (2) the *thermoreceptive senses*, which detect heat and cold; and (3) the *pain sense*, which is activated by factors that damage the tissues.

This chapter deals with the mechanoreceptive tactile and position senses. In Chapter 104 the thermoreceptive and pain senses are discussed. The tactile senses include *touch, pressure, vibration,* and *tickle* senses, and the position senses include *static position* and *rate of movement* senses.

Other Classifications of Somatic Sensations. Somatic sensations are also often grouped together in other classes, as follows.

Exteroreceptive sensations are those from the surface of the body. *Proprioceptive sensations* are those relating to the physical state of the body, including position sensations, tendon and muscle sensations, pressure sensations from the bottom of the feet, and even the sensation of equilibrium (which is often considered a "special" sensation rather than a somatic sensation).

Visceral sensations are those from the viscera of the body; in using this term, one usually refers specifically to sensations from the internal organs.

Deep sensations are those that come from deep tissues, such as from fasciae, muscles, and bone. These sensations include mainly "deep" pressure, pain, and vibration.

Detection and Transmission of Tactile Sensations

Interrelations Among the Tactile Sensations of Touch, Pressure, and Vibration. Although touch, pressure, and vibration are frequently classified as separate sensations, they are all detected by the same types of receptors. There are three principal differences among them: (1) touch sensation generally results from stimulation of tactile receptors in the skin or in tissues immediately beneath the skin; (2) pressure sensation generally results from deformation of deeper tissues; and (3) vibration sensation results from rapidly repetitive sensory signals, but some of the same types of receptors as those for touch and pressure are used.

Tactile Receptors. There are at least six entirely different types of tactile receptors, but many more similar to these also exist. Some were shown in Figure 102-1; their special characteristics are the following.

First, some *free nerve endings*, which are found everywhere in the skin and in many other tissues, can detect touch and pressure. For instance, even light contact with the cornea of the eye, which contains no other type of nerve ending besides free nerve endings, can nevertheless elicit touch and pressure sensations.

Second, a touch receptor with great sensitivity is the *Meissner corpuscle* (illustrated in Figure 102-1), an elongated encapsulated nerve ending of a large (type Aβ) myelinated sensory nerve fiber. Inside the capsulation are many branching terminal nerve filaments. These corpuscles are present in the nonhairy parts of the skin and are particularly abundant in the fingertips, lips, and other areas of the skin where one's ability to discern spatial locations of touch sensations is highly developed. Meissner corpuscles adapt in a fraction of a second after they are stimulated, which means that they are particularly sensitive to movement of objects over the surface of the skin, as well as to low-frequency vibration.

Third, the fingertips and other areas that contain large numbers of Meissner corpuscles usually also contain large numbers of *expanded tip tactile receptors*, one type of which is *Merkel discs*, shown in Figure 103-1. The hairy parts of the skin also contain moderate numbers of expanded tip receptors, even though they have almost no Meissner corpuscles. These receptors differ from Meissner corpuscles in that they transmit an initially strong but partially adapting signal and then a continuing weaker signal

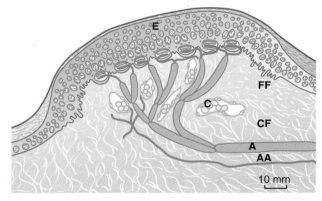

Figure 103-1 An Iggo dome receptor. Note the multiple numbers of Merkel discs connecting to a single large myelinated fiber and abutting tightly the undersurface of the epithelium. AA, nonmyelinated axon; C, capillary; CF, course bundles of collagen fibers; E, thickened epidermis of the touch corpuscle; FF, fine bundles of collagen fibers. *From Iggo, A., Muir, A.R., 1969. The structure and function of a slowly adapting touch corpuscle in hairy skin. J. Physiol. 200, 763.*

that adapts only slowly. Therefore, they are responsible for giving steady-state signals that allow one to determine continuous touch of objects against the skin.

Merkel discs are often grouped together in a receptor organ called the *Iggo dome receptor*, which projects upward against the underside of the epithelium of the skin, as is also shown in Figure 103-1. This upward projection causes the epithelium at this point to protrude outward, thus creating a dome and constituting an extremely sensitive receptor. Also note that the entire group of Merkel discs is innervated by a single large myelinated nerve fiber (type Aβ). These receptors, along with the Meissner corpuscles discussed earlier, play extremely important roles in localizing touch sensations to specific surface areas of the body and in determining the texture of what is felt.

Fourth, slight movement of any hair on the body stimulates a nerve fiber entwining its base. Thus, each hair and its basal nerve fiber, called the *hair end organ*, are also touch receptors. A receptor adapts readily and, like Meissner corpuscles, detects mainly (1) movement of objects on the surface of the body or (2) initial contact with the body.

Fifth, located in the deeper layers of the skin and also in still deeper internal tissues are many *Ruffini endings*, which are multibranched, encapsulated endings, as shown in Figure 102-1. These endings adapt very slowly and, therefore, are important for signaling continuous states of deformation of the tissues, such as heavy prolonged touch and pressure signals. They are also found in joint capsules and help to signal the degree of joint rotation.

Sixth, Pacinian corpuscles, which were discussed in detail in Chapter 102, lie both immediately beneath the skin and deep in the fascial tissues of the body. They are stimulated only by rapid local compression of the tissues because they adapt in a few hundredths of a second. Therefore, they are particularly important for detecting tissue vibration or other rapid changes in the mechanical state of the tissues.

Transmission of Tactile Signals in Peripheral Nerve Fibers. Almost all specialized sensory receptors, such as Meissner corpuscles, Iggo dome receptors, hair receptors, Pacinian corpuscles, and Ruffini endings, transmit their signals in type Aβ nerve fibers that have transmission velocities ranging from 30 to 70 m/second. Conversely, free nerve ending tactile receptors transmit

signals mainly by way of the small type Aδ myelinated fibers that conduct at velocities of only 5–30 m/second.

Some tactile free nerve endings transmit by way of type C unmyelinated fibers at velocities from a fraction of a meter up to 2 m/second; these nerve endings send signals into the spinal cord and lower brainstem, probably subserving mainly the sensation of tickle.

Thus, the more critical types of sensory signals—those that help to determine precise localization on the skin, minute gradations of intensity, or rapid changes in sensory signal intensity—are all transmitted in more rapidly conducting types of sensory nerve fibers. Conversely, the cruder types of signals, such as pressure, poorly localized touch, and especially tickle, are transmitted by way of much slower, very small nerve fibers that require much less space in the nerve bundle than the fast fibers.

DETECTION OF VIBRATION

All tactile receptors are involved in detection of vibration, although different receptors detect different frequencies of vibration. Pacinian corpuscles can detect signal vibrations from 30 to 800 cycles/second because they respond extremely rapidly to minute and rapid deformations of the tissues. They also transmit their signals over type Aβ nerve fibers, which can transmit as many as 1000 impulses/second. Low-frequency vibrations from 2 up to 80 cycles/second, in contrast, stimulate other tactile receptors, especially Meissner corpuscles, which adapt less rapidly adapting than Pacinian corpuscles.

DETECTION OF TICKLE AND ITCH BY MECHANORECEPTIVE FREE NERVE ENDINGS

Neurophysiological studies have demonstrated the existence of very sensitive, rapidly adapting mechanoreceptive free nerve endings that elicit only the tickle and itch sensations. Furthermore, these endings are found almost exclusively in superficial layers of the skin, which is also the only tissue from which the tickle and itch sensations usually can be elicited. These sensations are transmitted by very small type C, unmyelinated fibers similar to those that transmit the aching, slow type of pain.

The purpose of the itch sensation is presumably to call attention to mild surface stimuli such as a flea crawling on the skin or a fly about to bite, and the elicited signals then activate the scratch reflex or other maneuvers that rid the host of the irritant. Itch can be relieved by scratching if this removes the irritant or if the scratch is strong enough to elicit pain. The pain signals are believed to suppress the itch signals in the cord by lateral inhibition, as described in Chapter 104.

Sensory Pathways for Transmitting Somatic Signals into the Central Nervous System

Almost all sensory information from the somatic segments of the body enters the spinal cord through the dorsal roots of the spinal nerves. However, from the entry point into the cord and then to the brain, the sensory signals are carried through one of two alternative sensory pathways: (1) the *dorsal column–medial lemniscal system* or (2) the *anterolateral system*. These two systems come back together partially at the level of the thalamus.

The dorsal column–medial lemniscal system, as its name implies, carries signals upward to the medulla of the brain mainly in the *dorsal columns* of the cord. Then, after the signals synapse and cross to the opposite side in the medulla, they continue upward through the brainstem to the thalamus by way of the *medial lemniscus*.

Conversely, signals in the anterolateral system, immediately after entering the spinal cord from the dorsal spinal nerve roots, synapse in the dorsal horns of the spinal gray matter, and then cross to the opposite side of the cord and ascend through the anterior and lateral white columns of the cord. They terminate at all levels of the lower brainstem and in the thalamus.

The dorsal column–medial lemniscal system is composed of large, myelinated nerve fibers that transmit signals to the brain at velocities of 30–110 m/second, whereas the anterolateral system is composed of smaller myelinated fibers that transmit signals at velocities ranging from a few meters per second up to 40 m/second.

Another difference between the two systems is that the dorsal column–medial lemniscal system has a high degree of spatial orientation of the nerve fibers with respect to their origin, whereas the anterolateral system has much less spatial orientation. These differences immediately characterize the types of sensory information that can be transmitted by the two systems. That is, sensory information that must be transmitted rapidly with temporal and spatial fidelity is transmitted mainly in the dorsal column–medial lemniscal system; that which does not need to be transmitted rapidly or with great spatial fidelity is transmitted mainly in the anterolateral system.

The anterolateral system has a special capability that the dorsal system does not have– that is the ability to transmit a broad spectrum of sensory modalities—such as pain, warmth, cold, and crude tactile sensations. Most of these sensory modalities are discussed in detail in Chapters 102 and 104. The dorsal system is limited to discrete types of mechanoreceptive sensations.

With this differentiation in mind, we can now list the types of sensations transmitted in the two systems.

Dorsal Column—Medial Lemniscal System
1. Touch sensations requiring a high degree of localization of the stimulus
2. Touch sensations requiring transmission of fine gradations of intensity
3. Phasic sensations, such as vibratory sensations
4. Sensations that signal movement against the skin
5. Position sensations from the joints
6. Pressure sensations related to fine degrees of judgment of pressure intensity

Anterolateral System
1. Pain
2. Thermal sensations, including both warmth and cold sensations
3. Crude touch and pressure sensations capable only of crude localizing ability on the surface of the body
4. Tickle and itch sensations
5. Sexual sensations

Transmission in the Dorsal Column– Medial Lemniscal System

ANATOMY OF THE DORSAL COLUMN–MEDIAL LEMNISCAL SYSTEM

Upon entering the spinal cord through the spinal nerve dorsal roots, the large myelinated fibers from the specialized

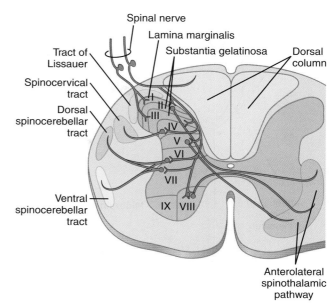

Figure 103-2 Cross-section of the spinal cord, showing the anatomy of the cord gray matter and of ascending sensory tracts in the white columns of the spinal cord.

mechanoreceptors divide almost immediately to form a *medial branch* and a *lateral branch*, shown by the right-hand fiber entering through the spinal root in Figure 103-2. The medial branch turns medially first and then upward in the dorsal column, proceeding by way of the dorsal column pathway all the way to the brain.

The lateral branch enters the dorsal horn of the cord gray matter, and then divides many times to provide terminals that synapse with local neurons in the intermediate and anterior portions of the cord gray matter. These local neurons in turn serve three functions: (1) a major share of them give off fibers that enter the dorsal columns of the cord and then travel upward to the brain; (2) many of their fibers are very short and terminate locally in the spinal cord gray matter to elicit local spinal cord reflexes, which are discussed in Chapter 111; (3) others give rise to the spinocerebellar tracts, which we discuss in Chapter 116 in relation to the function of the cerebellum.

Dorsal Column—Medial Lemniscal Pathway. Note in Figure 103-3 that nerve fibers entering the dorsal columns pass uninterrupted up to the dorsal medulla, where they synapse in the *dorsal column nuclei* (the *cuneate* and *gracile nuclei*). From there, *second-order neurons* decussate immediately to the opposite side of the brainstem and continue upward through the *medial lemnisci* to the thalamus. In this pathway through the brainstem, each medial lemniscus is joined by additional fibers from the *sensory nuclei of the trigeminal nerve*; these fibers subserve the same sensory functions for the head that the dorsal column fibers subserve for the body.

In the thalamus, the medial lemniscal fibers terminate in the thalamic sensory relay area called the *ventrobasal complex*. From the ventrobasal complex, *third-order nerve fibers* project, as shown in Figure 103-4, mainly to the *postcentral gyrus* of the *cerebral cortex*, which is called *somatic sensory area I* (as shown in Figure 105-2, these fibers also project to a smaller area in the lateral parietal cortex called *somatic sensory area II*).

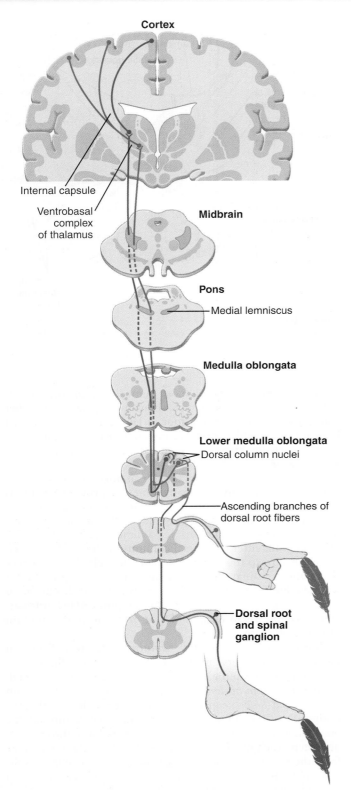

Figure 103-3   The dorsal column–medial lemniscal pathway for transmitting critical types of tactile signals.

Spatial Orientation of the Nerve Fibers in the Dorsal Column–Medial Lemniscal System

One of the distinguishing features of the dorsal column–medial lemniscal system is a distinct spatial orientation of nerve fibers from the individual parts of the body that is maintained

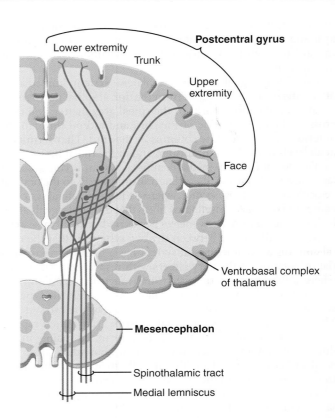

Figure 103-4   Projection of the dorsal column–medial lemniscal system through the thalamus to the somatosensory cortex. *Modified from Brodal, A., 1969. Neurological Anatomy in Relation to Clinical Medicine. Oxford University Press, New York, by permission of Oxford University Press.*

throughout. For instance, in the dorsal columns of the spinal cord the fibers from the lower parts of the body lie toward the center of the cord, whereas those that enter the cord at progressively higher segmental levels form successive layers laterally.

In the thalamus, distinct spatial orientation is still maintained, with the tail end of the body represented by the most lateral portions of the ventrobasal complex and the head and face represented by the medial areas of the complex. Because of the crossing of the medial lemnisci in the medulla, the left side of the body is represented in the right side of the thalamus and the right side of the body is represented in the left side of the thalamus.

JUDGMENT OF STIMULUS INTENSITY

Weber–Fechner Principle—Detection of "Ratio" of Stimulus Strength. In the mid-1800s, Weber first and Fechner later proposed the principle that *gradations of stimulus strength are discriminated approximately in proportion to the logarithm of stimulus strength.* That is, a person already holding 30 g weight in his or her hand can barely detect an additional 1-g increase in weight. And, when already holding 300 g, he or she can barely detect a 10-g increase in weight. Thus, in this instance, the *ratio* of the change in stimulus strength required for detection remains essentially constant, about 1–30, which is what the logarithmic principle means. To express this principle mathematically:

$$\text{Interpreted signal strength} = \log(\text{stimulus}) + \text{constant}$$

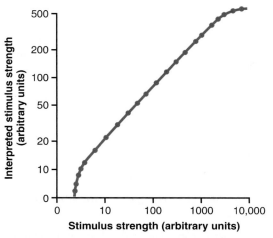

Figure 103-5 Graphical demonstration of the "power law" relation between actual stimulus strength and strength that the psyche interprets it to be. Note that the power law does not hold at either very weak or very strong stimulus strengths.

More recently, it has become evident that the Weber–Fechner principle is quantitatively accurate only for higher intensities of visual, auditory, and cutaneous sensory experience and applies only poorly to most other types of sensory experience. Yet the Weber–Fechner principle is still a good one to remember because it emphasizes that the greater the background sensory intensity, the greater an additional change must be for the psyche to detect the change.

Power Law. Another attempt by physiopsychologists to find a good mathematical relation is the following formula, known as the power law:

$$\text{Interpreted signal strength} = K \times (\text{stimulus} - k)^y$$

In this formula, the exponent y and the constants K and k are different for each type of sensation.

When this power law relation is plotted on a graph using double logarithmic coordinates, as shown in Figure 103-5, and when appropriate quantitative values for y, K, and k are found, a linear relation can be attained between interpreted stimulus strength and actual stimulus strength over a large range for almost any type of sensory perception.

POSITION SENSES

The *position senses* are frequently also called *proprioceptive senses*. They can be divided into two subtypes: (1) *static position sense*, which means conscious perception of the orientation of the different parts of the body with respect to one another, and (2) *rate of movement sense*, also called *kinesthesia* or *dynamic proprioception*.

Position Sensory Receptors. Knowledge of position, both static and dynamic, depends on knowing the degrees of angulation of all joints in all planes and their rates of change. Therefore, multiple different types of receptors help to determine joint angulation and are used together for position sense. Both skin tactile receptors and deep receptors near the joints are used. In the case of the fingers, where skin receptors are in great abundance, as much as half of position recognition is believed to be detected through the skin receptors. Conversely, for most of the larger joints of the body, deep receptors are more important.

For determining joint angulation in midranges of motion, the *muscle spindles* are among the most important receptors are the *muscle spindles*. They are also exceedingly important in helping to control muscle movement, as we shall see in Chapter 113. When the angle of a joint is changing, some muscles are being stretched while others are loosened, and the net stretch information from the spindles is transmitted into the computational system of the spinal cord and higher regions of the dorsal column system for deciphering joint angulations.

At the extremes of joint angulation, stretch of the ligaments and deep tissues around the joints is an additional important factor in determining position. Types of sensory endings used for this are the Pacinian corpuscles, Ruffini endings, and receptors similar to the Golgi tendon receptors found in muscle tendons.

The Pacinian corpuscles and muscle spindles are especially adapted for detecting rapid rates of change. It is likely that these are the receptors most responsible for detecting rate of movement.

Transmission of Less Critical Sensory Signals in the Anterolateral Pathway

The anterolateral pathway for transmitting sensory signals up the spinal cord and into the brain, in contrast to the dorsal column pathway, transmits sensory signals that do not require highly discrete localization of the signal source and do not require discrimination of fine gradations of intensity. These types of signals include pain, heat, cold, crude tactile, tickle, itch, and sexual sensations. In Chapter 104, pain and temperature sensations are discussed specifically.

ANATOMY OF THE ANTEROLATERAL PATHWAY

The *spinal cord anterolateral fibers* originate mainly in dorsal horn laminae I, IV, V, and VI (see Figure 103-2). These laminae are where many of the dorsal root sensory nerve fibers terminate after entering the cord.

As shown in Figure 103-6, the anterolateral fibers cross immediately in the *anterior commissure* of the cord to the opposite *anterior* and *lateral white columns*, where they turn upward toward the brain by way of the *anterior spinothalamic* and *lateral spinothalamic tracts*.

The upper terminus of the two spinothalamic tracts is mainly twofold: (1) throughout the *reticular nuclei of the brainstem* and (2) in two different nuclear complexes of the thalamus, the *ventrobasal complex* and the *intralaminar nuclei*. In general, the tactile signals are transmitted mainly into the ventrobasal complex, terminating in some of the same thalamic nuclei where the dorsal column tactile signals terminate. From here, the signals are transmitted to the somatosensory cortex along with the signals from the dorsal columns.

Conversely, only a small fraction of the pain signals project directly to the ventrobasal complex of the thalamus. Instead, most pain signals terminate in the reticular nuclei of the brainstem and from there are relayed to the intralaminar nuclei of the thalamus where the pain signals are further processed, as discussed in greater detail in Chapter 104.

Characteristics of Transmission in the Anterolateral Pathway. In general, the same principles apply to transmission in the anterolateral pathway as in the dorsal column–medial lemniscal system, except for the following differences: (1) the velocities

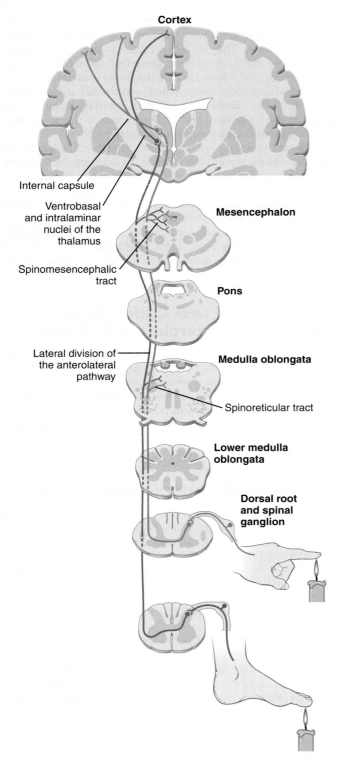

Figure 103-6   Anterior and lateral divisions of the anterolateral sensory pathway.

of transmission are only one-third to one-half of those in the dorsal column–medial lemniscal system, ranging between 8 and 40 m/second; (2) the degree of spatial localization of signals is poor; (3) the gradations of intensities are also far less accurate, with most of the sensations being recognized in 10–20 gradations of strength, rather than as many as 100 gradations for the

dorsal column system; and (4) the ability to transmit rapidly changing or rapidly repetitive signals is poor.

Thus, it is evident that the anterolateral system is a cruder type of transmission system than the dorsal column–medial lemniscal system. Even so, certain modalities of sensation are transmitted only in this system and not at all in the dorsal column–medial lemniscal system. They are pain, temperature, tickle, itch, and sexual sensations, in addition to crude touch and pressure.

Some Special Aspects of Somatosensory Function

FUNCTION OF THE THALAMUS IN SOMATIC SENSATION

When the somatosensory cortex of a human being is destroyed, that person loses most critical tactile sensibilities, but a slight degree of crude tactile sensibility does return. Therefore, it must be assumed that the thalamus (as well as other lower centers) has a slight ability to discriminate tactile sensation, even though

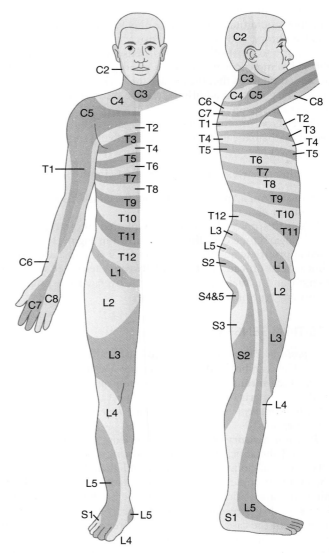

Figure 103-7   Dermatomes. *Modified from Grinker, R.R., Sahs, A.L., 1966. Neurology, sixth ed. Charles C. Thomas, Springfield, IL. Courtesy Charles C. Thomas, Publisher, Ltd., Springfield, IL.*

the thalamus normally functions mainly to relay this type of information to the cortex.

Conversely, loss of the somatosensory cortex has little effect on one's perception of pain sensation and only a moderate effect on the perception of temperature. Therefore, the lower brainstem, the thalamus, and other associated basal regions of the brain are believed to play dominant roles in discrimination of these sensibilities. It is interesting that these sensibilities appeared very early in the phylogenetic development of animals, whereas the critical tactile sensibilities and the somatosensory cortex were late developments.

SEGMENTAL FIELDS OF SENSATION—DERMATOMES

Each spinal nerve innervates a "segmental field" of the skin called a *dermatome*. The different dermatomes are shown in Figure 103-7. They are shown in the figure as if there were distinct borders between the adjacent dermatomes, which is far from true because much overlap exists from segment to segment.

Figure 103-7 shows that the anal region of the body lies in the dermatome of the most distal cord segment, dermatome S5. In the embryo, this is the tail region and the most distal portion of the body. The legs originate embryologically from the lumbar and upper sacral segments (L2 to S3), rather than from the distal sacral segments, which is evident from the dermatomal map. One can use a dermatomal map as shown in Figure 103-7 to determine the level in the spinal cord at which a cord injury has occurred when the peripheral sensations are disturbed by the injury.

THE LAW OF PROJECTION

The law of projection states that stimulating any afferent nerve fiber carrying sensory information to the brain, along its path, will give the impression of the specific stimulus to the brain. On reaching the brain normally responding to some specific type of stimulus (its adequate stimulus), the brain interprets action potentials in it as carrying information relating to the adequate stimulus.

BIBLIOGRAPHY

Alonso JM, Swadlow HA: Thalamocortical specificity and the synthesis of sensory cortical receptive fields, *J. Neurophysiol.* 94(26), 2005.

Bautista DM, Wilson SR, Hoon MA: Why we scratch an itch: the molecules, cells and circuits of itch, *Nat. Neurosci.* 17:175, 2014.

Bosco G, Poppele RE: Proprioception from a spinocerebellar perspective, *Physiol. Rev.* 81:539, 2001.

Chalfie M: Neurosensory mechanotransduction, *Nat. Rev. Mol. Cell Biol.* 10:44, 2009.

Fontanini A, Katz DB: Behavioral states, network states, and sensory response variability, *J. Neurophysiol.* 100:1160, 2008.

Haines DE: *Fundamental Neuroscience for Basic and Clinical Applications*, third ed., Philadelphia, 2006, Churchill Livingstone, Elsevier.

Hsiao S: Central mechanisms of tactile shape perception, *Curr. Opin. Neurobiol.* 18:418, 2008.

Johansson RS, Flanagan JR: Coding and use of tactile signals from the fingertips in object manipulation tasks, *Nat. Rev. Neurosci.* 10:345, 2009.

Kandel ER, Schwartz JH, Jessell TM: *Principles of Neural Science*, fourth ed., New York, 2000, McGraw-Hill.

Proske U, Gandevia SC: The proprioceptive senses: their roles in signaling body shape, body position and movement, and muscle force, *Physiol. Rev.* 92:1651, 2012.

104
Pain and Temperature

LEARNING OBJECTIVES

- Describe the theories of pain.
- Describe the pathways of pain transmission.
- Describe the pain suppression mechanisms.
- Explain referred pain and visceral pain.
- Describe the transmission of thermal sensations.

GLOSSARY OF TERMS

- **Hyperalgesia:** Increased sensitivity to pain
- **Neospinothalamic tract:** The evolutionarily newer pain pathway carrying sharp "fast" pain sensations in the anterolateral tract
- **Nociception:** The neural processes of detecting and processing noxious stimuli
- **Paleospinothalamic tract:** The evolutionarily older pathway carrying diffuse "slow" pain sensations in the anterolateral tract

Many ailments of the body cause pain. Furthermore, the ability to diagnose different diseases depends to a great extent on a physician's knowledge of the different qualities of pain. For these reasons, the first part of this chapter is devoted mainly to pain and to the physiological bases of some associated clinical phenomena.

Pain occurs whenever tissues are being damaged, and it causes the individual to react to remove the pain stimulus. Even such simple activities as sitting for a long time on the ischium can cause tissue destruction because of lack of blood flow to the skin where it is compressed by the weight of the body. When the skin becomes painful as a result of the ischemia, the person normally shifts weight subconsciously. However a person who has lost the pain sense, as after spinal cord injury, fails to feel the pain and, therefore, fails to shift. This situation soon results in total breakdown and desquamation of the skin at the areas of pressure.

Types of Pain and their Qualities—Fast Pain and Slow Pain

Pain has been classified into two major types: *fast pain* and *slow pain*. Fast pain is felt within about 0.1 second after a pain stimulus is applied, whereas slow pain begins only after 1 second or more and then increases slowly over many seconds and sometimes even minutes. During the course of this chapter, we shall see that the conduction pathways for these two types of pain are different and that each of them has specific qualities.

Fast pain is also described by many alternative names, such as *sharp pain*, *pricking pain*, *acute pain*, and *electric pain*. This type of pain is felt when a needle is stuck into the skin, when the skin is cut with a knife, or when the skin is acutely burned. It is

also felt when the skin is subjected to electric shock. Fast-sharp pain is not felt in most deep tissues of the body.

Slow pain also goes by many names, such as *slow burning pain*, *aching pain*, *throbbing pain*, *nauseous pain*, and *chronic pain*. This type of pain is usually associated with *tissue destruction*. It can lead to prolonged, almost unbearable suffering. Slow pain can occur both in the skin and in almost any deep tissue or organ.

Pain Receptors and their Stimulation

Pain Receptors Are Free Nerve Endings. The pain receptors in the skin and other tissues are all free nerve endings. They are widespread in the superficial layers of the *skin*, as well as in certain internal tissues, such as the *periosteum*, the *arterial walls*, the *joint surfaces*, and the *falx* and *tentorium* in the cranial vault. Most other deep tissues are only sparsely supplied with pain endings; nevertheless, any widespread tissue damage can summate to cause the slow-chronic-aching type of pain in most of these areas.

Three Types of Stimuli Excite Pain Receptors—Mechanical, Thermal, and Chemical. Pain can be elicited by multiple types of stimuliwhich are classified as *mechanical*, *thermal*, and *chemical pain stimuli*. In general, fast pain is elicited by the mechanical and thermal types of stimuli, whereas slow pain can be elicited by all three types.

Some of the chemicals that excite the chemical type of pain are *bradykinin*, *serotonin*, *histamine*, *potassium ions*, *acids*, *acetylcholine*, and *proteolytic enzymes*. In addition, *prostaglandins* and *substance P* enhance the sensitivity of pain endings but do not directly excite them. The chemical substances are especially important in stimulating the slow, suffering type of pain that occurs after tissue injury.

Nonadapting Nature of Pain Receptors. In contrast to most other sensory receptors of the body, pain receptors adapt very little and sometimes not at all. In fact, under some conditions, excitation of pain fibers becomes progressively greater, especially for slow-aching-nauseous pain, as the pain stimulus continues. This increase in sensitivity of the pain receptors is called *hyperalgesia*. One can readily understand the importance of this failure of pain receptors to adapt because it allows the pain to keep the person apprised of a tissue-damaging stimulus as long as it persists.

RATE OF TISSUE DAMAGE AS A STIMULUS FOR PAIN

The average person begins to perceive pain when the skin is heated above 45°C, as shown in Figure 104-1. This is also the temperature at which the tissues begin to be damaged by heat; indeed, the tissues are eventually destroyed if the temperature

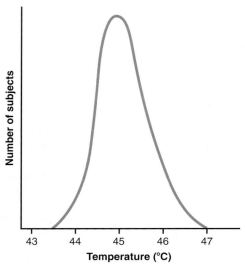

Figure 104-1   Distribution curve obtained from a large number of persons showing the minimal skin temperature that will cause pain. *Modified from Hardy, D.J., 1956. Nature of pain. J. Clin. Epidemiol. 4, 22.*

remains above this level indefinitely. Therefore, it is immediately apparent that pain resulting from heat is closely correlated with the *rate at which damage to the tissues is occurring* and not with the total damage that has already occurred.

The intensity of pain is also closely correlated with the *rate of tissue damage* from causes other than heat, such as bacterial infection, tissue ischemia, tissue contusion, and so forth.

Special Importance of Chemical Pain Stimuli During Tissue Damage. Extracts from damaged tissue cause intense pain when injected beneath the normal skin. Most of the chemicals listed earlier that excite the chemical pain receptors can be found in these extracts. One chemical that seems to be more painful than others is *bradykinin*. Researchers have suggested that bradykinin might be the agent most responsible for causing pain after tissue damage. Also, the intensity of the pain felt correlates with the local increase in potassium ion concentration or the increase in proteolytic enzymes that directly attack the nerve endings and excite pain by making the nerve membranes more permeable to ions.

Tissue Ischemia as a Cause of Pain. When blood flow to a tissue is blocked, the tissue often becomes very painful within a few minutes. The greater the rate of metabolism of the tissue, the more rapidly the pain appears. For instance, if a blood pressure cuff is placed around the upper arm and inflated until the arterial blood flow ceases, exercise of the forearm muscles sometimes can cause muscle pain within 15–20 seconds. In the absence of muscle exercise, the pain may not appear for 3–4 minutes even though the muscle blood flow remains zero.

One of the suggested causes of pain during ischemia is accumulation of large amounts of lactic acid in the tissues, formed as a consequence of anaerobic metabolism (metabolism without oxygen). It is also probable that other chemical agents, such as bradykinin and proteolytic enzymes, are formed in the tissues because of cell damage and that these, in addition to lactic acid, stimulate the pain nerve endings.

Muscle Spasm as a Cause of Pain. Muscle spasm is also a common cause of pain, and it is the basis of many clinical pain

syndromes. This pain probably results partially from the direct effect of muscle spasm in stimulating mechanosensitive pain receptors, but it might also result from the indirect effect of muscle spasm to compress the blood vessels and cause ischemia. The spasm also increases the rate of metabolism in the muscle tissue, thus making the relative ischemia even greater, creating ideal conditions for the release of chemical pain-inducing substances.

Dual Pathways for Transmission of Pain Signals into the Central Nervous System

Even though all pain receptors are free nerve endings, these endings use two separate pathways for transmitting pain signals into the central nervous system. The two pathways mainly correspond to the two types of pain—a *fast-sharp pain pathway* and a *slow-chronic pain pathway*.

Peripheral Pain Fibers—"Fast" and "Slow" Fibers. The fast-sharp pain signals are elicited by either mechanical or thermal pain stimuli. They are transmitted in the peripheral nerves to the spinal cord by small type Aδ fibers at velocities between 6 and 30 m/second. Conversely, the slow-chronic type of pain is elicited mostly by chemical types of pain stimuli but sometimes by persisting mechanical or thermal stimuli. This slow-chronic pain is transmitted to the spinal cord by type C fibers at velocities between 0.5 and 2 m/second.

Because of this double system of pain innervation, a sudden painful stimulus often gives a "double" pain sensation: a fast-sharp pain that is transmitted to the brain by the Aδ fiber pathway, followed a second or so later by a slow pain that is transmitted by the C fiber pathway. The sharp pain apprises the person rapidly of a damaging influence and, therefore, plays an important role in making the person react immediately to remove himself or herself from the stimulus. The slow pain tends to become greater over time. This sensation eventually produces intolerable pain and makes the person keep trying to relieve the cause of the pain.

Upon entering the spinal cord from the dorsal spinal roots, the pain fibers terminate on relay neurons in the dorsal horns. Here again, there are two systems for processing the pain signals on their way to the brain, as shown in Figures 104-2 and 104-3.

DUAL PAIN PATHWAYS IN THE CORD AND BRAINSTEM—THE NEOSPINOTHALAMIC TRACT AND THE PALEOSPINOTHALAMIC TRACT

Upon entering the spinal cord, the pain signals take two pathways to the brain, through (1) the *neospinothalamic tract* and (2) the *paleospinothalamic tract*.

Neospinothalamic Tract for Fast Pain. The fast type Aδ pain fibers transmit mainly mechanical and acute thermal pain. They terminate mainly in lamina I (lamina marginalis) of the dorsal horns, as shown in Figure 104-2, and there they excite second-order neurons of the neospinothalamic tract. These second-order neurons give rise to long fibers that cross immediately to the opposite side of the cord through the anterior commissure and then turn upward, passing to the brain in the anterolateral columns.

Termination of the Neospinothalamic Tract in the Brainstem and Thalamus. A few fibers of the neospinothalamic tract terminate in the reticular areas of the brainstem, but most pass

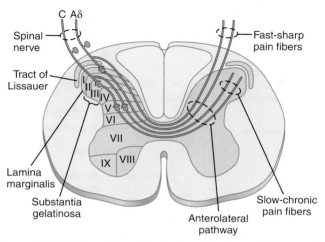

Figure 104-2 Transmission of both "fast-sharp" and "slow-chronic" pain signals into and through the spinal cord on their way to the brain. Aδ fibers transmit fast-sharp pain, and C fibers transmit slowchronic pain.

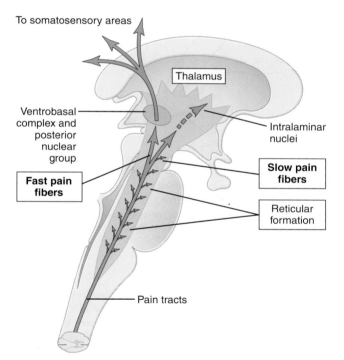

Figure 104-3 Transmission of pain signals into the brainstem, thalamus, and cerebral cortex by way of the *fast pricking pain pathway* and the *slow burning pain pathway.*

all the way to the thalamus without interruption, terminating in the *ventrobasal complex* along with the dorsal column–medial lemniscal tract for tactile sensations, as was discussed in Chapter 103. A few fibers also terminate in the posterior nuclear group of the thalamus. From these thalamic areas, the signals are transmitted to other basal areas of the brain, as well as to the somatosensory cortex.

Capability of the Nervous System to Localize Fast Pain in the Body. The fast-sharp type of pain can be localized much more exactly in the different parts of the body than can slow-chronic pain. However, when only pain receptors are stimulated, without the simultaneous stimulation of tactile receptors, even fast pain may be poorly localized, often only within 10 cm or

so of the stimulated area. Yet when tactile receptors that excite the dorsal column–medial lemniscal system are simultaneously stimulated, the localization can be nearly exact.

Glutamate, the Probable Neurotransmitter of the Type Aδ Fast Pain Fibers. It is believed that *glutamate* is the neurotransmitter substance secreted in the spinal cord at the type Aδ pain nerve fiber endings. Glutamate is one of the most widely used excitatory transmitters in the central nervous system, usually having a duration of action lasting for only a few milliseconds.

Paleospinothalamic Pathway for Transmitting Slow-Chronic Pain. The paleospinothalamic pathway is a much older system and transmits pain mainly from the peripheral slow-chronic type C pain fibers, although it does transmit some signals from type Aδ fibers as well. In this pathway, the peripheral fibers terminate in the spinal cord almost entirely in laminae II and III of the dorsal horns, which together are called the *substantia gelatinosa,* as shown by the lateral most dorsal root type C fiber in Figure 104-2. Most of the signals then pass through one or more additional short-fiber neurons within the dorsal horns themselves before entering mainly lamina V, also in the dorsal horn. Here the last neurons in the series give rise to long axons that mostly join the fibers from the fast pain pathway, passing first through the anterior commissure to the opposite side of the cord, and then upward to the brain in the anterolateral pathway.

Substance P, the Probable Slow-Chronic Neurotransmitter of Type C Nerve Endings. Research suggests that type C pain fiber terminals entering the spinal cord release both glutamate transmitter and substance P transmitter. The glutamate transmitter acts instantaneously and lasts for only a few milliseconds. Substance P is released much more slowly, building up in concentration over a period of seconds or even minutes. In fact, it has been suggested that the "double" pain sensation one feels after a pinprick might result partly from the fact that the glutamate transmitter gives a faster pain sensation, whereas the substance P transmitter gives a more lagging sensation. Regardless of the yet unknown details, it seems clear that glutamate is the neurotransmitter most involved in transmitting fast pain into the central nervous system, and substance P is concerned with slow-chronic pain.

Projection of the Paleospinothalamic Pathway (Slow-Chronic Pain Signals) into the Brainstem and Thalamus. The slow-chronic paleospinothalamic pathway terminates widely in the brainstem, in the large shaded area shown in Figure 104-3. Only one-tenth to one-fourth of the fibers pass all the way to the thalamus. Instead, most terminate in one of three areas: (1) the *reticular nuclei* of the medulla, pons, and mesencephalon; (2) the *tectal area* of the mesencephalon deep to the superior and inferior colliculi; or (3) the *periaqueductal gray region* surrounding the aqueduct of Sylvius. These lower regions of the brain appear to be important for feeling the suffering types of pain, because animals whose brains have been sectioned above the mesencephalon to block pain signals from reaching the cerebrum still have undeniable evidence of suffering when any part of the body is traumatized. From the brainstem pain areas, multiple short-fiber neurons relay the pain signals upward into the intralaminar and ventrolateral nuclei of the thalamus and into certain portions of the hypothalamus and other basal regions of the brain.

Poor Capability of the Nervous System to Precisely Localize the Source of Pain Transmitted in the Slow-Chronic Pathway. Localization of pain transmitted by way of the paleospinothalamic pathway is imprecise. For instance, slow-chronic pain can usually be localized only to a major part of the body, such as to one arm or leg but not to a specific point on the arm or leg. This phenomenon is in keeping with the multisynaptic, diffuse connectivity of this pathway. It explains why patients often have serious difficulty in localizing the source of some chronic types of pain.

Function of the Reticular Formation, Thalamus, and Cerebral Cortex in the Appreciation of Pain. Complete removal of the somatic sensory areas of the cerebral cortex does not prevent pain perception. Therefore, it is likely that pain impulses entering the brainstem reticular formation, the thalamus, and the other lower brain centers cause conscious perception of pain. This does not mean that the cerebral cortex has nothing to do with normal pain appreciation; electrical stimulation of cortical somatosensory areas does cause a human being to perceive mild pain from about 3% of the points stimulated. However, it is believed that the cortex plays an especially important role in interpreting pain quality, even though pain perception might be principally the function of lower centers.

Special Capability of Pain Signals to Arouse Overall Brain Excitability. Electrical stimulation in the *reticular areas of the brainstem* and in the *intralaminar nuclei of the thalamus*, the areas where the slow-suffering type of pain terminates, has a strong arousal effect on nervous activity throughout the entire brain. In fact, these two areas constitute part of the brain's principal "arousal system," which is discussed in Chapter 123. This explains why it is almost impossible for a person to sleep when he or she is in severe pain.

Surgical Interruption of Pain Pathways. When a person has severe and intractable pain (sometimes resulting from rapidly spreading cancer), it is necessary to relieve the pain. To provide pain relief, the pain nervous pathways can be cut at any one of several points. If the pain is in the lower part of the body, a *cordotomy* in the thoracic region of the spinal cord often relieves the pain for a few weeks to a few months. To perform a cordotomy, the spinal cord on the side opposite to the pain is partially cut in its *anterolateral quadrant* to interrupt the anterolateral sensory pathway.

A cordotomy is not always successful in relieving pain, for two reasons. First, many pain fibers from the upper part of the body do not cross to the opposite side of the spinal cord until they have reached the brain, and the cordotomy does not transect these fibers. Second, pain frequently returns several months later, partly as a result of sensitization of other pathways that normally are too weak to be effectual (eg, sparse pathways in the dorsolateral cord). Another experimental operative procedure to relieve pain has been to cauterize specific pain areas in the intralaminar nuclei in the thalamus, which often relieves suffering types of pain while leaving intact one's appreciation of "acute" pain, an important protective mechanism.

Pain Suppression ("Analgesia") System in the Brain and Spinal Cord

The degree to which a person reacts to pain varies tremendously. This variation results partly from a capability of the brain itself to suppress input of pain signals to the nervous system by activating a pain control system called an *analgesia system*.

The analgesia system is shown in Figure 104-4. It consists of three major components: (1) The *periaqueductal gray* and *periventricular areas* of the mesencephalon and upper pons surround the aqueduct of Sylvius and portions of the third and fourth ventricles. Neurons from these areas send signals to (2) the *raphe magnus nucleus*, a thin midline nucleus located in the

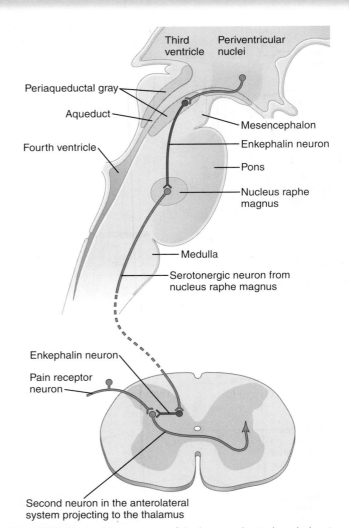

Figure 104-4   Analgesia system of the brain and spinal cord, showing (1) inhibition of incoming pain signals at the cord level and (2) presence of *enkephalin-secreting neurons* that suppress pain signals in both the cord and the brainstem.

lower pons and upper medulla, and the *nucleus reticularis paragigantocellularis*, located laterally in the medulla. From these nuclei, second-order signals are transmitted down the dorsolateral columns in the spinal cord to (3) a *pain inhibitory complex located in the dorsal horns of the spinal cord.* At this point, the analgesia signals can block the pain before it is relayed to the brain.

Electrical stimulation either in the periaqueductal gray area or in the raphe magnus nucleus can suppress many strong pain signals entering by way of the dorsal spinal roots. Also, stimulation of areas at still higher levels of the brain that excite the periaqueductal gray area can suppress pain. Some of these areas are (1) the *periventricular nuclei in the hypothalamus*, lying adjacent to the third ventricle, and (2) to a lesser extent, the *medial forebrain bundle*, also in the hypothalamus.

Several transmitter substances are involved in the analgesia system; especially involved are *enkephalin* and *serotonin*. Many nerve fibers derived from the periventricular nuclei and from the periaqueductal gray area secrete enkephalin at their endings. Thus, as shown in Figure 104-4, the endings of many fibers in the raphe magnus nucleus release enkephalin when stimulated.

Fibers originating in this area send signals to the dorsal horns of the spinal cord to secrete serotonin at their endings.

The serotonin causes local cord neurons to secrete enkephalin as well. The enkephalin is believed to cause both *presynaptic* and *postsynaptic inhibition* of incoming type C and type Aδ pain fibers where they synapse in the dorsal horns.

Thus, the analgesia system can block pain signals at the initial entry point to the spinal cord. In fact, it can also block many local cord reflexes that result from pain signals, especially withdrawal reflexes described in Chapter 114.

BRAIN'S OPIATE SYSTEM—ENDORPHINS AND ENKEPHALINS

More than 40 years ago it was discovered that injection of minute quantities of morphine either into the periventricular nucleus around the third ventricle or into the periaqueductal gray area of the brainstem causes an extreme degree of analgesia. In subsequent studies, morphine-like agents, mainly the opiates, have been found to act at many other points in the analgesia system, including the dorsal horns of the spinal cord. Because most drugs that alter excitability of neurons do so by acting on synaptic receptors, it was assumed that the "morphine receptors" of the analgesia system must be receptors for some morphine-like neurotransmitter that is naturally secreted in the brain. Therefore, an extensive search was undertaken for the natural opiate of the brain. About a dozen such opiate-like substances have now been found at different points of the nervous system. All are breakdown products of three large protein molecules: *proopiomelanocortin, proenkephalin,* and *prodynorphin.* Among the more important of these opiate-like substances are *β-endorphin, met-enkephalin, leu-enkephalin,* and *dynorphin.*

The two enkephalins are found in the brainstem and spinal cord, in the portions of the analgesia system described earlier, and β-endorphin is present in both the hypothalamus and the pituitary gland. Dynorphin is found mainly in the same areas as the enkephalins, but in much lower quantities.

Thus, although the details of the brain's opiate system are not completely understood, *activation of the analgesia system* by nervous signals entering the periaqueductal gray and periventricular areas, or *inactivation of pain pathways* by morphine-like drugs, can almost totally suppress many pain signals entering through the peripheral nerves.

INHIBITION OF PAIN TRANSMISSION BY SIMULTANEOUS TACTILE SENSORY SIGNALS

Another important event in the saga of pain control was the discovery that stimulation of large-type Aβ sensory fibers from peripheral tactile receptors can depress transmission of pain signals from the same body area. This effect presumably results from local lateral inhibition in the spinal cord. It explains why such simple maneuvers as rubbing the skin near painful areas are often effective in relieving pain and it probably also explains why liniments are often useful for pain relief.

This mechanism and the simultaneous psychogenic excitation of the central analgesia system are probably also the basis of pain relief by *acupuncture.*

TREATMENT OF PAIN BY ELECTRICAL STIMULATION

Several clinical procedures have been developed for suppressing pain with use of electrical stimulation. Stimulating electrodes are placed on selected areas of the skin or, on occasion, implanted over the spinal cord, supposedly to stimulate the dorsal sensory columns.

In some patients, electrodes have been placed stereotaxically in appropriate intralaminar nuclei of the thalamus or in the periventricular or periaqueductal area of the diencephalon. The patient can then personally control the degree of stimulation. Dramatic relief has been reported in some instances. Also, pain relief has been reported to last for as long as 24 hours after only a few minutes of stimulation.

Referred Pain

Often a person feels pain in a part of the body that is fairly remote from the tissue causing the pain. This phenomenon is called *referred pain.* For instance, pain in one of the visceral organs often is referred to an area on the body surface. Knowledge of the different types of referred pain is important in clinical diagnosis because in many visceral ailments the only clinical sign is referred pain.

Mechanism of Referred Pain. Figure 104-5 shows the probable mechanism by which most pain is referred. In the figure, branches of visceral pain fibers are shown to synapse in the spinal cord on the same second-order neurons (1 and 2) that receive pain signals from the skin. When the visceral pain fibers are stimulated, pain signals from the viscera are conducted through at least some of the same neurons that conduct pain signals from the skin, and the person has the feeling that the sensations originate in the skin.

Visceral Pain

Pain from the different viscera of the abdomen and chest is one of the few criteria that can be used for diagnosing visceral inflammation, visceral infectious disease, and other visceral ailments. Often, the viscera have sensory receptors for no other modalities of sensation besides pain. Also, visceral pain differs from surface pain in several important aspects.

One of the most important differences between surface pain and visceral pain is that highly localized types of damage to the viscera seldom cause severe pain. For instance, a surgeon can cut the gut entirely in two in a patient who is awake without causing significant pain. Conversely, any stimulus that causes *diffuse*

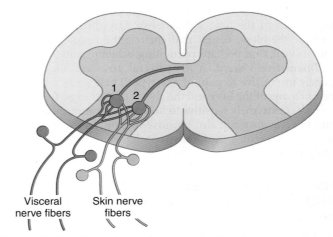

Figure 104-5 Mechanism of referred pain and referred hyperalgesia. Neurons 1 and 2 receive pain signals from the skin as well as from the viscera.

Visceral nerve fibers

Skin nerve fibers

stimulation of pain nerve endings throughout a viscus causes pain that can be severe. For instance, ischemia caused by occluding the blood supply to a large area of gut stimulates many diffuse pain fibers at the same time and can result in extreme pain.

CAUSES OF TRUE VISCERAL PAIN

Any stimulus that excites pain nerve endings in diffuse areas of the viscera can cause visceral pain. Such stimuli include ischemia of visceral tissue, chemical damage to the surfaces of the viscera, spasm of the smooth muscle of a hollow viscus, excess distention of a hollow viscus, and stretching of the connective tissue surrounding or within the viscus. Essentially all visceral pain that originates in the thoracic and abdominal cavities is transmitted through small type C pain fibers and, therefore, can transmit only the chronic-aching-suffering type of pain.

Ischemia. Ischemia causes visceral pain in the same way that it does in other tissues, presumably because of the formation of acidic metabolic end products or tissue-degenerative products such as bradykinin, proteolytic enzymes, or others that stimulate pain nerve endings.

Chemical Stimuli. On occasion, damaging substances leak from the gastrointestinal tract into the peritoneal cavity. For instance, proteolytic acidic gastric juice may leak through a ruptured gastric or duodenal ulcer. This juice causes widespread digestion of the visceral peritoneum, thus stimulating broad areas of pain fibers. The pain is usually excruciatingly severe.

Spasm of a Hollow Viscus. Spasm of a portion of the gut, the gallbladder, the bile duct, the ureter, or any other hollow viscus can cause pain, possibly by mechanical stimulation of the pain nerve endings. Another possibility is that the spasm may cause diminished blood flow to the muscle, combined with the muscle's increased metabolic need for nutrients, thus causing severe pain.

Often pain from a spastic viscus occurs in the form of *cramps*, with the pain increasing to a high degree of severity and then subsiding. This process continues intermittently, once every few minutes. The intermittent cycles result from periods of contraction of smooth muscle. For instance, each time a peristaltic wave travels along an overly excitable spastic gut, a cramp occurs. The cramping type of pain frequently occurs in persons with appendicitis, gastroenteritis, constipation, menstruation, parturition, gallbladder disease, or ureteral obstruction.

Overdistention of a Hollow Viscus. Extreme overfilling of a hollow viscus also can result in pain, presumably because of overstretch of the tissues themselves. Overdistention can also collapse the blood vessels that encircle the viscus or that pass into its wall, thus perhaps promoting ischemic pain.

Insensitive Viscera. A few visceral areas are almost completely insensitive to pain of any type. These areas include the parenchyma of the liver and the alveoli of the lungs. Yet the liver *capsule* is extremely sensitive to both direct trauma and stretch, and the *bile ducts* are also sensitive to pain. In the lungs, even though the alveoli are insensitive, both the *bronchi* and the *parietal pleura* are very sensitive to pain.

LOCALIZATION OF VISCERAL PAIN—"VISCERAL" AND THE "PARIETAL" PAIN TRANSMISSION PATHWAYS

Pain from the different viscera is frequently difficult to localize for several reasons. First, the patient's brain does not know from firsthand experience that the different internal organs exist; therefore, any pain that originates internally can be localized only generally. Second, sensations from the abdomen and thorax are transmitted through two pathways to the central nervous system—the *true visceral pathway* and the *parietal pathway*. True visceral pain is transmitted via pain sensory fibers within the autonomic nerve bundles, and the sensations are *referred* to surface areas of the body often far from the painful organ. Conversely, parietal sensations are conducted *directly* into local spinal nerves from the parietal peritoneum, pleura, or pericardium, and these sensations are usually *localized directly over the painful area*.

Localization of Referred Pain Transmitted via Visceral Pathways. When visceral pain is referred to the surface of the body, the person generally localizes it in the dermatomal segment from which the visceral organ originated in the embryo, not necessarily where the visceral organ now lies. For instance, the heart originated in the neck and upper thorax, so the heart's visceral pain fibers pass upward along the sympathetic sensory nerves and enter the spinal cord between segments C-3 and T-5. Therefore, as shown in Figure 104-6, pain from the heart is referred to the side of the neck, over the shoulder, over the pectoral muscles, down the arm, and into the substernal area of the upper chest. These are the areas of the body surface that send their own somatosensory nerve fibers into the C-3 to T-5 cord segments. Most frequently, the pain is on the left side rather than on the right because the left side of the heart is much more frequently involved in coronary disease than is the right side.

The stomach originated approximately from the seventh to ninth thoracic segments of the embryo. Therefore, stomach pain is referred to the anterior epigastrium above the umbilicus, which is the surface area of the body subserved by the seventh through ninth thoracic segments. Figure 104-6 shows several other surface areas to which visceral pain is referred from other organs, representing in general the areas in the embryo from which the respective organs originated.

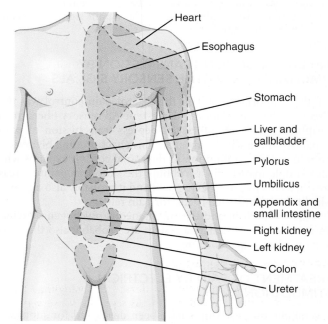

Figure 104-6 Surface areas of referred pain from different visceral organs.

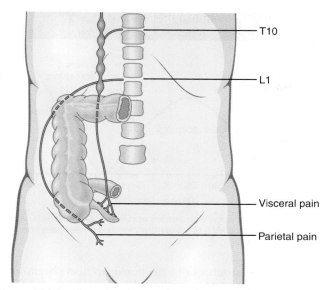

Figure 104-7 Visceral and parietal transmission of pain signals from the appendix.

Parietal Pathway for Transmission of Abdominal and Thoracic Pain. Pain from the viscera is frequently localized to two surface areas of the body at the same time because of the dual transmission of pain through the referred visceral pathway and the direct parietal pathway. Thus, Figure 104-7 shows dual transmission from an inflamed appendix. Pain impulses pass first from the appendix through visceral pain fibers located within sympathetic nerve bundles, and then into the spinal cord at about T-10 or T-11; this pain is referred to an area around the umbilicus and is of the aching, cramping type. Pain impulses also often originate in the parietal peritoneum where the inflamed appendix touches or is adherent to the abdominal wall. These impulses cause pain of the sharp type directly over the irritated peritoneum in the right lower quadrant of the abdomen.

Some Clinical Abnormalities of Pain and Other Somatic Sensations

HYPERALGESIA—HYPERSENSITIVITY TO PAIN

A pain nervous pathway sometimes becomes excessively excitablewhich gives rise to *hyperalgesia*,. Possible causes of hyperalgesia are (1) excessive sensitivity of the pain receptors, which is called *primary hyperalgesia*, and (2) facilitation of sensory transmission, which is called *secondary hyperalgesia*.

An example of primary hyperalgesia is the extreme sensitivity of sunburned skin, which results from sensitization of the skin pain endings by local tissue products from the burn—perhaps histamine, prostaglandins, and others. Secondary hyperalgesia frequently results from lesions in the spinal cord or the thalamus. Several of these lesions are discussed in subsequent sections.

HERPES ZOSTER (SHINGLES)

Occasionally *herpes virus* infects a dorsal root ganglion. This causes severe pain in the dermatomal segment subserved by the ganglion, thus eliciting a segmental type of pain that circles halfway around the body. The disease is called *herpes zoster*, or "shingles," because of a skin eruption that often ensues.

The cause of the pain is presumably infection of the pain neuronal cells in the dorsal root ganglion by the virus. In addition to causing pain, the virus is carried by neuronal cytoplasmic flow outward through the neuronal peripheral axons to their cutaneous origins. Here the virus causes a rash that vesiculates within a few days and then crusts over within another few days, all of this occurring within the dermatomal area served by the infected dorsal root.

TIC DOULOUREUX

Lancinating or stabbing type of pain occasionally occurs in some people over one side of the face in the sensory distribution area (or part of the area) of the fifth or ninth nerves; this phenomenon is called *tic douloureux* (or *trigeminal neuralgia* or *glossopharyngeal neuralgia*). The pain feels like sudden electrical shocks, and it may appear for only a few seconds at a time or may be almost continuous. Often it is set off by exceedingly sensitive trigger areas on the surface of the face, in the mouth, or inside the throat—almost always by a mechanoreceptive stimulus rather than a pain stimulus. For instance, when the patient swallows a bolus of food, as the food touches a tonsil, it might set off a severe lancinating pain in the mandibular portion of the fifth nerve.

The pain of tic douloureux can usually be blocked by surgically cutting the peripheral nerve from the hypersensitive area. The sensory portion of the fifth nerve is often sectioned immediately inside the cranium, where the motor and sensory roots of the fifth nerve separate from each other, so that the motor portions, which are necessary for many jaw movements, can be spared while the sensory elements are destroyed. This operation leaves the side of the face anesthetic, which may be annoying. Furthermore, sometimes the operation is unsuccessful, indicating that the lesion that causes the pain might be in the sensory nucleus in the brainstem and not in the peripheral nerves.

BROWN–SÉQUARD SYNDROME

If the spinal cord is transected entirely, all sensations and motor functions distal to the segment of transection are blocked, but if the spinal cord is transected on only one side, the *Brown–Séquard syndrome* occurs. The effects of such transection can be predicted from knowledge of the cord fiber tracts shown in Figure 104-8. All motor functions are blocked on the side of the transection in all segments below the level of the transection. Yet only some of the modalities of sensation are lost on the transected side, and others are lost on the opposite side. The

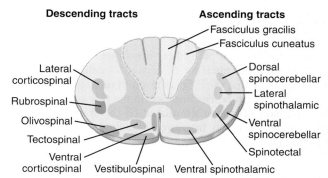

Figure 104-8 Cross-section of the spinal cord, showing principal ascending tracts on the right and principal descending tracts on the left.

sensations of pain, heat, and cold—sensations served by the spinothalamic pathway—are lost *on the opposite side of the body* in all dermatomes two to six segments below the level of the transection. By contrast, the sensations that are transmitted only in the dorsal and dorsolateral columns—kinesthetic and position sensations, vibration sensation, discrete localization, and two-point discrimination—are lost *on the side of the transection* in all dermatomes below the level of the transection. Discrete "light touch" is impaired on the side of the transection because the principal pathway for the transmission of light touch, the dorsal column, is transected. That is, the fibers in this column do not cross to the opposite side until they reach the medulla of the brain. "Crude touch," which is poorly localized, still persists because of partial transmission in the opposite spinothalamic tract.

Thermal Sensations

THERMAL RECEPTORS AND THEIR EXCITATION

The human being can perceive different gradations of cold and heat, from *freezing cold* to *cold* to *cool* to *indifferent* to *warm* to *hot* to *burning hot.*

Thermal gradations are discriminated by at least three types of sensory receptors: cold receptors, warmth receptors, and pain receptors. The pain receptors are stimulated only by extreme degrees of heat or cold and, therefore, are responsible, along with the cold and warmth receptors, for "freezing cold" and "burning hot" sensations.

The cold and warmth receptors are located immediately under the skin at discrete separated *spots.* Most areas of the body have 3–10 times as many cold spots as warmth spots, and the number in different areas of the body varies from 15 to 25 cold spots/cm^2 in the lips to 3–5 cold spots/cm^2 in the finger to less than 1 cold spot/cm^2 in some broad surface areas of the trunk.

Although psychological tests show that the existence of distinctive warmth nerve endings is quite certain, they have not been identified histologically. They are presumed to be free nerve endings because warmth signals are transmitted mainly over type C nerve fibers at transmission velocities of only 0.4–2 m/second.

A definitive cold receptor, has been identified. It is a special, small type Aδ myelinated nerve ending that branches several times, the tips of which protrude into the bottom surfaces of basal epidermal cells. Signals are transmitted from these receptors via type Aδ nerve fibers at velocities of about 20 m/second. Some cold sensations are believed to be transmitted in type C nerve fibers as well, which suggests that some free nerve endings also might function as cold receptors.

Stimulation of Thermal Receptors—Sensations of Cold, Cool, Indifferent, Warm, and Hot. Figure 104-9 shows the effects of different temperatures on the responses of four types of nerve fibers: (1) a pain fiber stimulated by cold, (2) a cold fiber, (3) a warmth fiber, and (4) a pain fiber stimulated by heat. Note especially that these fibers respond differently at different levels of temperature. For instance, in the *very* cold region, only the cold-pain fibers are stimulated (if the skin becomes even colder so that it nearly freezes or actually does freeze, these fibers cannot be stimulated). As the temperature rises to +10 to 15°C, the cold-pain impulses cease, but the cold receptors begin to be stimulated, reaching peak stimulation at about 24°C and fading out slightly above 40°C. Above about 30°C, the warmth receptors begin to be stimulated, but these also fade out at about

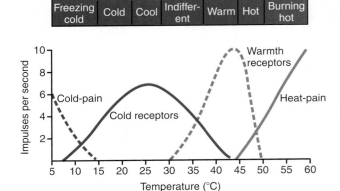

Figure 104-9 Discharge frequencies at different skin temperatures of a *cold-pain fiber*, a *cold fiber*, a *warmth fiber*, and a *heat-pain fiber.*

49°C. Finally, at around 45°C, the heat-pain fibers begin to be stimulated by heat and, paradoxically, some of the cold fibers begin to be stimulated again, possibly because of damage to the cold endings caused by the excessive heat.

One can understand from Figure 104-9 that a person determines the different gradations of thermal sensations by the relative degrees of stimulation of the different types of endings. One can also understand why extreme degrees of both cold and heat can be painful and why both these sensations, when intense enough, may give almost the same quality of sensation—that is, freezing cold and burning hot sensations feel almost alike.

Stimulatory Effects of Rising and Falling Temperature— Adaptation of Thermal Receptors. When a cold receptor is suddenly subjected to an abrupt fall in temperature, it becomes strongly stimulated at first, but this stimulation fades rapidly during the first few seconds and progressively more slowly during the next 30 minutes or more. In other words, the receptor "adapts" to a great extent, but never 100%.

Thus, it is evident that the thermal senses respond markedly to *changes in temperature*, in addition to being able to respond to steady states of temperature. This means that when the temperature of the skin is actively falling, a person feels much colder than when the temperature remains cold at the same level. Conversely, if the temperature is actively rising, the person feels much warmer than he or she would at the same temperature if it were constant. The response to changes in temperature explains the extreme degree of heat one feels on first entering a tub of hot water and the extreme degree of cold felt on going from a heated room to the out-of-doors on a cold day.

Mechanism of Stimulation of Thermal Receptors

It is believed that the cold and warmth receptors are stimulated by changes in their metabolic rates, and that these changes result from the fact that temperature alters the rate of intracellular chemical reactions more than twofold for each 10°C change. In other words, thermal detection probably results not from direct physical effects of heat or cold on the nerve endings but from chemical stimulation of the endings as modified by temperature.

Spatial Summation of Thermal Sensations. Because the number of cold or warm endings in any one surface area of the body is slight, it is difficult to judge gradations of temperature when small skin areas are stimulated. However, when a large skin area is stimulated all at once, the thermal signals from the entire area summate. For instance, rapid changes in temperature as little as 0.01°C can be detected if this change affects the entire surface of the body simultaneously. Conversely, temperature changes 100 times as great often will not be detected when the affected skin area is only 1 cm² in size.

TRANSMISSION OF THERMAL SIGNALS IN THE NERVOUS SYSTEM

In general, thermal signals are transmitted in pathways parallel to those for pain signals. Upon entering the spinal cord, the signals travel for a few segments upward or downward in the *tract of Lissauer* and then terminate mainly in laminae I, II, and III of the dorsal horns—the same as for pain. After a small amount of processing by one or more cord neurons, the signals enter long, ascending thermal fibers that cross to the opposite anterolateral sensory tract and terminate in both (1) the reticular areas of the brainstem and (2) the ventrobasal complex of the thalamus.

A few thermal signals are also relayed to the cerebral somatic sensory cortex from the ventrobasal complex. Occasionally a neuron in cortical somatic sensory area I has been found by microelectrode studies to be directly responsive to either cold or warm stimuli on a specific area of the skin. However, removal of the entire cortical postcentral gyrus in the human being reduces but does not abolish the ability to distinguish gradations of temperature.

BIBLIOGRAPHY

Akerman S, Holland PR, Goadsby PJ: Diencephalic and brainstem mechanisms in migraine, *Nat. Rev. Neurosci.* 12:570, 2011.

Almeida TF, Roizenblatt S, Tufik S: Afferent pain pathways: a neuroanatomical review, *Brain Res.* 1000:40, 2004.

Bandell M, Macpherson LJ, Patapoutian A: From chills to chilis: mechanisms for thermosensation and chemesthesis via thermoTRPs, *Curr. Opin. Neurobiol.* 17:490, 2007.

Denk F, McMahon SB, Tracey I: Pain vulnerability: a neurobiological perspective, *Nat. Neurosci.* 17:192, 2014.

Gebhart GF: Descending modulation of pain, *Neurosci. Biobehav. Rev.* 27:729, 2004.

Kandel ER, Schwartz JH, Jessell TM: *Principles of Neural Science*, fourth ed., New York, 2000, McGraw-Hill.

McKemy DD: Temperature sensing across species, *Pflugers Arch.* 454:777, 2007.

Mendell JR, Sahenk Z: Clinical practice: painful sensory neuropathy, *N. Engl. J. Med.* 348:1243, 2003.

Sandkühler J: Models and mechanisms of hyperalgesia and allodynia, *Physiol. Rev.* 89:707, 2009.

Schepers RJ, Ringkamp M: Thermoreceptors and thermosensitive afferents, *Neurosci. Biobehav. Rev.* 34:177, 2010.

White FA, Jung H, Miller RJ: Chemokines and the pathophysiology of neuropathic pain, *Proc. Natl. Acad. Sci. U. S. A.* 104:20151, 2007.

Zubrzycka M, Janecka A: Substance P: transmitter of nociception (minireview), *Endocr. Regul.* 34:195, 2000.

105

Somatosensory Cortex

LEARNING OBJECTIVES

- Describe the somatosensory areas of the cortex.
- Describe the spatial orientation in the cortex and the sensory homunculus.
- Name the layers of the somatosensory cortex and enumerate their functions.
- Describe the functions of the sensory cortex.
- Describe the effects of a lesion of the sensory cortex.

GLOSSARY OF TERMS

- **Amorphosynthesis:** Lack of awareness of somatic sensation from the opposite side of the body
- **Astereognosis:** Inability to identify an object by touch without looking at it
- **Brodmann areas:** Areas of the cortex defined in a numbered fashion, based on neuronal organization
- **Parietal cortex:** Part of the cortex behind the frontal lobe, which integrates sensory information

Before discussing the role of the cerebral cortex in somatic sensation, we need to give an orientation to the various areas of the cortex. Figure 105-1 is a map of the human cerebral cortex, showing that it is divided into about 50 distinct areas called *Brodmann areas* based on histological structural differences. This map is important because virtually all neurophysiologists and neurologists use it to refer by number to many of the different functional areas of the human cortex.

Note in Figure 105-1 the large *central fissure* (also called *central sulcus*) that extends horizontally across the brain. In general, sensory signals from all modalities of sensation terminate in the cerebral cortex immediately posterior to the central fissure. Generally, the anterior half of the *parietal lobe* is concerned almost entirely with reception and interpretation of *somatosensory signals* but the posterior half of the parietal lobe provides still higher levels of interpretation.

Visual signals terminate in the occipital lobe, and auditory signals terminate in the temporal lobe.

Conversely, the portion of the cerebral cortex anterior to the central fissure and constituting the posterior half of the frontal lobe is called the *motor cortex* and is devoted almost entirely to control of muscle contractions and body movements. A major share of this motor control is in response to somatosensory signals received from the sensory portions of the cortex, which keep the motor cortex informed at each instant about the positions and motions of the different body parts.

Somatosensory Areas I and II

Figure 105-2 shows two separate sensory areas in the anterior parietal lobe called *somatosensory area I* and *somatosensory*

area II. The reason for this division into two areas is that a distinct and separate spatial orientation of the different parts of the body is found in each of these two areas. However, somatosensory area I is so much more extensive and so much more important than somatosensory area II that in popular usage the term "somatosensory cortex" almost always means area I.

Somatosensory area I has a high degree of localization of the different parts of the body, as shown by the names of virtually all parts of the body in Figure 105-2. By contrast, localization is poor in somatosensory area II, although roughly, the face is represented anteriorly, the arms centrally, and the legs posteriorly.

Much less is known about the function of somatosensory area II. It is known that signals enter this area from the brainstem, transmitted upward from both sides of the body. In addition, many signals come secondarily from somatosensory area I, as well as from other sensory areas of the brain, even from the visual and auditory areas. Projections from somatosensory area I are required for function of somatosensory area II. However, removal of parts of somatosensory area II has no apparent effect on the response of neurons in somatosensory area I. Thus, much of what we know about somatic sensation appears to be explained by the functions of somatosensory area I.

Spatial Orientation of Signals from Different Parts of the Body in Somatosensory Area I

Somatosensory area I lies immediately behind the central fissure, located in the postcentral gyrus of the human cerebral cortex (in Brodmann areas 3, 1, and 2).

Figure 105-3 shows a cross-section through the brain at the level of the *postcentral gyrus*, demonstrating representations of the different parts of the body in separate regions of somatosensory area I. This representation is called a homunculus. Note, however, that each lateral side of the cortex receives sensory information almost exclusively from the opposite side of the body.

Some areas of the body are represented by large areas in the somatic cortex—the lips the greatest of all, followed by the face and thumb—whereas the trunk and lower part of the body are represented by relatively small areas. The sizes of these areas are directly proportional to the number of specialized sensory receptors in each respective peripheral area of the body. For instance, a great number of specialized nerve endings are found in the lips and thumb, whereas only a few are present in the skin of the body trunk.

Note also that the head is represented in the most lateral portion of somatosensory area I, and the lower part of the body is represented medially.

Layers of the Somatosensory Cortex and their Function

The cerebral cortex contains *six* layers of neurons, beginning with layer I next to the brain surface and extending progressively deeper to layer VI, shown in Figure 105-4. As would be

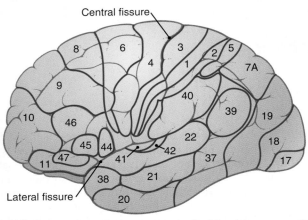

Figure 105-1 Structurally distinct areas, called *Brodmann areas*, of the human cerebral cortex. Note specifically areas *1, 2,* and *3*, which constitute *primary somatosensory area I,* and areas 5 and 7, which constitute the *somatosensory association area.*

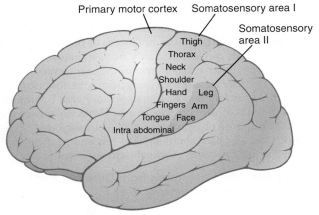

Figure 105-2 Two somatosensory cortical areas, somatosensory areas I and II.

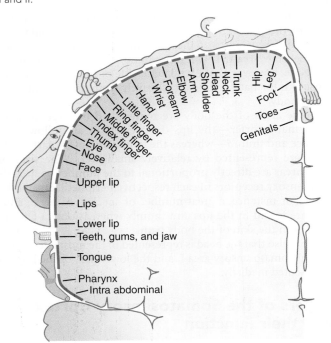

Figure 105-3 Representation of the different areas of the body in somatosensory area I of the cortex. *From Penfield, W., Rasmussen, T., 1968. Cerebral Cortex of Man: A Clinical Study of Localization of Function. Hafner, New York.*

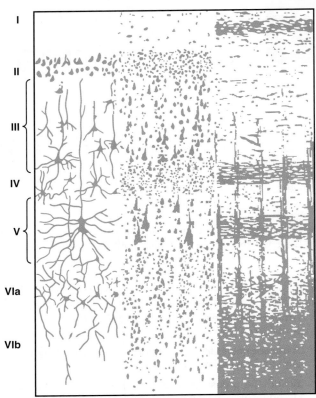

Figure 105-4 Structure of the cerebral cortex, showing (*I*) molecular layer; (*II*) external granular layer; (*III*) layer of small pyramidal cells; (*IV*) internal granular layer; (*V*) large pyramidal cell layer; and (*VI*) layer of fusiform or polymorphic cells. *From Ranson, S.W., Clark, S.L., 1959. Anatomy of the Nervous System. W.B. Saunders, Philadelphia.*

expected, the neurons in each layer perform functions different from those in other layers. Some of these functions are as follows:

1. The incoming sensory signal excites neuronal layer IV first; the signal then spreads toward the surface of the cortex and also toward deeper layers.
2. Layers I and II receive diffuse, nonspecific input signals from lower brain centers that facilitate specific regions of the cortex; this system is described in Chapter 126. This input mainly controls the overall level of excitability of the respective regions stimulated.
3. The neurons in layers II and III send axons to related portions of the cerebral cortex on the opposite side of the brain through the *corpus callosum.*
4. The neurons in layers V and VI send axons to the deeper parts of the nervous system. Those in layer V are generally larger and project to more distant areas, such as to the basal ganglia, brainstem, and spinal cord, where they control signal transmission. From layer VI, especially large numbers of axons extend to the thalamus, providing signals from the cerebral cortex that interact with and help to control the excitatory levels of incoming sensory signals entering the thalamus.

Functions of Somatosensory Area I

Widespread bilateral excision of somatosensory area I causes loss of the following types of sensory judgment:

1. The person is unable to localize discretely the different sensations in the different parts of the body. However,

he or she can localize these sensations crudely, such as to a particular hand, to a major level of the body trunk, or to one of the legs. Thus, it is clear that the brainstem, thalamus, or parts of the cerebral cortex not normally considered to be concerned with somatic sensations can perform some degree of localization.

2. The person is unable to judge critical degrees of pressure against the body.
3. The person is unable to judge the weights of objects.
4. The person is unable to judge shapes or forms of objects. This condition is called *astereognosis*.
5. The person is unable to judge texture of materials because this type of judgment depends on highly critical sensations caused by movement of the fingers over the surface to be judged.

Note that in the list nothing has been said about loss of pain and temperature sense. In the specific absence of only somatosensory area I, appreciation of these sensory modalities is still preserved in both quality and intensity. But the sensations are poorly localized, indicating that pain and temperature *localization* depend greatly on the topographical map of the body in somatosensory area I to localize the source.

Somatosensory Association Areas

Brodmann areas 5 and 7 of the cerebral cortex, located in the parietal cortex behind somatosensory area I (see Figure 105-1), play important roles in deciphering deeper meanings of the sensory information in the somatosensory areas. Therefore, these areas are called *somatosensory association areas*.

Electrical stimulation in a somatosensory association area can occasionally cause an awake person to experience a complex body sensation, sometimes even the "feeling" of an object such as a knife or a ball. Therefore, it seems clear that the somatosensory association area combines information arriving from multiple points in the primary somatosensory area to decipher its meaning. This occurrence also fits with the anatomical arrangement of the neuronal tracts that enter the somatosensory association area because it receives signals from (1) somatosensory area I, (2) the ventrobasal nuclei of the thalamus, (3) other areas of the thalamus, (4) the visual cortex, and (5) the auditory cortex.

EFFECT OF REMOVING THE SOMATOSENSORY ASSOCIATION AREA—AMORPHOSYNTHESIS

When the somatosensory association area is removed on one side of the brain, the person loses the ability to recognize complex objects and complex forms felt on the opposite side of the body. In addition, he or she loses most of the sense of form of his or her own body or body parts on the opposite side. In fact, the person is mainly oblivious to the opposite side of the body—that is, forgets that it is there. This condition is also called *neglect*. Therefore, the person also often forgets to use the other side for motor functions as well. Likewise, when feeling objects, the person tends to recognize only one side of the object and forgets that the other side even exists. This complex sensory deficit is called *amorphosynthesis*. The contralateral loss of the ability to recognize objects by touch without visual input is called astereognosis; this in turn requires a capacity for two-point discrimination, as described later.

Overall Characteristics of Signal Transmission and Analysis in the Dorsal Column–Medial Lemniscal–Cortical System

BASIC NEURONAL CIRCUIT IN THE DORSAL COLUMN–MEDIAL LEMNISCAL SYSTEM

The lower part of Figure 105-5 shows the basic organization of the neuronal circuit of the spinal cord dorsal column pathway, demonstrating that at each synaptic stage, divergence occurs. The upper curves of the figure show that the cortical neurons that discharge to the greatest extent are those in a central part of the cortical "field" for each respective receptor. Thus, a weak stimulus causes only the central-most neurons to fire. A stronger stimulus causes still more neurons to fire, but those in the center discharge at a considerably more rapid rate than do those farther away from the center.

TWO-POINT DISCRIMINATION

A method frequently used to test tactile discrimination is to determine a person's so-called "two-point" discriminatory ability. In this test, two needles are pressed lightly against the skin at the same time, and the person determines whether one point or two points of stimulus are felt or one point. On the tips of the fingers, a person can normally distinguish two separate points even when the needles are as close together as 1–2 mm.

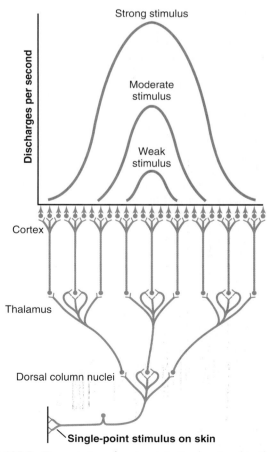

Figure 105-5 Transmission of a pinpoint stimulus signal to the cerebral cortex.

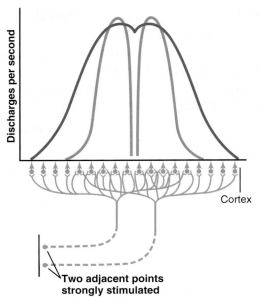

Figure 105-6 Transmission of signals to the cortex from two adjacent pinpoint stimuli. The blue curve represents the pattern of cortical stimulation without "surround" inhibition, and the two red curves represent the pattern when "surround" inhibition does occur.

However, on the person's back, the needles usually must be as far apart as 30–70 mm before two separate points can be detected. The reason for this difference is the different numbers of specialized tactile receptors in the two areas.

Figure 105-6 shows the mechanism by which the dorsal column pathway (as well as all other sensory pathways) transmits two-point discriminatory information. This figure shows two adjacent points on the skin that are strongly stimulated, as well as the areas of the somatosensory cortex (greatly enlarged) that are excited by signals from the two stimulated points. The blue curve shows the spatial pattern of cortical excitation when both skin points are stimulated simultaneously. Note that the resultant zone of excitation has two separate peaks. These two peaks, separated by a valley, allow the sensory cortex to detect the presence of two stimulatory points, rather than a single point. The capability of the sensorium to distinguish this presence of two points of stimulation is strongly influenced by another mechanism, *lateral inhibition*, as explained in the next section.

EFFECT OF LATERAL INHIBITION (ALSO CALLED *SURROUND INHIBITION*) TO INCREASE THE DEGREE OF CONTRAST IN THE PERCEIVED SPATIAL PATTERN

As pointed out in Chapters 103 and 104, virtually every sensory pathway, when excited, gives rise simultaneously to lateral *inhibitory* signals; these inhibitory signals spread to the sides of the excitatory signal and inhibit adjacent neurons. For instance, consider an excited neuron in a dorsal column nucleus. Aside from the central excitatory signal, short lateral pathways transmit inhibitory signals to the surrounding neurons–that is, these signals pass through additional interneurons that secrete an inhibitory transmitter.

The importance of *lateral inhibition* is that it blocks lateral spread of the excitatory signals and, therefore, increases the degree of contrast in the sensory pattern perceived in the cerebral cortex.

In the case of the dorsal column system, lateral inhibitory signals occur at each synaptic level—for instance, in (1) the dorsal column nuclei of the medulla, (2) the ventrobasal nuclei of the thalamus, and (3) the cortex itself. At each of these levels, the lateral inhibition helps to block lateral spread of the excitatory signal. As a result, the peaks of excitation stand out, and much of the surrounding diffuse stimulation is blocked. This effect is demonstrated by the two red curves in Figure 105-6, showing complete separation of the peaks when the intensity of lateral inhibition is great.

TRANSMISSION OF RAPIDLY CHANGING AND REPETITIVE SENSATIONS

The dorsal column system is also of particular importance in apprising the sensorium of rapidly changing peripheral conditions. Based on recorded action potentials, this system can recognize changing stimuli that occur in as little as 1/400 of a second.

VIBRATORY SENSATION

Vibratory signals are rapidly repetitive and can be detected as vibration up to 700 cycles/second. The higher-frequency vibratory signals originate from the Pacinian corpuscles in the skin and deeper tissues, but lower-frequency signals (below about 200 second^{-1}) can originate from Meissner corpuscles as well. These signals are transmitted only in the dorsal column pathway. For this reason, application of vibration (eg, from a "tuning fork") to different peripheral parts of the body is an important tool used by neurologists for testing functional integrity of the dorsal columns.

BIBLIOGRAPHY

Alonso JM, Swadlow HA: Thalamocortical specificity and the synthesis of sensory cortical receptive fields, *J. Neurophysiol.* 94:26, 2005.

Baker SN: Oscillatory interactions between sensorimotor cortex and the periphery, *Curr. Opin. Neurobiol.* 17:649, 2007.

Cohen YE, Andersen RA: A common reference frame for movement plans in the posterior parietal cortex, *Nat. Rev. Neurosci.* 3:553, 2002.

Fontanini A, Katz DB: Behavioral states, network states, and sensory response variability, *J. Neurophysiol.* 100:1160, 2008.

Fox K: Experience-dependent plasticity mechanisms for neural rehabilitation in somatosensory cortex, *Philos. Trans. R. Soc. Lond. B Biol. Sci.* 364:369, 2009.

Hsiao S: Central mechanisms of tactile shape perception, *Curr. Opin. Neurobiol.* 18:418, 2008.

Kaas JH, Qi HX, Burish MJ, et al: Cortical and subcortical plasticity in the brains of humans, primates, and rats after damage to sensory afferents in the dorsal columns of the spinal cord, *Exp. Neurol.* 209:407, 2008.

Kandel ER, Schwartz JH, Jessell TM: *Principles of Neural Science*, fourth ed., New York, 2000, McGraw-Hill.

PART II

Special Senses

ANURA KURPAD

106

Taste and Smell

The senses of taste and smell allow us to separate undesirable or even lethal foods from those that are pleasant to eat and nutritious. In additon, they elicit physiological responses that are involved in the digestion and utilization of foods. The sense of smell also allows animals to recognize the proximity of other animals or even individual animals. Finally, both senses are strongly tied to primitive emotional and behavioral functions of our nervous systems. In this chapter, we discuss how taste and smell stimuli are detected and how they are encoded in neural signals transmitted to the brain.

Sense of Taste

Taste is mainly a function of the *taste buds* in the mouth, but it is common experience that one's sense of smell also contributes strongly to taste perception. In addition, the texture of food, as detected by tactual senses of the mouth, and the presence of substances in the food that stimulate pain endings, such as pepper, greatly alter the taste experience. The importance of taste lies in the fact that it allows a person to select food in accord with desires and often in accord with the body tissues' metabolic need for specific substances.

PRIMARY SENSATIONS OF TASTE

The identities of the specific chemicals that excite different taste receptors are not all known. Even so, psychophysiological and neurophysiological studies have identified at least 13 probable chemical receptors in the taste cells, as follows: 2 sodium receptors, 2 potassium receptors, 1 chloride receptor, 1 adenosine receptor, 1 inosine receptor, 2 sweet receptors, 2 bitter receptors, 1 glutamate receptor, and 1 hydrogen ion receptor.

For practical analysis of taste, the aforementioned receptor capabilities have also been grouped into five general categories called the *primary sensations of taste*. They are *sour*, *salty*, *sweet*, *bitter*, and "*umami.*"

A person can perceive hundreds of different tastes. They are all thought to be combinations of the elementary taste sensations, just as all the colors we can see are combinations of the three primary colors, as described in Chapter 109.

Sour Taste. The sour taste is caused by acids, that is, by the hydrogen ion concentration, and the intensity of this taste sensation is approximately proportional to the *logarithm of the hydrogen ion concentration*(i.e., the more acidic the food, the stronger the sour sensation becomes).

Salty Taste. The salty taste is elicited by ionized salts, mainly by the sodium ion concentration. The quality of the taste varies somewhat from one salt to another because some salts elicit other taste sensations in addition to saltiness. The cations of the salts, especially sodium cations, are mainly responsible for the salty taste, but the anions also contribute to a lesser extent.

Sweet Taste. The sweet taste is not caused by any single class of chemicals. Some of the types of chemicals that cause this taste include sugars, glycols, alcohols, aldehydes, ketones, amides, esters, some amino acids, some small proteins, sulfonic acids, halogenated acids, and inorganic salts of lead and beryllium. Note specifically that most of the substances that cause a sweet taste are organic chemicals. It is especially interesting that slight changes in the chemical structure, such as addition of a simple radical, can often change the substance from sweet to bitter.

Bitter Taste. The bitter taste, like the sweet taste, is not caused by any single type of chemical agent. Here again, the substances that give the bitter taste are almost entirely organic substances. Two particular classes of substances are especially likely to cause bitter taste sensations: (1) long-chain organic substances that contain nitrogen and (2) alkaloids. The alkaloids include many of the drugs used in medicines, such as quinine, caffeine, strychnine, and nicotine.

Some substances that initially taste sweet have a bitter aftertaste. This characteristic is true of saccharin, which makes this substance objectionable to some people.

The bitter taste, when it occurs in high intensity, usually causes the person or animal to reject the food. This reaction is undoubtedly an important function of the bitter taste sensation because many deadly toxins found in poisonous plants are alkaloids, and virtually all of these alkaloids cause an intensely bitter taste, usually followed by rejection of the food.

Umami Taste. Umami is a Japanese word (meaning "delicious") designates a pleasant taste sensation that is qualitatively different from sour, salty, sweet, or bitter. Umami is the dominant taste of food containing *L-glutamate*, such as meat extracts and aging cheese, and some physiologists consider it to be a separate, fifth category of primary taste stimuli.

A taste receptor for L-glutamate may be related to one of the glutamate receptors that are also expressed in neuronal synapses of the brain. However, the precise molecular mechanisms responsible for umami taste are still unclear.

Threshold for Taste

The threshold for stimulation of the sour taste by hydrochloric acid averages 0.0009 N; for stimulation of the salty taste by sodium chloride, 0.01 M; for the sweet taste by sucrose, 0.01 M; and for the bitter taste by quinine, 0.000008 M. Note especially how much more sensitive the bitter taste sense is than all the others, which would be expected, because this sensation provides an important protective function against many dangerous toxins in food.

Table 106-1 gives the relative taste indices (the reciprocals of the taste thresholds) of different substances. In this table, the intensities of four of the primary sensations of taste are referred, respectively, to the intensities of the taste of hydrochloric acid, quinine, sucrose, and sodium chloride, each of which is arbitrarily chosen to have a taste index of 1.

Taste Blindness. Some people are taste blind for certain substances, especially for different types of thiourea compounds. A substance used frequently by psychologists for demonstrating taste blindness is *phenylthiocarbamide*, for which about 15–30% of all people exhibit taste blindness; the exact percentage depends on the method of testing and the concentration of the substance.

TASTE BUD AND ITS FUNCTION

Figure 106-1 shows a taste bud, which has a diameter of about 1/30 mm and a length of about 1/16 mm. The taste bud is composed of about 50 modified epithelial cells, some of which are supporting cells called *sustentacular cells* and others of which are *taste cells*. The taste cells are continually being replaced by mitotic division of surrounding epithelial cells, so some taste cells are young cells. Others are mature cells that lie toward the

TABLE 106-1	Relative Taste Indices of Different Substances						
Sour Substances	**Index**	**Bitter Substances**	**Index**	**Sweet Substances**	**Index**	**Salty Substances**	**Index**
Hydrochloric acid	1	Quinine	1	Sucrose	1	NaCl	1
Formic acid	1.1	Brucine	11	1-Propoxy-2-amino-4-nitrobenzene	5000	NaF	2
Chloracetic acid	0.9	Strychnine	3.1	Saccharin	675	CaCl$_2$	1
Acetylacetic acid	0.85	Nicotine	1.3	Chloroform	40	NaBr	0.4
Lactic acid	0.85	Phenylthiourea	0.9	Fructose	1.7	NaI	0.35
Tartaric acid	0.7	Caffeine	0.4	Alanine	1.3	LiCl	0.4
Malic acid	0.6	Veratrine	0.2	Glucose	0.8	NH$_4$Cl	2.5
Potassium H tartrate	0.58	Pilocarpine	0.16	Maltose	0.45	KCl	0.6
Acetic acid	0.55	Atropine	0.13	Galactose	0.32		
Citric acid	0.46	Cocaine	0.02	Lactose	0.3		
Carbonic acid	0.06	Morphine	0.02				

NaCl, sodium chloride; NaF, sodium fluoride; CaCl$_2$, calcium chloride; NaBr, sodium bromide; NaI, sodium iodide; LiCl, lithium chloride; NH$_4$Cl, ammonium chloride; KCl, potassium chloride.
Data from Pfaffman, C., 1959. Handbook of Physiology, vol. 1. Williams & Wilkins, Baltimore, p. 507.

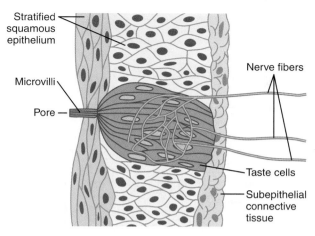

Figure 106-1 Taste bud.

center of the bud; these soon break up and dissolve. The life span of each taste cell is about 10 days in lower mammals but is unknown for humans.

The outer tips of the taste cells are arranged around a minute *taste pore*, shown in Figure 106-1. From the tip of each taste cell several *microvilli* or *taste hairs* protrude outward into the taste pore to approach the cavity of the mouth. These microvilli provide the receptor surface for taste.

Interwoven around the bodies of the taste cells is a branching terminal network of *taste nerve fibers* that are stimulated by the taste receptor cells. Some of these fibers invaginate into folds of the taste cell membranes. Many vesicles form beneath the cell membrane near the fibers. It is believed that these vesicles contain a neurotransmitter substance that is released through the cell membrane to excite the nerve fiber endings in response to taste stimulation.

Location of the Taste Buds. The taste buds are found on three types of papillae of the tongue, as follows: (1) a large number of taste buds are on the walls of the troughs that surround the circumvallate papillae, which form a V line on the surface of the posterior tongue; (2) moderate numbers of taste buds are on the fungiform papillae over the flat anterior surface of the tongue; and (3) moderate numbers are on the foliate papillae located in the folds along the lateral surfaces of the tongue. Additional taste buds are located on the palate, and a few are found on the tonsillar pillars, on the epiglottis, and even in the proximal esophagus. Adults have 3000–10,000 taste buds, and children have a few more. Beyond the age of 45 years, many taste buds degenerate, causing taste sensitivity to decrease in old age.

Specificity of Taste Buds for a Primary Taste Stimulus. Microelectrode studies from single taste buds show that each taste bud usually *responds mostly to one of the five primary taste stimuli when the taste substance is in low concentration.* However at high concentration, most buds can be excited by two or more of the primary taste stimuli, as well as by a few other taste stimuli that do not fit into the "primary" categories.

Mechanism of Stimulation of Taste Buds

Receptor Potential. The membrane of the taste cell, like that of most other sensory receptor cells, is negatively charged on the inside with respect to the outside. Application of a taste substance to the taste hairs causes partial loss of this negative potential—that is, the taste cell becomes *depolarized*. In most

instances, the decrease in potential, within a wide range, is approximately proportional to the logarithm of concentration of the stimulating substance. This *change in electrical potential* in the taste cell is called the *receptor potential* for taste.

The mechanism by which most stimulating substances react with the taste villi to initiate the receptor potential is by binding of the taste chemical to a protein receptor molecule that lies on the outer surface of the taste receptor cell near to or protruding through a villus membrane. This action, in turn, opens ion channels, which allows positively charged sodium ions or hydrogen ions to enter and depolarize the normal negativity of the cell. Then the taste chemical is gradually washed away from the taste villus by the saliva, which removes the stimulus.

The type of receptor protein in each taste villus determines the type of taste that will be perceived. For sodium ions and hydrogen ions, which elicit salty and sour taste sensations, respectively, the receptor proteins open specific ion channels in the apical membranes of the taste cells, thereby activating the receptors. However, for the sweet and bitter taste sensations, the portions of the receptor protein molecules that protrude through the apical membranes activate *second-messenger transmitter substances* inside the taste cells, and these second messengers cause intracellular chemical changes that elicit the taste signals.

Generation of Nerve Impulses by the Taste Bud. On first application of the taste stimulus, the rate of discharge of the nerve fibers from taste buds rises to a peak in a small fraction of a second but then adapts within the next few seconds back to a lower, steady level as long as the taste stimulus remains. Thus, a strong immediate signal is transmitted by the taste nerve, and a weaker continuous signal is transmitted as long as the taste bud is exposed to the taste stimulus.

TRANSMISSION OF TASTE SIGNALS INTO THE CENTRAL NERVOUS SYSTEM

Figure 106-2 shows the neuronal pathways for transmission of taste signals from the tongue and pharyngeal region into the central nervous system. Taste impulses from the anterior two-thirds of the tongue pass first into the *lingual nerve*, then through the *chorda tympani* into the *facial nerve*, and finally into the *tractus solitarius* in the brainstem. Taste sensations from the circumvallate papillae on the back of the tongue and from other posterior regions of the mouth and throat are transmitted through the *glossopharyngeal nerve* also into the *tractus solitarius*, but at a slightly more posterior level. Finally, a few taste signals are transmitted into the *tractus solitarius* from the base of the tongue and other parts of the pharyngeal region by way of the *vagus nerve*.

All taste fibers synapse in the posterior brainstem in the *nuclei of the tractus solitarius*. These nuclei send second-order neurons to a small area of the *ventral posterior medial nucleus of the thalamus*, located slightly medial to the thalamic terminations of the facial regions of the dorsal column–medial lemniscal system. From the thalamus, third-order neurons are transmitted to the *lower tip of the postcentral gyrus in the parietal cerebral cortex*, where it curls *deep into the Sylvian fissure*, and into the adjacent *opercular insular area*. This area lies slightly lateral, ventral, and rostral to the area for tongue tactile signals in cerebral somatic area I. From this description of the taste pathways, it is evident that they closely parallel the somatosensory pathways from the tongue.

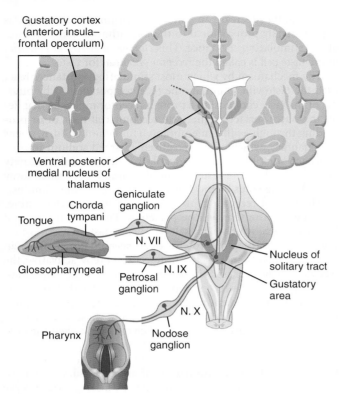

Figure 106-2 Transmission of taste signals into the central nervous system.

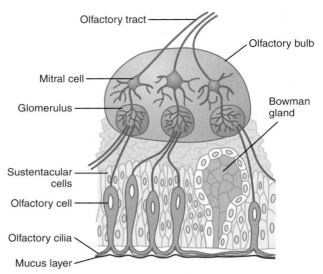

Figure 106-3 Organization of the olfactory membrane and olfactory bulb, and connections to the olfactory tract.

Taste Reflexes Are Integrated in the Brainstem. From the tractus solitarius, many taste signals are transmitted within the brainstem itself directly into the *superior* and *inferior salivatory nuclei*, and these areas transmit signals to the submandibular, sublingual, and parotid glands to help control the secretion of saliva during the ingestion and digestion of food.

Rapid Adaptation of Taste. Everyone is familiar with the fact that taste sensations adapt rapidly, often almost completely within a minute or so of continuous stimulation. Yet from electrophysiological studies of taste nerve fibers, it is clear that adaptation of the taste buds themselves usually accounts for no more than about half of this rapid taste adaptation. Therefore, the final extreme degree of adaptation that occurs in the sensation of taste almost certainly occurs in the central nervous system, mechanisms are not known. At any rate, it is a mechanism different from that of many other sensory systems, which adapts almost entirely at the receptors.

Disorders of Taste. Disorders of taste are either those that involve a loss of the ability to taste or those linked to a distorted sensation of taste. Loss of the ability to taste is called ageusia, while a reduced ability to taste is called hypogeusia. A distorted sense of taste is called dysgeusia. These conditions can occur due to advanced age or medications, and constitute an important threat to the quality of life.

Sense of Smell

Smell is the least understood of our senses partly because the sense of smell is a subjective phenomenon that cannot be studied with ease in lower animals. Another complicating problem is that the sense of smell is poorly developed in human beings compared with the sense of smell in many lower animals.

OLFACTORY MEMBRANE

The olfactory membrane, the histology of which is shown in Figure 106-3, lies in the superior part of each nostril. Medially, the olfactory membrane folds downward along the surface of the superior septum; laterally, it folds over the superior turbinate and even over a small portion of the upper surface of the middle turbinate. In each nostril, the olfactory membrane has a surface area of about 2.4 cm^2.

Olfactory Cells Are the Receptor Cells for Smell Sensation. The *olfactory cells* (see Figure 106-3), are actually bipolar nerve cells derived originally from the central nervous system. There are about 100 million of these cells in the olfactory epithelium interspersed among *sustentacular cells*, as shown in Figure 106-3. The mucosal end of the olfactory cell forms a knob from which 4–25 *olfactory hairs* (also called *olfactory cilia*), measuring 0.3 μm in diameter and up to 200 μm in length, project into the mucus that coats the inner surface of the nasal cavity. These projecting olfactory cilia form a dense mat in the mucus, and it is these cilia that react to odors in the air and stimulate the olfactory cells, as discussed later. Spaced among the olfactory cells in the olfactory membrane are many small *Bowman glands* that secrete mucus onto the surface of the olfactory membrane.

STIMULATION OF THE OLFACTORY CELLS

Mechanism of Excitation of the Olfactory Cells. The portion of each olfactory cell that responds to the olfactory chemical stimuli is the *olfactory cilia*. The odorant substance, upon coming in contact with the olfactory membrane surface, first diffuses into the mucus that covers the ciliaand then it binds with *receptor proteins* in the membrane of each cilium (Figure 106-4). Each receptor protein is actually a long molecule that threads its way through the membrane about seven times, folding inward and outward. The odorant binds with the portion of the receptor protein that folds to the outside. The inside of the folding protein, is coupled to a *G-protein*, itself a combination of three subunits. Upon excitation of the receptor protein, an *alpha* subunit breaks away from the G-protein and activates *adenylyl cyclase*, which is attached to the inside of the ciliary membrane near the receptor cell body. The activated cyclase, in turn, converts many

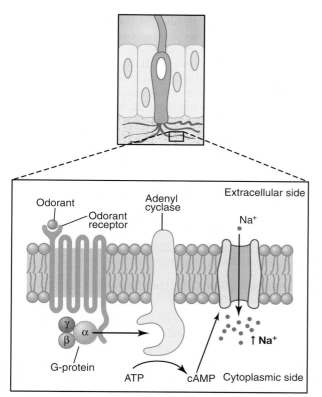

Figure 106-4 Summary of olfactory signal transduction. Binding of the odorant to a G-coupled protein receptor causes activation of adenylate cyclase, which converts adenosine triphosphate (ATP) to cyclic adenosine monophosphate (cAMP). The cAMP activates a gated sodium channel that increases sodium influx and depolarizes the cell, exciting the olfactory neuron and transmitting action potentials to the central nervous system.

molecules of intracellular *adenosine triphosphate* into *cyclic adenosine monophosphate* (cAMP). Finally, this cAMP activates another nearby membrane protein, a *gated sodium ion channel*, which opens its "gate" and allows large numbers of sodium ions to pour through the membrane into the receptor cell cytoplasm. The sodium ions increase the electrical potential in the positive direction inside the cell membrane, thus exciting the olfactory neuron and transmitting action potentials into the central nervous system by way of the *olfactory nerve*.

The importance of this mechanism for activating olfactory nerves is that it greatly multiplies the excitatory effect of even the weakest odorant. To summarize: (1) activation of the receptor protein by the odorant substance activates the G-protein complex which, in turn, (2) activates multiple molecules of adenylyl cyclase inside the olfactory cell membrane,which (3) causes the formation of many times more molecules of cAMP and finally (4) the cAMP opens still many times more sodium ion channels. Therefore, even a minute concentration of a specific odorant initiates a cascading effect that opens extremely large numbers of sodium channels. This process accounts for the exquisite sensitivity of the olfactory neurons to even the slightest amount of odorant.

In addition to the basic chemical mechanism by which the olfactory cells are stimulated, several physical factors affect the degree of stimulation. First, only volatile substances that can be sniffed into the nostrils can be smelled. Second, the stimulating substance must be at least slightly water soluble so that it can pass through the mucus to reach the olfactory cilia. Third,

it is helpful for the substance to be at least slightly lipid soluble, presumably because lipid constituents of the cilium are a weak barrier to nonlipid-soluble odorants.

Membrane Potentials and Action Potentials in Olfactory Cells. The membrane potential inside unstimulated olfactory cells, as measured by microelectrodes, averages about -55 mV. At this potential, most of the cells generate continuous action potentials at a very slow rate, varying from once every 20 seconds up to two or three per second.

Most odorants cause *depolarization* of the olfactory cell membrane, decreasing the negative potential in the cell from the normal level of -55 to -30 mV or less—that is, changing the voltage in the positive direction. Along with this, the number of action potentials increases to 20–30 second^{-1}, which is a high rate for the minute olfactory nerve fibers.

Over a wide range, the rate of olfactory nerve impulses changes approximately in proportion to the logarithm of the stimulus strength, which demonstrates that the olfactory receptors obey principles of transduction similar to those of other sensory receptors.

Rapid Adaptation of Olfactory Sensations. The olfactory receptors adapt about 50% in the first second or so after stimulation. Thereafter, they adapt very little and very slowly. Yet we all know from our own experience that smell sensations adapt almost to extinction within a minute or so after entering a strongly odorous atmosphere. Because this psychological adaptation is far greater than the degree of adaptation of the receptors, it is almost certain that most of the additional adaptation occurs within the central nervous systemwhich seems to be true for the adaptation of taste sensations as well.

The following neuronal mechanism for the adaptation ispostulated: Large numbers of centrifugal nerve fibers pass from the olfactory regions of the brain backward along the olfactory tract and terminate on special inhibitory cells in the olfactory bulb, the *granule cells*. It has been postulated that after the onset of an olfactory stimulus, the central nervous system quickly develops strong feedback inhibition to suppress relay of the smell signals through the olfactory bulb.

Search for the Primary Sensations of Smell

In the past, most physiologists were convinced that the many smell sensations are subserved by a few rather discrete primary sensations, in the same way that vision and taste are subserved by a few select primary sensations. On the basis of psychological studies, one attempt to classify these sensations is the following:

1. camphoraceous
2. musky
3. floral
4. pepperminty
5. ethereal
6. pungent
7. putrid

It is certain that this list does not represent the true primary sensations of smell. In recent years, multiple clues, including specific studies of the genes that encode for the receptor proteins, suggest the existence of at least 100 primary sensations of smell—a marked contrast to only 3 primary sensations of color detected by the eyes and only 5 primary sensations of taste detected by the tongue. Some studies suggest that there may be as many as 1000 different types of odorant receptors. Further support for the many primary sensations of smell is that people have been found who have *odor blindness* for single substances; such discrete odor blindness has been identified for more than

50 different substances. It is presumed that odor blindness for each substance represents lack of the appropriate receptor protein in olfactory cells for that particular substance.

"Affective Nature of Smell". Smell, even more so than taste, has the affective quality of either *pleasantness* or *unpleasantness*and thus, smell is probably even more important than taste for the selection of food. Indeed, a person who has previously eaten food that disagreed with him or her is often nauseated by the smell of that same food on a second occasion. Conversely, perfume of the right quality can be a powerful stimulant of human emotions. In addition, in some animals odors are the primary excitant of sexual drive.

Threshold for Smell. One of the principal characteristics of smell is the minute quantity of stimulating agent in the air that can elicit a smell sensation. For instance, the substance *methylmercaptan* can be smelled when only one 25 trillionth of a gram is present in each milliliter of air. Because of this very low threshold, this substance is mixed with natural gas to give the gas an odor that can be detected when even small amounts of gas leak from a pipeline.

Transmission of Smell Signals into the Central Nervous System. The olfactory portions of the brain were among the first brain structures developed in primitive animals, and much of the remainder of the brain developed around these olfactory beginnings. In fact, part of the brain that originally subserved olfaction later evolved into the basal brain structures that control emotions and other aspects of human behavior; we call this system the *limbic system*, as discussed in Chapter 124.

Transmission of Olfactory Signals into the Olfactory Bulb. The *olfactory bulb* is shown in Figure 106-5. The olfactory nerve fibers leading backward from the bulb are called *cranial nerve I*, or the *olfactory tract*. In reality, both the tract and the bulb are an anterior outgrowth of brain tissue from the base of the brain; the bulbous enlargement at its end, the *olfactory bulb*, lies over the *cribriform plate*, separating the brain cavity from the upper reaches of the nasal cavity. The cribriform plate has multiple small perforations through which an equal number of small nerves pass upward from the olfactory membrane in

the nasal cavity to enter the olfactory bulb in the cranial cavity. Figure 106-3 demonstrates the close relation between the *olfactory cells* in the olfactory membrane and the olfactory bulb, showing short axons from the olfactory cells terminating in multiple globular structures within the olfactory bulb called *glomeruli*. Each bulb has several thousand such glomeruli, each of which is the terminus for about 25,000 axons from olfactory cells. Each glomerulus also is the terminus for dendrites from about 25 large *mitral cells* and about 60 smaller *tufted cells*, the cell bodies of which lie in the olfactory bulb superior to the glomeruli. These dendrites receive synapses from the olfactory cell neurons, and the mitral and tufted cells send axons through the olfactory tract to transmit olfactory signals to higher levels in the central nervous system.

Some research has suggested that different glomeruli respond to different odors. It is possible that specific glomeruli are the real clue to the analysis of different odor signals transmitted into the central nervous system.

Primitive and Newer Olfactory Pathways into the Central Nervous System

The olfactory tract enters the brain at the anterior junction between the mesencephalon and cerebrum; there, the tract divides into two pathways, as shown in Figure 106-5, one passing medially into the *medial olfactory area* of the brainstem and the other passing laterally into the *lateral olfactory area*. The medial olfactory area represents a very primitive olfactory system, whereas the lateral olfactory area is the input to (1) a less old olfactory system and (2) a newer system.

The Primitive Olfactory System—The Medial Olfactory Area. The medial olfactory area consists of a group of nuclei located in the midbasal portions of the brain immediately anterior to the hypothalamus. Most conspicuous are the *septal nuclei*, which are midline nuclei that feed into the hypothalamus and other primitive portions of the brain's limbic system. This is the brain area most concerned with basic behavior (described in Chapter 124).

The importance of this medial olfactory area is best understood by considering what happens in animals when the lateral olfactory areas on both sides of the brain are removed and only the medial system remains. The removal of these areas hardly affects the more primitive responses to olfaction, such as licking the lips, salivation, and other feeding responses caused by the smell of food or by basic emotional drives associated with smell. Conversely, removal of the lateral areas abolishes the more complicated olfactory conditioned reflexes.

The Less Old Olfactory System—The Lateral Olfactory Area. The lateral olfactory area is composed mainly of the *prepyriform* and *pyriform cortex* plus the *cortical portion of the amygdaloid nuclei*. From these areas, signal pathways pass into almost all portions of the limbic system, especially into less primitive portions such as the hippocampus, which seem to be most important for learning to like or dislike certain foods depending on one's experiences with them. For instance, it is believed that this lateral olfactory area and its many connections with the limbic behavioral system cause a person to develop an absolute aversion to foods that have caused nausea and vomiting.

An important feature of the lateral olfactory area is that many signal pathways from this area also feed directly into an *older part of the cerebral cortex* called the *paleocortex* in the *anteromedial portion of the temporal lobe*. This area is the only area

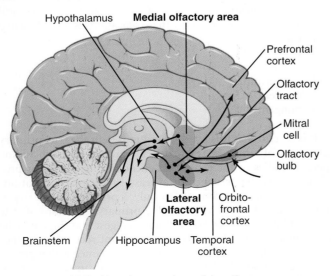

Figure 106-5 Neural connections of the olfactory system.

Labels in figure: Hypothalamus · Medial olfactory area · Prefrontal cortex · Olfactory tract · Mitral cell · Olfactory bulb · Lateral olfactory area · Orbito-frontal cortex · Brainstem · Hippocampus · Temporal cortex

of the entire cerebral cortex where sensory signals pass directly to the cortex without passing first through the thalamus.

The Newer Pathway. A newer olfactory pathway that passes through the thalamus, passing to the dorsomedial thalamic nucleus, and then passing to the lateroposterior quadrant of the orbitofrontal cortex has been found. On the basis of studies in monkeys, this newer system probably helps in the conscious analysis of odor.

Summary. Thus, there appears to be a *primitive* olfactory system that subserves the basic olfactory reflexes, a *less old* system that provides automatic but partially learned control of food intake and aversion to toxic and unhealthy foods, and a *newer* system that is comparable to most of the other cortical sensory systems and is used for conscious perception and analysis of olfaction.

DISORDERS OF SMELL

Disorders of smell, like those of taste, are either those that involve a loss of ability to smell or those linked to a distorted sensation of smell. Loss of the ability to smell is called anosmia, while a reduced ability to smell is called hyposmia. A distorted sense of smell is called dysosmia or parosmia, particularly when an unpleasant perception of an odor is present. Disorders of smell and taste go hand in hand in the perception of a patient; this is not surprising, since both taste and smell are involved in the perception of flavor.

BIBLIOGRAPHY

Auffarth B: Understanding smell—the olfactory stimulus problem, *Neurosci. Biobehav. Rev.* 37:1667, 2013.

Bermudez-Rattoni F: Molecular mechanisms of taste-recognition memory, *Nat. Rev. Neurosci.* 5:209, 2004.

Chandrashekar J, Hoon MA, Ryba NJ, et al: The receptors and cells for mammalian taste, *Nature* 444:288, 2006.

Giessel AJ, Datta SR: Olfactory maps, circuits and computations, *Curr. Opin. Neurobiol.* 24:120, 2014.

Keller A, Vosshall LB: Better smelling through genetics: mammalian odor perception, *Curr. Opin. Neurobiol.* 18:364, 2008.

Lowe G: Electrical signaling in the olfactory bulb, *Curr. Opin. Neurobiol.* 13:476, 2003.

Mandairon N, Linster C: Odor perception and olfactory bulb plasticity in adult mammals, *J. Neurophysiol.* 101:2204, 2009.

Margolskee RF: Molecular mechanisms of bitter and sweet taste transduction, *J. Biol. Chem.* 277:1, 2002.

Matthews HR, Reisert J: Calcium, the two-faced messenger of olfactory transduction and adaptation, *Curr. Opin. Neurobiol.* 13:469, 2003.

Menini A, Lagostena L, Boccaccio A: Olfaction: from odorant molecules to the olfactory cortex, *News Physiol. Sci.* 19:101, 2004.

Mori K, Takahashi YK, Igarashi KM, et al: Maps of odorant molecular features in the mammalian olfactory bulb, *Physiol. Rev.* 86:409, 2006.

Roper SD: Signal transduction and information processing in mammalian taste buds, *Pflugers Arch.* 454:759, 2007.

Simon SA, de Araujo IE, Gutierrez R, et al: The neural mechanisms of gustation: a distributed processing code, *Nat. Rev. Neurosci.* 7:890, 2006.

Smith DV, Margolskee RF: Making sense of taste, *Sci. Am.* 284:32, 2001.

Hearing

This chapter describes the mechanisms by which the ear receives sound waves, discriminates their frequencies, and transmits auditory information into the central nervous system, where its meaning is deciphered. Sound is transmitted to the middle ear through the external ear. There is no modification or distortion of the sound waves as they pass through the external ear (unless there is some physical obstruction such as wax), and it is at the middle ear where sound is amplified.

Middle Ear

CONDUCTION OF SOUND FROM THE TYMPANIC MEMBRANE TO THE COCHLEA

Figure 107-1 shows the *tympanic membrane* (commonly called the *eardrum*) and the *ossicles*, which conduct sound from the tympanic membrane through the middle ear to the *cochlea* (the inner ear). Attached to the tympanic membrane is the *handle* of the *malleus*. The malleus is bound to the *incus* by minute ligaments, so whenever the malleus moves, the incus moves with it. The opposite end of the incus articulates with the stem of the *stapes*, and the *faceplate* of the stapes lies against the *membranous labyrinth* of the cochlea in the opening of the *oval window*.

The tip end of the handle of the malleus is attached to the center of the tympanic membrane, and this point of attachment is constantly pulled by the *tensor tympani muscle*, which keeps the tympanic membrane tensed. This tension allows sound vibrations on *any* portion of the tympanic membrane to be transmitted to the ossicles, which would not be true if the membrane were lax.

The ossicles of the middle ear are suspended by ligaments in such a way that the combined malleus and incus act as a single lever, having its fulcrum approximately at the border of the tympanic membrane.

The articulation of the incus with the stapes causes the stapes to push forward on the oval window and on the cochlear fluid on the other side of the window every time the tympanic membrane moves inward, and to pull backward on the fluid every time the malleus moves outward.

The middle ear has several functions that are listed in Box 107-1.

"Impedance Matching" by the Ossicular System. The amplitude of movement of the stapes faceplate with each sound vibration is only three-fourths as much as the amplitude of the handle of the malleus. Therefore, the ossicular lever system does not increase the movement distance of the stapes, as is commonly believed. Instead, the system actually reduces the distance but increases the *force* of movement about 1.3 times. In addition, the surface area of the tympanic membrane is about 55 mm^2, whereas the surface area of the stapes averages 3.2 mm^2. This 17-fold difference times the 1.3-fold ratio of the lever system causes about 22 times as much *total force* to be exerted on the fluid of the cochlea as is exerted by the sound waves against the tympanic membrane. Because fluid has far greater inertia than air does, increased amounts of force are necessary to cause vibration in the fluid. Therefore, the tympanic membrane and ossicular system provide *impedance matching* between the sound waves in air and the sound vibrations in the fluid of the cochlea. Indeed, the impedance matching is about 50–75% of perfect for sound frequencies between 300 and 3000 cycles/second, which allows utilization of most of the energy in the incoming sound waves.

In the absence of the ossicular system and tympanic membrane, sound waves can still travel directly through the air of the middle ear and enter the cochlea at the oval window. However, the sensitivity for hearing is then 15–20 dB less than for ossicular transmission—equivalent to a decrease from a medium to a barely perceptible voice level.

Attenuation of Sound by Contraction of the Tensor Tympani and Stapedius Muscles. When loud sounds are transmitted through the ossicular system and from there into the central nervous system, a reflex occurs after a latent period of only 40–80 milliseconds to cause contraction of the *stapedius muscle* and, to a lesser extent, the *tensor tympani muscle*. The tensor tympani muscle pulls the handle of the malleus inward while the stapedius muscle pulls the stapes outward. These two forces oppose each other and thereby cause the entire ossicular system to develop increased rigidity, thus greatly reducing the ossicular conduction of low-frequency sound, mainly frequencies below 1000 cycles/second.

This *attenuation reflex* can reduce the intensity of lower-frequency sound transmission by 30–40 dB, which is about the same difference as that between a loud voice and a whisper. The function of this mechanism is believed to be twofold:

1. to *protect* the cochlea from damaging vibrations caused by excessively loud sound;

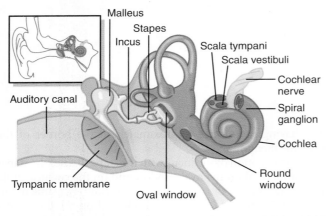

Figure 107-1 Tympanic membrane, ossicular system of the middle ear, and inner ear.

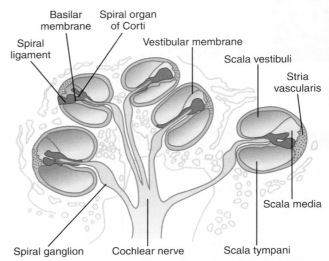

Figure 107-2 Cochlea. *Modified from Drake RL, Vogl AW, Mitchell AWM: Gray's Anatomy for Students, ed 2, Philadelphia, 2010, Elsevier.*

BOX 107-1 FUNCTIONS OF MIDDLE EAR

1. Conduction of sound from air in the external ear to fluid in the inner ear
2. Impedance matching to amplify sound
3. Protection from loud sounds—attenuation reflex
4. Efficient transmission—critical damping of tympanic membrane to mask low-frequency sounds and effectively transmit sounds in the vocal frequency range

---

2. to *mask* low-frequency sounds in loud environments. Masking usually removes a major share of the background noise and allows a person to concentrate on sounds above 1000 cycles/second, where most of the pertinent information in voice communication is transmitted.

Another function of the tensor tympani and stapedius muscles is to decrease a person's hearing sensitivity to his or her own speech. This effect is activated by collateral nerve signals transmitted to these muscles at the same time that the brain activates the voice mechanism.

TRANSMISSION OF SOUND THROUGH BONE

Because the inner ear, the *cochlea*, is embedded in a bony cavity in the temporal bone, called the *bony labyrinth*, vibrations of the entire skull can cause fluid vibrations in the cochlea itself. Therefore, under appropriate conditions, a tuning fork or an electronic vibrator placed on any bony protuberance of the skull, but especially on the mastoid process near the ear, causes the person to hear the sound. However, the energy available even in loud sound in the air is not sufficient to cause hearing via bone conduction unless a special electromechanical sound-amplifying device is applied to the bone.

Cochlea

FUNCTIONAL ANATOMY OF THE COCHLEA

The cochlea is a system of coiled tubes, shown in Figure 107-1 and in cross-section in Figures 107-2 and 107-3. It consists of three tubes coiled side by side: (1) the *scala vestibuli*, (2) the *scala media*, and (3) the *scala tympani*. The scala vestibuli and scala media are separated from each other by *Reissner membrane* (also called the *vestibular membrane*), shown in Figure 107-3; the scala tympani and scala media are separated from each other by the

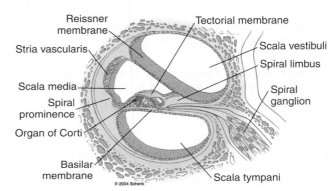

Figure 107-3 Section through one of the turns of the cochlea.

basilar membrane. On the surface of the basilar membrane lies the *organ of Corti*, which contains a series of electromechanically sensitive cells, the *hair cells*. They are the receptive end organs that generate nerve impulses in response to sound vibrations.

Figure 107-4 diagrams the functional parts of the uncoiled cochlea for conduction of sound vibrations. First, note that Reissner membrane is missing from this figure. This membrane is so thin and so easily moved that it does not obstruct the passage of sound vibrations from the scala vestibuli into the scala media. Therefore, as far as fluid conduction of sound is concerned, the scala vestibuli and scala media are considered to be a single chamber. (The importance of Reissner membrane is to maintain a special kind of fluid in the scala media that is required for normal function of the sound-receptive hair cells, as discussed later in the chapter.)

Sound vibrations enter the scala vestibuli from the faceplate of the stapes at the oval window. The faceplate covers this window and is connected with the window's edges by a loose annular ligament so that it can move inward and outward with the sound vibrations. Inward movement causes the fluid to move forward in the scala vestibuli and scala media, and outward movement causes the fluid to move backward.

Basilar Membrane and Resonance in the Cochlea. The basilar membrane is a fibrous membrane that separates the scala media from the scala tympani. It contains 20,000–30,000 *basilar fibers* that project from the bony center of the cochlea, the

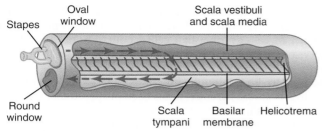

Figure 107-4 Movement of fluid in the cochlea after forward thrust of the stapes.

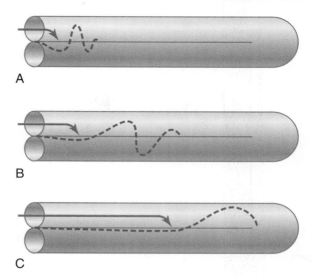

Figure 107-5 "Traveling waves" along the basilar membrane for (A) high-frequency, (B) medium-frequency, and (C) low-frequency sounds.

modiolus, toward the outer wall. These fibers are stiff, elastic, reed-like structures that are fixed at their basal ends in the central bony structure of the cochlea (the modiolus) but are not fixed at their distal ends, except that the distal ends are embedded in the loose basilar membrane. Because the fibers are stiff and free at one end, they can vibrate like the reeds of a harmonica.

The *lengths* of the basilar fibers *increase* progressively beginning at the oval window and going from the base of the cochlea to the apex, increasing from a length of about 0.04 mm near the oval and round windows to 0.5 mm at the tip of the cochlea (the "helicotrema"), a 12-fold increase in length.

The *diameters* of the fibers, however, *decrease* from the oval window to the helicotrema, so their overall stiffness decreases more than 100-fold. As a result, the stiff, short fibers near the oval window of the cochlea vibrate best at a very high frequency, whereas the long, limber fibers near the tip of the cochlea vibrate best at a low frequency.

Thus, *high-frequency resonance* of the basilar membrane occurs near the base, where the sound waves enter the cochlea through the oval window. But *low-frequency resonance* occurs near the helicotrema, mainly because of the less stiff fibers but also because of increased "loading" with extra masses of fluid that must vibrate along the cochlear tubules.

TRANSMISSION OF SOUND WAVES IN THE COCHLEA—"TRAVELING WAVE"

When the foot of the stapes moves inward against the *oval* window, the *round* window must bulge outward because the cochlea is bounded on all sides by bony walls. The initial effect of a sound wave entering at the oval window is to cause the basilar membrane at the base of the cochlea to bend in the direction of the round window. However, the elastic tension that is built up in the basilar fibers as they bend toward the round window initiates a fluid wave that "travels" along the basilar membrane toward the helicotrema, as shown in Figure 107-5. Figure 107-5A shows movement of a high-frequency wave down the basilar membrane; Figure 107-5B, shows a medium-frequency wave; and Figure 107-5C, shows a very low-frequency wave. Movement of the wave along the basilar membrane is comparable to the movement of a pressure wave along the arterial walls, which is discussed in Chapter 42; it is also comparable to a wave that travels along the surface of a pond.

Pattern of Vibration of the Basilar Membrane for Different Sound Frequencies. Note in Figure 107-5 the different patterns of transmission for sound waves of different frequencies. Each wave is relatively weak at the outset but becomes strong when it reaches the portion of the basilar membrane that has a natural resonant frequency equal to the respective sound frequency.

At this point, the basilar membrane can vibrate back and forth with such ease that the energy in the wave is dissipated. Consequently, the wave dies at this point and fails to travel the remaining distance along the basilar membrane. Thus, a high-frequency sound wave travels only a short distance along the basilar membrane before it reaches its resonant point and dies, a medium-frequency sound wave travels about halfway and then dies, and a very low-frequency sound wave travels the entire distance along the membrane.

Another feature of the traveling wave is that it travels fast along the initial portion of the basilar membrane but becomes progressively slower as it goes farther into the cochlea. The cause of this difference is the high coefficient of elasticity of the basilar fibers near the oval window and a progressively decreasing coefficient farther along the membrane. This rapid initial transmission of the wave allows the high-frequency sounds to travel far enough into the cochlea to spread out and separate from one another on the basilar membrane. Without this rapid initial transmission, all the high-frequency waves would be bunched together within the first millimeter or so of the basilar membrane, and their frequencies could not be discriminated.

FUNCTION OF THE ORGAN OF CORTI

The organ of Corti, shown in Figures 107-3 and 107-6, is the receptor organ that generates nerve impulses in response to vibration of the basilar membrane. Note that the organ of Corti lies on the surface of the basilar fibers and basilar membrane. The actual sensory receptors in the organ of Corti are two specialized types of nerve cells called *hair cells*—a single row of *internal* (or "inner") *hair cells*, numbering about 3500 and measuring about 12 μm in diameter, and 3 or 4 rows of *external* (or "outer") *hair cells*, numbering about 12,000 and having diameters of only about 8 μm. The bases and sides of the hair cells synapse with a network of cochlear nerve endings. Between 90 and 95% of these endings terminate on the inner hair cells, emphasizing their special importance for the detection of sound.

The nerve fibers stimulated by the hair cells lead to the *spiral ganglion of Corti,* which lies in the modiolus (center) of the cochlea. The spiral ganglion neuronal cells send axons—a total of about 30,000—into the *cochlear nerve* and then into the central

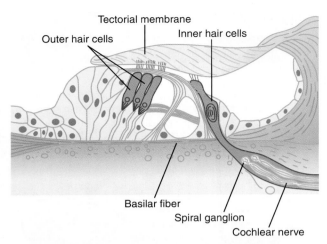

Figure 107-6 Organ of Corti, showing especially the hair cells and the tectorial membrane pressing against the projecting hairs.

nervous system at the level of the upper medulla. The relation of the organ of Corti to the spiral ganglion and to the cochlear nerve is shown in Figure 107-2.

Excitation of the Hair Cells. Note in Figure 107-6 that minute hairs, or *stereocilia*, project upward from the hair cells and either touch or are embedded in the surface gel coating of the *tectorial membrane*, which lies above the stereocilia in the scala media. These hair cells are similar to the hair cells found in the macula and cristae ampullaris of the vestibular apparatus, which are discussed in Chapter 115. Bending of the hairs in one direction depolarizes the hair cells, and bending in the opposite direction hyperpolarizes them. This in turn excites the auditory nerve fibers synapsing with their bases.

Figure 107-7 shows the mechanism by which vibration of the basilar membrane excites the hair endings. The outer ends of the hair cells are fixed tightly in a rigid structure composed of a flat plate, called the *reticular lamina*, supported by triangular *rods of Corti*, which are attached tightly to the basilar fibers. The basilar fibers, the rods of Corti, and the reticular lamina move as a rigid unit.

Upward movement of the basilar fiber rocks the reticular lamina upward and *inward* toward the modiolus. Then, when the basilar membrane moves downward, the reticular lamina rocks downward and *outward*. The inward and outward motion causes the hairs on the hair cells to shear back and forth against the tectorial membrane. Thus, the hair cells are excited whenever the basilar membrane vibrates.

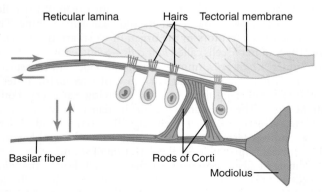

Figure 107-7 Stimulation of the hair cells by to-and-fro movement of the hairs projecting into the gel coating of the tectorial membrane.

Auditory Signals Are Transmitted Mainly by the Inner Hair Cells. Even though there are three to four times as many outer hair cells as inner hair cells, about 90% of the auditory nerve fibers are stimulated by the inner cells rather than by the outer cells.Nonetheless, if the outer cells are damaged while the inner cells remain fully functional, a large amount of hearing loss occurs. Therefore, it has been proposed that the outer hair cells in some way control the sensitivity of the inner hair cells at different sound pitches, a phenomenon called "tuning" of the receptor system. In support of this concept, a large number of retrograde nerve fibers pass from the brainstem to the vicinity of the outer hair cells. Stimulating these nerve fibers can actually cause shortening of the outer hair cells and possibly also change their degree of stiffness. These effects suggest a retrograde nervous mechanism for control of the ear's sensitivity to different sound pitches, activated through the outer hair cells.

Hair Cell Receptor Potentials and Excitation of Auditory Nerve Fibers. The stereocilia (i.e. the "hairs" protruding from the ends of the hair cells) are stiff structures because each has a rigid protein framework. Each hair cell has about 100 stereocilia on its apical border. These stereocilia become progressively longer on the side of the hair cell away from the modiolus, and the tops of the shorter stereocilia are attached by thin filaments to the back sides of their adjacent longer stereocilia. Therefore, whenever the cilia are bent in the direction of the longer ones, the tips of the smaller stereocilia are tugged outward from the surface of the hair cell. This causes a mechanical transduction that opens 200–300 cation-conducting channels, allowing rapid movement of positively charged potassium ions from the surrounding scala media fluid into the stereocilia, which causes depolarization of the hair cell membrane.

Endocochlear Potential. To explain even more fully the electrical potentials generated by the hair cells, we need to explain another electrical phenomenon called the *endocochlear potential*: The scala media is filled with a fluid called *endolymph*, in contradistinction to the *perilymph* present in the scala vestibuli and scala tympani. The scala vestibuli and scala tympani communicate directly with the subarachnoid space around the brain, so the perilymph is almost identical to cerebrospinal fluid. Conversely, the endolymph that fills the scala media is an entirely different fluid secreted by the *stria vascularis*, a highly vascular area on the outer wall of the scala media. Endolymph contains a high concentration of potassium and a low concentration of sodium, which is exactly opposite to the contents of perilymph.

An electrical potential of about +80 mV exists all the time between endolymph and perilymph, with positivity inside the scala media and negativity outside. This is called the *endocochlear potential*, and it is generated by continual secretion of positive potassium ions into the scala media by the stria vascularis.

The importance of the endocochlear potential is that the tops of the hair cells project through the reticular lamina and are bathed by the endolymph of the scala media, whereas perilymph bathes the lower bodies of the hair cells. Furthermore, the hair cells have a negative intracellular potential of −70 mV with respect to the perilymph but −150 mV with respect to the endolymph at their upper surfaces where the hairs project through the reticular lamina and into the endolymph. It is believed that this high electrical potential at the tips of the stereocilia sensitizes the cell an extra amount, thereby increasing its ability to respond to the slightest sound.

DETERMINATION OF SOUND FREQUENCY— THE "PLACE" AND "VOLLEY" PRINCIPLE

From earlier discussions in this chapter (see the section: Transmission of Sound Waves in the Cochlea—"Traveling Wave"), it is apparent that low-frequency sounds cause maximal activation of the basilar membrane near the apex of the cochlea, and high-frequency sounds activate the basilar membrane near the base of the cochlea. Intermediate-frequency sounds activate the membrane at intermediate distances between the two extremes. Furthermore, there is spatial organization of the nerve fibers in the cochlear pathway, all the way from the cochlea to the cerebral cortex. Recording of signals in the auditory tracts of the brainstem and in the auditory receptive fields of the cerebral cortex shows that specific brain neurons are activated by specific sound frequencies. Therefore, the *major* method used by the nervous system to detect different sound frequencies is to determine the positions along the basilar membrane that are most stimulatedwhich is called the *place principle* for the determination of sound frequency.

Referring again to Figure 107-8, one can see that the distal end of the basilar membrane at the helicotrema is stimulated by all sound frequencies below 200 cycles/second. Therefore, it has been difficult to understand from the place principle how one can differentiate between low sound frequencies in the range of 200 down to 20. These low frequencies have been postulated to be discriminated mainly by the so-called *volley* or *frequency principle*. That is, low-frequency sounds, from 20 to 1500–2000 cycles/second, can cause volleys of nerve impulses synchronized at the same frequencies, and these volleys are transmitted by the cochlear nerve into the cochlear nuclei of the brain. It is further suggested that the cochlear nuclei can distinguish the different frequencies of the volleys. In fact, destruction of the entire apical half of the cochlea, which destroys the basilar membrane where all lower-frequency sounds are normally detected, does not totally eliminate discrimination of the lower-frequency sounds.

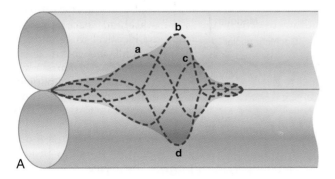

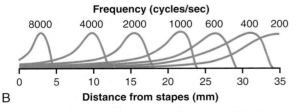

Figure 107-8 (A) Amplitude pattern of vibration of the basilar membrane for a medium-frequency sound; (B) amplitude patterns for sounds of frequencies between 200 and 8000 cycles/second, showing the points of maximum amplitude on the basilar membrane for the different frequencies.

DETERMINATION OF LOUDNESS

Loudness is determined by the auditory system in at least three ways.

First, as the sound becomes louder, the amplitude of vibration of the basilar membrane and hair cells also increases so that the hair cells excite the nerve endings at more rapid rates.

Second, as the amplitude of vibration increases, it causes more and more of the hair cells on the fringes of the resonating portion of the basilar membrane to become stimulated, thus causing *spatial summation* of impulses—that is, transmission through many nerve fibers rather than through only a few.

Third, the outer hair cells do not become stimulated significantly until vibration of the basilar membrane reaches high intensity, and stimulation of these cells presumably apprises the nervous system that the sound is loud.

Detection of Changes in Loudness—The Power Law. As pointed out in Chapter 102, a person interprets changes in intensity of sensory stimuli approximately in proportion to an inverse power function of the actual intensity. In the case of sound, the interpreted sensation changes approximately in proportion to the cube root of the actual sound intensity. To express this concept in another way, the ear can discriminate differences in sound intensity from the softest whisper to the loudest possible noise, representing an *approximately 1 trillion times* increase in sound energy or 1 million times increase in amplitude of movement of the basilar membrane. Yet the ear interprets this much difference in sound level as approximately a 10,000-fold change. Thus, the scale of intensity is greatly "compressed" by the sound perception mechanisms of the auditory system which allows a person to interpret differences in sound intensities over a far wider range than would be possible were it not for compression of the intensity scale.

Decibel Unit. Because of the extreme changes in sound intensities that the ear can detect and discriminate, sound intensities are usually expressed in terms of the logarithm of their actual intensities. A 10-fold increase in sound energy is called 1 *bel*, and 0.1 bel is called 1 *dB*. One decibel represents an actual increase in sound energy of 1.26 times.

Another reason for using the decibel system to express changes in loudness is that, in the usual sound intensity range for communication, the ears can barely distinguish an approximately 1-dB *change* in sound intensity.

Threshold for Hearing Sound at Different Frequencies. Figure 107-9 shows the pressure thresholds at which sounds of different frequencies can barely be heard by the ear. This figure demonstrates that a 3000-cycle-per-second sound can be heard even when its intensity is as low as 70 dB below 1 dyne/cm^2 sound pressure level, which is one ten-millionth microwatt per square centimeter. Conversely, a 100-cycle-per-second sound can be detected only if its intensity is 10,000 times as great as this.

Frequency Range of Hearing. The frequencies of sound that a young person can hear are between 20 and 20,000 cycles/second. However, referring again to Figure 107-9, we see that the sound range depends to a great extent on loudness. If the loudness is 60 dB below 1 dyne/cm^2 sound pressure level, the sound range is 500–5000 cycles/second; only with intense sounds can the complete range of 20–20,000 cycles be achieved. In old age, this frequency range is usually shortened to 50–8000 cycles/second or less, as discussed later in this chapter.

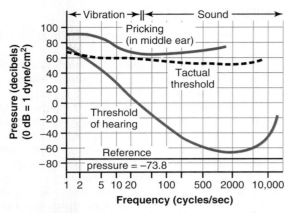

Figure 107-9 Relation of the threshold of hearing and of somesthetic perception (pricking and tactual threshold) to the sound energy level at each sound frequency.

Central Auditory Mechanisms

AUDITORY NERVOUS PATHWAYS

Figure 107-10 shows the major auditory pathways. Nerve fibers from the *spiral ganglion of Corti* enter the *dorsal* and *ventral cochlear nuclei* located in the upper part of the medulla. At this point, all the fibers synapse, and second-order neurons pass mainly to the opposite side of the brainstem to terminate in the *superior olivary nucleus*. A few second-order fibers also pass to the superior olivary nucleus on the same side.

From the superior olivary nucleus, the auditory pathway passes upward through the *lateral lemniscus*. Some of the fibers terminate in the *nucleus of the lateral lemniscus*, but many bypass this nucleus and travel on to the inferior colliculus, where all or almost all the auditory fibers synapse. From there, the pathway passes to the *medial geniculate nucleus*, where all the fibers do synapse. Finally, the pathway proceeds by way of the *auditory radiation* to the *auditory cortex*, located mainly in the superior gyrus of the temporal lobe.

Several important points should be noted. First, signals from both ears are transmitted through the pathways of both sides of the brain, with a preponderance of transmission in the contralateral pathway. In at least three places in the brainstem, crossing over occurs between the two pathways: (1) in the trapezoid body, (2) in the commissure between the two nuclei of the lateral lemnisci, and (3) in the commissure connecting the two inferior colliculi.

Second, many collateral fibers from the auditory tracts pass directly into the *reticular activating system of the brainstem*. This system projects diffusely upward in the brainstem and downward into the spinal cord and activates the entire nervous system in response to loud sounds. Other collaterals go to the *vermis of the cerebellum*, which is also activated instantaneously in the event of a sudden noise.

Third, a high degree of spatial orientation is maintained in the fiber tracts from the cochlea all the way to the cortex. In fact, there are *three spatial patterns* for termination of the different sound frequencies in the cochlear nuclei, *two patterns* in the inferior colliculi, *one precise pattern* for discrete sound frequencies in the auditory cortex, and *at least five other less precise patterns* in the auditory cortex and auditory association areas.

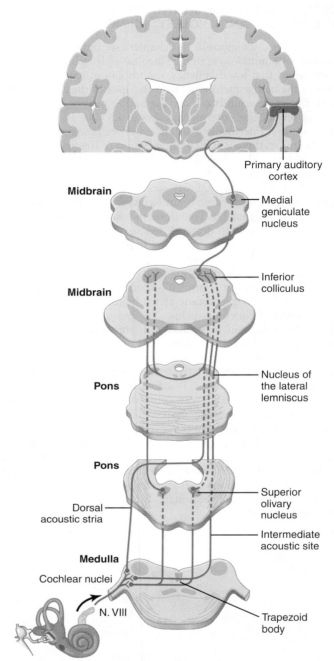

Figure 107-10 Auditory nervous pathways.

FUNCTION OF THE CEREBRAL CORTEX IN HEARING

The projection area of auditory signals to the cerebral cortex is shown in Figure 107-11, which demonstrates that the auditory cortex not only lies principally on the *supratemporal plane of the superior temporal gyrus* but also extends onto the *lateral side of the temporal lobe*, over much of the *insular cortex*, and even onto the lateral portion of the *parietal operculum*.

Two separate subdivisions are shown in Figure 107-11: the *primary auditory cortex* and the *auditory association cortex* (also called the *secondary auditory cortex*). The primary auditory cortex is directly excited by projections from the medial geniculate

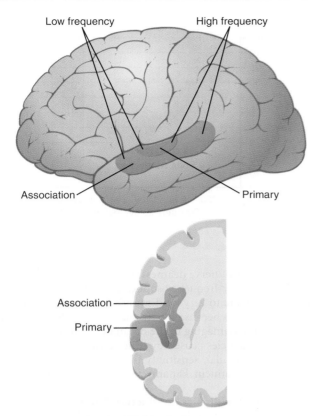

Figure 107-11 Auditory cortex.

body, whereas the auditory association areas are excited secondarily by impulses from the primary auditory cortex, as well as by some projections from thalamic association areas adjacent to the medial geniculate body.

Destruction of both primary auditory cortices in the human being greatly reduces one's sensitivity for hearing. Destruction of one side only slightly reduces hearing in the opposite ear; it does not cause deafness in the ear because of many crossover connections from side to side in the auditory neural pathway. However, it does affect one's ability to localize the source of a sound because comparative signals in both cortices are required for the localization function.

Lesions that affect the auditory association areas but not the primary auditory cortex do not decrease a person's ability to hear and differentiate sound tones, or even to interpret at least simple patterns of sound. However, the person is often unable to interpret the *meaning* of the sound heard. For instance, lesions in the posterior portion of the superior temporal gyrus, which is called Wernicke area and is part of the auditory association cortex, often make it impossible for a person to interpret the meanings of words even though he or she hears them perfectly well and can even repeat them. These functions of the auditory association areas and their relation to the overall intellectual functions of the brain are discussed in more detail in Chapter 126.

DETERMINATION OF THE DIRECTION FROM WHICH SOUND COMES

A person determines the horizontal direction from which sound comes by two principal means: (1) the time lag between the entry of sound into one ear and its entry into the opposite ear, and (2) the difference between the intensities of the sounds in the two ears.

The first mechanism functions best at frequencies below 3000 cycles/second, and the second mechanism operates best at higher frequencies because the head is a greater sound barrier at these frequencies. The time lag mechanism discriminates direction much more exactly than the intensity mechanism because it does not depend on extraneous factors but only on the exact interval of time between two acoustical signals. If a person is looking straight toward the source of the sound, the sound reaches both ears at exactly the same instant, whereas if the right ear is closer to the sound than the left ear is, the sound signals from the right ear enter the brain ahead of those from the left ear.

The two aforementioned mechanisms cannot tell whether the sound is emanating from in front of or behind the person or from above or below. This discrimination is achieved mainly by the *pinnae* of the two ears. The shape of the pinna changes the *quality* of the sound entering the ear, depending on the direction from which the sound comes. It changes the quality by emphasizing specific sound frequencies from the different directions.

CENTRIFUGAL SIGNALS FROM THE CENTRAL NERVOUS SYSTEM TO LOWER AUDITORY CENTERS

Retrograde pathways have been demonstrated at each level of the auditory nervous system from the cortex to the cochlea in the ear. The final pathway is mainly from the superior olivary nucleus to the sound-receptor hair cells in the organ of Corti.

These retrograde fibers are inhibitory. Indeed, direct stimulation of discrete points in the olivary nucleus has been shown to inhibit specific areas of the organ of Corti, reducing their sound sensitivities 15–20 dB. One can readily understand how this mechanism could allow a person to direct his or her attention to sounds of particular qualities while rejecting sounds of other qualities. This characteristic is readily demonstrated when one listens to a single instrument in a symphony orchestra.

Hearing Abnormalities

TYPES OF DEAFNESS

Deafness is usually divided into two types: (1) that caused by impairment of the cochlea, the auditory nerve, or the central nervous system circuits from the ear, which is usually classified as "nerve deafness," and (2) that caused by impairment of the physical structures of the ear that conduct sound itself to the cochlea, which is usually called "conduction deafness."

If either the cochlea or the auditory nerve is destroyed, the person becomes permanently deaf. However, if the cochlea and nerve are still intact but the tympanum–ossicular system has been destroyed or ankylosed ("frozen" in place by fibrosis or calcification), sound waves can still be conducted into the cochlea by means of bone conduction from a sound generator applied to the skull over the ear.

Audiometer. To determine the nature of hearing disabilities, an "audiometer" is used. This instrument is an earphone connected to an electronic oscillator capable of emitting pure tones ranging from low frequencies to high frequencies, and it is

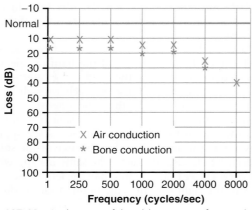

Figure 107-12 Audiogram of the old-age type of nerve deafness.

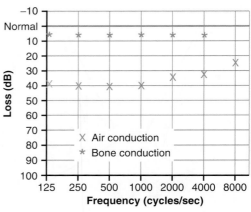

Figure 107-13 Audiogram of air conduction deafness resulting from middle ear sclerosis.

calibrated so that zero-intensity-level sound at each frequency is the loudness that can barely be heard by the normal ear. A calibrated volume control can increase the loudness above the zero level. If the loudness must be increased to 30 dB above normal before it can be heard, the person is said to have a *hearing loss* of 30 dB at that particular frequency.

In performing a hearing test using an audiometer, one tests about 8–10 frequencies covering the auditory spectrum, and the hearing loss is determined for each of these frequencies. Then the so-called *audiogram* is plotted, as shown in Figures 107-12 and 107-13, depicting hearing loss at each of the frequencies in the auditory spectrum. The audiometer, in addition to being equipped with an earphone for testing air conduction by the ear, is equipped with a mechanical vibrator for testing bone conduction from the mastoid process of the skull into the cochlea.

Audiogram in Nerve Deafness. In nerve deafness, which includes damage to the cochlea, the auditory nerve, or the central nervous system circuits from the ear, the person has loss of ability to hear sound as tested by both air conduction and bone conduction. An audiogram depicting partial nerve deafness is shown in Figure 107-12. In this figure, the deafness is mainly for high-frequency sound. Such deafness could be caused by damage to the base of the cochlea. This type of deafness occurs to some extent in almost all older people.

Other patterns of nerve deafness frequently occur as follows: (1) deafness for low-frequency sounds caused by excessive and prolonged exposure to very loud sounds (e.g., a rock band or a jet airplane engine) because low-frequency sounds are usually louder and more damaging to the organ of Corti, and (2) deafness for all frequencies caused by drug sensitivity of the organ of Corti—in particular, sensitivity to some antibiotics such as streptomycin, gentamicin, kanamycin, and chloramphenicol.

Audiogram for Middle Ear Conduction Deafness. A common type of deafness is caused by fibrosis in the middle ear after repeated infection or by fibrosis that occurs in the hereditary disease called *otosclerosis*. In either case, the sound waves cannot be transmitted easily through the ossicles from the tympanic membrane to the oval window. Figure 107-13 shows an audiogram from a person with "middle ear air conduction deafness." In this case, bone conduction is essentially normal, but conduction through the ossicular system is greatly depressed at all frequencies, but more so at low frequencies. In some instances of conduction deafness, the faceplate of the stapes becomes "ankylosed" by bone overgrowth to the edges of the oval window. In this case the person becomes totally deaf for ossicular conduction but can regain almost normal hearing by the surgical removal of the stapes and its replacement with a minute Teflon or metal prosthesis that transmits the sound from the incus to the oval window.

BIBLIOGRAPHY

Bizley JK, Cohen YE: The what, where and how of auditory-object perception, *Nat. Rev. Neurosci.* 14:693, 2013.

Dahmen JC, King AJ: Learning to hear: plasticity of auditory cortical processing, *Curr. Opin. Neurobiol.* 17:456, 2007.

Dallos P: Cochlear amplification, outer hair cells and prestin, *Curr. Opin. Neurobiol.* 18:370, 2008.

Frolenkov GI, Belyantseva IA, Friedman TB, et al: Genetic insights into the morphogenesis of inner ear hair cells, *Nat. Rev. Genet.* 5:489, 2004.

Géléoc GS, Holt JR: Sound strategies for hearing restoration, *Science* 344:1241062, 2014.

Glowatzki E, Grant L, Fuchs P: Hair cell afferent synapses, *Curr. Opin. Neurobiol.* 18:389, 2008.

Griffiths TD, Warren JD, Scott SK, et al: Cortical processing of complex sound: a way forward? *Trends Neurosci.* 27:181, 2004.

Hudspeth AJ: Making an effort to listen: mechanical amplification in the ear, *Neuron* 59:530, 2008.

King AJ, Nelken I: Unraveling the principles of auditory cortical processing: can we learn from the visual system? *Nat. Neurosci.* 12:698, 2009.

Nelken I: Processing of complex sounds in the auditory system, *Curr. Opin. Neurobiol.* 18:413, 2008.

Papsin BC, Gordon KA: Cochlear implants for children with severe-to-profound hearing loss, *N. Engl. J. Med.* 357:2380, 2007.

Rauschecker JP, Shannon RV: Sending sound to the brain, *Science* 295:1025, 2002.

Read HL, Winer JA, Schreiner CE: Functional architecture of auditory cortex, *Curr. Opin. Neurobiol.* 12:433, 2002.

Robles L, Ruggero MA: Mechanics of the mammalian cochlea, *Physiol. Rev.* 81:1305, 2001.

Syka J: Plastic changes in the central auditory system after hearing loss, restoration of function, and during learning, *Physiol. Rev.* 82:601, 2002.

Weinberger NM: Specific long-term memory traces in primary auditory cortex, *Nat. Rev. Neurosci.* 5:279, 2004.

108

Optics of Vision

Physical Principles of Optics

Understanding the optical system of the eyerequires familiarity with the basic principles of optics, including the physics of light refraction, focusing, depth of focus, and so forth. A brief review of these physical principles is therefore presented; followed by discussion of the optics of the eye.

REFRACTION OF LIGHT

Refractive Index of a Transparent Substance. Light rays travel through air at a velocity of about 300,000 km/second, but they travel much slower through transparent solids and liquids. The refractive index of a transparent substance is the *ratio* of the velocity of light in air to the velocity in the substance. The refractive index of air is 1.00. Thus, if light travels through a particular type of glass at a velocity of 200,000 km/second, the refractive index of this glass is 300,000 divided by 200,000 or 1.50.

Refraction of Light Rays at an Interface Between Two Media with Different Refractive Indices. When light rays traveling forward in a beam (as shown in Figure 108-1A) strike an interface that is *perpendicular* to the beam, the rays enter the second medium without deviating from their course. The only effect that occurs is decreased velocity of transmission and shorter wavelength, as shown in the figure by the shorter distances between wave fronts.

If the light rays pass through an angulated interface as shown in Figure 108-1B, the rays bend if the refractive indices of the two media are different from each other. In this figure, the light rays are leaving air, which has a refractive index of 1.00, and are entering a block of glass having a refractive index of 1.50. When the beam first strikes the angulated interface, the lower edge of the beam enters the glass ahead of the upper edge. The wave front in the upper portion of the beam continues to travel at a velocity

of 300,000 km/second, while that which entered the glass travels at a velocity of 200,000 km/second. This difference in velocity causes the upper portion of the wave front to move ahead of the lower portion so that the wave front is no longer vertical but is angulated to the right. Because *the direction in which light travels is always perpendicular to the plane of the wave front*, the direction of travel of the light beam bends downward.

This bending of light rays at an angulated interface is known as *refraction*. Note particularly that the degree of refraction increases as a function of (1) the ratio of the two refractive indices of the two transparent media and (2) the degree of angulation between the interface and the entering wave front.

APPLICATION OF REFRACTIVE PRINCIPLES TO LENSES

Convex Lens Focuses Light Rays. Figure 108-2 shows parallel light rays entering a convex lens. The light rays passing through the center of the lens strike the lens exactly perpendicular to the lens surface and, therefore, pass through the lens without being refracted. Toward either edge of the lens, however, the light rays strike a progressively more angulated interface. The outer rays bend more and more toward the center, which is called *convergence* of the rays. Half the bending occurs when the rays enter the lens and half occurs as the rays exit from the opposite side. If the lens has exactly the proper curvature, parallel light rays passing through each part of the lens will be bent exactly enough so that all the rays will pass through a single point, which is called the *focal point*.

Concave Lens Diverges Light Rays. Figure 108-3 shows the effect of a concave lens on parallel light rays. The rays that enter the center of the lens strike an interface that is perpendicular to the beam and, therefore, do not refract. The rays at the edge of

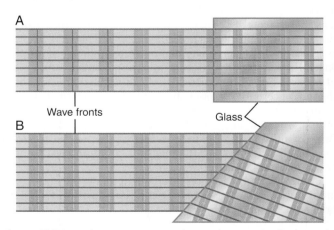

Figure 108-1 Light rays entering a glass surface perpendicular to the light rays (A) and a glass surface angulated to the light rays (B). This figure demonstrates that the distance between waves after they enter the glass is shortened to about two-thirds that in air. It also shows that light rays striking an angulated glass surface are bent.

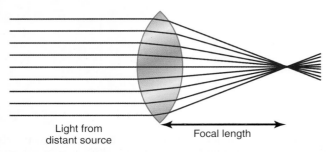

Figure 108-2 Bending of light rays at each surface of a convex spherical lens, showing that parallel light rays are focused to a *focal point*.

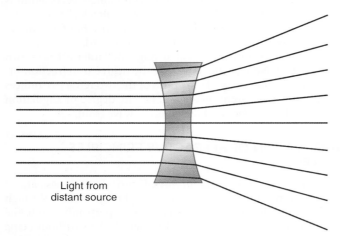

Figure 108-3 Bending of light rays at each surface of a concave spherical lens, showing that parallel light rays are *diverged*.

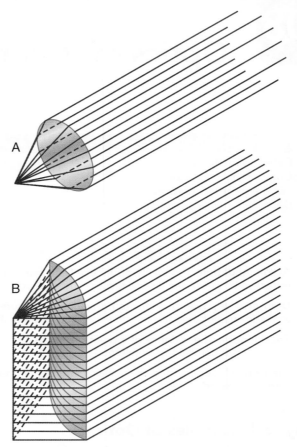

Figure 108-4 (A) *Point focus* of parallel light rays by a spherical convex lens; (B) *line focus* of parallel light rays by a cylindrical convex lens.

the lens enter the lens ahead of the rays in the center. This is opposite to the effect in the convex lens, and it causes the peripheral light rays to *diverge* from the light rays that pass through the center of the lens. Thus, the concave lens *diverges* light rays, but the convex lens *converges* light rays.

Cylindrical Lens Bends Light Rays in Only One Plane—Comparison with Spherical Lenses. Figure 108-4 shows both a convex *spherical* lens and a convex *cylindrical* lens. Note that the cylindrical lens bends light rays from the two sides of the lens but not from the top or the bottom—that is, bending occurs in one plane but not the other. Thus, parallel light rays are bent to a *focal line*. Conversely, light rays that pass through the spherical lens are refracted at all edges of the lens (in both planes) toward the central ray, and all the rays come to a *focal point*.

The cylindrical lens is well demonstrated by a test tube full of water. If the test tube is placed in a beam of sunlight and a piece of paper is brought progressively closer to the opposite side of the tube, a certain distance will be found at which the light rays come to a *focal line*. The spherical lens is demonstrated by an ordinary magnifying glass. If such a lens is placed in a beam of sunlight and a piece of paper is brought progressively closer to the lens, the light rays will impinge on a common focal point at an appropriate distance.

Concave cylindrical lenses *diverge* light rays in only one plane in the same manner that *convex* cylindrical lenses *converge* light rays in one plane.

FOCAL LENGTH OF A LENS

The distance beyond a convex lens at which *parallel* rays converge to a common focal point is called the *focal length* of the

lens. The diagram at the top of Figure 108-5 demonstrates this focusing of parallel light rays.

In the middle diagram, the light rays that enter the convex lens are not parallel but are *diverging* because the origin of the light is a point source not far away from the lens itself. Because these rays are diverging outward from the point source, it can be seen from the diagram that they do not focus at the same distance away from the lens as do parallel rays. In other words, when rays of light that are already diverging enter a convex lens, the distance of focus on the other side of the lens is farther from the lens than is the focal length of the lens for parallel rays.

The bottom diagram of Figure 108-5 shows light rays that are diverging toward a convex lens that has far greater curvature than that of the other two lenses in the figure. In this diagram, the distance from the lens at which the light rays come to focus is exactly the same as that from the lens in the first diagram, in which the lens is less convex but the rays entering it are parallel. This demonstrates that both parallel rays and diverging rays can be focused at the same distance beyond a lens, provided the lens changes its convexity.

The relation of focal length of the lens, distance of the point source of light, and distance of focus is expressed by the following formula:

$$\frac{1}{f} = \frac{1}{a} + \frac{1}{b}$$

where f is the focal length of the lens for parallel rays, a is the distance of the point source of light from the lens, and b is the distance of focus on the other side of the lens.

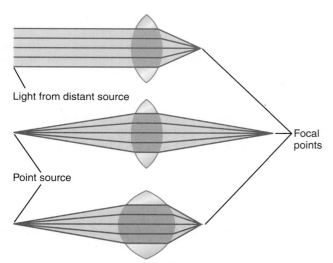

Figure 108-5 The two upper lenses of this figure have the same focal length, but the light rays entering the top lens are parallel, whereas those entering the middle lens are diverging; the effect of parallel versus diverging rays on the focal distance is shown. The bottom lens has far more refractive power than either of the other two lenses (ie, has a much shorter focal length), demonstrating that the stronger the lens is, the nearer to the lens the point focus is.

FORMATION OF AN IMAGE BY A CONVEX LENS

Figure 108-6A shows a convex lens with two-point sources of light to the left. Because light rays pass through the center of a convex lens without being refracted in either direction, the light rays from each point source of light are shown to come to a point focus on the opposite side of the lens *directly in line with the point source and the center of the lens*.

Any object in front of the lens is, in reality, a mosaic of point sources of light. Some of these points are very bright, and some are very weak, and they vary in color. Each point source of light on the object comes to a separate point focus on the opposite side of the lens in line with the lens center. If a white sheet of paper is placed at the focus distance from the lens, one can see an image of the object, as demonstrated in Figure 108-6B. However, this image is upside down with respect to the original object, and the two lateral sides of the image are reversed. The lens of a camera focuses images on film via this method.

MEASUREMENT OF THE REFRACTIVE POWER OF A LENS—"DIOPTER"

The more a lens bends light rays, the greater is its "refractive power." This refractive power is measured in terms of *diopters*. The refractive power in diopters of a convex lens is equal to 1 m divided by its focal length. Thus, a spherical lens that converges parallel light rays to a focal point 1 m beyond the lens has a refractive power of +1 D, as shown in Figure 108-7. If the lens is capable of bending parallel light rays twice as much as a lens with a power of +1 D, it is said to have a strength of +2 D, and the light rays come to a focal point 0.5 m beyond the lens. A lens capable of converging parallel light rays to a focal point only 10 cm (0.10 m) beyond the lens has a refractive power of +10 D.

The refractive power of concave lenses cannot be stated in terms of the focal distance beyond the lens because the light rays diverge, rather than focus to a point. However, if a concave lens diverges light rays at the same rate that a 1-D convex lens converges them, the concave lens is said to have a dioptric strength of −1. Likewise, if the concave lens diverges light rays as much as a +10-D lens converges them, this lens is said to have a strength of −10 D.

The strengths of cylindrical lenses are computed in the same manner as the strengths of spherical lenses, except that the *axis* of the cylindrical lens must be stated in addition to its strength. If a cylindrical lens focuses parallel light rays to a line focus 1 m beyond the lens, it has a strength of +1 D. Conversely, if a cylindrical lens of a concave type *diverges* light rays as much as a +1-D cylindrical lens *converges* them, it has a strength of −1 D. If the focused line is horizontal, its axis is said to be 0 degree. If it is vertical, its axis is 90 degrees.

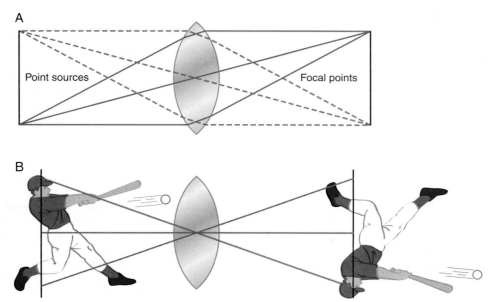

Figure 108-6 (A) Two-point sources of light focused at two separate points on opposite sides of the lens; (B) formation of an image by a convex spherical lens.

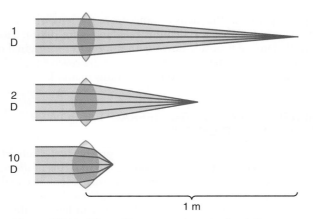

Figure 108-7   Effect of lens strength on the focal distance.

Optics of the Eye

THE EYE AS A CAMERA

The eye, shown in Figure 108-8, is optically equivalent to the usual photographic camera. It has a lens system, a variable aperture system (the pupil), and a retina that corresponds to the film. The lens system of the eye is composed of four refractive interfaces: (1) the interface between air and the anterior surface of the cornea, (2) the interface between the posterior surface of the cornea and the aqueous humor, (3) the interface between the aqueous humor and the anterior surface of the lens of the eye, and (4) the interface between the posterior surface of the lens and the vitreous humor. The internal index of air is 1; the cornea, 1.38; the aqueous humor, 1.33; the crystalline lens (on average), 1.40; and the vitreous humor, 1.34.

CONSIDERATION OF ALL REFRACTIVE SURFACES OF THE EYE AS A SINGLE LENS—THE "REDUCED" EYE

If all the refractive surfaces of the eye are algebraically added together and then considered to be one single lens, the optics of the normal eye may be simplified and represented schematically as a "reduced eye." This representation is useful in simple calculations. In the reduced eye, a single refractive surface is considered to exist, with its central point 17 mm in front of the retina and a total refractive power of 59 D when the lens is accommodated for distant vision.

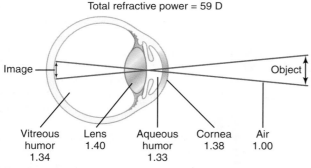

Total refractive power = 59 D

Image — Object

Vitreous humor 1.34 | Lens 1.40 | Aqueous humor 1.33 | Cornea 1.38 | Air 1.00

Figure 108-8   The eye as a camera. The numbers are the refractive indices.

About two-thirds of the 59 D of refractive power of the eye is provided by the anterior surface of the cornea (*not* by the eye lens). The principal reason for this phenomenon is that the refractive index of the cornea is markedly different from that of air, whereas the refractive index of the eye lens is not greatly different from the indices of the aqueous humor and vitreous humor.

The total refractive power of the internal lens of the eye, as it normally lies in the eye surrounded by fluid on each side, is only 20 D, about one-third the total refractive power of the eye. However, the importance of the internal lens is that, in response to nervous signals from the brain, *its curvature can be increased* markedly to provide "accommodation," which is discussed later in the chapter.

Formation of an Image on the Retina. In the same manner that a glass lens can focus an image on a sheet of paper, the lens system of the eye can focus an image on the retina. The image is inverted and reversed with respect to the object. However, the mind perceives objects in the upright position despite the upside-down orientation on the retina because the brain is trained to consider an inverted image as normal.

MECHANISM OF "ACCOMMODATION"

In children, the refractive power of the lens of the eye can be increased voluntarily from 20 to about 34 D which is an "accommodation" of 14 D. To make this accomodation, the shape of the lens is changed from that of a moderately convex lens to that of a very convex lens.

In a young person, the lens is composed of a strong elastic capsule filled with viscous, proteinaceous, but transparent fluid. When the lens is in a relaxed state with no tension on its capsule, it assumes an almost spherical shape, owing mainly to the elastic retraction of the lens capsule. However, as shown in Figure 108-9, about 70 *suspensory ligaments* attach radially around the lens, pulling the lens edges toward the outer circle of the eyeball. These ligaments are constantly tensed by their attachments at the anterior border of the choroid and retina. The tension on the ligaments causes the lens to remain relatively flat under normal conditions of the eye.

Also located at the lateral attachments of the lens ligaments to the eyeball is the *ciliary muscle*, which itself has two separate sets of smooth muscle fibers—*meridional fibers* and *circular fibers*. The meridional fibers extend from the peripheral ends of the suspensory ligaments to the corneoscleral junction. When these muscle fibers contract, the *peripheral insertions* of the lens ligaments are pulled medially toward the edges of the cornea, thereby releasing the 'ligaments' tension on the lens. The circular fibers are arranged circularly all the way around the ligament attachments so that when they contract, a sphincter-like action occurs, decreasing the diameter of the circle of ligament attachments; this action also allows the ligaments to pull less on the lens capsule.

Thus, contraction of either set of smooth muscle fibers in the ciliary muscle relaxes the ligaments to the lens capsule, and the lens assumes a more spherical shape, like that of a balloon, because of the natural elasticity of the lens capsule.

These changes in the curvature of the lens can be observed experimentally by holding a lit object in front of the eye, and observing the reflections of this object on the curved surfaces of the cornea and the lens. Three reflected images can be observed: the first and second are upright images on the corneal

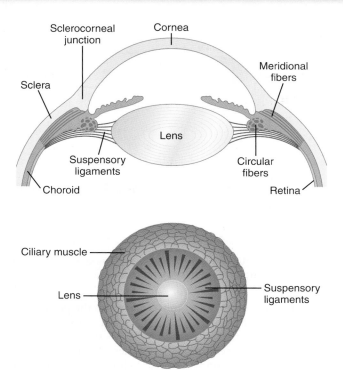

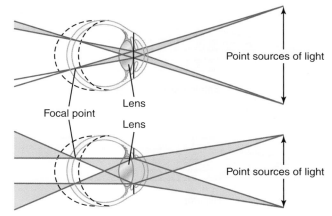

Figure 108-10 Effect of small (*top*) and large (*bottom*) pupillary apertures on "depth of focus."

Figure 108-9 Mechanism of accommodation (focusing).

and anterior lens surface, respectively, while a third dim, inverted image can be observed on the posterior surface of the lens. When the subject focuses the eye on a near object, the second reflection becomes brighter and smaller, indicating an increase in the curvature of the anterior surface of the lens. These images are called Purkinje–Sanson images, and allow one to observe changes in the lens during accommodation.

Accommodation Is Controlled by Parasympathetic Nerves. The ciliary muscle is controlled almost entirely by parasympathetic nerve signals transmitted to the eye through the third cranial nerve from the third nerve nucleus in the brainstem, as explained in Chapter 110. Stimulation of the parasympathetic nerves contracts both sets of ciliary muscle fibers, which relaxes the lens ligaments, thus allowing the lens to become thicker and increase its refractive power. With this increased refractive power, the eye focuses on objects nearer than when the eye has less refractive power. Consequently, as a distant object moves toward the eye, the number of parasympathetic impulses impinging on the ciliary muscle must be progressively increased for the eye to keep the object constantly in focus. (Sympathetic stimulation has an additional effect in relaxing the ciliary muscle, but this effect is so weak that it plays almost no role in the normal accommodation mechanism; the neurology of this mechanism is discussed in Chapter 110.)

Presbyopia—Loss of Accommodation by the Lens. As a person grows older, the lens grows larger and thicker and becomes far less elastic, partly because of progressive denaturation of the lens proteins. The ability of the lens to change shape decreases with age. The power of accommodation decreases from about 14 D in a child to less than 2 D by the time a person reaches 45–50 yearsand to essentially 0 D at age 70 years. Thereafter, the lens remains almost totally nonaccommodating, a condition known as "presbyopia."

Once a person has reached the state of presbyopia, each eye remains focused permanently at an almost constant distance; this distance depends on the physical characteristics of each person's eyes. The eyes can no longer accommodate for both near and far vision. To see clearly both in the distance and nearby, an older person must wear bifocal glasses with the upper segment focused for far-seeing and the lower segment focused for near-seeing (eg, for reading).

PUPILLARY DIAMETER

The major function of the iris is to increase the amount of light that enters the eye during darkness and to decrease the amount of light that enters the eye in daylight. The reflexes for controlling this mechanism are considered in Chapter 110.

The amount of light that enters the eye through the pupil is proportional to the *area* of the pupil or to the *square of the diameter* of the pupil. The pupil of the human eye can become as small as about 1.5 mm and as large as 8 mm in diameter. The quantity of light entering the eye can change about 30-fold as a result of changes in pupillary aperture.

"Depth of Focus" of the Lens System Increases with Decreasing Pupillary Diameter. Figure 108-10 shows two eyes that are exactly alike except for the diameters of the pupillary apertures. In the upper eye, the pupillary aperture is small, and in the lower eye, the aperture is large. In front of each of these two eyes are two small point sources of light; light from each passes through the pupillary aperture and focuses on the retina. Consequently, in both eyes, the retina sees two spots of light in perfect focus. It is evident from the diagrams, however, that if the retina is moved forward or backward to an out-of-focus position, the size of each spot will not change much in the upper eye, but in the lower eye the size of each spot will increase greatly, becoming a "blur circle." In other words, the upper lens system has far greater *depth of focus* than does the bottom lens system. When a lens system has great depth of focus, the retina can be displaced considerably from the focal plane or the lens strength can change considerably from normal and the image will still remain nearly in sharp focus, whereas when a lens system has a "shallow" depth of focus, moving the retina only slightly away from the focal plane causes extreme blurring.

The greatest possible depth of focus occurs when the pupil is extremely small. The reason for this is that, with a very small aperture, almost all the rays pass through the center of the lens, and the central-most rays are always in focus, as explained earlier.

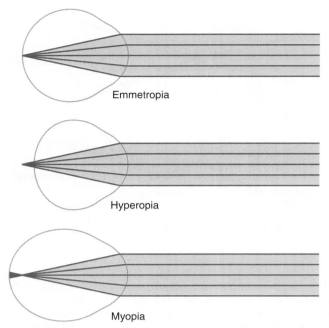

Figure 108-11   Parallel light rays focus on the retina in emmetropia, behind the retina in hyperopia, and in front of the retina in myopia.

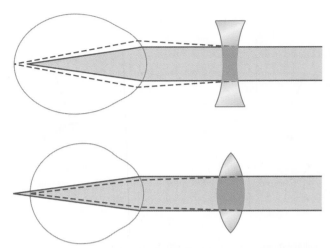

Figure 108-12   Correction of myopia with a concave lens(*top*), and correction of hyperopia with a convex lens(*bottom*).

ERRORS OF REFRACTION

Emmetropia (Normal Vision). As shown in Figure 108-11, the eye is considered to be normal, or "emmetropic," if parallel light rays *from distant objects* are in sharp focus on the retina *when the ciliary muscle is completely relaxed.* This means that the emmetropic eye can see all distant objects clearly with its ciliary muscle relaxed. However, to focus objects at close range, the eye must contract its ciliary muscle and thereby provide appropriate degrees of accommodation.

Hyperopia (Farsightedness). Hyperopia, which is also known as "farsightedness," is usually due to either an eyeball that is too short or, occasionally, a lens system that is too weak. In this condition, as seen in the middle panel of Figure 108-11, parallel light rays are not bent sufficiently by the relaxed lens system to come to focus by the time they reach the retina. To overcome this abnormality, the ciliary muscle must contract to increase the strength of the lens. By using the mechanism of accommodation, a farsighted person is capable of focusing distant objects on the retina. If the person has used only a small amount of strength in the ciliary muscle to accommodate for the distant objects, he or she still has much accommodative power left, and objects closer and closer to the eye can also be focused sharply until the ciliary muscle has contracted to its limit. In old age, when the lens becomes "presbyopic," a farsighted person is often unable to accommodate the lens sufficiently to focus even distant objects, much less near objects.

Myopia (Nearsightedness). In myopia, or "nearsightedness," when the ciliary muscle is completely relaxed, the light rays coming from distant objects are focused in front of the retina, as shown in the bottom panel of Figure 108-11. This condition is usually due to too long an eyeball, but it also can result from too much refractive power in the lens system of the eye.

No mechanism exists by which the eye can decrease the strength of its lens to less than that which exists when the ciliary muscle is completely relaxed. A myopic person has no mechanism by which to focus distant objects sharply on the retina. However, as an object moves nearer to the person's eye, it finally gets close enough that its image can be focused. Then, when the object comes still closer to the eye, the person can use the mechanism of accommodation to keep the image focused clearly. A myopic person has a definite limiting "far point" for clear vision.

Correction of Myopia and Hyperopia Through Use of Lenses. If the refractive surfaces of the eye have too much refractive power, as in *myopia*, this excessive refractive power can be neutralized by placing in front of the eye a concave spherical lens, which will diverge rays. Such correction is demonstrated in the upper diagram of Figure 108-12.

Conversely, in a person who has *hyperopia*—that is, someone who has too weak a lens system—the abnormal vision can be corrected by adding refractive power using a convex lens in front of the eye. This correction is demonstrated in the lower diagram of Figure 108-12.

One usually determines the strength of the concave or convex lens needed for clear vision by "trial and error"—that is, by trying first a strong lens and then a stronger or weaker lens until the one that gives the best visual acuity is found.

Astigmatism. Astigmatism is a refractive error of the eye that causes the visual image in one plane to focus at a different distance from that of the plane at right angles. Astigmatism most often results from too great a curvature of the cornea in one plane of the eye. An example of an astigmatic lens would be a lens surface like that of an egg lying sidewise to the incoming light. The degree of curvature in the plane through the long axis of the egg is not nearly as great as the degree of curvature in the plane through the short axis.

Because the curvature of the astigmatic lens along one plane is less than the curvature along the other plane, light rays striking the peripheral portions of the lens in one plane are not bent nearly as much as the rays striking the peripheral portions of the other plane. This effect is demonstrated in Figure 108-13, which shows rays of light originating from a point source and passing through an oblong, astigmatic lens. The light rays in the vertical plane, indicated by plane BD, are refracted greatly by the astigmatic lens because of the greater curvature in the vertical direction than in the horizontal direction. By contrast, the light rays in the horizontal plane, indicated by plane AC, are not bent nearly as much as the light rays in vertical plane BD.

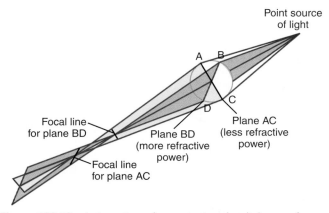

Figure 108-13 Astigmatism, demonstrating that light rays focus at one focal distance in one focal plane (*plane AC*) and at another focal distance in the plane at a right angle (*plane BD*).

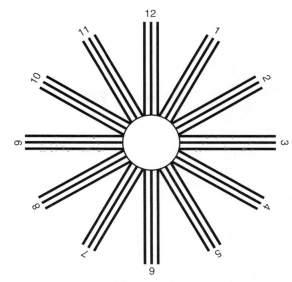

Figure 108-14 Chart composed of parallel black bars at different angular orientations for determining the axis of astigmatism.

It is obvious that light rays passing through an astigmatic lens do not all come to a common focal point because the light rays passing through one plane focus far in front of those passing through the other plane.

The accommodative power of the eye can never compensate for astigmatism because, during accommodation, the curvature of the eye lens changes approximately equally in both planes; therefore, in astigmatism, each of the two planes requires a different degree of accommodation. Thus, without the aid of glasses, a person with astigmatism never sees in sharp focus.

Correction of Astigmatism with a Cylindrical Lens. One may consider an astigmatic eye as having a lens system made up of two cylindrical lenses of different strengths and placed at right angles to each other. To correct for astigmatism, the usual procedure is to find a spherical lens by trial and error that corrects the focus in one of the two planes of the astigmatic lens. Then an additional cylindrical lens is used to correct the remaining error in the remaining plane. To do this, both the *axis* and the *strength* of the required cylindrical lens must be determined.

Several methods exist for determining the axis of the abnormal cylindrical component of the lens system of an eye. One of these methods is based on the use of parallel black bars of the type shown in Figure 108-14. Some of these parallel bars are vertical, some are horizontal, and some are at various angles to the vertical and horizontal axes. After placing various spherical lenses in front of the astigmatic eye, a strength of lens that causes sharp focus of one set of parallel bars but does not correct the fuzziness of the set of bars at right angles to the sharp bars is usually found. It can be shown from the physical principles of optics discussed earlier in this chapter that the *axis* of the *out-of-focus* cylindrical component of the optical system is parallel to the bars that are fuzzy. Once this axis is found, the examiner tries progressively stronger and weaker positive or negative *cylindrical* lenses, the axes of which are placed in line with the out-of-focus bars, until the patient sees all the crossed bars with equal clarity. When this goal has been accomplished, the examiner directs the optician to grind a special lens combining both the spherical correction and the cylindrical correction at the appropriate axis.

Cataracts—Opaque Areas in the Lens

"Cataracts" are an especially common eye abnormality that occurs mainly in older people. A cataract is a cloudy or opaque area or areas in the lens. In the early stage of cataract formation, the proteins in some of the lens fibers become denatured. Later, these same proteins coagulate to form opaque areas in place of the normal transparent protein fibers.

When a cataract has obscured light transmission so greatly that it seriously impairs vision, the condition can be corrected by surgical removal of the lens. When the lens is removed, the eye loses a large portion of its refractive power, which must be replaced by placing a powerful convex lens in front of the eye; usually, however, an artificial plastic lens is implanted in the eye in place of the removed lens.

VISUAL ACUITY

Theoretically, light from a distant point source, when focused on the retina, should be infinitely small. However, because the lens system of the eye is never perfect, such a retinal spot ordinarily has a total diameter of about 11 μm, even with maximal resolution of the normal eye optical system. The spot is brightest in its center and shades off gradually toward the edges, as shown by the two-point images in Figure 108-15.

The average diameter of the cones in the *fovea* of the retina—the central part of the retina, where vision is most highly developed—is about 1.5 μm, which is one-seventh the diameter of the spot of light. Nevertheless, because the spot of light has a bright center point and shaded edges, a person can normally distinguish two separate points if their centers lie up to 2 μm apart on the retina, which is slightly greater than the width of a foveal cone. This discrimination between points is also shown in Figure 108-15.

The normal visual acuity of the human eye for discriminating between point sources of light is about 25 seconds of arc. That is, when light rays from two separate points strike the eye with an angle of at least 25 seconds between them, they can usually be recognized as two points instead of one. This means that a person with normal visual acuity looking at two bright pinpoint spots of light 10 m away can barely distinguish the spots as separate entities when they are 1.5–2 mm apart.

The fovea is less than 0.5 mm (<500 μm) in diameter, which means that maximum visual acuity occurs in less than 2 degrees

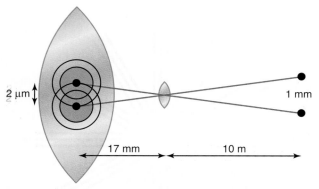

Figure 108-15   Maximum visual acuity for two-point sources of light.

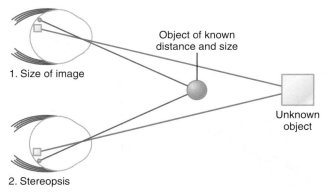

Figure 108-16   Perception of distance by the size of the image on the retina (*1*) and as a result of stereopsis (*2*).

of the visual field. Outside this foveal area, the visual acuity becomes progressively poorer, decreasing more than 10-fold as the periphery is approached. This is caused by the connection of more and more rods and cones to each optic nerve fiber in the nonfoveal, more peripheral parts of the retina, as discussed in Chapter 110.

Clinical Method for Stating Visual Acuity. The chart for testing eyes usually consists of letters of different sizes placed 20 ft. away from the person being tested. If the person can see well the letters of a size that he or she should be able to see at 20 ft., the person is said to have 20/20 vision—that is, normal vision. If the person can see only letters that he or she should be able to see at 200 ft., the person is said to have 20/200 vision. In other words, the clinical method for expressing visual acuity is to use a mathematical fraction that expresses the ratio of two distances, which is also the ratio of one's visual acuity to that of a person with normal visual acuity.

DETERMINATION OF DISTANCE OF AN OBJECT FROM THE EYE—"DEPTH PERCEPTION"

A person normally perceives distance by three main means: (1) the sizes of the images of known objects on the retina, (2) the phenomenon of moving parallax, and (3) the phenomenon of stereopsis. This ability to determine distance is called *depth perception.*

Determination of Distance by Sizes of Retinal Images of Known Objects. If one knows that a person being viewed is 6 ft. tall, one can determine how far away the person is simply by the size of the person's image on the retina. One does not consciously think about the size, but the brain has learned to calculate automatically from image sizes the distances of objects when the dimensions are known.

Determination of Distance by Moving Parallax. Another important means by which the eyes determine distance is that of moving parallax. If a person looks off into the distance with the eyes completely still, he or she perceives no moving parallax, but when the person moves his or her head to one side or the other, the images of close-by objects move rapidly across the retinas, while the images of distant objects remain almost completely stationary. For instance, by moving the head 1 in. to the side when the object is only 1 in. in front of the eye, the image moves almost all the way across the retinas, whereas the image of an object 200 ft. away from the eyes does not move perceptibly. Thus, by using this mechanism of moving parallax, one can tell the *relative distances* of different objects even though only one eye is used.

Determination of Distance by Stereopsis—Binocular Vision. Another method by which one perceives parallax is that of "binocular vision." Because one eye is a little more than 2 in. to one side of the other eye, the images on the two retinas are different from each other. For instance, an object 1 in. in front of the nose forms an image on the left side of the retina of the left eye but on the right side of the retina of the right eye, whereas a small object 20 ft. in front of the nose has its image at closely corresponding points in the centers of the two retinas. This type of parallax is demonstrated in Figure 108-16, which shows the images of a red spot and a yellow square actually reversed on the two retinas because they are at different distances in front of the eyes. This gives a type of parallax that is present all the time when both eyes are being used. It is almost entirely this binocular parallax (or *stereopsis*) that gives a person with two eyes far greater ability to judge relative distances *when objects are nearby* than a person who has only one eye. However, stereopsis is virtually useless for depth perception at distances beyond 50–200 ft.

OPHTHALMOSCOPE

The ophthalmoscope is an instrument through which an observer can look into another person's eye and see the retina with clarity. Although the ophthalmoscope appears to be a relatively complicated instrument, its principles are simple. The basic components are shown in Figure 108-17 and can be explained as follows.

If a bright spot of light is on the retina of an *emmetropic eye*, light rays from this spot diverge toward the lens system of

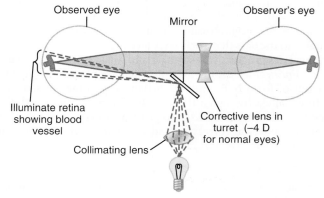

Figure 108-17   Optical system of the ophthalmoscope.

the eye. After passing through the lens system, they are parallel with one another because the retina is located one focal length distance behind the lens system. Then, when these parallel rays pass into an emmetropic eye of another person, they focus again to a point focus on the retina of the second person, because his or her retina is also one focal length distance behind the lens. Any spot of light on the retina of the observed eye projects to a focal spot on the retina of the observing eye. Thus, if the retina of one person is made to emit light, the image of his or her retina will be focused on the retina of the observer, provided the two eyes are emmetropic and are simply looking into each other.

If the refractive power of either the observed eye or the observer's eye is abnormal, it is necessary to correct the refractive power for the observer to see a sharp image of the observed retina. The usual ophthalmoscope has a series of very small lenses mounted on a turret so that the turret can be rotated from one lens to another until the correction for abnormal refraction is made by selecting a lens of appropriate strength. In normal young adults, natural accommodative reflexes occur, causing an approximate +2-D increase in strength of the lens of each eye. To correct for this, it is necessary that the lens turret be rotated to approximately −4-D correction.

Fluid System of the Eye—Intraocular Fluid

The eye is filled with *intraocular fluid*, which maintains sufficient pressure in the eyeball to keep it distended. Figure 108-18 demonstrates that this fluid can be divided into two portions—*aqueous humor*, which lies in front of the lens, and *vitreous humor*, which is between the posterior surface of the lens and the retina. The aqueous humor is a freely flowing fluid, whereas the vitreous humor, sometimes called the *vitreous body*, is a gelatinous mass held together by a fine fibrillar network composed primarily of greatly elongated proteoglycan molecules. Both water and dissolved substances can *diffuse* slowly in the vitreous humor, but there is little *flow* of fluid.

Aqueous humor is continually being formed and reabsorbed. The balance between formation and reabsorption of aqueous

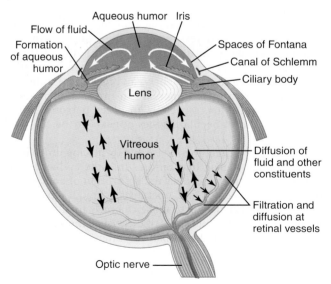

Figure 108-18 Formation and flow of fluid in the eye.

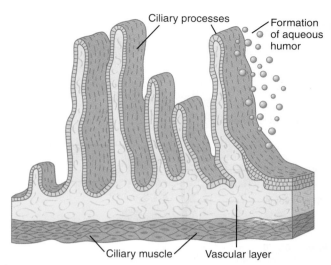

Figure 108-19 Anatomy of the ciliary processes. Aqueous humor is formed on surfaces.

humor regulates the total volume and pressure of the intraocular fluid.

FORMATION OF AQUEOUS HUMOR BY THE CILIARY BODY

Aqueous humor is formed in the eye *at an average rate of 2–3 μL each minute*. Essentially all of it is secreted by the *ciliary processes*, which are linear folds projecting from the *ciliary body* into the space behind the iris where the lens ligaments and ciliary muscle attach to the eyeball. A cross-section of these ciliary processes is shown in Figure 108-19, and their relation to the fluid chambers of the eye can be seen in Figure 108-18. Because of their folded architecture, the total surface area of the ciliary processes is about 6 cm^2 in each eye—a large area, considering the small size of the ciliary body. The surfaces of these processes are covered by highly secretory epithelial cells, and immediately beneath them is a highly vascular area.

Aqueous humor is formed almost entirely as an active secretion by the epithelium of the ciliary processes. Secretion begins with active transport of sodium ions into the spaces between the epithelial cells. The sodium ions pull chloride and bicarbonate ions along with them to maintain electrical neutrality. Then all these ions together cause osmosis of water from the blood capillaries lying below into the same epithelial intercellular spaces, and the resulting solution washes from the spaces of the ciliary processes into the anterior chamber of the eye. In addition, several nutrients are transported across the epithelium by active transport or facilitated diffusion; they include amino acids, ascorbic acid, and glucose.

OUTFLOW OF AQUEOUS HUMOR FROM THE EYE

After aqueous humor is formed by the ciliary processes, it first flows, as shown in Figure 108-18, *through the pupil into the anterior chamber of the eye*. From here, the fluid flows *anterior to the lens* and into the *angle between the cornea and the iris*, then through a meshwork of *trabeculae*, finally entering the *canal of Schlemm*, which empties into extraocular veins. Figure 108-20 demonstrates the anatomical structures at this iridocorneal

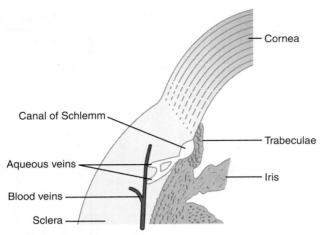

Figure 108-20 Anatomy of the iridocorneal angle, showing the system for outflow of aqueous humor from the eyeball into the conjunctival veins.

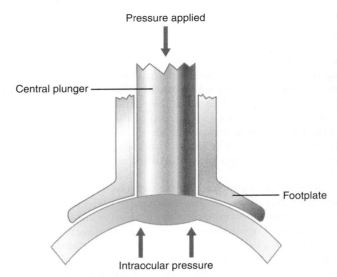

Figure 108-21 Principles of the tonometer.

angle, showing that the spaces between the trabeculae extend all the way from the anterior chamber to the canal of Schlemm. The canal of Schlemm is a thin-walled vein that extends circumferentially all the way around the eye. Its endothelial membrane is so porous that even large protein molecules, as well as small particulate matter up to the size of red blood cells, can pass from the anterior chamber into the canal of Schlemm. Even though the canal of Schlemm is actually a venous blood vessel, so much aqueous humor normally flows into it that it is filled only with aqueous humor rather than with blood. The small veins that lead from the canal of Schlemm to the larger veins of the eye usually contain only aqueous humor, and they are called *aqueous veins.*

INTRAOCULAR PRESSURE

The average normal intraocular pressure is about 15 mmHg, with a range from 12 to 20 mmHg.

Measuring Intraocular Pressure by Tonometry. Because it is impractical to pass a needle into a patient's eye to measure intraocular pressure, this pressure is measured clinically by using a "tonometer," the principle of which is shown in Figure 108-21. The cornea of the eye is anesthetized with a local anesthetic, and the footplate of the tonometer is placed on the cornea. A small force is then applied to a central plunger, causing the part of the cornea beneath the plunger to be displaced inward. The amount of displacement is recorded on the scale of the tonometer, and this is calibrated in terms of intraocular pressure.

Regulation of Intraocular Pressure. Intraocular pressure remains constant in the normal eye, usually within ±2 mmHg of its normal level, which averages about 15 mmHg. The level of this pressure is determined mainly by the resistance to outflow of aqueous humor from the anterior chamber into the canal of Schlemm. This outflow resistance results from the meshwork of trabeculae through which the fluid must percolate on its way from the lateral angles of the anterior chamber to the wall of the canal of Schlemm. These trabeculae have minute openings of only 2–3 μm. The rate of fluid flow into the canal increases markedly as the pressure rises. At

about 15 mmHg in the normal eye, the amount of fluid leaving the eye by way of the canal of Schlemm usually averages 2.5 μL/minute and equals the inflow of fluid from the ciliary body. The pressure normally remains at about this level of 15 mmHg.

"Glaucoma"— Causes High Intraocular Pressure and Is a Principal Cause of Blindness. Glaucoma is one of the most common causes of blindness. It is a disease of the eye in which the intraocular pressure becomes pathologically high, sometimes rising acutely to 60–70 mmHg. Pressures above 25–30 mmHg can cause loss of vision when maintained for long periods. Extremely high pressures can cause blindness within days or even hours. As the pressure rises, the axons of the optic nerve are compressed where they leave the eyeball at the optic disc. This compression is believed to block axonal flow of cytoplasm from the retinal neuronal cell bodies into the optic nerve fibers leading to the brain. The result is lack of appropriate nutrition of the fibers, which eventually causes death of the involved fibers. It is possible that compression of the retinal artery, which enters the eyeball at the optic disc, also adds to the neuronal damage by reducing nutrition to the retina.

In most cases of glaucoma, the abnormally high pressure results from increased resistance to fluid outflow through the trabecular spaces into the canal of Schlemm at the iridocorneal junction. For instance, in acute eye inflammation, white blood cells and tissue debris can block these trabecular spaces and cause an acute increase in intraocular pressure. In chronic conditions, especially in older persons, fibrous occlusion of the trabecular spaces appears to be the likely culprit.

Glaucoma can sometimes be treated by placing drops in the eye that contain a drug that diffuses into the eyeball and reduces the secretion or increases the absorption of aqueous humor. When drug therapy fails, operative techniques to open the spaces of the trabeculae or to make channels to allow fluid to flow directly from the fluid space of the eyeball into the subconjunctival space outside the eyeball can often effectively reduce the pressure.

BIBLIOGRAPHY

Buznego C, Trattler WB: Presbyopia-correcting intraocular lenses, *Curr. Opin. Ophthalmol.* 20:13, 2009.

Candia OA, Alvarez LJ: Fluid transport phenomena in ocular epithelia, *Prog. Retin. Eye Res.* 27:197, 2008.

Congdon NG, Friedman DS, Lietman T: Important causes of visual impairment in the world today, *JAMA* 290:2057, 2003.

De Groef L, Van Hove I, Dekeyster E, et al: MMPs in the trabecular meshwork: promising targets for future glaucoma therapies? *Invest. Ophthalmol. Vis. Sci.* 54:7756, 2013.

Khaw PT, Shah P, Elkington AR: Glaucoma—1: diagnosis, *BMJ* 328:97, 2004.

Krag S, Andreassen TT: Mechanical properties of the human lens capsule, *Prog. Retin. Eye Res.* 22:749, 2003.

Kwon YH, Fingert JH, Kuehn MH, et al: Primary open-angle glaucoma, *N. Engl. J. Med.* 360:1113, 2009.

Mathias RT, Rae JL, Baldo GJ: Physiological properties of the normal lens, *Physiol. Rev.* 77:21, 1997.

Schwartz K, Budenz D: Current management of glaucoma, *Curr. Opin. Ophthalmol.* 15:119, 2004.

Smith G: The optical properties of the crystalline lens and their significance, *Clin. Exp. Optom.* 86:3, 2003.

Tan JC, Peters DM, Kaufman PL: Recent developments in understanding the pathophysiology of elevated intraocular pressure, *Curr. Opin. Ophthalmol.* 17:168, 2006.

Weinreb RN, Aung T, Medeiros FA: The pathophysiology and treatment of glaucoma: a review, *JAMA* 311:1901, 2014.

109

The Retina

The retina is the light-sensitive portion of the eye that contains (1) the *cones*, which are responsible for color vision, and (2) the *rods*, which can detect dim light and are mainly responsible for black and white vision, and vision in the dark. When either rods or cones are excited, signals are transmitted first through successive layers of neurons in the retina and, finally, into optic nerve fibers and the cerebral cortex. Under low-light conditions, vision is mainly served by the rods and this is called scotopic vision. Under well-lit conditions, the cones primarily serve vision, when color can easily be discriminated; this is called photopic vision. In this chapter we explain the mechanisms by which the rods and cones detect light and color and convert the visual image into optic nerve signals.

Anatomy and Function of the Structural Elements of the Retina

Layers of the Retina. Figure 109-1A shows the functional components of the retina, which are arranged in layers from the outside to the inside as follows: (1) pigmented layer, (2) layer of rods and cones projecting to the pigment, (3) outer nuclear layer containing the cell bodies of the rods and cones, (4) outer plexiform layer, (5) inner nuclear layer, (6) inner plexiform layer, (7) ganglionic layer, (8) layer of optic nerve fibers, and

(9) inner limiting membrane. These are represented in a simple manner in Figure 109-1B.

After light passes through the lens system of the eye and then through the vitreous humor, it *enters the retina from the inside of the eye* (see Figure 109-1); that is, it passes first through the ganglion cells and then through the plexiform and nuclear layers before it finally reaches the layer of rods and cones located all the way on the outer edge of the retina. This distance is a thickness of several hundred micrometers; visual acuity is decreased by this passage through such nonhomogeneous tissue. However, in the *central foveal region of the retina*, as discussed subsequently, the inside layers are pulled aside to decrease this loss of acuity.

Foveal Region of the Retina and its Importance in Acute Vision. The *fovea* is a minute area in the center of the retina, shown in Figure 109-2, occupying a total area a little more than 1 mm^2; it is especially capable of acute and detailed vision. The *central fovea*, only 0.3 mm in diameter, is composed almost entirely of cones. These cones have a special structure that aids their detection of detail in the visual image that is, the foveal cones have especially long and slender bodies, in contradistinction to the much fatter cones located more peripherally in the retina. Also, in the foveal region the blood vessels, ganglion cells, inner nuclear layer of cells, and plexiform layers are all displaced to one side rather than resting directly on top of the cones which allows light to pass unimpeded to the cones.

Rods and Cones. Figure 109-3 is a diagrammatic representation of the essential components of a photoreceptor (either a rod or a cone). As shown in Figure 109-4, the outer segment of the cone is conical in shape. In general, the rods are narrower and longer than the cones, but this is not always the case. In the peripheral portions of the retina, the rods are 2–5 μm in diameter, whereas the cones are 5–8 μm in diameter; in the central part of the retina, in the fovea, there are rods, and the cones are slender and have a diameter of only 1.5 μm.

The major functional segments of either a rod or a cone are shown in Figure 109-3: (1) the *outer segment*, (2) the *inner segment*, (3) the *nucleus*, and (4) the *synaptic body*. The light-sensitive photochemical is found in the outer segment. In the case of the rods, this photochemical is *rhodopsin*; in the cones, it is one of the three "color" photochemicals, usually called simply *color pigments*, which functions almost exactly the same as rhodopsin except for differences in spectral sensitivity.

Note the large numbers of *discs* in the *outer segments* of the rods and cones in Figures 109-3 and 109-4. Each disc is actually an infolded shelf of cell membrane. There are as many as 1000 discs in each rod or cone.

Both rhodopsin and the color pigments are conjugated proteins. They are incorporated into the membranes of the discs in the form of transmembrane proteins. The concentrations of these photosensitive pigments in the discs are so great that the pigments themselves constitute about 40% of the entire mass of the outer segment.

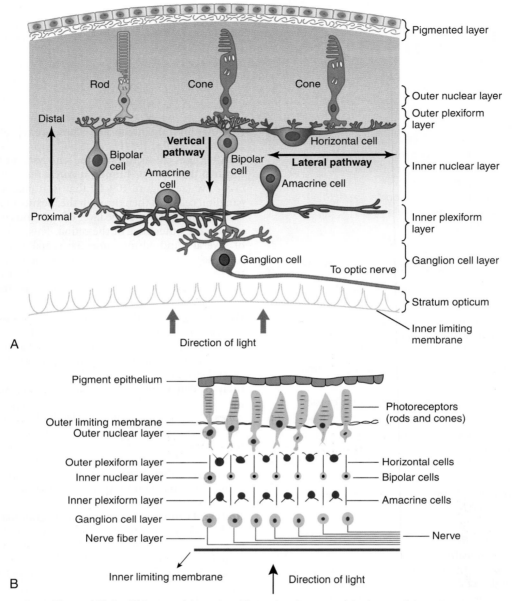

Pigmented layer

Rod

Cone

Cone

Outer nuclear layer

Distal

Outer plexiform layer

Vertical pathway

Horizontal cell

Bipolar cell

Bipolar cell

Lateral pathway

Inner nuclear layer

Amacrine cell

Amacrine cell

Proximal

Inner plexiform layer

Ganglion cell

Ganglion cell layer

To optic nerve

Stratum opticum

Inner limiting membrane

A

Direction of light

Pigment epithelium

Photoreceptors (rods and cones)

Outer limiting membrane
Outer nuclear layer

Outer plexiform layer

Horizontal cells

Inner nuclear layer

Bipolar cells

Inner plexiform layer

Amacrine cells

Ganglion cell layer

Nerve fiber layer

Nerve

Inner limiting membrane

Direction of light

B

Figure 109-1   (A) Layers of the retina; (B) simple schematic of the layers of the retina.

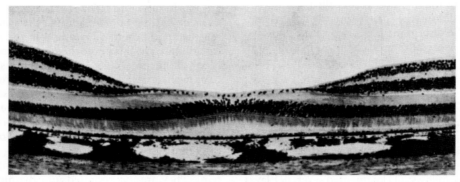

Figure 109-2   Photomicrograph of the macula and of the fovea in its center. Note that the inner layers of the retina are pulled to the side to decrease interference with light transmission. *From Fawcett, D.W., 1986. Bloom and Fawcett: A Textbook of Histology, 11th ed. W.B. Saunders, Philadelphia; courtesy H. Mizoguchi.*

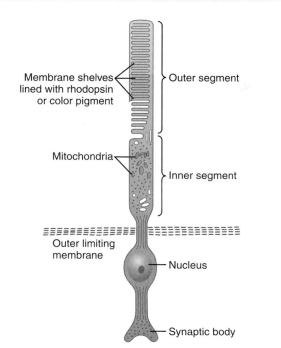

Figure 109-3 Schematic drawing of the functional parts of the rods and cones.

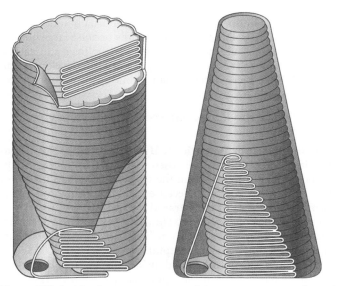

Figure 109-4 Membranous structures of the outer segments of a rod (*left*) and a cone (*right*). *Courtesy Dr. Richard Young.*

The *inner segment* of the rod or cone contains the usual cytoplasm with cytoplasmic organelles. Especially important are the mitochondria, which, as explained later, play the important role of providing energy for function of the photoreceptors.

The *synaptic body* is the portion of the rod or cone that connects with subsequent neuronal cells, the *horizontal* and *bipolar cells*, which represent the next stages in the vision chain.

Pigment Layer of the Retina. The black pigment *melanin* in the pigment layer prevents light reflection throughout the globe of the eyeball which is extremely important for clear vision. This pigment performs the same function in the eye as the black coloring inside the bellows of a camera. Without it, light rays

would be reflected in all directions within the eyeball and would cause diffuse lighting of the retina rather than the normal contrast between dark and light spots required for formation of precise images.

The importance of melanin in the pigment layer is well illustrated by its absence in *albinos*, people who are hereditarily lacking in melanin pigment in all parts of their bodies. When an albino enters a bright room, light that impinges on the retina is reflected in all directions inside the eyeball by the unpigmented surfaces of the retina and by the underlying sclera, so a single discrete spot of light that would normally excite only a few rods or cones is reflected everywhere and excites many receptors. Therefore, the visual acuity of albinos, even with the best optical correction, is seldom better than 20/100 to 20/200 rather than the normal 20/20 values.

The pigment layer also stores large quantities of *vitamin A*. This vitamin A is exchanged back and forth through the cell membranes of the outer segments of the rods and cones, which themselves are embedded in the pigment. We show later that vitamin A is an important precursor of the photosensitive chemicals of the rods and cones.

Blood Supply of the Retina—The Central Retinal Artery and the Choroid. The nutrient blood supply for the internal layers of the retina is derived from the central retinal artery, which enters the eyeball through the center of the optic nerve and then divides *to supply the entire inside retinal surface.* Thus, the inner layers of the retina have their own blood supply independent of the other structures of the eye.

However, the outermost layer of the retina is adherent to the *choroid,* which is also a highly vascular tissue lying between the retina and the sclera. The outer layers of the retina, especially the outer segments of the rods and cones, depend mainly on diffusion from the choroid blood vessels for their nutrition, especially for their oxygen.

Retinal Detachment. The neural retina occasionally *detaches from the pigment epithelium.* In some instances, the cause of such detachment is injury to the eyeball that allows fluid or blood to collect between the neural retina and the pigment epithelium. Detachment is occasionally caused by contracture of fine collagenous fibrils in the vitreous humor, which pull areas of the retina toward the interior of the globe.

Partly because of diffusion across the detachment gap and partly because of the independent blood supply to the neural retina through the retinal artery, the detached retina can resist degeneration for days and can become functional again if it is surgically replaced in its normal relation with the pigment epithelium. If it is not replaced soon, however, the retina will be destroyed and will be unable to function even after surgical repair.

Photochemistry of Vision

Both rods and cones contain chemicals that decompose on exposure to light and, in the process, excite the nerve fibers leading from the eye. The light-sensitive chemical in the *rods* is called *rhodopsin;* the light-sensitive chemicals in the *cones,* called *cone pigments* or *color pigments,* have compositions only slightly different from that of rhodopsin.

In this section, we discuss principally the photochemistry of rhodopsin, but the same principles can be applied to the cone pigments.

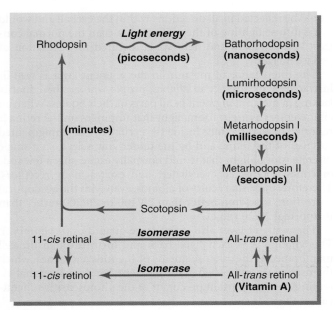

Figure 109-5 Rhodopsin–retinal visual cycle in the rod, showing decomposition of rhodopsin during exposure to light and subsequent slow re-formation of rhodopsin by the chemical processes.

RHODOPSIN–RETINAL VISUAL CYCLE, AND EXCITATION OF THE RODS

Rhodopsin and its Decomposition by Light Energy. The outer segment of the rod that projects into the pigment layer of the retina has a concentration of about 40% of the light-sensitive pigment called *rhodopsin* or *visual purple*. This substance is a combination of the protein *scotopsin* and the carotenoid pigment *retinal* (also called "retinene"). Furthermore, the retinal is a particular type called 11-*cis* retinal. This *cis* form of retinal is important because only this form can bind with scotopsin to synthesize rhodopsin.

When light energy is absorbed by rhodopsin, the rhodopsin begins to decompose within a very small fraction of a second, as shown at the top of Figure 109-5. The cause of this rapid decomposition is photoactivation of electrons in the retinal portion of the rhodopsin, which leads to instantaneous change of the *cis* form of retinal into an all-*trans* form that has the same chemical structure as the *cis* form but a different physical structure—it is a straight molecule rather than an angulated molecule. Because the three-dimensional orientation of the reactive sites of the all-*trans* retinal no longer fits with the orientation of the reactive sites on the protein *scotopsin*, the all-*trans* retinal begins to pull away from the scotopsin. The immediate product is *bathorhodopsin*, which is a partially split combination of the all-*trans* retinal and scotopsin. Bathorhodopsin is extremely unstable and decays in nanoseconds to *lumirhodopsin*. This product then decays in microseconds to *metarhodopsin I*, then in about a millisecond to *metarhodopsin II*, and finally, much more slowly (in seconds), into the completely split products *scotopsin* and all-*trans* retinal.

It is the metarhodopsin II, also called *activated rhodopsin*, that excites electrical changes in the rods, and the rods then transmit the visual image into the central nervous system in the form of optic nerve action potential, as we discuss later.

Re-formation of Rhodopsin. The first stage in re-formation of rhodopsin, as shown in Figure 109-5, is to reconvert the all-*trans* retinal into 11-*cis* retinal. This process requires metabolic energy

and is catalyzed by the enzyme *retinal isomerase*. Once the 11-*cis* retinal is formed, it automatically recombines with the scotopsin to re-form rhodopsin, which then remains stable until its decomposition is again triggered by absorption of light energy.

Role of Vitamin A for Formation of Rhodopsin. Note in Figure 109-5 that there is a second chemical route by which all-*trans* retinal can be converted into 11-*cis* retinal. This second route is by conversion of the all-*trans* retinal first into all-*trans* retinol, which is one form of vitamin A. Then the all-*trans* retinol is converted into 11-*cis* retinol under the influence of the enzyme isomerase. Finally, the 11-*cis* retinol is converted into 11-*cis* retinal, which combines with scotopsin to form new rhodopsin.

Vitamin A is present both in the cytoplasm of the rods and in the pigment layer of the retina. Therefore, vitamin A is normally always available to form new retinal when needed. Conversely, when there is excess retinal in the retina, it is converted back into vitamin A, thus reducing the amount of light-sensitive pigment in the retina. We shall see later that this interconversion between retinal and vitamin A is especially important in long-term adaptation of the retina to different light intensities.

Night Blindness. Night blindness occurs in persons with severe vitamin A deficiency because without vitamin A, the amounts of retinal and rhodopsin that can be formed are severely depressed. This condition is called *night blindness* because the amount of light available at night is too little to permit adequate vision in vitamin A–deficient persons.

For night blindness to occur, a person usually must remain on a vitamin A–deficient diet for months because large quantities of vitamin A are normally stored in the liver and can be made available to the eyes. Once night blindness develops, it can sometimes be reversed in less than 1 hour by intravenous injection of vitamin A.

Excitation of the Rod when Rhodopsin Is Activated by Light

The Rod Receptor Potential Is Hyperpolarizing, Not Depolarizing. When the rod is exposed to light, the resulting receptor potential is different from the receptor potentials in almost all other sensory receptors because excitation of the rod causes *increased negativity* of the intrarod membrane potential, which is a state of *hyperpolarization,*. This is exactly opposite to the decreased negativity (the process of "depolarization") that occurs in almost all other sensory receptors.

How does activation of rhodopsin cause hyperpolarization? The answer is that *when rhodopsin decomposes, it decreases the rod membrane conductance for sodium ions in the outer segment of the rod.* This causes hyperpolarization of the entire rod membrane in the following way.

Figure 109-6 shows movement of sodium and potassium ions in a complete electrical circuit through the inner and outer segments of the rod. The inner segment continually pumps sodium from inside the rod to the outside and potassium ions are pumped to the inside of the cell. Potassium ions leak out of the cell through nongated potassium channels that are confined to the inner segment of the rod. As in other cells, this sodium–potassium pump creates a negative potential on the inside of the entire cell. However, the outer segment of the rod, where the photoreceptor discs are located, is entirely different; here, the rod membrane, in the *dark* state, is leaky to sodium ions that flow through cyclic guanosine monophosphate (cGMP)–gated channels. In the dark state, cGMP levels are high, permitting

A

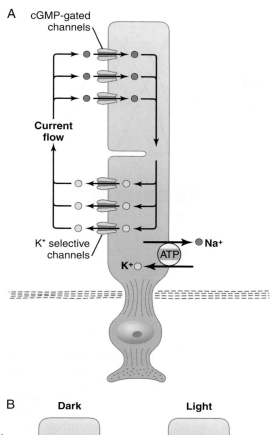

Figure 109-6 (A) Sodium flows into a photoreceptor (eg, rod) through cGMP-gated channels. Potassium flows out of the cell through nongated potassium channels. A sodium–potassium pump maintains steady levels of sodium and potassium inside the cell. (B) In the dark, cGMP levels are high and the sodium channels are open. In the light, cGMP levels are reduced and the sodium channels close, causing the cell to hyperpolarize. *ATP*, adenosine triphosphate; *cGMP*, cyclic guanosine monophosphate.

B

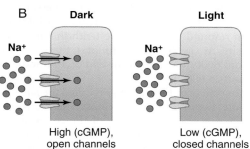

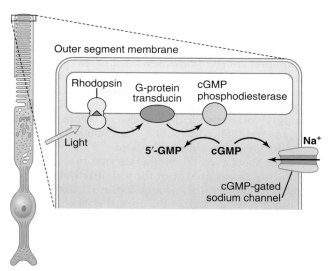

Figure 109-7 Phototransduction in the outer segment of the photoreceptor (rod or cone) membrane. When light hits the photoreceptor (eg, rod cell), the light-absorbing retinal portion of rhodopsin is activated. This stimulates transducin, a G-protein, which then activates cGMP phosphodiesterase. This enzyme catalyzes the degradation of cGMP into 5'-GMP. The reduction in cGMP then causes closure of the sodium channels, which, in turn, causes hyperpolarization of the photoreceptor. *cGMP*, cyclic guanosine monophosphate.

the reduction in cGMP closes the cGMP-gated sodium channels and reduces the inward sodium current. Sodium ions continue to be pumped outward through the membrane of the inner segment. Thus, more sodium ions now leave the rod than leak back in. Because they are positive ions, their loss from inside the rod creates increased negativity inside the membrane, and the greater the amount of light energy striking the rod, the greater the electronegativity becomes—that is, the greater is the degree of *hyperpolarization*. At maximum light intensity, the membrane potential approaches −70 to −80 mV, which is near the equilibrium potential for potassium ions across the membrane.

Mechanism by which Rhodopsin Decomposition Decreases Membrane Sodium Conductance—The Excitation "Cascade". Under optimal conditions, a single photon of light, the smallest possible quantal unit of light energy, can cause a receptor potential of about 1 mV in a rod. Only 30 photons of light will cause half saturation of the rod. How can such a small amount of light cause such great excitation? The answer is that the photoreceptors have an extremely sensitive chemical cascade that amplifies the stimulatory effects about a millionfold, as follows:

1. The *photon activates an electron* in the 11-*cis* retinal portion of the rhodopsin; this activation leads to the formation of *metarhodopsin II*, which is the active form of rhodopsin, as already discussed and shown in Figure 109-5.
2. The *activated rhodopsin* functions as an enzyme to activate many molecules of *transducin*, a protein present in an inactive form in the membranes of the discs and cell membrane of the rod.
3. The *activated transducin* activates many more molecules of *phosphodiesterase*.
4. *Activated phosphodiesterase* is another enzyme; it immediately hydrolyzes many molecules of *cGMP*, thus destroying it. Before being destroyed, the cGMP had been bound with the sodium channel protein of the rod's outer

positively charged sodium ions to continually leak back to the inside of the rod and thereby neutralize much of the negativity on the inside of the entire cell. Thus, *under normal dark conditions, when the rod is not excited, there is reduced electronegativity* inside the membrane of the rod, measuring about −40 mV rather than the usual −70 to −80 mV found in most sensory receptors.

When the rhodopsin in the outer segment of the rod is exposed to light, it is activated and begins to decompose. The cGMP-gated sodium channels are then closed, and the outer segment membrane conductance of sodium to the interior of the rod is reduced by a three-step process (Figure 109-7): (1) light is absorbed by the rhodopsin, causing photoactivation of the electrons in the retinal portion, as previously described; (2) the activated rhodopsin stimulates a G-protein called *transducin*, which then activates cGMP phosphodiesterase (an enzyme that catalyzes the breakdown of cGMP to 5'-cGMP); and (3)

membrane in a way that "splints" it in the open state. However in light, hydrolyzation of the cGMP by phosphodiesterase this removes the splinting and allows the sodium channels to close. Several hundred channels close for each originally activated molecule of rhodopsin. Because the sodium flux through each of these channels has been extremely rapid, flow of more than a million sodium ions is blocked by the channel closure before the channel opens again. This diminution of sodium ion flow is what excites the rod, as already discussed.

5. Within about a second, another enzyme, *rhodopsin kinase*, which is always present in the rod, inactivates the activated rhodopsin (the metarhodopsin II), and the entire cascade reverses back to the normal state with open sodium channels.

Thus, the rods have developed an important chemical cascade that amplifies the effect of a single photon of light to cause movement of millions of sodium ions. This mechanism explains the extreme sensitivity of the rods under dark conditions.

The cones are about 30–300 times less sensitive than the rods, but even this degree of sensitivity allows color vision at any intensity of light greater than extremely dim twilight.

Photochemistry of Color Vision by the Cones

We previously was pointed out that the photochemicals in the cones have almost exactly the same chemical composition as that of rhodopsin in the rods. The only difference is that the protein portions, or the opsins—called *photopsins* in the cones—are slightly different from the scotopsin of the rods. The *retinal* portion of all the visual pigments is exactly the same in the cones as in the rods. The color-sensitive pigments of the cones, therefore, are combinations of retinal and photopsins.

In the discussion of color vision later in the chapter, it will become evident that only one of three types of color pigments is present in each of the different cones, thus making the cones selectively sensitive to different colors: blue, green, or red. These color pigments are called, respectively, *blue-sensitive pigment*, *green-sensitive pigment*, and *red-sensitive pigment*. The absorption characteristics of the pigments in the three types of cones show peak absorbencies at light wavelengths of 445, 535, and 570 nm, respectively. These wavelengths are also the wavelengths for peak light sensitivity for each type of cone, which begins to explain how the retina differentiates the colors. The approximate absorption curves for these three pigments are shown in Figure 109-8. Also shown is the absorption curve for the rhodopsin of the rods, with a peak at 505 nm.

AUTOMATIC REGULATION OF RETINAL SENSITIVITY—LIGHT AND DARK ADAPTATION

If a person has been in bright light for hours, large portions of the photochemicals in both the rods and the cones will have been reduced to retinal and opsins. Furthermore, much of the retinal of both the rods and the cones will have been converted into vitamin A. Because of these two effects, the concentrations of the photosensitive chemicals remaining in the rods and cones are considerably reduced, and the sensitivity of the eye to light is correspondingly reduced. This process is called *light adaptation*.

Conversely, if a person remains in darkness for a long time, the retinal and opsins in the rods and cones are converted back into the light-sensitive pigments. Furthermore, vitamin A is converted back into retinal to increase light-sensitive pigments, the final limit being determined by the amount of opsins in

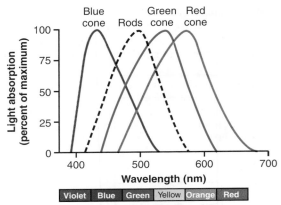

Figure 109-8 Light absorption by the pigment of the rods and by the pigments of the three color-receptive cones of the human retina. *Data from curves recorded by Marks, W.B., Dobelle, W.H., MacNichol Jr., E.F. 1964. Visual pigments of single primate cones. Science 143, 1181, and by Brown, P.K., Wald, G., 1964. Visual pigments in single rods and cones of the human retina: direct measurements reveal mechanisms of human night and color vision. Science 144, 45. American Association for the Advancement of Science.*

the rods and cones to combine with the retinal. This process is called *dark adaptation*.

Figure 109-9 shows the course of dark adaptation when a person is exposed to total darkness after having been exposed to bright light for several hours. Note that the sensitivity of the retina is very low upon first entering the darkness, but within 1 minute the sensitivity has already increased 10-fold—that is, the retina can respond to light of one-tenth the previously required intensity. At the end of 20 minutes, the sensitivity has increased about 6000-fold, and at the end of 40 minutes, it has increased about 25,000-fold.

The resulting curve of Figure 109-9 is called the *dark adaptation curve*. Note, the inflection in the curve. The early portion of the curve is caused by adaptation of the cones because all the chemical events of vision, including adaptation, occur about four times as rapidly in cones as in rods. However, the cones do not achieve anywhere near the same degree of sensitivity change in darkness as the rods do. Therefore, despite rapid adaptation, the cones cease adapting after only a few minutes, whereas the slowly adapting rods continue to adapt for many minutes and

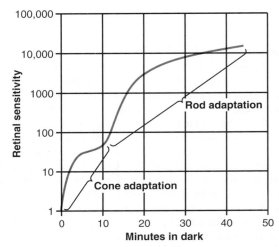

Figure 109-9 Dark adaptation, demonstrating the relation of cone adaptation to rod adaptation.

even hours, with their sensitivity increasing tremendously. Additionally sensitivity of the rods is caused by neuronal signal convergence of 100 or more rods onto a single ganglion cell in the retina; these rods summate to increase their sensitivity, as discussed later in the chapter.

Other Mechanisms of Light and Dark Adaptation. In addition to adaptation caused by changes in concentrations of rhodopsin or color photochemicals, the eye has two other mechanisms for light and dark adaptation. The first is a *change in pupillary size,* as discussed in Chapter 108. This change can cause adaptation of approximately 30-fold within a fraction of a second because of changes in the amount of light allowed through the pupillary opening.

The other mechanism is *neural adaptation,* involving the neurons in the successive stages of the visual chain in the retina itself and in the brain. That is, when light intensity first increases, the signals transmitted by the bipolar cells, horizontal cells, amacrine cells, and ganglion cells are all intense. However, most of these signals decrease rapidly at different stages of transmission in the neural circuit. Although the degree of adaptation is only a fewfold rather than the many thousandfold that occurs during adaptation of the photochemical system, neural adaptation occurs in a fraction of a second, in contrast to the many minutes to hours required for full adaptation by the photochemicals.

Color Vision

From the preceding sections, we learned that different cones are sensitive to different colors of light. This section is a discussion of the mechanisms by which the retina detects the different gradations of color in the visual spectrum.

TRICOLOR MECHANISM OF COLOR DETECTION

All theories of color vision are based on the well-known observation that the human eye can detect almost all gradations of colors when only red, green, and blue monochromatic lights are appropriately mixed in different combinations. The wavelengths of these colors are 700, 530, and 470 nm, respectively, although a range exists (see Figure 109-8).

Spectral Sensitivities of the Three Types of Cones. On the basis of color vision tests, the spectral sensitivities of the three types of cones in humans have proved to be essentially the same as the light absorption curves for the three types of pigment found in the cones. These curves are shown in Figure 109-8 and slightly differently in Figure 109-10. They can explain most of the phenomena of color vision.

Interpretation of Color in the Nervous System. In Figure 109-10, one can see that an orange monochromatic light with a wavelength of 580 nm stimulates the red cones to a value of about 99 (99% of the peak stimulation at optimum wavelength); it stimulates the green cones to a value of about 42, but the blue cones are not stimulated at all. Thus, the ratios of stimulation of the three types of cones in this instance are 99:42:0. The nervous system interprets this set of ratios as the sensation of orange. Conversely, a monochromatic blue light with a wavelength of 450 nm stimulates the red cones to a stimulus value of 0, the green cones to a value of 0, and the blue cones to a value of 97. This set of ratios—0:0:97—is interpreted by the nervous system as blue. Likewise, ratios of 83:83:0 are interpreted as yellow, and ratios of 31:67:36 are interpreted as green.

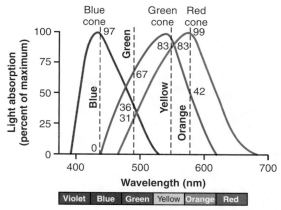

Figure 109-10 Demonstration of the degree of stimulation of the different color-sensitive cones by monochromatic lights of four colors: blue, green, yellow, and orange.

Perception of White Light. About equal stimulation of all the red, green, and blue cones gives one the sensation of seeing white. Yet there is no single wavelength of light corresponding to white; instead, white is a combination of all the wavelengths of the spectrum. Furthermore, the perception of white can be achieved by stimulating the retina with a proper combination of only three chosen colors that stimulate the respective types of cones about equally.

COLOR BLINDNESS

Red–Green Color Blindness. When a single group of color-receptive cones is missing from the eye, the person is unable to distinguish some colors from others. For instance, one can see in Figure 109-10 that green, yellow, orange, and red colors, which are the colors between the wavelengths of 525 and 675 nm, are normally distinguished from one another by the red and green cones. If either of these two cones is missing, the person cannot use this mechanism for distinguishing these four colors; the person is especially unable to distinguish red from green and is therefore said to have *red–green color blindness.*

A person with loss of red cones is called a *protanope;* the overall visual spectrum is noticeably shortened at the long-wavelength end because of a lack of the red cones. A color-blind person who lacks green cones is called a *deuteranope;* this person has a perfectly normal visual spectral width because red cones are available to detect the long-wavelength red color.

Red–green color blindness is a genetic disorder that occurs almost exclusively in males. That is, genes in the female X chromosome code for the respective cones. Yet color blindness almost never occurs in females because at least one of the two X chromosomes almost always has a normal gene for each type of cone. Because the male has only one X chromosome, a missing gene can lead to color blindness.

Because the X chromosome in the male is always inherited from the mother, never from the father, color blindness is passed from mother to son, and the mother is said to be a *color blindness carrier;* about 8% of all women are color blindness carriers.

Blue Weakness. Only rarely are blue cones missing, although sometimes they are underrepresented, which is a genetically inherited condition giving rise to the phenomenon called *blue weakness.*

Color Test Charts. A rapid method for determining color blindness is based on the use of spot charts such as those shown

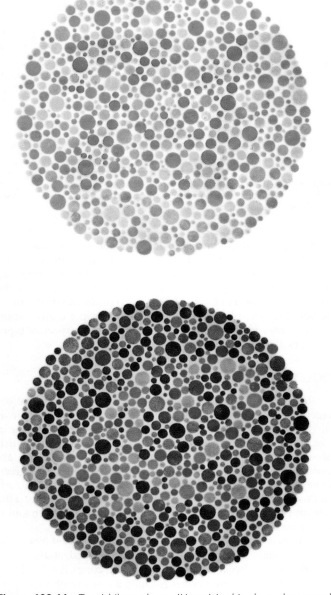

Figure 109-11   Two Ishihara charts. (*Upper*) In this chart, the normal person reads "74," but the red–green color-blind person reads "21." (*Lower*) In this chart, the red-blind person (protanope) reads "2," but the green-blind person (deuteranope) reads "4." The normal person reads "42." *From Ishihara's Tests for Colour Blindness. Kanehara & Co., Tokyo, but tests for color blindness cannot be conducted with this material. For accurate testing, the original plates should be used.*

in Figure 109-11. These charts are arranged with a confusion of spots of several different colors. In the top chart, a person with normal color vision reads "74," whereas the red–green color-blind person reads "21." In the bottom chart, a person with normal color vision reads "42," whereas a red-blind person reads "2," and a green-blind person reads "4."

If one studies these charts while at the same time observing the spectral sensitivity curves of the different cones depicted in Figure 109-10, it can be readily understood how excessive emphasis can be placed on spots of certain colors by color-blind people.

Neural Function of the Retina

Figure 109-12 presents the essentials of the retina's neural connections, showing at the left the circuit in the peripheral retina and at the right the circuit in the foveal retina. The different neuronal cell types are as follows:

1. the photoreceptors—the *rods* and *cones*—which transmit signals to the outer plexiform layer, where they synapse with bipolar cells and horizontal cells;
2. the *horizontal cells*, which transmit signals horizontally in the outer plexiform layer from the rods and cones to bipolar cells;
3. the *bipolar cells*, which transmit signals vertically from the rods, cones, and horizontal cells to the inner plexiform layer, where they synapse with ganglion cells and amacrine cells;
4. the *amacrine cells*, which transmit signals in two directions, either directly from bipolar cells to ganglion cells or horizontally within the inner plexiform layer from axons of the bipolar cells to dendrites of the ganglion cells or to other amacrine cells;
5. the *ganglion cells*, which transmit output signals from the retina through the optic nerve into the brain.

A sixth type of neuronal cell in the retina, which is not very prominent and is not shown in the figure, is the *interplexiform* cell. This cell transmits signals in the retrograde direction from the inner plexiform layer to the outer plexiform layer. These signals are inhibitory and are believed to control lateral spread of visual signals by the horizontal cells in the outer plexiform layer. Their role may be to help control the degree of contrast in the visual image.

The Visual Pathway from the Cones to the Ganglion Cells Functions Differently from the Rod Pathway. As is true for many of our other sensory systems, the retina has both an old type of vision based on rod vision and a new type of vision based on cone vision. The neurons and nerve fibers that conduct the visual signals for cone vision are considerably larger than those that conduct the visual signals for rod vision, and the signals are conducted to the brain two to five times as rapidly. Also, the circuitry for the two systems is slightly different, as follows.

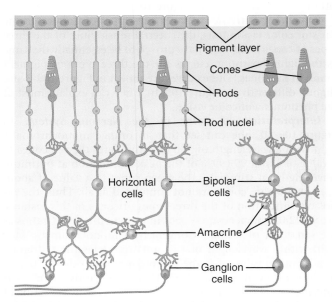

Figure 109-12   Neural organization of the retina: peripheral area to the left, foveal area to the right.

To the right in Figure 109-12 is the visual pathway from the *foveal portion of the retina*, representing the new, fast cone system. This illustration shows three neurons in the direct pathway: (1) cones, (2) bipolar cells, and (3) ganglion cells. In addition, horizontal cells transmit inhibitory signals laterally in the outer plexiform layer, and amacrine cells transmit signals laterally in the inner plexiform layer.

To the left in Figure 109-12 are the neural connections for the peripheral retina, where both rods and cones are present. Three bipolar cells are shown; the middle of these connects only to rods, representing the type of visual system present in many lower animals. The output from the bipolar cell passes only to amacrine cells, which relay the signals to the ganglion cells. Thus, for pure rod vision, there are four neurons in the direct visual pathway: (1) rods, (2) bipolar cells, (3) amacrine cells, and (4) ganglion cells. In addition, horizontal and amacrine cells provide lateral connectivity.

The other two bipolar cells shown in the peripheral retinal circuitry of Figure 109-12 connect with both rods and cones; the outputs of these bipolar cells pass both directly to ganglion cells and by way of amacrine cells.

Transmission of Most Signals Occurs in the Retinal Neurons by Electrotonic Conduction, Not by Action Potentials. The only retinal neurons that always transmit visual signals by means of action potentials are the ganglion cells, and they send their signals all the way to the brain through the optic nerve. Occasionally, action potentials have also been recorded in amacrine cells, although the importance of these action potentials is questionable. Otherwise, all the retinal neurons conduct their visual signals by *electrotonic conduction*, which can be explained as follows.

Electrotonic conduction means direct flow of electric current, not action potentials, in the neuronal cytoplasm and nerve axons from the point of excitation all the way to the output synapses. Even in the rods and cones, conduction from their outer segments, where the visual signals are generated, to the synaptic bodies is by electrotonic conduction. That is, when hyperpolarization occurs in response to light in the outer segment of a rod or a cone, almost the same degree of hyperpolarization is conducted by direct electric current flow in the cytoplasm all the way to the synaptic body, and no action potential is required. Then, when the transmitter from a rod or cone stimulates a bipolar cell or horizontal cell, once again the signal is transmitted from the input to the output by direct electric current flow, not by action potentials.

The importance of electrotonic conduction is that it allows *graded conduction* of signal strength. Thus, for the rods and cones, the strength of the hyperpolarizing output signal is directly related to the intensity of illumination; the signal is not all or none, as would be the case for each action potential.

Lateral Inhibition to Enhance Visual Contrast—Function of the Horizontal Cells

The horizontal cells, shown in Figure 109-12, connect laterally between the synaptic bodies of the rods and cones, and also connect with the dendrites of the bipolar cells. The outputs of the horizontal cells *are always inhibitory*. Therefore, this lateral connection provides the same phenomenon of lateral inhibition that is important in other sensory systems—that is, helping to ensure transmission of visual patterns with proper visual contrast. This phenomenon is demonstrated in Figure 109-13, which shows a minute spot of light focused on the retina. The visual pathway from the central-most area where the light

strikes is excited, whereas an area to the side is inhibited. In other words, instead of the excitatory signal spreading widely in the retina because of spreading dendritic and axonal trees in the plexiform layers, transmission through the horizontal cells puts a stop to this spread by providing lateral inhibition in the surrounding areas. This process is essential to allow high visual accuracy in transmitting contrast borders in the visual image.

Some of the amacrine cells probably provide additional lateral inhibition and further enhancement of visual contrast in the inner plexiform layer of the retina as well.

Depolarizing and Hyperpolarizing Bipolar Cells

Two types of bipolar cells provide opposing excitatory and inhibitory signals in the visual pathway: (1) the *depolarizing bipolar cell* and (2) the *hyperpolarizing bipolar cell*. That is, some bipolar cells depolarize when the rods and cones are excited, and others hyperpolarize.

There are two possible explanations for this difference. One explanation is that the two bipolar cells are of entirely different types—with one responding by depolarizing in response to the glutamate neurotransmitter released by the rods and cones, and the other responding by hyperpolarizing. The other possibility is that one of the bipolar cells receives direct excitation from the rods and cones, whereas the other receives its signal indirectly through a horizontal cell. Because the horizontal cell is an inhibitory cell, this would reverse the polarity of the electrical response.

Regardless of the mechanism for the two types of bipolar responses, the importance of this phenomenon is that it allows half the bipolar cells to transmit positive signals and the other half to transmit negative signals. We shall see later that both positive and negative signals are used in transmitting visual information to the brain.

Another important aspect of this reciprocal relation between depolarizing and hyperpolarizing bipolar cells is that it provides a second mechanism for lateral inhibition, in addition to the horizontal cell mechanism. Because depolarizing and hyperpolarizing bipolar cells lie immediately against each other, this provides a mechanism for separating contrast borders in the visual image, even when the border lies exactly between two adjacent photoreceptors. In contrast, the horizontal cell mechanism for lateral inhibition operates over a much greater distance.

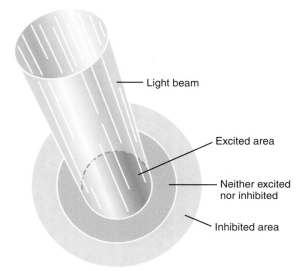

— Light beam

— Excited area

— Neither excited nor inhibited

— Inhibited area

Figure 109-13 Excitation and inhibition of a retinal area caused by a small beam of light, demonstrating the principle of lateral inhibition.

Amacrine Cells and their Functions

About 30 types of amacrine cells have been identified by morphological or histochemical means. The functions of about half a dozen types of amacrine cells have been characterized, and all of them are different.

- One type of amacrine cell is part of the direct pathway for rod vision—that is, from rod to bipolar cells to amacrine cells to ganglion cells.
- Another type of amacrine cell responds strongly at the onset of a continuing visual signal, but the response dies rapidly.
- Other amacrine cells respond strongly at the offset of visual signals, but, again, the response fades quickly.
- Still other amacrine cells respond when a light is turned either on or off, signaling simply a change in illumination, irrespective of direction.
- Another type of amacrine cell responds to movement of a spot across the retina in a specific direction; therefore, these amacrine cells are said to be *directionally sensitive*.

In a sense, then, many or most amacrine cells are interneurons that help analyze visual signals before they ever leave the retina.

GANGLION CELLS AND OPTIC NERVE FIBERS

Each retina contains about 100 million rods and 3 million cones; yet the number of ganglion cells is only about 1.6 million. Thus, an average of 60 rods and 2 cones converge on each ganglion cell and the optic nerve fiber leading from the ganglion cell to the brain.

However, major differences exist between the peripheral retina and the central retina. As one approaches the fovea, fewer rods and cones converge on each optic fiber, and the rods and cones also become more slender. These effects progressively increase the acuity of vision in the central retina. In the center, in the *central fovea*, there are only slender cones—about 35,000 of them—and no rods. Also, the number of optic nerve fibers leading from this part of the retina is almost exactly equal to the number of cones, as shown to the right in Figure 109-12. This phenomenon explains the high degree of visual acuity in the central retina in comparison with the much poorer acuity peripherally.

Another difference between the peripheral and central portions of the retina is the much greater sensitivity of the peripheral retina to weak light, which occurs partly because rods are 30–300 times more sensitive to light than cones. However, this greater sensitivity is further magnified by the fact that as many as 200 rods converge on a single optic nerve fiber in the more peripheral portions of the retina, and thus signals from the rods summate to give even more intense stimulation of the peripheral ganglion cells and their optic nerve fibers.

There are three distinct types of ganglion cells, designated W, X, and Y cells. Each of these serves a different function.

BIBLIOGRAPHY

Artemyev NO: Light-dependent compartmentalization of transducin in rod photoreceptors, *Mol. Neurobiol.* 37:44, 2008.

Bloomfield SA, Völgyi B: The diverse functional roles and regulation of neuronal gap junctions in the retina, *Nat. Rev. Neurosci.* 10:495, 2009.

Bowmaker JK: Evolution of vertebrate visual pigments, *Vision Res.* 48:2022, 2008.

Carroll J: Focus on molecules: the cone opsins, *Exp. Eye Res.* 86:865, 2008.

D'Amico DJ: Clinical practice. Primary retinal detachment, *N. Engl. J. Med.* 359:2346, 2008.

Dhande OS, Huberman AD: Retinal ganglion cell maps in the brain: implications for visual processing, *Curr. Opin. Neurobiol.* 24:133, 2014.

Gegenfurtner KR, Kiper DC: Color vision, *Annu. Rev. Neurosci.* 26:181, 2003.

Hardie RC: Phototransduction: shedding light on translocation, *Curr. Biol.* 13:R775, 2003.

Kandel ER, Schwartz JH, Jessell TM: *Principles of Neural Science*, fourth ed, New York, 2000, McGraw-Hill.

Luo DG, Xue T, Yau KW: How vision begins: an odyssey, *Proc. Natl. Acad. Sci. U. S. A.* 105:9855, 2008.

Masland RH: The neuronal organization of the retina, *Neuron* 76:266, 2012.

Solomon SG, Lennie P: The machinery of colour vision, *Nat. Rev. Neurosci.* 8:276, 2007.

Wensel TG: Signal transducing membrane complexes of photoreceptor outer segments, *Vision Res.* 48:2052, 2008.

110

Visual Pathways and Central Processing

Figure 110-1 shows the principal visual pathways from the two retinas to the *visual cortex*. The visual nerve signals leave the retinas through the *optic nerves*. At the *optic chiasm*, the optic nerve fibers from the nasal halves of the retinas cross to the opposite sides, where they join the fibers from the opposite temporal retinas to form the *optic tracts*. The fibers of each optic tract then synapse in the *dorsal lateral geniculate nucleus* of the thalamus, and from there, *geniculocalcarine fibers* pass by way of the *optic radiation* (also called the *geniculocalcarine tract*) to the *primary visual cortex* in the *calcarine fissure* area of the medial occipital lobe.

Visual fibers also pass to several older areas of the brain: (1) from the optic tracts to the *suprachiasmatic nucleus of the hypothalamus*, presumably to control circadian rhythms that synchronize various physiological changes of the body with night and day; (2) into the *pretectal nuclei* in the midbrain, to elicit reflex movements of the eyes to focus on objects of importance and to activate the pupillary light reflex; (3) into the *superior colliculus*, to control rapid directional movements of the two eyes; and (4) into the *ventral lateral geniculate nucleus* of the thalamus and surrounding basal regions of the brain, presumably to help control some of the body's behavioral functions.

Thus, the visual pathways can be divided roughly into an *old system* to the midbrain and base of the forebrain and a *new*

system for direct transmission of visual signals into the visual cortex located in the occipital lobes. In humans, the new system is responsible for perception of virtually all aspects of visual form, colors, and other conscious vision. Conversely, in many primitive animals, even visual form is detected by the older system, using the superior colliculus in the same manner that the visual cortex is used in mammals.

FUNCTION OF THE DORSAL LATERAL GENICULATE NUCLEUS OF THE THALAMUS

The optic nerve fibers of the new visual system terminate in the *dorsal lateral geniculate nucleus*, located at the dorsal end of the thalamus and also called the *lateral geniculate body*, as shown in Figure 110-1. The dorsal lateral geniculate nucleus serves two principal functions: First, it relays visual information from the optic tract to the *visual cortex* by way of the *optic radiation* (also called the *geniculocalcarine tract*). This relay function is so accurate that there is exact point-to-point transmission with a high degree of spatial fidelity all the way from the retina to the visual cortex.

Half the fibers in each optic tract after passing the optic chiasm are derived from one eye and half are derived from the other eye, representing corresponding points on the two retinas. However, the signals from the two eyes are kept apart in the dorsal lateral geniculate nucleus. This nucleus is composed of six nuclear layers. Layers II, III, and V (from ventral to dorsal) receive signals from the lateral half of the ipsilateral retina, whereas layers I, IV, and VI receive signals from the medial half of the retina of the opposite eye. The respective retinal areas of the two eyes connect with neurons that are superimposed over one another in the paired layers, and similar parallel transmission is preserved all the way to the visual cortex.

The second major function of the dorsal lateral geniculate nucleus is to "gate" the transmission of signals to the visual cortex—that is, to control how much of the signal is allowed to pass to the cortex. The nucleus receives gating control signals from two major sources: (1) *corticofugal fibers* returning in a backward direction from the primary visual cortex to the lateral geniculate nucleus and (2) *reticular areas of the mesencephalon*. Both of these sources are inhibitory and, when stimulated, can turn off transmission through selected portions of the dorsal lateral geniculate nucleus. Both of these gating circuits help highlight the visual information that is allowed to pass.

Finally, the dorsal lateral geniculate nucleus is divided in another way: (1) Layers I and II are called *magnocellular layers* because they contain large neurons. These neurons receive their input almost entirely from the large *type M retinal ganglion cells*. This magnocellular system provides a *rapidly conducting* pathway to the visual cortex. However, this system is color blind, transmitting only black-and-white information. Also, its point-to-point transmission is poor because there are not many M ganglion cells, and their dendrites spread widely in the retina. (2) Layers III–VI are called *parvocellular layers* because they

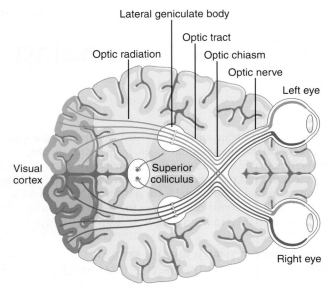

Figure 110-1   Principal visual pathways from the eyes to the visual cortex. *Modified from Polyak, S.L., 1941. The Retina. University of Chicago, Chicago.*

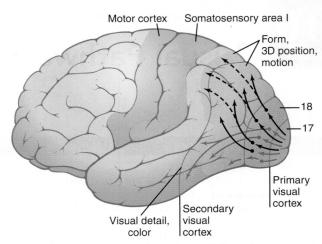

Figure 110-3   Transmission of visual signals from the primary visual cortex into secondary visual areas on the lateral surfaces of the occipital and parietal cortices. Note that the signals representing form, third-dimensional position, and motion are transmitted mainly into the superior portions of the occipital lobe and posterior portions of the parietal lobe. By contrast, the signals for visual detail and color are transmitted mainly into the anteroventral portion of the occipital lobe and the ventral portion of the posterior temporal lobe.

contain large numbers of small- to medium-sized neurons. These neurons receive their input almost entirely from the *type P retinal ganglion cells* that transmit color and convey accurate point-to-point spatial information, but at only a moderate velocity of conduction rather than at high velocity.

Organization and Function of the Visual Cortex

Figures 110-2 and 110-3 show the *visual cortex*, which is located primarily on the medial aspect of the occipital lobes. Like the cortical representations of the other sensory systems, the visual cortex is divided into a *primary visual cortex* and *secondary visual areas*.

Primary Visual Cortex. The primary visual cortex (see Figure 110-2) lies in the *calcarine fissure area*, extending forward from the *occipital pole* on the *medial* aspect of each occipital

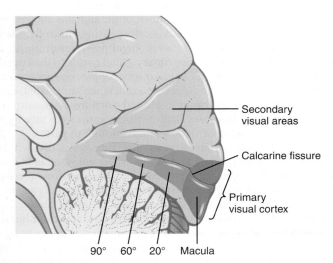

Figure 110-2   Visual cortex in the *calcarine fissure area* of the *medial* occipital cortex.

cortex. This area is the terminus of direct visual signals from the eyes. Signals from the macular area of the retina terminate near the occipital pole, as shown in Figure 110-2, whereas signals from the more peripheral retina terminate at or in concentric half circles anterior to the pole but still along the calcarine fissure on the medial occipital lobe. The upper portion of the retina is represented superiorly and the lower portion is represented inferiorly.

Note in the figure the large area that represents the macula. It is to this region that the retinal fovea transmits its signals. The fovea is responsible for the highest degree of visual acuity. Based on retinal area, the fovea has several hundred times as much representation in the primary visual cortex as do the most peripheral portions of the retina.

The primary visual cortex is also called *visual area I* or the *striate cortex* because this area has a grossly striated appearance.

Secondary Visual Areas of the Cortex. The secondary visual areas, also called *visual association areas*, lie lateral, anterior, superior, and inferior to the primary visual cortex. Most of these areas also fold outward over the lateral surfaces of the occipital and parietal cortex, as shown in Figure 110-3. Secondary signals are transmitted to these areas for analysis of visual meanings. For instance, on all sides of the primary visual cortex is *Brodmann area 18* (see Figure 110-3), which is where virtually all signals from the primary visual cortex pass next. Therefore, Brodmann area 18 is called *visual area II*, or simply V-2. The other, more distant secondary visual areas have specific designations—V-3, V-4, and so forth—up to more than a dozen areas. The importance of all these areas is that various aspects of the visual image are progressively dissected and analyzed.

THE PRIMARY VISUAL CORTEX HAS SIX MAJOR LAYERS

Like almost all other portions of the cerebral cortex, the primary visual cortex has six distinct layers, as shown in Figure 110-4. Also, as is true for the other sensory systems, the

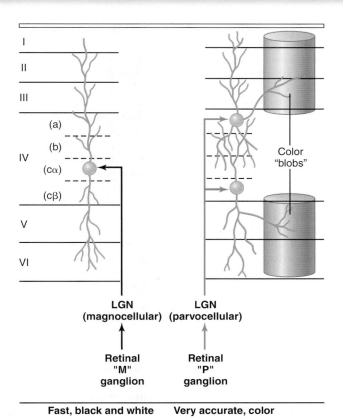

Figure 110-4   Six layers of the primary visual cortex. The connections shown on the left side of the figure originate in the magnocellular layers of the lateral geniculate nucleus (LGN) and transmit rapidly changing black-and-white visual signals. The pathways to the right originate in the parvocellular layers (layers III–VI) of the LGN; they transmit signals that depict accurate spatial detail, as well as color. Note especially the areas of the visual cortex called "color blobs," which are necessary for detection of color.

geniculocalcarine fibers terminate mainly in layer IV but this layer is also organized into subdivisions. The rapidly conducted signals from the M retinal ganglion cells terminate in layer IVcα, and from there they are relayed vertically both outward toward the cortical surface and inward toward deeper levels.

The visual signals from the medium-sized optic nerve fibers, derived from the P ganglion cells in the retina, also terminate in layer IV, but at points different from the M signals. They terminate in layers IVa and IVcβ, the shallowest and deepest portions of layer IV, shown to the left in Figure 110-4. From there, these signals are transmitted vertically both toward the surface of the cortex and to deeper layers. It is these P ganglion pathways that transmit the accurate point-to-point type of vision, as well as color vision.

Vertical Neuronal Columns in the Visual Cortex. The visual cortex is organized structurally into several million vertical columns of neuronal cells, with each column having a diameter of 30–50 μm. The same vertical columnar organization is found throughout the cerebral cortex for the other senses as well (and also in the motor and analytical cortical regions). Each column represents a functional unit. One can roughly calculate that each of the visual vertical columns has perhaps 1000 or more neurons.

After the optic signals terminate in layer IV, they are further processed as they spread both outward and inward along each vertical column unit. This processing is believed to decipher

separate bits of visual information at successive stations along the pathway. The signals that pass outward to layers I, II, and III eventually transmit signals for short distances laterally in the cortex. Conversely, the signals that pass inward to layers V and VI excite neurons that transmit signals much greater distances.

"Color Blobs" in the Visual Cortex. Interspersed among the primary visual columns, as well as among the columns of some of the secondary visual areas, are special column-like areas called *color blobs*. They receive lateral signals from adjacent visual columns and are activated specifically by color signals. Therefore, these blobs are presumably the primary areas for deciphering color.

Interaction of Visual Signals from the Two Separate Eyes. Recall that visual signals from the two separate eyes are relayed through separate neuronal layers in the lateral geniculate nucleus. These signals remain separated from each other when they arrive in layer IV of the primary visual cortex. In fact, layer IV is interlaced with stripes of neuronal columns, with each stripe about 0.5 mm wide; the signals from one eye enter the columns of every other stripe, alternating with signals from the second eye. This cortical area deciphers whether the respective areas of the two visual images from the two separate eyes are "in register" with each other—that is, whether corresponding points from the two retinas fit with each other. In turn, the deciphered information is used to adjust the directional gaze of the separate eyes so that they will fuse with each other (i.e., be brought into "register"). The information observed about degree of register of images from the two eyes also allows a person to distinguish the distance of objects by the mechanism of *stereopsis*.

Neuronal Patterns of Stimulation During Analysis of the Visual Image

Analysis of Contrasts in the Visual Image. If a person looks at a blank wall, only a few neurons in the primary visual cortex will be stimulated, regardless of whether the illumination of the wall is bright or weak. Therefore, what does the primary visual cortex detect? To answer this question, let us now place on the wall a large solid cross, as shown to the left in Figure 110-5. To the right is shown the spatial pattern of the most excited neurons in the visual cortex. *Note that the areas of maximum excitation occur along the sharp borders of the visual pattern.* Thus, the visual signal in the primary visual cortex is concerned mainly with *contrasts* in the visual scene, rather than with noncontrasting areas. We noted in Chapter 109 that this is also true of most of the retinal ganglion because equally stimulated adjacent retinal receptors mutually inhibit one another. However at any border in the visual scene where there is a change from dark to light or light to dark, mutual inhibition does not occur, and the intensity

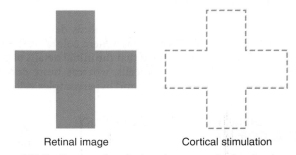

Retinal image   Cortical stimulation

Figure 110-5   Pattern of excitation that occurs in the visual cortex in response to a retinal image of a dark cross.

of stimulation of most neurons is proportional to the *gradient of contrast*—that is, the greater the sharpness of contrast and the greater the intensity difference between light and dark areas, the greater is the degree of stimulation.

Visual Cortex Also Detects Orientation of Lines and Borders—"Simple" Cells. The visual cortex detects not only the existence of lines and borders in the different areas of the retinal image but also the direction of orientation of each line or border—that is, whether it is vertical or horizontal or lies at some degree of inclination. This capability is believed to result from linear organizations of mutually inhibiting cells that excite second-order neurons when inhibition occurs all along a line of cells where there is a contrast edge. Thus, for each such orientation of a line, specific neuronal cells are stimulated. A line oriented in a different direction excites a different set of cells. These neuronal cells are called *simple cells*. They are found mainly in layer IV of the primary visual cortex.

Detection of Line Orientation when a Line Is Displaced Laterally or Vertically in the Visual Field—"Complex" Cells. As the visual signal progresses farther away from layer IV, some neurons respond to lines that are oriented in the same direction but are not position specific. That is, even if a line is displaced moderate distances laterally or vertically in the field, the same few neurons will still be stimulated if the line has the same direction. These cells are called *complex cells*.

Detection of Lines of Specific Lengths, Angles, or Other Shapes. Some neurons in the outer layers of the primary visual columns, as well as neurons in some secondary visual areas, are stimulated only by lines or borders of specific lengths, by specific angulated shapes, or by images that have other characteristics. That is, these neurons detect still higher orders of information from the visual scene. Thus, as one goes farther into the analytical pathway of the visual cortex, progressively more characteristics of each visual scene are deciphered.

DETECTION OF COLOR

Color is detected in much the same way that lines are detected: by means of color contrast. For instance, a red area is often contrasted against a green area, a blue area against a red area, or a green area against a yellow area. All these colors can also be contrasted against a white area within the visual scene. In fact, this contrasting against white is believed to be mainly responsible for the phenomenon called "color constancy"; that is, when the color of an illuminating light changes, the color of the "white" changes with the light, and appropriate computation in the brain allows red to be interpreted as red even though the illuminating light has changed the color entering the eyes.

The mechanism of color contrast analysis depends on the fact that contrasting colors, called "opponent colors," excite specific neuronal cells. It is presumed that the initial details of color contrast are detected by simple cells, whereas more complex contrasts are detected by complex and hypercomplex cells.

EFFECT OF REMOVING THE PRIMARY VISUAL CORTEX

Removal of the primary visual cortex in the human being causes loss of conscious vision, that is, blindness. However,

psychological studies demonstrate that such "blind" people can still, at times, react subconsciously to changes in light intensity, to movement in the visual scene, or, rarely, even to some gross patterns of vision. These reactions include turning the eyes, turning the head, and avoidance. This vision is believed to be subserved by neuronal pathways that pass from the optic tracts mainly into the superior colliculi and other portions of the older visual system.

Cortical blindness is the term given to the loss of vision caused by lesions in the visual area of the occipital cortex. In these patients, the eye appears normal but there is a loss of conscious vision as described earlier. Typically, this type of lesion is caused by ischemic damage subsequent to blocks in the posterior cerebral artery. In such patients, there may also be a sparing of the macular region (also called macular sparing), owing to collateral supply to this area of the visual cortex by the middle cerebral artery.

Fields of Vision; Perimetry

The *field of vision* is the visual area seen by an eye at a given instant. The area seen to the nasal side is called the *nasal field of vision*, and the area seen to the lateral side is called the *temporal field of vision*.

To diagnose blindness in specific portions of the retina, one charts the field of vision for each eye by a process called *perimetry*. This charting is performed by having the subject look with one eye toward a central spot directly in front of the eye; the other eye is closed. A small dot of light or a small object is then moved back and forth in all areas of the field of vision, and the subject indicates when the spot of light or object can and cannot be seen. The field of vision for the left eye is plotted as shown in Figure 110-6. In all perimetry charts, a *blind spot* caused by lack of rods and cones in the retina over the *optic disc* is found about 15 degrees lateral to the central point of vision, as shown in the figure.

Abnormalities in the Fields of Vision. Occasionally, blind spots are found in portions of the field of vision other than the optic disc area. Such blind spots called *scotomata* are frequently

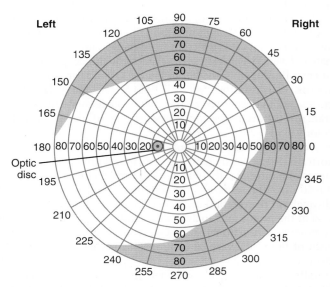

Figure 110-6 Perimetry chart, showing the field of vision for the left eye. The red circle shows the blind spot.

TABLE 110-1	Lesions in the Optic Pathway and their Outcomes
Site of Lesion	**Outcome**
Optic nerve	Ipsilateral complete anopsia (blindness)
Optic chiasm	Bitemporal hemianopsia
Optic tract	Contralateral homonymous hemianopsia
Visual cortex	Contralateral homonymous hemianopsia with macular sparing

caused by damage to the optic nerve resulting from glaucoma (too much fluid pressure in the eyeball), allergic reactions in the retina, or toxic conditions such as lead poisoning or excessive use of tobacco.

Another condition that can be diagnosed by perimetry is *retinitis pigmentosa*. In this disease, portions of the retina degenerate and excessive melanin pigment is deposited in the degenerated areas. Retinitis pigmentosa usually causes blindness in the peripheral field of vision first and then gradually encroaches on the central areas.

Effect of Lesions in the Optic Pathway on the Fields of Vision (Table 110-1). Destruction of an entire *optic nerve* causes blindness of the affected eye.

Destruction of the *optic chiasm* prevents the crossing of impulses from the nasal half of each retina to the opposite optic tract. Therefore, the nasal half of each retina is blinded, which means that the person is blind in the temporal field of vision for each eye *because the image of the field of vision is inverted on the retina* by the optical system of the eye; this condition is called *bitemporal hemianopsia*. Such lesions frequently result from tumors of the pituitary gland pressing upward from the sella turcica on the bottom of the optic chiasm.

Interruption of an *optic tract* denervates the corresponding half of each retina on the same side as the lesion; as a result, neither eye can see objects to the opposite side of the head. This condition is known as *homonymous hemianopsia*.

Eye Movements and their Control

To make full use of the visual abilities of the eyes, almost equally as important as interpretation of the visual signals from the eyes is the cerebral control system for directing the eyes toward the object to be viewed.

Muscular Control of Eye Movements. The eye movements are controlled by three pairs of muscles, shown in Figure 110-7: (1) the *medial* and *lateral recti*, (2) the *superior* and *inferior recti*, and (3) the *superior* and *inferior obliques*. The medial and lateral recti contract to move the eyes from side to side. The superior and inferior recti contract to move the eyes upward or downward. The oblique muscles function mainly to rotate the eyeballs to keep the visual fields in the upright position.

Neural Pathways for Control of Eye Movements. Figure 110-7 also shows brainstem nuclei for the third, fourth, and sixth cranial nerves and their connections with the peripheral nerves to the ocular muscles. Also shown are interconnections among the brainstem nuclei by way of the nerve tract called the *medial longitudinal fasciculus*. Each of the three sets of muscles to each eye is *reciprocally* innervated so that one muscle of the pair relaxes while the other contracts.

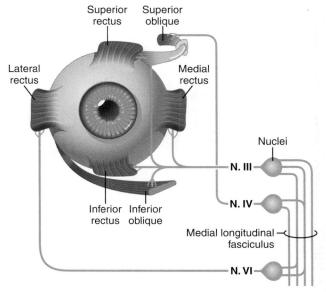

Figure 110-7 Anterior view of the right eye showing extraocular muscles of the eye and their innervation. N., nerve.

Figure 110-8 demonstrates cortical control of the oculomotor apparatus, showing spread of signals from visual areas in the occipital cortex through occipitotectal and occipitocollicular tracts to the pretectal and superior colliculus areas of the brainstem. From both the pretectal and the superior colliculus areas, the oculomotor control signals pass to the brainstem nuclei of the oculomotor nerves. Strong signals are also transmitted from the body's equilibrium control centers in the brainstem into the oculomotor system (from the vestibular nuclei by way of the medial longitudinal fasciculus).

Superior Colliculi Are Mainly Responsible for Turning the Eyes and Head Toward a Visual Disturbance

Even after the visual cortex has been destroyed, a sudden visual disturbance in a lateral area of the visual field often causes immediate turning of the eyes in that direction. This turning does not occur if the superior colliculi have also been destroyed. To support this function, the various points of the retina are represented topographically in the superior colliculi in the same way as in the primary visual cortex, although with less accuracy. Even so, the principal direction of a flash of light in a peripheral retinal field is mapped by the colliculi, and secondary signals are transmitted to the oculomotor nuclei to turn the eyes. To help in this directional movement of the eyes, the superior colliculi also have topological maps of somatic sensations from the body and acoustic signals from the ears.

The optic nerve fibers from the eyes to the colliculi, which are responsible for these rapid turning movements, are branches from the rapidly conducting M fibers, with one branch going to the visual cortex and the other going to the superior colliculi.

In addition to causing the eyes to turn toward a visual disturbance, signals are relayed from the superior colliculi through the *medial longitudinal fasciculus* to other levels of the brainstem to cause turning of the whole head and even of the whole body toward the direction of the disturbance. Other types of nonvisual disturbances, such as strong sounds or even stroking of the side of the body, cause similar turning of the eyes, head,

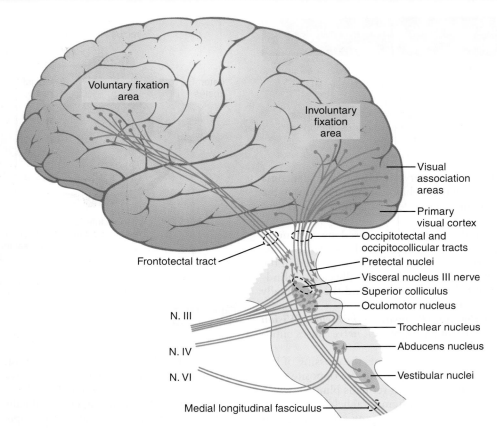

Figure 110-8 Neural pathways for control of conjugate movement of the eyes. N., nerve.

and body, but only if the superior colliculi are intact. Therefore, the superior colliculi play a global role in orienting the eyes, head, and body with respect to external disturbances, whether they are visual, auditory, or somatic.

Strabismus

Strabismus, also called *squint* or *cross-eye*, means lack of fusion of the eyes in one or more of the visual coordinates: horizontal, vertical, or rotational. The basic types of strabismus are shown in Figure 110-9: (1) *horizontal strabismus*, (2) *torsional strabismus*, and (3) *vertical strabismus*. Combinations of two or even all three of the different types of strabismus often occur.

Strabismus is often caused by abnormal "set" of the fusion mechanism of the visual system. That is, in a young child's early efforts to fixate the two eyes on the same object, one of the eyes fixates satisfactorily while the other fails to do so, or they both fixate satisfactorily but never simultaneously. Soon the patterns of conjugate movements of the eyes become abnormally "set" in the neuronal control pathways themselves, so the eyes never fuse.

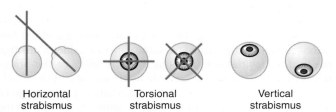

Figure 110-9 Basic types of strabismus.

Autonomic Control of Accommodation and Pupillary Aperture

Autonomic Nerves to the Eyes. The eye is innervated by both parasympathetic and sympathetic nerve fibers, as shown in Figure 110-10. The parasympathetic preganglionic fibers arise in the *Edinger–Westphal nucleus* (the visceral nucleus portion of the third cranial nerve) and then pass in the *third nerve* to the *ciliary ganglion*, which lies immediately behind the eye. There, the preganglionic fibers synapse with postganglionic parasympathetic neurons, which in turn send fibers through *ciliary nerves* into the eyeball. These nerves excite (1) the ciliary muscle that controls focusing of the eye lens and (2) the sphincter of the iris that constricts the pupil.

The sympathetic innervation of the eye originates in the *intermediolateral horn cells* of the first thoracic segment of the spinal cord. From there, sympathetic fibers enter the sympathetic chain and pass upward to the *superior cervical ganglion*, where they synapse with postganglionic neurons. Postganglionic sympathetic fibers from these then spread along the surfaces of the carotid artery and successively smaller arteries until they reach the eye. There, the sympathetic fibers innervate the radial fibers of the iris (which open the pupil), as well as several extraocular muscles of the eye, which are discussed subsequently in relation to Horner syndrome.

CONTROL OF ACCOMMODATION (FOCUSING THE EYES)

The accommodation mechanism—that is, the mechanism that focuses the lens system of the eye—is essential for a high degree

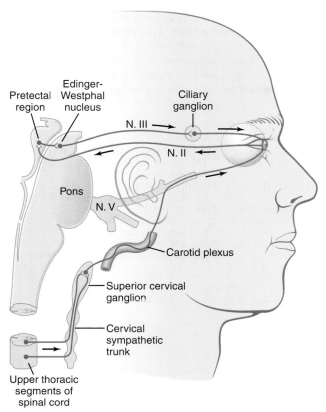

Figure 110-10 Autonomic innervation of the eye, showing also the reflex arc of the light reflex. N., nerve. *Modified from Ranson, S.W., Clark, S.L., 1959. Anatomy of the Nervous System: its Development and Function, 10th ed. W.B. Saunders, Philadelphia.*

3. *Because the fovea lies in a hollowed-out depression that is slightly deeper than the remainder of the retina, the clarity of focus in the depth of the fovea is different from the clarity of focus on the edges.* This difference may also give clues about which way the strength of the lens needs to be changed.
4. *The degree of accommodation of the lens oscillates slightly all the time at a frequency up to twice per second.* The visual image becomes clearer when the oscillation of the lens strength is changing in the appropriate direction and becomes poorer when the lens strength is changing in the wrong direction. This could give a rapid clue as to which way the strength of the lens needs to change to provide appropriate focus.

The brain cortical areas that control accommodation closely parallel those that control fixation movements of the eyes. Analysis of the visual signals in Brodmann cortical areas 18 and 19 and transmission of motor signals to the ciliary muscle occur through the pretectal area in the brainstem, then through the *Edinger–Westphal nucleus*, and finally by way of parasympathetic nerve fibers to the eyes.

CONTROL OF PUPILLARY DIAMETER

Stimulation of the parasympathetic nerves also excites the pupillary sphincter muscle, thereby decreasing the pupillary aperture; this process is called *miosis*. Conversely, stimulation of the sympathetic nerves excites the radial fibers of the iris and causes pupillary dilation, which is called *mydriasis*.

Pupillary Light Reflex. When light is shone into the eyes, the pupils constrict, a reaction called the *pupillary light reflex*. The direct pupillary reflex is observed when constriction of the pupil is observed in the eye that the light is shone on. The consensual pupillary reflex occurs when the pupil of the other eye also constricts, at the same time. The neuronal pathway for this reflex is demonstrated by the upper two black arrows in Figure 110-10. When light impinges on the retina, a few of the resulting impulses pass from the optic nerves to the pretectal nuclei. From here, secondary impulses pass to the *Edinger–Westphal nucleus* and, finally, back through *parasympathetic nerves* to constrict the sphincter of the iris. Conversely, in darkness, the reflex becomes inhibited, which results in dilation of the pupil.

The function of the light reflex is to help the eye adapt extremely rapidly to changing light conditions, as explained in Chapter 108. The limits of pupillary diameter are about 1.5 mm on the small side and 8 mm on the large side. Therefore, because light brightness on the retina increases with the square of pupillary diameter, the range of light and dark adaptation that can be brought about by the pupillary reflex is about 30–1—that is, up to as much as 30 times change in the amount of light entering the eye.

Pupillary Reflexes or Reactions in Central Nervous System Disease. A few central nervous system diseases damage nerve transmission of visual signals from the retinas to the Edinger–Westphal nucleus, thus sometimes blocking the pupillary reflexes. Such blocks may occur as a result of *central nervous system syphilis, alcoholism, encephalitis*, and so forth. The block usually occurs in the pretectal region of the brainstem, although it can result from destruction of some small fibers in the optic nerves.

The final nerve fibers in the pathway through the pretectal area to the Edinger–Westphal nucleus are mostly of the inhibitory type. When their inhibitory effect is lost, the nucleus

of visual acuity. Accommodation results from contraction or relaxation of the eye ciliary muscle. Contraction causes increased refractive power of the lens, as explained in Chapter 108, and relaxation causes decreased power. How does a person adjust accommodation to keep the eyes in focus all the time?

Accommodation of the lens is regulated by a negative feedback mechanism that automatically adjusts the refractive power of the lens to achieve the highest degree of visual acuity. When the eyes have been focused on some far object and must then suddenly focus on a near object, the lens usually accommodates for best acuity of vision within less than 1 second. Although the precise control mechanism that causes this rapid and accurate focusing of the eye is unclear, the following features are known.

First, when the eyes suddenly change distance of the fixation point, the lens changes its strength in the proper direction to achieve a new state of focus within a fraction of a second. Second, different types of clues help to change the lens strength in the proper direction:

1. *Chromatic aberration* appears to be important. That is, red light rays focus slightly posteriorly to blue light rays because the lens bends blue rays more than red rays. The eyes appear to be able to detect which of these two types of rays is in better focus, and this clue relays information to the accommodation mechanism with regard to whether to make the lens stronger or weaker.
2. When the eyes fixate on a near object, the eyes must converge. The neural mechanisms for *convergence cause a simultaneous signal to strengthen the lens of the eye.*

becomes chronically active, causing the pupils to remain mostly constricted, in addition to their failure to respond to light.

Yet the pupils can constrict a little more if the Edinger–Westphal nucleus is stimulated through some other pathway. For instance, when the eyes fixate on a near object, the signals that cause accommodation of the lens and those that cause convergence of the two eyes cause a mild degree of pupillary constriction at the same time. This phenomenon is called the *pupillary reaction to accommodation*. A pupil that fails to respond to light but does respond to accommodation and is also very small (an *Argyll Robertson pupil*) is an important diagnostic sign of central nervous system disease such as syphilis.

BIBLIOGRAPHY

Bridge H, Cumming BG: Representation of binocular surfaces by cortical neurons, *Curr. Opin. Neurobiol.* 18:425, 2008.

Derrington AM, Webb BS: Visual system: how is the retina wired up to the cortex? *Curr. Biol.* 14:R14, 2004.

Espinosa JS, Stryker MP: Development and plasticity of the primary visual cortex, *Neuron* 75:230, 2012.

Kandel ER, Schwartz JH, Jessell TM: *Principles of Neural Science*, fourth ed., New York, 2000, McGraw-Hill.

Katzner S, Weigelt S: Visual cortical networks: of mice and men, *Curr. Opin. Neurobiol.* 23:202, 2013.

Kingdom FA: Perceiving light versus material, *Vision Res.* 48:2090, 2008.

Klier EM, Angelaki DE: Spatial updating and the maintenance of visual constancy, *Neuroscience* 156:801, 2008.

Luna B, Velanova K, Geier CF: Development of eye-movement control, *Brain Cogn.* 68:293, 2008.

Martinez-Conde S, Macknik SL, Hubel DH: The role of fixational eye movements in visual perception, *Nat. Rev. Neurosci.* 5:229, 2004.

Nassi JJ, Callaway EM: Parallel processing strategies of the primate visual system, *Nat. Rev. Neurosci.* 10:360, 2009.

Parker AJ: Binocular depth perception and the cerebral cortex, *Nat. Rev. Neurosci.* 8:379, 2007.

Peelen MV, Downing PE: The neural basis of visual body perception, *Nat. Rev. Neurosci.* 8:636, 2007.

PART III

Motor System

ANURA KURPAD

Introduction to the Motor System: Spinal Cord

Sensory information is integrated at all levels of the nervous system and causes appropriate motor responses that begin in the spinal cord with relatively simple muscle reflexes, extend into the brainstem with more complicated responses, and finally extend to the cerebrum, where the most complicated muscle skills are controlled.

In this chapter, we discuss spinal cord control of muscle function. Without the special neuronal circuits of the cord, even the most complex motor control systems in the brain could not cause any purposeful muscle movement. For example, there is no neuronal circuit anywhere in the brain that causes the specific to-and-fro movements of the legs that are required in walking. Instead, the circuits for these movements are in the cord and the brain simply sends *command* signals to the spinal cord to set into motion the walking process.

Let us not belittle the role of the brain. The brain gives directions that control the sequential cord activities— for example, to promote turning movements when they are required, to lean the body forward during acceleration, to change the movements from walking to jumping as needed, and to monitor continuously and control equilibrium. All this is done through "analytical" and "command" signals generated in the brain. However the many neuronal circuits of the spinal cord that are the objects of the commands are also required. These circuits provide all but a small fraction of the direct control of the muscles.

Organization of the Spinal Cord for Motor Functions

The cord gray matter is the integrative area for the cord reflexes. Figure 111-1 shows the typical organization of the cord gray matter in a single cord segment. Sensory signals enter the cord almost entirely through the sensory roots, also know as the

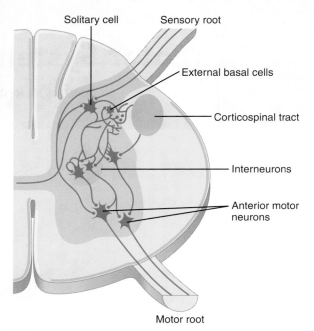

Figure 111-1 Connections of peripheral sensory fibers and cortico-spinal fibers with the interneurons and anterior motor neurons of the spinal cord.

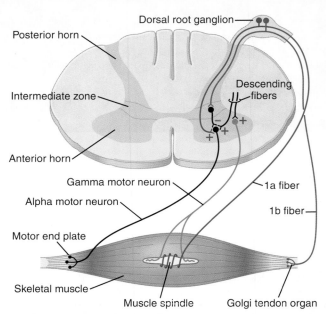

Figure 111-2 Peripheral sensory fibers and anterior motor neurons innervating skeletal muscle.

posterior or *dorsal roots*. After entering the cord, every sensory signal travels to two separate destinations: One branch of the sensory nerve terminates almost immediately in the gray matter of the cord and elicits local segmental cord reflexes and other local effects, and another branch transmits signals to higher levels of the nervous system—that is, to higher levels in the cord itself, to the brainstem, or even to the cerebral cortex, as described in Chapters 103 and 104.

Each segment of the spinal cord (at the level of each spinal nerve) has several million neurons in its gray matter. Aside from the sensory relay neurons discussed in Chapters 103 and 104, the other neurons are of two types: (1) *anterior motor neurons* and (2) *interneurons*.

Anterior Motor Neurons. Located in each segment of the anterior horns of the cord gray matter are several thousand neurons that are 50–100% larger than most of the others and are called *anterior motor neurons* (Figure 111-2). They give rise to the nerve fibers that leave the cord by way of the anterior roots and directly innervate the skeletal muscle fibers. The neurons are of two types, *alpha motor neurons* and *gamma motor neurons*.

Alpha Motor Neurons. The alpha motor neurons give rise to large type A alpha (Aα) motor nerve fibers, averaging 14 μm in diameter; these fibers branch many times after they enter the muscle and innervate the large skeletal muscle fibers. Stimulation of a single alpha nerve fiber excites anywhere from three to several hundred skeletal muscle fibers, which are collectively called the *motor unit*. Transmission of nerve impulses into skeletal muscles and their stimulation of the muscle motor units are discussed in Chapter 12.

Gamma Motor Neurons. Along with the alpha motor neurons, which excite contraction of the skeletal muscle fibers, about one-half as many much smaller *gamma motor neurons* are located in the spinal cord anterior horns. These gamma motor

neurons transmit impulses through much smaller type A gamma (Aγ) motor nerve fibers, averaging 5 μm in diameter, which go to small, special skeletal muscle fibers called *intrafusal fibers*, shown in Figures 111-2 and 111-3. These fibers constitute the middle of the *muscle spindle*, which helps control basic muscle "tone," as discussed later in this chapter.

Interneurons. Interneurons are present in all areas of the cord gray matter—in the dorsal horns, the anterior horns, and the intermediate areas between them, as shown in Figure 111-1. These cells are about 30 times as numerous as the anterior motor neurons. They are small and highly excitable, often exhibiting spontaneous activity and capable of firing as rapidly as 1500 times/second. They have many interconnections with one another, and many of them also synapse directly with the anterior motor neurons, as shown in Figure 111-1. The interconnections among the interneurons and anterior motor neurons are responsible for most of the integrative functions of the spinal cord that are discussed in the remainder of this chapter.

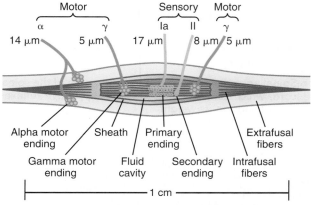

Figure 111-3 Muscle spindle, showing its relation to the large extrafusal skeletal muscle fibers. Note also both motor and sensory innervation of the muscle spindle.

Essentially all the different types of neuronal circuits are found in the interneuron pool of cells of the spinal cord, including *diverging*, *converging*, *repetitive-discharge*, and other types of circuits. In this chapter, we examine many applications of these different circuits in the performance of specific reflex actions by the spinal cord.

Only a few incoming sensory signals from the spinal nerves or signals from the brain terminate directly on the anterior motor neurons. Instead, almost all these signals are transmitted first through interneurons, where they are appropriately processed. Thus, in Figure 111-1, the corticospinal tract from the brain is shown to terminate almost entirely on spinal interneurons, where the signals from this tract are combined with signals from other spinal tracts or spinal nerves before finally converging on the anterior motor neurons to control muscle function.

Renshaw Cells Transmit Inhibitory Signals to Surrounding Motor Neurons. Also located in the anterior horns of the spinal cord, in close association with the motor neurons, are a large number of small neurons called *Renshaw cells*. Almost immediately after the anterior motor neuron axon leaves the body of the neuron, collateral branches from the axon pass to adjacent Renshaw cells. Renshaw cells are *inhibitory cells* that transmit inhibitory signals to the surrounding motor neurons. Thus, stimulation of each motor neuron tends to inhibit adjacent motor neurons, an effect called *lateral inhibition*. This effect is important for the following major reason: The motor system uses this lateral inhibition to focus, or sharpen, its signals in the same way that the sensory system uses the same principle to allow unabated transmission of the primary signal in the desired direction while suppressing the tendency for signals to spread laterally.

Multisegmental Connections from One Spinal Cord Level to Other Levels—Propriospinal Fibers

More than half of all the nerve fibers that ascend and descend in the spinal cord are *propriospinal fibers*. These fibers run from one segment of the cord to another. In addition, as the sensory fibers enter the cord from the posterior cord roots, they bifurcate and branch both up and down the spinal cord; some of the branches transmit signals to only a segment or two, whereas others transmit signals to many segments. These ascending and descending propriospinal fibers of the cord provide pathways for the multisegmental reflexes described later in this chapter, including reflexes that coordinate simultaneous movements in the forelimbs and hind limbs.

Autonomic Reflexes in the Spinal Cord

Many types of segmental autonomic reflexes are integrated in the spinal cord, most of which are discussed in other chapters. Briefly, these reflexes include (1) changes in vascular tone resulting from changes in local skin heat (see Chapter 128); (2) sweating, which results from localized heat on the surface of the body (see Chapter 128); (3) intestinointestinal reflexes that control some motor functions of the gut (see Chapter 65); (4) peritoneointestinal reflexes that inhibit gastrointestinal motility in response to peritoneal irritation (see Chapter 75); and (5) evacuation reflexes for emptying the full bladder (see Chapter 83) or the colon (see Chapter 74). In addition, all the segmental reflexes can at times be elicited simultaneously in the form of the so-called *mass reflex*, described next.

Mass Reflex. In a spinal animal or human being, sometimes the spinal cord suddenly becomes excessively active, causing massive discharge in large portions of the cord. The usual stimulus that causes this excess activity is a strong pain stimulus to the skin or excessive filling of a viscus, such as overdistention of the bladder or the gut. Regardless of the type of stimulus, the resulting reflex, called the *mass reflex*, involves large portions or even all of the cord. The effects are as follows: (1) a major portion of the body's skeletal muscles goes into strong flexor spasm; (2) the colon and bladder are likely to evacuate; (3) the arterial pressure often rises to maximal values, sometimes to a systolic pressure well over 200 mmHg; and (4) large areas of the body break out into profuse sweating.

Because the mass reflex can last for minutes, it presumably results from activation of great numbers of reverberating circuits that excite large areas of the cord at once. This mechanism is similar to the mechanism of epileptic seizures, which involve reverberating circuits that occur in the brain instead of in the cord.

Spinal Cord Transection and Spinal Shock

When the spinal cord is suddenly transected in the upper neck, at first, essentially all cord functions, including the cord reflexes, immediately become depressed to the point of total silence, a reaction called *spinal shock*. The reason for this reaction is that normal activity of the cord neurons depends to a great extent on continual tonic excitation by the discharge of nerve fibers entering the cord from higher centers, particularly discharge transmitted through the reticulospinal tracts, vestibulospinal tracts, and corticospinal tracts.

After a few hours to a few weeks, the spinal neurons gradually regain their excitability. This seems to be a natural characteristic of neurons everywhere in the nervous system—that is, after they lose their source of facilitatory impulses, they increase their own natural degree of excitability to make up at least partially for the loss. In most nonprimates, excitability of the cord centers returns essentially to normal within a few hours to a day or so, but in human beings, the return is often delayed for several weeks and occasionally is never complete; conversely, sometimes recovery is excessive, with resultant hyperexcitability of some or all cord functions. Nevertheless, the recovery of reflexes is insufficient to bear the weight of the person, and hence it is not possible to stand unsupported. In terms of postural reflexes, this is the feature of the so-called *spinal animal*.

Some of the spinal functions specifically affected during or after spinal shock are the following:

1. At onset of spinal shock, the arterial blood pressure falls almost instantly and drastically—sometimes to as low as 40 mmHg—thus demonstrating that sympathetic nervous system activity becomes blocked almost to extinction. The pressure ordinarily returns to normal within a few days, even in human beings.

2. All skeletal muscle reflexes integrated in the spinal cord are blocked during the initial stages of shock. In lower animals, a few hours to a few days are required for these reflexes to return to normal; in human beings, 2 weeks to several months are sometimes required. In both animals and humans, some reflexes may eventually become hyperexcitable, particularly if a few facilitatory pathways remain intact between the brain and the cord while the

remainder of the spinal cord is transected. The first reflexes to return are the stretch reflexes, followed in order by the progressively more complex reflexes: flexor reflexes, postural antigravity reflexes, and remnants of stepping reflexes.

3. The sacral reflexes for control of bladder and colon evacuation are suppressed in human beings for the first few weeks after cord transection, but in most cases they eventually return. These effects are discussed in Chapters 74 and 83.

Hemisection of the Cord

A hemisection of the cord, that is, transection of half the cord on any one side, can occur due to injury or an expanding tumor of the cord, and leads to a unique set of signs in the patient. These are an ipsilateral (on the same side of the lesion) upper motor neuron paralysis below the lesion, due to interruption of the corticospinal tract, which supplies the anterior horn motor cells on the same side below that level. It may also be possible to demonstrate a lower motor neuron paralysis ipsilaterally at the level of the lesion. There is also a loss of superficial reflexes, and loss of proprioception, two-point discrimination, and vibratory sense ipsilaterally, due to interruption of the posterior white columns (fasciculus gracilis/cuneatus).

However, pain and temperature sensation is lost on the opposite (contralateral) side below the lesion, due to interruption of the lateral spinothalamic tract whose fibers originated on the side opposite the lesion but which crossed in the anterior white commissure. This presentation is also called the Brown–Séquard syndrome.

Tabes Dorsalis

Tabes dorsalis is a disorder of the spinal cord due to demyelination of the dorsal columns. These columns carry the sensations of fine touch, vibration, and position. The condition occurs as a result of untreated syphilis, and is quite rare presently. There is a decreased tone of muscles with diminished tendon reflexes, a loss of coordination, and a characteristic high stepping gait, since the patient is unable to sense the position of the foot in relation to the ground, while stepping.

Syringomyelia

Syringomyelia is another disorder of the spinal cord due to the formation of a fluid-filled cavity in the central cord. This expanding cavity in the center of the cord puts pressure particularly on nerves that cross at this point, which are the afferent nerves carrying pain and temperature sensation to the anterolateral tract. The primary symptom is therefore a loss of thermal and crude pain sensations. The cavity or cyst can be congenital, or acquired, due to trauma or infections, and is also called a *syrinx*.

BIBLIOGRAPHY

Dietz V, Fouad K: Restoration of sensorimotor functions after spinal cord injury, *Brain* 137:654, 2014.

Frigon A: Reconfiguration of the spinal interneuronal network during locomotion in vertebrates, *J. Neurophysiol.* 101:2201, 2009.

Goulding M: Circuits controlling vertebrate locomotion: moving in a new direction, *Nat. Rev. Neurosci.* 10:507, 2009.

Grillner S: The motor infrastructure: from ion channels to neuronal networks, *Nat. Rev. Neurosci.* 4:573, 2003.

Kandel ER, Schwartz JH, Jessell TM: *Principles of Neural Science*, fourth ed., New York, 2000, McGraw-Hill.

Rossignol S, Barrière G, Alluin O, et al: Re-expression of locomotor function after partial spinal cord injury, *Physiology (Bethesda)* 24:127, 2009.

Rossignol S, Barrière G, Frigon A, et al: Plasticity of locomotor sensorimotor interactions after peripheral and/or spinal lesions, *Brain Res. Rev.* 57:228, 2008.

Cortical and Brainstem Control of Motor Function: The Pyramidal Tract

Most "voluntary" movements initiated by the cerebral cortex are achieved when the cortex activates "patterns" of function stored in lower brain areas—the cord, brainstem, basal ganglia, and cerebellum. These lower centers, in turn, send specific control signals to the muscles.

For a few types of movements, however, the cortex has almost a direct pathway to the anterior motor neurons of the cord, bypassing some motor centers on the way. This is especially true for control of the fine dexterous movements of the fingers and hands. This chapter and Chapter 113 explain the interplay among the different motor areas of the brain and spinal cord to provide overall synthesis of voluntary motor function.

Motor Cortex and Corticospinal (Pyramidal) Tract

Figure 112-1 shows the functional areas of the cerebral cortex. Anterior to the central cortical sulcus, occupying approximately the posterior one-third of the frontal lobes, is the *motor cortex*. Posterior to the central sulcus is the *somatosensory cortex* (an area discussed in detail in Chapter 105), which feeds the motor cortex many of the signals that initiate motor activities.

The motor cortex is divided into three subareas, each of which has its own topographical representation of muscle groups and specific motor functions: (1) the *primary motor cortex*, (2) the *premotor area*, and (3) the *supplementary motor area*.

PRIMARY MOTOR CORTEX

The primary motor cortex, shown in Figure 112-1, lies in the first convolution of the frontal lobes anterior to the central sulcus. It begins laterally in the Sylvian fissure, spreads superiorly to the uppermost portion of the brain, and then dips deep into the longitudinal fissure. (This area is the same as area 4 in Brodmann's classification of the brain cortical areas, shown in Figure 105-1.)

Figure 112-1 lists the approximate topographical representations of the different muscle areas of the body in the primary motor cortex, beginning with the face and mouth region near the Sylvian fissure; the arm and hand area, in the midportion of the primary motor cortex; the trunk, near the apex of the brain; and the leg and foot areas, in the part of the primary motor cortex that dips into the longitudinal fissure. This topographical organization is demonstrated even more graphically in Figure 112-2, which shows the degrees of representation of the different muscle areas as mapped by Penfield and Rasmussen. This mapping was done by electrically stimulating the different areas of the motor cortex in human beings who were undergoing neurosurgical operations. Note that more than one-half of the entire primary motor cortex is concerned with controlling the muscles of the hands and the muscles of speech. Point stimulation in these hand and speech motor areas on rare occasion causes contraction of a single muscle; but most often, stimulation contracts a group of muscles. To express this in another way, excitation of a single motor cortex neuron usually excites a specific movement rather than one specific muscle. To do this, it excites a "pattern" of separate muscles, each of which contributes its own direction and strength of muscle movement.

PREMOTOR AREA

The premotor area, also shown in Figure 112-1, lies 1–3 cm anterior to the primary motor cortex. It extends inferiorly into the Sylvian fissure and superiorly into the longitudinal fissure, where it abuts the supplementary motor area, which has functions similar to those of the premotor area. The topographical organization of the premotor cortex is roughly the same as that of the primary motor cortex, with the mouth and face areas located most laterally; as one moves upward, the hand, arm, trunk, and leg areas are encountered.

Nerve signals generated in the premotor area cause much more complex "patterns" of movement than the discrete patterns generated in the primary motor cortex. For instance, the pattern may be to position the shoulders and arms so that the hands are properly oriented to perform specific tasks. To achieve these results, the most anterior part of the premotor area first develops a "motor image" of the total muscle movement that is to be performed. Then, in the posterior premotor cortex, this image excites each successive pattern of muscle

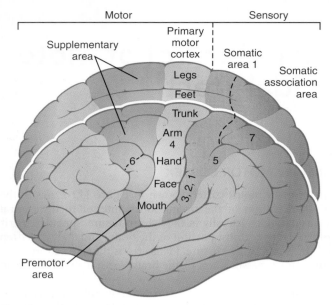

Figure 112-1   Motor and somatosensory functional areas of the cerebral cortex. The numbers 4, 5, 6, and 7 are Brodmann cortical areas, as explained in Chapter 105.

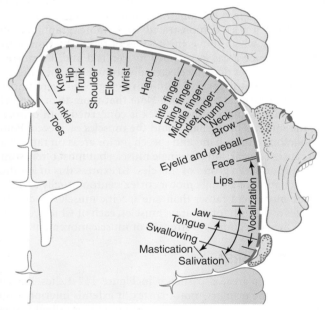

Figure 112-2   Degree of representation of the different muscles of the body in the motor cortex. *Modified from Penfield, W., Rasmussen, T., 1968. The Cerebral Cortex of Man: A Clinical Study of Localization of Function. Hafner, New York.*

activity required to achieve the image. This posterior part of the premotor cortex sends its signals either directly to the primary motor cortex to excite specific muscles or, often, by way of the basal ganglia and thalamus back to the primary motor cortex.

SUPPLEMENTARY MOTOR AREA

The supplementary motor area has yet another topographical organization for the control of motor function. It lies mainly in the longitudinal fissure but extends a few centimeters onto the superior frontal cortex. Contractions elicited by stimulating

this area are often bilateral rather than unilateral. For instance, stimulation frequently leads to bilateral grasping movements of both hands simultaneously; these movements are perhaps rudiments of the hand functions required for climbing. In general, this area functions in concert with the premotor area to provide body-wide attitudinal movements, fixation movements of the different segments of the body, positional movements of the head and eyes, and so forth, as background for the finer motor control of the arms and hands by the premotor area and primary motor cortex.

SOME SPECIALIZED AREAS OF MOTOR CONTROL FOUND IN THE HUMAN MOTOR CORTEX

A few highly specialized motor regions of the human cerebral cortex (shown in Figure 112-3) control specific motor functions. These regions have been localized either by electrical stimulation or by noting the loss of motor function when destructive lesions occur in specific cortical areas. Some of the more important regions are described in the following sections.

Broca Area (Motor Speech Area). Figure 112-3 shows a premotor area labeled "word formation" lying immediately anterior to the primary motor cortex and immediately above the Sylvian fissure. This region is called *Broca area.* Damage to it does not prevent a person from vocalizing but makes it impossible for the person to speak whole words rather than uncoordinated utterances or an occasional simple word such as "no" or "yes." A closely associated cortical area also causes appropriate respiratory function, so respiratory activation of the vocal cords can occur simultaneously with the movements of the mouth and tongue during speech. Thus, the premotor neuronal activities related to speech are highly complex.

"Voluntary" Eye Movement Field. In the premotor area immediately above Broca area is a locus for controlling voluntary eye movements. Damage to this area prevents a person from *voluntarily* moving the eyes toward different objects. Instead, the eyes tend to lock involuntarily onto specific objects, an effect controlled by signals from the occipital visual cortex, as explained in Chapter 110. This frontal area also controls eyelid movements such as blinking.

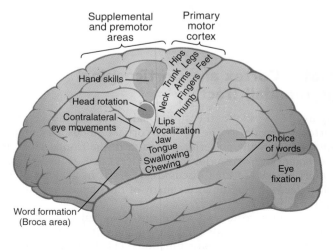

Figure 112-3   Representation of the different muscles of the body in the motor cortex and location of other cortical areas responsible for specific types of motor movements.

TRANSMISSION OF SIGNALS FROM THE MOTOR CORTEX TO THE MUSCLES

Motor signals are transmitted directly from the cortex to the spinal cord through the *corticospinal tract* and indirectly through multiple accessory pathways that involve the *basal ganglia, cerebellum,* and various *nuclei of the brainstem.* In general, the direct pathways are concerned more with discrete and detailed movements, especially of the distal segments of the limbs, particularly the hands and fingers.

Corticospinal (Pyramidal) Tract

The most important output pathway from the motor cortex is the *corticospinal tract,* also called the *pyramidal tract,* shown in Figure 112-4. The corticospinal tract originates about 30% from the primary motor cortex, 30% from the premotor and supplementary motor areas, and 40% from the somatosensory areas posterior to the central sulcus.

After leaving the cortex, it passes through the posterior limb of the internal capsule (between the caudate nucleus and the putamen of the basal ganglia) and then downward through the brainstem, forming the *pyramids of the medulla.* The

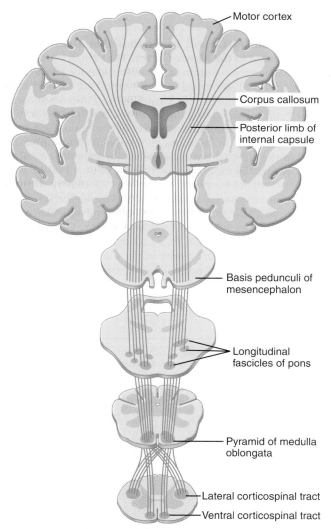

Figure 112-4 Corticospinal (pyramidal) tract. *Modified from Ranson, S.W., Clark, S.L., 1959. Anatomy of the Nervous System. W.B. Saunders, Philadelphia.*

Labels: Motor cortex; Corpus callosum; Posterior limb of internal capsule; Basis pedunculi of mesencephalon; Longitudinal fascicles of pons; Pyramid of medulla oblongata; Lateral corticospinal tract; Ventral corticospinal tract

majority of the pyramidal fibers then cross in the lower medulla to the opposite side and descend into the *lateral corticospinal tracts* of the cord, finally terminating principally on the interneurons in the intermediate regions of the cord gray matter; a few terminate on sensory relay neurons in the dorsal horn, and a very few terminate directly on the anterior motor neurons that cause muscle contraction.

A few of the fibers do not cross to the opposite side in the medulla but pass ipsilaterally down the cord in the *ventral corticospinal tracts.* Many, if not most, of these fibers eventually cross to the opposite side of the cord either in the neck or in the upper thoracic region. These fibers may be concerned with control of bilateral postural movements by the supplementary motor cortex.

The most impressive fibers in the pyramidal tract are a population of large myelinated fibers with a mean diameter of 16 µm. These fibers originate from *giant pyramidal cells,* called *Betz cells,* that are found only in the primary motor cortex. The Betz cells are about 60 µm in diameter, and their fibers transmit nerve impulses to the spinal cord at a velocity of about 70 m/second, the most rapid rate of transmission of any signals from the brain to the cord. There are about 34,000 of these large Betz cell fibers in each corticospinal tract. The total number of fibers in each corticospinal tract is more than 1 million, so these large fibers represent only 3% of the total. The other 97% are mainly fibers smaller than 4 µm in diameter that conduct background tonic signals to the motor areas of the cord.

Other Fiber Pathways from the Motor Cortex. The motor cortex gives rise to large numbers of additional, mainly small, fibers that go to deep regions in the cerebrum and brainstem, including the following:

1. The axons from the giant Betz cells send short collaterals back to the cortex itself. These collaterals are believed to inhibit adjacent regions of the cortex when the Betz cells discharge, thereby "sharpening" the boundaries of the excitatory signal.

2. A large number of fibers pass from the motor cortex into the *caudate nucleus* and *putamen.* From there, additional pathways extend into the brainstem and spinal cord, as discussed in Chapter 118, mainly to control body postural muscle contractions.

3. A moderate number of motor fibers pass to *red nuclei* of the midbrain. From these nuclei, additional fibers pass down the cord through the *rubrospinal tract.*

4. A moderate number of motor fibers deviate into the *reticular substance* and *vestibular nuclei* of the brainstem; from there, signals go to the cord by way of *reticulospinal* and *vestibulospinal tracts,* and others go to the cerebellum by way of *reticulocerebellar* and *vestibulocerebellar tracts.*

5. A tremendous number of motor fibers synapse in the pontile nuclei, which give rise to the *pontocerebellar fibers,* carrying signals into the cerebellar hemispheres.

6. Collaterals also terminate in the *inferior olivary nuclei,* and from there, secondary *olivocerebellar fibers* transmit signals to multiple areas of the cerebellum.

Thus, the basal ganglia, brainstem, and cerebellum all receive strong motor signals from the corticospinal system every time a signal is transmitted down the spinal cord to cause a motor activity.

"EXTRAPYRAMIDAL" SYSTEM

The term *extrapyramidal motor system* has been used in clinical circles to denote all the portions of the brain and brainstem that contribute to motor control but are not part of the direct corticospinal–pyramidal system. These portions include pathways through the basal ganglia, the reticular formation of the brainstem, the vestibular nuclei, and often the red nuclei. This group of motor control areas is such an all-inclusive and diverse group that it is difficult to ascribe specific neurophysiological functions to the extrapyramidal system as a whole. In fact, the pyramidal and extrapyramidal systems are extensively interconnected and interact to control movement. For these reasons, the term "extrapyramidal" is being used less often both clinically and physiologically.

Effect of Lesions in the Motor Cortex or in the Corticospinal Pathway—The "Stroke"

The motor control system can be damaged by the common abnormality called a "stroke." A stroke is caused by either a ruptured blood vessel that hemorrhages into the brain or thrombosis of one of the major arteries supplying blood to the brain. In either case, the result is loss of blood supply to the cortex or to the corticospinal tract where it passes through the internal capsule between the caudate nucleus and the putamen. Also, experiments have been performed in animals to selectively remove different parts of the motor cortex.

Lesion in the Internal Capsule. Since the corticospinal tract passes through a relatively small area in the internal capsule, lesions here, due to inadequate blood supply, for example, are accompanied by a dramatic loss of function on the opposite side of the body. Interruptions in the pyramidal tract here lead to a condition called hemiplegia or hemiparesis, in which there is a paralysis or weakness on the entire opposite side. This is also called an upper motor neuron paralysis, in contrast to a lower motor neuron paralysis, which occurs due to damage anywhere distal to the anterior horn cells. Table 112-1 lists differences between an upper and lower motor neuron paralysis. In the hemiplegia due to the upper motor neuron lesion, there is usually no atrophy of the muscles, but a marked stiffness or spasticity is observed (see the subsequent text), along with heightened tendon reflexes.

Removal of the Primary Motor Cortex (Area Pyramidalis). Removal of a portion of the primary motor cortex—the area that contains the giant Betz pyramidal cells—causes varying degrees of paralysis of the represented muscles. If the sublying

TABLE 112-1	Difference Between Upper and Lower Motor Neuron Paralysis	
Upper Motor Neuron Paralysis	**Lower Motor Neuron Paralysis**
Generally affects whole groups of muscles—such as hemiplegia, paraplegia, or monoplegia	Single muscles affected
No atrophy	Severe atrophy
No fasciculations	Fasciculations present
Rigidity	Flaccid paralysis
Increased tendon reflexes	Absent tendon reflexes
Extensor plantar reflex (Babinski sign)	Normal, if present

caudate nucleus and adjacent premotor and supplementary motor areas are not damaged, gross postural and limb "fixation" movements can still occur, but there is *loss of voluntary control of discrete movements of the distal segments of the limbs, especially of the hands and fingers.* This does not mean that the hand and finger muscles cannot contract; rather, the *ability to control the fine movements is gone.* From these observations, one can conclude that the area pyramidalis is essential for voluntary initiation of finely controlled movements, especially of the hands and fingers.

Muscle Spasticity Caused by Lesions that Damage Large Areas Adjacent to the Motor Cortex. The primary motor cortex normally exerts a continual tonic stimulatory effect on the motor neurons of the spinal cord; when this stimulatory effect is removed, *hypotonia* results. Most lesions of the motor cortex, especially those caused by a *stroke,* involve not only the primary motor cortex but also adjacent parts of the brain such as the basal ganglia. In these instances, *muscle spasm* almost invariably occurs in the afflicted muscle areas on the *opposite side* of the body (because the motor pathways cross to the opposite side). This spasm results mainly from damage to accessory pathways from the nonpyramidal portions of the motor cortex. These pathways normally inhibit the vestibular and reticular brainstem motor nuclei. When these nuclei cease their state of inhibition (ie, are "disinhibited"), they become spontaneously active and cause excessive spastic tone in the involved muscles. This spasticity is that which normally accompanies a "stroke" in a human being.

BIBLIOGRAPHY

Harrison TC, Murphy TH: Motor maps and the cortical control of movement, *Curr. Opin. Neurobiol.* 24:88, 2014.

Horak FB: Postural compensation for vestibular loss, *Ann. N. Y. Acad. Sci.* 1164(76), 2009.

Lemon RN: Descending pathways in motor control, *Annu. Rev. Neurosci.* 31:195, 2008.

Levine AJ, Lewallen KA, Pfaff SL: Spatial organization of cortical and spinal neurons controlling

motor behavior, *Curr. Opin. Neurobiol.* 22:812, 2012.

Nachev P, Kennard C, Husain M: Functional role of the supplementary and pre-supplementary motor areas, *Nat. Rev. Neurosci.* 9:856, 2008.

Nielsen JB, Cohen LG: The Olympic brain. Does corticospinal plasticity play a role in acquisition of skills required for high-performance sports? *J. Physiol.* 586:65, 2008.

Nishitani N, Schürmann M, Amunts K, et al: Broca's region: from action to language, *Physiology (Bethesda)* 20:60, 2005.

Schieber MH: Motor control: basic units of cortical output? *Curr. Biol.* 14:R353, 2004.

GLOSSARY OF TERMS

- **Clasp knife reflex:** A rapid decrease in resistance when attempting to flex a joint (characteristic of an upper motor neuron lesion)

- **Golgi tendon organ:** Sensory receptor located at the myotendinous junction, which detects the force of muscle contraction (provides the sensory component of the Golgi tendon reflex)

- **Spindle:** Sensory receptors located within the muscle, which detect changes in the length of muscle (provide the sensory component of the deep tendon reflex)

Muscle Sensory Receptors—Muscle Spindles and Golgi Tendon Organs—And their Roles in Muscle Control

Proper control of muscle function requires not only excitation of the muscle by spinal cord anterior motor neurons but also continuous feedback of sensory information from each muscle to the spinal cord, indicating the functional status of each muscle at each instant. That is, what is the length of the muscle, what is its instantaneous tension, and how rapidly is its length or tension changing? To provide this information, the muscles and their tendons are supplied abundantly with two special types of sensory receptors: (1) *muscle spindles* (see Figure 111-2), which are distributed throughout the belly of the muscle and send information to the nervous system about muscle length or rate of change of length, and (2) *Golgi tendon organs* (see Figures 111-2 and 113-5), which are located in the muscle tendons and transmit information about tendon tension or rate of change of tension.

The signals from these two receptors are almost entirely for the purpose of intrinsic muscle control. They operate almost completely at a subconscious level. Even so, they transmit tremendous amounts of information not only to the spinal cord but also to the cerebellum and even to the cerebral cortex, helping each of these portions of the nervous system function to control muscle contraction.

RECEPTOR FUNCTION OF THE MUSCLE SPINDLE

Structure and Motor Innervation of the Muscle Spindle. The organization of the muscle spindle is shown in Figure 111-3. Each spindle is 3–10 mm long. It is built around 3–12 tiny *intrafusal muscle fibers* that are pointed at their ends and attached to the glycocalyx of the surrounding large *extrafusal* skeletal muscle fibers.

Each intrafusal muscle fiber is a tiny skeletal muscle fiber. However, the central region of each of these fibers—that is, the area midway between its two ends—has few or no actin and myosin filaments. Therefore, this central portion does not contract when the ends do. Instead, it functions as a sensory receptor, as described later. The end portions that do contract are excited by small *gamma motor nerve fibers* that originate from small type A gamma motor neurons in the anterior horns of the spinal cord, as described earlier. These gamma motor nerve fibers are also called *gamma efferent fibers*, in contradistinction to the large *alpha efferent fibers* (type Aα nerve fibers) that innervate the extrafusal skeletal muscle.

Sensory Innervation of the Muscle Spindle. The receptor portion of the muscle spindle is its central portion. In this area, the intrafusal muscle fibers do not have myosin and actin contractile elements. As shown in Figure 111-3 and in more detail in Figure 113-1, sensory fibers originate in this area and are stimulated by stretching of this midportion of the spindle. One can readily see that the muscle spindle receptor can be excited in two ways:

1. Lengthening the whole muscle stretches the midportion of the spindle and, therefore, excites the receptor.
2. Even if the length of the entire muscle does not change, contraction of the end portions of the spindle's intrafusal fibers stretches the midportion of the spindle and therefore excites the receptor.

Two types of sensory endings, the *primary afferent* and *secondary afferent endings,* are found in this central receptor area of the muscle spindle.

Primary Ending. In the center of the receptor area, a large sensory nerve fiber encircles the central portion of each intrafusal fiber, forming the so-called *primary afferent ending* or *annulospiral ending*. This nerve fiber is a type Ia fiber averaging 17 μm in diameter, and it transmits sensory signals to the spinal cord at a velocity of 70–120 m/second, as rapidly as any type of nerve fiber in the entire body.

Secondary Ending. Usually one but sometimes two smaller sensory nerve fibers—type II fibers with an average diameter of 8 μm—innervate the receptor region on one or both sides of the primary ending, as shown in Figures 111-3 and 113-1. This sensory ending is called the *secondary afferent ending*; sometimes it encircles the intrafusal fibers in the same way that the type Ia fiber does, but often it spreads like branches on a bush.

Division of the Intrafusal Fibers into Nuclear Bag and Nuclear Chain Fibers—Dynamic and Static Responses of the

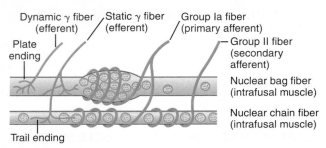

Figure 113-1 Details of nerve connections from the nuclear bag and nuclear chain muscle spindle fibers. *Modified from Stein, R.B., 1974. Peripheral control of movement. Physiol. Rev. 54, 225.*

Muscle Spindle. There are also two types of muscle spindle intrafusal fibers: (1) *nuclear bag muscle fibers* (one to three in each spindle), in which several muscle fiber nuclei are congregated in expanded "bags" in the central portion of the receptor area, as shown by the top fiber in Figure 113-1, and (2) *nuclear chain fibers* (three to nine), which are about half as large in diameter and half as long as the nuclear bag fibers, and have nuclei aligned in a chain throughout the receptor area, as shown by the bottom fiber in the figure. The primary sensory nerve ending (the 17-μm sensory fiber) is excited by both the nuclear bag intrafusal fibers *and* the nuclear chain fibers. Conversely, the secondary ending (the 8-μm sensory fiber) is usually excited only by nuclear chain fibers. These relations are shown in Figure 113-1.

Response of Both the Primary and the Secondary Endings to the Length of the Receptor—"Static" Response. When the receptor portion of the muscle spindle is stretched *slowly*, the number of impulses transmitted from both the primary and the secondary endings increases almost directly in proportion to the degree of stretching and the endings continue to transmit these impulses for several minutes. This effect is called the *static response* of the spindle receptor, meaning simply that both the primary and secondary endings continue to transmit their signals for at least several minutes if the muscle spindle remains stretched.

Response of the Primary Ending (but Not the Secondary Ending) to Rate of Change of Receptor Length—"Dynamic" Response. When the length of the spindle receptor increases suddenly, the primary ending (but not the secondary ending) is stimulated powerfully. This stimulus of the primary ending is called the *dynamic response*, which means that the primary ending responds extremely actively to a rapid *rate of change* in spindle length. Even when the length of a spindle receptor increases only a fraction of a micrometer for only a fraction of a second, the primary receptor transmits tremendous numbers of excess impulses to the large 17-μm sensory nerve fiber, *but only while the length is actually increasing*. As soon as the length stops increasing, this extra rate of impulse discharge returns to the level of the much smaller static response that is still present in the signal.

Conversely, when the spindle receptor shortens, exactly opposite sensory signals occur. Thus, the primary ending sends extremely strong signals, either positive or negative, to the spinal cord to apprise it of any change in length of the spindle receptor.

Control of Intensity of the Static and Dynamic Responses by the Gamma Motor Nerves. The gamma motor nerves to the muscle spindle can be divided into two types: *gamma-dynamic* (*gamma-d*) and *gamma-static* (*gamma-s*). The first of these gamma motor nerves excites mainly the nuclear bag intrafusal fibers, and the second excites mainly the nuclear chain intrafusal

fibers. When the gamma-d fibers excite the nuclear bag fibers, the dynamic response of the muscle spindle becomes tremendously enhanced, whereas the static response is hardly affected. Conversely, stimulation of the gamma-s fibers, which excite the nuclear chain fibers, enhances the static response while having little influence on the dynamic response. Subsequent paragraphs illustrate that these two types of muscle spindle responses are important in different types of muscle control.

Continuous Discharge of the Muscle Spindles Under Normal Conditions. Normally, when there is some degree of gamma nerve excitation, the muscle spindles emit sensory nerve impulses continuously. Stretching the muscle spindles increases the rate of firing, whereas shortening the spindle decreases the rate of firing. Thus, the spindles can send to the spinal cord either *positive signals* (increased numbers of impulses to indicate stretch of a muscle) or *negative signals* (reduced numbers of impulses to indicate that the muscle is unstretched).

MUSCLE STRETCH REFLEX

The simplest manifestation of muscle spindle function is the *muscle stretch reflex*. Whenever a muscle is stretched suddenly, excitation of the spindles causes reflex contraction of the large skeletal muscle fibers of the stretched muscle and also of closely allied synergistic muscles.

Neuronal Circuitry of the Stretch Reflex. Figure 113-2 demonstrates the basic circuit of the muscle spindle stretch reflex, showing a type Ia proprioceptor nerve fiber originating in a muscle spindle and entering a dorsal root of the spinal cord. A branch of this fiber then goes directly to the anterior horn of the cord gray matter and synapses with anterior motor neurons that send motor nerve fibers back to the same muscle from which the muscle spindle fiber originated. Thus, this is a *monosynaptic pathway* that allows a reflex signal to return with the shortest possible time delay back to the muscle after excitation of the spindle. Most type II fibers from the muscle spindle terminate on multiple interneurons in the cord gray matter, and these transmit delayed signals to the anterior motor neurons or serve other functions.

Dynamic Stretch and Static Stretch Reflexes. The stretch reflex can be divided into two components: the dynamic stretch

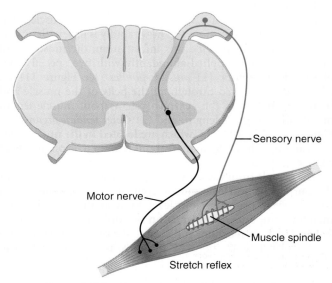

Figure 113-2 Neuronal circuit of the stretch reflex.

reflex and the static stretch reflex. The *dynamic stretch reflex* is elicited by potent dynamic signals transmitted from the primary sensory endings of the muscle spindles, caused by rapid stretch or unstretch. That is, when a muscle is suddenly stretched or unstretched, a strong signal is transmitted to the spinal cord, which causes an instantaneous strong reflex contraction (or decrease in contraction) of the same muscle from which the signal originated. Thus, *the reflex functions to oppose sudden changes in muscle length.*

The dynamic stretch reflex is over within a fraction of a second after the muscle has been stretched (or unstretched) to its new length, but then a weaker *static stretch reflex* continues for a prolonged period thereafter. This reflex is elicited by the continuous static receptor signals transmitted by both primary and secondary endings. The importance of the static stretch reflex is that it causes the degree of muscle contraction to remain reasonably constant, except when the person's nervous system specifically wills otherwise.

"Damping" Function of the Dynamic and Static Stretch Reflexes in Smoothing Muscle Contraction

An especially important function of the stretch reflex is its ability to prevent oscillation or jerkiness of body movements, which is a *damping*, or smoothing, function.

Signals from the spinal cord are often transmitted to a muscle in an unsmooth form, increasing in intensity for a few milliseconds, then decreasing in intensity, then changing to another intensity level, and so forth. When the muscle spindle apparatus is not functioning satisfactorily, the muscle contraction is jerky during the course of such a signal. This effect is demonstrated in Figure 113-3. In curve A, the muscle spindle reflex of the excited muscle is intact. Note that the contraction is relatively smooth, even though the motor nerve to the muscle is excited at a slow frequency of only eight signals per second. Curve B illustrates the same experiment in an animal whose muscle spindle sensory nerves had been sectioned 3 months earlier. Note the unsmooth muscle contraction. Thus, curve A graphically demonstrates the damping mechanism's ability to smooth muscle contractions, even though the primary input signals to the muscle motor system may themselves be jerky. This effect can also be called a *signal averaging* function of the muscle spindle reflex.

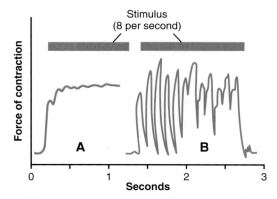

Figure 113-3   Muscle contraction caused by a spinal cord signal under two conditions: (*curve A*) in a normal muscle and (*curve B*) in a muscle whose muscle spindles were denervated by section of the posterior roots of the cord 82 days previously. Note the smoothing effect of the muscle spindle reflex in *curve A*. Modified from Creed, R.S., et al., 1932. *Reflex Activity of the Spinal Cord. Oxford University Press, New York.*

ROLE OF THE MUSCLE SPINDLE IN VOLUNTARY MOTOR ACTIVITY

To understand the importance of the gamma efferent system, one should recognize that 31% of all the motor nerve fibers to the muscle are the small type A gamma efferent fibers rather than large type A alpha motor fibers. Whenever signals are transmitted from the motor cortex or from any other area of the brain to the alpha motor neurons, in most instances the gamma motor neurons are stimulated simultaneously, an effect called *coactivation* of the alpha and gamma motor neurons. This effect causes both the extrafusal skeletal muscle fibers and the muscle spindle intrafusal muscle fibers to contract at the same time.

The purpose of contracting the muscle spindle intrafusal fibers at the same time that the large skeletal muscle fibers contract is twofold: First, it keeps the length of the receptor portion of the muscle spindle from changing during the course of the whole muscle contraction. Therefore, coactivation keeps the muscle spindle reflex from opposing the muscle contraction. Second, it maintains the proper damping function of the muscle spindle, regardless of any change in muscle length. For instance, if the muscle spindle did not contract and relax along with the large muscle fibers, the receptor portion of the spindle would sometimes be flail and sometimes be overstretched, in neither instance operating under optimal conditions for spindle function.

Brain Areas for Control of the Gamma Motor System

The gamma efferent system is excited specifically by signals from the *bulboreticular facilitatory* region of the brainstem and, secondarily, by impulses transmitted into the bulboreticular area from (1) the *cerebellum*, (2) the *basal ganglia*, and (3) the *cerebral cortex*.

Little is known about the precise mechanisms of control of the gamma efferent system. However, because the bulboreticular facilitatory area is particularly concerned with antigravity contractions, and because the antigravity muscles have an especially high density of muscle spindles, emphasis is given to the importance of the gamma efferent mechanism for damping the movements of the different body parts during walking and running.

CLINICAL APPLICATIONS OF THE STRETCH REFLEX

Almost every time a clinician performs a physical examination on a patient, he or she elicits multiple stretch reflexes. The purpose is to determine how much background excitation, or "tone," the brain is sending to the spinal cord. This reflex is elicited as follows.

Knee Jerk and Other Muscle Jerks Can Be Used to Assess Sensitivity of Stretch Reflexes. Clinically, a method used to determine the sensitivity of the stretch reflexes is to elicit the knee jerk and other muscle jerks. The knee jerk can be elicited by simply striking the patellar tendon with a reflex hammer; this action instantaneously stretches the quadriceps muscle and excites a *dynamic stretch reflex* that causes the lower leg to "jerk" forward. The upper part of Figure 113-4 shows a myogram from the quadriceps muscle recorded during a knee jerk.

Similar reflexes can be obtained from almost any muscle of the body either by striking the tendon of the muscle or by striking the belly of the muscle itself. In other words, sudden

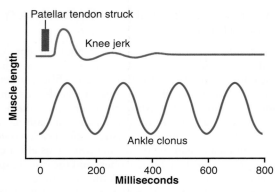

Figure 113-4   Myograms recorded from the quadriceps muscle during elicitation of the knee jerk (*above*) and from the gastrocnemius muscle during ankle clonus (*below*).

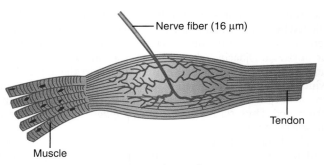

Figure 113-5   Golgi tendon organ.

stretch of muscle spindles is all that is required to elicit a dynamic stretch reflex.

The muscle jerks are used by neurologists to assess the degree of facilitation of spinal cord centers. When large numbers of facilitatory impulses are being transmitted from the upper regions of the central nervous system into the cord, the muscle jerks are greatly exaggerated. Conversely, if the facilitatory impulses are depressed or abrogated, the muscle jerks are considerably weakened or absent. These reflexes are used most frequently in determining the presence or absence of muscle spasticity caused by lesions in the motor areas of the brain or diseases that excite the bulboreticular facilitatory area of the brainstem. Ordinarily, large *lesions in the motor areas of the cerebral cortex* but not in the lower motor control areas (especially lesions caused by strokes or brain tumors) cause greatly exaggerated muscle jerks in the muscles on the opposite side of the body.

Clonus—Oscillation of Muscle Jerks. Under some conditions, the muscle jerks can oscillate, a phenomenon called *clonus* (see lower myogram, Figure 113-4). Oscillation can be explained particularly well in relation to ankle clonus, as follows.

If a person standing on the tip ends of the feet suddenly drops his or her body downward and stretches the gastrocnemius muscles, stretch reflex impulses are transmitted from the muscle spindles into the spinal cord. These impulses reflexively excite the stretched muscle, which lifts the body up again. After a fraction of a second, the reflex contraction of the muscle dies out and the body falls again, thus stretching the spindles a second time. Again, a dynamic stretch reflex lifts the body, but this too dies out after a fraction of a second, and the body falls once more to begin a new cycle. In this way, the stretch reflex of the gastrocnemius muscle continues to oscillate, often for long periods, which is clonus.

Clonus ordinarily occurs only when the stretch reflex is highly sensitized by facilitatory impulses from the brain. For instance, in a decerebrate animal, in which the stretch reflexes are highly facilitated, clonus develops readily. To determine the degree of facilitation of the spinal cord, neurologists test patients for clonus by suddenly stretching a muscle and applying a steady stretching force to it. If clonus occurs, the degree of facilitation is certain to be high.

GOLGI TENDON REFLEX

Golgi Tendon Organ Helps Control Muscle Tension. The Golgi tendon organ, shown in Figure 113-5, is an encapsulated sensory receptor through which muscle tendon fibers

pass. About 10–15 muscle fibers are usually connected to each Golgi tendon organ, and the organ is stimulated when this small bundle of muscle fibers is "tensed" by contracting or stretching the muscle. Thus, the major difference in excitation of the Golgi tendon organ versus the muscle spindle is that *the spindle detects muscle length and changes in muscle length*, whereas *the tendon organ detects muscle tension* as reflected by the tension in itself.

The tendon organ, like the primary receptor of the muscle spindle, has both a *dynamic response* and a *static response*, reacting intensely when the muscle tension suddenly increases (the dynamic response) but settling down within a fraction of a second to a lower level of steady-state firing that is almost directly proportional to the muscle tension (the static response). Thus, Golgi tendon organs provide the nervous system with instantaneous information on the degree of tension in each small segment of each muscle.

Transmission of Impulses from the Tendon Organ into the Central Nervous System. Signals from the tendon organ are transmitted through large, rapidly conducting type Ib nerve fibers that average 16 μm in diameter, only slightly smaller than those from the primary endings of the muscle spindle. These fibers, like those from the primary spindle endings, transmit signals both into local areas of the cord and, after synapsing in a dorsal horn of the cord, through long fiber pathways such as the spinocerebellar tracts into the cerebellum and through still other tracts to the cerebral cortex. The local cord signal excites a single *inhibitory* interneuron that inhibits the anterior motor neuron. This local circuit directly inhibits the individual muscle without affecting adjacent muscles. The relation between signals to the brain and function of the cerebellum and other parts of the brain for muscle control is discussed in Chapter 116.

The Tendon Reflex Prevents Excessive Tension on the Muscle

When the Golgi tendon organs of a muscle tendon are stimulated by increased tension in the connecting muscle, signals are transmitted to the spinal cord to cause reflex effects in the respective muscle. This reflex is entirely *inhibitory*. Thus, this reflex provides a *negative feedback* mechanism that prevents the development of too much tension on the muscle.

When tension on the muscle and, therefore, on the tendon becomes extreme, the inhibitory effect from the tendon organ can be so great that it leads to a sudden reaction in the spinal cord that causes instantaneous relaxation of the entire muscle. This effect is called the *lengthening reaction*; it is probably a protective mechanism to prevent tearing of the muscle or avulsion of the tendon from its attachments to the bone.

Possible Role of the Tendon Reflex to Equalize Contractile Force among the Muscle Fibers. Another likely function of the Golgi tendon reflex is to equalize contractile forces of the separate muscle fibers. That is, the fibers that exert excess tension become inhibited by the reflex, whereas those that exert too little tension become more excited because of the absence of reflex inhibition. This phenomenon spreads the muscle load over all the fibers and prevents damage in isolated areas of a muscle where small numbers of fibers might be overloaded.

BIBLIOGRAPHY

Dietz V: Proprioception and locomotor disorders, *Nat. Rev. Neurosci.* 3:781, 2002.

Dietz V, Sinkjaer T: Spastic movement disorder: impaired reflex function and altered muscle mechanics, *Lancet Neurol.* 6:725, 2007.

Duysens J, Clarac F, Cruse H: Load-regulating mechanisms in gait and posture: comparative aspects, *Physiol. Rev.* 80:83, 2000.

Frigon A: Reconfiguration of the spinal interneuronal network during locomotion in vertebrates, *J. Neurophysiol.* 101:2201, 2009.

Goulding M: Circuits controlling vertebrate locomotion: moving in a new direction, *Nat. Rev. Neurosci.* 10:507, 2009.

Grillner S: The motor infrastructure: from ion channels to neuronal networks, *Nat. Rev. Neurosci.* 4:573, 2003.

Kandel ER, Schwartz JH, Jessell TM: *Principles of Neural Science*, fourth ed., New York, 2000, McGraw-Hill.

Kiehn O: Locomotor circuits in the mammalian spinal cord, *Annu. Rev. Neurosci.* 29:279, 2006.

Prochazka A, Ellaway P: Sensory systems in the control of movement, *Compr. Physiol.* 2:2615, 2012.

114 Motor Reflexes

LEARNING OBJECTIVES

- Describe reflex action.
- List the components of reflex arc with a diagram.
- Describe monosynaptic and multisynaptic reflexes.
- List the properties of reflexes.

GLOSSARY OF TERMS

- **Reciprocal inhibition:** When muscles acting on one side of a joint relax to allow the muscles acting on the other side of the joint to contract
- **Reflex:** Involuntary and nearly instantaneous motor response to a stimulus

Reflexes

Reflex actions are based on a sequence of events involving a receptor, an afferent neuron or arc, an efferent neuron or arc, and an effector. This is a typical monosynaptic reflex, that is, there is only one synapse (and consequently little delay in transmission) within the pathway. An example of such a reflex is the myotatic reflex, and the combination of the receptor (muscle spindle), afferent sensory nerve, efferent motor nerve, and the effector (striated muscle fiber) is called a myotatic unit. There may be other neurons that exist between the afferent and efferent arms of the reflex, and these are called connectors or internuncial neurons (Figure 114-1). Consequently, depending on the number of internuncial cells, these could be disynaptic or multisynaptic.

Reflexes are classified based on their pathways passing through segments of the spinal cord or based on a clinical approach. Based on a segmental approach, there are segmental, intersegmental, and suprasegmental reflexes. A segmental reflex passes through a single segment of the spinal cord, while intersegmental reflexes have ascending or descending paths in the spinal cord. An example of a segmental reflex is the tendon reflex, while superficial reflexes are usually intersegmental. Suprasegmental reflexes have long pathways that involve different nuclei above the level of the spinal cord.

Clinically, reflexes are classified based on where they are elicited—superficial, deep, and visceral. Examples of these are the plantar reflex, the tendon reflexes, and the papillary reflex, respectively. Sometimes, a reflex may be altered in pathological states; an example is the Babinski reflex, which is an altered plantar reflex. This is called a pathological reflex.

PROPERTIES OF REFLEXES

As explained earlier, reflexes have defined structures, and their properties vary depending on their classification. Therefore, monosynaptic reflexes are very fast (of the order of 0.5 millisecond), while multisynaptic reflexes are slower with a latency of a few milliseconds. Reciprocal innervations occur, meaning that the excitation due to the reflex on one set of muscles is accompanied by inhibition on the other. For example, this means that flexion and extension cannot simultaneously be accomplished on the same limb. This reciprocal innervation reflects an organization of the nervous system at this spinal level, and extends to the contralateral side as well, where a flexor reflex on one side is accompanied by an inhibition of the same reflex and an augmentation of the opposing muscle reflex on the opposite side (see Table 114-1).

Flexor Reflex and the Withdrawal Reflexes

In the spinal or decerebrate animal, almost any type of cutaneous sensory stimulus from a limb is likely to cause the flexor muscles of the limb to contract, thereby withdrawing the limb from the stimulating object. This reflex is called the *flexor reflex*.

In its classic form, the flexor reflex is elicited most powerfully by stimulation of pain endings, such as by a pinprick, heat, or a wound, for which reason it is also called a *nociceptive reflex*, or simply a *pain reflex*. Stimulation of touch receptors can also elicit a weaker and less prolonged flexor reflex.

If some part of the body other than one of the limbs is painfully stimulated, that part will similarly be *withdrawn from the stimulus*, but the reflex may not be confined to flexor muscles, even though it is basically the same type of reflex. Therefore, the many patterns of these reflexes in the different areas of the body are called *withdrawal reflexes*.

Neuronal Mechanism of the Flexor Reflex. The left-hand portion of Figure 114-2 shows the neuronal pathways for the flexor reflex. In this instance, a painful stimulus is applied to the hand; as a result, the flexor muscles of the upper arm become excited, thus withdrawing the hand from the painful stimulus.

The pathways for eliciting the flexor reflex do not pass directly to the anterior motor neurons but instead pass first into the spinal cord interneuron pool of neurons and only secondarily to the motor neurons. The shortest possible circuit is a three- or four-neuron pathway; however, most of the signals of the reflex traverse many more neurons and involve the following basic types of circuits: (1) diverging circuits to spread the reflex to the necessary muscles for withdrawal; (2) circuits to inhibit the antagonist muscles, called *reciprocal inhibition circuits*; and (3) circuits to cause *afterdischarge* that lasts many fractions of a second after the stimulus is over.

Figure 114-3 shows a typical myogram from a flexor muscle during a flexor reflex. Within a few milliseconds after a pain nerve begins to be stimulated, the flexor response appears. Then, in the next few seconds, the reflex begins to *fatigue*, which is characteristic of essentially all complex integrative reflexes of the spinal cord. Finally, after the stimulus is over, the contraction of the muscle returns toward the baseline, but because of afterdischarge, it takes many milliseconds for this contraction to

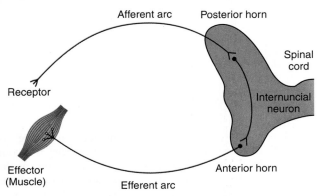

Figure 114-1 Components of reflex arc.

TABLE 114-1	**Properties of Reflexes**

1. The principle of convergence: increased (facilitation) or decreased (occlusion) discharge into the reflex arc could occur
2. The principle of divergence: one single afferent nerve can excite a large number of spinal neurons leading to a greater reflex response
3. Posttetanic potentiation: repetitive stimulation of the afferent nerve prior to applying a single stimulus elicits a greater reflex response. This potentiation becomes less depending on how much time interval there is between the conditioning burst of repetitive stimuli and the single stimulus
4. Rebound: inhibition is followed by a state of increased excitation
5. Renshaw inhibition: negative feedback control that damps down reflex discharges

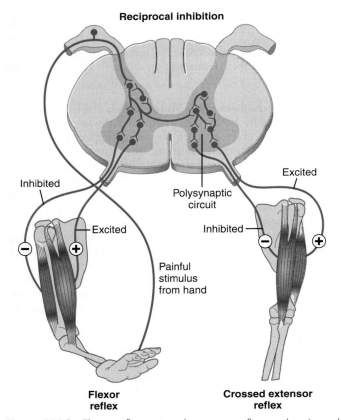

Figure 114-2 Flexor reflex, crossed extensor reflex, and reciprocal inhibition.

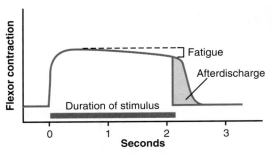

Figure 114-3 Myogram of the flexor reflex showing rapid onset of the reflex, an interval of fatigue, and, finally, afterdischarge after the input stimulus is over.

occur. The duration of afterdischarge depends on the intensity of the sensory stimulus that elicited the reflex; a weak tactile stimulus causes almost no afterdischarge, but after a strong pain stimulus, the afterdischarge may last for a second or more.

The afterdischarge that occurs in the flexor reflex almost certainly results from both types of repetitive discharge circuits discussed in Chapter 102. Electrophysiological studies indicate that immediate afterdischarge, lasting for about 6–8 milliseconds, results from repetitive firing of the excited interneurons themselves. Also, prolonged afterdischarge occurs after strong pain stimuli, almost certainly resulting from recurrent pathways that initiate oscillation in reverberating interneuron circuits. These, in turn, transmit impulses to the anterior motor neurons, sometimes for several seconds after the incoming sensory signal is over.

Thus, the flexor reflex is appropriately organized to withdraw a pained or otherwise irritated part of the body from a stimulus. Further, because of afterdischarge, the reflex can hold the irritated part away from the stimulus for 0.1–3 seconds after the irritation is over. During this time, other reflexes and actions of the central nervous system can move the entire body away from the painful stimulus.

Pattern of Withdrawal During Flexor Reflex. The pattern of withdrawal that results when the flexor reflex is elicited depends on which sensory nerve is stimulated. Thus, a pain stimulus on the inward side of the arm elicits not only contraction of the flexor muscles of the arm but also contraction of abductor muscles to pull the arm outward. In other words, the integrative centers of the cord cause the muscles to contract that can most effectively remove the pained part of the body away from the object causing the pain. Although this principle applies to any part of the body, it is especially applicable to the limbs because of their highly developed flexor reflexes.

Crossed Extensor Reflex

About 0.2–0.5 second after a stimulus elicits a flexor reflex in one limb, the opposite limb begins to extend. This reflex is called the *crossed extensor reflex*. Extension of the opposite limb can push the entire body away from the object causing the painful stimulus in the withdrawn limb.

Neuronal Mechanism of the Crossed Extensor Reflex. The right-hand portion of Figure 114-2 shows the neuronal circuit responsible for the crossed extensor reflex, demonstrating that signals from sensory nerves cross to the opposite side of the cord

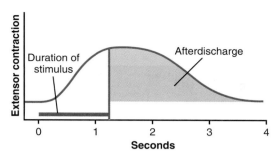

Figure 114-4 Myogram of a crossed extensor reflex showing slow onset but prolonged afterdischarge.

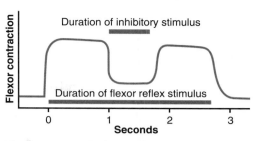

Figure 114-5 Myogram of a flexor reflex showing reciprocal inhibition caused by an inhibitory stimulus from a stronger flexor reflex on the opposite side of the body.

to excite extensor muscles. Because the crossed extensor reflex usually does not begin until 200–500 milliseconds after onset of the initial pain stimulus, it is certain that many interneurons are involved in the circuit between the incoming sensory neuron and the motor neurons of the opposite side of the cord responsible for the crossed extension. After the painful stimulus is removed, the crossed extensor reflex has an even longer period of afterdischarge than does the flexor reflex. Again, it is presumed that this prolonged afterdischarge results from reverberating circuits among the interneuronal cells.

Figure 114-4 shows a typical myogram recorded from a muscle involved in a crossed extensor reflex. This myogram demonstrates the relatively long latency before the reflex begins and the long afterdischarge at the end of the stimulus. The prolonged afterdischarge is of benefit in holding the pained area of the body away from the painful object until other nervous reactions cause the entire body to move away.

Reciprocal Inhibition and Reciprocal Innervation

We previously pointed out that excitation of one group of muscles is often associated with inhibition of another group. For instance, when a stretch reflex excites one muscle, it often simultaneously inhibits the antagonist muscles, which is the phenomenon of *reciprocal inhibition*, and the neuronal circuit that causes this reciprocal relation is called *reciprocal innervation*. Likewise, reciprocal relations often exist between the muscles on the two sides of the body, as exemplified by the flexor and extensor muscle reflexes described earlier.

Figure 114-5 shows a typical example of reciprocal inhibition. In this instance, a moderate but prolonged flexor reflex is elicited from one limb of the body; while this reflex is still being elicited, a stronger flexor reflex is elicited in the limb on the opposite side of the body. This stronger reflex sends reciprocal inhibitory signals to the first limb and depresses its degree of flexion. Finally, removal of the stronger reflex allows the original reflex to reassume its previous intensity.

Spinal Cord Reflexes that Cause Muscle Spasm

In human beings, local muscle spasm is often observed. In many, if not most, instances, localized pain is the cause of the local spasm.

Muscle Spasm Resulting from a Broken Bone. One type of clinically important spasm occurs in muscles that surround a broken bone. The spasm results from pain impulses initiated from the broken edges of the bone, which cause the muscles that surround the area to contract tonically. Pain relief obtained by injecting a local anesthetic at the broken edges of the bone relieves the spasm; a deep general anesthetic of the entire body, such as ether anesthesia, also relieves the spasm.

Abdominal Muscle Spasm in Persons with Peritonitis. Another type of local spasm caused by cord reflexes is abdominal spasm resulting from irritation of the parietal peritoneum by peritonitis. Here again, relief of the pain caused by the peritonitis allows the spastic muscle to relax. The same type of spasm often occurs during surgical operations; for instance, during abdominal operations, pain impulses from the parietal peritoneum often cause the abdominal muscles to contract extensively, sometimes extruding the intestines through the surgical wound. For this reason, deep anesthesia is usually required for intraabdominal operations.

Muscle Cramps. Another type of local spasm is the typical muscle cramp. Any local irritating factor or metabolic abnormality of a muscle, such as severe cold, lack of blood flow, or overexercise, can elicit pain or other sensory signals transmitted from the muscle to the spinal cord, which in turn cause reflex feedback muscle contraction. The contraction is believed to stimulate the same sensory receptors even more, which causes the spinal cord to increase the intensity of contraction. Thus, positive feedback develops, so a small amount of initial irritation causes more and more contraction until a full-blown muscle cramp ensues.

BIBLIOGRAPHY

Dietz V, Sinkjaer T: Spastic movement disorder: impaired reflex function and altered muscle mechanics, *Lancet Neurol.* 6:725, 2007.

Glover JC: Development of specific connectivity between premotor neurons and motoneurons in the brain stem and spinal cord, *Physiol. Rev.* 80:615, 2000.

Kandel ER, Schwartz JH, Jessell TM: *Principles of Neural Science*, fourth ed., New York, 2000, McGraw-Hill.

Kiehn O: Development and functional organization of spinal locomotor circuits, *Curr. Opin. Neurobiol.* 21:100, 2011.

Marchand-Pauvert V, Iglesias C: Properties of human spinal interneurones: normal and dystonic control, *J. Physiol.* 586:1247, 2008.

Rekling JC, Funk GD, Bayliss DA, et al: Synaptic control of motoneuronal excitability, *Physiol. Rev.* 80:767, 2000.

115

Regulation of Tone and Posture

Conceptually, it is useful to consider that there are levels of control of posture within the nervous system. At the lowest level, the spinal level, local reflexes act to maintain tone within muscles, while at a higher, bulbar level, nuclei in the medulla and pons act to enhance the tone of muscles that are involved in keeping the animal upright, or the antigravity muscles. An animal that has had a transection of the brainstem at the level of the pons will therefore be able to "stand upright" due to this phenomenon, but not in any functional way.

Support of the Body Against Gravity—Roles of the Reticular and Vestibular Nuclei

Figure 115-1 shows the locations of the reticular and vestibular nuclei in the brainstem.

EXCITATORY–INHIBITORY ANTAGONISM BETWEEN PONTINE AND MEDULLARY RETICULAR NUCLEI

The reticular nuclei are divided into two major groups: (1) *pontine reticular nuclei*, located slightly posteriorly and laterally in the pons and extending into the mesencephalon, and (2) *medullary reticular nuclei*, which extend through the entire medulla, lying ventrally and medially near the midline. These two sets of nuclei function mainly antagonistically to each other, with the pontine exciting the antigravity muscles and the medullary relaxing these same muscles.

ROLE OF THE VESTIBULAR NUCLEI TO EXCITE THE ANTIGRAVITY MUSCLES

All the *vestibular nuclei*, shown in Figure 115-1, function in association with the pontine reticular nuclei to control the antigravity muscles. The vestibular nuclei transmit strong excitatory signals to the antigravity muscles by way of the *lateral* and *medial vestibulospinal tracts* in the anterior columns of the spinal cord, as shown in Figure 115-2. Without this support of the vestibular nuclei, the pontine reticular system would lose much of its excitation of the axial antigravity muscles.

The specific role of the vestibular nuclei, however, is to *selectively* control the excitatory signals to the different antigravity muscles to maintain equilibrium *in response to signals from the vestibular apparatus*. We discuss this concept more fully later in Chapter 117.

THE DECEREBRATE ANIMAL DEVELOPS SPASTIC RIGIDITY

To study the effect of the brainstem on posture, an experimental animal model called the decerebrate animal can be studied, in which the brainstem is interrupted between the superior colliculi and the vestibular nuclei, that is, the vestibular nuclei connections with the cerebellum are intact, as well as the pontine and medullary reticular systems. This model is called the Sherrington model of decerebration, and was performed in mammals whose natural posture required the use of antigravity muscles, such as cats. The postoperative animal develops a condition called decerebrate rigidity with a characteristic attitude of extended limbs that allows it to be placed in an erect posture, since the extended limbs could support the weight of the body (see the subsequent text). The neck was also extended against gravity, meaning that the tonic neck reflexes were intact. However, the animal could not right itself when pushed over. A key feature of this decerebrate animal was that when the dorsal roots of the spinal cord were cut (deafferentation), the rigidity disappeared, showing that the cause of the rigidity was a hyperactive stretch reflex in the antigravity muscles. This hyperactivity was caused by an increased stimulation of the γ-motor neurons by facilitatory areas of the reticular formation in the brainstem, below the level of the interruption. There is normally a strong input to the medullary reticular nuclei from the cerebral cortex, the red nuclei, and the basal ganglia. Lacking this input, the medullary reticular inhibitor system becomes nonfunctional; full overactivity of the pontine excitatory system occurs and rigidity develops. We shall see later that other causes of rigidity occur in other neuromotor diseases, especially lesions of the basal ganglia.

In man, with large lesions in the midbrain area, a similar picture is observed, with all four extremities rigidly extended. Since the operation to transect the brainstem at the level of the colliculi was a major one, with a high chance of death of the animal, a less invasive approach was to ligate or tie off the basilar arteries by a less traumatic buccal approach.

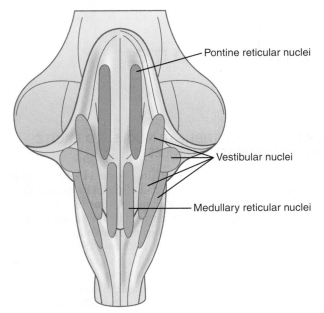

Figure 115-1   Locations of the reticular and vestibular nuclei in the brainstem.

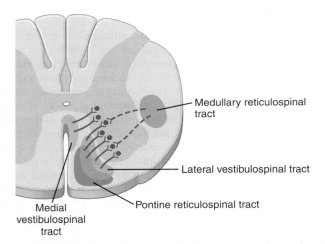

Figure 115-2   Vestibulospinal and reticulospinal tracts descending in the spinal cord to excite (*solid lines*) or inhibit (*dashed lines*) the anterior motor neurons that control the body's axial musculature.

This procedure was called ischemic decerebration, and was described by Pollock and Davis. Ischemic decerebrate animals also exhibit the same rigidity, but this is *not* abolished by deafferentation, and suggests that there is another cause for the rigidity. This was found to be due to an increased direct stimulation of the α-motor neuron because of ischemic damage to the cerebellum and consequent disinhibition of the vestibular nucleus.

Postural and Locomotive Reflexes of the Cord

Positive Supportive Reaction. Pressure on the footpad of a decerebrate animal causes the limb to extend against the pressure applied to the foot. Indeed, this reflex is so strong that if an animal whose spinal cord has been transected for several months—that is, after the reflexes have become exaggerated—is placed on its feet, the reflex often stiffens the limbs sufficiently to support the weight of the body. This reflex is called the *positive supportive reaction*.

The positive supportive reaction involves a complex circuit in the interneurons similar to the circuits responsible for the flexor and crossed extensor reflexes. The locus of the pressure on the pad of the foot determines the direction in which the limb will extend; pressure on one side causes extension in that direction, an effect called the *magnet reaction*. This reaction helps keep an animal from falling to that side.

Cord "Righting" Reflexes. When a spinal animal is laid on its side, it will make uncoordinated movements to try to raise itself to the standing position. This reflex is called the *cord righting reflex*. Such a reflex demonstrates that some relatively complex reflexes associated with posture are integrated in the spinal cord. Indeed, an animal with a well-healed transected thoracic cord between the levels for forelimb and hindlimb innervation can right itself from the lying position and even walk using its hind limbs in addition to its forelimbs. In the case of an opossum with a similar transection of the thoracic cord, the walking movements of the hind limbs are hardly different from those in a normal opossum, except that the hindlimb walking movements are not synchronized with those of the forelimbs.

STEPPING AND WALKING MOVEMENTS

Rhythmical stepping movements are frequently observed in the limbs of spinal animals. Indeed, even when the lumbar portion of the spinal cord is separated from the remainder of the cord and a longitudinal section is made down the center of the cord to block neuronal connections between the two sides of the cord and between the two limbs, each hind limb can still perform individual stepping functions. Forward flexion of the limb is followed a second or so later by backward extension. Then flexion occurs again, and the cycle is repeated over and over.

This oscillation back and forth between flexor and extensor muscles can occur even after the sensory nerves have been cut, and it seems to result mainly from mutually reciprocal inhibition circuits within the matrix of the cord itself, oscillating between the neurons controlling agonist and antagonist muscles.

The sensory signals from the footpads and from the position sensors around the joints play a strong role in controlling foot pressure and frequency of stepping when the foot is allowed to walk along a surface. In fact, the cord mechanism for control of stepping can be even more complex. For instance, if the top of the foot encounters an obstruction during forward thrust, the forward thrust will stop temporarily; then, in rapid sequence, the foot will be lifted higher and proceed forward to be placed over the obstruction. This is the *stumble reflex*. Thus, the cord is an intelligent walking controller.

BIBLIOGRAPHY

Duysens J, Clarac F, Cruse H: Load-regulating mechanisms in gait and posture: comparative aspects, *Physiol. Rev.* 80:83, 2000.

Frigon A: Reconfiguration of the spinal interneuronal network during locomotion in vertebrates, *J. Neurophysiol.* 101:2201, 2009.

Goulding M: Circuits controlling vertebrate locomotion: moving in a new direction, *Nat. Rev. Neurosci.* 10:507, 2009.

Horak FB: Postural compensation for vestibular loss, *Ann. N. Y. Acad. Sci.* 1164:76, 2009.

Ivanenko YP, Poppele RE, Lacquaniti F: Distributed neural networks for controlling human locomotion: lessons from normal and SCI subjects, *Brain Res. Bull.* 78:13, 2009.

Kandel ER, Schwartz JH, Jessell TM: *Principles of Neural Science*, fourth ed., New York, 2000, McGraw-Hill.

Kiehn O: Locomotor circuits in the mammalian spinal cord, *Annu. Rev. Neurosci.* 29:279, 2006.

Pearson KG: Generating the walking gait: role of sensory feedback, *Prog. Brain Res.* 143:123, 2004.

Rekling JC, Funk GD, Bayliss DA, et al: Synaptic control of motoneuronal excitability, *Physiol. Rev.* 80:767, 2000.

Cerebellum

Cerebellum and its Motor Functions

Aside from the areas in the cerebral cortex that stimulate muscle contraction, two other brain structures are also essential for normal motor function: the *cerebellum* and the *basal ganglia*. Neither of these structures can control muscle function by itself. Instead, these structures *always function in association with other systems of motor control*.

The cerebellum plays major roles in the timing of motor activities and in rapid, smooth progression from one muscle movement to the next. It also helps control the intensity of muscle contraction when the muscle load changes and controls the necessary instantaneous interplay between agonist and antagonist muscle groups.

The cerebellum, illustrated in Figures 116-1 and 116-2, has long been called a *silent area* of the brain, principally because electrical excitation of the cerebellum does not cause any conscious sensation and rarely causes any motor movement. Removal of the cerebellum, however, causes body movements to become highly abnormal. The cerebellum is especially vital during rapid muscular activities such as running, typing, playing the piano, and even talking. Loss of this area of the brain can cause almost total lack of coordination of these activities even though its loss does not cause paralysis of any muscles.

How is it that the cerebellum can be so important when it has no direct ability to cause muscle contraction? The answer is that it helps *sequence the motor activities* and also *monitors and makes corrective adjustments in the body's motor activities while they are being executed so that they will conform to the motor signals directed by the cerebral motor cortex and other parts of the brain.*

The cerebellum receives continuously updated information about the desired sequence of muscle contractions from the brain motor control areas; it also receives continuous sensory information from the peripheral parts of the body, giving sequential changes in the status of each part of the body—its position, rate of movement, forces acting on it, and so forth. The cerebellum then *compares* the actual movements as depicted by the peripheral sensory feedback information with the movements intended by the motor system. If the two do not compare favorably, then instantaneous subconscious corrective signals are transmitted back into the motor system to increase or decrease the levels of activation of specific muscles.

The cerebellum also aids the cerebral cortex in planning the next sequential movement, a fraction of a second in advance of the current movement, which is still being executed, thus helping the person to progress smoothly from one movement to the next. Also, it learns by its mistakes—that is, if a movement does not occur exactly as intended, the cerebellar circuit learns to make a stronger or weaker movement the next time. To make this adjustment, *changes occur in the excitability of appropriate cerebellar neurons, thus bringing subsequent muscle contractions into better correspondence with the intended movements.*

ANATOMICAL AND FUNCTIONAL AREAS OF THE CEREBELLUM

Anatomically, the cerebellum is divided into three lobes by two deep fissures, as shown in Figures 116-1 and 116-2: (1) the *anterior lobe*, (2) the *posterior lobe*, and (3) the *flocculonodular lobe*. The flocculonodular lobe is the oldest of all portions of the cerebellum; it developed along with (and functions with) the vestibular system in controlling body equilibrium, as discussed in Chapter 117.

Longitudinal Functional Divisions of the Anterior and Posterior Lobes. From a functional point of view, the anterior and posterior lobes are organized not by lobes but along the longitudinal axis, as demonstrated in Figure 116-2, which shows a posterior view of the human cerebellum after the lower end of the posterior cerebellum has been rolled downward from its normally hidden position. Note down the center of the cerebellum a narrow band called the *vermis*, which is separated from the remainder of the cerebellum by shallow grooves. Most cerebellar control functions for muscle movements of the *axial body, neck, shoulders, and hips* are located in this area.

To each side of the vermis is a large, laterally protruding *cerebellar hemisphere*, and each of these hemispheres is divided into an *intermediate zone* and a *lateral zone*.

The intermediate zone of the hemisphere is concerned with controlling muscle contractions in the distal portions of the upper and lower limbs, especially the hands, fingers, feet, and toes.

The lateral zone of the hemisphere operates at a much more remote level because this area joins with the cerebral cortex in

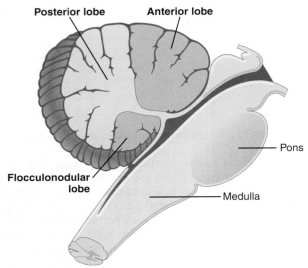

Figure 116-1 Anatomical lobes of the cerebellum, as seen from the lateral side.

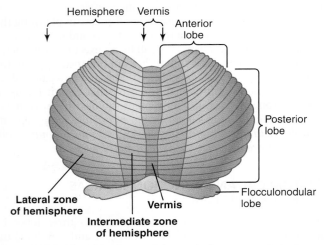

Figure 116-2 Functional parts of the cerebellum as seen from the posteroinferior view, with the inferior-most portion of the cerebellum rolled outward to flatten the surface.

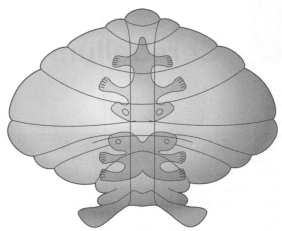

Figure 116-3 Somatosensory projection areas in the cerebellar cortex.

the overall planning of sequential motor movements. Without this lateral zone, most discrete motor activities of the body lose their appropriate timing and sequencing and therefore become uncoordinated, as we discuss more fully later in this chapter.

Topographical Representation of the Body in the Vermis and Intermediate Zones. In the same manner that the cerebral sensory cortex, motor cortex, basal ganglia, red nuclei, and reticular formation all have topographical representations of the different parts of the body, so does the vermis and intermediate zones of the cerebellum. Figure 116-3 shows two such representations. Note that the axial portions of the body lie in the vermis part of the cerebellum, whereas the limbs and facial regions lie in the intermediate zones. These topographical representations receive afferent nerve signals from all the respective parts of the body, as well as from corresponding topographical motor areas in the cerebral cortex and brainstem. In turn, they send motor signals back to the same respective topographical areas of the cerebral motor cortex, as well as to topographical areas of the red nucleus and reticular formation in the brainstem.

Note that the large lateral portions of the cerebellar hemispheres *do not* have topographical representations of the body. These areas of the cerebellum receive input signals almost exclusively from the cerebral cortex, especially the premotor areas of the frontal cortex and from the somatosensory and other sensory association areas of the parietal cortex. It is believed that this connectivity with the cerebral cortex allows the lateral portions of the cerebellar hemispheres to play important roles in planning and coordinating the body's *rapid* sequential muscular activities that occur one after another within fractions of a second.

NEURONAL CIRCUIT OF THE CEREBELLUM

The human cerebellar cortex is actually a large folded sheet, about 17 cm wide by 120 cm long, with the folds lying crosswise, as shown in Figures 116-2 and 116-3. Each fold is called a *folium.* Lying deep beneath the folded mass of cerebellar cortex are *deep cerebellar nuclei.*

Input Pathways to the Cerebellum

Afferent Pathways from Other Parts of the Brain. The basic input pathways to the cerebellum are shown in Figure 116-4. An extensive and important afferent pathway is the *corticopontocerebellar pathway,* which originates in the *cerebral motor* and *premotor cortices* and also in the *cerebral somatosensory cortex.* It passes by way of the *pontile nuclei* and *pontocerebellar tracts* mainly to the lateral divisions of the cerebellar hemispheres on the opposite side of the brain from the cerebral areas.

In addition, important afferent tracts originate in each side of the brainstem. These tracts include (1) an extensive *olivocerebellar tract,* which passes from the *inferior olive* to all parts of the cerebellum and is excited in the olive by fibers from the *cerebral motor cortex, basal ganglia,* widespread areas of the *reticular formation,* and *spinal cord;* (2) *vestibulocerebellar fibers,* some of which originate in the vestibular apparatus itself and others from the brainstem vestibular nuclei with almost all of these fibers terminating in the *flocculonodular lobe* and *fastigial nucleus* of the cerebellum; and (3) *reticulocerebellar fibers,* which originate in different portions of the brainstem reticular formation and terminate in the midline cerebellar areas (mainly in the vermis).

Afferent Pathways from the Periphery. The cerebellum also receives important sensory signals directly from the peripheral

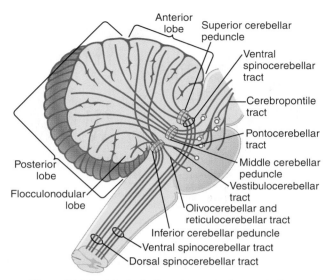

Figure 116-4 Principal *afferent* tracts to the cerebellum.

parts of the body mainly through four tracts on each side, two of which are located dorsally in the cord and two ventrally. The two most important of these tracts are shown in Figure 116-5: the *dorsal spinocerebellar tract* and the *ventral spinocerebellar tract*. The dorsal tract enters the cerebellum through the inferior cerebellar peduncle and terminates in the vermis and intermediate zones of the cerebellum on the same side as its origin. The ventral tract enters the cerebellum through the superior cerebellar peduncle, but it terminates in both sides of the cerebellum.

The signals transmitted in the dorsal spinocerebellar tracts come mainly from the muscle spindles and to a lesser extent from other somatic receptors throughout the body, such as

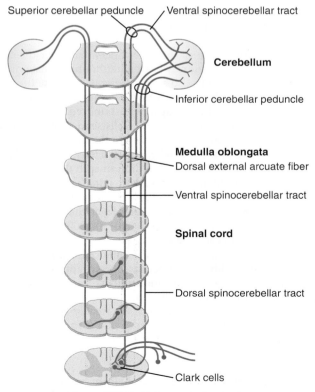

Figure 116-5 Spinocerebellar tracts.

Golgi tendon organs, large tactile receptors of the skin, and joint receptors. All these signals apprise the cerebellum of the momentary status of (1) muscle contraction, (2) degree of tension on the muscle tendons, (3) positions and rates of movement of the parts of the body, and (4) forces acting on the surfaces of the body.

The ventral spinocerebellar tracts receive much less information from the peripheral receptors. Instead, they are excited mainly by motor signals arriving in the anterior horns of the spinal cord from (1) the brain through the corticospinal and rubrospinal tracts and (2) the internal motor pattern generators in the cord itself. Thus, this ventral fiber pathway tells the cerebellum which motor signals have arrived at the anterior horns; this feedback is called the *efference copy* of the anterior horn motor drive.

The spinocerebellar pathways can transmit impulses at velocities up to 120 m/second, which is the most rapid conduction in any pathway in the central nervous system. This speed is important for instantaneous appraisal of the cerebellum of changes in peripheral muscle actions.

In addition to signals from the spinocerebellar tracts, signals are transmitted into the cerebellum from the body periphery through the spinal dorsal columns to the dorsal column nuclei of the medulla and are then relayed to the cerebellum. Likewise, signals are transmitted up the spinal cord through the *spinoreticular pathway* to the reticular formation of the brainstem and also through the *spinoolivary pathway* to the inferior olivary nucleus. Signals are then relayed from both of these areas to the cerebellum. Thus, the cerebellum continually collects information about the movements and positions of all parts of the body even though it is operating at a subconscious level.

Output Signals from the Cerebellum

Deep Cerebellar Nuclei and the Efferent Pathways. Located deep in the cerebellar mass on each side are three *deep cerebellar nuclei—the dentate, interposed, and fastigial.* (The *vestibular nuclei* in the medulla also function in some respects as if they were deep cerebellar nuclei because of their direct connections with the cortex of the flocculonodular lobe.) All the deep cerebellar nuclei receive signals from two sources: (1) the cerebellar cortex and (2) the deep sensory afferent tracts to the cerebellum.

Each time an input signal arrives in the cerebellum, it divides and goes in two directions: (1) directly to one of the cerebellar deep nuclei and (2) to a corresponding area of the cerebellar cortex overlying the deep nucleus. Then, a fraction of a second later, the cerebellar cortex relays an *inhibitory* output signal to the deep nucleus. Thus, all input signals that enter the cerebellum eventually end in the deep nuclei in the form of initial excitatory signals followed a fraction of a second later by inhibitory signals. From the deep nuclei, output signals leave the cerebellum and are distributed to other parts of the brain.

The general plan of the major efferent pathways leading out of the cerebellum is shown in Figure 116-6 and consists of the following pathways:

1. A pathway that originates in the *midline structures of the cerebellum* (the *vermis*) and then passes through the *fastigial nuclei* into the *medullary* and *pontile regions of the brainstem*. This circuit functions in close association with the equilibrium apparatus and brainstem vestibular nuclei to control equilibrium, as well as in association with the reticular formation of the brainstem to control the postural attitudes of the body. It is discussed in detail in Chapter 117 in relation to equilibrium.

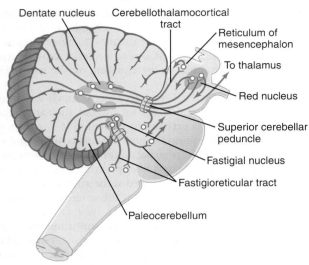

Figure 116-6 Principal *efferent* tracts from the cerebellum.

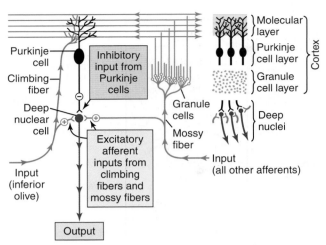

Figure 116-7 Deep nuclear cells receive excitatory and inhibitory inputs. The left side of this figure shows the basic neuronal circuit of the cerebellum, with excitatory neurons shown in *red* and the Purkinje cell (an inhibitory neuron) shown in *black*. To the right is shown the physical relationship of the deep cerebellar nuclei to the cerebellar cortex with its three layers.

2. A pathway that originates in (a) the intermediate zone of the cerebellar hemisphere and then passes through (b) the interposed nucleus to (c) the ventrolateral and ventroanterior nuclei of the thalamus and then to (d) the cerebral cortex to (e) several midline structures of the thalamus and then to (f) the basal ganglia and (g) the red nucleus and reticular formation of the upper portion of the brainstem. This complex circuit mainly helps coordinate the reciprocal contractions of agonist and antagonist muscles in the peripheral portions of the limbs, especially in the hands, fingers, and thumbs.

3. A pathway that begins in the cerebellar cortex of the lateral zone of the cerebellar hemisphere and then passes to the dentate nucleus, next to the ventrolateral and ventroanterior nuclei of the thalamus, and, finally, to the cerebral cortex. This pathway plays an important role in helping coordinate sequential motor activities initiated by the cerebral cortex.

Functional Unit of the Cerebellar Cortex— The Purkinje and Deep Nuclear Cells

The cerebellum has about 30 million nearly identical functional units, 1 of which is shown to the left in Figure 116-7. This functional unit centers on a single, very large *Purkinje cell* and on a corresponding *deep nuclear cell*.

To the top and right in Figure 116-7, the three major layers of the cerebellar cortex are shown: the *molecular layer, Purkinje cell layer*, and *granule cell layer*. Beneath these cortical layers, in the center of the cerebellar mass, are the deep cerebellar nuclei that send output signals to other parts of the nervous system.

Neuronal Circuit of the Functional Unit. Also shown in the left half of Figure 116-7 is the neuronal circuit of the functional unit, which is repeated with little variation 30 million times in the cerebellum. The output from the functional unit is from a *deep nuclear cell*. This cell is continually under both excitatory and inhibitory influences. The excitatory influences arise from direct connections with afferent fibers that enter the cerebellum from the brain or the periphery. The inhibitory influence arises entirely from the Purkinje cell in the cortex of the cerebellum.

The afferent inputs to the cerebellum are mainly of two types, one called the *climbing fiber type* and the other called the *mossy fiber type*.

The climbing fibers *all originate from the inferior olives of the medulla*. There is one climbing fiber for about 5–10 Purkinje cells. After sending branches to several deep nuclear cells, the climbing fiber continues all the way to the outer layers of the cerebellar cortex, where it makes about 300 synapses with the soma and dendrites of each Purkinje cell. This climbing fiber is distinguished by the fact that a single impulse in it will always cause a single, prolonged (up to 1 second), peculiar type of action potential in each Purkinje cell with which it connects, beginning with a strong spike and followed by a trail of weakening secondary spikes. This action potential is called the *complex spike*.

The mossy fibers are all the other fibers that enter the cerebellum from multiple sources–the higher brain, brainstem, and spinal cord. These fibers also send collaterals to excite the deep nuclear cells. They then proceed to the granule cell layer of the cortex, where they, also, synapse with hundreds to thousands of *granule cells*. In turn, the granule cells send extremely small axons, less than 1 μm in diameter, up to the molecular layer on the outer surface of the cerebellar cortex. Here the axons divide into two branches that extend 1–2 mm in each direction parallel to the folia. Many millions of these *parallel nerve fibers* exist because there are some 500–1000 granule cells for every one Purkinje cell. It is into this molecular layer that the dendrites of the Purkinje cells project and 80,000–200,000 of the parallel fibers synapse with each Purkinje cell.

The mossy fiber input to the Purkinje cell is quite different from the climbing fiber input because the synaptic connections are weak, so large numbers of mossy fibers must be stimulated simultaneously to excite the Purkinje cell. Furthermore, activation usually takes the form of a much weaker short-duration Purkinje cell action potential called a *simple spike*, rather than the prolonged complex action potential caused by climbing fiber input.

Other Inhibitory Cells in the Cerebellum. In addition to the deep nuclear cells, granule cells, and Purkinje cells, two other types of neurons are located in the cerebellum: *basket cells* and *stellate cells*, which are inhibitory cells with short axons. Both the basket cells and the stellate cells are located in the molecular layer of the cerebellar cortex, lying among and stimulated by the small parallel fibers. These cells in turn send their axons at right angles across the parallel fibers and cause *lateral inhibition* of adjacent Purkinje cells, thus sharpening the signal in the same manner that lateral inhibition sharpens contrast of signals in many other neuronal circuits of the nervous system.

FUNCTION OF THE CEREBELLUM IN OVERALL MOTOR CONTROL

The nervous system uses the cerebellum to coordinate motor control functions at three levels:
1. The *vestibulocerebellum*. This level consists principally of the small flocculonodular cerebellar lobes that lie under the posterior cerebellum and adjacent portions of the vermis. It provides neural circuits for most of the body's equilibrium movements.
2. The *spinocerebellum*. This level consists of most of the vermis of the posterior and anterior cerebellum plus the adjacent intermediate zones on both sides of the vermis. It provides the circuitry for coordinating mainly movements of the distal portions of the limbs, especially the hands and fingers.
3. The *cerebrocerebellum*. This level consists of the large lateral zones of the cerebellar hemispheres, lateral to the intermediate zones. It receives virtually all its input from the cerebral motor cortex and adjacent premotor and somatosensory cortices of the cerebrum. It transmits its output information in the upward direction back to the brain, functioning in a feedback manner with the cerebral cortical sensorimotor system to plan sequential voluntary body and limb movements. These movements are planned as much as tenths of a second in advance of the actual movements. This process is called development of "motor imagery" of movements to be performed.

The Vestibulocerebellum Functions in Association with the Brainstem and Spinal Cord to Control Equilibrium and Postural Movements

The vestibulocerebellum originated phylogenetically at about the same time that the vestibular apparatus in the inner ear developed. Furthermore, as discussed in Chapter 117, loss of the flocculonodular lobes and adjacent portions of the vermis of the cerebellum, which constitute the vestibulocerebellum, causes extreme disturbance of equilibrium and postural movements.

In people with vestibulocerebellar dysfunction, equilibrium is far more disturbed *during performance of rapid motions* than during stasis, especially when these movements involve *changes in direction* of movement and stimulate the semicircular ducts. This phenomenon suggests that the vestibulocerebellum is important in controlling balance between agonist and antagonist muscle contractions of the spine, hips, and shoulders during *rapid changes* in body positions as required by the vestibular apparatus.

One of the major problems in controlling balance is the amount of time required to transmit position signals and velocity of movement signals from the different parts of the body to the brain. Even when the most rapidly conducting sensory pathways are used, up to 120 m/second in the spinocerebellar afferent tracts, the delay for transmission from the feet to the brain is still 15–20 milliseconds. The feet of a person running rapidly can move as much as 10 in. during that time. Therefore, it is never possible for return signals from the peripheral parts of the body to reach the brain at the same time that the movements actually occur. How, then, is it possible for the brain to know when to stop a movement and to perform the next sequential act when the movements are performed rapidly? The answer is that the signals from the periphery tell the brain how rapidly and in which directions the body parts are moving. It is then the function of the vestibulocerebellum to *calculate in advance* from these rates and directions where the different parts will be during the next few milliseconds. The results of these calculations are the key to the brain's progression to the next sequential movement.

Thus, during control of equilibrium, it is presumed that information from both the body periphery and the vestibular apparatus is used in a typical feedback control circuit to provide *anticipatory correction* of postural motor signals necessary for maintaining equilibrium even during extremely rapid motion, including rapidly changing directions of motion.

Spinocerebellum—Feedback Control of Distal Limb Movements by Way of the Intermediate Cerebellar Cortex and the Interposed Nucleus

As shown in Figure 116-8, the intermediate zone of each cerebellar hemisphere receives two types of information when a movement is performed: (1) information from the cerebral motor cortex and from the midbrain red nucleus, telling the cerebellum the *intended sequential plan of movement* for the next few fractions of a second, and (2) feedback information from the peripheral parts of the body, especially from the distal proprioceptors of the limbs, telling the cerebellum what *actual movements* result.

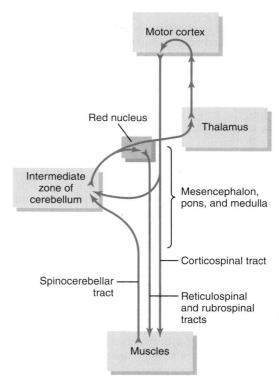

Figure 116-8 Cerebral and cerebellar control of voluntary movements, involving especially the intermediate zone of the cerebellum.

After the intermediate zone of the cerebellum has compared the intended movements with the actual movements, the deep nuclear cells of the interposed nucleus send *corrective* output signals (1) back to the *cerebral motor cortex* through relay nuclei in the *thalamus* and (2) to the *magnocellular portion* (the lower portion) *of the red nucleus* that gives rise to the *rubrospinal tract*. The rubrospinal tract in turn joins the corticospinal tract in innervating the lateral-most motor neurons in the anterior horns of the spinal cord gray matter, the neurons that control the distal parts of the limbs, particularly the hands and fingers.

This part of the cerebellar motor control system provides smooth, coordinated movements of the agonist and antagonist muscles of the distal limbs for performing acute purposeful patterned movements. The cerebellum seems to compare the "intentions" of the higher levels of the motor control system, as transmitted to the intermediate cerebellar zone through the corticopontocerebellar tract, with the "performance" by the respective parts of the body, as transmitted back to the cerebellum from the periphery. In fact, the ventral spinocerebellar tract even transmits back to the cerebellum an "efference" copy of the actual motor control signals that reach the anterior motor neurons, and this information is also integrated with the signals arriving from the muscle spindles and other proprioceptor sensory organs, transmitted principally in the dorsal spinocerebellar tract. Similar comparator signals also go to the inferior olivary complex; if the signals do not compare favorably, the olivary–Purkinje cell system along with possibly other cerebellar learning mechanisms eventually corrects the motions until they perform the desired function.

Function of the Cerebellum to Prevent Overshoot and to "Damp" Movements. Almost all movements of the body are "pendular." For instance, when an arm is moved, momentum develops, and the momentum must be overcome before the movement can be stopped. Because of momentum, all pendular movements have a tendency to *overshoot*. If overshooting occurs in a person whose cerebellum has been destroyed, the conscious centers of the cerebrum eventually recognize this occurrence and initiate a movement in the reverse direction to attempt to bring the arm to its intended position. However the arm, by virtue of its momentum, overshoots once more in the opposite direction, and appropriate corrective signals must again be instituted. Thus, the arm oscillates back and forth past its intended point for several cycles before it finally fixes on its mark. This effect is called an *action tremor* or *intention tremor*.

If the cerebellum is intact, appropriate learned, subconscious signals stop the movement precisely at the intended point, thereby preventing the overshoot and the tremor. *This activity is the basic characteristic of a damping system.* All control systems regulating pendular elements that have inertia must have damping circuits built into the mechanisms. For motor control by the nervous system, the cerebellum provides most of this damping function.

Cerebellar Control of Ballistic Movements. Most rapid movements of the body, such as the movements of the fingers in typing, occur so rapidly that it is not possible to receive feedback information either from the periphery to the cerebellum or from the cerebellum back to the motor cortex before the movements are over. These movements are called *ballistic movements*, meaning that the entire movement is preplanned and set into motion to go a specific distance and then to stop. Another important example is the saccadic movements of the eyes, in which

the eyes jump from one position to the next when reading or when looking at successive points along a road as a person is moving in a car.

Much can be understood about the function of the cerebellum by studying the changes that occur in these ballistic movements when the cerebellum is removed. Three major changes occur: (1) the movements are slow to develop and do not have the extra onset surge that the cerebellum usually provides, (2) the force developed is weak, and (3) the movements are slow to turn off, usually allowing the movement to go well beyond the intended mark. Therefore, in the absence of the cerebellar circuit, the motor cortex has to think extra hard to turn ballistic movements on and again has to think hard and take extra time to turn the movement off. Thus, the automatism of ballistic movements is lost.

Considering once again the circuitry of the cerebellum, one sees that it is beautifully organized to perform this biphasic, first excitatory and then delayed inhibitory function that is required for preplanned rapid ballistic movements. Also, the built-in timing circuits of the cerebellar cortex are fundamental to this particular ability of the cerebellum.

Cerebrocerebellum—Function of the Large Lateral Zone of the Cerebellar Hemisphere to Plan, Sequence, and Time Complex Movements

In human beings, the lateral zones of the two cerebellar hemispheres are highly developed and greatly enlarged. This characteristic goes along with human abilities to plan and perform intricate sequential patterns of movement, especially with the hands and fingers, and to speak. Yet the large lateral zones of the cerebellar hemispheres have no direct input of information from the peripheral parts of the body. In addition, almost all communication between these lateral cerebellar areas and the cerebral cortex is not with the primary cerebral motor cortex but instead with the *premotor area* and *primary* and *association somatosensory areas*.

Even so, destruction of the lateral zones of the cerebellar hemispheres along with their deep nuclei, the dentate nuclei, can lead to extreme incoordination of complex purposeful movements of the hands, fingers, and feet and of the speech apparatus. This condition has been difficult to understand because of lack of direct communication between this part of the cerebellum and the primary motor cortex. However, experimental studies suggest that these portions of the cerebellum are concerned with two other important but indirect aspects of motor control: (1) the planning of sequential movements and (2) the "timing" of the sequential movements.

Planning of Sequential Movements. The planning of sequential movements requires that the lateral zones of the hemispheres communicate with both the premotor and sensory portions of the cerebral cortex, and it requires two-way communication between these cerebral cortex areas with corresponding areas of the basal ganglia. It seems that the "plan" of sequential movements actually begins in the sensory and premotor areas of the cerebral cortex, and from there the plan is transmitted to the lateral zones of the cerebellar hemispheres. Then, amid much two-way traffic between the cerebellum and the cerebral cortex, appropriate motor signals provide transition from one sequence of movements to the next.

An interesting observation that supports this view is that many neurons in the cerebellar dentate nuclei display the activity pattern for the sequential movement that is yet to come while the present movement is still occurring. Thus, the lateral cerebellar zones appear to be involved not with what movement is happening at a given moment but with *what will be happening during the next sequential movement* a fraction of a second or perhaps even seconds later.

To summarize, one of the most important features of normal motor function is one's ability to progress smoothly from one movement to the next in orderly succession. In the absence of the large lateral zones of the cerebellar hemispheres, this capability is seriously disturbed for rapid movements.

Timing Function for Sequential Movements. Another important function of the lateral zones of the cerebellar hemispheres is to provide appropriate timing for each succeeding movement. In the absence of these cerebellar zones, one loses the subconscious ability to predict how far the different parts of the body will move in a given time. Without this timing capability, the person becomes unable to determine when the next sequential movement needs to begin. As a result, the succeeding movement may begin too early or, more likely, too late. Therefore, lesions in the lateral zones of the cerebellum cause complex movements (eg, those required for writing, running, or even talking) to become incoordinate and lacking ability to progress in orderly sequence from one movement to the next. Such cerebellar lesions are said to cause *failure of smooth progression of movements*.

Summary of Integrated Functions of the Cerebellum

The cerebellum functions with all levels of muscle control. It functions with the spinal cord especially to enhance the stretch reflex, so when a contracting muscle encounters an unexpectedly heavy load, a long stretch reflex signal transmitted all the way through the cerebellum and back again to the cord strongly enhances the load-resisting effect of the basic stretch reflex.

At the brainstem level, the cerebellum functions to make the postural movements of the body, especially the rapid movements required by the equilibrium system, smooth and continuous and without abnormal oscillations.

At the cerebral cortex level, the cerebellum operates in association with the cortex to provide many accessory motor functions, especially to provide extra motor force for turning on muscle contraction rapidly at the start of a movement. Near the end of each movement, the *cerebellum* turns on antagonist muscles at exactly the right time and with proper force to stop the movement at the intended point. Furthermore, there is good physiological evidence that all aspects of this turn-on/turn-off patterning by the cerebellum can be learned with experience.

The cerebellum functions with the cerebral cortex at still another level of motor control: It helps to program in advance muscle contractions that are required for smooth progression from a present rapid movement in one direction to the next rapid movement in another direction, with all this occurring in a fraction of a second. The neural circuit for this passes from the cerebral cortex to the large lateral zones of the cerebellar hemispheres and then back to the cerebral cortex.

The cerebellum functions mainly when rapid muscle movements are required. Without the cerebellum, slow and calculated movements can still occur, but it is difficult for the corticospinal system to achieve rapid and changing intended movements to execute a particular goal or especially to progress smoothly from one rapid movement to the next.

CLINICAL ABNORMALITIES OF THE CEREBELLUM

Destruction of small portions of the lateral cerebellar *cortex* seldom causes detectable abnormalities in motor function. In fact, several months after as much as one-half of the lateral cerebellar cortex on one side of the brain has been removed, if the deep cerebellar nuclei are not removed along with the cortex, the motor functions of the animal appear to be almost normal *as long as the animal performs all movements slowly*. Thus, the remaining portions of the motor control system are capable of compensating to a great extent for loss of parts of the cerebellum.

To cause serious and continuing dysfunction of the cerebellum, the cerebellar lesion usually must involve one or more of the deep cerebellar nuclei—the *dentate, interposed,* or *fastigial nuclei.* Tests of cerebellar function include the testing of coordination of movements (ataxia) and the gait, inspection for tremors, tests for tone (hypotonia), and tests of rapidly alternating movements (dysdiadochokinesis). These are described in the following.

Dysmetria and Ataxia. Two of the most important symptoms of cerebellar disease are *dysmetria* and *ataxia.* In the absence of the cerebellum, the subconscious motor control system cannot predict how far movements will go. Therefore, the movements ordinarily overshoot their intended mark; then the conscious portion of the brain overcompensates in the opposite direction for the succeeding compensatory movement. This effect is called *dysmetria*, and it results in uncoordinated movements that are called *ataxia.* Dysmetria and ataxia can also result from *lesions in the spinocerebellar tracts* because feedback information from the moving parts of the body to the cerebellum is essential for cerebellar timing of movement termination.

Past Pointing. Past pointing means that in the absence of the cerebellum, a person ordinarily moves the hand or some other moving part of the body considerably beyond the point of intention. This movement results from the fact that normally the cerebellum initiates most of the motor signal that turns off a movement after it is begun; if the cerebellum is not available to initiate this motor signal, the movement ordinarily goes beyond the intended mark. Therefore, past pointing is actually a manifestation of dysmetria.

Failure of Progression

Dysdiadochokinesia—Inability to Perform Rapid Alternating Movements. When the motor control system fails to predict where the different parts of the body will be at a given time, it "loses" perception of the parts during rapid motor movements. As a result, the succeeding movement may begin much too early or much too late, so no orderly "progression of movement" can occur. One can demonstrate this effect readily by having a patient with cerebellar damage turn one hand upward and downward at a rapid rate. The patient rapidly "loses" all perception of the instantaneous position of the hand during any portion of the movement. As a result, a series of stalled attempted but jumbled movements occurs instead of the normal coordinate upward and downward motions. This condition is called *dysdiadochokinesia.*

Dysarthria—Failure of Progression in Talking. Another example in which failure of progression occurs is in talking because the formation of words depends on rapid and orderly succession of individual muscle movements in the larynx, mouth, and respiratory system. Lack of coordination among these structures and the inability to adjust in advance either the intensity of sound or the duration of each successive sound causes jumbled vocalization, with some syllables loud, some weak, some held for long intervals, and some held for short intervals, with resultant speech that is often unintelligible. This condition is called *dysarthria*.

Intention Tremor. When a person who has lost the cerebellum performs a voluntary act, the movements tend to oscillate, especially when they approach the intended mark, first overshooting the mark, and then vibrating back and forth several times before settling on the mark. This reaction is called an *intention tremor* or an *action tremor*, and it results from cerebellar overshooting and failure of the cerebellar system to "damp" the motor movements.

Cerebellar Nystagmus—Tremor of the Eyeballs. *Cerebellar nystagmus* is tremor of the eyeballs that usually occurs when one attempts to fixate the eyes on a scene to one side of the head. This off-center type of fixation results in rapid, tremulous movements of the eyes rather than steady fixation, and it is another manifestation of the failure of damping by the cerebellum. It occurs especially when the flocculonodular lobes of the cerebellum are damaged; in this instance it is also associated with loss of equilibrium because of dysfunction of the pathways through the flocculonodular cerebellum from the semicircular ducts.

Hypotonia—Decreased Tone of the Musculature. Loss of the deep cerebellar nuclei, particularly of the dentate and interposed nuclei, causes decreased tone of the peripheral body musculature on the side of the cerebellar lesion. The hypotonia results from loss of cerebellar facilitation of the motor cortex and brainstem motor nuclei by tonic signals from the deep cerebellar nuclei.

BIBLIOGRAPHY

Bastian AJ: Learning to predict the future: the cerebellum adapts feedforward movement control, *Curr. Opin. Neurobiol.* 16:645, 2006.

Chadderton P, Schaefer AT, Williams SR, Margrie TW: Sensory-evoked synaptic integration in cerebellar and cerebral cortical neurons, *Nat. Rev. Neurosci.* 15:71, 2014.

Cheron G, Servais L, Dan B: Cerebellar network plasticity: from genes to fast oscillation, *Neuroscience* 153:1, 2008.

Fuentes CT, Bastian AJ: 'Motor cognition'—what is it and is the cerebellum involved? *Cerebellum* 6:232, 2007.

Heck DH, De Zeeuw CI, Jaeger D, et al: The neuronal code(s) of the cerebellum, *J. Neurosci.* 33:17603, 2013.

Kandel ER, Schwartz JH, Jessell TM: *Principles of Neural Science*, fourth ed., New York, 2000, McGraw-Hill.

Ramnani N: The primate cortico-cerebellar system: anatomy and function, *Nat. Rev. Neurosci.* 7:511, 2006.

Ullsperger M, Danielmeier C, Jocham G: Neurophysiology of performance monitoring and adaptive behavior, *Physiol. Rev.* 94:35, 2014.

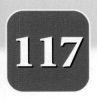

Vestibular Apparatus

Maintenance of Equilibrium

The vestibular apparatus, as shown in Figure 117-1, is the sensory organ for detecting sensations of equilibrium. It is encased in a system of bony tubes and chambers located in the petrous portion of the temporal bone, called the *bony labyrinth*. Within this system are membranous tubes and chambers called the *membranous labyrinth*. The membranous labyrinth is the functional part of the vestibular apparatus.

The top of Figure 117-1 shows the membranous labyrinth. It is composed mainly of the *cochlea* (ductus cochlearis); three *semicircular canals*; and two large chambers, the *utricle* and *saccule*. The cochlea is the major sensory organ for hearing (see Chapter 107) and has little to do with equilibrium. However, the *semicircular canals*, the *utricle*, and the *saccule* are all integral parts of the equilibrium mechanism.

"MACULAE"—SENSORY ORGANS OF THE UTRICLE AND SACCULE FOR DETECTING ORIENTATION OF THE HEAD WITH RESPECT TO GRAVITY

Located on the inside surface of each utricle and saccule, shown in the top diagram of Figure 117-1, is a small sensory area slightly greater than 2 mm in diameter called a *macula*. The *macula of the utricle* lies mainly in the *horizontal plane* on the inferior surface of the utricle and plays an important role in determining orientation of the head when the head is upright. Conversely, the *macula of the saccule* is located mainly in a *vertical plane* and signals head orientation when the person is lying down.

Each macula is covered by a gelatinous layer in which many small calcium carbonate crystals called *statoconia* are embedded. Also in the macula are thousands of *hair cells*, one of which is shown in Figure 117-2; these hair cells project *cilia* up into the gelatinous layer. The bases and sides of the hair cells synapse with sensory endings of the *vestibular nerve*.

The calcified statoconia have a *specific gravity* two to three times the specific gravity of the surrounding fluid and tissues. The weight of the statoconia bends the cilia in the direction of gravitational pull.

DIRECTIONAL SENSITIVITY OF THE HAIR CELLS—KINOCILIUM

Each hair cell has 50–70 small cilia called *stereocilia*, plus one large cilium, the *kinocilium*, as shown in Figure 117-2. The kinocilium is always located to one side, and the stereocilia become progressively shorter toward the other side of the cell. Minute filamentous attachments, almost invisible even to the electron microscope, connect the tip of each stereocilium to the next longer stereocilium and, finally, to the kinocilium.

Because of these attachments, when the stereocilia and kinocilium bend in the direction of the kinocilium, the filamentous attachments tug in sequence on the stereocilia, pulling them outward from the cell body. This movement opens several hundred fluid channels in the neuronal cell membrane around the bases of the stereocilia, and these channels are capable of conducting large numbers of positive ions. Therefore, positive ions pour into the cell from the surrounding endolymphatic fluid, causing *receptor membrane depolarization*. Conversely, bending the pile of stereocilia in the opposite direction (backward to the kinocilium) reduces the tension on the attachments; this movement closes the ion channels, thus causing *receptor hyperpolarization*.

Under normal resting conditions, the nerve fibers leading from the hair cells transmit continuous nerve impulses at a rate of about 100 $second^{-1}$. When the stereocilia are bent toward the kinocilium, the impulse traffic increases, often to several hundred per second; conversely, bending the cilia away from the kinocilium decreases the impulse traffic, often turning it off completely. Therefore, as the orientation of the head in space changes and the weight of the statoconia bends the cilia, appropriate signals are transmitted to the brain to control equilibrium.

In each macula, each of the hair cells is oriented in a different direction so that some of the hair cells are stimulated when the head bends forward, some are stimulated when it bends backward, others are stimulated when it bends to one side, and so forth. Therefore, a different pattern of excitation occurs in the macular nerve fibers for each orientation of the head in the

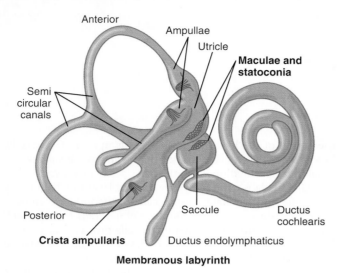

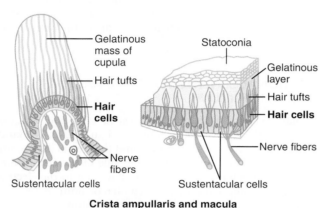

Figure 117-1 Membranous labyrinth and organization of the crista ampullaris and the macula.

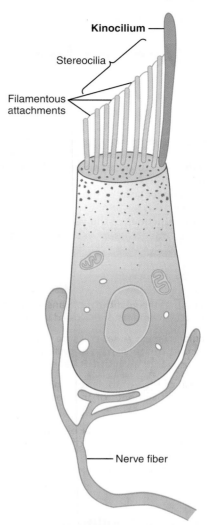

Figure 117-2 Hair cell of the equilibrium apparatus and its synapses with the vestibular nerve.

gravitational field. It is this "pattern" that apprises the brain of the head's orientation in space.

SEMICIRCULAR DUCTS

The three semicircular ducts in each vestibular apparatus, known as the *anterior*, *posterior*, and *lateral (horizontal) semicircular ducts*, are arranged at right angles to one another so that they represent all three planes in space. When the head is bent forward about 30 degrees, the lateral semicircular ducts are approximately horizontal with respect to the surface of the Earth; the anterior ducts are in vertical planes that project *forward and 45 degrees outward*, whereas the posterior ducts are in vertical planes that project *backward and 45 degrees outward*.

Each semicircular duct has an enlargement at one of its ends called the *ampulla*, and the ducts and ampulla are filled with a fluid called *endolymph*. Flow of this fluid through one of the ducts and through its ampulla excites the sensory organ of the ampulla in the following manner: Figure 117-3 shows in each ampulla a small crest called a *crista ampullaris*. On top of this crista is a loose gelatinous tissue mass, the *cupula*. When a person's head begins to rotate in any direction, the inertia of the fluid in one or more of the semicircular ducts causes the fluid to remain stationary while the semicircular duct rotates with the head. This process causes fluid to flow from the duct and

through the ampulla, bending the cupula to one side, as demonstrated by the position of the colored cupula in Figure 117-3. Rotation of the head in the opposite direction causes the cupula to bend to the opposite side.

Into the cupula are projected hundreds of cilia from hair cells located on the ampullary crest. The kinocilia of these hair cells are all oriented in the same direction in the cupula, and bending the cupula in that direction causes depolarization of the hair cells, whereas bending it in the opposite direction hyperpolarizes the cells. Then, from the hair cells, appropriate signals are sent by way of the *vestibular nerve* to apprise the central nervous system of a *change in rotation* of the head and the *rate of change* in each of the three planes of space.

CENTRAL CONNECTIONS OF THE VESTIBULAR SYSTEM

The vestibular nerve carries information from the utricle, saccule, and semicircular canals to the brainstem, after passing through Scarpa ganglion in the internal auditory canal. These vestibular afferents connect with the vestibular nucleus in the brainstem, which has four parts: the lateral (Deiters nucleus), medial (Schwalbe nucleus), superior (Bechterew nucleus), and

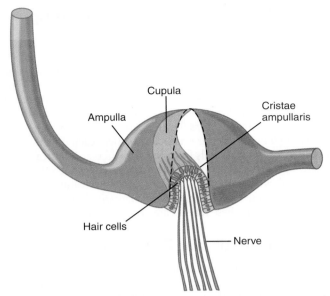

Figure 117-3 Movement of the cupula and its embedded hairs at the onset of rotation.

descending (spinal vestibular nucleus). There is also an afferent projection to the flocculonodular lobe of the cerebellum.

The central connections of the vestibular afferents serve a diverse array of functions, which coordinate balance and position with movements of the upper body, head and neck, as well as righting reflexes. They also integrate with other important areas of the brain such as the cerebellum and the reticular formation. The lateral vestibular nucleus takes part in coordinating the righting reflexes on the same side, through the vestibulospinal pathway. The projection of this nucleus to the motor neurons of the spinal cord, along with those from the medial vestibular nucleus through the medial longitudinal fasciculus, is important for the maintenance of tone, particularly in extensor muscles for posture control. The medial vestibular nucleus also takes part in coordinating movements of the head and neck with the conjugate eye movement, through its connections with the medial longitudinal fasciculus. The superior vestibular nucleus is involved in transmitting information from the semicircular canals for conjugate ocular reflexes. The descending vestibular nucleus has the main integrative function with the cerebellum, reticular formation, and the contralateral vestibular nucleus. This integration is necessary for eye movements and position.

Functions of the Vestibular System

FUNCTION OF THE UTRICLE AND SACCULE IN THE MAINTENANCE OF STATIC EQUILIBRIUM

It is especially important that the hair cells are all oriented in different directions in the maculae of the utricles and saccules so that with different positions of the head, different hair cells become stimulated. The "patterns" of stimulation of the different hair cells apprise the brain of the position of the head with respect to the pull of gravity. In turn, the vestibular, cerebellar, and reticular motor nerve systems of the brain excite appropriate postural muscles to maintain proper equilibrium.

This utricle and saccule system functions extremely effectively for maintaining equilibrium when the head is in the near-vertical position. Indeed, a person can determine as little as half a degree of disequilibrium when the body leans from the precise upright position.

DETECTION OF LINEAR ACCELERATION BY THE UTRICLE AND SACCULE MACULAE

When the body is suddenly thrust forward—that is, when the body accelerates—the statoconia, which have greater mass inertia than the surrounding fluid, fall backward on the hair cell cilia, and information of disequilibrium is sent into the nervous centers, causing the person to feel as though he or she were falling backward. This sensation automatically causes the person to lean forward until the resulting anterior shift of the statoconia exactly equals the tendency for the statoconia to fall backward because of the acceleration. At this point, the nervous system senses a state of proper equilibrium and leans the body forward no farther. Thus, the maculae operate to maintain equilibrium during linear acceleration in exactly the same manner as they operate during static equilibrium.

The maculae *do not* operate for the detection of linear *velocity*. When runners first begin to run, they must lean far forward to keep from falling backward because of initial *acceleration*, but once they have achieved running speed, if they were running in a vacuum, they would not have to lean forward. When running in air, they lean forward to maintain equilibrium only because of air resistance against their bodies; in this instance, it is not the maculae that make them lean but air pressure acting on pressure end organs in the skin, which initiate appropriate equilibrium adjustments to prevent falling.

Detection of Head Rotation by the Semicircular Ducts

When the head suddenly begins to rotate in any direction (called *angular acceleration*), the endolymph in the semicircular ducts, because of its inertia, tends to remain stationary while the semicircular ducts turn. This mechanism causes relative fluid flow in the ducts in the direction opposite to head rotation.

Figure 117-4 shows a typical discharge signal from a single hair cell in the crista ampullaris when an animal is rotated for 40 seconds, demonstrating that (1) even when the cupula is in its resting position, the hair cell emits a tonic discharge of about 100 impulses/second; (2) when the animal begins to rotate, the hairs bend to one side and the rate of discharge increases greatly; and (3) with continued rotation, the excess discharge of the hair cell gradually subsides back to the resting level during the next few seconds.

The reason for this adaptation of the receptor is that within the first few seconds of rotation, back resistance to the flow of fluid in the semicircular duct and past the bent cupula causes the endolymph to begin rotating as rapidly as the semicircular canal itself; then, in another 5–20 seconds, the cupula slowly returns to its resting position in the middle of the ampulla because of its own elastic recoil.

When the rotation suddenly stops, exactly opposite effects take place: The endolymph continues to rotate while the semicircular duct stops. This time, the cupula bends in the opposite direction, causing the hair cell to stop discharging entirely. After another few seconds, the endolymph stops moving and the cupula gradually returns to its resting position, thus allowing hair cell discharge to return to its normal tonic level, as shown to the

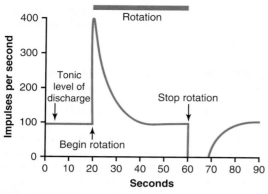

Figure 117-4   Response of a hair cell when a semicircular canal is stimulated first by the onset of head rotation and then by stopping rotation.

Vestibular Mechanisms for Stabilizing the Eyes

When a person changes his or her direction of movement rapidly or even leans the head sideways, forward, or backward, it would be impossible to maintain a stable image on the retinas unless the person had some automatic control mechanism to stabilize the direction of the eyes' gaze. In addition, the eyes would be of little use in detecting an image unless they remained "fixed" on each object long enough to gain a clear image. Fortunately, each time the head is suddenly rotated, signals from the semicircular ducts cause the eyes to rotate in a direction equal and opposite to the rotation of the head. This movement results from reflexes transmitted through the *vestibular nuclei* and the *medial longitudinal fasciculus* to the *oculomotor nuclei*. These reflexes are described in Chapter 110.

Tests for Vestibular Function

Vestibular function is tested by rotating the head, by placing the person in a revolving chair, wherein nystagmus movements can be observed and timed after the rotation stops. Another clinically used test is caloric stimulation, by the placement of warm water in the ear. This has the advantage of unilateral testing, and is due to the warming of the vestibular fluid that causes convection currents, and by placing the head in different positions, so that at least one canal is in the horizontal plane (with no effect of convectional movement), more precise evaluations can be achieved.

right in Figure 117-4. Thus, the semicircular duct transmits a signal of one polarity when the head *begins* to rotate and of opposite polarity when it *stops* rotating.

Removal of the flocculonodular lobes of the cerebellum prevents normal detection of semicircular duct signals but has less effect on detecting macular signals. It is especially interesting that the cerebellum serves as a "predictive" organ for most rapid movements of the body, as well as for those having to do with equilibrium. These other functions of the cerebellum are discussed in Chapter 116.

BIBLIOGRAPHY

Angelaki DE, Cullen KE: Vestibular system: the many facets of a multimodal sense, *Annu. Rev. Neurosci.* 31:125, 2008.

Cullen KE, Roy JE: Signal processing in the vestibular system during active versus passive head movements, *J. Neurophysiol.* 91:1919, 2004.

Horak FB: Postural compensation for vestibular loss, *Ann. N. Y. Acad. Sci.* 1164:76, 2009.
Pierrot-Deseilligny C: Effect of gravity on vertical eye position, *Ann. N. Y. Acad. Sci.* 1164:155, 2009.

118

Basal Ganglia

LEARNING OBJECTIVES

- List components of the basal ganglia and describe their connections.
- Describe functions of the basal ganglia.
- List clinical disorders of the basal ganglia.
- Describe the pathophysiology and clinical features of parkinsonism and its treatment.

GLOSSARY OF TERMS

- **Akinesia:** Difficulty or inability to initiate purposeful movement, seen in Parkinson disease

- **Athetosis:** Abnormal involuntary movement disorder with convoluted, writhing movements of the fingers, arms, legs, and neck (lesion usually in the corpus striatum)

- **Caudate nucleus:** Present within each hemisphere of the brain, sited on top of the thalamus [the caudate nucleus (cauda = head in Latin) resembles a C-shape]

- **Chorea:** Abnormal involuntary movement disorder, or dyskinesia (derived from the Greek word for dance)

- **Globus pallidus:** Latin = pale globe, also known as paleostriatum (connected to the subthalamus and part of the extrapyramidal motor system)

- **Hemiballismus:** Rare abnormal movement disorder, with violent movements of the limb, and due to lesions usually in the subthalamic nucleus

- **Huntington's disease:** Genetic cause of chorea with an abnormality on chromosome 4

- **Internal capsule:** Contains both ascending and descending axons, and is an area of white matter in the brain that separates the caudate nucleus and the thalamus from the lenticular nucleus

- **Parkinson's disease:** Disorder of the basal ganglia in the substantia nigra, with symptoms of a characteristic tremor, rigidity, and akinesia

- **Putamen:** Together with caudate nucleus forms the striatum (the putamen has connections to the substantia nigra and globus pallidus)

- **Substantia nigra:** Has projections to the caudate and putamen (it is thought to be the site of the lesion in Parkinson disease or paralysis agitans; this is due to degeneration of the melanin-containing cells in the substantia nigra, which produce dopamine normally)

- **Subthalamic nucleus:** Small lens-shaped nucleus in the brain (lesions of this nucleus produce hemiballismus)

The basal ganglia help plan and control complex patterns of muscle movement. They control relative intensities of the separate movements, directions of movements, and sequencing of multiple successive and parallel movements to achieve specific complicated motor goals. This chapter explains the basic functions of the cerebellum and basal ganglia and discusses the overall brain mechanisms for achieving intricate coordination of total motor activity.

The basal ganglia, like the cerebellum, constitute another *accessory motor system* that functions usually not by itself but in close association with the cerebral cortex and corticospinal motor control system. In fact, the basal ganglia receive most of their input signals from the cerebral cortex itself and also return almost all their output signals back to the cortex.

Figure 118-1 shows the anatomical relations of the basal ganglia to other structures of the brain. On each side of the brain, these ganglia consist of the *caudate nucleus*, *putamen*, *globus pallidus*, *substantia nigra*, and *subthalamic nucleus*. They are located mainly lateral to and surrounding the thalamus, occupying a large portion of the interior regions of both cerebral hemispheres. Almost all motor and sensory nerve fibers connecting the cerebral cortex and spinal cord pass through the space that lies between the major masses of the basal ganglia, the *caudate nucleus* and the *putamen*. This space is called the *internal capsule* of the brain. It is important for our current discussion because of the intimate association between the basal ganglia and the corticospinal system for motor control.

Neuronal Circuitry of the Basal Ganglia. The anatomical connections between the basal ganglia and the other brain elements that provide motor control are complex, as shown in Figure 118-2. To the left is shown the motor cortex, thalamus, and associated brainstem and cerebellar circuitry. To the right is the major circuitry of the basal ganglia system, showing the tremendous interconnections among the basal ganglia plus extensive input and output pathways between the other motor regions of the brain and the basal ganglia.

In the next few sections we concentrate especially on two major circuits, the *putamen circuit* and the *caudate circuit*.

Function of the Basal Ganglia in Executing Patterns of Motor Activity—The Putamen Circuit

One of the principal roles of the basal ganglia in motor control is to function in association with the corticospinal system to control *complex patterns of motor activity*. An example is the writing of letters of the alphabet. When the basal ganglia sustain serious damage, the cortical system of motor control can no longer provide these patterns. Instead, one's writing becomes crude, as if one were learning how to write for the first time.

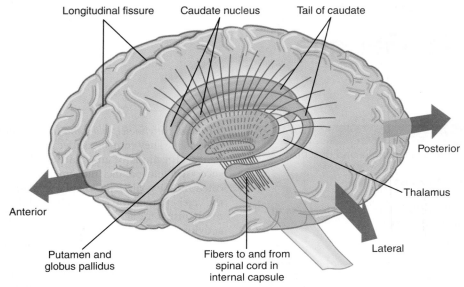

Figure 118-1 Anatomical relations of the basal ganglia to the cerebral cortex and thalamus, shown in three-dimensional view. *Modified from Guyton, A.C., 1992. Basic Neuroscience: Anatomy and Physiology. W.B. Saunders, Philadelphia.*

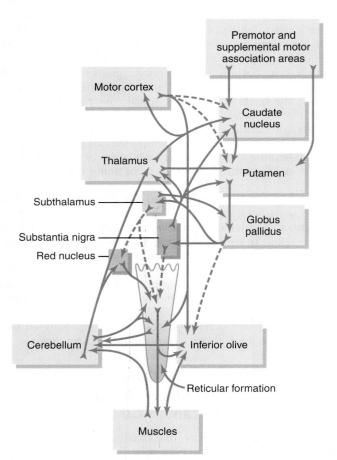

Figure 118-2 Relation of the basal ganglial circuitry to the corticospinal–cerebellar system for movement control.

Other patterns that require the basal ganglia are cutting paper with scissors, hammering nails, shooting a basketball through a hoop, passing a football, throwing a baseball, the movements of shoveling dirt, most aspects of vocalization, controlled movements of the eyes, and virtually any other of our skilled movements, most of them performed subconsciously.

Neural Pathways of the Putamen Circuit. Figure 118-3 shows the principal pathways through the basal ganglia for executing learned patterns of movement. They begin mainly in the premotor and supplementary areas of the motor cortex, and in the somatosensory areas of the sensory cortex. Next they pass to the putamen (mainly bypassing the caudate nucleus), then to the internal portion of the globus pallidus, next to the ventroanterior and ventrolateral relay nuclei of the thalamus, and finally return to the cerebral primary motor cortex and to portions of the premotor and supplementary cerebral areas closely associated with the primary motor cortex. Thus, *the putamen circuit has its inputs mainly from the parts of the brain adjacent to the primary motor cortex* but not much from the primary motor

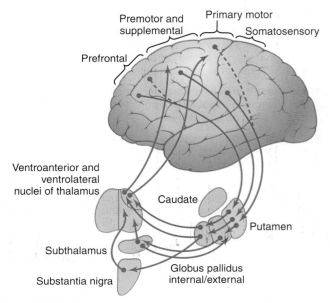

Figure 118-3 Putamen circuit through the basal ganglia for subconscious execution of learned patterns of movement.

cortex itself. Then, its outputs go mainly back to the *primary motor cortex* or closely associated *premotor* and *supplementary* cortex. Functioning in close association with this primary putamen circuit are ancillary circuits that pass from the putamen through the external globus pallidus, the subthalamus, and the substantia nigra—finally returning to the motor cortex by way of the thalamus.

Abnormal Function in the Putamen Circuit: Athetosis, Hemiballismus, and Chorea. How does the putamen circuit function to help execute patterns of movement? Little is known about this function. However, when a portion of the circuit is damaged or blocked, certain patterns of movement become severely abnormal. For instance, lesions in the *globus pallidus* frequently lead to spontaneous and often continuous *writing movements* of a hand, an arm, the neck, or the face. These movements are called *athetosis*.

A lesion in the *subthalamus* often leads to sudden *flailing movements* of an entire limb, a condition called *hemiballismus*.

Multiple small lesions in the *putamen* lead to *flicking movements* in the hands, face, and other parts of the body, called *chorea*.

Lesions of the *substantia nigra* lead to the common and extremely severe disease of *rigidity*, *akinesia*, and *tremors* known as *Parkinson's disease*, which we discuss in more detail later in this chapter.

Role of the Basal Ganglia for Cognitive Control of Sequences of Motor Patterns—The Caudate Circuit

The term *cognition* means the thinking processes of the brain, using both sensory input to the brain and information already stored in memory. Most of our motor actions occur as a consequence of thoughts generated in the mind, a process called *cognitive control of motor activity*. The caudate nucleus plays a major role in this cognitive control of motor activity.

The neural connections between the caudate nucleus and the corticospinal motor control system, shown in Figure 118-4, are somewhat different from those of the putamen circuit. Part of the reason for this difference is that the caudate nucleus, as shown in Figure 118-1, extends into all lobes of the cerebrum, beginning anteriorly in the frontal lobes, then passing posteriorly through the parietal and occipital lobes, and finally curving forward again like the letter "C" into the temporal lobes. Furthermore, the caudate nucleus receives large amounts of its input from the *association areas* of the cerebral cortex overlying the caudate nucleus, mainly areas that also integrate the different types of sensory and motor information into usable thought patterns.

After the signals pass from the cerebral cortex to the caudate nucleus, they are next transmitted to the *internal globus pallidus*, then to the *relay nuclei of the ventroanterior and ventrolateral thalamus*, and finally back to the *prefrontal, premotor, and supplementary motor areas* of the cerebral cortex, but with almost none of the returning signals passing directly to the primary motor cortex. Instead, the returning signals go to the accessory motor regions in the premotor and supplementary motor areas that are concerned with putting together sequential patterns of movement lasting 5 or more seconds instead of exciting individual muscle movements.

A good example of this phenomenon would be a person seeing a lion approach and then responding instantaneously and

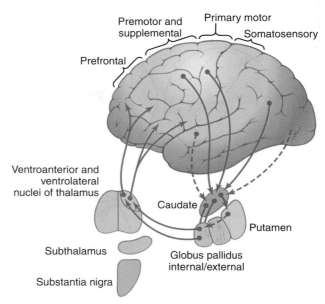

Figure 118-4 Caudate circuit through the basal ganglia for cognitive planning of sequential and parallel motor patterns to achieve specific conscious goals.

automatically by (1) turning away from the lion, (2) beginning to run, and (3) even attempting to climb a tree. Without the cognitive functions, the person might not have the instinctive knowledge, without thinking for too long a time, to respond quickly and appropriately. Thus, cognitive control of motor activity determines subconsciously, and within seconds, which patterns of movement will be used together to achieve a complex goal that might itself last for many seconds.

Function of the Basal Ganglia to Change the Timing and to Scale the Intensity of Movements

Two important capabilities of the brain in controlling movement are to (1) determine how rapidly the movement is to be performed and (2) control how large the movement will be. For instance, a person may write the letter "a" slowly or rapidly. Also, he or she may write a small "a" on a piece of paper or a large "A" on a chalkboard. Regardless of the choice, the proportional characteristics of the letter remain nearly the same.

In patients with severe lesions of the basal ganglia, these timing and scaling functions are poor; in fact, sometimes they are nonexistent. Here again, the basal ganglia do not function alone; rather they function in close association with the cerebral cortex. One especially important cortical area is the posterior parietal cortex, which is the locus of the spatial coordinates for motor control of all parts of the body, as well as for the relation of the body and its parts to all its surroundings. Damage to this area does not produce simple deficits of sensory perception, such as loss of tactile sensation, blindness, or deafness. Instead, lesions of the posterior parietal cortex produce an inability to accurately perceive objects through normally functioning sensory mechanisms, a condition called *agnosia*. Figure 118-5 shows how a person with a lesion in the right posterior parietal cortex might try to copy drawings. In these cases, the patient's ability to copy the left side of the drawings is severely impaired. Also, such a person will always try to avoid using his or her left arm, left hand, or other portions of his or her left body for the

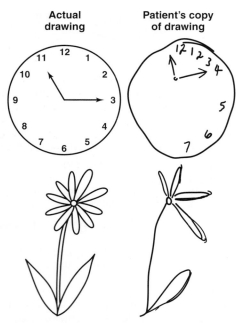

Actual drawing   **Patient's copy of drawing**

Figure 118-5   Illustration of drawings that might be made by a person who has *neglect syndrome* caused by severe damage in his or her right posterior parietal cortex compared with the actual drawing the patient was requested to copy. Note that the person's ability to copy the left side of the drawings is severely impaired.

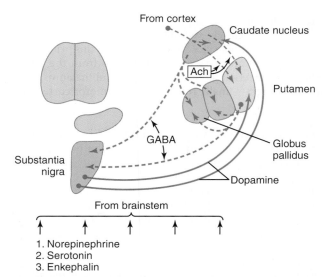

1. Norepinephrine
2. Serotonin
3. Enkephalin

Figure 118-6   Neuronal pathways that secrete different types of neurotransmitter substances in the basal ganglia. *Ach*, acetylcholine; *GABA*, gamma-aminobutyric acid.

performance of tasks, or even to wash this side of the body (*personal neglect syndrome*), almost not knowing that these parts of his or her body exist.

Because the caudate circuit of the basal ganglial system functions mainly with association areas of the cerebral cortex such as the posterior parietal cortex, presumably the timing and scaling of movements are functions of this caudate cognitive motor control circuit. However, our understanding of function in the basal ganglia is still so imprecise that much of what is conjectured in the last few sections is analytical deduction rather than proven fact.

Functions of Specific Neurotransmitter Substances in the Basal Ganglial System

Figure 118-6 demonstrates the interplay of several specific neurotransmitters that are known to function within the basal ganglia, showing (1) *dopamine* pathways from the substantia nigra to the caudate nucleus and putamen, (2) *gamma-aminobutyric acid* (*GABA*) pathways from the caudate nucleus and putamen to the globus pallidus and substantia nigra, (3) *acetylcholine* pathways from the cortex to the caudate nucleus and putamen, and (4) multiple general pathways from the brainstem that secrete *norepinephrine, serotonin, enkephalin,* and several other neurotransmitters in the basal ganglia, as well as in other parts of the cerebrum. In addition to all these are *multiple glutamate pathways* that provide most of the excitatory signals (not shown in the figure) that balance out the large numbers of inhibitory signals transmitted especially by the dopamine, GABA, and serotonin inhibitory transmitters. We have more to say about some of these neurotransmitter and hormonal systems in subsequent sections when we discuss diseases of the basal ganglia, as well as in subsequent chapters when we discuss behavior, sleep, wakefulness, and functions of the autonomic nervous system.

For the present, it should be remembered that the neurotransmitter GABA functions as an inhibitory agent. Therefore, GABA neurons in the feedback loops from the cortex through the basal ganglia and then back to the cortex make virtually all these loops *negative feedback loops*, rather than positive feedback loops, thus lending stability to the motor control systems. Dopamine also functions as an inhibitory neurotransmitter in most parts of the brain, so it also functions as a stabilizer under some conditions.

Summary of Integrated Functions of the Basal Ganglia

The basal ganglia are essential to motor control in ways entirely different from those of the cerebellum. Their most important functions are (1) to help the cortex execute subconscious but *learned patterns of movement* and (2) to help plan multiple parallel and sequential patterns of movement that the mind must put together to accomplish a purposeful task.

Other functions included relate to facilitating types of complex motor patterns such as those for writing all the different letters of the alphabet, for throwing a ball, and for typing. Also, the basal ganglia are required to modify these patterns for writing small or writing very large, thus controlling dimensions of the patterns.

At a still higher level of control is another combined cerebral and basal ganglia circuit, beginning in the thinking processes of the cerebrum to provide overall sequential steps of action for responding to each new situation, such as planning one's immediate motor response to an assailant or one's sequential response to an unexpectedly fond embrace.

Clinical Syndromes Resulting from Damage to the Basal Ganglia

Aside from *athetosis* and *hemiballismus*, which have already been mentioned in relation to lesions in the globus pallidus and subthalamus, two other major diseases result from damage in the basal ganglia. These deseases are *Parkinson's disease* and *Huntington's disease*.

PARKINSON'S DISEASE

Parkinson's disease, which is also known as *paralysis agitans*, results from widespread destruction of the portion of the substantia nigra (the pars compacta) that sends dopamine-secreting nerve fibers to the caudate nucleus and putamen. The disease is characterized by (1) rigidity of much of the musculature of the body; (2) involuntary tremor of the involved areas even when the person is resting at a fixed rate of three to six cycles per second; (3) serious difficulty in initiating movement, called *akinesia*; (4) postural instability caused by impaired postural reflexes, leading to poor balance and falls; and (5) other motor symptoms including dysphagia (impaired ability to swallow), speech disorders, gait disturbances, and fatigue.

The causes of these abnormal motor effects are unknown. However, the dopamine secreted in the caudate nucleus and putamen is an inhibitory transmitter; therefore, destruction of the dopaminergic neurons in the substantia nigra of the parkinsonian patient theoretically would allow the caudate nucleus and putamen to become overly active and possibly cause continuous output of excitatory signals to the corticospinal motor control system. These signals could overly excite many or all of the muscles of the body, thus leading to *rigidity*.

Some of the feedback circuits might easily *oscillate* because of high feedback gains after loss of their inhibition, leading to the *tremor* of Parkinson's disease. This tremor is quite different from that of cerebellar disease because it occurs during all waking hours and therefore is an *involuntary tremor*, in contradistinction to cerebellar tremor, which occurs only when the person performs intentionally initiated movements and therefore is called *intention tremor*.

The *akinesia* that occurs in Parkinson's disease is often much more distressing to the patient than are the symptoms of muscle rigidity and tremor, because a person with severe parkinsonism, must exert the highest degree of concentration to perform even the simplest movement. The mental effort, even mental anguish, which is necessary to make the desired movements, is often at the limit of the patient's willpower. Then, when the movements do occur, they are usually stiff and staccato in character instead of smooth. The cause of this akinesia is still speculative. However, dopamine secretion in the limbic system, especially in the *nucleus accumbens*, is often decreased along with its decrease in the basal ganglia. It has been suggested that this decrease might reduce the psychic drive for motor activity so greatly that akinesia results.

Treatment with L-Dopa. Administration of the drug *L-Dopa* to patients with Parkinson's disease usually ameliorates many of the symptoms, especially the rigidity and akinesia. The reason for this amelioration is believed to be that L-Dopa is converted in the brain into dopamine, and the dopamine then restores the normal balance between inhibition and excitation in the caudate nucleus and putamen. Administration of dopamine does not have the same effect because dopamine has a chemical structure that will not allow it to pass through the blood–brain barrier; the slightly different structure of L-Dopa allows it to pass through this barrier.

Treatment with L-Deprenyl. Another treatment for Parkinson's disease is the drug L-deprenyl. This drug inhibits monoamine oxidase, which is responsible for destruction of most of the dopamine after it has been secreted. Therefore, any dopamine that is released remains in the basal ganglial tissues for a longer time. In addition, for reasons that are not understood, this treatment helps to slow destruction of the dopamine-secreting neurons in the substantia nigra. Therefore, appropriate combinations of L-Dopa therapy along with L-deprenyl therapy usually provide much better treatment than use of one of these drugs alone.

HUNTINGTON'S DISEASE (HUNTINGTON'S CHOREA)

Huntington's disease is an autosomal dominant hereditary disorder that usually begins causing symptoms at age 30–40 years. It is characterized at first by flicking movements in individual muscles and then progressive severe distortional movements of the entire body. In addition, severe dementia develops along with the motor dysfunctions.

The abnormal movements of Huntington's disease are believed to be caused by the loss of most of the cell bodies of the GABA-secreting neurons in the caudate nucleus and putamen and the loss of acetylcholine-secreting neurons in many parts of the brain. The axon terminals of the GABA neurons normally inhibit portions of the globus pallidus and substantia nigra. This loss of inhibition is believed to allow spontaneous outbursts of globus pallidus and substantia nigra activity that cause the distortional movements.

Dementia in persons with Huntington's disease probably does not result from the loss of GABA neurons but from the loss of acetylcholine-secreting neurons, perhaps especially in the thinking areas of the cerebral cortex.

The abnormal gene that causes Huntington's disease has been found; it has a many-times-repeating codon, CAG, that codes for multiple extra *glutamine* amino acids in the molecular structure of an abnormal neuronal cell protein called *huntington* that causes the symptoms. How this protein causes the disease effects is now the question for major research efforts.

WHAT DRIVES US TO ACTION?

What is it that arouses us from inactivity and sets into play our trains of movement? We are beginning to learn about the motivational systems of the brain. Basically, the brain has an older core located beneath, anterior, and lateral to the thalamus—including the hypothalamus, amygdala, hippocampus, septal region anterior to the hypothalamus and thalamus, and even old regions of the thalamus and cerebral cortex—all of which function together to initiate most motor and other functional activities of the brain. These areas are collectively called the *limbic system* of the brain. We discuss this system in detail in Chapter 124.

BIBLIOGRAPHY

Breakefield XO, Blood AJ, Li Y, et al: The pathophysiological basis of dystonias, *Nat. Rev. Neurosci.* 9:222, 2008.

Corti O, Lesage S, Brice A: What genetics tells us about the causes and mechanisms of Parkinson's disease, *Physiol. Rev.* 91:1161, 2011.

DeKosky ST, Marek K: Looking backward to move forward: early detection of neurodegenerative disorders, *Science* 302:830, 2003.

Kandel ER, Schwartz JH, Jessell TM: *Principles of Neural Science*, fourth ed., New York, 2000, McGraw-Hill.

Kreitzer AC, Malenka RC: Striatal plasticity and basal ganglia circuit function, *Neuron* 60:543, 2008.

Lees AJ, Hardy J, Revesz T: Parkinson's disease, *Lancet* 373:2055, 2009.

Li JY, Plomann M, Brundin P: Huntington's disease: a synaptopathy? *Trends Mol. Med.* 9:414, 2003.

Nambu A: Seven problems on the basal ganglia, *Curr. Opin. Neurobiol.* 18:595, 2008.

Okun MS: Deep-brain stimulation for Parkinson's disease, *N. Engl. J. Med.* 367:1529, 2012.

Rosas HD, Salat DH, Lee SY, et al: Complexity and heterogeneity: what drives the ever-changing brain in Huntington's disease? *Ann. N. Y. Acad. Sci.* 1147:196, 2008.

Sethi KD: Tremor, *Curr. Opin. Neurol.* 16:481, 2003.

PART IV

Other Functions and Activities of the Brain

MARIO VAZ

The Autonomic Nervous System

The *autonomic nervous system* is the portion of the nervous system that controls most visceral functions of the body. This system helps to control arterial pressure, gastrointestinal motility, gastrointestinal secretion, urinary bladder emptying, sweating, body temperature, and many other activities. Some of these activities are controlled almost entirely and some only partially by the autonomic nervous system.

One of the most striking characteristics of the autonomic nervous system is the rapidity and intensity with which it can change visceral functions. For instance, within 3–5 seconds it can increase the heart rate to twice normal, and within 10–15 seconds the arterial pressure can be doubled. At the other extreme, the arterial pressure can be decreased low enough within 10–15 seconds to cause fainting. Sweating can begin within seconds, and the urinary bladder may empty involuntarily, also within seconds.

General Organization of the Autonomic Nervous System

The autonomic nervous system is activated mainly by centers located in the *spinal cord*, *brainstem*, and *hypothalamus*. In addition, portions of the cerebral cortex, especially of the limbic cortex, can transmit signals to the lower centers and in this way can influence autonomic control.

The autonomic nervous system also often operates through *visceral reflexes*. That is, subconscious sensory signals from visceral organs can enter the autonomic ganglia, the brainstem, or the hypothalamus and then return *subconscious reflex responses* directly back to the visceral organs to control their activities.

The efferent autonomic signals are transmitted to the various organs of the body through two major subdivisions called the *sympathetic nervous system* and the *parasympathetic nervous*

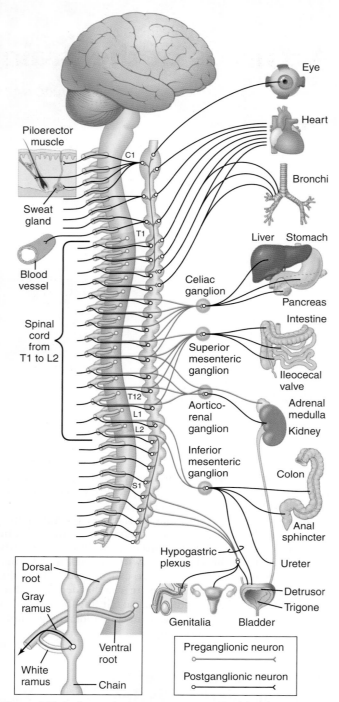

Figure 119-1 Sympathetic nervous system. The black lines represent postganglionic fibers, and the red lines show preganglionic fibers.

system, the characteristics of which are described in the following sections.

Physiological Anatomy of the Sympathetic Nervous System.
Figure 119-1 shows the general organization of the peripheral portions of the sympathetic nervous system. Shown specifically in the figure are (1) one of the two *paravertebral sympathetic chains of ganglia* that are interconnected with the spinal nerves on the side of the vertebral column, (2) *prevertebral ganglia* (the *celiac, superior mesenteric, aorticorenal, inferior mesenteric*, and

hypogastric), and (3) nerves extending from the ganglia to the different internal organs.

The sympathetic nerve fibers originate in the spinal cord along with spinal nerves between cord segments T1 and L2, and pass first into the *sympathetic chain* and then to the tissues and organs that are stimulated by the sympathetic nerves.

Preganglionic and Postganglionic Sympathetic Neurons.
The sympathetic nerves are different from skeletal motor nerves in the following way: Each sympathetic pathway from the cord to the stimulated tissue is composed of two neurons, a *preganglionic neuron* and a *postganglionic neuron*, in contrast to only a single neuron in the skeletal motor pathway. The cell body of each preganglionic neuron lies in the *intermediolateral horn* of the spinal cord; its fiber passes through *a ventral root* of the cord into the corresponding *spinal nerve* as shown in Figure 119-2.

Immediately after the spinal nerve leaves the spinal canal, the preganglionic sympathetic fibers leave the spinal nerve and pass through a *white ramus* into one of the *ganglia* of the *sympathetic chain*. The fibers then take one of three courses: (1) they can synapse with postganglionic sympathetic neurons in the ganglion that they enter; (2) they can pass upward or downward in the chain and synapse in one of the other ganglia of the chain; or (3) they can pass for variable distances through the chain and then through one of the *sympathetic nerves* radiating outward from the chain, finally synapsing in a *peripheral sympathetic ganglion*.

The postganglionic sympathetic neuron thus originates either in one of the sympathetic chain ganglia or in one of the peripheral sympathetic ganglia. From either of these two sources, the postganglionic fibers then travel to their destinations in the various organs.

Sympathetic Nerve Fibers in the Skeletal Nerves. Some of the postganglionic fibers pass back from the sympathetic chain into the spinal nerves through *gray rami* at all levels of the cord, as shown in Figure 119-2. These sympathetic fibers are all very

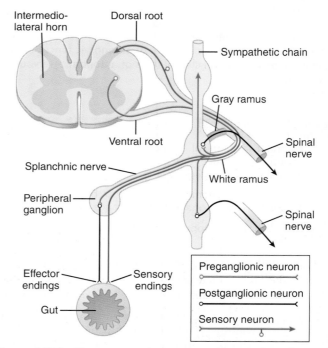

Figure 119-2 Nerve connections among the spinal cord, spinal nerves, sympathetic chain, and peripheral sympathetic nerves.

small type C fibers, and they extend to all parts of the body by way of the skeletal nerves. They control the blood vessels, sweat glands, and piloerector muscles of the hairs. About 8% of the fibers in the average skeletal nerve are sympathetic fibers, a fact that indicates their great importance.

Segmental Distribution of the Sympathetic Nerve Fibers. The sympathetic pathways that originate in the different segments of the spinal cord are not necessarily distributed to the same part of the body as the somatic spinal nerve fibers from the same segments. Instead, the *sympathetic fibers from cord segment T1 generally pass (1) up the sympathetic chain to terminate in the head; (2) from T2 to terminate in the neck; (3) from T3, T4, T5, and T6 into the thorax; (4) from T7, T8, T9, T10, and T11 into the abdomen; and (5) from T12, L1, and L2 into the legs.* This distribution is only approximate and overlaps greatly.

The distribution of sympathetic nerves to each organ is determined partly by the locus in the embryo from which the organ originated. For instance, the heart receives many sympathetic nerve fibers from the neck portion of the sympathetic chain because the heart originated in the neck of the embryo before translocation into the thorax. Likewise, the abdominal organs receive most of their sympathetic innervation from the lower thoracic spinal cord segments because most of the primitive gut originated in this area.

PHYSIOLOGICAL ANATOMY OF THE PARASYMPATHETIC NERVOUS SYSTEM

The *parasympathetic nervous system* is shown in Figure 119-3, which demonstrates that parasympathetic fibers leave the central nervous system through cranial nerves III, VII, IX, and X; additional parasympathetic fibers leave the lowermost part of the spinal cord through the second and third sacral spinal nerves, and occasionally the first and fourth sacral nerves. About 75% of all parasympathetic nerve fibers are in the *vagus nerves* (cranial nerve X), passing to the entire thoracic and abdominal regions of the body. Therefore, a physiologist speaking of the parasympathetic nervous system often thinks mainly of the two vagus nerves. The vagus nerves supply parasympathetic nerves to the heart, lungs, esophagus, stomach, entire small intestine, proximal half of the colon, liver, gallbladder, pancreas, kidneys, and upper portions of the ureters.

Parasympathetic fibers in the *third cranial nerve* go to the pupillary sphincter and ciliary muscle of the eye. Fibers from the *seventh cranial nerve* pass to the lacrimal, nasal, and submandibular glands, and fibers from the *ninth cranial nerve* go to the parotid gland.

The sacral parasympathetic fibers are in the *pelvic nerves*, which pass through the spinal nerve sacral plexus on each side of the cord at the S2 and S3 levels. These fibers then distribute to the descending colon, rectum, urinary bladder, and lower portions of the ureters. Also, this sacral group of parasympathetics supplies nerve signals to the external genitalia to cause erection.

Preganglionic and Postganglionic Parasympathetic Neurons. The parasympathetic system, like the sympathetic system, has both preganglionic and postganglionic neurons. However, except in the case of a few cranial parasympathetic nerves, the *preganglionic fibers* pass uninterrupted all the way to the organ that is to be controlled. The *postganglionic neurons* are located in the wall of the organ. The preganglionic fibers synapse with these neurons, and extremely short postganglionic fibers, a fraction of a millimeter to several centimeters in length, leave the neurons to innervate the tissues of the organ. This location of

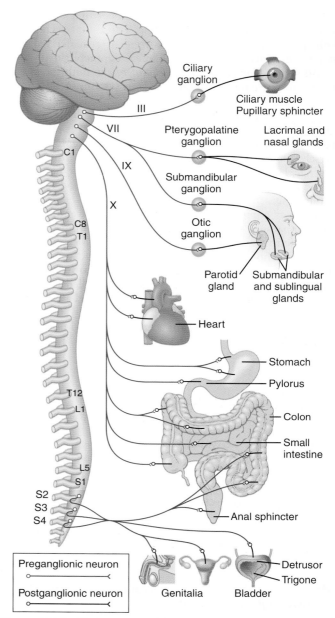

Figure 119-3   The parasympathetic nervous system. The blue lines represent preganglionic fibers and the black lines show postganglionic fibers.

the parasympathetic postganglionic neurons in the visceral organ is quite different from the arrangement of the sympathetic ganglia because the cell bodies of the sympathetic postganglionic neurons are almost always located in the ganglia of the sympathetic chain or in various other discrete ganglia in the abdomen, rather than in the excited organ.

Basic Characteristics of Sympathetic and Parasympathetic Function

CHOLINERGIC AND ADRENERGIC FIBERS—SECRETION OF ACETYLCHOLINE OR NOREPINEPHRINE

The sympathetic and parasympathetic nerve fibers secrete mainly one or the other of two synaptic transmitter substances, *acetylcholine* or *norepinephrine*. The fibers that secrete acetylcholine are said to be *cholinergic*. Those that secrete norepinephrine are said to be *adrenergic*, a term derived from *adrenalin*, which is an alternate name for epinephrine.

All *preganglionic neurons* are *cholinergic* in both the sympathetic and the parasympathetic nervous systems. Acetylcholine or acetylcholine-like substances, when applied to the ganglia, will excite both sympathetic and parasympathetic postganglionic neurons. Either *all or almost all of the postganglionic neurons of the parasympathetic system are also cholinergic*. Conversely, *most of the postganglionic sympathetic neurons are adrenergic*. However, the postganglionic sympathetic nerve fibers to the sweat glands, and perhaps to a very few blood vessels, are cholinergic.

Thus, *all or virtually all* of the terminal nerve endings of the parasympathetic system secrete *acetylcholine*. Almost all of the sympathetic nerve endings secrete *norepinephrine*, but a few secrete acetylcholine. These neurotransmitters in turn act on the different organs to cause respective parasympathetic or sympathetic effects. Therefore, acetylcholine is called a *parasympathetic transmitter* and norepinephrine is called a *sympathetic transmitter*.

The molecular structures of acetylcholine and norepinephrine are the following:

Acetylcholine

Norepinephrine

Mechanisms of Transmitter Secretion and Removal at Postganglionic Endings

Secretion of Acetylcholine and Norepinephrine by Postganglionic Nerve Endings. A few of the postganglionic autonomic nerve endings, especially those of the parasympathetic nerves, are similar to but much smaller than those of the skeletal neuromuscular junction. However, many of the parasympathetic nerve fibers and almost all the sympathetic fibers merely touch the effector cells of the organs that they innervate as they pass by, or in some instances, they terminate in connective tissue located adjacent to the cells that are to be stimulated. Where these filaments touch or pass over or near the cells to be stimulated, they usually have bulbous enlargements called *varicosities*; it is in these varicosities that the transmitter vesicles of acetylcholine or norepinephrine are synthesized and stored. Also in the varicosities are large numbers of mitochondria that supply adenosine triphosphate, which is required to energize acetylcholine or norepinephrine synthesis.

When an action potential spreads over the terminal fibers, the depolarization process increases the permeability of the fiber membrane to calcium ions, allowing these ions to diffuse into the nerve terminals or nerve varicosities. The calcium ions

in turn cause the terminals or varicosities to empty their contents to the exterior. Thus, the transmitter substance is secreted.

Synthesis of Acetylcholine, its Destruction After Secretion, and its Duration of Action. Acetylcholine is synthesized in the terminal endings and varicosities of the cholinergic nerve fibers where it is stored in vesicles in highly concentrated form until it is released. The basic chemical reaction of this synthesis is the following:

$$\text{Acetyl-CoA} + \text{choline} \xrightarrow[\text{acetyltran sferase}]{\text{choline}} \text{acetylcholine}$$

Once acetylcholine is secreted into a tissue by a cholinergic nerve ending, it persists in the tissue for a few seconds while it performs its nerve signal transmitter function. Then it is split into an *acetate ion* and *choline*, catalyzed by the enzyme *acetylcholinesterase* that is bound with collagen and glycosaminoglycans in the local connective tissue. This mechanism is the same as that for acetylcholine signal transmission and subsequent acetylcholine destruction that occurs at the neuromuscular junctions of skeletal nerve fibers. The choline that is formed is then transported back into the terminal nerve ending, where it is used again and again for synthesis of new acetylcholine.

Synthesis of Norepinephrine, its Removal, and its Duration of Action. Synthesis of norepinephrine begins in the axoplasm of the terminal nerve endings of adrenergic nerve fibers but is completed inside the secretory vesicles.

After secretion of norepinephrine by the terminal nerve endings, it is removed from the secretory site in three ways: (1) reuptake into the adrenergic nerve endings by an active transport process—accounting for removal of 50–80% of the secreted norepinephrine; (2) diffusion away from the nerve endings into the surrounding body fluids and then into the blood—accounting for removal of most of the remaining norepinephrine; and (3) destruction of small amounts by tissue enzymes (one of these enzymes is *monoamine oxidase*, which is found in the nerve endings, and another is *catechol-O-methyltransferase*, which is present diffusely in the tissues).

Ordinarily, the norepinephrine secreted directly into a tissue remains active for only a few seconds, demonstrating that its reuptake and diffusion away from the tissue are rapid. However, the norepinephrine and epinephrine secreted into the blood by the adrenal medullae remain active until they diffuse into some tissue, where they can be destroyed by catechol-O-methyltransferase; this action occurs mainly in the liver. Therefore, when secreted into the blood, both norepinephrine and epinephrine remain active for 10–30 seconds, but their activity declines to extinction over 1 to several minutes.

RECEPTORS ON THE EFFECTOR ORGANS

Before acetylcholine, norepinephrine, or epinephrine secreted at an autonomic nerve ending can stimulate an effector organ, it must first bind with specific *receptors* on the effector cells. The receptor is on the outside of the cell membrane, bound as a prosthetic group to a protein molecule that penetrates all the way through the cell membrane. Binding of the transmitter substance with the receptor causes a conformational change in the structure of the protein molecule. In turn, the altered protein molecule excites or inhibits the cell, most often by (1) causing a change in cell membrane permeability to one or more ions or (2) activating or inactivating an enzyme attached to the other end of the receptor protein, where it protrudes into the interior of the cell.

Two Principal Types of Acetylcholine Receptors—Muscarinic and Nicotinic Receptors. Acetylcholine activates mainly two types of *receptors*, which are called *muscarinic* and *nicotinic* receptors. The reason for these names is that muscarine, a poison from toadstools, activates only muscarinic receptors and will not activate nicotinic receptors, whereas nicotine activates only nicotinic receptors. Acetylcholine activates both of them.

Muscarinic receptors, which use G proteins as their signaling mechanism, are found on all effector cells that are stimulated by the postganglionic cholinergic neurons of either the parasympathetic nervous system or the sympathetic system.

Nicotinic receptors are ligand-gated ion channels found in autonomic ganglia at the synapses between the preganglionic and postganglionic neurons of both the sympathetic and parasympathetic systems. [Nicotinic receptors are also present at many nonautonomic nerve endings—eg, at the neuromuscular junctions in skeletal muscle (discussed in Chapter 12).]

An understanding of the two types of receptors is especially important because specific drugs are frequently used as medicine to stimulate or block one or the other of the two types of receptors.

Adrenergic Receptors—Alpha and Beta Receptors. Two major classes of adrenergic receptors also exist; they are called *alpha receptors* and *beta receptors*. There are two major types of alpha receptors, alpha$_1$ and alpha$_2$, which are linked to different G proteins. The beta receptors are divided into *beta$_1$*, *beta$_2$*, and *beta$_3$* receptors because certain chemicals affect only certain beta receptors. The beta receptors also sue G proteins for signaling.

Norepinephrine and epinephrine, both of which are secreted into the blood by the adrenal medulla, have slightly different effects in exciting the alpha and beta receptors. Norepinephrine excites mainly alpha receptors but excites the beta receptors to a lesser extent as well. Epinephrine excites both types of receptors approximately equally. Therefore, the relative effects of norepinephrine and epinephrine on different effector organs are determined by the types of receptors in the organs. If they are all beta receptors, epinephrine will be the more effective excitant.

Table 92-1 lists the distribution of alpha and beta receptors in some of the organs and systems controlled by the sympathetic nerves. Note that certain alpha functions are excitatory, whereas others are inhibitory. Likewise, certain beta functions are excitatory and others are inhibitory. Therefore, alpha and beta receptors are not necessarily associated with excitation or inhibition but simply with the affinity of the hormone for the receptors in the given effector organ.

A synthetic hormone chemically similar to epinephrine and norepinephrine, *isopropyl norepinephrine*, has an extremely strong action on beta receptors but essentially no action on alpha receptors.

EXCITATORY AND INHIBITORY ACTIONS OF SYMPATHETIC AND PARASYMPATHETIC STIMULATION

Table 119-1 lists the effects on different visceral functions of the body caused by stimulating either the parasympathetic nerves or the sympathetic nerves. Note again that *sympathetic stimulation causes excitatory effects in some organs but inhibitory effects in others. Likewise, parasympathetic stimulation causes excitation in some organs but inhibition in others.* Also, when sympathetic stimulation excites a particular organ, parasympathetic stimulation sometimes inhibits it, demonstrating that the two systems occasionally act reciprocally to each other. However, most organs are dominantly controlled by one or the other of the two systems.

There is no generalization one can use to explain whether sympathetic or parasympathetic stimulation will cause excitation or inhibition of a particular organ. Therefore, to understand sympathetic and parasympathetic function, one must learn all the separate functions of these two nervous systems on each organ, as listed in Table 119-1.

Intramural Nerve Plexus of the Gastrointestinal System. The gastrointestinal system has its own intrinsic set of nerves known as the *intramural plexus* or the *intestinal enteric nervous system*, located in the walls of the gut. Also, both parasympathetic and sympathetic stimulation originating in the brain can affect gastrointestinal activity mainly by increasing or decreasing specific actions in the gastrointestinal intramural plexus. Parasympathetic stimulation, in general, increases the overall degree of activity of the gastrointestinal tract by promoting peristalsis and relaxing the sphincters, thus allowing rapid propulsion of contents along the tract. This propulsive effect is associated with simultaneous increases in rates of secretion by many of the gastrointestinal glands, described earlier.

Normal motility functions of the gastrointestinal tract are not very dependent on sympathetic stimulation. However, strong sympathetic stimulation inhibits peristalsis and increases the tone of the sphincters. The net result is greatly slowed propulsion of food through the tract and sometimes decreased secretion as well—even to the extent of sometimes causing constipation.

Heart. In general, sympathetic stimulation increases the overall activity of the heart. This effect is accomplished by increasing both the rate and force of heart contraction.

Parasympathetic stimulation causes mainly opposite effects—decreased heart rate and strength of contraction. To express these effects in another way, sympathetic stimulation increases the effectiveness of the heart as a pump, as required during heavy exercise, whereas parasympathetic stimulation decreases heart pumping, allowing the heart to rest between bouts of strenuous activity.

Systemic Blood Vessels. Most systemic blood vessels, especially those of the abdominal viscera and skin of the limbs, are constricted by sympathetic stimulation. Parasympathetic stimulation has almost no effects on most blood vessels. Under some conditions, the beta function of the sympathetics causes vascular dilation instead of the usual sympathetic vascular constriction, but this dilation occurs rarely except after drugs have paralyzed the sympathetic alpha vasoconstrictor effects, which, in most blood vessels, are usually far dominant over the beta effects.

Effect of Sympathetic and Parasympathetic Stimulation on Arterial Pressure. The arterial pressure is determined by two factors: propulsion of blood by the heart and resistance to flow of blood through the peripheral blood vessels. Sympathetic stimulation increases both propulsion by the heart and resistance to flow, which usually causes a marked *acute* increase in arterial pressure but often very little change in long-term pressure unless the sympathetics also stimulate the kidneys to retain salt and water at the same time.

Conversely, moderate parasympathetic stimulation via the vagal nerves decreases pumping by the heart but has virtually no effect on vascular peripheral resistance. Therefore, the usual effect is a slight decrease in arterial pressure. However, *very*

TABLE 119-1	Autonomic Effects on Various Organs of the Body	
Organ	Effect of Sympathetic Stimulation	Effect of Parasympathetic Stimulation
Eye		
Pupil	Dilated	Constricted
Ciliary muscle	Slight relaxation (far vision)	Constricted (near vision)
Glands	Vasoconstriction and slight secretion	Stimulation of copious secretion (containing many enzymes for enzyme-secreting glands)
Nasal		
Lacrimal		
Parotid		
Submandibular		
Gastric		
Pancreatic		
Sweat glands	Copious sweating (cholinergic)	Sweating on palms of hands
Apocrine glands	Thick, odoriferous secretion	None
Blood vessels	Most often constricted	Most often little or no effect
Heart		
Muscle	Increased rate. Increased force of contraction	Slowed rate
Coronaries	Dilated (β_2); constricted (α)	Decreased force of contraction (especially of atria)
Lungs		
Bronchi	Dilated	Constricted
Blood vessels	Mildly constricted	? Dilated
Gut		
Lumen	Decreased peristalsis and tone	Increased peristalsis and tone
Sphincter	Increased tone (most times)	Relaxed (most times)
Liver	Glucose released	Slight glycogen synthesis
Gallbladder and bile ducts	Relaxed	Contracted
Kidney	Decreased urine output and increased renin secretion	None
Bladder		
Detrusor	Relaxed (slight)	Contracted
Trigone	Contracted	Relaxed
Penis	Ejaculation	Erection
Systemic arterioles		
Abdominal viscera	Constricted	None
Muscle	Constricted (adrenergic α)	None
Skin	Dilated (adrenergic $\beta2$) Dilated (cholinergic) Constricted	None
Blood		
Coagulation	Increased	None
Glucose	Increased	None
Lipids	Increased	None
Basal metabolism	Increased up to 100%	None
Adrenal medullary secretion	Increased	None
Mental activity	Increased	None
Piloerector muscles	Contracted	None
Skeletal muscle	Increased glycogenolysis Increased strength	None
Fat cells	Lipolysis	None

strong vagal parasympathetic stimulation can almost stop or occasionally actually stop the heart entirely for a few seconds and cause temporary loss of all or most arterial pressure.

Effects of Sympathetic and Parasympathetic Stimulation on Other Functions of the Body. Because of the great importance of the sympathetic and parasympathetic control systems, they are discussed many times in this text in relation to multiple body functions. In general, most of the entodermal structures, such as the ducts of the liver, gallbladder, ureter, urinary bladder, and bronchi, are inhibited by sympathetic stimulation but excited by parasympathetic stimulation. Sympathetic stimulation also has multiple metabolic effects such as release of glu-

cose from the liver, and an increase in blood glucose concentration, glycogenolysis in both liver and muscle, skeletal muscle strength, basal metabolic rate, and mental activity. Finally, the sympathetics and parasympathetics are involved in execution of the male and female sexual acts, as explained in Chapter 97.

RELATION OF STIMULUS RATE TO DEGREE OF SYMPATHETIC AND PARASYMPATHETIC EFFECT

A special difference between the autonomic nervous system and the skeletal nervous system is that only a low frequency of stimulation is required for full activation of autonomic effectors. In general, only one nerve impulse every few seconds suffices to maintain normal sympathetic or parasympathetic effect, and full activation occurs when the nerve fibers discharge 10–20 times/second. This rate compares with full activation in the skeletal nervous system at 50–500 or more impulses/second.

SYMPATHETIC AND PARASYMPATHETIC "TONE"

The autonomic nervous system is continuously active at rest and this constitutes the *resting tone*. Sympathetic tone normally keeps almost all the systemic arterioles constricted to about one-half their maximum diameter. By increasing the degree of sympathetic stimulation above normal, these vessels can be constricted even more; conversely, by decreasing the stimulation below normal, the arterioles can be dilated. If it were not for the continual background sympathetic tone, the sympathetic system could cause only vasoconstriction, never vasodilation.

Another interesting example of tone is the background "tone" of the parasympathetics in the gastrointestinal tract. Surgical removal of the parasympathetic supply to most of the gut by cutting the vagus nerves can cause serious and prolonged gastric and intestinal "atony" with resulting blockage of much of the normal gastrointestinal propulsion and consequent serious constipation, thus demonstrating that parasympathetic tone to the gut is normally very much required. This tone can be decreased by the brain, thereby inhibiting gastrointestinal motility, or it can be increased, thereby promoting increased gastrointestinal activity.

Effect of Loss of Sympathetic or Parasympathetic Tone After Denervation. Immediately after a sympathetic or parasympathetic nerve is cut, the innervated organ loses its sympathetic or parasympathetic tone. In many blood vessels, for instance, cutting the sympathetic nerves results in substantial vasodilation within 5–30 seconds. However, over minutes, hours, days, or weeks, *intrinsic tone* in the smooth muscle of the vessels increases—that is, increased tone caused by increased smooth muscle contractile force that is *not* the result of sympathetic stimulation but of chemical adaptations in the smooth muscle fibers themselves. This intrinsic tone eventually restores almost normal vasoconstriction.

Essentially the same effects occur in most other effector organs whenever sympathetic or parasympathetic tone is lost. That is, intrinsic compensation soon develops to return the function of the organ almost to its normal basal level. However, in the parasympathetic system, the compensation sometimes requires many months. For instance, loss of parasympathetic tone to the heart after cardiac vagotomy increases the heart rate to 160 beats/minute in a dog, and this rate will still be partially elevated 6 months later.

DENERVATION SUPERSENSITIVITY OF SYMPATHETIC AND PARASYMPATHETIC ORGANS AFTER DENERVATION

During the first week or so after a sympathetic or parasympathetic nerve is destroyed, the innervated organ becomes more sensitive to injected norepinephrine or acetylcholine, respectively. This effect is demonstrated in Figure 119-4, which shows that blood flow in the forearm before removal of the sympathetics is about 200 mL/minute; a test dose of norepinephrine causes only a slight depression in flow lasting a minute or so. Then the stellate ganglion is removed, and normal sympathetic tone is lost. At first, the blood flow rises markedly because of

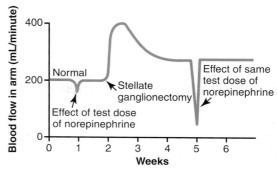

Figure 119-4 The effect of sympathectomy on blood flow in the arm, and the effect of a test dose of norepinephrine before and after sympathectomy, showing *supersensitization* of the vasculature to norepinephrine.

the lost vascular tone, but over a period of days to weeks the blood flow returns much of the way back toward normal because of a progressive increase in the intrinsic tone of the vascular musculature itself, thus partially compensating for the loss of sympathetic tone. Then another test dose of norepinephrine is administered, and the blood flow decreases much more than before, demonstrating that the blood vessels have become about two to four times as responsive to norepinephrine as previously. This phenomenon is called *denervation supersensitivity*. It occurs in both sympathetic and parasympathetic organs but to a far greater extent in some organs than in others, occasionally increasing the response more than 10-fold.

Mechanism of Denervation Supersensitivity. The cause of denervation supersensitivity is only partially known. Part of the answer is that the number of receptors in the postsynaptic membranes of the effector cells increases—sometimes manyfold—when norepinephrine or acetylcholine is no longer released at the synapses, a process called "upregulation" of the receptors. Therefore, when a dose of the hormone is now injected into the circulating blood, the effector reaction is vastly enhanced.

Stimulation of Discrete Organs in Some Instances and Mass Stimulation in Other Instances by the Sympathetic and Parasympathetic Systems

The Sympathetic System Sometimes Responds by Mass Discharge. In some instances, almost all portions of the sympathetic nervous system discharge simultaneously as a complete unit, a phenomenon called *mass discharge*. This frequently occurs when the hypothalamus is activated by fright or severe pain. The result is a widespread reaction throughout the body called the *alarm* or *stress response*, which is discussed shortly.

At other times, activation occurs in isolated portions of the sympathetic nervous system. Important examples are the following: (1) During the process of heat regulation, the sympathetics control sweating and blood flow in the skin without affecting other organs innervated by the sympathetics. (2) Many "local reflexes" involving sensory afferent fibers travel centrally in the peripheral nerves to the sympathetic ganglia and spinal cord and cause highly localized reflex responses. For instance, heating a skin area causes local vasodilation and enhanced local sweating, whereas cooling causes opposite effects. (3) Many of the sympathetic reflexes that control gastrointestinal functions operate by way of nerve pathways that do not even enter the spinal cord, merely passing from the gut mainly to the paravertebral ganglia, and then back to the gut through sympathetic nerves to control motor or secretory activity.

THE PARASYMPATHETIC SYSTEM USUALLY CAUSES SPECIFIC LOCALIZED RESPONSES

Control functions by the parasympathetic system are often highly specific. For instance, parasympathetic cardiovascular reflexes usually act only on the heart to increase or decrease its rate of beating. Likewise, other parasympathetic reflexes cause secretion mainly by the mouth glands and in other instances secretion is mainly by the stomach glands. Finally, the rectal emptying reflex does not affect other parts of the bowel to a major extent.

Yet there is often association between closely allied parasympathetic functions. For instance, although salivary secretion can occur independently of gastric secretion, these two also often occur together, and pancreatic secretion frequently occurs at the same time. Also, the rectal emptying reflex often initiates a urinary bladder emptying reflex, resulting in simultaneous emptying of both the bladder and the rectum. Conversely, the bladder emptying reflex can help initiate rectal emptying.

"ALARM" OR "STRESS" RESPONSE OF THE SYMPATHETIC NERVOUS SYSTEM

The sympathetic stress response characterized by a *mass discharge* of the sympathetic system has been described earlier in Chapter 92. In addition, the sympathetic system is especially strongly activated in many emotional states. For instance, in the state of *rage*, which is elicited to a great extent by stimulating the hypothalamus, signals are transmitted downward through the reticular formation of the brainstem and into the spinal cord to cause massive sympathetic discharge; most aforementioned sympathetic events ensue immediately. This is called the sympathetic *alarm reaction*. It is also called the *fight-or-flight reaction* because an animal in this state decides almost instantly whether to stand and fight or to run. In either event, the sympathetic alarm reaction makes the animal's subsequent activities vigorous.

MEDULLARY, PONTINE, AND MESENCEPHALIC CONTROL OF THE AUTONOMIC NERVOUS SYSTEM

Many neuronal areas in the brainstem reticular substance and along the course of the tractus solitarius of the medulla, pons, and mesencephalon, as well as in many special nuclei (Figure 119-5), control different autonomic functions such as arterial pressure, heart rate, glandular secretion in the gastrointestinal tract, gastrointestinal peristalsis, and degree of contraction of the urinary bladder. Control of each of these is discussed at appropriate points in this text. Some of the *most important factors controlled in the brainstem are arterial pressure, heart rate, and respiratory rate.* Indeed, transection of the brainstem above the midpontine level allows basal control of arterial pressure to continue as before but prevents its modulation by higher nervous centers such as the hypothalamus. Conversely, transection immediately below the medulla causes the arterial pressure to fall to less than one-half normal.

Closely associated with the cardiovascular regulatory centers in the brainstem are the medullary and pontine centers for

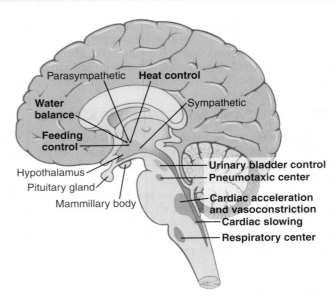

Figure 119-5 Autonomic control areas in the brainstem and hypothalamus.

regulation of respiration, which are discussed in Chapter 62. Although regulation of respiration is not considered to be an autonomic function, it is one of the *involuntary* functions of the body.

Control of Brainstem Autonomic Centers by Higher Areas. Signals from the hypothalamus and even from the cerebrum can affect the activities of almost all the brainstem autonomic control centers. For instance, stimulation in appropriate areas mainly of the posterior hypothalamus can activate the medullary cardiovascular control centers strongly enough to increase arterial pressure to more than twice normal. Likewise, other hypothalamic centers control body temperature, increase or decrease salivation and gastrointestinal activity, and cause bladder emptying. To some extent, therefore, the autonomic centers in the brainstem act as relay stations for control activities initiated at higher levels of the brain, especially in the hypothalamus.

In Chapter 123, it is pointed out also that many of our behavioral responses are mediated through (1) the hypothalamus, (2) the reticular areas of the brainstem, and (3) the autonomic nervous system. Indeed, some higher areas of the brain can alter function of the whole autonomic nervous system or of portions of it strongly enough to cause severe autonomic-induced disease such as peptic ulcer of the stomach or duodenum, constipation, heart palpitation, or even heart attack.

Pharmacology of the Autonomic Nervous System

DRUGS THAT ACT ON ADRENERGIC EFFECTOR ORGANS—SYMPATHOMIMETIC DRUGS

From the foregoing discussion, it is obvious that intravenous injection of norepinephrine causes essentially the same effects throughout the body as sympathetic stimulation. Therefore, norepinephrine is called a *sympathomimetic* or *adrenergic drug.* *Epinephrine* and *methoxamine* are also sympathomimetic drugs, and there are many others. They differ from one another in the degree to which they stimulate different sympathetic effector organs and in their duration of action. Norepinephrine and epinephrine have actions as short as 1–2 minutes, whereas the actions of some other commonly used sympathomimetic drugs last for 30 minutes to 2 hours.

Important drugs that stimulate specific adrenergic receptors are *phenylephrine* (alpha receptors), *isoproterenol* (beta receptors), and *albuterol* (only beta$_2$ receptors).

Drugs that Cause Release of Norepinephrine from Nerve Endings

Certain drugs have an indirect sympathomimetic action instead of directly exciting adrenergic effector organs. These drugs include *ephedrine, tyramine,* and *amphetamine.* Their effect is to cause release of norepinephrine from its storage vesicles in the sympathetic nerve endings. The released norepinephrine in turn causes the sympathetic effects.

Drugs that Block Adrenergic Activity. Adrenergic activity can be blocked at several points in the stimulatory process, as follows:

1. The synthesis and storage of norepinephrine in the sympathetic nerve endings can be prevented. The best known drug that causes this effect is *reserpine.*
2. Release of norepinephrine from the sympathetic endings can be blocked. This effect can be caused by *guanethidine.*
3. The sympathetic *alpha* receptors can be blocked. Two drugs that block both alpha$_1$ and alpha$_2$ adrenergic receptors are *phenoxybenzamine* and *phentolamine.* Selective alpha$_1$ adrenergic blockers include *prazosin* and *terazosin,* whereas *yohimbine* blocks alpha$_2$ receptors.
4. The sympathetic *beta* receptors can be blocked. A drug that blocks beta$_1$ and beta$_2$ receptors is *propranolol.* Drugs that block mainly beta$_1$ receptors are *atenolol, nebivolol,* and *metoprolol.*
5. Sympathetic activity can be blocked by drugs that block transmission of nerve impulses through the autonomic ganglia. They are discussed in a later section, but an important drug for blockade of both sympathetic and parasympathetic transmission through the ganglia is *hexamethonium.*

DRUGS THAT ACT ON CHOLINERGIC EFFECTOR ORGANS

Parasympathomimetic Drugs (Cholinergic Drugs). Acetylcholine injected intravenously usually does not cause exactly the same effects throughout the body as parasympathetic stimulation because most of the acetylcholine is destroyed by cholinesterase in the blood and body fluids before it can reach all the effector organs. Yet a number of other drugs that are not so rapidly destroyed can produce typical widespread parasympathetic effects; they are called *parasympathomimetic drugs.*

Two commonly used parasympathomimetic drugs are *pilocarpine* and *methacholine.* They act directly on the muscarinic type of cholinergic receptors.

Drugs that Have a Parasympathetic Potentiating Effect— Anticholinesterase Drugs. Some drugs do not have a direct effect on parasympathetic effector organs but do potentiate the effects of the naturally secreted acetylcholine at the parasympathetic endings. They are the same drugs as those discussed in Chapter 12 that potentiate the effect of acetylcholine at the neuromuscular junction. These drugs include *neostigmine, pyridostigmine,* and *ambenonium.* They inhibit acetylcholinesterase, thus *preventing rapid destruction of the acetylcholine* liberated at parasympathetic nerve endings. As a consequence, the quantity of acetylcholine increases with successive stimuli and the degree of action also increases.

Drugs that Block Cholinergic Activity at Effector Organs— Antimuscarinic Drugs. *Atropine* and similar drugs, such as *homatropine* and *scopolamine, block the action of acetylcholine on the muscarinic type of cholinergic effector organs.* These drugs *do not* affect the nicotinic action of acetylcholine on the postganglionic neurons or on skeletal muscle.

DRUGS THAT STIMULATE OR BLOCK SYMPATHETIC AND PARASYMPATHETIC POSTGANGLIONIC NEURONS

Drugs that Stimulate Autonomic Postganglionic Neurons. The preganglionic neurons of both the parasympathetic and the sympathetic nervous systems secrete acetylcholine at their endings, and the acetylcholine in turn stimulates the postganglionic neurons. Furthermore, injected acetylcholine can also stimulate the postganglionic neurons of both systems, thereby causing at the same time both sympathetic and parasympathetic effects throughout the body.

Nicotine is another drug that can stimulate postganglionic neurons in the same manner as acetylcholine because the membranes of these neurons all contain the *nicotinic type of acetylcholine receptor.* Therefore, drugs that cause autonomic effects by stimulating postganglionic neurons are called *nicotinic drugs.* Some other drugs, such as *methacholine,* have both nicotinic and muscarinic actions, whereas *pilocarpine* has only muscarinic actions.

Nicotine excites both the sympathetic and parasympathetic postganglionic neurons at the same time, resulting in strong sympathetic vasoconstriction in the abdominal organs and limbs but at the same time resulting in parasympathetic effects such as increased gastrointestinal activity.

Ganglionic Blocking Drugs. Drugs that block impulse transmission from the autonomic preganglionic neurons to the postganglionic neurons include *tetraethyl ammonium ion, hexamethonium ion,* and *pentolinium.* These drugs block acetylcholine stimulation of the postganglionic neurons in both the sympathetic and the parasympathetic systems simultaneously. They are often used for blocking sympathetic activity but seldom for blocking parasympathetic activity because their effects of sympathetic blockade usually far overshadow the effects of parasympathetic blockade. The ganglionic blocking drugs especially can reduce the arterial pressure rapidly, but they are not very useful clinically because their effects are difficult to control.

Disorders of the Autonomic Nervous Systems

It is beyond the scope of this book to describe the wide range of autonomic disorders that the medical student will encounter in a hospital setting. However, autonomic dysfunction is not uncommon. It is, for instance, seen in a variety of situations, including the following, among others:

- aging
- long-standing diabetes mellitus
- Parkinson disease
- chronic renal disease
- nutritional deficiencies as, for instance, with vitamin B$_{12}$
- infectious diseases including HIV, leprosy, Chagas disease, etc.

TESTS OF THE AUTONOMIC NERVOUS SYSTEM

There are various tests that are used to evaluate the autonomic nervous system. These vary in complexity and the ease with which they can be used in a clinical setting. Some are used primarily in research. The following tests are not exhaustive but provide some examples:

1. *Tests of autonomic reflexes.* In principle, a stimulus is provided and easily measurable physiological parameters such as the heart rate and blood pressure are monitored. Some of the tests differentiate sympathetic and parasympathetic system involvement. The tests include:
   a. Valsalva maneuver
   b. postural stress (lying to standing)
   c. timed deep breathing
   d. inspiratory gasp
   e. sustained isometric contraction
2. *Biochemical tests.* These include measuring the neurotransmitter norepinephrine and/or its metabolites in plasma/urine. Acetylcholine is not easily measured because it is rapidly broken down by cholinesterases.
3. *Heart rate variability.* This requires the continuous recording of heart rate over a period of time with subsequent mathematical analysis of the data.

BIBLIOGRAPHY

Cannon WB: Organization for physiological homeostasis, *Physiol. Rev.* 9:399, 1929.

Dajas-Bailador F, Wonnacott S: Nicotinic acetylcholine receptors and the regulation of neuronal signalling, *Trends Pharmacol. Sci.* 25:317, 2004.

DiBona GF: Sympathetic nervous system and hypertension, *Hypertension* 61:556, 2013.

Eisenhofer G, Kopin IJ, Goldstein DS: Catecholamine metabolism: a contemporary view with implications for physiology and medicine, *Pharmacol. Rev.* 56:331, 2004.

Goldstein DS, Sharabi Y: Neurogenic orthostatic hypotension: a pathophysiological approach, *Circulation* 119:139, 2009.

Hall JE, da Silva AA, do Carmo JM, et al: Obesity-induced hypertension: role of sympathetic nervous system, leptin, and melanocortins, *J. Biol. Chem.* 285(23):17271, 2010.

Kvetnansky R, Sabban EL, Palkovits M: Catecholaminergic systems in stress: structural and molecular genetic approaches, *Physiol. Rev.* 89:535, 2009.

Lymperopoulos A, Rengo G, Koch WJ: Adrenergic nervous system in heart failure: pathophysiology and therapy, *Circ. Res.* 113:739, 2013.

Malpas SC: Sympathetic nervous system overactivity and its role in the development of cardiovascular disease, *Physiol. Rev.* 90:513, 2010.

Mancia G, Grassi G: The autonomic nervous system and hypertension, *Circ. Res.* 114:1804, 2014.

Taylor EW, Jordan D, Coote JH: Central control of the cardiovascular and respiratory systems and their interactions in vertebrates, *Physiol. Rev.* 79:855, 1999.

Ulrich-Lai YM, Herman JP: Neural regulation of endocrine and autonomic stress responses, *Nat. Rev. Neurosci.* 10:397, 2009.

Functions of the Hypothalamus

The hypothalamus, despite its small size of only a few cubic centimeters (weighing only about 4 g), has two-way communicating pathways with all levels of the limbic system. In turn, the hypothalamus and its closely allied structures send output signals in three directions: (1) backward and downward to the brainstem, mainly into the reticular areas of the mesencephalon, pons, and medulla and from these areas into the peripheral nerves of the autonomic nervous system; (2) upward toward many higher areas of the diencephalon and cerebrum, especially to the anterior thalamus and limbic portions of the cerebral cortex; and (3) into the hypothalamic infundibulum to control or partially control most of the secretory functions of both the posterior and the anterior pituitary glands.

Thus, the hypothalamus, which represents less than 1% of the brain mass, is one of the most important of the control pathways of the limbic system. It controls most of the vegetative and endocrine functions of the body and many aspects of emotional behavior.

Vegetative and Endocrine Control Functions of the Hypothalamus

The different hypothalamic mechanisms for controlling multiple functions of the body are so important that they are discussed in different chapters throughout this text. For instance, the role of the hypothalamus to help regulate water conservation is discussed in Chapter 81, temperature regulation in Chapter 128, and endocrine control in Chapters 85, 87, and 88. To illustrate the organization of the hypothalamus as a functional unit, let us summarize the more important of its vegetative and endocrine functions here as well.

Figures 120-1 and 120-2 show enlarged sagittal and coronal views of the hypothalamus. Take a few minutes to study these diagrams, especially Figure 120-1, to see the multiple activities that are excited or inhibited when respective hypothalamic nuclei are stimulated. In addition to the centers shown in Figure 120-1, a large *lateral hypothalamic* area (shown in Figure 120-2) is present on each side of the hypothalamus. The lateral areas are especially important in controlling thirst, hunger, and many of the emotional drives.

A word of caution must be issued when studying these diagrams because the areas that cause specific activities are not nearly as accurately localized as suggested in the figures. Also, it is not known whether the effects noted in the figures result from stimulation of specific control nuclei or merely from activation of fiber tracts leading from or to control nuclei located elsewhere. With this caution in mind, we can give the following general description of the vegetative and control functions of the hypothalamus.

Cardiovascular Regulation. Stimulation of different areas throughout the hypothalamus can cause many neurogenic effects on the cardiovascular system, including changes in arterial pressure and heart rate. In general, stimulation in the *posterior* and *lateral hypothalamus* increases the arterial pressure and heart rate, whereas stimulation in the *preoptic area* often has opposite effects, causing a decrease in both heart rate and arterial pressure. These effects are transmitted mainly through specific cardiovascular control centers in the reticular regions of the pons and medulla.

Body Temperature Regulation. The anterior portion of the hypothalamus, especially the *preoptic area*, is concerned with regulation of body temperature. An increase in temperature of the blood flowing through this area increases activity of temperature-sensitive neurons, whereas a decrease in temperature decreases their activity. In turn, these neurons control mechanisms for increasing or decreasing body temperature. A summary of the role of the hypothalamus in temperature regulation is presented in Figure 120-3.

Body Water Regulation. The hypothalamus regulates body water in two ways: (1) by creating the sensation of thirst, which drives the animal or person to drink water, and (2) by controlling the excretion of water into the urine. An area called the *thirst center* is located in the lateral hypothalamus. When the fluid electrolytes in either this center or closely allied areas become too concentrated, the animal develops an intense desire to drink water; it will search out the nearest source of water and drink enough to return the electrolyte concentration of the thirst center to normal.

Control of renal excretion of water is vested mainly in the *supraoptic* nuclei. When the body fluids become too concentrated, the neurons of these areas become stimulated. Nerve fibers from these neurons project downward through the infundibulum of the hypothalamus into the posterior pituitary gland, where the nerve endings secrete the hormone *antidiuretic hormone*

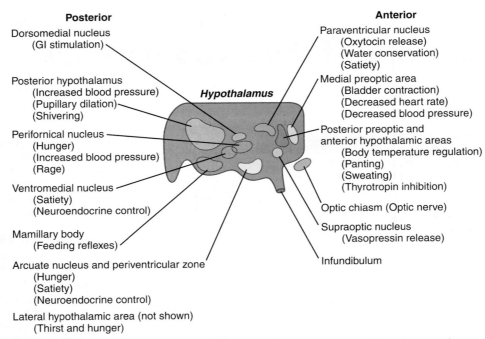

Figure 120-1   Control centers of the hypothalamus (sagittal view). *GI*, gastrointestinal.

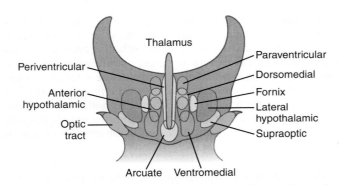

Figure 120-2   Coronal view of the hypothalamus, showing the mediolateral positions of the respective hypothalamic nuclei.

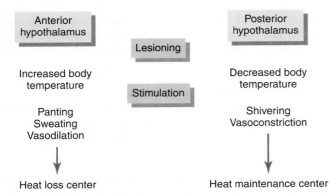

Figure 120-3   Role of hypothalamus in temperature regulation.

(also called *vasopressin*). This hormone is then absorbed into the blood and transported to the kidneys, where it acts on the collecting ducts of the kidneys to cause increased reabsorption of water. This action decreases loss of water into the urine but allows continuing excretion of electrolytes, thus decreasing the concentration of the body fluids back toward normal. These

functions are presented in Chapter 79. A summary of the regulation of water balance is presented in Figure 120-4.

Regulation of Uterine Contractility and of Milk Ejection from the Breasts. Stimulation of the *paraventricular nuclei* causes their neuronal cells to secrete the hormone *oxytocin*. Secretion of oxytocin in turn causes increased contractility of the uterus, as well as contraction of the myoepithelial cells surrounding the alveoli of the breasts, which then causes the alveoli to empty their milk through the nipples.

At the end of pregnancy, especially large quantities of oxytocin are secreted and this secretion helps to promote labor contractions that expel the baby. Then, whenever the baby suckles the mother's breast, a reflex signal from the nipple to the posterior hypothalamus also causes oxytocin release and the oxytocin now performs the necessary function of contracting the ductules of the breast, thereby expelling milk through the nipples so that the baby can nourish itself. These functions are discussed in Chapter 99.

Gastrointestinal and Feeding Regulation. Stimulation of several areas of the hypothalamus causes an animal to experience extreme hunger, a voracious appetite, and an intense desire to search for food. One area associated with hunger is the *lateral hypothalamic area.* Conversely, damage to this area on both sides of the hypothalamus causes the animal to lose desire for food, sometimes causing lethal starvation.

A center that opposes the desire for food, called the *satiety center,* is located in the *ventromedial nuclei.* When this center is stimulated electrically, an animal that is eating food suddenly stops eating and shows complete indifference to food. However, if this area is destroyed bilaterally, the animal cannot be satiated; instead, its hypothalamic hunger centers become overactive, so it has a voracious appetite, resulting eventually in tremendous obesity. The *arcuate nucleus* of the hypothalamus contains at least two different types of neurons that, when stimulated, lead to either increased or decreased appetite. Another area of the

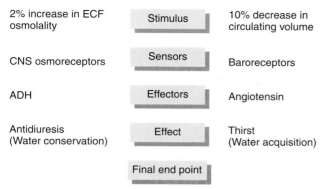

Figure 120-4 Role of hypothalamus in water balance. *ADH*, antidiuretic hormone; *CNS*, central nervous system; *ECF*, extracellular fluid.

hypothalamus that enters into overall control of gastrointestinal activity is the *mammillary bodies*, which control at least partially the patterns of many feeding reflexes, such as licking the lips and swallowing.

Hypothalamic Control of Circadian Rhythms. A large number of physiological rhythms (body temperature, sleep–wakefulness, cortisol secretion among a host of others) in the body run to a cyclical pattern that is approximately 25 hours long. These rhythms are *entrained* to 24 hours due to environmental signals such as light and darkness. These signals are called *zeitgebers*. The *suprachiasmatic* nucleus of the hypothalamus is believed to be responsible for the rhythmicity of these circadian cycles.

Hypothalamic Control of Endocrine Hormone Secretion by the Anterior Pituitary Gland. Stimulation of certain areas of the hypothalamus also causes the *anterior* pituitary gland to secrete its endocrine hormones. This subject is discussed in detail in Chapters 85 and 87. Briefly, the basic mechanisms are as follows.

The anterior pituitary gland receives its blood supply mainly from blood that flows first through the lower part of the hypothalamus and then through the anterior pituitary vascular sinuses. As the blood courses through the hypothalamus before reaching the anterior pituitary, specific *releasing* and *inhibitory hormones* are secreted into the blood by various hypothalamic nuclei. These hormones are then transported via the blood to the anterior pituitary gland, where they act on the glandular cells to control release of specific anterior pituitary hormones.

Summary. Several areas of the hypothalamus control specific vegetative and endocrine functions. The functions of these areas are still not completely understood, so the specification given earlier of different areas for different hypothalamic functions is still partially tentative.

Behavioral Functions of the Hypothalamus and Associated Limbic Structures

Effects Caused by Stimulation of the Hypothalamus. In addition to the vegetative and endocrine functions of the hypothalamus, stimulation of or lesions in the hypothalamus often have profound effects on emotional behavior of animals and human beings.

Some of the behavioral effects of stimulation are the following:

1. Stimulation in the *lateral hypothalamus* not only causes thirst and eating, as discussed earlier, but also increases the general level of activity of the animal, sometimes leading to overt rage and fighting, as discussed subsequently.
2. Stimulation in the *ventromedial nucleus* and surrounding areas mainly causes effects opposite to those caused by lateral hypothalamic stimulation—that is, a sense of *satiety, decreased eating,* and *tranquility.*
3. Stimulation of a *thin zone of periventricular nuclei,* located immediately adjacent to the third ventricle (or also stimulation of the central gray area of the mesencephalon that is continuous with this portion of the hypothalamus), usually leads to *fear* and *punishment reactions.*
4. *Sexual drive* can be stimulated from several areas of the hypothalamus, especially the most anterior and most posterior portions.

Effects Caused by Hypothalamic Lesions. Lesions in the hypothalamus, in general, cause effects opposite to those caused by stimulation. For instance:

1. Bilateral lesions in the lateral hypothalamus will decrease drinking and eating almost to zero, often leading to lethal starvation. These lesions cause extreme *passivity* of the animal as well, with loss of most of its overt drives.
2. Bilateral lesions of the ventromedial areas of the hypothalamus cause effects that are mainly opposite to those caused by lesions of the lateral hypothalamus: excessive drinking and eating, as well as hyperactivity and often frequent bouts of extreme rage on the slightest provocation.

Stimulation or lesions in other regions of the limbic system, especially in the amygdala, the septal area, and areas in the mesencephalon, often cause effects similar to those elicited from the hypothalamus.

BIBLIOGRAPHY

Joels M, Verkuyl JM, Van Riel E: Hippocampal and hypothalamic function after chronic stress, *Ann. N. Y. Acad. Sci.* 1007:367, 2003.

Kandel ER, Schwartz JH, Jessell TM: *Principles of Neural Science,* fourth ed., New York, 2000, McGraw-Hill.

LeDoux JE: Emotion circuits in the brain, *Annu. Rev. Neurosci.* 23:155, 2000.

Lumb BM: Hypothalamic and midbrain circuitry that distinguishes between escapable and inescapable pain, *News Physiol. Sci.* 19:22, 2004.

Morton GJ, Meek TH, Schwartz MW: Neurobiology of food intake in health and disease, *Nat. Rev. Neurosci.* 15:367, 2014.

Ulrich-Lai YM, Herman JP: Neural regulation of endocrine and autonomic stress responses, *Nat. Rev. Neurosci.* 10:397, 2009.

Woods SC, D'Alessio DA: Central control of body weight and appetite, *J. Clin. Endocrinol. Metab.* 93(11 Suppl. 1):S37, 2008.

121

Cerebrospinal Fluid

LEARNING OBJECTIVES

- State the sites of production and removal of cerebrospinal fluid (CSF).
- Describe the composition of CSF in relation to plasma.
- List the functions of CSF.
- List the structural features of the blood–brain barrier.
- Describe the different types of hydrocephalus.
- List the uses of a lumbar puncture.

GLOSSARY OF TERMS

- **Blood–brain barrier:** An anatomical and physiological barrier between the blood and the brain parenchyma
- **Blood–cerebrospinal fluid barrier:** Located at the choroid plexus where despite the fenestrated nature of the choroid plexus capillaries, a barrier is provided by the epithelial cells, which are joined together by tight junctions
- **Hydrocephalus:** An abnormal increase in the ventricles of the brain due to accumulation of excess fluid
- **Lumbar puncture:** Access to the subarachnoid space in the lumbar area (between L3 and L4) using a needle
- **Papilloedema:** Swelling of the optic nerve at the optic disc because of an increase in intracranial pressure
- **Subarachnoid space:** The space between the arachnoid and pia mater, which contains cerebrospinal fluid

The entire cerebral cavity enclosing the brain and spinal cord has a capacity of about 1600–1700 mL. About 150 mL of this capacity is occupied by *cerebrospinal fluid* (CSF) and the remainder by the brain and cord. This fluid, as shown in Figure 121-1, is present in the *ventricles of the brain*, in the *cisterns around the outside of the brain*, and in the *subarachnoid space around both the brain and the spinal cord*. All these chambers are connected with one another, and the pressure of the fluid is maintained at a surprisingly constant level.

Cushioning Function of the Cerebrospinal Fluid

A major function of the CSF is to cushion the brain within its solid vault. The brain and the CSF have about the same specific gravity (with only about a 4% difference), so the brain simply floats in the fluid. Therefore, a blow to the head, if it is not too intense, moves the entire brain simultaneously with the skull, causing no one portion of the brain to be momentarily contorted by the blow.

Contrecoup. When a blow to the head is extremely severe, it may not damage the brain on the side of the head where the blow is struck but is likely to damage the opposite side. This phenomenon is known as "contrecoup," and the reason for this effect is the following: When the blow is struck, the fluid on the struck side is so incompressible that as the skull moves, the fluid pushes the brain at the same time in unison with the skull. On the side opposite to the area that is struck, the sudden movement of the whole skull causes the skull to pull away from the brain momentarily because of the brain's inertia, creating for a split second a vacuum space in the cranial vault in the area opposite to the blow. Then, when the skull is no longer being accelerated by the blow, the vacuum suddenly collapses and the brain strikes the inner surface of the skull.

The poles and the inferior surfaces of the frontal and temporal lobes, where the brain comes into contact with bony protuberances in the base of the skull, are often the sites of injury and *contusions* (bruises) after a severe blow to the head, such as that experienced by a boxer. If the contusion occurs on the same side as the impact injury, it is a *coup injury*; if it occurs on the opposite side, the contusion is a *contrecoup injury*.

Coup and contrecoup injuries can also be caused by rapid acceleration or deceleration alone in the absence of physical impact due to a blow to the head. In these instances the brain may bounce off the wall of the skull causing a coup injury and then also bounce off the opposite side causing a contrecoup contusion. Such injuries are thought to occur, for example, in "shaken baby syndrome" or sometimes in vehicular accidents.

The functions of the CSF including that discussed earlier are listed in Box 121-1.

Formation, Flow, and Absorption of Cerebrospinal Fluid

CSF is formed at a rate of about 500 mL each day, which is three to four times as much as the total volume of fluid in the entire CSF system. There are three means by which CSF is produced:

- About two-thirds or more of this fluid originates as *secretion from the choroid plexuses* in the four ventricles, *mainly in the two lateral ventricles*.
- Additional small amounts of fluid are secreted by the ependymal surfaces of all the ventricles and by the arachnoidal membranes.
- A small amount comes from the brain through the perivascular spaces that surround the blood vessels passing through the brain.

The arrows in Figure 121-1 show that the main channels of fluid flow from the *choroid plexuses* and then through the CSF system. The fluid secreted in the *lateral ventricles* passes first into the *third ventricle*; then, after addition of minute amounts of fluid from the third ventricle, it flows downward along the *aqueduct of Sylvius* into the *fourth ventricle*, where still another minute amount of fluid is added. Finally, the fluid passes out of the fourth ventricle through three small openings, *two lateral*

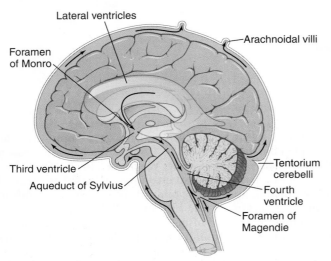

Figure 121-1 The arrows show the pathway of cerebrospinal fluid (CSF) flow from the choroid plexuses in the lateral ventricles to the arachnoidal villi protruding into the dural sinuses.

BOX 121-1   FUNCTIONS OF THE CEREBROSPINAL FLUID

- Mechanical cushion
- Excretory: removal of harmful brain metabolites
- Buffer
- Medium for nutrient exchanges
- Regulatory: medium for transferring signals through regulatory factors

---

foramina of Luschka and a *midline foramen of Magendie*, entering the *cisterna magna*, a fluid space that lies behind the medulla and beneath the cerebellum.

The cisterna magna is continuous with the *subarachnoid space* that surrounds the entire brain and spinal cord. Almost all the CSF then flows upward from the cisterna magna through the subarachnoid spaces surrounding the cerebrum. From here, the fluid flows into and through multiple *arachnoidal villi* that project into the large sagittal venous sinus and other venous sinuses of the cerebrum. Thus, any extra fluid empties into the venous blood through pores of these villi.

Secretion by the Choroid Plexus. The *choroid plexus*, a section of which is shown in Figure 121-2, is a cauliflower-like growth of blood vessels covered by a thin layer of epithelial cells. This plexus projects into the temporal horn of each lateral ventricle, the posterior portion of the third ventricle, and the roof of the fourth ventricle.

Secretion of fluid into the ventricles by the choroid plexus depends mainly on active transport of sodium ions through the epithelial cells lining the outside of the plexus. The sodium ions in turn pull along large amounts of chloride ions as well because the positive charge of the sodium ion attracts the chloride ion's negative charge. The two ions combined increase the quantity of osmotically active sodium chloride in the CSF, which then causes almost immediate osmosis of water through the membrane, thus providing the fluid of the secretion.

Less important transport processes move small amounts of glucose into the CSF and both potassium and bicarbonate ions

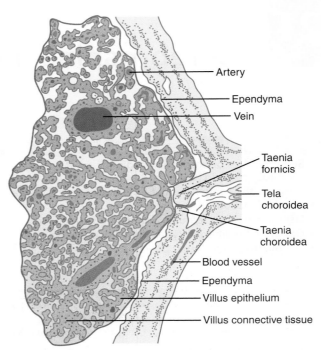

Figure 121-2 Choroid plexus in a lateral ventricle.

out of the CSF into the capillaries. The resultant composition of the CSF is the following:

- osmotic pressure, approximately equal to that of plasma;
- sodium ion concentration, also approximately equal to that of plasma;
- chloride ion, about 15% greater than in plasma;
- potassium ion, approximately 40% less;
- glucose, about 30% less;
- almost protein and cell free.

Absorption of Cerebrospinal Fluid Through the Arachnoidal Villi. The *arachnoidal villi* are microscopic finger-like inward projections of the arachnoidal membrane through the walls and into the venous sinuses. Conglomerates of these villi form macroscopic structures called *arachnoidal granulations* that can be seen protruding into the sinuses. The endothelial cells covering the villi have been shown by electron microscopy to have vesicular passages directly through the bodies of the cells large enough to allow relatively free flow of (1) CSF, (2) dissolved protein molecules, and (3) even particles as large as red and white blood cells into the venous blood.

Perivascular Spaces and Cerebrospinal Fluid. The large arteries and veins of the brain lie on the surface of the brain but their ends penetrate inward, carrying with them a layer of *pia mater*, the membrane that covers the brain, as shown in Figure 121-3. The pia is only loosely adherent to the vessels, so a space, the *perivascular space*, exists between it and each vessel. Therefore, perivascular spaces follow both the arteries and the veins into the brain as far as the arterioles and venules go.

Lymphatic Function of the Perivascular Spaces. As is true elsewhere in the body, a small amount of protein leaks out of the brain capillaries into the interstitial spaces of the brain. Because no true lymphatics are present in brain tissue, excess protein in the brain tissue leaves the tissue flowing with fluid

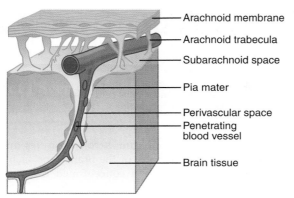

Figure 121-3 Drainage of a perivascular space into the subarachnoid space. *Modified from Ranson, S.W., Clark, S.L., 1959. Anatomy of the Nervous System. W.B. Saunders, Philadelphia.*

- Arachnoid membrane
- Arachnoid trabecula
- Subarachnoid space
- Pia mater
- Perivascular space
- Penetrating blood vessel
- Brain tissue

through the perivascular spaces into the subarachnoid spaces. Upon reaching the subarachnoid spaces, the protein then flows with the CSF, to be absorbed through the *arachnoidal villi* into the large cerebral veins. Therefore, perivascular spaces, in effect, are a specialized lymphatic system for the brain.

In addition to transporting fluid and proteins, the perivascular spaces transport extraneous particulate matter out of the brain. For instance, whenever infection occurs in the brain, dead white blood cells and other infectious debris are carried away through the perivascular spaces.

Cerebrospinal Fluid Pressure

The normal pressure in the CSF system *when one is lying in a horizontal position* averages 130 mm H_2O (10 mmHg), although this pressure may be as low as 65 mm H_2O or as high as 195 mm H_2O even in the normal healthy person.

Regulation of Cerebrospinal Fluid Pressure by the Arachnoidal Villi. The normal rate of CSF formation remains nearly constant, so changes in fluid formation are seldom a factor in pressure control. Conversely, the arachnoidal villi function like "valves" that allow CSF and its contents to flow readily into the blood of the venous sinuses while not allowing blood to flow backward in the opposite direction. Normally, this valve action of the villi allows CSF to begin to flow into the blood when CSF pressure is about 1.5 mmHg greater than the pressure of the blood in the venous sinuses. Then, if the CSF pressure rises still higher, the valves open more widely. Under normal conditions, the CSF pressure almost never rises more than a few millimeters of mercury higher than the pressure in the cerebral venous sinuses.

High Cerebrospinal Fluid Pressure in Pathological Conditions of the Brain. Often a large *brain tumor* elevates the CSF pressure by decreasing reabsorption of the CSF back into the blood. As a result, the CSF pressure can rise to as much as 500 mm H_2O (37 mmHg) or about four times normal.

The CSF pressure also rises considerably when *hemorrhage* or *infection* occurs in the cranial vault. In both these conditions, large numbers of red and/or white blood cells suddenly appear in the CSF and can cause serious blockage of the small absorption channels through the arachnoidal villi. This also sometimes elevates the CSF pressure to 400–600 mm H_2O (about four times normal).

Some babies are born with high CSF pressure, which is often caused by abnormally high resistance to fluid reabsorption through the arachnoidal villi, resulting either from too few arachnoidal villi or from villi with abnormal absorptive properties. This is discussed later in connection with *hydrocephalus*.

Obstruction to Flow of Cerebrospinal Fluid Can Cause Hydrocephalus

"Hydrocephalus" means excess water in the cranial vault. This condition is frequently divided into:

- *Communicating hydrocephalus*: fluid flows readily from the ventricular system into the subarachnoid space.
- *Noncommunicating hydrocephalus*: fluid flow out of one or more of the ventricles is blocked.

Usually the *noncommunicating* type of hydrocephalus is caused by a *block in the aqueduct of Sylvius*, resulting from *atresia* (closure) before birth in many babies or from blockage by a brain tumor at any age. As fluid is formed by the choroid plexuses in the two lateral and the third ventricles, the volumes of these three ventricles increase greatly, which flattens the brain into a thin shell against the skull. In neonates, the increased pressure also causes the whole head to swell because the skull bones have not yet fused.

The *communicating* type of hydrocephalus is usually caused by blockage of fluid flow in the subarachnoid spaces around the basal regions of the brain or by blockage of the arachnoidal villi where the fluid is normally absorbed into the venous sinuses. Fluid therefore collects both on the outside of the brain and to a lesser extent inside the ventricles. This will also cause the head to swell tremendously if it occurs in infancy when the skull is still pliable and can be stretched, and it can damage the brain at any age. A therapy for many types of hydrocephalus is surgical placement of a silicone tube shunt all the way from one of the brain ventricles to the peritoneal cavity where the excess fluid can be absorbed into the blood.

Blood–Cerebrospinal Fluid and Blood–Brain Barriers

It has already been pointed out that the concentrations of several important constituents of CSF are not the same as in extracellular fluid elsewhere in the body. Furthermore, many large molecules hardly pass at all from the blood into the CSF or into the interstitial fluids of the brain, even though these same substances pass readily into the usual interstitial fluids of the body. Therefore, it is said that barriers, called the *blood–CSF barrier* and the *blood–brain barrier*, exist between the blood and the CSF and brain fluid, respectively.

Barriers exist both at the choroid plexus and at the tissue capillary membranes in essentially all areas of the brain parenchyma *except in some areas of the hypothalamus, pineal gland*, and *area postrema*, where substances diffuse with greater ease into the tissue spaces. The ease of diffusion in these areas is important because they have sensory receptors that respond to specific changes in the body fluids, such as changes in osmolality and in glucose concentration, as well as receptors for peptide hormones that regulate thirst, such as angiotensin II. The blood–brain barrier also has specific carrier molecules that facilitate transport of hormones, such as leptin, from the blood into the hypothalamus where they bind to specific receptors that control other functions such as appetite and sympathetic nervous system activity.

In general, the blood–CSF and blood–brain barriers are highly permeable to water, carbon dioxide, oxygen, and most lipid-soluble substances such as alcohol and anesthetics; slightly permeable to electrolytes such as sodium, chloride, and potassium; and almost totally impermeable to plasma proteins and most nonlipid-soluble large organic molecules. Therefore, the blood–CSF and blood–brain barriers often make it impossible to achieve effective concentrations of therapeutic drugs, such as protein antibodies and nonlipid-soluble drugs, in the CSF or parenchyma of the brain.

The cause of the low permeability of the blood–CSF and blood–brain barriers is the manner in which the endothelial cells of the brain tissue capillaries are joined to one another. They are joined by so-called *tight junctions*. That is, the membranes of the adjacent endothelial cells are tightly fused rather than having large slit pores between them, as is the case for most other capillaries of the body. The blood–brain barrier thus has several features that are summarized in Box 121-2.

Brain Edema

One of the most serious complications of abnormal cerebral fluid dynamics is the development of *brain edema*. Because the brain is encased in a solid cranial vault, accumulation of extra edema fluid compresses the blood vessels, often causing seriously decreased blood flow and destruction of brain tissue. The decreased cerebral blood flow also decreases oxygen delivery. This increases the permeability of the capillaries, allowing still more fluid leakage. It also turns off the sodium pumps of the neuronal tissue cells, thus allowing these cells to swell in addition.

BOX 121-2 FEATURES OF BLOOD–BRAIN BARRIER

- Tight junctions
- Endothelial cells that are not fenestrated
- Closely associated layer of astrocytes
- Specific degradation enzymes
- Decreased vesicles in endothelial cells
- Increased density of mitochondria

Once these processes have begun, heroic measures must be used to prevent total destruction of the brain. One such measure is to infuse intravenously a concentrated osmotic substance, such as a concentrated mannitol solution, which pulls fluid by osmosis from the brain tissue and breaks up the vicious circles. Another procedure is to remove fluid quickly from the lateral ventricles of the brain by means of ventricular needle puncture, thereby relieving the intracerebral pressure.

Lumbar Puncture

Access to the CSF in a hospital is obtained by inserting a needle into the subarachnoid space between the L3 and L4 vertebrae. This spot is ideal because the spinal cord terminates well above this (at L1). The needle is inserted with the patient lying on their side and in "fetal" position, since this allows maximum separation of the vertebrae and allows the needle to be inserted more easily.

There are various reasons why a lumbar puncture may be performed. These include:
- obtaining CSF for diagnostic purposes as in meningitis
- administering spinal anesthesia
- administering other drugs

BIBLIOGRAPHY

Chesler M: Regulation and modulation of pH in the brain, *Physiol. Rev.* 83:1183, 2003.

Damkier HH, Brown PD, Praetorius J: Cerebrospinal fluid secretion by the choroid plexus, *Physiol. Rev.* 93:1847, 2013.

Johnston M, Papaiconomou C: Cerebrospinal fluid transport: a lymphatic perspective, *News Physiol. Sci.* 17:227, 2002.

Kahle KT, Simard JM, Staley KJ, et al: Molecular mechanisms of ischemic cerebral edema: role of electroneutral ion transport, *Physiology (Bethesda)* 24:257, 2009.

Paulson OB: Blood–brain barrier, brain metabolism and cerebral blood flow, *Eur. Neuropsychopharmacol.* 12:495, 2002.

122

Electroencephalography and Epilepsy

Electrical recordings from the surface of the brain or even from the outer surface of the head demonstrate that there is continuous electrical activity in the brain. Both the intensity and the patterns of this electrical activity are determined by the level of excitation of different parts of the brain resulting from *sleep, wakefulness,* or brain disorders such as *epilepsy* or even *psychoses.* The undulations in the recorded electrical potentials, shown in Figure 122-1, are called *brain waves,* and the entire record is called an electroencephalogram (EEG).

The intensities of brain waves recorded from the surface of the scalp range from 0 to 200 µV, and their frequencies range from once every few seconds to 50 or more per second. The character of the waves is dependent on the degree of activity in respective parts of the cerebral cortex, and the waves change markedly between the states of wakefulness and sleep and coma.

Much of the time, the brain waves are irregular and no specific pattern can be discerned in the EEG. At other times, distinct patterns do appear, some of which are characteristic of specific abnormalities of the brain such as epilepsy, which is discussed later.

Electroencephalography

TYPES OF EEG WAVES

In healthy people, most waves in the EEG can be classified as *alpha, beta, theta,* and *delta waves,* which are shown in Figure 122-1.

Alpha waves are rhythmical waves that occur at frequencies between 8 and 13 cycles/second and are found in the EEGs of almost all healthy adults when they are awake and in a quiet, resting state of cerebration. These waves occur most intensely in the occipital region but can also be recorded from the parietal and frontal regions of the scalp. Their voltage is usually about 50 µV. During deep sleep, the alpha waves disappear.

When the awake person's attention is directed to some specific type of mental activity, the alpha waves are replaced by asynchronous, higher-frequency but lower-voltage *beta waves.* Figure 122-2 shows the effect on the alpha waves of simply opening the eyes in bright light and then closing the eyes. Note that the visual sensations cause immediate cessation of the alpha waves and that these waves are replaced by low-voltage, asynchronous beta waves.

Beta waves occur at frequencies greater than 14 cycles/second and as high as 80 cycles/second. They are recorded mainly from the parietal and frontal regions during specific activation of these parts of the brain.

Theta waves have frequencies between 4 and 7 cycles/second. They occur normally in the parietal and temporal regions in children, but they also occur during emotional stress in some adults, particularly during disappointment and frustration. Theta waves also occur in many brain disorders, often in degenerative brain states.

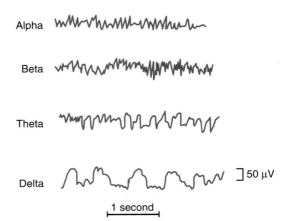

Figure 122-1 Different types of *brain waves* in the normal electroencephalogram.

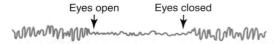

Figure 122-2   Replacement of the *alpha* rhythm by an asynchronous, low-voltage *beta* rhythm when the eyes are opened.

Delta waves include all the waves of the EEG with frequencies less than 3.5 cycles/second, and they often have voltages two to four times greater than most other types of brain waves. They occur in very deep sleep, in infancy, and in persons with serious organic brain disease. They also occur in the cortex of animals that have had subcortical transections in which the cerebral cortex is separated from the thalamus. Therefore, delta waves can occur strictly in the cortex independent of activities in lower regions of the brain.

ORIGIN OF BRAIN WAVES

The discharge of a single neuron or single nerve fiber in the brain can never be recorded from the surface of the head. Instead, many thousands or even millions of neurons or fibers *must fire synchronously*; only then will the potentials from the individual neurons or fibers summate enough to be recorded all the way through the skull. Thus, the intensity of the brain waves from the scalp is determined mainly by the numbers of neurons and fibers that fire *in synchrony* with one another, not by the total level of electrical activity in the brain. In fact, strong *nonsynchronous* nerve signals often nullify one another in the recorded brain waves because of opposing polarities. This phenomenon is demonstrated in Figure 122-2, which shows, when the eyes were closed, synchronous discharge of many neurons in the cerebral cortex at a frequency of about 12 second^{-1}, thus causing *alpha waves*. Then, when the eyes were opened, the activity of the brain increased greatly, but synchronization of the signals became so little that the brain waves mainly nullified one another. The resultant effect was low-voltage waves of generally high but irregular frequency, the *beta waves*.

Origin of Alpha Waves. Alpha waves will *not* occur in the cerebral cortex without cortical connections with the thalamus. Conversely, stimulation in the nonspecific layer of *reticular nuclei* that surround the thalamus or in "diffuse" nuclei deep inside the thalamus often sets up electrical waves in the thalamocortical system at a frequency between 8 and 13 second^{-1}, which is the natural frequency of the alpha waves. Therefore, it is believed that the alpha waves result from spontaneous feedback oscillation in this diffuse thalamocortical system, possibly including the reticular activating system in the brainstem as well. This oscillation presumably causes both the periodicity of the alpha waves and the synchronous activation of literally millions of cortical neurons during each wave.

Origin of Delta Waves. Transection of the fiber tracts from the thalamus to the cerebral cortex, which blocks thalamic activation of the cortex and thereby eliminates the alpha waves, nevertheless does not block delta waves in the cortex. This indicates that some synchronizing mechanism can occur in the cortical neuronal system by itself—mainly independent of lower structures in the brain—to cause the delta waves.

Delta waves also occur during deep slow-wave sleep, which suggests that the cortex then is mainly released from the activating influences of the thalamus and other lower centers.

EFFECT OF VARYING LEVELS OF CEREBRAL ACTIVITY ON THE FREQUENCY OF THE EEG

There is a general correlation between level of cerebral activity and average frequency of the EEG rhythm, with the average frequency increasing progressively with higher degrees of activity. This is demonstrated in Figure 122-3, which shows the existence of delta waves in surgical anesthesia, and deep sleep; theta waves in psychomotor states; alpha waves during relaxed states; and beta waves during periods of intense mental activity or fright. *During periods of mental activity, the waves usually become asynchronous rather than synchronous, so the voltage falls considerably despite markedly increased cortical activity*, as shown in Figure 122-2.

HOW IS EEG MEASURED AND WHAT IS ITS USE?

The number and placement of electrodes on the surface of the scalp varies depending on the purpose of the recording. The EEG is typically recorded with the patient lying down comfortably with the eyes closed for about 30 minutes. Longer durations of recordings can be made as, for instance, with sleep studies. In addition, the EEG may also be recorded during responses to various stimuli including photic stimuli and hyperventilation.

One of the recordings commonly made during the EEG is that of "*alpha block.*" The EEG recording when the individual is resting with the eyes closed, but awake, shows a typical alpha rhythm. When the individual opens their eyes, irregular, low-voltage activity is recorded—this is called alpha block or alerting/arousal response. The EEG pattern reverts back to an alpha rhythm when the individual closes their eyes. This is depicted in Figure 122-2.

EEG has many clinical uses and some of these are listed as follows:

- epilepsy (this is discussed in greater detail later in the chapter)
- sleep studies (this is discussed in greater detail in Chapter 123)
- evaluation of patients who are comatose
- as part of the evaluation of brain death

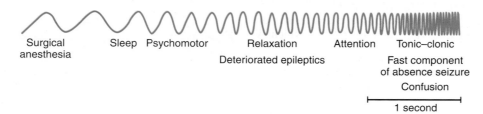

Figure 122-3   Effect of varying degrees of cerebral activity on the basic rhythm of the electroencephalogram.

Seizures and Epilepsy

Seizures are temporary disruptions of brain function caused by uncontrolled excessive neuronal activity. Depending on the distribution of neuronal discharges, seizure manifestations can range from experiential phenomena that are barely noticeable to dramatic convulsions.

Epilepsy is a chronic condition of *recurrent seizures* that can also vary from brief and nearly undetectable symptoms to periods of vigorous shaking and convulsions. Epilepsy is not a single disease. Its clinical symptoms are heterogeneous and reflect multiple underlying causes and pathophysiological mechanisms that cause cerebral dysfunction and injury, such as trauma, tumors, infection, or degenerative changes. Hereditary factors appear to be important, although a specific cause cannot be identified in many patients and several factors may coexist, reflecting an acquired brain pathology and genetic predisposition. Epilepsy is estimated to affect approximately 1% of the population, or 65 million people worldwide.

Epileptic seizures can be classified into two major types: (1) *focal seizures* (also called *partial seizures*) that are limited to a focal area of one cerebral hemisphere and (2) *generalized seizures* that diffusely involve both hemispheres of the cerebral cortex. However, partial seizures may sometimes evolve into generalized seizures.

FOCAL (PARTIAL) EPILEPTIC SEIZURES

Focal epileptic seizures begin in a small localized region of the cerebral cortex or deeper structures of the cerebrum and brainstem and have clinical manifestations that reflect the function of the affected brain area. Most often, focal epilepsy results from some localized organic lesion or functional abnormality, such as (1) scar tissue in the brain that pulls on the adjacent neuronal tissue, (2) a tumor that compresses an area of the brain, (3) a destroyed area of brain tissue, or (4) congenitally deranged local circuitry.

These lesions can promote extremely rapid discharges in the local neurons; when the discharge rate rises above several hundred per second, synchronous waves begin to spread over adjacent cortical regions. These waves presumably result from *localized reverberating circuits* that may gradually recruit adjacent areas of the cortex into the epileptic discharge zone. The process spreads to adjacent areas at a rate as slow as a few millimeters a minute to as fast as several centimeters per second.

Focal seizures can spread locally from a focus or more remotely to the contralateral cortex and subcortical areas of the brain through projections to the thalamus, which has widespread connections to both hemispheres. When such a wave of excitation spreads over the motor cortex, it causes a progressive "march" of muscle contractions throughout the opposite side of the body, beginning most characteristically in the mouth region and marching progressively downward to the legs but at other times marching in the opposite direction. This phenomenon is called *Jacksonian march*.

A focal epileptic attack may remain confined to a single area of the brain, often the temporal lobe, but in some instances strong signals spread from the focal region and the person may lose consciousness. Complex partial seizures may also begin with an aura followed by impaired consciousness and strange repetitive movements (*automatisms*), such as chewing or lip smacking. After recovery from the seizure the person may have no memory of the attack, except for the aura. The time after the

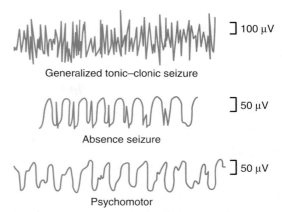

Figure 122-4 Electroencephalograms in different types of epilepsy.

seizure, prior to the return of normal neurological function, is called the *postictal period*.

Psychomotor, temporal lobe, and limbic seizures are terms that have been used in the past to describe many of the behaviors that are now classified as complex partial seizures. However, these terms are not synonymous. Complex partial seizures can arise from regions other than the temporal lobe and do not always involve the limbic system. Also, automatisms (the "psychomotor" element) are not always present in complex partial seizures. Attacks of this type frequently involve part of the limbic portion of the brain, such as the hippocampus, the amygdala, the septum, and/or portions of the temporal cortex. The lowest tracing of Figure 122-4 demonstrates a typical EEG during a psychomotor seizure, showing a low-frequency rectangular wave with a frequency between 2 and 4 second^{-1} and with occasional superimposed 14-second^{-1} waves.

GENERALIZED SEIZURES

Generalized epileptic seizures are characterized by diffuse, excessive, and uncontrolled neuronal discharges that at the outset spread rapidly and simultaneously to both cerebral hemispheres through interconnections between the thalamus and cortex. However, it is sometimes difficult clinically to distinguish between a primary generalized seizure and a focal seizure that rapidly spreads.

Generalized Tonic–Clonic (Grand Mal) Seizures

Generalized tonic–clonic seizures, previously called *grand mal seizures*, are characterized by an abrupt loss of consciousness and extreme neuronal discharges in all areas of the brain cerebral cortex, the deeper parts of the cerebrum, and even the brainstem. Also, discharges transmitted all the way into the spinal cord sometimes cause generalized *tonic seizures* of the entire body, followed toward the end of the attack by alternating tonic and spasmodic muscle contractions called *tonic–clonic seizures*. Often the person bites or "swallows" his or her tongue and may have difficulty breathing, sometimes to the extent that cyanosis occurs. Also, signals transmitted from the brain to the viscera frequently cause urination and defecation.

The usual generalized tonic–clonic seizure lasts from a few seconds to 3–4 minutes. It is also characterized by *postseizure depression* of the entire nervous system; the person remains in stupor for 1 to many minutes after the seizure attack is over and then often remains severely fatigued and asleep for hours thereafter.

The top recording of Figure 122-4 shows a typical EEG from almost any region of the cortex during the tonic phase of generalized tonic–clonic seizure. This demonstrates that high-voltage, high-frequency discharges occur over the entire cortex. Furthermore, the same type of discharge occurs on both sides of the brain at the same time, demonstrating that the abnormal neuronal circuitry responsible for the attack strongly involves the basal regions of the brain that drive the two halves of the cerebrum simultaneously.

Absence Seizures (Petit Mal Seizures)

Absence seizures, formerly called *petit mal seizures*, usually be-gin in childhood or early adolescence and account for 15–20% of epilepsy cases in children. Absence seizures almost certainly involve the thalamocortical brain activating system. They are usually characterized by 3–30 seconds of unconsciousness or diminished consciousness, during which time the person of-ten stares and has twitch-like contractions of muscles, usually in the head region, especially blinking of the eyes; this phase is followed by a rapid return of consciousness and resumption of previous activities. This total sequence is called the *absence syndrome* or *absence epilepsy*.

The brain wave pattern in mailpersons with absence sei-zure epilepsy is demonstrated by the middle recording of Figure 122-4, which is typified by a *spike and dome pattern*. The spike and dome can be recorded over most or all of the cerebral cortex, showing that the seizure involves much or most of the thalamocortical activating system of the brain. In fact, animal studies suggest that it results from oscillation of (1) inhibitory thalamic reticular neurons [which are *inhibitory* gamma-aminobutyric acid (GABA)–producing neurons] and (2) *excit-atory* thalamocortical and corticothalamic neurons.

TREATMENT OF EPILEPSY

Most of the currently available drugs used to treat epilepsy appear to block the initiation or spread of seizures, although the precise mode of action for some drugs is unknown or may involve multiple actions. Some of the major effects of various antiepileptic drugs include (1) blockade of voltage-dependent sodium channels (eg, carbamazepine and phenytoin); (2) altered calcium currents (eg, ethosuximide); (3) an increase in GABA activity (eg, phenobarbital and benzodiazepines); (4) inhibition of receptors for glutamate, the most prevalent excitatory neu-rotransmitter (eg, perampanel); and (5) multiple mechanisms of action (eg, valproate and topiramate, which block voltage-dependent sodium channels and increase GABA levels in the brain). The choice of antiepileptic drug recommended by cur-rent guidelines depends on the type of seizure, the age of the patient, and other factors, but correction of the underlying cause of the seizures is the best option when possible.

Epilepsy can usually be controlled with the appropriate medication. However, when the epilepsy is medically intractable and does not respond to treatments, the EEG can sometimes be used to localize abnormal spiking waves originating in areas of organic brain disease that predispose to focal epileptic attacks. Once such a focal point is found, surgical excision of the focus frequently prevents future attacks.

BIBLIOGRAPHY

Goldberg EM, Coulter DA: Mechanisms of epilepto-genesis: a convergence on neural circuit dysfunc-tion, *Nat. Rev. Neurosci.* 14:337, 2013.

Jacob TC, Moss SJ, Jurd R: GABA(A) receptor traf-ficking and its role in the dynamic modulation of neuronal inhibition, *Nat. Rev. Neurosci.* 9:331, 2008.

McCormick DA, Contreras D: On the cellular and network bases of epileptic seizures, *Annu. Rev. Physiol.* 63:815, 2001.

Steinlein OK: Genetic mechanisms that underlie epilepsy, *Nat. Rev. Neurosci.* 5:400-408, 2004.

123

Sleep

LEARNING OBJECTIVES

- List the stages of sleep.
- List the features of different stages of sleep.
- Describe the physiological basis of sleep.
- List the essential features of common sleep disorders.

GLOSSARY OF TERMS

- **Hypersomnias:** Disorders of excessive sleep, include obstructive sleep apnea and narcolepsy, among others

- **Insomnia:** Any impairment in the depth, duration, or restorative properties of sleep, resulting in a "want" of sleep

- **Nocturnal enuresis:** Involuntary urination during sleep in children over the age of 5 years

- **REM (paradoxical, desynchronized) sleep:** A stage in sleep characterized by rapid eye movement, dreams, irregular heart rate and respiration, and increased brain activity

- **Sleep spindles:** Episodic burst of electrical activity that characterize the EEG pattern in non-REM sleep (stage 2)

- **Somnambulism:** Sleep walking

Sleep is defined as unconsciousness from which a person can be aroused by sensory or other stimuli. It is to be distinguished from *coma*, which is unconsciousness from which a person cannot be aroused. There are multiple stages of sleep, from very light sleep to very deep sleep. Sleep researchers also divide sleep into two entirely different types of sleep that have different qualities, as described in the following section.

Two Types of Sleep—Slow-Wave Sleep and Rapid Eye Movement Sleep

Each night, a person goes through stages of two major types of sleep that alternate with each other (Figure 123-1). These types are called (1) *rapid eye movement sleep* (REM sleep), in which the eyes undergo rapid movements despite the fact that the person is still asleep, and (2) *slow-wave sleep* or *non-REM (NREM) sleep*, in which the brain waves are strong and of low frequency, as we discuss later.

REM sleep occurs in episodes that occupy about 25% of the sleep time in young adults; each episode normally recurs about every 90 minutes. This type of sleep is not so restful, and it is often associated with vivid dreaming.

Figure 123-1 summarizes a single sleep episode of approximately 8 hours. The figure indicates that:

- There are multiple alternating cycles of slow-wave and REM sleep.

- The depth of sleep progressively decreases with each cycle. Thus when individuals initially go to sleep, they achieve stage 4 of slow-wave sleep but in later cycles they may achieve only stage 3 or stage 2.
- The duration of REM sleep with each successive sleep cycle progressively increases.

Changes in the EEG at Different Stages of Wakefulness and Sleep. Figure 123-1 also shows electroencephalography (EEG) patterns from a typical person in different stages of wakefulness and sleep. Alert wakefulness is characterized by high-frequency *beta waves*, whereas quiet wakefulness is usually associated with *alpha waves*, as demonstrated by the first two EEGs of the figure.

Slow-wave sleep is divided into four stages. In the first stage, a stage of light sleep, the voltage of the EEG waves becomes low. This is broken by "*sleep spindles*" (ie, short spindle-shaped bursts of alpha waves that occur periodically). In stages 2, 3, and 4 of slow-wave sleep, the frequency of the EEG becomes progressively slower until it reaches a frequency of only one to three waves per second in stage 4; these are *delta waves*.

Finally, the bottom record in Figure 123-1 shows the EEG during REM sleep. It is often difficult to tell the difference between this brain wave pattern and that of an awake, active person. The waves are irregular and of high frequency, which are normally suggestive of desynchronized nervous activity as found in the awake state. Therefore, REM sleep is frequently called *desynchronized sleep* because there is lack of synchrony in the firing of the neurons despite significant brain activity.

REM SLEEP (PARADOXICAL SLEEP, DESYNCHRONIZED SLEEP)

In a normal night of sleep, bouts of REM sleep lasting 5–30 minutes usually appear on the average every 90 minutes. When the person is extremely sleepy, each bout of REM sleep is short and may even be absent. As the person becomes more rested through the night, the durations of the REM bouts increase.

REM sleep has several important characteristics:

1. It is an active form of sleep usually associated with active bodily muscle movements.
2. The person is even more difficult to arouse by sensory stimuli than during deep slow-wave sleep.
3. People usually awaken spontaneously in the morning during an episode of REM sleep.
4. Muscle tone throughout the body is exceedingly depressed, indicating strong inhibition of the spinal muscle control areas.
5. Heart rate and respiratory rate usually become irregular, which is characteristic of the dream state.
6. Despite the extreme inhibition of the peripheral muscles, irregular muscle movements do occur in addition to the rapid movements of the eyes.
7. The brain is highly active in REM sleep, and overall brain metabolism may be increased as much as 20%. An EEG

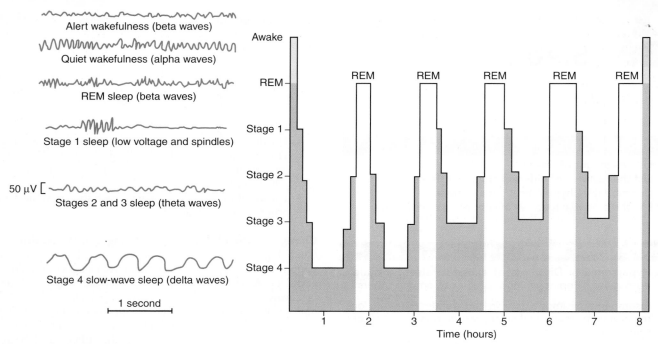

Figure 123-1 Progressive change in the characteristics of the brain waves during alert wakefulness, rapid eye movement (*REM*) sleep, and stages 1–4 of sleep.

shows a pattern of brain waves similar to those that occur during wakefulness. This type of sleep is also called *paradoxical sleep* because it is a paradox that a person can still be asleep despite marked activity in the brain.

8. This phase of sleep is associated with dreaming.

In summary, REM sleep is a type of sleep in which the brain is quite active. However, the person is not fully aware of his or her surroundings, and therefore he or she is truly asleep.

SLOW-WAVE SLEEP

We can understand the characteristics of deep slow-wave sleep by remembering the last time we were kept awake for more than 24 hours and the deep sleep that occurred during the first hour after going to sleep. This sleep is exceedingly restful and is associated with decreases in both peripheral vascular tone and many other vegetative functions of the body. For instance, 10–30% decreases occur in blood pressure, respiratory rate, and basal metabolic rate.

Although slow-wave sleep is frequently called "dreamless sleep," dreams and sometimes even nightmares do occur during slow-wave sleep. The difference between the dreams that occur in slow-wave sleep and those that occur in REM sleep is that those of REM sleep are associated with more bodily muscle activity. Also, the dreams of slow-wave sleep are usually not remembered because consolidation of the dreams in memory does not occur.

Basic Theories of Sleep

Sleep Is Caused by an Active Inhibitory Process. An earlier theory of sleep was that the excitatory areas of the upper brainstem, the *reticular activating system*, simply became fatigued during the waking day and became inactive as a result. An important experiment changed this thinking to the current view that *sleep is caused by an active inhibitory process* because

it was discovered that transecting the brainstem at the level of the midpons creates a brain cortex that never goes to sleep. In other words, a center located below the midpontile level of the brainstem appears to be required to cause sleep by inhibiting other parts of the brain.

NEURONAL CENTERS, NEUROHUMORAL SUBSTANCES, AND MECHANISMS THAT CAN CAUSE SLEEP—A POSSIBLE SPECIFIC ROLE FOR SEROTONIN

Stimulation of several specific areas of the brain can produce sleep with characteristics near those of natural sleep. Some of these areas are the following:

1. The most conspicuous stimulation area for causing almost natural sleep is the *raphe nuclei in the lower half of the pons and in the medulla*. These nuclei comprise a thin sheet of special neurons located in the midline. Nerve fibers from these nuclei spread locally in the brainstem reticular formation and also upward into the thalamus, hypothalamus, most areas of the limbic system, and even the neocortex of the cerebrum. In addition, fibers extend downward into the spinal cord, terminating in the posterior horns, where they can inhibit incoming sensory signals, including pain, as discussed in Chapter 104. Many nerve endings of fibers from these raphe neurons secrete *serotonin*. When a drug that blocks the formation of serotonin is administered to an animal, the animal often cannot sleep for the next several days. Therefore, it has been assumed that serotonin is a transmitter substance associated with production of sleep.

2. Stimulation of some areas in the *nucleus of the tractus solitarius* can also cause sleep. This nucleus is the termination in the medulla and pons for visceral sensory signals entering by way of the vagus and glossopharyngeal nerves.

3. Sleep can be promoted by stimulation of several regions in the diencephalon, including (a) the rostral part of the hypothalamus, mainly in the suprachiasmal area, and (b) an occasional area in the diffuse nuclei of the thalamus.

Lesions in Sleep-Promoting Centers Can Cause Intense Wakefulness

Discrete lesions in the *raphe nuclei* lead to a high state of wakefulness. This phenomenon is also true of bilateral lesions in the *medial rostral suprachiasmal area in the anterior hypothalamus.* In both instances, the excitatory reticular nuclei of the mesencephalon and upper pons seem to become released from inhibition, thus causing intense wakefulness. Indeed, sometimes lesions of the anterior hypothalamus can cause such intense wakefulness that the animal actually dies of exhaustion.

Other Possible Transmitter Substances Related to Sleep

Experiments have shown that the cerebrospinal fluid and the blood or urine of animals that have been kept awake for several days contain a substance or substances that will cause sleep when injected into the brain ventricular system of another animal. One likely substance has been identified as *muramyl peptide*, a low-molecular-weight substance that accumulates in the cerebrospinal fluid and urine in animals kept awake for several days. When only micrograms of this sleep-producing substance are injected into the third ventricle, almost natural sleep occurs within a few minutes and the animal may stay asleep for several hours. Another substance that has similar effects in causing sleep is a nonapeptide isolated from the blood of sleeping animals. Still a third sleep factor, not yet identified molecularly, has been isolated from the neuronal tissues of the brainstem of animals kept awake for days. It is possible that prolonged wakefulness causes progressive accumulation of a sleep factor or factors in the brainstem or cerebrospinal fluid that lead(s) to sleep.

Possible Cause of REM Sleep

It is not understood why slow-wave sleep is broken periodically by REM sleep. However, drugs that mimic the action of acetylcholine increase the occurrence of REM sleep. Therefore, it has been postulated that the large acetylcholine-secreting neurons in the upper brainstem reticular formation might, through their extensive efferent fibers, activate many portions of the brain. This mechanism theoretically could cause the excess activity that occurs in certain brain regions in REM sleep, even though the signals are not channeled appropriately in the brain to cause normal conscious awareness that is characteristic of wakefulness.

CYCLE BETWEEN SLEEP AND WAKEFULNESS

The preceding discussions have merely identified neuronal areas, transmitters, and mechanisms that are related to sleep; they have not explained the cyclical, reciprocal operation of the sleep–wakefulness cycle. There is as yet no definitive explanation. Therefore, we might suggest the following possible mechanism for causing the sleep–wakefulness cycle.

When the sleep centers are *not* activated, the mesencephalic and upper pontile reticular activating nuclei are released from inhibition, which allows the reticular activating nuclei to become spontaneously active. This spontaneous activity in turn excites both the cerebral cortex and the peripheral nervous system, both of which send numerous *positive feedback* signals back to the same reticular activating nuclei to activate them still further. Therefore, once wakefulness begins, it has a natural tendency to sustain itself because of all this positive feedback activity.

Then, after the brain remains activated for many hours, even the neurons in the activating system presumably become fatigued. Consequently, the positive feedback cycle between the mesencephalic reticular nuclei and the cerebral cortex fades and the sleep-promoting effects of the sleep centers take over, leading to rapid transition from wakefulness back to sleep.

This overall theory could explain the rapid transitions from sleep to wakefulness and from wakefulness to sleep. It could also explain arousal, that is, the insomnia that occurs when a person's mind becomes preoccupied with a thought, and the wakefulness that is produced by bodily physical activity.

Orexin Neurons Are Important in Arousal and Wakefulness. *Orexin* (also called *hypocretin*) is produced by neurons in the hypothalamus that provide excitatory input to many other areas of the brain where there are orexin receptors. Orexin neurons are most active during waking and almost stop firing during slow-wave and REM sleep. Loss of orexin signaling as a result of defective orexin receptors or destruction of orexin-producing neurons causes *narcolepsy*, a sleep disorder characterized by overwhelming daytime drowsiness and sudden attacks of sleep that can occur even when a person is talking or working. Patients with narcolepsy may also experience a sudden loss of muscle tone (*cataplexy*) that can be partial or even severe enough to cause paralysis during the attack. These observations point to an important role for orexin neurons in maintaining wakefulness, but their contribution to the normal daily cycle between sleep and wakefulness is unclear.

Sleep Has Important Physiological Functions

There is little doubt that sleep has important functions. It exists in all mammals and after total deprivation there is usually a period of "catch-up" or "rebound" sleep; after selective deprivation of REM or slow-wave sleep, there is also a selective rebound of these specific stages of sleep. Even mild sleep restriction over a few days may degrade cognitive and physical performance, overall productivity, and the health of a person. The essential role of sleep in homeostasis is perhaps most vividly demonstrated by the fact that rats deprived of sleep for 2–3 weeks may actually die. Despite the obvious importance of sleep, our understanding of why sleep is an essential part of life is still limited.

Sleep causes two major types of physiological effects: first, effects on the nervous system, and second, effects on other functional systems of the body. The nervous system effects seem to be by far the more important because any person who has a transected spinal cord in the neck (and therefore has no sleep–wakefulness cycle below the transection) shows no harmful effects in the body beneath the level of transection that can be attributed directly to a sleep–wakefulness cycle.

Lack of sleep certainly does affect the functions of the central nervous system. Prolonged wakefulness is often associated with progressive malfunction of the thought processes and sometimes even causes abnormal behavioral activities. We are all familiar with the increased sluggishness of thought that occurs toward the end of a prolonged wakeful period, but in addition, a person can become irritable or even psychotic after forced wakefulness. Therefore, we can assume that sleep in multiple ways restores both normal levels of brain activity and normal "balance" among the different functions of the central nervous system.

Sleep has been postulated to serve many functions including (1) neural maturation, (2) facilitation of learning or memory, (3) cognition, (4) clearance of metabolic waste products generated by neural activity in the awake brain, and (5) conservation of metabolic energy. There is some evidence for each of these functions, but evidence supporting each of these ideas has been challenged. We might postulate that *the principal value of sleep is to restore natural balances among the neuronal centers*. The specific physiological functions of sleep, however, remain a mystery, and are the subject of much research.

Disorders of Sleep

There are a whole range of sleep disorders, which can be broadly characterized into four groups:

1. *Insomnias* are disorders of initiating or maintaining sleep such that the individual feels a want of sleep. In many cases insomnia may occur without an identifiable cause (primary) but it is also seen in depression and anxiety disorders, and with excessive drug or alcohol use.
2. *Hypersomnias* encompass a number of disorders characterized by excessive sleep. These include:
   a. *Obstructive sleep apnea*, an increasingly recognized disorder where the individual complains of increased daytime sleepiness. Males are affected more than females and obesity is common. Family members may report that the affected individual usually snores loudly and that this is punctuated by loud obstructive gasps. It is during this phase that the individual shows transient falls in oxygen saturation.
   b. *Narcolepsy* is a condition that often sets in early in childhood or in adolescence and is lifelong. It is characterized by uncontrolled daytime sleepiness and the individual reports having to take frequent naps of 10- to 20-minute duration.
3. Disorders of the sleep–wake schedule are often seen with jet lag and in shift workers who periodically work days and then nights.
4. *Parasomnias* are a broad range of disorders associated with sleep and include *somnambulism* (sleep walking), *enuresis* (bed wetting), nightmares, and night terrors.

BIBLIOGRAPHY

Brown RE, Basheer R, McKenna JT, et al: Control of sleep and wakefulness, *Physiol. Rev.* 92:1087, 2012.

Buysse DJ: Insomnia, *JAMA* 309:706, 2013.

Cirelli C: The genetic and molecular regulation of sleep: from fruit flies to humans, *Nat. Rev. Neurosci.* 10:549, 2009.

Kilduff TS, Lein ES, de la Iglesia H, et al: New developments in sleep research: molecular genetics, gene expression, and systems neurobiology, *J. Neurosci.* 28:11814, 2008.

Krueger JM, Rector DM, Roy S, et al: Sleep as a fundamental property of neuronal assemblies, *Nat. Rev. Neurosci.* 9:910, 2008.

Luppi PH, Clément O, Fort P: Paradoxical (REM) sleep genesis by the brainstem is under hypothalamic control, *Curr. Opin. Neurobiol.* 23:786, 2013.

Peever J, Luppi PH, Montplaisir J: Breakdown in REM sleep circuitry underlies REM sleep behavior disorder, *Trends Neurosci.* 37:279, 2014.

Rasch B, Born J: About sleep's role in memory, *Physiol. Rev.* 93:681, 2013.

Sakurai T: Orexin deficiency and narcolepsy, *Curr. Opin. Neurobiol.* 23:760, 2013.

Saper CB: The central circadian timing system, *Curr. Opin. Neurobiol.* 23:747, 2013.

Stickgold R, Walker MP: Sleep-dependent memory triage: evolving generalization through selective processing, *Nat. Neurosci.* 16:139, 2013.

Tononi G, Cirelli C: Staying awake puts pressure on brain arousal systems, *J. Clin. Invest.* 117:3648, 2007.

124

The Limbic System and Behavior

LEARNING OBJECTIVES

- List the anatomical structures comprising the limbic system.
- Describe the role of the limbic system in reward, punishment, and behavior.
- List the functions of the following structures:
  - hippocampus
  - amygdala
- Describe the role of neurohormonal systems in depression and psychoses.

GLOSSARY OF TERMS

- **Klüver–Bucy syndrome:** A syndrome observed following bilateral temporal lobe lesions and characterized by excessive oral tendencies, hypersexuality, and rage, among other features

- **Neocortex:** The six-layered cortex comprising the most recently evolved part of the brain of mammals involved in higher cognitive function

- **Reticular activating (excitatory) system:** A diffuse system from the brainstem upwards that is associated with arousal, attentiveness, and sleep

- **Sham rage:** Undirected anger in experimental animals as seen with stimulation of the lateral hypothalamus and amygdala and ablation of the prefrontal cortex

In this chapter, we deal first with the mechanisms that control activity levels in the different parts of the brain. Then we discuss the causes of motivational drives, especially motivational control of the learning process, and feelings of pleasure and punishment. These functions of the nervous system are performed mainly by the basal regions of the brain, which together are loosely called the *limbic system*, meaning the "border" system.

Activating—Driving Systems of the Brain

Without continuous transmission of nerve signals from the lower brain into the cerebrum, the cerebrum becomes useless. In fact, severe compression of the brainstem at the juncture between the mesencephalon and cerebrum, as sometimes results from a pineal tumor, often causes the person to enter into unremitting coma lasting for the remainder of his or her life.

Nerve signals in the brainstem activate the cerebral part of the brain in two ways: (1) by directly stimulating a background level of neuronal activity in wide areas of the brain and (2) by activating neurohormonal systems that release specific facilitatory or inhibitory hormone-like neurotransmitters into selected areas of the brain.

CONTROL OF CEREBRAL ACTIVITY BY CONTINUOUS EXCITATORY SIGNALS FROM THE BRAINSTEM

Reticular Excitatory Area of the Brainstem

Figure 124-1 shows a general system for controlling the activity level of the brain. The central driving component of this system is an excitatory area located in the *reticular substance of the pons and mesencephalon*. This area is also known by the name *bulboreticular facilitatory area*. We also discuss this area in Chapter 115 because it is the same brainstem reticular area that transmits facilitatory signals *downward to the spinal cord* to maintain tone in the antigravity muscles and to control levels of activity of the spinal cord reflexes. In addition to these downward signals, this area also sends a profusion of signals in the upward direction. Most of these signals go first to the thalamus, where they excite a different set of neurons that transmit nerve signals to all regions of the cerebral cortex, as well as to multiple subcortical areas.

The signals passing through the thalamus are of two types. One type is rapidly transmitted action potentials that excite the cerebrum for only a few milliseconds. These signals originate from large neuronal cell bodies that lie throughout the brainstem reticular area. Their nerve endings release the neurotransmitter *acetylcholine*, which serves as an excitatory agent, that lasts for only a few milliseconds before it is destroyed.

The second type of excitatory signal originates from large numbers of small neurons spread throughout the brainstem reticular excitatory area. Again, most of these signals pass to the thalamus, but this time through small, slowly conducting fibers that synapse mainly in the intralaminar nuclei of the thalamus and in the reticular nuclei over the surface of the thalamus. From here, additional small fibers are distributed throughout the cerebral cortex. The excitatory effect caused by this system of fibers can build up progressively for many seconds to a minute or more, which suggests that its signals are especially important for controlling the longer-term background excitability level of the brain.

Excitation of the Excitatory Area by Peripheral Sensory Signals. The level of activity of the excitatory area in the brainstem, and therefore the level of activity of the entire brain, is determined to a great extent by the number and type of sensory signals that enter the brain from the periphery. Pain signals in particular increase activity in this excitatory area and therefore strongly excite the brain to attention.

The importance of sensory signals in activating the excitatory area is demonstrated by the effect of cutting the brainstem above the point where the fifth cerebral nerves enter the pons. These nerves are the highest nerves entering the brain that transmit significant numbers of somatosensory signals into the brain. When all these input sensory signals are gone, the level of activity in the brain excitatory area diminishes abruptly, and the brain proceeds instantly to a state of greatly reduced activity,

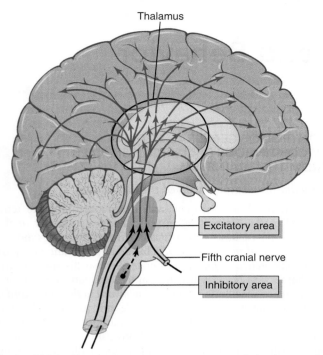

Thalamus

Excitatory area

Fifth cranial nerve

Inhibitory area

Figure 124-1 The excitatory–activating system of the brain. Also shown is an inhibitory area in the medulla that can inhibit or depress the activating system.

approaching a permanent state of coma. However, when the brainstem is transected *below* the fifth nerves, which leaves much input of sensory signals from the facial and oral regions, the coma is averted.

Increased Activity of the Excitatory Area Caused by Feedback Signals Returning from the Cerebral Cortex. Not only do excitatory signals pass to the cerebral cortex from the bulboreticular excitatory area of the brainstem, but feedback signals also return from the cerebral cortex back to this same area. Therefore, any time the cerebral cortex becomes activated by either brain thought processes or motor processes, signals are sent from the cortex to the brainstem excitatory area, which in turn sends still more excitatory signals to the cortex. This process helps to maintain the level of excitation of the cerebral cortex or even to enhance it. This mechanism of *positive feedback* allows any beginning activity in the cerebral cortex to support still more activity, thus leading to an "awake" mind.

The Thalamus Is a Distribution Center that Controls Activity in Specific Regions of the Cortex. As pointed out in Chapter 126, almost every area of the cerebral cortex connects with its own highly specific area in the thalamus. Therefore, electrical stimulation of a specific point in the thalamus generally activates its own specific small region of the cortex. Furthermore, signals regularly reverberate back and forth between the thalamus and the cerebral cortex, with the thalamus exciting the cortex and the cortex then reexciting the thalamus by way of return fibers. It has been suggested that the thinking process establishes long-term memories by activating such back-and-forth reverberation of signals.

Whether the thalamus also functions to call forth specific memories from the cortex or to activate specific thought processes is still unclear, but the thalamus does have appropriate neuronal circuitry for these purposes.

A Reticular Inhibitory Area Is Located in the Lower Brainstem

Figure 124-1 shows another area that is important in controlling brain activity—the reticular *inhibitory area*, located medially and ventrally in the medulla. In Chapter 115, we learned that this area can inhibit the reticular facilitatory area of the upper brainstem and thereby decrease activity in the superior portions of the brain as well. One of the mechanisms for this activity is to excite *serotonergic neurons*, which in turn secrete the inhibitory neurohormone *serotonin* at crucial points in the brain. We discuss this concept in more detail later.

NEUROHORMONAL CONTROL OF BRAIN ACTIVITY

Aside from direct control of brain activity by specific transmission of nerve signals from the lower brain areas to the cortical regions of the brain, still another physiological mechanism is often used to control brain activity. This mechanism is to secrete *excitatory* or *inhibitory neurotransmitter hormonal agents* into the substance of the brain. These neurohormones often persist for minutes or hours and thereby provide long periods of control, rather than just instantaneous activation or inhibition.

Figure 124-2 shows three neurohormonal systems that have been studied in detail in the rat brain: (1) a *norepinephrine system*, (2) a *dopamine system*, and (3) a *serotonin system*.

Neurohormonal Systems in the Human Brain. Figure 124-3 shows the brainstem areas in the human brain for activating four neurohormonal systems, the same three discussed for the rat and one other, the *acetylcholine system*. Some of the specific functions of these systems are as follows:

1. *The locus ceruleus and the norepinephrine system.* The locus ceruleus is a small area located bilaterally and posteriorly at the juncture between the pons and mesencephalon. Nerve fibers from this area spread throughout the brain, the same as shown for the rat in the top frame of Figure 124-2, and they secrete *norepinephrine*. The norepinephrine generally excites the brain to increased activity. However, it has inhibitory effects in a few brain areas because of inhibitory receptors at certain neuronal synapses. Chapter 123 describes how this system probably plays an important role in causing dreaming, thus leading to a type of sleep called rapid eye movement (REM) sleep.

2. *The substantia nigra and the dopamine system.* The substantia nigra is discussed in Chapter 118 in relation to the basal ganglia. It lies anteriorly in the superior mesencephalon, and its neurons send nerve endings mainly to the caudate nucleus and putamen of the cerebrum, where they secrete *dopamine*. Other neurons located in adjacent regions also secrete dopamine, but they send their endings into more ventral areas of the brain, especially to the hypothalamus and the limbic system. The dopamine is believed to act as an inhibitory transmitter in the basal ganglia, but in some other areas of the brain it is possibly excitatory. Also, remember from Chapter 118 that destruction of the dopaminergic neurons in the substantia nigra is the basic cause of Parkinson disease.

3. *The raphe nuclei and the serotonin system.* In the midline of the pons and medulla are several thin nuclei called the raphe nuclei. Many of the neurons in these nuclei secrete *serotonin*. They send fibers into the diencephalon and a few fibers to the cerebral cortex; still other fibers descend

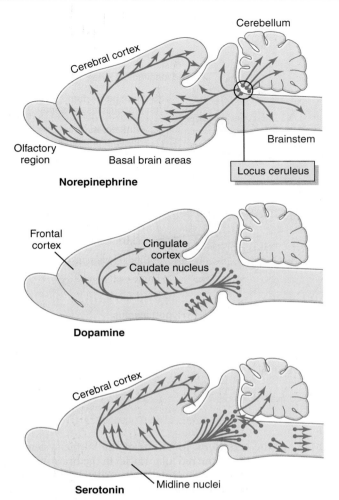

Norepinephrine

Dopamine

Serotonin

Figure 124-2 Three neurohormonal systems that have been mapped in the rat brain: a *norepinephrine system*, a *dopamine system*, and a *serotonin system. Modified from Kandel, E.R., Schwartz, J.H. (Eds.), 1985. Principles of Neural Science, second ed. Elsevier, New York.*

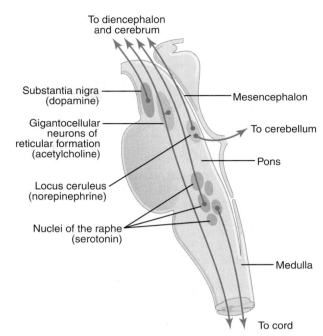

Figure 124-3 Multiple centers in the brainstem, the neurons of which secrete different transmitter substances (specified in parentheses). These neurons send control signals upward into the diencephalon and cerebrum and downward into the spinal cord.

acid (GABA), glutamate, vasopressin, adrenocorticotropic hormone, α-melanocyte–stimulating hormone (α-MSH), neuropeptide-Y (NPY), epinephrine, histamine, endorphins, angiotensin II, and neurotensin. Thus, there are multiple neurohormonal systems in the brain, the activation of each of which plays its own role in controlling a different quality of brain function.

Limbic System

The word "limbic" means "border." Originally, the term "limbic" was used to describe the border structures around the basal regions of the cerebrum, but as we have learned more about the functions of the limbic system, the term *limbic system* has been expanded to mean the entire neuronal circuitry that controls emotional behavior and motivational drives.

A major part of the limbic system is the *hypothalamus,* the functions of which are discussed in Chapter 120.

Functional Anatomy of the Limbic System

Figure 124-4 shows the anatomical structures of the limbic system, demonstrating that they are an interconnected complex of basal brain elements. Located in the middle of all these structures is the extremely small *hypothalamus,* which from a physiological point of view is one of the central elements of the limbic system. Figure 124-5 illustrates schematically this key position of the hypothalamus in the limbic system and shows surrounding it other subcortical structures of the limbic system, including the *septum, paraolfactory area, anterior nucleus of the thalamus, portions of the basal ganglia, hippocampus,* and *amygdala.*

Surrounding the subcortical limbic areas is the *limbic cortex,* composed of a ring of cerebral cortex on each side of the brain

to the spinal cord. The serotonin secreted at the cord fiber endings has the ability to suppress pain, which was discussed in Chapter 104. The serotonin released in the diencephalon and cerebrum almost certainly plays an essential inhibitory role to help cause normal sleep, as we discussed in Chapter 123.

4. *The gigantocellular neurons of the reticular excitatory area and the acetylcholine system.* We previously discussed the gigantocellular neurons (*giant cells*) in the reticular excitatory area of the pons and mesencephalon. The fibers from these large cells divide immediately into two branches, one passing upward to the higher levels of the brain and the other passing downward through the reticulospinal tracts into the spinal cord. The neurohormone secreted at their terminals is *acetylcholine.* In most places, the acetylcholine functions as an excitatory neurotransmitter. Activation of these acetylcholine neurons leads to an acutely awake and excited nervous system.

Other Neurotransmitters and Neurohormonal Substances Secreted in the Brain. Without describing their function, the following is a partial list of still other neurohormonal substances that function either at specific synapses or by release into the fluids of the brain: enkephalins, gamma-aminobutyric

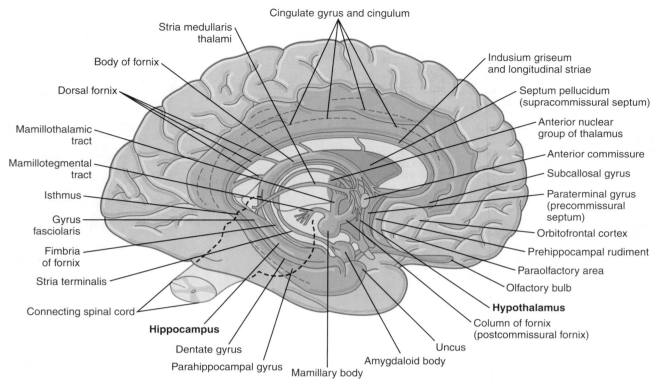

Figure 124-4   Anatomy of the limbic system, shown in the dark pink area. *Modified from Warwick, R., Williams, P.L., 1973. Gray's Anatomy, 35th British ed. Longman Group Ltd., London.*

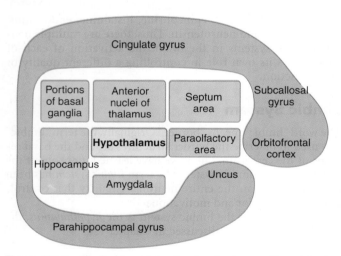

Figure 124-5   The limbic system, showing the key position of the hypothalamus.

(1) beginning in the *orbitofrontal area* on the ventral surface of the frontal lobes, (2) extending upward into the *subcallosal gyrus*, (3) then over the top of the corpus callosum onto the medial aspect of the cerebral hemisphere in the *cingulate gyrus*, and finally (4) passing behind the corpus callosum and downward onto the ventromedial surface of the temporal lobe to the *parahippocampal gyrus* and *uncus*.

Thus, on the medial and ventral surfaces of each cerebral hemisphere is a ring of mostly *paleocortex* that surrounds a group of deep structures intimately associated with overall behavior and emotions. In turn, this ring of limbic cortex functions as a two-way communication and association linkage between the *neocortex* and the lower limbic structures.

Many of the behavioral functions of the limbic system are also mediated through the reticular nuclei in the brainstem and their associated nuclei. We pointed out earlier in this chapter that stimulation of the excitatory portion of this reticular formation can cause high degrees of cerebral excitability while also increasing the excitability of much of the spinal cord synapses. An important route of communication between the limbic system and the brainstem is the *medial forebrain bundle*, which extends from the septal and orbitofrontal regions of the cerebral cortex downward through the middle of the hypothalamus to the brainstem reticular formation. This bundle carries fibers in both directions, forming a trunk line communication system. A second route of communication is through short pathways among the reticular formation of the brainstem, thalamus, hypothalamus, and most other contiguous areas of the basal brain.

"REWARD" AND "PUNISHMENT" FUNCTION OF THE LIMBIC SYSTEM

From the discussion thus far, it is already clear that several limbic structures are particularly concerned with the *affective* nature of sensory sensations—that is, whether the sensations are *pleasant* or *unpleasant*. These affective qualities are also called *reward* or *punishment*, or *satisfaction* or *aversion*. Electrical stimulation of certain limbic areas pleases or satisfies the animal, whereas electrical stimulation of other regions causes terror, pain, fear, defense, escape reactions, and all the other elements of punishment. The degrees of stimulation of these two oppositely responding systems greatly affect the behavior of the animal.

Reward Centers

Experimental studies in monkeys have used electrical stimulators to map out the reward and punishment centers of the brain.

Through use of this procedure, the major reward centers have been found to be located *along the course of the medial forebrain bundle*, especially in the *lateral* and *ventromedial nuclei of the hypothalamus*. It is strange that the lateral nucleus should be included among the reward areas—indeed, it is one of the most potent of all—because even stronger stimuli in this area can cause rage. However, this phenomenon occurs in many areas, with weaker stimuli giving a sense of reward and stronger ones a sense of punishment. Less potent reward centers, which are perhaps secondary to the major ones in the hypothalamus, are found in the septum, the amygdala, certain areas of the thalamus and basal ganglia, and extending downward into the basal tegmentum of the mesencephalon.

Punishment Centers

The most potent areas for punishment and escape tendencies have been found in the central gray area surrounding the aqueduct of Sylvius in the mesencephalon and extending upward into the periventricular zones of the hypothalamus and thalamus. Less potent punishment areas are found in some locations in the amygdala and hippocampus. It is particularly interesting that stimulation in the punishment centers can frequently inhibit the reward and pleasure centers completely, demonstrating that *punishment and fear can take precedence over pleasure and reward.*

Association of Rage with Punishment Centers

An emotional pattern that involves the punishment centers of the hypothalamus and other limbic structures, and that has also been well characterized, is the *rage pattern*, described as follows.

Strong stimulation of the punishment centers of the brain, especially in the *periventricular zone of the hypothalamus* and in the *lateral hypothalamus*, causes the animal to (1) develop a defense posture, (2) extend its claws, (3) lift its tail, (4) hiss, (5) spit, (6) growl, and (7) develop piloerection, wide-open eyes, and dilated pupils. Furthermore, even the slightest provocation causes an immediate savage attack. This behavior is what one would expect from an animal being severely punished, and it is a pattern of behavior called *rage*.

Fortunately, in the normal animal, the rage phenomenon is held in check mainly by inhibitory signals from the ventromedial nuclei of the hypothalamus. In addition, portions of the hippocampi and anterior limbic cortex, especially in the anterior cingulate gyri and subcallosal gyri, help suppress the rage phenomenon.

Placidity and Tameness. Exactly the opposite emotional behavior patterns occur when the reward centers are stimulated: placidity and tameness.

IMPORTANCE OF REWARD OR PUNISHMENT ON BEHAVIOR

Almost everything that we do is related in some way to reward and punishment. If we are doing something that is rewarding, we continue to do it; if it is punishing, we cease to do it. Therefore, the reward and punishment centers undoubtedly constitute one of the most important of all the controllers of our bodily activities, our drives, our aversions, and our motivations.

Importance of Reward or Punishment in Learning and Memory—Habituation Versus Reinforcement. Animal experiments have shown that a sensory experience that causes neither reward nor punishment is hardly remembered at all.

Electrical recordings from the brain show that a newly experienced sensory stimulus almost always excites multiple areas in the cerebral cortex. However, if the sensory experience does not elicit a sense of either reward or punishment, repetition of the stimulus over and over leads to almost complete extinction of the cerebral cortical response, that is, the animal becomes *habituated* to that specific sensory stimulus and thereafter ignores it.

If the stimulus *does* cause reward or punishment rather than indifference, the cerebral cortical response becomes progressively more and more intense during repeated stimulation instead of fading away, and the response is said to be *reinforced*. An animal builds up strong memory traces for sensations that are either rewarding or punishing but, conversely, develops complete habituation to indifferent sensory stimuli.

It is evident that the reward and punishment centers of the limbic system have much to do with selecting the information that we learn, usually throwing away more than 99% of it and selecting less than 1% for retention.

Specific Functions of Other Parts of the Limbic System

FUNCTIONS OF THE HIPPOCAMPUS

The hippocampus is the elongated portion of the cerebral cortex that folds inward to form the ventral surface of much of the inside of the lateral ventricle. One end of the hippocampus abuts the amygdaloid nuclei, and along its lateral border it fuses with the parahippocampal gyrus, which is the cerebral cortex on the ventromedial outside surface of the temporal lobe.

The hippocampus (and its adjacent temporal and parietal lobe structures, all together called the *hippocampal formation*) has numerous but mainly indirect connections with many portions of the cerebral cortex, as well as with the basal structures of the limbic system—the amygdala, hypothalamus, septum, and mammillary bodies. Almost any type of sensory experience causes activation of at least some part of the hippocampus, and the hippocampus in turn distributes many outgoing signals to the anterior thalamus, hypothalamus, and other parts of the limbic system, especially through the *fornix*, a major communicating pathway. Thus, the hippocampus is an additional channel through which incoming sensory signals can initiate behavioral reactions for different purposes. As in other limbic structures, stimulation of different areas in the hippocampus can cause almost any of the different behavioral patterns such as pleasure, rage, passivity, or excess sex drive.

Another feature of the hippocampus is that it can become hyperexcitable. For instance, weak electrical stimuli can cause focal epileptic seizures in small areas of the hippocampi. These seizures often persist for many seconds after the stimulation is over, suggesting that the hippocampi can perhaps give off prolonged output signals even under normal functioning conditions. During hippocampal seizures, the person experiences various psychomotor effects, including olfactory, visual, auditory, tactile, and other types of hallucinations that cannot be suppressed as long as the seizure persists, even though the person has not lost consciousness and knows these hallucinations to be unreal. Probably one of the reasons for this hyperexcitability of the hippocampi is that they have a different type of cortex from that elsewhere in the cerebrum, with only three nerve cell layers in some of its areas instead of the six layers found elsewhere.

Role of the Hippocampus in Learning

Anterograde Amnesia After Bilateral Removal of the Hippocampi. Portions of the hippocampi have been surgically removed bilaterally in a few human beings for treatment of epilepsy. These people can recall most previously learned memories satisfactorily. However, they often can learn essentially no new information that is based on verbal symbolism. In fact, they often cannot even learn the names of people with whom they come in contact every day. Yet they can remember for a moment or so what transpires during the course of their activities. Thus, they are capable of short-term memory for seconds up to 1 or 2 minutes, although their ability to establish memories lasting longer than a few minutes is either completely or almost completely abolished. This is the phenomenon called *anterograde amnesia*.

Theoretical Function of the Hippocampus in Learning. The hippocampus originated as part of the olfactory cortex. In many lower animals, this cortex plays essential roles in determining whether the animal will eat a particular food, whether the smell of a particular object suggests danger, or whether the odor is sexually inviting, thus making decisions that are of life-or-death importance. Very early in evolutionary development of the brain, the hippocampus presumably became a critical decision-making neuronal mechanism, determining the importance of the incoming sensory signals. Once this critical decision-making capability had been established, presumably the remainder of the brain also began to call on the hippocampus for decision making. Therefore, if the hippocampus signals that a neuronal input is important, the information is likely to be committed to memory.

Thus, a person rapidly becomes habituated to indifferent stimuli but learns assiduously any sensory experience that causes either pleasure or pain. But what is the mechanism by which this occurs? It has been suggested that the hippocampus provides the drive that causes translation of short-term memory into long-term memory—that is, the hippocampus transmits signals that seem to make the mind *rehearse over and over* the new information until permanent storage takes place. Whatever the mechanism, without the hippocampi, *consolidation* of long-term memories of the verbal or symbolic thinking type is poor or does not take place.

FUNCTIONS OF THE AMYGDALA

The amygdala is a complex of multiple small nuclei located immediately beneath the cerebral cortex of the medial anterior pole of each temporal lobe. It has abundant bidirectional connections with the hypothalamus, as well as with other areas of the limbic system.

In lower animals, the amygdala is concerned to a great extent with olfactory stimuli and their interrelations with the limbic brain. Indeed, it is pointed out in Chapter 106 that one of the major divisions of the olfactory tract terminates in a portion of the amygdala called the *corticomedial nuclei*, which lies immediately beneath the cerebral cortex in the olfactory pyriform area of the temporal lobe. In the human being, another portion of the amygdala, the *basolateral nuclei*, has become much more highly developed than the olfactory portion and plays important roles in many behavioral activities not generally associated with olfactory stimuli.

The amygdala receives neuronal signals from all portions of the limbic cortex, as well as from the neocortex of the temporal, parietal, and occipital lobes—especially from the auditory and visual association areas. Because of these multiple connections, the amygdala has been called the "window" through which the limbic system sees the place of the person in the world. In turn, the amygdala transmits signals (1) back into these same cortical areas, (2) into the hippocampus, (3) into the septum, (4) into the thalamus, and (5) especially into the hypothalamus.

Effects of Stimulating the Amygdala. In general, stimulation in the amygdala can cause almost all the same effects as those elicited by direct stimulation of the hypothalamus, plus other effects. Effects initiated from the amygdala and then sent through the hypothalamus include (1) increases or decreases in arterial pressure; (2) increases or decreases in heart rate; (3) increases or decreases in gastrointestinal motility and secretion; (4) defecation or micturition; (5) pupillary dilation or, rarely, constriction; (6) piloerection; and (7) secretion of various anterior pituitary hormones, especially the gonadotropins and adrenocorticotropic hormone.

Aside from these effects mediated through the hypothalamus, amygdala stimulation can also cause several types of involuntary movement. These types include (1) tonic movements, such as raising the head or bending the body; (2) circling movements; (3) occasionally clonic, rhythmical movements; and (4) different types of movements associated with olfaction and eating, such as licking, chewing, and swallowing.

In addition, stimulation of certain amygdaloid nuclei can cause a pattern of rage, escape, punishment, severe pain, and fear similar to the rage pattern elicited from the hypothalamus, as described earlier. Stimulation of other amygdaloid nuclei can give reactions of reward and pleasure.

Finally, excitation of still other portions of the amygdala can cause sexual activities that include erection, copulatory movements, ejaculation, ovulation, uterine activity, and premature labor.

Effects of Bilateral Ablation of the Amygdala—The Klüver–Bucy Syndrome. When the anterior parts of both temporal lobes are destroyed in a monkey, this procedure removes portions not only of temporal cortex but also of the amygdalas that lie inside these parts of the temporal lobes. This removal causes changes in behavior called the *Klüver–Bucy syndrome*, which is demonstrated by an animal that (1) is not afraid of anything, (2) has extreme curiosity about everything, (3) forgets rapidly, (4) has a tendency to place everything in its mouth and sometimes even tries to eat solid objects, and (5) often has a sex drive so strong that it attempts to copulate with immature animals, animals of the wrong sex, or even animals of a different species. Although similar lesions in human beings are rare, afflicted people respond in a manner not too different from that of the monkey.

Overall Function of the Amygdalas. The amygdalas seem to be behavioral awareness areas that operate at a semiconscious level. They also seem to project into the limbic system one's current status in relation to both surroundings and thoughts. On the basis of this information, the amygdala is believed to make the person's behavioral response appropriate for each occasion. Figure 124-6 summarizes some of these roles of the amygdala.

FUNCTION OF THE LIMBIC CORTEX

The most poorly understood portion of the limbic system is the ring of cerebral cortex called the *limbic cortex* that surrounds the subcortical limbic structures. This cortex functions as a transitional zone through which signals are transmitted from the remainder of the brain cortex into the limbic system and also in the opposite direction. Therefore, the limbic cortex in effect functions as a cerebral *association area for control of behavior*.

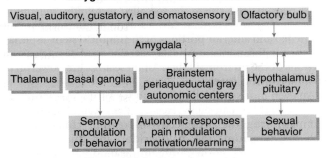

Amygdala: Connections and functions

Figure 124-6   Role of amygdala.

Stimulation of the different regions of the limbic cortex has failed to give any real idea of their functions. However, many behavioral patterns can be elicited by stimulation of specific portions of the limbic cortex. Likewise, ablation of some limbic cortical areas can cause persistent changes in an animal's behavior, as follows.

Ablation of the Anterior Temporal Cortex. When the anterior temporal cortex is ablated bilaterally, the amygdalas are almost invariably damaged as well and, as discussed earlier in this chapter, Klüver–Bucy syndrome occurs. The animal especially develops consummatory behavior: it investigates any and all objects, has intense sex drives toward inappropriate animals or even inanimate objects, and loses all fear—and thus develops tameness as well.

Ablation of the Posterior Orbital Frontal Cortex. Bilateral removal of the posterior portion of the orbital frontal cortex often causes an animal to develop insomnia associated with intense motor restlessness; the animal becomes unable to sit still, and moves about continuously.

Ablation of the Anterior Cingulate Gyri and Subcallosal Gyri. The anterior cingulate gyri and the subcallosal gyri are the portions of the limbic cortex that communicate between the prefrontal cerebral cortex and the subcortical limbic structures. Destruction of these gyri bilaterally releases the rage centers of the septum and hypothalamus from prefrontal inhibitory influence. Therefore, the animal can become vicious and much more subject to fits of rage than normally.

Summary. Until further information is available, it is perhaps best to state that the cortical regions of the limbic system occupy intermediate associative positions between the functions of the specific areas of the cerebral cortex and functions of the subcortical limbic structures for control of behavioral patterns. Thus, in the anterior temporal cortex, one especially finds gustatory and olfactory behavioral associations. In the parahippocampal gyri, there is a tendency for complex auditory associations and complex thought associations derived from Wernicke area of the posterior temporal lobe. In the middle and posterior cingulate cortex, there is reason to believe that sensorimotor behavioral associations occur.

Depression and Manic–Depressive Psychoses—Decreased Activity of the Norepinephrine and Serotonin Neurotransmitter Systems

Much evidence has accumulated suggesting that *mental depression psychosis* might be caused by *diminished formation in the brain of norepinephrine or serotonin, or both.* (New evidence has implicated still other neurotransmitters.) Depressed patients experience symptoms of grief, unhappiness, despair, and misery. In addition, they often lose their appetite and sex drive, and have severe insomnia. Often associated with these symptoms is a state of psychomotor agitation despite the depression.

Moderate numbers of *norepinephrine-secreting neurons* are located in the brainstem, especially in the *locus ceruleus.* These neurons send fibers upward to most parts of the brain limbic system, thalamus, and cerebral cortex. Also, many *serotonin-producing neurons* located in the *midline raphe nuclei* of the lower pons and medulla send fibers to many areas of the limbic system, and to some other areas of the brain.

A principal reason for believing that depression might be caused by diminished activity of norepinephrine- and serotonin-secreting neurons is that drugs that block secretion of norepinephrine and serotonin, such as reserpine, frequently cause depression. Conversely, about 70% of depressive patients can be treated effectively with drugs that increase the excitatory effects of norepinephrine and serotonin at the nerve endings—for instance, (1) *monoamine oxidase inhibitors,* which block destruction of norepinephrine and serotonin once they are formed, and (2) *tricyclic antidepressants,* such as *imipramine* and *amitriptyline,* which block reuptake of norepinephrine and serotonin by nerve endings so that these transmitters remain active for longer periods after secretion.

Some patients with mental depression alternate between depression and mania, which is called either *bipolar disorder* or *manic–depressive psychosis,* and fewer patients exhibit only mania without the depressive episodes. Drugs that diminish the formation or action of norepinephrine and serotonin, such as lithium compounds, can be effective in treating the manic phase of the condition.

It is presumed that the norepinephrine and serotonin systems normally provide drive to the limbic areas of the brain to increase a person's sense of well-being, and to create happiness, contentment, good appetite, appropriate sex drive, and psychomotor balance—although too much of a good thing can cause mania. In support of this concept is the fact that pleasure and reward centers of the hypothalamus and surrounding areas receive large numbers of nerve endings from the norepinephrine and serotonin systems.

Schizophrenia—Possible Exaggerated Function of Part of the Dopamine System

Schizophrenia comes in many varieties. One of the most common types is seen in the person who hears voices and has delusions, intense fear, or other types of feelings that are unreal. Many schizophrenics are highly paranoid, with a sense of persecution from outside sources. They may develop incoherent speech, dissociation of ideas, and abnormal sequences of thought, and they are often withdrawn, sometimes with abnormal posture and even rigidity.

There are reasons to believe that schizophrenia results from one or more of three possibilities: (1) multiple areas in the cerebral cortex *prefrontal lobes* in which neural signals have become blocked or where processing of the signals becomes dysfunctional because many synapses normally excited by the neurotransmitter *glutamate* lose their responsiveness to this transmitter; (2) excessive excitement of a group of neurons that secrete *dopamine* in the behavioral centers of the brain, including in the frontal lobes; and/or (3) abnormal function of a crucial part of the brain's *limbic behavioral control system centered around the hippocampus.*

The reason for believing that the prefrontal lobes are involved in schizophrenia is that a schizophrenic-like pattern of mental activity can be induced in monkeys by making multiple minute lesions in widespread areas of the prefrontal lobes.

Dopamine has been implicated as a possible cause of schizophrenia because schizophrenic-like symptoms develop in many patients with schizophrenia when they are treated with the drug called L-Dopa. This drug releases dopamine in the brain, which is advantageous for treating Parkinson disease, but at the same time it depresses various portions of the prefrontal lobes and other related areas.

It has been suggested that in persons with schizophrenia excess dopamine is secreted by a group of dopamine-secreting neurons whose cell bodies lie in the ventral tegmentum of the mesencephalon, medial and superior to the substantia nigra. These neurons give rise to the so-called *mesolimbic dopaminergic system* that projects nerve fibers and dopamine secretion into the medial and anterior portions of the limbic system, especially into the hippocampus, amygdala, anterior caudate nucleus, and portions of the prefrontal lobes. All these areas are powerful behavioral control centers.

An even more compelling reason for believing that schizophrenia might be caused by excess production of dopamine is that many drugs that are effective in treating schizophrenia—such as chlorpromazine, haloperidol, and thiothixene—all either decrease secretion of dopamine at dopaminergic nerve endings or decrease the effect of dopamine on subsequent neurons.

Finally, possible involvement of the hippocampus in schizophrenia was discovered when it was learned that *in persons with schizophrenia, the hippocampus is often reduced in size*, especially in the dominant hemisphere.

BIBLIOGRAPHY

Bird CM, Burgess N: The hippocampus and memory: insights from spatial processing, *Nat. Rev. Neurosci.* 9:182, 2008.

Craddock N, Sklar P: Genetics of bipolar disorder, *Lancet* 381:1654, 2013.

LeDoux JE: Coming to terms with fear, *Proc. Natl. Acad. Sci. U. S. A.* 111:2871, 2014.

Loy CT, Schofield PR, Turner AM, Kwok JB: Genetics of dementia, *Lancet* 383:828, 2014.

Marek R, Strobel C, Bredy TW, Sah P: The amygdala and medial prefrontal cortex: partners in the fear circuit, *J. Physiol.* 591:2381, 2013.

Maren S, Phan KL, Liberzon I: The contextual brain: implications for fear conditioning, extinction and psychopathology, *Nat. Rev. Neurosci.* 14:417, 2013.

Neves G, Cooke SF, Bliss TV: Synaptic plasticity, memory and the hippocampus: a neural network approach to causality, *Nat. Rev. Neurosci.* 9:65, 2008.

Pessoa L: On the relationship between emotion and cognition, *Nat. Rev. Neurosci.* 9:148, 2008.

Roozendaal B, McEwen BS, Chattarji S: Stress, memory and the amygdala, *Nat. Rev. Neurosci.* 10:423, 2009.

Russo SJ, Nestler EJ: The brain reward circuitry in mood disorders, *Nat. Rev. Neurosci.* 14:609, 2013.

Russo SJ, Murrough JW, Han MH, et al: Neurobiology of resilience, *Nat. Neurosci.* 15:1475, 2012.

Sah P, Faber ES, Lopez De Armentia M, Power J: The amygdaloid complex: anatomy and physiology, *Physiol. Rev.* 83:803, 2003.

Sara SJ: The locus coeruleus and noradrenergic modulation of cognition, *Nat. Rev. Neurosci.* 10:211, 2009.

Ulrich-Lai YM, Herman JP: Neural regulation of endocrine and autonomic stress responses, *Nat. Rev. Neurosci.* 10:397, 2009.

LEARNING OBJECTIVES

- Describe the key features of classical and operant conditioning.
- List the different stages of memory storage.
- Describe the biochemical processes involved in memory storage.
- Describe the various types of amnesia.
- Describe the features of Alzheimer disease.

GLOSSARY OF TERMS

- **Anterograde amnesia:** Inability to establish new long-term memories

- **Classical (Pavlovian) conditioning:** The process by which a subject responds to a neutral stimulus ("the bell," later called the conditioned stimulus) that is repeatedly presented in association with an unconditioned stimulus ("the food") to elicit a desired response ("salivation," the unconditioned response) until the neutral stimulus alone elicits the same response (now called the conditioned response)

- **Habituation:** A decrease in the behavioral response to a repeated nonnoxious stimulus

- **Operant conditioning:** The process of learning by which the likelihood of a specific behavior is increased by negative or positive reinforcement

- **Retrograde amnesia:** Inability to recall memories from the past

- **Sensitization:** An increased behavioral response to a wide variety of stimuli following an intense or noxious stimulus

Psychological tests have shown that prefrontal lobectomized lower animals presented with successive bits of sensory information fail to keep track of these bits even in temporary memory, probably because they are distracted so easily that they cannot hold thoughts long enough for memory storage to take place.

This ability of the prefrontal areas to keep track of many bits of information simultaneously and to cause recall of this information instantaneously as it is needed for subsequent thoughts is called the brain's "working memory" which may explain the many functions of the brain that we associate with higher intelligence. In fact, studies have shown that the prefrontal areas are divided into separate segments for storing different types of temporary memory, such as one area for storing shape and form of an object or a part of the body and another for storing movement.

By combining all these temporary bits of working memory, we have the abilities to (1) prognosticate; (2) plan for the future; (3) delay action in response to incoming sensory signals so that the sensory information can be weighed until the best course of response is decided; (4) consider the consequences of motor actions before they are performed; (5) solve complicated mathematical, legal, or philosophical problems; (6) correlate all avenues of information in diagnosing rare diseases; and (7) control our activities in accord with moral laws.

Learning

Learning is often described as the process of *"acquiring"* knowledge while *memory is the process of "storing" knowledge.* Conditioning is one of the ways in which learning can be studied.

1. *Classical conditioning* was first described by Pavlov in his famous dog–food–bell experiment. When a dog is presented with food, the dog salivates. In this case the food constitutes an unconditional stimulus and salivation, an unconditional response. When a bell is rung, a dog orients itself to the sound but does not salivate. Pavlov showed that if the bell was followed by the presentation of food repetitively, then the dog salivated, but importantly, when the food was removed, continued to do so. Thus, the bell was now followed by salivation; the bell in this situation constitutes the conditioned stimulus and the salivation, the conditioned response. There are several important characteristics of classical conditioning:
   a. The conditioned stimulus (bell) must precede the unconditioned stimulus (food).
   b. The two stimuli must be given in close proximity of each other.
   c. Repeated pairing of stimuli is required to elicit conditioning.
   d. Unconditional stimuli can be either:
      1) Rewarding: *appetitive* (as in the food)
      2) Noxious: *defensive* (as with an electric shock)
   e. Classical conditioning can undergo *extinction*, that is, loss of prior learning.
2. *Operant conditioning* is otherwise called trial and error conditioning or Skinnerian conditioning after Skinner. In order to understand this, picture a rat in a cage with a lever in one corner that when pressed results in the release of a pellet of food. The rat explores its cage and presses the lever as part of its exploratory behavior; this results in the release of a pellet of food. Over a period of time, the association between the lever and the food becomes apparent. In this case the food is an appetitive stimulus, but as in classical or Pavlovian conditioning, noxious stimuli can also be used.

Thoughts, Consciousness, and Memory

Our most difficult problem in discussing consciousness, thoughts, memory, and learning is that we do not know the neural mechanisms of a thought and we know little about the mechanisms of memory. We know that destruction of large portions of the cerebral cortex does not prevent a person from having thoughts, but it does reduce the *depth* of the thoughts and also the *degree* of awareness of the surroundings.

Each thought certainly involves simultaneous signals in many portions of the cerebral cortex, thalamus, limbic system, and reticular formation of the brainstem. Some basic thoughts probably depend almost entirely on lower centers; the thought of pain is probably a good example because electrical stimulation of the human cortex seldom elicits anything more than mild pain, whereas stimulation of certain areas of the hypothalamus, amygdala, and mesencephalon can cause excruciating pain. Conversely, a type of thought pattern that does require large involvement of the cerebral cortex is that of vision because loss of the visual cortex causes complete inability to perceive visual form or color.

We might formulate a provisional definition of a thought in terms of neural activity as follows: A thought results from a "pattern" of stimulation of many parts of the nervous system at the same time, probably involving most importantly the cerebral cortex, thalamus, limbic system, and upper reticular formation of the brainstem. This theory is called the *holistic theory* of thoughts. The stimulated areas of the limbic system, thalamus, and reticular formation are believed to determine the general nature of the thought, giving it such qualities as pleasure, displeasure, pain, comfort, crude modalities of sensation, localization to gross areas of the body, and other general characteristics. However, specific stimulated areas of the cerebral cortex determine discrete characteristics of the thought, such as (1) specific localization of sensations on the surface of the body and of objects in the fields of vision, (2) the feeling of the texture of silk, (3) visual recognition of the rectangular pattern of a concrete block wall, and (4) other individual characteristics that enter into one's overall awareness of a particular instant. *Consciousness* can perhaps be described as our continuing stream of awareness of either our surroundings or our sequential thoughts.

MEMORY—ROLES OF SYNAPTIC FACILITATION AND SYNAPTIC INHIBITION

Memories are stored in the brain by changing the basic sensitivity of synaptic transmission between neurons as a result of previous neural activity. The new or facilitated pathways are called *memory traces*. They are important because once the traces are established, they can be selectively activated by the thinking mind to reproduce the memories.

Experiments in lower animals have demonstrated that memory traces can occur at all levels of the nervous system. Even spinal cord reflexes can change at least slightly in response to repetitive cord activation, and these reflex changes are part of the memory process. Also, long-term memories result from changed synaptic conduction in lower brain centers. However, most memory that we associate with intellectual processes is based on memory traces in the cerebral cortex.

Positive and Negative Memory—"Sensitization" or "Habituation" of Synaptic Transmission. Although we often think of memories as being *positive* recollections of previous thoughts or experiences, probably the greater share of our memories is *negative*, not positive. That is, our brain is inundated with sensory information from all our senses. If our minds attempted to remember all this information, the memory capacity of the brain would be rapidly exceeded.

Fortunately, the brain has the capability to ignore information that is of no consequence. This capability results from *inhibition* of the synaptic pathways for this type of information; the resulting effect is called *habituation*, which is a type of *negative* memory.

Conversely, for incoming information that causes important consequences such as pain or pleasure, the brain has a different automatic capability of enhancing and storing the memory traces, which is *positive* memory. It results from *facilitation* of the synaptic pathways, and the process is called *memory sensitization*. As we discuss later, special areas in the basal limbic regions of the brain determine whether information is important or unimportant and make the subconscious decision about whether to store the thought as a *sensitized* memory trace or to suppress it.

Classification of Memories. We know that some memories last for only a few seconds, whereas others last for hours, days, months, or years. For the purpose of discussing these types of memories, let us use a common classification that divides memories into (1) *short-term memory*, which includes memories that last for seconds or at most minutes unless they are converted into longer-term memories; (2) *intermediate long-term memories*, which last for days to weeks but then fade away; and (3) *long-term memory*, which, once stored, can be recalled up to years or even a lifetime later.

In addition to this general classification of memories, we also discussed earlier (in connection with the prefrontal lobes) another type of memory, called "working memory," which includes mainly short-term memory that is used during the course of intellectual reasoning but is terminated as each stage of the problem is resolved.

Memories are frequently classified according to the type of information that is stored. One of these classifications divides memory into *declarative memory* and *skill memory*, as follows:

1. *Declarative memory* basically means memory of the various details of an integrated thought, such as memory of an important experience that includes (a) memory of the surroundings, (b) memory of time relationships, (c) memory of causes of the experience, (d) memory of the meaning of the experience, and (e) memory of one's deductions that were left in the person's mind.
2. *Skill memory* is frequently associated with motor activities of the person's body, such as all the skills developed for hitting a tennis ball, including automatic memories to (a) sight the ball, (b) calculate the relationship and speed of the ball to the racquet, and (c) deduce rapidly the motions of the body, the arms, and the racquet required to hit the ball as desired—with all of these skills activated instantly based on previous learning of the game—and then moving on to the next stroke of the game while forgetting the details of the previous stroke.

SHORT-TERM MEMORY

Short-term memory is typified by one's memory of 7–10 numerals in a telephone number (or 7–10 other discrete facts) for a few seconds to a few minutes at a time but lasting only as long as the person continues to think about the numbers or facts.

Many physiologists have suggested that this short-term memory is caused by continual neural activity resulting from nerve signals that travel around and around a temporary memory trace in a *circuit of reverberating neurons*. It has not yet been possible to prove this theory. Another possible explanation of short-term memory is *presynaptic facilitation or inhibition*, which occurs at synapses that lie on terminal nerve fibrils immediately before these fibrils synapse with a subsequent neuron. The neurotransmitter chemicals secreted at such terminals frequently cause facilitation or inhibition lasting for seconds up to several minutes. Circuits of this type could lead to short-term memory.

INTERMEDIATE LONG-TERM MEMORY

Intermediate long-term memories may last for many minutes or even weeks. They will eventually be lost unless the memory traces are activated enough to become more permanent; then they are classified as long-term memories. Experiments in primitive animals have demonstrated that memories of the intermediate long-term type can result from temporary chemical or physical changes, or both, in either the synapse presynaptic terminals or the synapse postsynaptic membrane, changes that can persist for a few minutes up to several weeks. These mechanisms are so important that they deserve special description.

Memory Based on Chemical Changes in Presynaptic Terminals or Postsynaptic Neuronal Membranes

Figure 125-1 shows a mechanism of memory studied especially by Kandel and his colleagues that can cause memories lasting from a few minutes up to 3 weeks in the large snail *Aplysia*. In Figure 125-1, there are two synaptic terminals. One terminal that is from a sensory input neuron terminates directly on the surface of the neuron that is to be stimulated and is called the *sensory terminal*. The other terminal, a *presynaptic ending* that lies on the surface of the sensory terminal, is called the *facilitator terminal*. When the sensory terminal is stimulated repeatedly, but without stimulation of the facilitator terminal, signal transmission at first is great, but it becomes less and less intense with repeated stimulation until transmission almost ceases. This phenomenon is *habituation*, as was explained previously. It is a type of *negative* memory that causes the neuronal circuit to lose its response to repeated events that are insignificant.

Conversely, if a noxious stimulus excites the facilitator terminal at the same time that the sensory terminal is stimulated, instead of the transmitted signal into the postsynaptic neuron becoming progressively weaker, the ease of transmission becomes stronger and stronger, and it will remain strong for minutes, hours, days, or, with more intense training, up to about 3 weeks even without further stimulation of the facilitator terminal. Thus, the noxious stimulus causes the memory pathway

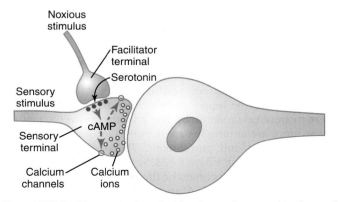

through the sensory terminal to become *facilitated* for days or weeks thereafter. It is especially interesting that even after habituation has occurred, this pathway can be converted back to a facilitated pathway with only a few noxious stimuli.

Molecular Mechanism of Intermediate Memory

Mechanism for Habituation. At the molecular level, the habituation effect in the sensory terminal results from progressive closure of calcium channels through the terminal membrane, although the cause of this calcium channel closure is not fully known. Nevertheless, much smaller than normal amounts of calcium ions can diffuse into the habituated terminal, and much less sensory terminal transmitter is therefore released because calcium entry is the principal stimulus for transmitter release.

Mechanism for Facilitation. In the case of facilitation, at least part of the molecular mechanism is believed to be the following:

1. Stimulation of the facilitator presynaptic terminal at the same time that the sensory terminal is stimulated causes *serotonin* release at the facilitator synapse on the surface of the sensory terminal.
2. The serotonin acts on *serotonin receptors* in the sensory terminal membrane, and these receptors activate the enzyme *adenyl cyclase* inside the membrane. The adenyl cyclase then causes formation of *cyclic adenosine monophosphate* (cAMP) also inside the sensory presynaptic terminal.
3. The cAMP activates a *protein kinase* that causes phosphorylation of a protein that itself is part of the potassium channels in the sensory synaptic terminal membrane; this in turn blocks the channels for potassium conductance. The blockage can last for minutes up to several weeks.
4. Lack of potassium conductance causes a greatly prolonged action potential in the synaptic terminal because flow of potassium ions out of the terminal is necessary for rapid recovery from the action potential.
5. The prolonged action potential causes prolonged activation of the calcium channels, allowing tremendous quantities of calcium ions to enter the sensory synaptic terminal. These calcium ions cause greatly increased transmitter release by the synapse, thereby markedly facilitating synaptic transmission to the subsequent neuron.

Thus, in a very indirect way, the associative effect of stimulating the facilitator terminal at the same time that the sensory terminal is stimulated causes prolonged increase in excitatory sensitivity of the sensory terminal, which establishes the memory trace. Studies by Byrne and colleagues, also in the snail *Aplysia*, have suggested still another mechanism of synaptic memory. Their studies have shown that stimuli from separate sources acting on a single neuron, under appropriate conditions, can cause long-term changes in *membrane properties of the postsynaptic neuron* instead of in the presynaptic neuronal membrane, but leading to essentially the same memory effects.

LONG-TERM MEMORY

No obvious demarcation exists between the more prolonged types of intermediate long-term memory and true long-term memory. The distinction is one of degree. However, long-term memory is generally believed to result from actual *structural changes*, instead of only chemical changes, at the synapses, and these changes enhance or suppress signal conduction. Again, let us recall experiments in primitive animals (where the nervous

Figure 125-1 Memory system that has been discovered in the snail *Aplysia*. cAMP, cyclic adenosine monophosphate.

systems are much easier to study) that have aided immensely in understanding possible mechanisms of long-term memory.

Structural Changes Occur in Synapses During Development of Long-Term Memory

Electron microscopic pictures taken from invertebrate animals have demonstrated multiple physical structural changes in many synapses during development of long-term memory traces. The structural changes will not occur if a drug is given that blocks protein synthesis in the presynaptic neuron, nor will the permanent memory trace develop. Therefore, it appears that development of true long-term memory depends on physically restructuring the synapses themselves in a way that changes their sensitivity for transmitting nervous signals.

The following important structural changes occur:
1. an increase in vesicle release sites for secretion of transmitter substance;
2. an increase in the number of transmitter vesicles released;
3. an increase in the number of presynaptic terminals;
4. changes in structures of the dendritic spines that permit transmission of stronger signals.

Thus, in several different ways, the structural capability of synapses to transmit signals appears to increase during establishment of true long-term memory traces.

Number of Neurons and their Connectivities Often Change Significantly During Learning

During the first few weeks, months, and perhaps even year or so of life, many parts of the brain produce a great excess of neurons and the neurons send out numerous axon branches to make connections with other neurons. If the new axons fail to connect with appropriate neurons, muscle cells, or gland cells, the new axons will dissolute within a few weeks. Thus, the number of neuronal connections is determined by specific *nerve growth factors* released retrogradely from the stimulated cells. Furthermore, when insufficient connectivity occurs, the entire neuron that is sending out the axon branches might eventually disappear.

Therefore, soon after birth, the principle of "use it or lose it" governs the final number of neurons and their connectivities in respective parts of the human nervous system. This is a type of learning. For example, if one eye of a newborn animal is covered for many weeks after birth, neurons in alternate stripes of the cerebral visual cortex—neurons normally connected to the covered eye—will degenerate, and the covered eye will remain either partially or totally blind for the remainder of life. Until recently, it was believed that very little "learning" is achieved in adult human beings and animals by modification of numbers of neurons in the memory circuits; however, recent research suggests that even adults use this mechanism at least to some extent.

CONSOLIDATION OF MEMORY

For short-term memory to be converted into long-term memory that can be recalled weeks or years later, it must become "consolidated." That is, the short-term memory if activated repeatedly will initiate chemical, physical, and anatomical changes in the synapses that are responsible for the long-term type of memory. This process requires 5–10 minutes for minimal consolidation and 1 hour or more for strong consolidation. For instance, if a strong sensory impression is made on the brain but is then followed within a minute or so by an electrically induced brain convulsion, the sensory experience will not be remembered. Likewise, brain concussion, sudden application of deep general anesthesia, or any other effect that temporarily blocks the dynamic function of the brain can prevent consolidation.

Consolidation and the time required for it to occur can probably be explained by the phenomenon of rehearsal of the short-term memory, as described in the following section.

Rehearsal Enhances the Transference of Short-Term Memory into Long-Term Memory. Studies have shown that rehearsal of the same information again and again in the mind accelerates and potentiates the degree of transfer of short-term memory into long-term memory, and therefore accelerates and enhances consolidation. The brain has a natural tendency to rehearse newfound information, especially newfound information that catches the mind's attention. Therefore, over a period of time, the important features of sensory experiences become progressively more and more fixed in the memory stores. This phenomenon explains why a person can remember small amounts of information studied in depth far better than large amounts of information studied only superficially. It also explains why a person who is wide awake can consolidate memories far better than a person who is in a state of mental fatigue.

New Memories Are Codified During Consolidation. One of the most important features of consolidation is that new memories are *codified* into different classes of information. During this process, similar types of information are pulled from the memory storage bins and used to help process the new information. The new and old are compared for similarities and differences, and part of the storage process is to store the information about these similarities and differences, rather than to store the new information unprocessed. Thus, during consolidation, the new memories are not stored randomly in the brain but are stored in direct association with other memories of the same type. This process is necessary for one to be able to "search" the memory store at a later date to find the required information.

Role of Specific Parts of the Brain in the Memory Process

The Hippocampus Promotes Storage of Memories—Anterograde Amnesia Occurs After Hippocampal Lesions Are Sustained. The hippocampus is the most medial portion of the temporal lobe cortex, where it folds first medially underneath the brain and then upward into the lower, inside surface of the lateral ventricle. The two hippocampi have been removed for the treatment of epilepsy in a few patients. This procedure does not seriously affect the person's memory for information stored in the brain before removal of the hippocampi. However, after removal, these people have virtually no capability thereafter for storing *verbal and symbolic types* of memories (declarative types of memory) in long-term memory, or even in intermediate memory lasting longer than a few minutes. Therefore, these people are unable to establish new long-term memories of those types of information that are the basis of intelligence. This condition is called *anterograde amnesia*.

But why are the hippocampi so important in helping the brain to store new memories? The probable answer is that the hippocampi are among the most important output pathways from the "reward" and "punishment." The role of the hippocampi is also discussed in Chapter 124. Sensory stimuli or thoughts that cause pain or aversion excite the limbic *punishment centers*, and stimuli that cause pleasure, happiness, or sense of reward excite the limbic *reward centers*. All these together provide the background mood and motivations of the person. Among these motivations is the drive in the brain to remember those experiences and thoughts that are either pleasant or unpleasant. The hippocampi especially and to a lesser degree the dorsal medial nuclei of the thalamus, another limbic structure, have proved especially important in making the decision about which of our thoughts are important enough on a basis of reward or punishment to be worthy of memory.

Retrograde Amnesia—Inability to Recall Memories from the Past. When retrograde amnesia occurs, the degree of amnesia for recent events is likely to be much greater than for events of the distant past. The reason for this difference is probably that the distant memories have been rehearsed so many times that the memory traces are deeply ingrained, and elements of these memories are stored in widespread areas of the brain.

In some people who have hippocampal lesions, some degree of retrograde amnesia occurs along with anterograde amnesia, which suggests that these two types of amnesia are at least partially related and that hippocampal lesions can cause both. However, damage in some thalamic areas may lead specifically to retrograde amnesia without causing significant anterograde amnesia. A possible explanation of this is that the thalamus may play a role in helping the person "search" the memory storehouses and thus "read out" the memories. That is, the memory process not only requires the storing of memories but also an ability to search and find the memory at a later date.

Hippocampi Are Not Important in Reflexive Learning. People with hippocampal lesions usually do not have difficulty in learning physical skills that do not involve verbalization or symbolic types of intelligence. For instance, these people can still learn the rapid hand and physical skills required in many types of sports. This type of learning is called *skill learning* or *reflexive learning*; it depends on physically repeating the required tasks over and over again, rather than on symbolic rehearsing in the mind.

Alzheimer Disease—Amyloid Plaques and Depressed Memory

Alzheimer disease is defined as premature aging of the brain, usually beginning in mid-adult life and progressing rapidly to extreme loss of mental powers—similar to that seen in very, very old age. The clinical features of Alzheimer disease include (1) an amnesic type of memory impairment, (2) deterioration of language, and (3) visuospatial deficits. Motor and sensory abnormalities, gait disturbances, and seizures are uncommon until the late phases of the disease. One consistent finding in Alzheimer disease is loss of neurons in the part of the limbic pathway that drives the memory process. Loss of this memory function is devastating.

Alzheimer disease is a progressive and fatal neurodegenerative disorder that results in impairment of the person's ability to perform activities of daily living, as well as a variety of neuropsychiatric symptoms and behavioral disturbances in the later stages of the disease. Patients with Alzheimer disease usually require continuous care within a few years after the disease begins.

Alzheimer disease is a common form of dementia in elderly persons, and more than 5 million people in the United States are estimated to be afflicted by this disorder. The percentage of persons with Alzheimer disease approximately doubles with every 5 years of age, with about 1% of 60-year-olds and about 30% of 85-year-olds having the disease.

Alzheimer Disease Is Associated with Accumulation of Brain Beta-Amyloid Peptide. Pathologically, one finds increased amounts of beta-amyloid peptide in the brains of patients with Alzheimer disease. The peptide accumulates in amyloid plaques, which range in diameter from 10 to several hundred micrometers and are found in widespread areas of the brain, including in the cerebral cortex, hippocampus, basal ganglia, thalamus, and even the cerebellum. Thus, Alzheimer disease appears to be a metabolic degenerative disease.

A key role for excess accumulation of beta-amyloid peptide in the pathogenesis of Alzheimer disease is suggested by the following observations: (1) all currently known mutations associated with Alzheimer disease increase the production of beta-amyloid peptide; (2) patients with trisomy 21 (Down syndrome) have three copies of the gene for amyloid precursor protein and develop neurological characteristics of Alzheimer disease by midlife; (3) patients who have abnormality of a gene that controls apolipoprotein E, a blood protein that transports cholesterol to the tissues, have accelerated deposition of amyloid and greatly increased risk for Alzheimer disease; (4) transgenic mice that overproduce the human amyloid precursor protein have learning and memory deficits in association with the accumulation of amyloid plaques; and (5) generation of antiamyloid antibodies in humans with Alzheimer disease appears to attenuate the disease process.

Vascular Disorders May Contribute to Progression of Alzheimer Disease. There is also accumulating evidence that cerebrovascular disease caused by *hypertension* and *atherosclerosis* may play a role in Alzheimer disease. Cerebrovascular disease is the second most common cause of acquired cognitive impairment and dementia, and likely contributes to cognitive decline in persons with Alzheimer disease. In fact, many of the common risk factors for cerebrovascular disease, such as hypertension, diabetes, and hyperlipidemia, are also recognized to greatly increase the risk for developing Alzheimer disease.

BIBLIOGRAPHY

Bloom GS: Amyloid-β and tau: the trigger and bullet in Alzheimer disease pathogenesis, *JAMA Neurol.* 71:505, 2014.

Euston DR, Gruber AJ, McNaughton BL: The role of medial prefrontal cortex in memory and decision making, *Neuron* 76:1057, 2012.

Flavell CR, Lambert EA, Winters BD, Bredy TW: Mechanisms governing the reactivation-dependent destabilization of memories and their role in extinction, *Front Behav. Neurosci.* 7:214, 2013.

Iadecola C: Neurovascular regulation in the normal brain and in Alzheimer's disease, *Nat. Rev. Neurosci.* 5:347, 2004.

Irwin DJ, Lee VM, Trojanowski JQ: Parkinson's disease dementia: convergence of α-synuclein, tau and amyloid-β pathologies, *Nat. Rev. Neurosci.* 14:626, 2013.

Kandel ER, Dudai Y, Mayford MR: The molecular and systems biology of memory, *Cell* 157:163, 2014.

LaBar KS, Cabeza R: Cognitive neuroscience of emotional memory, *Nat. Rev. Neurosci.* 7:54, 2006.

Lynch MA: Long-term potentiation and memory, *Physiol. Rev.* 84:87, 2004.

Ma WJ, Husain M, Bays PM: Changing concepts of working memory, *Nat. Neurosci.* 17:347, 2014.

Markowitsch HJ, Staniloiu A: Amnesic disorders, *Lancet* 380:1429, 2012.

Nader K, Hardt O: A single standard for memory: the case for reconsolidation, *Nat. Rev. Neurosci.* 10:224, 2009.

Osada T, Adachi Y, Kimura HM, et al: Towards understanding of the cortical network underlying associative memory, *Philos. Trans. R. Soc. Lond. B Biol. Sci.* 363:2187, 2008.

Rasch B, Born J: About sleep's role in memory, *Physiol. Rev.* 93:681, 2013.

Rizzolatti G, Cattaneo L, Fabbri-Destro M, Rozzi S: Cortical mechanisms underlying the organization of goal-directed actions and mirror neuron-based action understanding, *Physiol. Rev.* 94:655, 2014.

Rogerson T, Cai DJ, Frank A, et al: Synaptic tagging during memory allocation, *Nat. Rev. Neurosci.* 15:157, 2014.

Roth TL, Sweatt JD: Rhythms of memory, *Nat. Neurosci.* 11:993, 2008.

Stickgold R, Walker MP: Sleep-dependent memory triage: evolving generalization through selective processing, *Nat. Neurosci.* 16:139, 2013.

Tanji J, Hoshi E: Role of the lateral prefrontal cortex in executive behavioral control, *Physiol. Rev.* 88:37, 2008.

Tronson NC, Taylor JR: Molecular mechanisms of memory reconsolidation, *Nat. Rev. Neurosci.* 8:262, 2007.

van Strien NM, Cappaert NL, Witter MP: The anatomy of memory: an interactive overview of the parahippocampal–hippocampal network, *Nat. Rev. Neurosci.* 10:272, 2009.

Wilson DA, Linster C: Neurobiology of a simple memory, *J. Neurophysiol.* 100:2, 2008.

Zamarian L, Ischebeck A, Delazer M: Neuroscience of learning arithmetic—evidence from brain imaging studies, *Neurosci. Biobehav. Rev.* 33:909, 2009.

126

Cortical Function, Cerebral Lateralization, and Speech

LEARNING OBJECTIVES

- List the functions of the cortical association areas.
- Describe the areas in the brain involved in speech and language.
- List the types of aphasias and give the salient features of each.
- List the differences of the right and left cerebral hemispheres.

GLOSSARY OF TERMS

- **Aphasia:** Disorder of communication, either partial or complete, of spoken or written language, due to lesions in the brain

- **Cerebral lateralization:** Specific functions being more highly developed on one side of the brain or the other

- **Cortical association areas:** Cortical areas that receive and analyze signals simultaneously from multiple regions of both the motor and sensory cortices, as well as from subcortical structures

It is ironic that of all the parts of the brain, we know the least about the functions of the cerebral cortex, even though it is by far the largest portion of the nervous system. However, we do know the effects of damage or specific stimulation in various portions of the cortex. In the first part of this chapter, the known cortical functions are discussed and then basic theories of neuronal mechanisms involved in thought processes, memory, analysis of sensory information, and so forth are presented briefly.

Physiological Anatomy of the Cerebral Cortex

The functional part of the cerebral cortex is a thin layer of neurons covering the surface of all the convolutions of the cerebrum. This layer is only 2–5 mm thick, with a total area of about one-quarter of a square meter. The total cerebral cortex contains about 100 *billion* neurons.

Figure 126-1 shows the typical histological structure of the neuronal surface of the cerebral cortex, with its successive layers of different types of neurons. Most of the neurons are of three types: (1) *granular* (also called *stellate*), (2) *fusiform*, and (3) *pyramidal*, the last named for their characteristic pyramidal shape.

The *granular* neurons generally have short axons and, therefore, function mainly as interneurons that transmit neural signals only short distances within the cortex. Some are excitatory, releasing mainly the excitatory neurotransmitter *glutamate*, whereas others are inhibitory and release mainly the inhibitory neurotransmitter *gamma-aminobutyric acid* (GABA). The sensory areas of the cortex, as well as the association areas between sensory and motor areas, have large concentrations of these granule cells, suggesting a high degree of intracortical processing of incoming sensory signals within the sensory areas and association areas.

The *pyramidal* and *fusiform cells* give rise to almost all the output fibers from the cortex. The pyramidal cells, which are larger and more numerous than the fusiform cells, are the source of the long, large nerve fibers that go all the way to the spinal cord. The pyramidal cells also give rise to most of the large subcortical association fiber bundles that pass from one major part of the brain to another.

To the right in Figure 126-1 is shown the typical organization of nerve fibers within the different layers of the cerebral cortex. Note particularly the large number of *horizontal fibers* that extend between adjacent areas of the cortex, but note also the *vertical fibers* that extend to and from the cortex to lower areas of the brain and some all the way to the spinal cord or to distant regions of the cerebral cortex through long association bundles.

The functions of the specific layers of the somatosensory cortex are described in Chapter 105. By way of review, let us recall that most incoming specific sensory signals from the body terminate in cortical layer IV. Most of the output signals leave the cortex through neurons located in layers V and VI; the very large fibers to the brainstem and cord arise generally in layer V, and the tremendous numbers of fibers to the thalamus arise in layer VI. Layers I, II, and III perform most of the intracortical association functions, with especially large numbers of neurons in layers II and III making short horizontal connections with adjacent cortical areas.

Anatomical and Functional Relations of the Cerebral Cortex to the Thalamus and Other Lower Centers. All areas of the cerebral cortex have extensive to-and-fro efferent and afferent connections with deeper structures of the brain. It is important to emphasize the relation between the cerebral cortex and the thalamus. When the thalamus is damaged along with the cortex, the loss of cerebral function is far greater than when the cortex alone is damaged because thalamic excitation of the cortex is necessary for almost all cortical activity.

Figure 126-2 shows the areas of the cerebral cortex that connect with specific parts of the thalamus. These connections act in *two* directions, both from the thalamus to the cortex and then from the cortex back to essentially the same area of the thalamus. Furthermore, when the thalamic connections are cut, the functions of the corresponding cortical area become almost entirely lost. Therefore, the cortex operates in close association with the thalamus and can almost be considered both anatomically and functionally a unit with the thalamus: For this reason, the thalamus and the cortex together are sometimes called the

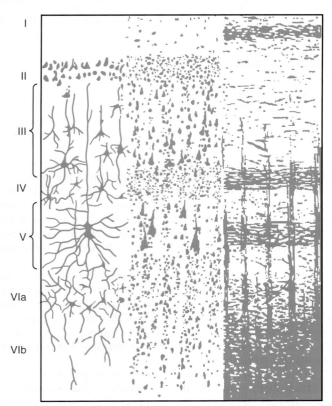

Figure 126-1 Structure of the cerebral cortex, showing the following layers: (*I*) molecular layer; (*II*) external granular layer; (*III*) layer of pyramidal cells; (*IV*) internal granular layer; (*V*) large pyramidal cell layer; and (*VI*) layer of fusiform or polymorphic cells. *Modifi ed from Ranson SW,Clark SL: Anatomy of the Nervous System. Philadelphia: WB Saunders, 1959.*

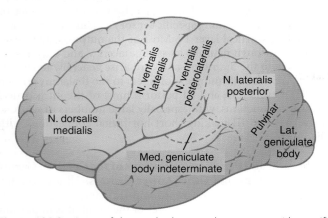

Figure 126-2 Areas of the cerebral cortex that connect with specific portions of the thalamus.

thalamocortical system. Almost all pathways from the sensory receptors and sensory organs to the cortex pass through the thalamus, with the principal exception of some sensory pathways of olfaction.

Functions of Specific Cortical Areas

Studies in human beings have shown that different cerebral cortical areas have separate functions. Figure 126-3 is a map of some of these functions as determined from electrical stimulation of the cortex in awake patients or during neurological examination of patients after portions of the cortex had been

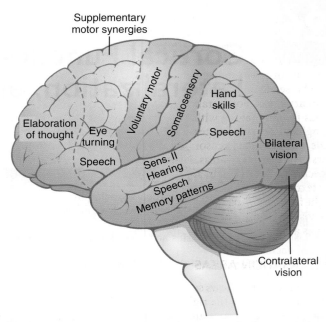

Figure 126-3 Functional areas of the human cerebral cortex as determined by electrical stimulation of the cortex during neurosurgical operations and by neurological examinations of patients with destroyed cortical regions. *Modified from Penfield, W., Rasmussen, T., 1968. The Cerebral Cortex of Man: A Clinical Study of Localization of Function. Hafner, New York.*

removed. The electrically stimulated patients told their thoughts evoked by the stimulation, and sometimes they experienced movements. Occasionally they spontaneously emitted a sound or even a word or gave some other evidence of the stimulation.

Putting large amounts of information together from many different sources gives a more general map, as shown in Figure 126-4. This figure shows the major primary and secondary premotor and supplementary motor areas of the cortex, as well as the major primary and secondary sensory areas for somatic sensation, vision, and hearing, all of which are discussed

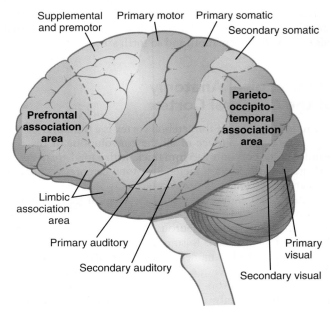

Figure 126-4 Locations of major association areas of the cerebral cortex, as well as primary and secondary motor and sensory areas.

in earlier chapters. The primary motor areas have direct connections with specific muscles for causing discrete muscle movements. The primary sensory areas detect specific sensations—visual, auditory, or somatic—transmitted directly to the brain from peripheral sensory organs.

The secondary areas make sense out of the signals in the primary areas. For instance, the supplementary and premotor areas function along with the primary motor cortex and basal ganglia to provide "patterns" of motor activity. On the sensory side, the secondary sensory areas, located within a few centimeters of the primary areas, begin to analyze the meanings of the specific sensory signals, such as (1) interpretation of the shape or texture of an object in one's hand; (2) interpretation of color, light intensity, directions of lines and angles, and other aspects of vision; and (3) interpretations of the meanings of sound tones and sequence of tones in the auditory signals.

ASSOCIATION AREAS

Figure 126-4 also shows several large areas of the cerebral cortex that do not fit into the rigid categories of primary and secondary motor and sensory areas. These areas are called *association areas* because they receive and analyze signals simultaneously from multiple regions of both the motor and sensory cortices, as well as from subcortical structures. Yet even the association areas have their specializations. Important association areas include (1) the *parieto-occipitotemporal association area*, (2) the *prefrontal association area*, and (3) the *limbic association area*.

Parieto-Occipitotemporal Association Area. The parieto-occipitotemporal association area lies in the large parietal and occipital cortical space bounded by the somatosensory cortex anteriorly, the visual cortex posteriorly, and the auditory cortex laterally. As would be expected, it provides a high level of interpretative meaning for signals from all the surrounding sensory areas. However, even the parieto-occipitotemporal association area has its own functional subareas, which are shown in Figure 126-5.

1. *Analysis of the spatial coordinates of the body.* An area beginning in the posterior parietal cortex and extending into the superior occipital cortex provides continuous analysis of the spatial coordinates of all parts of the body, as well as of the surroundings of the body. This area receives visual sensory information from the posterior occipital cortex and simultaneous somatosensory information from the anterior parietal cortex. From all this information, it computes the coordinates of the visual, auditory, and body surroundings.

2. *Wernicke area is important for language comprehension.* The major area for language comprehension, called *Wernicke area*, lies behind *the primary auditory cortex in the posterior part of the superior gyrus of the temporal lobe*. We discuss this area more fully later; it is the most important region of the entire brain for higher intellectual function because almost all such intellectual functions are language based.

3. *Angular gyrus area is needed for initial processing of visual language (reading).* Posterior to the language comprehension area, lying mainly in the anterolateral region of the occipital lobe, is a visual association area that feeds visual information conveyed by words read from a book into Wernicke area, the language comprehension area. This so-called *angular gyrus area* is needed to make meaning out of the visually perceived words. In its absence, a person can still have excellent language comprehension through hearing but not through reading.

4. *Area for naming objects.* In the most lateral portions of the anterior occipital lobe and posterior temporal lobe is an area for naming objects. The names are learned mainly through auditory input, whereas the physical natures of the objects are learned mainly through visual input. In turn, the names are essential for both auditory and visual language comprehension (*functions performed in Wernicke area located immediately superior to the auditory "names" region and anterior to the visual word processing area*).

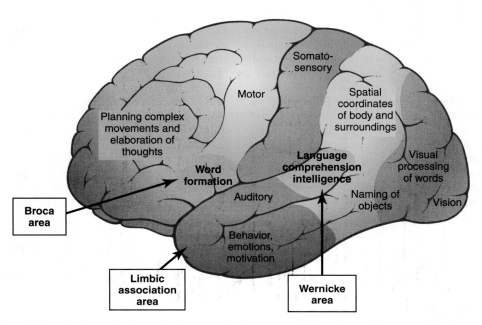

Figure 126-5 Map of specific functional areas in the cerebral cortex, showing especially Wernicke and Broca areas for language comprehension and speech production, which in 95% of all people are located in the left hemisphere.

Broca Area Provides the Neural Circuitry for Word Formation. *Broca area*, shown in Figure 126-5, is located partly in the posterior lateral prefrontal cortex and partly in the premotor area. It is here that plans and motor patterns for expressing individual words or even short phrases are initiated and executed. This area also works in close association with the Wernicke language comprehension center in the temporal association cortex, as we discuss more fully later in the chapter.

An especially interesting discovery is the following: When a person has already learned one language and then learns a new language, the area in the brain where the new language is stored is slightly removed from the storage area for the first language. If both languages are learned simultaneously, they are stored together in the same area of the brain.

Prefrontal Association Area. The prefrontal association area functions in close association with the motor cortex to plan complex patterns and sequences of motor movements. To aid in this function, it receives strong input through a massive subcortical bundle of nerve fibers connecting the parieto-occipitotemporal association area with the prefrontal association area. Through this bundle, the prefrontal cortex receives much preanalyzed sensory information, especially information on the spatial coordinates of the body that is necessary for planning effective movements. Much of the output from the prefrontal area into the motor control system passes through the caudate portion of the basal ganglia–thalamic feedback circuit for motor planning, which provides many of the sequential and parallel components of movement stimulation.

The *prefrontal association area* is also *essential to carrying out "thought" processes.* This characteristic presumably results from some of the same capabilities of the prefrontal cortex that allow it to plan motor activities. It seems to be capable of processing nonmotor and motor information from widespread areas of the brain and therefore to achieve nonmotor types of thinking, as well as motor types. In fact, the prefrontal association area is frequently described simply as important for *elaboration of thoughts*, and it is said to store on a short-term basis "working memories" that are used to combine new thoughts while they are entering the brain.

Higher Intellectual Functions of the Prefrontal Association Areas. For years, it has been taught that the prefrontal cortex is the locus of "higher intellect" in the human being, principally because the main difference between the brains of monkeys and of human beings is the great prominence of the human prefrontal areas. Yet efforts to show that the prefrontal cortex is more important in higher intellectual functions than other portions of the brain have not been successful. Indeed, destruction of the language comprehension area in the posterior superior temporal lobe (Wernicke area) and the adjacent angular gyrus region in the dominant hemisphere causes much more harm to the intellect than does destruction of the prefrontal areas. The prefrontal areas do, however, have less definable but nevertheless important intellectual functions of their own. These functions can best be explained by describing what happens to patients in whom the prefrontal areas have become damaged, as follows.

Several decades ago, before the advent of modern drugs for treating psychiatric conditions, it was discovered that some patients could receive significant relief from severe psychotic depression by severing the neuronal connections between the prefrontal areas of the brain and the remainder of the brain, that is, by a procedure called *prefrontal lobotomy*. This procedure was performed by inserting a blunt, thin-bladed knife through a small opening in the lateral frontal skull on each side of the head and slicing the brain at the back edge of the prefrontal lobes from top to bottom. Subsequent studies in these patients showed the following mental changes:

1. The patients lost their ability to solve complex problems.
2. They became unable to string together sequential tasks to reach complex goals.
3. They became unable to learn to do several parallel tasks at the same time.
4. Their level of aggressiveness decreased, sometimes markedly, and they often lost ambition.
5. Their social responses were often inappropriate for the occasion, often including loss of morals and little reticence in relation to sexual activity and excretion.
6. The patients could still talk and comprehend language, but they were unable to carry through any long trains of thought, and their moods changed rapidly from sweetness to rage to exhilaration to madness.
7. The patients could also still perform most of the usual patterns of motor function that they had performed throughout life, but often without purpose.

From this information, let us try to piece together a coherent understanding of the function of the prefrontal association areas.

Limbic Association Area. Figures 126-4 and 126-5 show still another association area called the *limbic association area*. This area is found in the anterior pole of the temporal lobe, in the ventral portion of the frontal lobe, and in the cingulate gyrus lying deep in the longitudinal fissure on the midsurface of each cerebral hemisphere. It is concerned primarily with *behavior*, *emotions*, and *motivation*. We discuss in Chapter 124 that the limbic cortex is part of a much more extensive system, the *limbic system*, that includes a complex set of neuronal structures in the midbasal regions of the brain. This limbic system provides most of the emotional drives for activating other areas of the brain and even provides motivational drive for the process of learning itself.

Area for Recognition of Faces. An interesting type of brain abnormality called *prosopagnosia* is the inability to recognize faces. This condition occurs in people who have extensive damage on the medial undersides of both occipital lobes and along the medioventral surfaces of the temporal lobes, as shown in Figure 126-6. Loss of these face recognition areas, strangely enough, results in little other abnormality of brain function.

One may wonder why so much of the cerebral cortex should be reserved for the simple task of face recognition. However, most of our daily tasks involve associations with other people, and thus one can see the importance of this intellectual function.

The occipital portion of this facial recognition area is contiguous with the visual cortex, and the temporal portion is closely associated with the limbic system that has to do with emotions, brain activation, and control of one's behavioral response to the environment.

COMPREHENSIVE INTERPRETATIVE FUNCTION OF THE POSTERIOR SUPERIOR TEMPORAL LOBE—"WERNICKE AREA" (A GENERAL INTERPRETATIVE AREA)

The somatic, visual, and auditory association areas all meet one another in the posterior part of the superior temporal lobe, shown in Figure 126-7, where the temporal, parietal, and

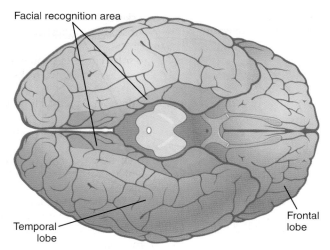

Figure 126-6 Facial recognition areas located on the underside of the brain in the medial occipital and temporal lobes. *Modified from Geschwind, N., 1979. Specializations of the human brain. Sci. Am. 241, 180.*

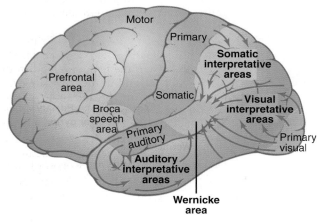

Figure 126-7 Organization of the somatic auditory and visual association areas into a general mechanism for interpretation of sensory experience. All of these feed also into *Wernicke area*, located in the posterosuperior portion of the temporal lobe. Note also the prefrontal area and *Broca speech area* in the frontal lobe.

occipital lobes all come together. This area of confluence of the different sensory interpretative areas is especially highly developed in the *dominant* side of the brain—the *left side* in almost all right-handed people—and it plays the greatest single role of any part of the cerebral cortex for the higher comprehension levels of brain function that we call *intelligence*. Therefore, this region has been called by different names suggestive of an area that has almost global importance: the *general interpretative area*, the *gnostic area*, the *knowing area*, the *tertiary association area*, and so forth. It is best known as *Wernicke area* in honor of the neurologist who first described its special significance in intellectual processes.

After severe damage in Wernicke area, a person might hear perfectly well and even recognize different words but still be unable to arrange these words into a coherent thought. Likewise, the person may be able to read words from the printed page but be unable to recognize the thought that is conveyed.

Electrical stimulation of Wernicke area in a conscious person occasionally causes a highly complex thought, particularly when the stimulation electrode is passed deep enough into the brain to approach the corresponding connecting

areas of the thalamus. The types of thoughts that might be experienced include complicated visual scenes that one might remember from childhood, auditory hallucinations such as a specific musical piece, or even a statement made by a specific person. For this reason, it is believed that activation of Wernicke area can call forth complicated memory patterns that involve more than one sensory modality even though most of the individual memories may be stored elsewhere. This belief is in accord with the importance of Wernicke area in interpreting the complicated meanings of different patterns of sensory experiences.

Angular Gyrus—Interpretation of Visual Information. The *angular gyrus* is the most inferior portion of the posterior parietal lobe, lying immediately behind Wernicke area and fusing posteriorly into the visual areas of the occipital lobe as well. If this region is destroyed while Wernicke area in the temporal lobe is still intact, the person can still interpret auditory experiences as usual, but the stream of visual experiences passing into Wernicke area from the visual cortex is mainly blocked. Therefore, the person may be able to see words and even know that they are words but not be able to interpret their meanings. This condition is called *dyslexia* or *word blindness*.

Let us again emphasize the global importance of Wernicke area for processing most intellectual functions of the brain. Loss of this area in an adult usually leads thereafter to a lifetime of almost demented existence.

Concept of the Dominant Hemisphere

The general interpretative functions of Wernicke area and the angular gyrus, as well as the functions of the speech and motor control areas, are usually much more highly developed in one cerebral hemisphere than in the other. Therefore, this hemisphere is called the *dominant hemisphere*. In about 95% of all people, the left hemisphere is the dominant one.

Even at birth, the area of the cortex that will eventually become Wernicke area is as much as 50% larger in the left hemisphere than in the right in more than one-half of neonates. Therefore, it is easy to understand why the left side of the brain might become dominant over the right side. However, if for some reason this left-side area is damaged or removed in very early childhood, the opposite side of the brain will usually develop dominant characteristics.

The following theory can explain the capability of one hemisphere to dominate the other hemisphere. The attention of the "mind" seems to be directed to one principal thought at a time. Presumably, because the left posterior temporal lobe at birth is usually slightly larger than the right lobe, the left side normally begins to be used to a greater extent than is the right side. Thereafter, because of the tendency to direct one's attention to the better developed region, the rate of learning in the cerebral hemisphere that gains the first start increases rapidly, whereas in the opposite, less-used side, learning remains less well developed. Therefore, the left side normally becomes dominant over the right side.

In about 95% of all people, the left temporal lobe and angular gyrus become dominant, and in the remaining 5%, either both sides develop simultaneously to have dual function or, more rarely, the right side alone becomes highly developed, with full dominance.

As discussed later in the chapter, the premotor speech area (Broca area), located far laterally in the intermediate frontal lobe, is also almost always dominant on the left side of the brain.

This speech area is responsible for formation of words by exciting simultaneously the laryngeal muscles, respiratory muscles, and muscles of the mouth.

The motor areas for controlling hands are also dominant in the left side of the brain in about 9 of 10 persons, thus causing right-handedness in most people.

Although the interpretative areas of the temporal lobe and angular gyrus, as well as many of the motor areas, are usually highly developed in only the left hemisphere, these areas receive sensory information from both hemispheres and are also capable of controlling motor activities in both hemispheres. For this purpose, they use mainly fiber pathways in the *corpus callosum* for communication between the two hemispheres. This unitary, cross-feeding organization prevents interference between the two sides of the brain; such interference could create havoc with both mental thoughts and motor responses.

Role of Language in the Function of Wernicke Area and in Intellectual Functions

A major share of our sensory experience is converted into its language equivalent before being stored in the memory areas of the brain and before being processed for other intellectual purposes. For instance, when we read a book, we do not store the visual images of the printed words but instead store the words themselves or their conveyed thoughts often in language form.

The sensory area of the dominant hemisphere for interpretation of language is Wernicke area, and this area is closely associated with both the primary and secondary hearing areas of the temporal lobe. This close relation probably results from the fact that the first introduction to language is by way of hearing. Later in life, when visual perception of language through the medium of reading develops, the visual information conveyed by written words is then presumably channeled through the angular gyrus, a visual association area, into the already developed Wernicke language interpretative area of the dominant temporal lobe.

FUNCTIONS OF THE PARIETO-OCCIPITOTEMPORAL CORTEX IN THE NONDOMINANT HEMISPHERE

When Wernicke area in the dominant hemisphere of an adult person is destroyed, the person normally loses almost all intellectual functions associated with language or verbal symbolism, such as the ability to read, the ability to perform mathematical operations, and even the ability to think through logical problems. Many other types of interpretative capabilities, some of which use the temporal lobe and angular gyrus regions of the opposite hemisphere, are retained.

Psychological studies in patients with damage to the nondominant hemisphere have suggested that this hemisphere may be especially important for understanding and interpreting music, nonverbal visual experiences (especially visual patterns), spatial relations between the person and their surroundings, the significance of "body language" and intonations of people's voices, and probably many somatic experiences related to use of the limbs and hands. Thus, even though we speak of the "dominant" hemisphere, this dominance is primarily for language-based intellectual functions; the so-called nondominant hemisphere might actually be dominant for some other types of intelligence.

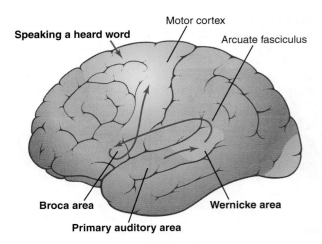

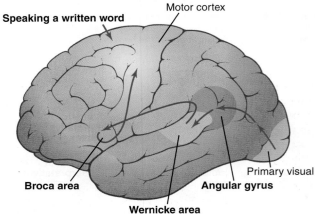

Figure 126-8   Brain pathways for (*top*) perceiving a heard word and then speaking the same word and (*bottom*) perceiving a written word and then speaking the same word. *Modified from Geschwind, N., 1979. Specializations of the human brain. Sci. Am. 241, 180.*

Function of the Brain in Communication—Language Input and Language Output

One of the most important differences between human beings and other animals is the facility with which human beings can communicate with one another. Furthermore, because neurological tests can easily assess the ability of a person to communicate with others, we know more about the sensory and motor systems related to communication than about any other segment of brain cortex function. Therefore, we will review, with the help of anatomical maps of neural pathways in Figure 126-8, the function of the cortex in communication. From this examination, one will see immediately how the principles of sensory analysis and motor control apply to this art.

Communication has two aspects: the *sensory* (language input), involving the ears and eyes, and the *motor* (language output), involving vocalization and its control.

Sensory Aspects of Communication. We noted earlier in the chapter that destruction of portions of the *auditory* or *visual association areas* of the cortex can result in the inability to understand the spoken or written word. These effects are called, respectively, *auditory receptive aphasia* and *visual receptive aphasia* or, more commonly, *word deafness* and *word blindness* (also called *dyslexia*).

Wernicke Aphasia and Global Aphasia. Some people are capable of understanding either the spoken word or the written word but are *unable to interpret the thought* that is expressed. This condition results most frequently when *Wernicke area* in the *posterior superior temporal gyrus in the dominant hemisphere* is damaged or destroyed. Therefore, this type of aphasia is called *Wernicke aphasia.*

When the lesion in Wernicke area is widespread and extends (1) backward into the angular gyrus region, (2) inferiorly into the lower areas of the temporal lobe, and (3) superiorly into the superior border of the Sylvian fissure, the person is likely to be almost totally demented for language understanding or communication and therefore is said to have *global aphasia.*

Motor Aspects of Communication. The process of speech involves two principal stages of mentation: (1) formation in the mind of thoughts to be expressed, as well as choice of words to be used, and then (2) motor control of vocalization and the actual act of vocalization itself.

The formation of thoughts and even most choices of words are the function of sensory association areas of the brain. Again, it is Wernicke area in the posterior part of the superior temporal gyrus that is most important for this ability. Therefore, a person with either Wernicke aphasia or global aphasia is unable to formulate the thoughts that are to be communicated. Or, if the lesion is less severe, the person may be able to formulate the thoughts but unable to put together appropriate sequences of words to express the thought. The person sometimes is even fluent with words but the words are jumbled.

Loss of Broca Area Causes Motor Aphasia. Sometimes a person is capable of deciding what he or she wants to say but cannot make the vocal system emit words instead of noises. This effect, called *motor aphasia,* results from damage to *Broca speech area,* which lies in the *prefrontal* and *premotor* facial region of the cerebral cortex—about 95% of the time in the left hemisphere, as shown in Figures 126-5 and 126-8. The *skilled motor patterns* for control of the larynx, lips, mouth, respiratory system, and other accessory muscles of speech are all initiated from this area.

Articulation. Finally, we have the act of articulation, which means the muscular movements of the mouth, tongue, larynx, vocal cords, and so forth that are responsible for the intonations, timing, and rapid changes in intensities of the sequential sounds. The *facial and laryngeal regions of the motor cortex* activate these muscles, and the *cerebellum, basal ganglia,* and *sensory cortex* all help to control the sequences and intensities of muscle contractions, making liberal use of basal ganglia and cerebellar feedback mechanisms described in Chapters 116 and 118. Destruction of any of these regions can cause either total or partial inability to speak distinctly.

Summary. Figure 126-8 shows two principal pathways for communication. The upper half of the figure shows the pathway involved in hearing and speaking. This sequence is as follows: (1) reception in the primary auditory area of the sound signals that encode the words; (2) interpretation of the words in Wernicke area; (3) determination, also in Wernicke area, of the thoughts and the words to be spoken; (4) transmission of signals from Wernicke area to Broca area by way of the *arcuate fasciculus;* (5) activation of the skilled motor programs in Broca area for control of word formation; and (6) transmission of appropriate signals into the motor cortex to control the speech muscles.

The lower figure illustrates the comparable steps in reading and then speaking in response. The initial receptive area for the words is in the primary visual area rather than in the primary auditory area. The information then passes through early stages of interpretation in the *angular gyrus region* and finally reaches its full level of recognition in Wernicke area. From here, the sequence is the same as for speaking in response to the spoken word.

Function of the Corpus Callosum and Anterior Commissure to Transfer Thoughts, Memories, Training, and Other Information Between the Two Cerebral Hemispheres

Fibers in the *corpus callosum* provide abundant bidirectional neural connections between most of the respective cortical areas of the two cerebral hemispheres except for the anterior portions of the temporal lobes; these temporal areas, including especially the *amygdala,* are interconnected by fibers that pass through the *anterior commissure.*

Because of the tremendous number of fibers in the corpus callosum, it was assumed from the beginning that this massive structure must have some important function to correlate activities of the two cerebral hemispheres. However, when the corpus callosum was destroyed in laboratory animals, it was at first difficult to discern deficits in brain function. Therefore, for a long time, the function of the corpus callosum was a mystery. However, properly designed experiments have now demonstrated extremely important functions of the corpus callosum and anterior commissure.

One of the functions of the corpus callosum and the anterior commissure is to make information stored in the cortex of one hemisphere available to corresponding cortical areas of the opposite hemisphere. The following important examples illustrate such cooperation between the two hemispheres:

1. Cutting the corpus callosum blocks transfer of information from Wernicke area of the dominant hemisphere to the motor cortex on the opposite side of the brain. Therefore, the intellectual functions of Wernicke area, located in the left hemisphere, lose control over the right motor cortex that initiates voluntary motor functions of the left hand and arm, even though the usual subconscious movements of the left hand and arm are normal.

2. Cutting the corpus callosum prevents transfer of somatic and visual information from the right hemisphere into Wernicke area in the left dominant hemisphere. Therefore, somatic and visual information from the left side of the body frequently fails to reach this general interpretative area of the brain and therefore cannot be used for decision making.

3. Finally, people whose corpus callosum is completely sectioned have two entirely separate conscious portions of the brain. For example, in a teenage boy with a sectioned corpus callosum, only the left half of his brain could understand both the written word and the spoken word because the left side was the dominant hemisphere. Conversely, the right side of the brain could understand the written word but not the spoken word. Furthermore, the right cortex could elicit a motor action response to the written word without the left cortex ever knowing why the response was performed.

The effect was quite different when an emotional response was evoked in the right side of the brain: In this case, a subconscious emotional response occurred in the left side of the brain as well. This response undoubtedly occurred because the areas of the two sides of the brain for emotions, the anterior temporal cortices and adjacent areas, were still communicating with each other through the anterior commissure that was not sectioned. For instance, when the command "kiss" was written for the right half of his brain to see, the boy immediately and with full emotion said, "No way!" This response required function of Wernicke area and the motor areas for speech in the left hemisphere because these left-side areas were necessary to speak the words "No way!" When asked why he said this, however, the boy could not explain it. Thus, the two halves of the brain have independent capabilities for consciousness, memory storage, communication, and control of motor

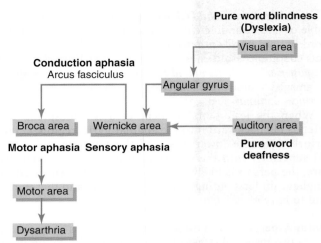

Figure 126-9   Speech: areas involved and associated disorders.

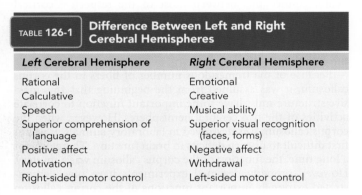

Left Cerebral Hemisphere	*Right* Cerebral Hemisphere
Rational	Emotional
Calculative	Creative
Speech	Musical ability
Superior comprehension of language	Superior visual recognition (faces, forms)
Positive affect	Negative affect
Motivation	Withdrawal
Right-sided motor control	Left-sided motor control

activities. The corpus callosum is required for the two sides to operate cooperatively at the superficial subconscious level, and the anterior commissure plays an important additional role in unifying the emotional responses of the two sides of the brain. Our understanding of cerebral lateralization has evolved based on "split brain" experiments such as those described earlier; a comparison of the right and left cerebral hemispheres is summarized in Table 126-1.

The areas involved with speech and the disorders of speech associated with these different areas are summarized in Figure 126-9.

BIBLIOGRAPHY

Bizley JK, Cohen YE: The what, where and how of auditory-object perception, *Nat. Rev. Neurosci.* 14:693, 2013.

Friederici AD: The brain basis of language processing: from structure to function, *Physiol. Rev.* 91:1357, 2011.

Hickok G, Poeppel D: The cortical organization of speech processing, *Nat. Rev. Neurosci.* 8:393, 2007.

Kandel ER, Schwartz JH, Jessell TM: *Principles of Neural Science*, fifth ed., New York, 2012, McGraw-Hill.

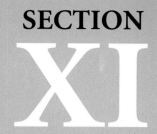

SECTION XI

Miscellaneous Topics

TONY RAJ

127 Components of Energy Expenditure

LEARNING OBJECTIVES

- List the components of 24-hour energy expenditure.
- List the determinants for basal metabolic rate.
- Describe the methods to measure metabolic rate.

GLOSSARY OF TERMS

- **Nonshivering thermogenesis:** A process that is stimulated by sympathetic nervous system activation, which releases norepinephrine and epinephrine, which in turn increases metabolic activity and heat generation

BOX 127-1   CONDITIONS TO BE MAINTAINED DURING BMR MEASUREMENT

1. The person must not have eaten food for at least 12 hours.
2. The BMR is determined after a night of restful sleep.
3. No strenuous activity is performed for at least 1 hour before the test.
4. All psychic and physical factors that cause excitement must be eliminated.
5. The temperature of the air must be comfortable and between 68 and 80°F.
6. No physical activity is permitted during the test.

Components of 24-Hour Energy Expenditure

The 24-hour daily energy expenditure (EE) has several components listed as follows:

1. basal metabolic rate (BMR; ~60%)
2. energy used for physical activity (~25%)
3. energy used for nonexercise activity (~7%)
4. thermogenic effect of food (~8%)

BASAL METABOLIC RATE—THE MINIMUM ENERGY EXPENDITURE FOR THE BODY TO EXIST

Even when a person is at complete rest, considerable energy is required to perform all the chemical reactions of the body. This minimum level of energy required to exist is called the *BMR* and accounts for about 50–70% of the daily EE in most sedentary persons (Figure 127-1).

Because the level of physical activity is highly variable among different persons, measurement of the BMR provides a useful means of comparing one person's metabolic rate with that of

another. The usual method for determining BMR is to measure the rate of oxygen utilization over a given period. The conditions for measuring BMR are listed in Box 127-1.

The BMR normally averages about 65–70 Calories/hour in an average 70-kg man. Although much of the BMR is accounted for by essential activities of the central nervous system, heart, kidneys, and other organs, the *variations* in BMR among different persons are related mainly to differences in the amount of skeletal muscle and body size.

Skeletal muscle, even under resting conditions, accounts for 20–30% of the BMR. For this reason, BMR is usually corrected for differences in body size by expressing it as Calories per hour per square meter of body surface area, calculated from height and weight. The average values for males and females of different ages are shown in Figure 127-2.

Much of the decline in BMR with increasing age is probably related to loss of muscle mass and replacement of muscle with adipose tissue, which has a lower rate of metabolism. Likewise, slightly lower BMRs in women, compared with those in men, are due partly to the lower percentage of muscle mass and higher percentage of adipose tissue in women.

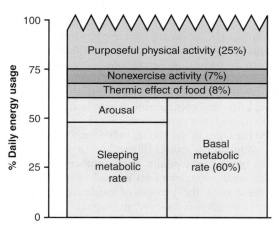

Figure 127-1   Components of energy expenditure.

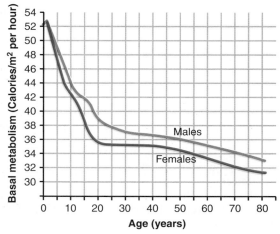

Figure 127-2   Normal basal metabolic rates at different ages for each gender.

Other Factors Can Influence the BMR

Thyroid Hormone Increases Metabolic Rate. When the thyroid gland secretes maximal amounts of thyroxine, the metabolic rate sometimes rises 50–100% above normal. Conversely, total loss of thyroid secretion decreases the metabolic rate to 40–60% of normal. Thyroxine increases the rates of the chemical reactions of many cells in the body and therefore increases metabolic rate.

Male Sex Hormone Increases Metabolic Rate. The male sex hormone testosterone can increase the metabolic rate about 10–15%. The female sex hormones may increase the BMR a small amount, but usually not enough to be significant. Much of this effect of the male sex hormone is related to its anabolic effect to increase skeletal muscle mass.

Growth Hormone Increases Metabolic Rate. Growth hormone can increase the metabolic rate by stimulating cellular metabolism and by increasing skeletal muscle mass. In adults with growth hormone deficiency, replacement therapy with recombinant growth hormone increases the BMR by about 20%.

Fever Increases Metabolic Rate. Fever, regardless of its cause, increases the chemical reactions of the body by an average of about 120% for every 10°C rise in temperature. This is discussed in more detail in Chapter 128.

Sleep Decreases Metabolic Rate. The metabolic rate decreases 10–15% below normal during sleep. This decrease is due to two principal factors: (1) decreased tone of the skeletal musculature during sleep and (2) decreased activity of the central nervous system.

Malnutrition Decreases Metabolic Rate. Prolonged malnutrition can decrease the metabolic rate 20–30%, presumably because of the paucity of food substances in the cells. In the final stages of many disease conditions, the inanition that accompanies the disease causes a marked decrease in metabolic rate, to the extent that the body temperature may fall several degrees shortly before death.

ENERGY USED FOR PHYSICAL ACTIVITIES

The factor that most dramatically increases metabolic rate is strenuous exercise. Short bursts of maximal muscle contraction in a single muscle can liberate as much as 100 times its normal resting amount of heat for a few seconds. For the entire body, maximal muscle exercise can increase the overall heat production of the body for a few seconds to about 50 times normal, or to about 20 times normal for more sustained exercise in a well-trained individual.

Table 127-1 shows the EE during different types of physical activity for an average 70-kg man. Because of the great variation in the amount of physical activity among individuals, this component of EE is the most important reason for the differences in caloric intake required to maintain energy balance. However, in industrialized countries where food supplies are generally plentiful, and the level of physical activity is often low, caloric intake often periodically exceeds EE, and the excess energy is stored mainly as fat.

Even in sedentary individuals who perform little or no daily exercise or physical work, significant energy is spent on

TABLE 127-1	Energy Expenditure During Different Types of Activity for a 70-kg Man[a]
Form of Activity	**Calories Per Hour**
Sleeping	65
Awake lying still	77
Sitting at rest	100
Standing relaxed	105
Dressing and undressing	118
Typewriting rapidly	140
Walking slowly (2.6 miles/hour)	200
Carpentry, metalworking, industrial painting	240
Sawing wood	480
Swimming	500
Running (5.3 miles/hour)	570
Walking up stairs rapidly	1100

[a]Extracted from data compiled by Professor M.S. Rose.

spontaneous physical activity required to maintain muscle tone and body posture and on other nonexercise activities such as "fidgeting." Together, these nonexercise activities account for about 7% of a person's daily energy usage.

ENERGY USED FOR PROCESSING FOOD— THERMOGENIC EFFECT OF FOOD

After a meal is ingested, the metabolic rate increases as a result of the different chemical reactions associated with digestion, absorption, and storage of food in the body. This increase is called the *thermogenic effect of food* because these processes require energy and generate heat.

After a meal that contains a large quantity of carbohydrates or fats, the metabolic rate usually increases about 4%. However, after a meal high in protein, the metabolic rate usually begins rising within an hour, reaching a maximum of about 30% above normal, and this rate lasts for 3–12 hours. This effect of protein on the metabolic rate is called the *specific dynamic action of protein*. The thermogenic effect of food accounts for about 8% of the total daily EE in many persons.

ENERGY USED FOR NONSHIVERING THERMOGENESIS—ROLE OF SYMPATHETIC STIMULATION

Although physical work and the thermogenic effect of food cause liberation of heat, these mechanisms are not aimed primarily at regulation of body temperature. Shivering provides a regulated means of producing heat by increasing muscle activity in response to cold stress, as discussed in Chapter 128. Another mechanism, *nonshivering thermogenesis*, can also produce heat in response to cold stress. This type of thermogenesis is stimulated by sympathetic nervous system activation, which releases norepinephrine and epinephrine, which in turn increase metabolic activity and heat generation.

In certain types of fat tissue, called *brown fat*, sympathetic nervous stimulation causes liberation of large amounts of heat. This type of fat contains large numbers of mitochondria and many small globules of fat instead of one large fat globule. In these cells, the process of oxidative phosphorylation in the mitochondria is mainly "uncoupled." That is, when the cells are stimulated by the sympathetic nerves, the mitochondria produce a large amount of heat but almost no adenosine triphosphate (ATP), so almost all the released oxidative energy immediately becomes heat.

A neonate has a considerable amount of brown fat, and maximal sympathetic stimulation can increase the child's metabolism more than 100%. The magnitude of this type of thermogenesis in an adult human, who has virtually no brown fat, is probably less than 15%, although this might increase significantly after cold adaptation.

Nonshivering thermogenesis may also serve as a buffer against obesity. Recent studies indicate that sympathetic nervous system activity is increased in obese persons who have a persistent excess caloric intake. The mechanism responsible for sympathetic activation in obese persons is uncertain, but it may be mediated partly through the effects of increased leptin, which activates proopiomelanocortin neurons in the hypothalamus. Sympathetic stimulation, by increasing thermogenesis, helps to limit excess weight gain.

METABOLIC RATE AND ITS MEASUREMENT

Heat Is the End Product of Almost All the Energy Released in the Body. In discussing many of the metabolic reactions in the preceding chapters, we noted that not all the energy in foods is transferred to ATP; instead, a large portion of this energy becomes heat. On average, 35% of the energy in foods becomes heat during ATP formation. Additional energy becomes heat as it is transferred from ATP to the functional systems of the cells, so even under optimal conditions, no more than 27% of all the energy from food is finally used by the functional systems. Even when 27% of the energy reaches the functional systems of the cells, most of this energy eventually becomes heat.

Essentially all the energy expended by the body is eventually converted into heat. The only significant exception occurs when the muscles are used to perform some form of work outside the body. For instance, when the muscles elevate an object to a height or propel the body up steps, a type of potential energy is created by raising a mass against gravity. However when external expenditure of energy is not taking place, all the energy released by the metabolic processes eventually becomes body heat.

The Calorie. Most often, the *Calorie* is the unit used to quantitatively discuss the metabolic rate of the body. It will be recalled that 1 *cal*—spelled with a small "c" and often called a *gram calorie*—is the quantity of heat required to raise the temperature of 1 g of water 1°C. The calorie is much too small a unit to use when referring to energy in the body. Consequently, the Calorie—spelled with a capital "C" and often called a *kilocalorie*, which is equivalent to 1000 cal—is the unit ordinarily used when discussing energy metabolism. More recently, kilojoules or megajoules are used to express EE.

MEASUREMENT OF THE WHOLE-BODY METABOLIC RATE

Direct Calorimetry Measures Heat Liberated from the Body. If a person is not performing any external work, the whole-body metabolic rate can be determined by simply measuring the total quantity of heat liberated from the body in a given time.

In determining the metabolic rate by direct calorimetry, one measures the quantity of heat liberated from the body in a large, specially constructed *calorimeter*. The subject is placed in an air chamber that is so well insulated that no heat can leak through the walls of the chamber. Heat formed by the subject's body warms the air of the chamber. However, the air temperature within the chamber is maintained at a constant level by forcing the air through pipes in a cool water bath. The rate of heat gain by the water bath, which can be measured with an accurate thermometer, is equal to the rate at which heat is liberated by the subject's body.

Direct calorimetry is physically difficult to perform and is used only for research purposes.

Indirect Calorimetry—The "Energy Equivalent" of Oxygen. Because more than 95% of the energy expended in the body is derived from reactions of oxygen with the different foods, the whole-body metabolic rate can also be calculated with a high degree of accuracy from the rate of oxygen utilization. When 1 L of oxygen is metabolized with glucose, 5.01 Calories of energy is released; when metabolized with starches, 5.06 Calories is released; with fat, 4.70 Calories; and with protein, 4.60 Calories.

These figures clearly demonstrate that the quantities of energy liberated per liter of oxygen consumed are nearly equivalent when different types of food are metabolized. For the average diet, the *quantity of energy liberated per liter of oxygen used in the body averages about 4.825 Calories*, which is called the *energy equivalent* of oxygen. By using this energy equivalent, one can calculate with a high degree of precision the rate of heat liberation in the body from the quantity of oxygen used in a given period.

If a person metabolizes only carbohydrates during the period of the metabolic rate determination, the calculated quantity of energy liberated, based on the value for the average energy equivalent of oxygen (4.825 Calories/L), would be about 4% too little. Conversely, if the person obtains most energy from fat, the calculated value would be about 4% too great. Table 127-2 summarizes the determinants of BMR.

Other methods to measure EE are heart rate (HR) monitoring and doubly labeled water (DLW) methods. In the HR monitoring method, because there is a linear relationship between HR and EE, this relationship is used as the basis for the measurement. However, due to physiological variations such as age, gender, body size, and nutritional status, the relationship between HR and EE must be calibrated for each individual measured.

The DLW method is based on a technique where individuals are administered two stable isotopic (nonradioactive) forms of water ($H_2^{18}O$ and ^2H_2O). The rate at which ^{18}O and ^2H disappear from the body is monitored for about 7–21 days. Based on the differential disappearance rates, CO_2 production is calculated and finally EE can be calculated. These methods can be used ideally in free living conditions and in field settings.

TABLE 127-2	Determinants of Basal Metabolic Rate
Determinants	
1. Hormones	Thyroid hormones increase BMR
	Testosterone increases BMR
	Growth hormone increases BMR
	Catecholamines increase BMR
2. Muscle mass	BMR increases with increase in muscle mass
3. Body size	BMR increases proportional to body size
4. Age	BMR decreases with age due to loss of muscle mass

BMR, basal metabolic rate.

BIBLIOGRAPHY

Cannon B, Nedergaard J: Nonshivering thermogenesis and its adequate measurement in metabolic studies, *J. Exp. Biol.* 214:242, 2011.

Chechi K, Carpentier AC, Richard D: Understanding the brown adipocyte as a contributor to energy homeostasis, *Trends Endocrinol. Metab.* 24:408, 2013.

Clapham JC: Central control of thermogenesis, *Neuropharmacology* 63:111, 2012.

Giralt M, Villarroya F: White, brown, beige/brite: different adipose cells for different functions? *Endocrinology* 154:2992, 2013.

Harper ME, Green K, Brand MD: The efficiency of cellular energy transduction and its implications for obesity, *Annu. Rev. Nutr.* 28:13, 2008.

Harper ME, Seifert EL: Thyroid hormone effects on mitochondrial energetics, *Thyroid* 18:145, 2008.

Kim B: Thyroid hormone as a determinant of energy expenditure and the basal metabolic rate, *Thyroid* 18:141, 2008.

Morrison SF, Madden CJ, Tupone D: Central neural regulation of brown adipose tissue thermogenesis and energy expenditure, *Cell Metab.* 19:741, 2014.

Morrison SF, Nakamura K, Madden CJ: Central control of thermogenesis in mammals, *Exp. Physiol.* 93:773, 2008.

Mullur R, Liu YY, Brent GA: Thyroid hormone regulation of metabolism, *Physiol. Rev.* 94:355, 2014.

Peirce V, Carobbio S, Vidal-Puig A: The different shades of fat, *Nature* 510:76, 2014.

Schoeller DA, Van Santen E: Measurement of energy expenditure in humans by doubly labeled water method, *J. Appl. Physiol. Respir. Environ. Exerc. Physiol.* 53(4):955, 1982.

Schutz Y, Weinsier RL, Hunter G: Assessment of free-living physical activity in humans: an overview of currently available and proposed new measures, *Obes. Res.* 9(6):368, 2001.

Silva JE: Thermogenic mechanisms and their hormonal regulation, *Physiol. Rev.* 86:435, 2006.

van Marken Lichtenbelt WD, Schrauwen P: Implications of nonshivering thermogenesis for energy balance regulation in humans, *Am. J. Physiol. Regul. Integr. Comp. Physiol.* 301:R285, 2011.

Viscarra JA, Ortiz RM: Cellular mechanisms regulating fuel metabolism in mammals: role of adipose tissue and lipids during prolonged food deprivation, *Metabolism* 62:889, 2013.

128

Body Temperature Regulation and Cutaneous Circulation

Normal Body Temperatures

Body Core Temperature and Skin Temperature. The temperature of the deep tissues of the body—the "core" of the body—usually remains very constant, within ±1°F (±0.6°C), except when a person has a febrile illness. The mechanisms for regulating body temperature represent a beautifully designed control system, which is discussed in this chapter.

The *skin temperature*, in contrast to the *core temperature*, rises and falls with the temperature of the surroundings. The skin temperature is important when we refer to the skin's ability to lose heat to the surroundings.

Normal Core Temperature. No single core temperature can be considered normal because measurements in many healthy people have shown a *range* of normal temperatures measured orally, as shown in Figure 128-1, from less than 97°F (36°C) to greater than 99.5°F (37.5°C). The average normal core temperature is generally considered to be between 98.0°F and 98.6°F when measured orally and about 1°F higher when measured rectally.

Body Temperature Is Controlled by Balancing Heat Production and Heat Loss

When the rate of heat production in the body is greater than the rate at which heat is being lost, heat builds up in the body and the body temperature rises. Conversely, when heat loss is greater, both body heat and body temperature decrease. Most of the remainder of this chapter is concerned with this balance between heat production and heat loss, and the mechanisms by which the body controls this production and loss.

HEAT PRODUCTION

Heat production is a principal by-product of metabolism. The most important factors that determine heat production are listed as follows:

1. basal rate of metabolism of all the cells of the body;
2. extra rate of metabolism caused by muscle activity, including muscle contractions caused by shivering;
3. extra metabolism caused by the effect of thyroxine (and, to a lesser extent, other hormones, such as growth hormone and testosterone) on the cells;
4. extra metabolism caused by the effect of epinephrine, norepinephrine, and sympathetic stimulation on the cells;
5. extra metabolism caused by increased chemical activity in the cells, especially when the cell temperature increases;
6. extra metabolism needed for digestion, absorption, and storage of food (thermogenic effect of food).

HEAT LOSS

Most of the heat produced in the body is generated in the deep organs, especially the liver, brain, and heart, and in the skeletal muscles during exercise. This heat is then transferred from the deeper organs and tissues to the skin, where it is lost to the air and other surroundings. Therefore, the rate at which heat is lost is determined almost entirely by two factors:

1. how rapidly heat can be conducted from where it is produced in the body core to the skin;
2. how rapidly heat can then be transferred from the skin to the surroundings.

Let us begin by discussing the system that insulates the core from the skin surface.

Insulator System of the Body

The skin, the subcutaneous tissues, and especially the fat of the subcutaneous tissues act together as a heat insulator for the body. The fat is important because it conducts heat only *one-third* as readily as other tissues.

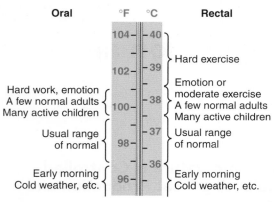

Figure 128-1 Estimated normal range of body "core" temperature. *Modified from DuBois, E.F., 1948. Fever. Charles C. Thomas, Springfield, IL.*

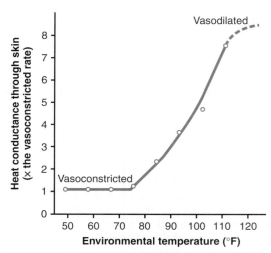

Figure 128-3 Effect of changes in the environmental temperature on heat conductance from the body core to the skin surface. *Modified from Benzinger, T.H., 1980. Heat and Temperature Fundamentals of Medical Physiology. Dowden, Hutchinson & Ross, New York.*

The insulation beneath the skin is an effective means of maintaining normal internal core temperature, even though it allows the temperature of the skin to approach the temperature of the surroundings.

CUTANEOUS CIRCULATION

Blood Flow to the Skin from the Body Core Provides Heat Transfer

When no blood is flowing from the heated internal organs to the skin, the insulating properties of the normal male body are about equal to three-quarters the insulating properties of a usual suit of clothes. In women, this insulation is even better. Blood vessels are distributed profusely beneath the skin. Especially important is a continuous venous plexus that is supplied by inflow of blood from the skin capillaries, shown in Figure 128-2. In the most exposed areas of the body—the hands, feet, and ears—blood is also supplied to the plexus directly from the small arteries through highly muscular *arteriovenous anastomoses*.

The rate of blood flow into the skin venous plexus can vary tremendously—from barely above zero to as great as 30% of the total cardiac output. A high rate of skin flow causes heat to be conducted from the core of the body to the skin with great efficiency, whereas reduction in the rate of skin flow can decrease the heat conduction from the core significantly.

Figure 128-3 shows quantitatively the effect of environmental air temperature on conductance of heat from the core to the skin surface and then conductance into the air, demonstrating an approximate eightfold increase in heat conductance between the fully vasoconstricted state and the fully vasodilated state.

Therefore, the skin is an effective *controlled "heat radiator" system*, and the flow of blood to the skin is a most effective mechanism for heat transfer from the body core to the skin.

Control of Heat Conduction to the Skin by the Sympathetic Nervous System. Heat conduction to the skin by the blood is controlled by the degree of vasoconstriction of the arterioles and the arteriovenous anastomoses that supply blood to the venous plexus of the skin. This vasoconstriction is controlled almost entirely by the sympathetic nervous system in response to changes in body core temperature and changes in environmental temperature. This is discussed later in the chapter in connection with control of body temperature by the hypothalamus.

Basic Physics of How Heat Is Lost from the Skin Surface

The various methods by which heat is lost from the skin to the surroundings are shown in Figure 128-4 and summarized in Box 128-1.

Radiation Causes Heat Loss in the Form of Infrared Rays. As shown in Figure 128-4, in a nude person sitting inside at normal room temperature, about 60% of total heat loss is by radiation.

Most infrared heat rays (a type of electromagnetic ray) that radiate from the body have wavelengths of 5–20 μm, 10–30 times the wavelengths of light rays. All objects that are not at absolute zero temperature radiate such rays. The human body radiates heat rays in all directions. Heat rays are also being radiated from the walls of rooms and other objects toward the body. If the temperature of the body is greater than the temperature of the surroundings, a greater quantity of heat is radiated from the body than is radiated to the body.

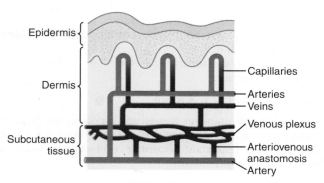

Figure 128-2 Skin circulation.

BOX 128-1   HEAT LOSS FROM THE BODY

1. Radiation ~60%
2. Conduction
   a. Conduction to air ~15%
   b. Conduction to objects ~3%
3. Evaporation ~22%

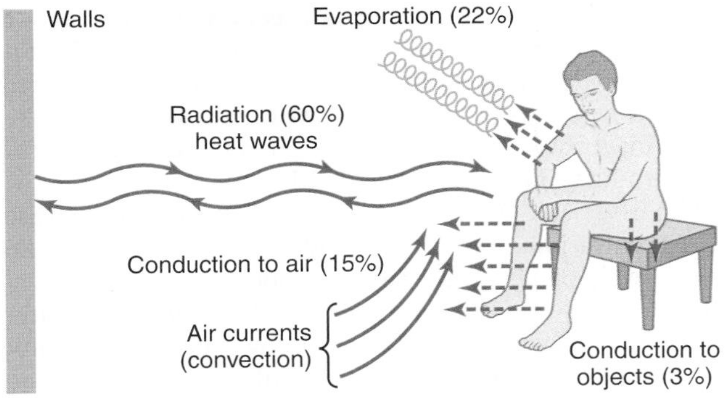

Figure 128-4 Mechanisms of heat loss from the body.

Conductive Heat Loss Occurs by Direct Contact with an Object. As shown in Figure 128-4, only minute quantities of heat, about 3%, are normally lost from the body by direct conduction from the surface of the body to *solid objects*, such as a chair or a bed. Loss of heat by *conduction to air*, however, represents a sizable proportion of the body's heat loss (about 15%) even under normal conditions.

Once the temperature of the air adjacent to the skin equals the temperature of the skin, no further loss of heat occurs in this way because now an equal amount of heat is conducted from the air to the body. Therefore, conduction of heat from the body to the air is self-limited *unless the heated air moves away from the skin*, so new, unheated air is continually brought in contact with the skin, a phenomenon called *air convection*.

Convective Heat Loss Results from Air Movement. The heat from the skin is first *conducted* to the air and then carried away by the convection air currents.

Therefore, in a nude person seated in a comfortable room without gross air movement, about 15% of his or her total heat loss occurs by conduction to the air and then by air convection away from the body.

Cooling Effect of Wind. When the body is exposed to wind, the layer of air immediately adjacent to the skin is replaced by new air much more rapidly than is normal, and heat loss by convection increases accordingly. The cooling effect of wind at low velocities is about proportional to the *square root of the wind velocity*. For instance, a wind of 4 miles/hour is about twice as effective for cooling as a wind of 1 mile/hour.

Conduction and Convection of Heat from a Person Suspended in Water. Water has a specific heat several thousand times as great as that of air, so each unit portion of water adjacent to the skin can absorb far greater quantities of heat than can be absorbed by air. Also, heat conductivity in water is very great in comparison with that in air. Therefore, the rate of heat loss to water is usually many times greater than the rate of heat loss to air if the temperature of the water is below body temperature.

Evaporation. When water evaporates from the body surface, 0.58 Calorie (kilocalorie) of heat is lost for each gram of water that evaporates. Even when a person is not sweating, water still evaporates *insensibly* from the skin and lungs at a rate of about 600–700 mL/day. This insensible evaporation causes continual heat loss at a rate of 16–19 Calories/hour. Insensible evaporation through the skin and lungs cannot be controlled for purposes

of temperature regulation because it results from continual diffusion of water molecules through the skin and respiratory surfaces. However, loss of heat by *evaporation of sweat* can be controlled by regulating the rate of sweating, which is discussed later in this chapter.

Evaporation Is a Necessary Cooling Mechanism at Very High Air Temperatures. As long as skin temperature is greater than the temperature of the surroundings, heat can be lost by radiation and conduction. However, when the temperature of the surroundings becomes greater than that of the skin, instead of losing heat, the body gains heat by both radiation and conduction. Under these conditions, *the only means by which the body can rid itself of heat is by evaporation.*

Therefore, anything that prevents adequate evaporation when the surrounding temperature is higher than the skin temperature will cause the internal body temperature to rise. This phenomenon occurs occasionally in human beings who are born with congenital absence of sweat glands who could develop heatstroke in tropical zones where the environmental temperature is high.

Clothing Reduces Conductive and Convective Heat Loss. Clothing entraps air next to the skin in the weave of the cloth, thereby increasing the thickness of the so-called *private zone* of air adjacent to the skin and also decreasing the flow of convection air currents. Consequently, the rate of heat loss from the body by conduction and convection is greatly depressed. A usual suit of clothes decreases the rate of heat loss to about half that from the nude body, but Arctic-type clothing can decrease this heat loss to as little as one-sixth.

The effectiveness of clothing in maintaining body temperature is almost completely lost when the clothing becomes wet because the high conductivity of water increases the rate of heat transmission through cloth 20-fold or more. Therefore, one of the most important factors for protecting the body against cold in Arctic regions is extreme caution against allowing the clothing to become wet.

Sweating and its Regulation by the Autonomic Nervous System

Stimulation of the anterior hypothalamus–preoptic area in the brain either electrically or by excess heat causes sweating. The nerve impulses from this area that cause sweating are transmitted in the autonomic pathways to the spinal cord and then through sympathetic outflow to the skin everywhere in the body.

Sweat glands are innervated by *cholinergic* nerve fibers (fibers that secrete acetylcholine but that run in the sympathetic nerves along with the adrenergic fibers). These glands can also be stimulated to some extent by epinephrine or norepinephrine circulating in the blood, even though the glands themselves do not have adrenergic innervation. This mechanism is important during exercise, when these hormones are secreted by the adrenal medullae and the body needs to lose excessive amounts of heat produced by the active muscles.

Mechanism of Sweat Secretion. In Figure 128-5, the sweat gland is shown to be a tubular structure consisting of two parts: (1) a deep subdermal *coiled portion* that secretes the sweat and (2) a *duct portion* that passes outward through the dermis and epidermis of the skin. As is true of so many other glands, the secretory portion of the sweat gland secretes a fluid called the

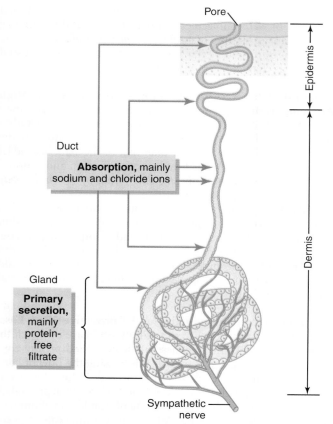

Figure 128-5 Sweat gland innervated by an acetylcholine-secreting sympathetic nerve. A *primary protein-free secretion* is formed by the glandular portion, but most of the electrolytes are reabsorbed in the duct, leaving a dilute, watery secretion.

primary secretion or *precursor secretion*; the concentrations of constituents in the fluid are then modified as the fluid flows through the duct.

The precursor secretion is an active secretory product of the epithelial cells lining the coiled portion of the sweat gland. Cholinergic sympathetic nerve fibers ending on or near the glandular cells elicit the secretion.

The composition of the precursor secretion is similar to that of plasma, except that it does not contain plasma proteins. The concentration of sodium is about 142 mEq/L and that of chloride is about 104 mEq/L, with much smaller concentrations of the other solutes of plasma. As this precursor solution flows through the duct portion of the gland, it is modified by reabsorption of most of the sodium and chloride ions.

Conversely, when the sweat glands are strongly stimulated by the sympathetic nervous system, large amounts of precursor secretion are formed, and the duct may reabsorb only slightly more than half the sodium chloride. Furthermore, the sweat flows through the glandular tubules so rapidly that little of the water is reabsorbed. Therefore, the other dissolved constituents of sweat are only moderately increased in concentration—urea is about twice that in the plasma, lactic acid about 4 times, and potassium about 1.2 times.

A significant loss of sodium chloride occurs in the sweat when a person is unacclimatized to heat. Much less electrolyte loss occurs, despite increased sweating capacity, once a person has become acclimatized.

Acclimatization of the Sweating Mechanism to Heat—The Role of Aldosterone. Although a normal, unacclimatized person seldom produces more than about 1 L of sweat per hour, when this person is exposed to hot weather for 1–6 weeks, he or she begins to sweat more profusely, often increasing maximum sweat production to as much as 2–3 L/hour.

Also associated with acclimatization is a further decrease in the concentration of sodium chloride in the sweat, which allows progressively better conservation of body salt. Most of this effect is caused by *increased secretion of aldosterone* by the adrenocortical glands, which results from a slight decrease in sodium chloride concentration in the extracellular fluid and plasma. An *unacclimatized* person who sweats profusely often loses 15–30 g of salt each day for the first few days. After 4–6 weeks of acclimatization, the loss is usually 3–5 g/day.

Other Mechanisms of Heat Loss in Lower Animals—Panting

See Box 128-2.

Regulation of Body Temperature—Role of the Hypothalamus

The temperature of the body is regulated almost entirely by nervous feedback mechanisms, and almost all these mechanisms operate through *temperature-regulating centers* located in the *hypothalamus*. For these feedback mechanisms to operate, there must also be temperature detectors to determine when the body temperature becomes either too high or too low.

ROLE OF THE ANTERIOR HYPOTHALAMIC–PREOPTIC AREA IN THERMOSTATIC DETECTION OF TEMPERATURE

The anterior hypothalamic–preoptic area contains large numbers of heat-sensitive neurons, as well as about one-third as many cold-sensitive neurons. These neurons are believed to function as temperature sensors for controlling body temperature. The heat-sensitive neurons increase their firing rate 2- to 10-fold in response to a 10°C increase in body temperature. The cold-sensitive neurons, by contrast, increase their firing rate when the body temperature falls.

BOX 128-2   LOSS OF HEAT BY PANTING

Many lower animals have little ability to lose heat from the surfaces of their bodies, for two reasons: (1) the surfaces are often covered with fur and (2) the skin of most of the lower animals is not supplied with sweat glands, which prevents most of the evaporative loss of heat from the skin. A substitute mechanism, the *panting* mechanism, is used by many lower animals as a means of dissipating heat.

The phenomenon of panting is "turned on" by the thermoregulator centers of the brain. That is, when the blood becomes overheated, the hypothalamus initiates neurogenic signals to decrease the body temperature. One of these signals initiates panting. The actual panting process is controlled by a *panting center* that is associated with the pneumotaxic respiratory center located in the pons.

When an animal pants, it breathes in and out rapidly, and thus large quantities of new air from the exterior come in contact with the upper portions of the respiratory passages. This mechanism cools the blood in the respiratory passage mucosa as a result of water evaporation from the mucosal surfaces.

When the preoptic area is heated, the skin all over the body immediately breaks out in a profuse sweat, whereas the skin blood vessels over the entire body become greatly dilated. This response is an immediate reaction to cause the body to lose heat, thereby helping to return the body temperature toward the normal level. In addition, any excess body heat production is inhibited. Therefore, it is clear that the *hypothalamic–preoptic area* has the capability to serve as a thermostatic body temperature control center.

DETECTION OF TEMPERATURE BY RECEPTORS IN THE SKIN AND DEEP BODY TISSUES

Although the signals generated by the temperature receptors of the hypothalamus are extremely powerful in controlling body temperature, receptors in other parts of the body play additional roles in temperature regulation. This is especially true of temperature receptors in the skin such as the *cold* and *warmth* receptors, and a few receptors in specific deep tissues of the body.

Due to the fact that the skin has far more cold receptors than warm receptors, the peripheral detection of temperature mainly concerns detecting cool and cold instead of warm temperatures.

Although the molecular mechanisms for sensing changes in temperature are not well understood, experimental studies suggest that the *transient receptor potential family of cation channels*, found in somatosensory neurons and epidermal cells, may mediate thermal sensation over a wide range of skin temperatures.

Deep body temperature receptors are found mainly in the *spinal cord*, in the *abdominal viscera*, and in or around the *great veins* in the upper abdomen and thorax. These deep receptors function differently from the skin receptors because they are exposed to the body core temperature rather than the body surface temperature. Yet, like the skin temperature receptors, they detect mainly cold rather than warmth. It is probable that both the skin and the deep body receptors are concerned with preventing *hypothermia*—that is, preventing low body temperature. The physiological response to a cold stimulus is summarized in Box 128-3.

POSTERIOR HYPOTHALAMUS INTEGRATES THE CENTRAL AND PERIPHERAL TEMPERATURE SENSORY SIGNALS

Even though many temperature sensory signals arise in peripheral receptors, these signals contribute to body temperature control mainly through the hypothalamus. The area of the hypothalamus that they stimulate is located bilaterally in the posterior hypothalamus approximately at the level of the mammillary bodies. The temperature sensory signals from the anterior hypothalamic–preoptic area are also transmitted into this posterior hypothalamic area. Here the signals from the preoptic area and the signals from elsewhere in the body are combined and integrated to control the heat-producing and heat-conserving reactions of the body.

NEURONAL EFFECTOR MECHANISMS THAT DECREASE OR INCREASE BODY TEMPERATURE

When the hypothalamic temperature centers detect that the body temperature is either too high or too low, they institute appropriate temperature-decreasing or temperature-increasing procedures. The reader is probably familiar with most of these procedures from personal experience, but special features are described in the following sections.

Temperature-Decreasing Mechanisms when the Body Is Too Hot

The temperature control system uses three important mechanisms to reduce body heat when the body temperature becomes too great:

1. *Vasodilation of skin blood vessels.* In almost all areas of the body, the skin blood vessels become intensely dilated. This dilation is caused by inhibition of the sympathetic centers in the posterior hypothalamus that cause vasoconstriction. Full vasodilation can increase the rate of heat transfer to the skin as much as eightfold.
2. *Sweating.* The effect of increased body temperature to cause sweating is demonstrated by the blue curve in Figure 128-6, which shows a sharp increase in the rate of evaporative heat loss resulting from sweating when the body core temperature rises above the critical level of 37°C (98.6°F). An additional 1°C increase in body temperature causes enough sweating to remove 10 times the basal rate of body heat production.
3. *Decrease in heat production.* The mechanisms that cause excess heat production, such as shivering and chemical thermogenesis, are strongly inhibited.

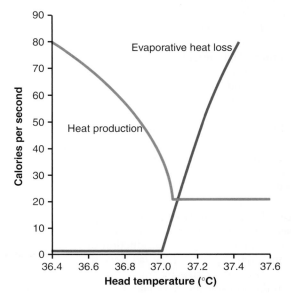

Figure 128-6 Effect of hypothalamic temperature on evaporative heat loss from the body and on heat production caused primarily by muscle activity and shivering. This figure demonstrates the extremely critical temperature level at which increased heat loss begins and heat production reaches a minimum stable level.

BOX 128-3   PHYSIOLOGICAL RESPONSE TO A COLD STIMULUS

When the skin of the whole body is exposed to cold, immediate reflex effects are invoked and begin to increase the temperature of the body in several ways:
1. By providing a strong stimulus to cause shivering, with a resultant increase in the rate of body heat production
2. By inhibiting the process of sweating, if this is already occurring
3. By promoting skin vasoconstriction to diminish loss of body heat from the skin

Temperature-Increasing Mechanisms when the Body Is Too Cold

When the body is too cold, the temperature control system institutes exactly opposite procedures. They are as follows:

1. *Skin vasoconstriction throughout the body.* This vasoconstriction is caused by stimulation of the posterior hypothalamic sympathetic centers.

2. *Piloerection.* Piloerection means hairs "standing on end." Sympathetic stimulation causes the arrector pili muscles attached to the hair follicles to contract, which brings the hairs to an upright stance. This mechanism is not important in human beings, but in many animals, upright projection of the hairs allows them to entrap a thick layer of "insulator air" next to the skin, so transfer of heat to the surroundings is greatly depressed.

3. *Increase in thermogenesis (heat production).* Heat production by the metabolic systems is increased by promoting shivering, sympathetic excitation of heat production, and thyroxine secretion. These methods of increasing heat require additional explanation, which is provided in the following sections.

Hypothalamic Stimulation of Shivering. Located in the dorsomedial portion of the posterior hypothalamus near the wall of the third ventricle is an area called the *primary motor center for shivering.* This area is normally inhibited by signals from the heat center in the anterior hypothalamic–preoptic area but is excited by cold signals from the skin and spinal cord. Therefore, as shown by the sudden increase in "heat production" (see the red curve in Figure 128-6), this center becomes activated when the body temperature falls even a fraction of a degree below a critical temperature level. It then transmits signals that cause shivering through bilateral tracts down the brainstem, into the lateral columns of the spinal cord, and finally to the anterior motor neurons. These signals are nonrhythmical and do not cause the actual muscle shaking. Instead, they increase the tone of the skeletal muscles throughout the body by facilitating the activity of the anterior motor neurons. When the tone rises above a certain critical level, shivering begins. *During maximum shivering, body heat production can rise to four to five times normal.*

Sympathetic "Chemical" Excitation of Heat Production. An increase in either sympathetic stimulation or circulating norepinephrine and epinephrine in the blood can rapidly increase the rate of cellular metabolism. This effect is called *chemical thermogenesis* or *nonshivering thermogenesis.* It results at least partially from the ability of norepinephrine and epinephrine to *uncouple* oxidative phosphorylation, which means that excess foodstuffs are oxidized and thereby release energy in the form of heat but do not cause adenosine triphosphate to be formed.

Increased Thyroxine Output as a Long-Term Cause of Increased Heat Production. Cooling the anterior hypothalamic–preoptic area also increases production of the neurosecretory hormone *thyrotropin-releasing hormone* by the hypothalamus. This hormone is carried by way of the hypothalamic portal veins to the anterior pituitary gland, where it stimulates secretion of *thyroid-stimulating hormone.*

Thyroid-stimulating hormone in turn stimulates increased output of *thyroxine* by the thyroid gland, which activates uncoupling protein and increases the rate of cellular metabolism throughout the body, which is yet another mechanism of *chemical thermogenesis.*

Exposure of animals to extreme cold for several weeks can cause their thyroid glands to increase in size 20–40%. Isolated measurements have shown that metabolic rates increase in military personnel residing for several months in the Arctic; some of the Inuit (Eskimos), the indigenous people who inhabit the Arctic regions of Alaska, Canada, or Greenland, also have abnormally high basal metabolic rates. Further, the continuous stimulatory effect of cold on the thyroid gland may explain the much higher incidence of toxic thyroid goiters in people who live in cold climates than in those who live in warm climates.

"SET POINT" FOR TEMPERATURE CONTROL

In the example of Figure 128-6, it is clear that at a critical body core temperature of about 37.1°C (98.8°F), drastic changes occur in the rates of both heat loss and heat production. At temperatures above this level, the rate of heat loss is greater than that of heat production, so the body temperature falls and approaches the 37.1°C level. At temperatures below this level, the rate of heat production is greater than that of heat loss, so the body temperature rises and again approaches the 37.1°C level. This crucial temperature level is called the "set point" of the temperature control mechanism, that is, all the temperature control mechanisms continually attempt to bring the body temperature back to this set-point level.

BEHAVIORAL CONTROL OF BODY TEMPERATURE

Whenever the internal body temperature becomes too high, signals from the temperature-controlling areas in the brain give the person a psychic sensation of being overheated. Conversely, whenever the body becomes too cold, signals from the skin and probably also from some deep body receptors elicit the feeling of cold discomfort. Therefore, the person makes appropriate environmental adjustments to reestablish comfort, such as moving into a heated room or wearing well-insulated clothing in freezing weather. Behavioral control of temperature is a much more powerful system of body temperature control than most physiologists have acknowledged in the past. Indeed, it is the only really effective mechanism to maintain body heat control in severely cold environments.

LOCAL SKIN TEMPERATURE REFLEXES

When a person places a foot under a hot lamp and leaves it there for a short time, *local vasodilation* and mild *local sweating* occur. Conversely, placing the foot in cold water causes local vasoconstriction and local cessation of sweating. These reactions are caused by local effects of temperature directly on the blood vessels and also by local cord reflexes conducted from skin receptors to the spinal cord and back to the same skin area and the sweat glands. The *intensity* of these local effects is, in addition, controlled by the central brain temperature controller, so their overall effect is proportional to the hypothalamic heat control signal *times* the local signal. Such reflexes can help prevent excessive heat exchange from locally cooled or heated portions of the body.

Regulation of Internal Body Temperature Is Impaired by Cutting the Spinal Cord. If the spinal cord is severed in the neck above the sympathetic outflow from the cord, regulation of body temperature becomes extremely poor because the hypothalamus can no longer control either skin blood flow or the degree of sweating anywhere in the body. This is true even though the local temperature reflexes originating in the skin, spinal cord, and intraabdominal receptors still exist. These reflexes are extremely weak in comparison with hypothalamic control of body temperature.

In people with this condition, body temperature must be regulated principally by the patient's psychic response to cold and hot sensations in the head region—that is, by behavioral control of clothing and by moving into an appropriate warm or cold environment.

Abnormalities of Body Temperature Regulation

FEVER

Fever, which means a body temperature above the usual range of normal, can be caused by abnormalities in the brain or by toxic substances that affect the temperature-regulating centers. Some causes of fever (and also of subnormal body temperatures) are presented in Figure 128-7. They include bacterial or viral infections, brain tumors, and environmental conditions that may terminate in heatstroke.

Resetting the Hypothalamic Temperature-Regulating Center in Febrile Diseases—Effect of Pyrogens

Many proteins, breakdown products of proteins, and certain other substances, especially lipopolysaccharide toxins released from bacterial cell membranes, can cause the set point of the hypothalamic thermostat to rise. Substances that cause this effect are called *pyrogens*. Pyrogens released from toxic bacteria or those released from degenerating body tissues cause fever during disease conditions. Within a few hours after the set point has been increased, the body temperature also approaches this level, as shown in Figure 128-8.

Mechanism of Action of Pyrogens in Causing Fever—Role of Cytokines. Experiments in animals have shown that some pyrogens, when injected into the hypothalamus, can act directly

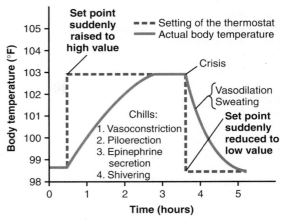

Figure 128-8 Effects of changing the set point of the hypothalamic temperature controller.

and immediately on the hypothalamic temperature-regulating center to increase its set point. Other pyrogens function indirectly and may require several hours of latency before causing their effects.

When bacteria or breakdown products of bacteria are present in the tissues or in the blood, they are *phagocytized by the blood leukocytes, by tissue macrophages, and by large granular killer lymphocytes*. All these cells digest the bacterial products and then release cytokines, a diverse group of peptide signaling molecules involved in the innate and adaptive immune responses. One of the most important of these cytokines in causing fever is *interleukin-1 (IL-1)*, also called *leukocyte pyrogen* or *endogenous pyrogen*. IL-1 is released from macrophages into the body fluids and, upon reaching the hypothalamus, almost immediately activates the processes to produce fever, sometimes increasing the body temperature a noticeable amount in only 8–10 minutes.

Several experiments have suggested that IL-1 causes fever by first inducing formation of one of the prostaglandins, mainly prostaglandin E_2, or a similar substance, which acts in the hypothalamus to elicit the fever reaction. When prostaglandin formation is blocked by drugs, the fever is either completely abrogated or at least reduced. In fact, this may be the explanation for the manner in which aspirin reduces fever because aspirin impedes the formation of prostaglandins from arachidonic acid. Drugs such as aspirin that reduce fever are called *antipyretics*.

Fever Caused by Brain Lesions. When a brain surgeon operates in the region of the hypothalamus, severe fever almost always occurs; rarely, the opposite effect, hypothermia, occurs, demonstrating both the potency of the hypothalamic mechanisms for body temperature control and the ease with which abnormalities of the hypothalamus can alter the set point of temperature control. Another condition that frequently causes prolonged high temperature is compression of the hypothalamus by a brain tumor.

CHARACTERISTICS OF FEBRILE CONDITIONS

Chills. When the set point of the hypothalamic temperature control center is suddenly changed from the normal level to higher than normal (as a result of tissue destruction, pyrogenic

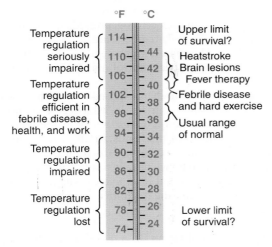

Figure 128-7 Body temperatures under different conditions. *(Modified from DuBois, E.F., 1948. Fever. Charles C. Thomas, Springfield, IL.)*

substances, or dehydration), the body temperature usually takes several hours to reach the new temperature set point.

Figure 128-8 demonstrates the effect of suddenly increasing the temperature set point to a level of 103°F. Because the blood temperature is now less than the set point of the hypothalamic temperature controller, the usual responses that cause elevation of body temperature occur. During this period, the person experiences chill and feels extremely cold, even though his or her body temperature may already be above normal. Also, the skin becomes cold because of vasoconstriction and the person shivers. Chills can continue until the body temperature reaches the hypothalamic set point of 103°F. Then the person no longer experiences chills but instead feels neither cold nor hot. As long as the factor that is causing the higher set point of the hypothalamic temperature controller is present, the body temperature is regulated more or less in the normal manner, but at the high-temperature set-point level.

Crisis or "Flush". If the factor that is causing the high temperature is removed, the set point of the hypothalamic temperature controller will be reduced to a lower value—perhaps even back to the normal level, as shown in Figure 128-8. In this instance, the body temperature is still 103°F, but the hypothalamus is attempting to regulate the temperature to 98.6°F. This situation is analogous to excessive heating of the anterior hypothalamic–preoptic area, which causes intense sweating and the sudden development of hot skin because of vasodilation everywhere. This sudden change of events in a febrile state is known as the "crisis" or, more appropriately, the "flush." In the days before the advent of antibiotics, the crisis was always anxiously awaited because once this occurred, the doctor assumed that the patient's temperature would soon begin falling.

Heatstroke

The upper limit of air temperature that one can stand depends to a great extent on whether the air is dry or wet. If the air is dry and sufficient convection air currents are flowing to promote rapid evaporation from the body, a person can withstand several hours of air temperature at 130°F. Conversely, if the air is 100% humidified or if the body is in water, the body temperature begins to rise whenever the environmental temperature rises above about 94°F. If the person is performing heavy work, the critical *environmental temperature* above which heatstroke is likely to occur may be as low as 85–90°F.

When the body temperature rises beyond a critical temperature, into the range of 105°F–108°F, heatstroke is likely to develop (Box 128-4).

These symptoms are often exacerbated by a degree of *circulatory shock* brought on by excessive loss of fluid and electrolytes in the sweat.

The hyperpyrexia is also exceedingly damaging to the body tissues, especially the brain, and is responsible for many of the effects. In fact, even a few minutes of very high body temperature can sometimes be fatal. For this reason, many authorities recommend immediate treatment of heatstroke by placing the

BOX 128-4 SYMPTOMS OF HEATSTROKE
1. Dizziness
2. Abdominal distress sometimes accompanied by vomiting
3. Delirium (sometimes)
4. Loss of consciousness (eventually)

person in a cold water bath. Because a cold water bath often induces uncontrollable shivering, with a considerable increase in the rate of heat production, others have suggested that sponge or spray cooling of the skin is likely to be more effective for rapidly decreasing the body core temperature.

Harmful Effects of High Temperature. The pathological findings in a person who dies of hyperpyrexia are local hemorrhages and parenchymatous degeneration of cells throughout the entire body, but especially in the brain. Once neuronal cells are destroyed, they can never be replaced. Also, damage to the liver, kidneys, and other organs can often be severe enough that failure of one or more of these organs eventually causes death, but sometimes not until several days after the heatstroke occurs.

Acclimatization to Heat. It can be extremely important to acclimatize people to extreme heat. Examples of people requiring acclimatization are soldiers on duty in the tropics and miners working in the 2-mile-deep gold mines of South Africa, where the temperature approaches body temperature and the humidity approaches 100%. A person exposed to heat for several hours each day while performing a reasonably heavy workload will develop increased tolerance to hot and humid conditions in 1–3 weeks.

Among the most important physiological changes that occur during this acclimatization process are an approximately twofold increase in the maximum rate of sweating, an increase in plasma volume, and diminished loss of salt in the sweat and urine to almost none; the last two effects result from increased secretion of aldosterone by the adrenal glands.

EXPOSURE OF THE BODY TO EXTREME COLD

Unless treated immediately, a person exposed to ice water for 20–30 minutes ordinarily dies because of heart standstill or heart fibrillation. By that time, the internal body temperature will have fallen to about 77°F. If warmed rapidly by the application of external heat, the person's life can often be saved.

Loss of Temperature Regulation at Low Temperatures. As noted in Figure 128-7, once the body temperature has fallen below about 85°F, the ability of the hypothalamus to regulate temperature is lost; it is greatly impaired even when the body temperature falls below about 94°F. Part of the reason for this diminished temperature regulation is that the rate of chemical heat production in each cell is depressed almost twofold for each 10°F decrease in body temperature. Also, sleepiness develops (later followed by coma), which depresses the activity of the central nervous system heat control mechanisms and prevents shivering.

Frostbite. When the body is exposed to extremely low temperatures, surface areas can freeze, which is a phenomenon called *frostbite*. Frostbite occurs especially in the lobes of the ears, and in the digits of the hands and feet. If the freeze has been sufficient to cause extensive formation of ice crystals in the cells, permanent damage usually results, such as permanent circulatory impairment and local tissue damage. Gangrene often follows thawing, and the frostbitten areas must be removed surgically.

Cold-Induced Vasodilation Is a Final Protection Against Frostbite at Almost Freezing Temperatures. When the temperature of tissues falls almost to freezing, the smooth muscle in the vascular wall becomes paralyzed because of the cold, and sudden vasodilation occurs, often manifested by a flush of the skin. This mechanism helps prevent frostbite by delivering warm blood to the skin. This mechanism is far less developed in humans than in most of lower animals that live in the cold all the time.

BIBLIOGRAPHY

Chechi K, Carpentier AC, Richard D: Understanding the brown adipocyte as a contributor to energy homeostasis, *Trends Endocrinol. Metab.* 24:408, 2013.

Clapham JC: Central control of thermogenesis, *Neuropharmacology* 63:111, 2012.

Crandall CG, González-Alonso J: Cardiovascular function in the heat-stressed human, *Acta Physiol. (Oxf.)* 199:407, 2010.

González-Alonso J, Crandall CG, Johnson JM: The cardiovascular challenge of exercising in the heat, *J. Physiol.* 586:45, 2008.

Katschinski DM: On heat and cells and proteins, *News Physiol. Sci.* 19:11, 2004.

Leon LR, Helwig BG: Heat stroke: role of the systemic inflammatory response, *J. Appl. Physiol.* 109:1980, 2010.

Morrison SF, Madden CJ, Tupone D: Central neural regulation of brown adipose tissue thermogenesis and energy expenditure, *Cell Metab.* 19:741, 2014.

Mullur R, Liu YY, Brent GA: Thyroid hormone regulation of metabolism, *Physiol. Rev.* 94:355, 2014.

Nakamura K: Central circuitries for body temperature regulation and fever, *Am. J. Physiol. Regul. Integr. Comp. Physiol.* 301:R1207, 2011.

Patapoutian A, Peier AM, Story GM, Viswanath V: ThermoTRP channels and beyond: mechanisms of temperature sensation, *Nat. Rev. Neurosci.* 4:529, 2003.

Romanovsky AA: Thermoregulation: some concepts have changed. Functional architecture of the thermoregulatory system, *Am. J. Physiol. Regul. Integr. Comp. Physiol.* 292:R37, 2007.

Schlader ZJ, Stannard SR, Mündel T: Human thermoregulatory behavior during rest and exercise—a prospective review, *Physiol. Behav.* 99:269, 2010.

Silva JE: Thermogenic mechanisms and their hormonal regulation, *Physiol. Rev.* 86:435, 2006.

Sladek CD, Johnson AK: Integration of thermal and osmotic regulation of water homeostasis: the role of TRPV channels, *Am. J. Physiol. Regul. Integr. Comp. Physiol.* 305:R669, 2013.

Tupone D, Madden CJ, Morrison SF: Autonomic regulation of brown adipose tissue thermogenesis in health and disease: potential clinical applications for altering BAT thermogenesis, *Front. Neurosci.* 8:14, 2014.

Note: Page numbers followed by "*f*" indicate figures, and "*t*" indicate tables.

Pregnanediol, 673
Pregnancy, 683
Pregnancy-induced hypertension, 688
Pregnancy, physiology of, 683
  anatomy/function of placenta, 685
  blastocyst implantation in uterus, 684
  diffusion of
    carbon dioxide, 686
    foodstuffs, 686
    oxygen through placental membrane, 685–686
  embryo, early nutrition of, 684
  estrogens secretion by placenta, 687
  excretion of waste products, 686
  fertilized ovum, transportation in fallopian
    tube, 683
  hormonal factors, 686
    human chorionic gonadotropin, 686
      fetal testes, 687
      function of, 687
    increased corticosteroid secretion, 688
    increased parathyroid gland secretion, 688
    increased thyroid gland secretion, 688
    pituitary secretion, 688
    relaxin, 688
  human chorionic somatomammotropin, 687–688
  maternal changes, 690
  maternal circulatory system, 689
    amniotic fluid, 689
    blood flow through placenta and maternal
      cardiac output, 689
    kidney function, 689
    maternal respiration, 689
    preeclampsia/eclampsia, 689
  metabolism, 688
  mother's body, 688
  nutrition, 688
  ovum
    into fallopian tube, 683
    fertilization of, 683
  progesterone secretion by placenta, 687
  weight gain in pregnant woman, 688
Preload, 177
Premature contractions, 199–200
  atrial, 199–200f
    premature beat, 200
  A-V nodal or A-V bundle, 200, 200f
  causes, 199
  ventricular, 200
Premature ventricular contractions
  vectorial analysis, 200
Premotor area, 791
pre-mRNA. See Precursor messenger RNA
  (pre-mRNA)
Preprohormones, 567
Preproinsulin, 638
Prerenal acute kidney injury, 553
Presbyopia, 761
Pressoreceptors, 264
Pressure buffer system, 266, 266f
Pressure difference, 366
Pressure diuresis, 271, 272f, 551, 556, 618
  aldosterone oversecretion and, 556, 618
  antidiuretic hormone and, 556
Pressure, flow, and resistance
  interrelationship between, 231, 232
Pressure gradient
  blood flow and, 231
  for venous return, 221
Pressure natriuresis, 271, 274, 556, 618, 619
  aldosterone oversecretion and, 618
    antidiuretic hormone and, 556
  obesity and, 554
Pressure pulse wave
  abnormal contours of, 255
  transmission of, 256–257, 256f
Pressure sensations, 719
  on footpads, equilibrium and, 806

Presynaptic inhibition, 709
Presynaptic facilitation, memory and, 863
Presynaptic inhibition, 709
Presynaptic neuron, 704, 710
Presynaptic terminals, 705
  temporal summation by, 717
Pretectal nuclei, visual fibers to, 779
Preverterbral ganglia, 828
Primary active transporter
  calcium ATPase, 504
  hydrogen ATPase, 504
  hydrogen-potassium ATPase, 504
  sodium-potassium ATPase, 503
Primary aldosteronism (Conn's syndrome), 628
Primary auditory cortex, 754–755
Primary hyperparathyroidism, 611–613
Primary motor cortex, 791
  removal of, 794
Primary sensations
  of smell, search for, 745
  of taste, 741–742
Primary visual cortex, 779, 780, 780f
  effect of removal of, 782
  six layers of, 780–781, 781f
Primitive and newer olfactory pathways
  into central nervous system, 746
Primitive olfactory system, 746
Primordial chordamesoderm, 33
Principal cells, renal, 524–525, 524f
  aldosterone and, 520–521
  potassium and, 524–525, 524f
Principal female hormones, synthesis of, 672
P-R interval, 192
  prolonged, 198–199, 198f
Procaine, 66
Procarboxypolypeptidase, 435
Procoagulants, 155
Proelastase, 455
Proerythroblast, 117, 119f
Profibrinolysin, 159
Progesterone, 664, 687
  breasts and, 674
  endometrium and, 664
  excretion of, by placenta, 672
  fallopian tubes and, 674
  fate of, 673
  functions of, 671–674
  insulin and, 642
  lobule-alveolar system and, 694
  in luteal phase, 667
  negative feedback effects of, 670, 670f
  secretion of, 686
  transport of, 672
  uterine contractility and, 691
  uterus and, secretory changes in, 674
Progestins, 671
  synthesis of, 672, 673f
Programmed cell death, 33
Prohormones, 567
  convertase, 626f
Prolactin, 579, 674, 688, 694–695
Prolactin inhibitory hormone (PIH), 579, 694, 695
Prolactin-inhibitory hormone, 694
Prometaphase, 31f, 32
Promoter, 24, 28
  transcription by, 29
Pronucleus
  female, 682
  male, 682, 682f
Pro-opiomelanocortin (POMC), 625, 626f
Prophase, 31f, 32
Proprioceptive sensations, 719
Propriospinal fibers, 789
Propulsive movements, 465. See also Peristalsis
  of colon, 465
  of small intestine, 470
Propylthiouracil, 598

thyroid hormone and, 598–599
Prosopagnosia, 870
Prostaglandin E₂ (PGE₂), 300
Prostaglandins, 561, 562, 574
  fertilization and, 654, 683
  fever and, 887
  glomerular filtration rate and, 499
  platelet synthesis of, 152
  in seminal vesicles, 654
Prostate gland, 651
  abnormalities of, 661
  cancer of, 661
  function of, 654
Protanope, 775
Proteases, 33, 77
Protein(s), 9, 16f, 453. See also Plasma proteins
  absorption, 455
    as amino acids, 455
    as bases, 531
    as dipeptides, 455
    as tripeptides, 455
  as buffers, 535
    hemoglobin as, 535
  catabolism of, 580, 639
  deficiency in, 582, 583f
  digestion, 453
    in stomach, 453
  degradation of, starvation on, 468
  depletion of
    diabetes mellitus and, 644–645
  deposition of
    estrogen and, 670–671
  digestion of, 453–455, 454f
    pancreatic enzymes in, 435
    pancreatic proteolytic enzymes in, 453
  formation of
    by granular endoplasmic reticulum, 17
  functional, 9
  hydrolysis, 453
  metabolism of, 440
  structural, 9
Protein C, 159
Protein channels, 36–37
  gating, 37–38, 37f
  selective permeability, 37–38
Protein hormones, 567
  secretory vesicles and, 567
Protein kinase, hormone action and, 574
Protein sparers, 480
Proteinuria, in minimal change nephropathy, 493
Proteoglycan filaments, 240, 240f
  fluid flow and, 57
  interstitial fluid pressure and, 57
  Proteoglycans, 605
  Proteolytic enzymes
  in acrosome, 653
Proteoses, 438, 453
Prothrombin, 155
  activator, 155
Prothrombin, 155–156
  decreased, 159–160
  to thrombin, conversion of, 155–156, 155f
Prothrombin activator, 155
  effect of Xa to form, 157
  formation of, 156–158
Prothrombin time, 161–162, 161f
Protoplasm, 9
Proximal tubule, 485, 504, 505, 514f
  reabsorption in, 503f
    of amino acids, 500
    of calcium, 528, 528f
    of glucose, 500
    of phosphate, 529
    of potassium, 524–525, 524f
    of sodium, 505
    of water, 506
  secretion by, 505f, 506